Pediatric
ICD-10-CM 2017

A MANUAL FOR PROVIDER-BASED CODING

• 2nd Edition •

American Academy of Pediatrics

Cindy Hughes, CPC, CFPC, Consulting Editor

Becky Dolan, MPH, CPC, CPEDC, Staff Editor

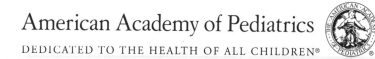

American Academy of Pediatrics

DEDICATED TO THE HEALTH OF ALL CHILDREN®

American Academy of Pediatrics Publishing Staff

Mark Grimes, *Director, Department of Publishing*

Alain Park, *Senior Product Development Editor*

Carrie Peters, *Editor, Professional and Clinical Publishing*

Leesa Levin-Doroba, *Manager, Publishing and Production Services*

Jason Crase, *Manager, Editorial Services*

Peg Mulcahy, *Manager, Art Direction and Production*

Mary Lou White, *Director, Department of Marketing and Sales*

Mary Jo Reynolds, *Marketing Manager, Practice Publications*

American Academy of Pediatrics Coding Staff

Becky Dolan, MPH, CPC, CPEDC

Teri Salus, MPA, CPC, CPEDC

Linda Walsh, MAB

Published by the American Academy of Pediatrics
141 Northwest Point Blvd
Elk Grove Village, IL 60007-1019
Telephone: 847/434-4000
Facsimile: 847/434-8000
www.aap.org

11-114

1 2 3 4 5 6 7 8 9 10

MA0800
ISBN: 978-1-61002-042-8
eBook: 978-1-61002-043-5
Library of Congress Control Number: 2016950531

Disclaimer

Every effort has been made to include all pediatric-relevant *International Classification of Diseases, 10th Revision, Clinical Modification* (*ICD-10-CM*) codes and their respective guidelines. It is the responsibility of the reader to use this manual as a companion to the official *ICD-10-CM* publication. Do not report new or revised *ICD-10-CM* codes until its published implementation date, at time of publication set for October 1, 2016. Further, it is the reader's responsibility to access the American Academy of Pediatrics (AAP) Coding at the AAP Web site (www.aap.org/coding) routinely to find any corrections due to errata in the published version.

Contents

Tabular List

CONTENTS

Foreword

The American Academy of Pediatrics (AAP) is pleased to publish this second edition of *Pediatric ICD-10-CM: A Manual for Provider-Based Coding,* a pediatric version of the *International Classification of Diseases, 10th Revision, Clinical Modification (ICD-10-CM)* manual. As we continue this new chapter in diagnostic coding, the AAP believes it vital to publish an *ICD-10-CM* manual that is more manageable for pediatric providers. The expansive nature of the code set from *International Classification of Diseases, Ninth Revision, Clinical Modification* to *ICD-10-CM* has overwhelmed many physicians, providers, and coders, so we have condensed the code set by only providing pediatric-relevant diagnoses and their corresponding codes. We have reduced the guidelines so that only those applicable to the physician or provider are included, while those only relevant to facilities are removed and can be located in the larger *ICD-10-CM* manual. Lastly, guidelines that exist for topic-specific chapters or specific codes can now be found in their respective tabular chapter or right where the specific code is listed. This will aid the user in identifying any chapter- or code-specific guidelines right where they are needed most. This should assist in reducing any coding errors caused by reporting services that go against the guidelines that were once solely kept in the front of the manual, away from applicable codes.

The AAP is committed to the clinical modification of the *ICD* code set and for the past several years has sent an AAP liaison, Jeffrey F. Linzer Sr, MD, FACEP, FAAP, to the *ICD* Coordination and Maintenance Committee Meeting, which is the semiannual meeting where all new *ICD* codes are presented as well as revisions to the tabular list, index, and guidelines. Having a dedicated expert liaison aids in presenting pediatric issues at the meeting. The AAP is also very pleased to continue its work with the *ICD* Editorial Advisory Board for *Coding Clinic for ICD-10-CM and ICD-10-PCS. Coding Clinic* is responsible for publishing *ICD* coding guidance and clarifications to supplement the *ICD-10-CM* manual. Dr Linzer sits on the Editorial Advisory Board to represent pediatric issues and is an expert on all *ICD-10-CM* matters.

The AAP will continue to support its members on issues regarding coding, and the Division of Health Care Finance at the AAP headquarters stands ready to assist with problem areas not adequately covered in this manual. The AAP Coding Hotline can be accessed through e-mail at aapcodinghotline@aap.org.

Acknowledgments

Pediatric ICD-10-CM: A Manual for Provider-Based Coding is the product of the efforts of many dedicated individuals. First and foremost, we must thank Cindy Hughes, CPC, CFPC, consulting editor, for her professional input and particularly for her ongoing work to make this manual more user-friendly.

We would also like to thank members of the American Academy of Pediatrics (AAP) Committee on Coding and Nomenclature, past and present, and the AAP Coding Publications Editorial Advisory Board. The members of these committees have contributed extensive time in reviewing and editing content of this manual.

Eileen D. Brewer, MD, FAAP

Jamie Calabrese, MD, CPC, FAAP

David M. Kanter, MD, CPC, FAAP

Edward A. Liechty, MD, FAAP

Jeffrey F. Linzer Sr, MD, FACEP, FAAP

Richard A. Molteni, MD, FAAP

Julia M. Pillsbury, DO, FAAP

Lynn Wegner, MD, FAAP

We would also like to extend a very special thank-you to members of various subspecialty sections of the AAP who contributed their expertise and knowledge to the development of the original manual.

Margaret Ikeda, MD, FAAP, Section on Infectious Diseases

Robert Squires, MD, FAAP, Section on Gastroenterology, Hepatology, and Nutrition

Kupper A. Wintergerst, MD, FAAP, Section on Endocrinology

Jane Lynch, MD, FAAP, Section on Endocrinology

Lastly, we would like to acknowledge the tireless work of Jeffrey F. Linzer Sr, MD, FACEP, FAAP. Dr Linzer is the official AAP liaison to the *ICD* Coordination and Maintenance Committee and member of the Editorial Advisory Board for *Coding Clinic for ICD-10-CM and ICD-10-PCS*. Dr Linzer is an advocate for pediatrics and pediatric conditions and ensures that our issues are heard. He is an advocate for all pediatric patients in helping codes get established for conditions that need to be tracked for purposes of research and quality. Dr Linzer keeps the AAP and pediatric issues at the forefront of diagnostic coding, and we are very grateful for his time and expertise!

How to Use This Manual

While attempting to stay true to the complete *International Classification of Diseases, 10th Revision, Clinical Modification* (*ICD-10-CM*) manual, *Pediatric ICD-10-CM: A Manual for Provider-Based Coding* is meant specifically for pediatrics and only includes those conditions more commonly seen in pediatrics. We have attempted to remove all adult-only conditions as well as those conditions not typically found in the United States. Because *ICD* classification is used worldwide, many conditions listed in the official manual are not found in this part of the world.

Guidelines that are relevant to all pediatric codes are still included. Note that some chapter-specific guidelines will appear at the beginning of the related chapter when they are overarching to most of that chapter. However, chapter-specific guidelines that are relevant only at specific category or code levels will be found at those category or code levels. The beginning of each chapter will reference the category(ies) or code(s) where the guidelines can be found.

We use our own abbreviations throughout that may not appear in *ICD-10-CM;* however, all abbreviations are defined on the inside front cover for easy access as you navigate through the manual.

While unspecified codes can still be found throughout and in certain instances will be the most appropriate code, we have removed nearly every code that uses unspecified laterality. We feel it is important that laterality is documented in nearly all conditions. You will see a footnote in those chapters where we have specifically left out laterality in nearly all conditions. If you need to report unspecified laterality for a condition and it is not listed in the chapter, refer to the full *ICD-10-CM* manual. Those codes will typically have a final character of 0 (zero) or 9.

Three-character codes still exist in *ICD-10-CM.* Those will be noted specifically throughout the chapters as well.

In an effort to keep the size of the manual manageable, some codes are only written out fully at the category or subcategory level. The category or subcategory will be notated with a semicolon (;) and the code will begin with a lowercase letter. For example

A37.0   Whooping cough due to Bordetella pertussis;
  A37.00 without pneumonia
  A37.01 with pneumonia

At the subcategory level (A37.0) you see the semicolon (;) and at the code levels (A37.00 and A37.01) the codes begin with a lowercase letter. Therefore, code A37.00 reads, "Whooping cough due to Bordetella pertussis without pneumonia."

ICD-10-CM Official Guidelines for Coding and Reporting
FY 2017

The Centers for Medicare and Medicaid Services (CMS) and the National Center for Health Statistics (NCHS), two departments within the U.S. Federal Government's Department of Health and Human Services (DHHS) provide the following guidelines for coding and reporting using the International Classification of Diseases, 10th Revision, Clinical Modification (*ICD-10-CM*). These guidelines should be used as a companion document to the official version of the *ICD-10-CM* as published on the NCHS website. The *ICD-10-CM* is a morbidity classification published by the United States for classifying diagnoses and reason for visits in all health care settings. The *ICD-10-CM* is based on the ICD-10, the statistical classification of disease published by the World Health Organization (WHO).

These guidelines have been approved by the four organizations that make up the Cooperating Parties for the *ICD-10-CM*: the American Hospital Association (AHA), the American Health Information Management Association (AHIMA), CMS, and NCHS.

These guidelines are a set of rules that have been developed to accompany and complement the official conventions and instructions provided within the *ICD-10-CM* itself. The instructions and conventions of the classification take precedence over guidelines. These guidelines are based on the coding and sequencing instructions in the Tabular List and Alphabetic Index of *ICD-10-CM*, but provide additional instruction. Adherence to these guidelines when assigning *ICD-10-CM* diagnosis codes is required under the Health Insurance Portability and Accountability Act (HIPAA). The diagnosis codes (Tabular List and Alphabetic Index) have been adopted under HIPAA for all healthcare settings. A joint effort between the healthcare provider and the coder is essential to achieve complete and accurate documentation, code assignment, and reporting of diagnoses and procedures. These guidelines have been developed to assist both the healthcare provider and the coder in identifying those diagnoses that are to be reported. The importance of consistent, complete documentation in the medical record cannot be overemphasized. Without such documentation accurate coding cannot be achieved. The entire record should be reviewed to determine the specific reason for the encounter and the conditions treated.

The term encounter is used for all settings, including hospital admissions. In the context of these guidelines, the term provider is used throughout the guidelines to mean physician or any qualified health care practitioner who is legally accountable for establishing the patient's diagnosis. Only this set of guidelines, approved by the Cooperating Parties, is official.

The guidelines are organized into sections. Section I includes the structure and conventions of the classification and general guidelines that apply to the entire classification, and chapter-specific guidelines that correspond to the chapters as they are arranged in the classification. Section II includes guidelines for selection of principal diagnosis for non-outpatient settings. Section III includes guidelines for reporting additional diagnoses in non-outpatient settings. Section IV is for outpatient coding and reporting. It is necessary to review all sections of the guidelines to fully understand all of the rules and instructions needed to code properly.

Section I. Conventions, general coding guidelines and chapter specific guidelines

The conventions, general guidelines and chapter-specific guidelines are applicable to all health care settings unless otherwise indicated. The conventions and instructions of the classification take precedence over guidelines.

A. Conventions for the *ICD-10-CM*

The conventions for the *ICD-10-CM* are the general rules for use of the classification independent of the guidelines. These conventions are incorporated within the Alphabetic Index and Tabular List of the *ICD-10-CM* as instructional notes.

1. The Alphabetic Index and Tabular List

The *ICD-10-CM* is divided into the Alphabetic Index, an alphabetical list of terms and their corresponding code, and the Tabular List, a structured list of codes divided into chapters based on body system or condition. The Alphabetic Index consists of the following parts: the Index of Diseases and Injury, the Index of External Causes of Injury, the Table of Neoplasms and the Table of Drugs and Chemicals.

See Section I.C2. General guidelines

See Section I.C.19. Adverse effects, poisoning, underdosing and toxic effects

2. Format and Structure

The *ICD-10-CM* Tabular List contains categories, subcategories and codes. Characters for categories, subcategories and codes may be either a letter or a number. All categories are 3 characters. A three-character category that has no further subdivision is equivalent to a code. Subcategories are either 4 or 5 characters. Codes may be 3, 4, 5, 6 or 7 characters. That is, each level of subdivision after a category is a subcategory. The final level of subdivision is a code. Codes that have applicable 7th characters are still referred to as codes, not subcategories. A code that has an applicable 7th character is considered invalid without the 7th character.

The *ICD-10-CM* uses an indented format for ease in reference.

3. Use of codes for reporting purposes

For reporting purposes only codes are permissible, not categories or subcategories, and any applicable 7th character is required.

4. Placeholder character

The *ICD-10-CM* utilizes a placeholder character "X". The "X" is used as a placeholder at certain codes to allow for future expansion. An example of this is at the poisoning, adverse effect and underdosing codes, categories T36-T50. Where a placeholder exists, the X must be used in order for the code to be considered a valid code.

5. 7th Characters

Certain *ICD-10-CM* categories have applicable 7th characters. The applicable 7th character is required for all codes within the category, or as the notes in the Tabular List instruct. The 7th character must always be the 7th character in the data field. If a code that requires a 7th character is not 6 characters, a placeholder X must be used to fill in the empty characters.

6. Abbreviations

a. Alphabetic Index abbreviations

NEC "Not elsewhere classifiable"—This abbreviation in the Alphabetic Index represents "other specified". When a specific code is not available for a condition, the Alphabetic Index directs the coder to the "other specified" code in the Tabular List.

NOS "Not otherwise specified"—This abbreviation is the equivalent of unspecified.

b. Tabular List abbreviations

NEC "Not elsewhere classifiable"—This abbreviation in the Tabular List represents "other specified". When a specific code is not available for a condition the Tabular List includes an NEC entry under a code to identify the code as the "other specified" code.

NOS "Not otherwise specified"—This abbreviation is the equivalent of unspecified.

7. Punctuation

[ ] Brackets are used in the Tabular List to enclose synonyms, alternative wording or explanatory phrases. Brackets are used in the Alphabetic Index to identify manifestation codes.

( ) Parentheses are used in both the Alphabetic Index and Tabular List to enclose supplementary words that may be present or absent in the statement of a disease or procedure without affecting the code number to which it is assigned. The terms within the parentheses are referred to as nonessential modifiers. The nonessential modifiers in the Alphabetic Index to Diseases apply to subterms following a main term except when a nonessential modifier and a subentry are mutually exclusive, the subentry takes precedence. For example, in the *ICD-10-CM* Alphabetic Index under the main term Enteritis, "acute" is a nonessential modifier and "chronic" is a subentry. In this case, the nonessential modifier "acute" does not apply to the subentry "chronic".

: Colons are used in the Tabular List after an incomplete term which needs one or more of the modifiers following the colon to make it assignable to a given category.

8. **Use of "and".**

   Refer to Section I.A.14 (page xiv). Use of the term "And"

9. **Other and Unspecified codes**

   a. **"Other" codes**

      Codes titled "other" or "other specified" are for use when the information in the medical record provides detail for which a specific code does not exist. Alphabetic Index entries with NEC in the line designate "other" codes in the Tabular List. These Alphabetic Index entries represent specific disease entities for which no specific code exists so the term is included within an "other" code.

   b. **"Unspecified" codes**

      Codes titled "unspecified" are for use when the information in the medical record is insufficient to assign a more specific code. For those categories for which an unspecified code is not provided, the "other specified" code may represent both other and unspecified.

      See Use of Sign/Symptom/Unspecified Codes, page xvii

10. **Includes Notes**

    This note appears immediately under a three character code title to further define, or give examples of, the content of the category.

11. **Inclusion terms**

    List of terms is included under some codes. These terms are the conditions for which that code is to be used. The terms may be synonyms of the code title, or, in the case of "other specified" codes, the terms are a list of the various conditions assigned to that code. The inclusion terms are not necessarily exhaustive. Additional terms found only in the Alphabetic Index may also be assigned to a code.

12. **Excludes Notes**

    The *ICD-10-CM* has two types of excludes notes. Each type of note has a different definition for use but they are all similar in that they indicate that codes excluded from each other are independent of each other.

    a. **Excludes1**

       A type 1 Excludes note is a pure excludes note. It means "NOT CODED HERE!" An Excludes1 note indicates that the code excluded should never be used at the same time as the code above the Excludes1 note. An Excludes1 is used when two conditions cannot occur together, such as a congenital form versus an acquired form of the same condition.

    b. **Excludes2**

       A type 2 Excludes note represents "Not included here". An excludes2 note indicates that the condition excluded is not part of the condition represented by the code, but a patient may have both conditions at the same time. When an Excludes2 note appears under a code, it is acceptable to use both the code and the excluded code together, when appropriate.

13. **Etiology/manifestation convention ("code first", "use additional code" and "in diseases classified elsewhere" notes)**

    Certain conditions have both an underlying etiology and multiple body system manifestations due to the underlying etiology. For such conditions, the *ICD-10-CM* has a coding convention that requires the underlying condition be sequenced first followed by the manifestation. Wherever such a combination exists, there is a "use additional code" note at the etiology code, and a "code first" note at the manifestation code. These instructional notes indicate the proper sequencing order of the codes, etiology followed by manifestation.

    In most cases the manifestation codes will have in the code title, "in diseases classified elsewhere." Codes with this title are a component of the etiology/ manifestation convention. The code title indicates that it is a manifestation code. "In diseases classified elsewhere" codes are never permitted to be used as first-listed or principal diagnosis codes. They must be used in conjunction with an underlying condition code and they must be listed following the underlying condition. See category F02, Dementia in other diseases classified elsewhere, for an example of this convention.

There are manifestation codes that do not have "in diseases classified elsewhere" in the title. For such codes, there is a "use additional code" note at the etiology code and a "code first" note at the manifestation code and the rules for sequencing apply.

In addition to the notes in the Tabular List, these conditions also have a specific Alphabetic Index entry structure. In the Alphabetic Index both conditions are listed together with the etiology code first followed by the manifestation codes in brackets. The code in brackets is always to be sequenced second.

An example of the etiology/manifestation convention is dementia in Parkinson's disease. In the Alphabetic Index, code G20 is listed first, followed by code F02.80 or F02.81 in brackets. Code G20 represents the underlying etiology, Parkinson's disease, and must be sequenced first, whereas codes F02.80 and F02.81 represent the manifestation of dementia in diseases classified elsewhere, with or without behavioral disturbance.

"Code first" and "Use additional code" notes are also used as sequencing rules in the classification for certain codes that are not part of an etiology/ manifestation combination.

See Section I.B.7. Multiple coding for a single condition.

14. "And"

The word "and" should be interpreted to mean either "and" or "or" when it appears in a title.

For example, cases of "tuberculosis of bones", "tuberculosis of joints" and "tuberculosis of bones and joints" are classified to subcategory A18.0, Tuberculosis of bones and joints.

15. "With"

The word "with" should be interpreted to mean "associated with" or "due to" when it appears in a code title, the Alphabetic Index, or an instructional note in the Tabular List.

The word "with" in the Alphabetic Index is sequenced immediately following the main term, not in alphabetical order.

16. "See" and "See Also"

The "see" instruction following a main term in the Alphabetic Index indicates that another term should be referenced. It is necessary to go to the main term referenced with the "see" note to locate the correct code.

A "see also" instruction following a main term in the Alphabetic Index instructs that there is another main term that may also be referenced that may provide additional Alphabetic Index entries that may be useful. It is not necessary to follow the "see also" note when the original main term provides the necessary code.

17. "Code also note"

A "code also" note instructs that two codes may be required to fully describe a condition, but this note does not provide sequencing direction.

18. Default codes

A code listed next to a main term in the *ICD-10-CM* Alphabetic Index is referred to as a default code. The default code represents that condition that is most commonly associated with the main term, or is the unspecified code for the condition. If a condition is documented in a medical record (for example, appendicitis) without any additional information, such as acute or chronic, the default code should be assigned.

B. General Coding Guidelines

1. Locating a code in the *ICD-10-CM*

To select a code in the classification that corresponds to a diagnosis or reason for visit documented in a medical record, first locate the term in the Alphabetic Index, and then verify the code in the Tabular List. Read and be guided by instructional notations that appear in both the Alphabetic Index and the Tabular List.

It is essential to use both the Alphabetic Index and Tabular List when locating and assigning a code. The Alphabetic Index does not always provide the full code. Selection of the full code, including laterality and any applicable 7th character can only be done in the Tabular List. A dash (-) at the end of an Alphabetic Index entry indicates that additional characters are required. Even if a dash is not included at the Alphabetic Index entry, it is necessary to refer to the Tabular List to verify that no 7th character is required.

2. Level of Detail in Coding

Diagnosis codes are to be used and reported at their highest number of characters available.

ICD-10-CM diagnosis codes are composed of codes with 3, 4, 5, 6 or 7 characters. Codes with three characters are included in *ICD-10-CM* as the heading of a category of codes that may be further subdivided by the use of fourth and/or fifth characters and/or sixth characters, which provide greater detail.

A three-character code is to be used only if it is not further subdivided. A code is invalid if it has not been coded to the full number of characters required for that code, including the 7th character, if applicable.

3. **Code or codes from A00.0 through T88.9, Z00–Z99.8**

The appropriate code or codes from A00.0 through T88.9, Z00–Z99.8 must be used to identify diagnoses, symptoms, conditions, problems, complaints or other reason(s) for the encounter/visit.

4. **Signs and symptoms**

Codes that describe symptoms and signs, as opposed to diagnoses, are acceptable for reporting purposes when a related definitive diagnosis has not been established (confirmed) by the provider. Chapter 18 of *ICD-10-CM*, Symptoms, Signs, and Abnormal Clinical and Laboratory Findings, Not Elsewhere Classified (codes R00.0–R99) contains many, but not all codes for symptoms.

See Use of Signs/Symptom/Unspecified Codes, page xvii

5. **Conditions that are an integral part of a disease process**

Signs and symptoms that are associated routinely with a disease process should not be assigned as additional codes, unless otherwise instructed by the classification.

6. **Conditions that are not an integral part of a disease process**

Additional signs and symptoms that may not be associated routinely with a disease process should be coded when present.

7. **Multiple coding for a single condition**

In addition to the etiology/manifestation convention that requires two codes to fully describe a single condition that affects multiple body systems, there are other single conditions that also require more than one code. "Use additional code" notes are found in the Tabular List at codes that are not part of an etiology/manifestation pair where a secondary code is useful to fully describe a condition. The sequencing rule is the same as the etiology/manifestation pair, "use additional code" indicates that a secondary code should be added.

For example, for bacterial infections that are not included in chapter 1, a secondary code from category B95, Streptococcus, Staphylococcus, and Enterococcus, as the cause of diseases classified elsewhere, or B96, Other bacterial agents as the cause of diseases classified elsewhere, may be required to identify the bacterial organism causing the infection. A "use additional code" note will normally be found at the infectious disease code, indicating a need for the organism code to be added as a secondary code.

"Code first" notes are also under certain codes that are not specifically manifestation codes but may be due to an underlying cause. When there is a "code first" note and an underlying condition is present, the underlying condition should be sequenced first.

"Code, if applicable, any causal condition first", notes indicate that this code may be assigned as a principal diagnosis when the causal condition is unknown or not applicable. If a causal condition is known, then the code for that condition should be sequenced as the principal or first-listed diagnosis.

Multiple codes may be needed for sequela, complication codes and obstetric codes to more fully describe a condition. See the specific guidelines for these conditions for further instruction.

8. **Acute and Chronic Conditions**

If the same condition is described as both acute (subacute) and chronic, and separate subentries exist in the Alphabetic Index at the same indentation level, code both and sequence the acute (subacute) code first.

9. **Combination Code**

A combination code is a single code used to classify:

Two diagnoses, or

A diagnosis with an associated secondary process (manifestation)

A diagnosis with an associated complication

Combination codes are identified by referring to subterm entries in the Alphabetic Index and by reading the inclusion and exclusion notes in the Tabular List.

Assign only the combination code when that code fully identifies the diagnostic conditions involved or when the Alphabetic Index so directs. Multiple coding should not be used when the classification provides a combination code that clearly identifies all of the elements documented in the diagnosis. When the combination code lacks necessary specificity in describing the manifestation or complication, an additional code should be used as a secondary code.

10. Sequela (Late Effects)

A sequela is the residual effect (condition produced) after the acute phase of an illness or injury has terminated. There is no time limit on when a sequela code can be used. The residual may be apparent early, such as in cerebral infarction, or it may occur months or years later, such as that due to a previous injury. Examples of sequela include: scar formation resulting from a burn, deviated septum due to a nasal fracture, and infertility due to tubal occlusion from old tuberculosis.Coding of sequela generally requires two codes sequenced in the following order: The condition or nature of the sequela is sequenced first. The sequela code is sequenced second.

An exception to the above guidelines are those instances where the code for the sequela is followed by a manifestation code identified in the Tabular List and title, or the sequela code has been expanded (at the fourth, fifth or sixth character levels) to include the manifestation(s). The code for the acute phase of an illness or injury that led to the sequela is never used with a code for the late effect.

Application of 7th characters refer to Chapter 19

11. Impending or Threatened Condition

Code any condition described at the time of discharge as "impending" or "threatened" as follows:

If it did occur, code as confirmed diagnosis. If it did not occur, reference the Alphabetic Index to determine if the condition has a subentry term for "impending" or "threatened" and also reference main term entries for "Impending" and for "Threatened." If the subterms are listed, assign the given code. If the subterms are not listed, code the existing underlying condition(s) and not the condition described as impending or threatened.

12. Reporting Same Diagnosis Code More than Once

Each unique *ICD-10-CM* diagnosis code may be reported only once for an encounter. This applies to bilateral conditions when there are no distinct codes identifying laterality or two different conditions classified to the same *ICD-10-CM* diagnosis code.

13. Laterality

Some *ICD-10-CM* codes indicate laterality, specifying whether the condition occurs on the left, right or is bilateral. If no bilateral code is provided and the condition is bilateral, assign separate codes for both the left and right side. If the side is not identified in the medical record, assign the code for the unspecified side.

14. Documentation for BMI, Non-pressure ulcers and Pressure Ulcer Stages

For the Body Mass Index (BMI), depth of non-pressure chronic ulcers and pressure ulcer stage codes, code assignment may be based on medical record documentation from clinicians who are not the patient's provider (i.e., physician or other qualified healthcare practitioner legally accountable for establishing the patient's diagnosis), since this information is typically documented by other clinicians involved in the care of the patient (e.g., a dietitian often documents the BMI and nurses often documents the pressure ulcer stages). However, the associated diagnosis (such as overweight, obesity, or pressure ulcer) must be documented by the patient's provider. If there is conflicting medical record documentation, either from the same clinician or different clinicians, the patient's attending provider should be queried for clarification.

The BMI codes should only be reported as secondary diagnoses. As with all other secondary diagnosis codes, the BMI codes should only be assigned when they meet the definition of a reportable additional diagnosis (see Section III, Reporting Additional Diagnoses).

15. Syndromes

Follow the Alphabetic Index guidance when coding syndromes. In the absence of Alphabetic Index guidance, assign codes for the documented manifestations of the syndrome. Additional codes for manifestations that are not an integral part of the disease process may also be assigned when the condition does not have a unique code.

16. Documentation of Complications of Care

Code assignment is based on the provider's documentation of the relationship between the condition and the care or procedure. The guideline extends to any complications of care, regardless of the chapter the code is located in. It is important to note that not all conditions that occur during or following medical care or surgery are classified as complications. There must be a cause-and-effect relationship between the care provided and the condition, and an indication in the documentation that it is a complication. Query the provider for clarification, if the complication is not clearly documented.

17. Borderline Diagnosis

If the provider documents a "borderline" diagnosis at the time of discharge, the diagnosis is coded as confirmed, unless the classification provides a specific entry (e.g., borderline diabetes). If a borderline condition has a specific index entry in *ICD-10-CM*, it should be coded as such. Since borderline conditions are not uncertain diagnoses, no distinction is made between the care setting (inpatient versus outpatient). Whenever the documentation is unclear regarding a borderline condition, coders are encouraged to query for clarification.

18. Use of Sign/Symptom/Unspecified Codes

Sign/symptom and "unspecified" codes have acceptable, even necessary, uses. While specific diagnosis codes should be reported when they are supported by the available medical record documentation and clinical knowledge of the patient's health condition, there are instances when signs/symptoms or unspecified codes are the best choices for accurately reflecting the healthcare encounter. Each healthcare encounter should be coded to the level of certainty known for that encounter.

If a definitive diagnosis has not been established by the end of the encounter, it is appropriate to report codes for sign(s) and/ or symptom(s) in lieu of a definitive diagnosis. When sufficient clinical information isn't known or available about a particular health condition to assign a more specific code, it is acceptable to report the appropriate "unspecified" code (e.g., a diagnosis of pneumonia has been determined, but not the specific type). Unspecified codes should be reported when they are the codes that most accurately reflects what is known about the patient's condition at the time of that particular encounter. It would be inappropriate to select a specific code that is not supported by the medical record documentation or conduct medically unnecessary diagnostic testing in order to determine a more specific code.

C. Chapter-Specific Coding Guidelines

Please refer to each chapter for information on specific guidelines.

Section II. Selection of Principle Diagnosis

Excluded as not relevant to provider-based coding refer to the full *ICD-10-CM* manual if needed

Section III. Reporting Additional Diagnoses

Excluded as not relevant to provider-based coding refer to the full *ICD-10-CM* manual if needed

Section IV. Diagnostic Coding and Reporting Guidelines for Outpatient Services

These coding guidelines for outpatient diagnoses have been approved for use by hospitals/ providers in coding and reporting hospital-based outpatient services and provider-based office visits.

Information about the use of certain abbreviations, punctuation, symbols, and other conventions used in the *ICD-10-CM* Tabular List (code numbers and titles), can be found in Section IA of these guidelines, under "Conventions Used in the Tabular List." **Section I.B. contains general guidelines that apply to the entire classification. Section I.C. contains chapter-specific guidelines that correspond to the chapters as they are arranged in the classification.** Information about the correct sequence to use in finding a code is also described in Section I.

The terms encounter and visit are often used interchangeably in describing outpatient service contacts and, therefore, appear together in these guidelines without distinguishing one from the other.

Though the conventions and general guidelines apply to all settings, coding guidelines for outpatient and provider reporting of diagnoses will vary in a number of instances from those for inpatient diagnoses, recognizing that:

A. Selection of first-listed condition

In the outpatient setting, the term first-listed diagnosis is used in lieu of principal diagnosis.

In determining the first-listed diagnosis the coding conventions of *ICD-10-CM*, as well as the general and disease specific guidelines take precedence over the outpatient guidelines.

Diagnoses often are not established at the time of the initial encounter/visit. It may take two or more visits before the diagnosis is confirmed.

The most critical rule involves beginning the search for the correct code assignment through the Alphabetic Index. Never begin searching initially in the Tabular List as this will lead to coding errors.

1. Outpatient Surgery

When a patient presents for outpatient surgery (same day surgery), code the reason for the surgery as the first-listed diagnosis (reason for the encounter), even if the surgery is not performed due to a contraindication.

2. Observation Stay

When a patient is admitted for observation for a medical condition, assign a code for the medical condition as the first-listed diagnosis.

When a patient presents for outpatient surgery and develops complications requiring admission to observation, code the reason for the surgery as the first reported diagnosis (reason for the encounter), followed by codes for the complications as secondary diagnoses.

B. Codes from A00.0 through T88.9, Z00–Z99

The appropriate code(s) from A00.0 through T88.9, Z00–Z99 must be used to identify diagnoses, symptoms, conditions, problems, complaints, or other reason(s) for the encounter/visit.

C. Accurate reporting of *ICD-10-CM* diagnosis codes

For accurate reporting of *ICD-10-CM* diagnosis codes, the documentation should describe the patient's condition, using terminology which includes specific diagnoses as well as symptoms, problems, or reasons for the encounter. There are *ICD-10-CM* codes to describe all of these.

D. Codes that describe symptoms and signs

Codes that describe symptoms and signs, as opposed to diagnoses, are acceptable for reporting purposes when a diagnosis has not been established (confirmed) by the provider. Chapter 18 of *ICD-10-CM*, Symptoms, Signs, and Abnormal Clinical and Laboratory Findings Not Elsewhere Classified (codes R00–R99) contain many, but not all codes for symptoms.

E. Encounters for circumstances other than a disease or injury

ICD-10-CM provides codes to deal with encounters for circumstances other than a disease or injury. The Factors Influencing Health Status and Contact with Health Services codes (Z00–Z99) are provided to deal with occasions when circumstances other than a disease or injury are recorded as diagnosis or problems.

See Chapter 21, Factors influencing health status and contact with health services.

F. Level of Detail in Coding

1. *ICD-10-CM* codes with 3, 4, 5, 6 or 7 characters

ICD-10-CM is composed of codes with 3, 4, 5, 6 or 7 characters. Codes with three characters are included in *ICD-10-CM* as the heading of a category of codes that may be further subdivided by the use of fourth, fifth, sixth or seventh characters to provide greater specificity.

2. Use of full number of *characters* required for a code

A three-character code is to be used only if it is not further subdivided. A code is invalid if it has not been coded to the full number of characters required for that code, including the 7th character, if applicable.

G. *ICD-10-CM* code for the diagnosis, condition, problem, or other reason for encounter/visit

List first the *ICD-10-CM* code for the diagnosis, condition, problem, or other reason for encounter/visit shown in the medical record to be chiefly responsible for the services provided. List additional codes that describe any coexisting conditions. In some cases the first-listed diagnosis may be a symptom when a diagnosis has not been established (confirmed) by the physician.

H. Uncertain diagnosis

<u>Do not code</u> diagnoses documented as "probable", "suspected," "questionable," "rule out," or "working diagnosis" or other similar terms indicating uncertainty. Rather, code the condition(s) to the highest degree of certainty for that encounter/visit, such as symptoms, signs, abnormal test results, or other reason for the visit.

I. Chronic diseases

Chronic diseases treated on an ongoing basis may be coded and reported as many times as the patient receives treatment and care for the condition(s)

J. Code all documented conditions that coexist

Code all documented conditions that coexist at the time of the encounter/visit, and require or affect patient care treatment or management. Do not code conditions that were previously treated and no longer exist. However, history codes (categories Z80–Z87) may be used as secondary codes if the historical condition or family history has an impact on current care or influences treatment.

K. Patients receiving diagnostic services only

For patients receiving diagnostic services only during an encounter/visit, sequence first the diagnosis, condition, problem, or other reason for encounter/visit shown in the medical record to be chiefly responsible for the outpatient services provided during the encounter/visit. Codes for other diagnoses (e.g., chronic conditions) may be sequenced as additional diagnoses.

For encounters for routine laboratory/radiology testing in the absence of any signs, symptoms, or associated diagnosis, assign Z01.89, Encounter for other specified special examinations. If routine testing is performed during the same encounter as a test to evaluate a sign, symptom, or diagnosis, it is appropriate to assign both the **Z** code and the code describing the reason for the non-routine test.

For outpatient encounters for diagnostic tests that have been interpreted by a physician, and the final report is available at the time of coding, code any confirmed or definitive diagnosis(es) documented in the interpretation. Do not code related signs and symptoms as additional diagnoses.

Please note: This differs from the coding practice in the hospital inpatient setting regarding abnormal findings on test results.

L. Patients receiving therapeutic services only

For patients receiving therapeutic services only during an encounter/visit, sequence first the diagnosis, condition, problem, or other reason for encounter/visit shown in the medical record to be chiefly responsible for the outpatient services provided during the encounter/visit. Codes for other diagnoses (e.g., chronic conditions) may be sequenced as additional diagnoses.

The only exception to this rule is that when the primary reason for the admission/encounter is chemotherapy or radiation therapy, the appropriate Z code for the service is listed first, and the diagnosis or problem for which the service is being performed listed second.

M. Patients receiving preoperative evaluations only

For patients receiving preoperative evaluations only, sequence first a code from subcategory Z01.81, Encounter for pre-procedural examinations, to describe the pre-op consultations. Assign a code for the condition to describe the reason for the surgery as an additional diagnosis. Code also any findings related to the pre-op evaluation.

N. Ambulatory surgery

For ambulatory surgery, code the diagnosis for which the surgery was performed. If the postoperative diagnosis is known to be different from the preoperative diagnosis at the time the diagnosis is confirmed, select the postoperative diagnosis for coding, since it is the most definitive.

O. Routine outpatient prenatal visits

See Chapter 15, Routine outpatient prenatal visits.

P. Encounters for general medical examinations with abnormal findings

The subcategories for encounters for general medical examinations, Z00.0-, provide codes for with and without abnormal findings. Should a general medical examination result in an abnormal finding, the code for general medical examination with abnormal finding should be assigned as the first-listed diagnosis. A secondary code for the abnormal finding should also be coded.

Q. Encounters for routine health screenings

See Chapter 21, Factors influencing health status and contact with health services, Screening

Alphabetic Index

Instructions are listed in *italic font.* The "*see*" instruction indicates it is necessary to reference another term while "*see also*" instruction indicates another main term may provide additional entries. It is not necessary to follow a "*see also*" instruction when the current entry directs to a code for the condition. "*Code*" or "*Code to*" directs to the appropriate reference for a condition.

Punctuation

[ ]—used to identify manifestation codes
( )—enclose nonessential words that do not affect code assignment
:—the colon identifies that a term is incomplete and requires additional modifying terms

A

Aarskog's syndrome Q87.1
Abandonment—*see* Maltreatment
Abasia (-astasia) (hysterical) F44.4
Abdomen, abdominal—*see also* condition
  acute R10.0
  angina K55.1
  muscle deficiency syndrome Q79.4
Abdominalgia—*see* Pain, abdominal
Abduction contracture, hip or other joint—*see* Contraction, joint
Aberrant (congenital)—*see also* Malposition, congenital
  artery (peripheral) Q27.8
    pulmonary Q25.79
  endocrine gland NEC Q89.2
  hepatic duct Q44.5
  parathyroid gland Q89.2
  pituitary gland Q89.2
  thymus (gland) Q89.2
  thyroid gland Q89.2
Abiotrophy R68.89
Abnormal, abnormality, abnormalities—*see also* Anomaly
  auditory perception H93.29-
  autosomes Q99.9
  bleeding time R79.1
  blood gas level R79.81
  blood pressure
    elevated R03.0
  chest sounds (friction) (rales) R09.89
  chemistry, blood R79.9
    C-reactive protein R79.82
    drugs—*see* Findings, abnormal, in blood
    gas level R79.81
    pancytopenia D61.818
    PTT R79.1
  chromosome, chromosomal Q99.9
    sex Q99.8
      female phenotype Q97.9
      male phenotype Q98.9
  clinical findings NEC R68.89
  coagulation D68.9
    newborn, transient P61.6
    profile R79.1
    time R79.1
  development, developmental Q89.9
    central nervous system Q07.9
  diagnostic imaging
    abdomen, abdominal region NEC R93.5
    bladder R93.41
    coronary circulation R93.1
    head R93.0
    heart R93.1
    kidney R93.42-
    lung (field) R91.8
    musculoskeletal system NEC R93.7
    renal pelvis R93.41
    retroperitoneum R93.5
    skull R93.0
    ureter R93.41
    urinary organs, specified R93.49
  echocardiogram R93.1
  feces (color) (contents) (mucus) R19.5
  gait—*see* Gait
    hysterical F44.4

Abnormal, abnormality, abnormalities, *continued*
  heart
    rate R00.9
      specified NEC R00.8
    shadow R93.1
  hemoglobin (disease) (*see also* Disease, hemoglobin) D58.2
    trait—*see* Trait, hemoglobin, abnormal
  loss of
    weight R63.4
  Mantoux test R76.11
  movement (disorder)—*see also* Disorder, movement
    involuntary R25.9
      spasm R25.2
      tremor R25.1
  neonatal screening P09
  palmar creases Q82.8
  partial thromboplastin time (PTT) R79.1
  percussion, chest (tympany) R09.89
  posture R29.3
  prothrombin time (PT) R79.1
  pulmonary
    artery, congenital Q25.79
    function, newborn P28.89
  pulsations in neck R00.2
  sinus venosus Q21.1
  specimen
    specified organ, system and tissue NOS R89.9
  sputum (amount) (color) (odor) R09.3
  stool (color) (contents) (mucus) R19.5
    bloody K92.1
    guaiac positive R19.5
  transport protein E88.09
  urination NEC R39.198
  urine (constituents) R82.90
    glucose R81
    hemoglobin R82.3
    microbiological examination (positive culture) R82.79
  white blood cells D72.9
    specified NEC D72.89
  X-ray examination—*see* Abnormal, diagnostic imaging
Abnormity (any organ or part)—*see* Anomaly
Abocclusion M26.29
  hemolytic disease (newborn) P55.1
Abortion (complete) (spontaneous) O03.9
  incomplete (spontaneous) O03.4
  missed O02.1
  spontaneous—*see* Abortion (complete) (spontaneous)
    threatened O20.0
  threatened (spontaneous) O20.0
  tubal O00.10
    with intrauterine pregnancy O00.11
Abramov-Fiedler myocarditis (acute isolated myocarditis) I40.1
Abrasion T14.8
  abdomen, abdominal (wall) S30.811
  alveolar process S00.512
  ankle S90.51-
  antecubital space—*see* Abrasion, elbow
  anus S30.817
  arm (upper) S40.81-
  auditory canal—*see* Abrasion, ear
  auricle—*see* Abrasion, ear
  axilla—*see* Abrasion, arm
  back, lower S30.810
  breast S20.11-
  brow S00.81
  buttock S30.810
  calf—*see* Abrasion, leg
  canthus—*see* Abrasion, eyelid
  cheek S00.81
    internal S00.512
  chest wall—*see* Abrasion, thorax
  chin S00.81
  clitoris S30.814
  cornea S05.0-
  costal region—*see* Abrasion, thorax
  dental K03.1
  digit (s)
    foot—*see* Abrasion, toe
    hand—*see* Abrasion, finger
  ear S00.41-
  elbow S50.31-

Abrasion, *continued*
  epididymis S30.813
  epigastric region S30.811
  epiglottis S10.11
  esophagus (thoracic) S27.818
    cervical S10.11
  eyebrow S00.21-
  eyelid S00.21-
  face S00.81
  finger (s) S60.41-
    index S60.41-
    little S60.41-
    middle S60.41-
    ring S60.41-
  flank S30.811
  foot (except toe(s) alone) S90.81
    toe—*see* Abrasion, toe
  forearm S50.81-
    elbow only—*see* Abrasion, elbow
  forehead S00.81
  genital organs, external
    male S30.815
  groin S30.811
  gum S00.512
  hand S60.51-
  head S00.91
    ear—*see* Abrasion, ear
    eyelid—*see* Abrasion, eyelid
    lip S00.511
    nose S00.31
    oral cavity S00.512
    scalp S00.01
    specified site NEC S00.81
  heel—*see* Abrasion, foot
  hip S70.21-
  inguinal region S30.811
  interscapular region S20.419
  jaw S00.81
  knee S80.21-
  labium (majus) (minus) S30.814
  larynx S10.11
  leg (lower) S80.81-
    knee—*see* Abrasion, knee
    upper—*see* Abrasion, thigh
  lip S00.511
  lower back S30.810
  lumbar region S30.810
  malar region S00.81
  mammary—*see* Abrasion, breast
  mastoid region S00.81
  mouth S00.512
  nail
    finger—*see* Abrasion, finger
    toe—*see* Abrasion, toe
  nape S10.81
  nasal S00.31
  neck S10.91
    specified site NEC S10.81
    throat S10.11
  nose S00.31
  occipital region S00.01
  oral cavity S00.512
  orbital region—*see* Abrasion, eyelid
  palate S00.512
  palm—*see* Abrasion, hand
  parietal region S00.01
  pelvis S30.810
  penis S30.812
  perineum
    female S30.814
    male S30.810
  periocular area—*see* Abrasion, eyelid
  phalanges
    finger—*see* Abrasion, finger
    toe—*see* Abrasion, toe
  pharynx S10.11
  pinna—*see* Abrasion, ear
  popliteal space—*see* Abrasion, knee
  prepuce S30.812
  pubic region S30.810
  pudendum
    female S30.816
    male S30.815

Abrasion, *continued*
  sacral region S30.810
  scalp S00.01
  scapular region—*see* Abrasion, shoulder
  scrotum S30.813
  shin—*see* Abrasion, leg
  shoulder S40.21
  skin NEC T14.8
  sternal region S20.319
  submaxillary region S00.81
  submental region S00.81
  subungual
    finger (s)—*see* Abrasion, finger
    toe (s)—*see* Abrasion, toe
  supraclavicular fossa S10.81
  supraorbital S00.81
  temple S00.81
  temporal region S00.81
  testis S30.813
  thigh S70.31-
  thorax, thoracic (wall) S20.91
    back S20.41-
    front S20.31-
  throat S10.11
  thumb S60.31-
  toe (s) (lesser) S90.416
    great S90.41-
  tongue S00.512
  tooth, teeth (dentifrice) (habitual) (hard tissues)
        (occupational) (ritual)
        (traditional) K03.1
  trachea S10.11
  tunica vaginalis S30.813
  tympanum, tympanic membrane—*see* Abrasion, ear
  uvula S00.512
  vagina S30.814
  vocal cords S10.11
  vulva S30.814
  wrist S60.81-
Abscess (connective tissue) (embolic) (fistulous) (metastatic)
        (multiple) (pernicious)
        (pyogenic) (septic)
        L02.91
  abdomen, abdominal
    cavity K65.1
    wall L02.211
  abdominopelvic K65.1
  accessory sinus—*see* Sinusitis
  alveolar K04.7
  anus K61.0
  apical (tooth) K04.7
  appendix K35.3
  areola (acute) (chronic) (nonpuerperal) N61.1
  axilla (region) L02.41
    lymph gland or node L04.2
  back (any part, except buttock) L02.212
  Bartholin's gland N75.1
  brain (any part) (cystic) (otogenic) G06.0
  breast (acute) (chronic) (nonpuerperal) N61.1
    newborn P39.0
  buccal cavity K12.2
  buttock L02.31
  cerebellum, cerebellar G06.0
    sequelae G09
  cecum K35.3
  cerebral (embolic) G06.0
    sequelae G09
  cervical (meaning neck) L02.11
    lymph gland or node L04.0
  cheek (external) L02.01
    inner K12.2
  chest J86.9
    with fistula J86.0
    wall L02.213
  chin L02.01
  circumtonsillar J36
  cranium G06.0
  dental K04.7
  dentoalveolar K04.7
  ear (middle)—*see also* Otitis, media, suppurative
    acute—*see* Otitis, media, suppurative, acute
    external H60.0-

Abscess, *continued*
  epididymis N45.4
  epidural G06.2
    brain G06.0
    spinal cord G06.1
  erysipelatous—*see* Erysipelas
  esophagus K20.8
  ethmoid (bone) (chronic) (sinus) J32.2
  extradural G06.2
    brain G06.0
      sequelae G09
    spinal cord G06.1
  eyelid H00.03-
  face (any part, except ear, eye and nose) L02.01
  foot L02.61-
  forehead L02.01
  frontal sinus (chronic) J32.1
  gallbladder K81.0
  gluteal (region) L02.31
  groin L02.214
  hand L02.51-
  head NEC L02.811
    face (any part, except ear, eye and nose) L02.01
  heel—*see* Abscess, foot
  iliac (region) L02.214
  ileocecal K35.3
  iliac (region) L02.214
    fossa K35.3
  inguinal (region) L02.214
    lymph gland or node L04.1
  intracranial G06.0
  intratonsillar J36
  knee—*see also* Abscess, lower limb
    joint M00.9
  lateral (alveolar) K04.7
  lingual K14.0
    tonsil J36
  lip K13.0
  loin (region) L02.211
  lower limb L02.41
  lumbar (tuberculous) A18.01
    nontuberculous L02.212
  lymph, lymphatic, gland or node (acute)—*see also*
        Lymphadenitis, acute
    mesentery I88.0
  marginal, anus K61.0
  maxilla, maxillary M27.2
    molar (tooth) K04.7
    premolar K04.7
    sinus (chronic) J32.0
  mons pubis L02.215
  mouth (floor) K12.2
  myocardium I40.0
  nasal J32.9
  navel L02.216
    newborn P38.9
      with mild hemorrhage P38.1
      without hemorrhage P38.9
  neck (region) L02.11
    lymph gland or node L04.0
  nipple N61.1
  nose (external) (fossa) (septum) J34.0
    sinus (chronic)—*see* Sinusitis
  otogenic G06.0
  palate (soft) K12.2
    hard M27.2
  parapharyngeal J39.0
  parietal (region) (scalp) L02.811
  parotid (duct) (gland) K11.3
    region K12.2
  pectoral (region) L02.213
  perianal K61.0
  periapical K04.7
  periappendicular K35.3
  pericardial I30.1
  pericecal K35.3
  perineum, perineal (superficial) L02.215
    urethra N34.0
  periodontal (parietal) K05.21
    apical K04.7
  peripharyngeal J39.0

Abscess, *continued*
  peripleuritic J86.9
    with fistula J86.0
  peritoneum, peritoneal (perforated) (ruptured) K65.1
    with appendicitis K35.3
  peritonsillar J36
  perityphlic K35.3
  phagedenic NOS L02.91
    chancroid A57
  pleura J86.9
    with fistula J86.0
  pilonidal L05.01
  postcecal K35.3
  postnasal J34.0
  postpharyngeal J39.0
  posttonsillar J36
  retropharyngeal J39.0
  root, tooth K04.7
  rupture (spontaneous) NOS L02.91
  scalp (any part) L02.811
  scrofulous (tuberculous) A18.2
  septal, dental K04.7
  sinus (accessory) (chronic) (nasal)—*see also* Sinusitis
    intracranial venous (any) G06.0
  specified site NEC L02.818
  sphenoidal (sinus) (chronic) J32.3
  subarachnoid G06.2
    brain G06.0
    spinal cord G06.1
  subcecal K35.3
  subcutaneous—*see also* Abscess, by site
  subdural G06.2
    brain G06.0
      sequelae G09
    spinal cord G06.1
  subgaleal L02.811
  sublingual K12.2
    gland K11.3
  submandibular (region) (space) (triangle) K12.2
    gland K11.3
  submaxillary (region) L02.01
    gland K11.3
  submental L02.01
    gland K11.3
  temple L02.01
  temporal region L02.01
  temporosphenoidal G06.0
  testes N45.4
  thyroid (gland) E06.0
  thorax J86.9
    with fistula J86.0
  tongue (staphylococcal) K14.0
  tonsil (s) (lingual) J36
  tonsillopharyngeal J36
  tooth, teeth (root) K04.7
  trunk L02.219
    abdominal wall L02.211
    back L02.212
    chest wall L02.213
    groin L02.214
    perineum L02.215
    umbilicus L02.216
  umbilicus L02.216
  upper
    limb L02.41-
  uvula K12.2
  vermiform appendix K35.3
  vulvovaginal gland N75.1
Absence (of) (organ or part) (complete or partial)
  albumin in blood E88.09
  alimentary tract (congenital) Q45.8
    upper Q40.8
  anus (congenital) Q42.3
    with fistula Q42.2
  aorta (congenital) Q25.41
  appendix, congenital Q42.8
  artery (congenital) (peripheral) Q27.8
    pulmonary Q25.79
    umbilical Q27.0
  atrial septum (congenital) Q21.1
  bile, biliary duct, congenital Q44.5
  corpus callosum Q04.0

Absence, *continued*
  digestive organ (s) or tract, congenital Q45.8
    acquired NEC Z90.49
    upper Q40.8
  endocrine gland (congenital) NEC Q89.2
    acquired E89.89
  family member (causing problem in home) NEC (*see also* Disruption, family) Z63.32
  fibrinogen (congenital) D68.2
    acquired D65
  gallbladder (acquired) Z90.49
    congenital Q44.0
  gamma globulin in blood D80.1
    hereditary D80.0
  genital organs
    acquired (female) (male) Z90.79
    female, congenital Q52.8
      external Q52.71
      internal NEC Q52.8
    male, congenital Q55.8
  genitourinary organs, congenital NEC
    female Q52.8
    male Q55.8
  ileum (acquired) Z90.49
    congenital Q41.2
  intestine (acquired) (small) Z90.49
    congenital Q41.9
      specified NEC Q41.8
    large Z90.49
      congenital Q42.9
        specified NEC Q42.8
  jejunum (acquired) Z90.49
    congenital Q41.1
  kidney (s) (acquired) Z90.5
    congenital Q60.2
      bilateral Q60.1
      unilateral Q60.0
  organ
    or site, congenital NEC Q89.8
    acquired NEC Z90.89
  parathyroid gland (acquired) E89.2
    congenital Q89.2
  pituitary gland (congenital) Q89.2
    acquired E89.3
  rectum (congenital) Q42.1
    with fistula Q42.0
    acquired Z90.49
  respiratory organ NOS Q34.9
  scrotum, congenital Q55.29
  septum
    atrial (congenital) Q21.1
  skull bone (congenital) Q75.8
    with
      anencephaly Q00.0
      encephalocele—*see* Encephalocele
      hydrocephalus Q03.9
        with spina bifida—*see* Spina bifida, by site, with hydrocephalus
      microcephaly Q02
  teeth, tooth (congenital) K00.0
    acquired (complete) K08.109
      class I K08.101
      class II K08.102
      class III K08.103
      class IV K08.104
      due to
        caries K08.139
          class I K08.131
          class II K08.132
          class III K08.133
          class IV K08.134
        periodontal disease K08.129
          class I K08.121
          class II K08.122
          class III K08.123
          class IV K08.124
      specified NEC K08.199
        class I K08.191
        class II K08.192
        class III K08.193
        class IV K08.194

Absence, *continued*
    trauma K08.119
      class I K08.111
      class II K08.112
      class III K08.113
      class IV K08.114
    partial K08.409
      class I K08.401
      class II K08.402
      class III K08.403
      class IV K08.404
      due to
        caries K08.439
          class I K08.431
          class II K08.432
          class III K08.433
          class IV K08.434
        periodontal disease K08.429
          class I K08.421
          class II K08.422
          class III K08.423
          class IV K08.424
      specified NEC K08.499
        class I K08.491
        class II K08.492
        class III K08.493
        class IV K08.494
      trauma K08.419
        class I K08.411
        class II K08.412
        class III K08.413
        class IV K08.414
  testes (congenital) Q55.0
    acquired Z90.79
  thymus gland Q89.2
  thyroid (gland) (acquired) E89.0
    cartilage, congenital Q31.8
    congenital E03.1
    tricuspid valve Q22.4
  transverse aortic arch, congenital Q25.49
  umbilical artery, congenital Q27.0

Absorption
  carbohydrate, disturbance K90.49
  chemical—*see* Table of Drugs and Chemicals
    through placenta (newborn) P04.9
      environmental substance P04.6
      nutritional substance P04.5
      obstetric anesthetic or analgesic drug P04.0
  drug NEC—*see* Table of Drugs and Chemicals
    addictive
      through placenta (newborn) P04.49
        cocaine P04.41
    medicinal
      through placenta (newborn) P04.1
    through placenta (newborn) P04.1
      obstetric anesthetic or analgesic drug P04.0
  fat, disturbance K90.49
    pancreatic K90.3
  noxious substance—*see* Table of Drugs and Chemicals
  protein, disturbance K90.49
  starch, disturbance K90.49
  toxic substance—*see* Table of Drugs and Chemicals
Abstinence symptoms, syndrome
  alcohol F10.239
  cocaine F14.23
  neonatal P96.1
  nicotine—*see* Dependence, drug, nicotine, with, withdrawal
  stimulant NEC F15.93
    with dependence F15.23
Abuse
  alcohol (nondependent) F10.10
    with
      anxiety disorder F10.180
      intoxication F10.129
        with delirium F10.121
        uncomplicated F10.120
      mood disorder F10.14
      other specified disorder F10.188
      counseling and surveillance Z71.41
  amphetamine (or related substance)—*see* Abuse, drug, stimulant NEC

Abuse, *continued*
  anxiolytic—*see* Abuse, drug, sedative
  barbiturates—*see* Abuse, drug, sedative
  caffeine—*see* Abuse, drug, stimulant NEC
  cannabis, cannabinoids—*see* Abuse, drug, cannabis
  child—*see* Maltreatment, child
  cocaine—*see* Abuse, drug, cocaine
  drug NEC (nondependent) F19.10
    amphetamine type—*see* Abuse, drug, stimulant NEC
    anxiolytics—*see* Abuse, drug, sedative
    barbiturates—*see* Abuse, drug, sedative
    caffeine—*see* Abuse, drug, stimulant NEC
    cannabis F12.10
      with
        intoxication F12.129
          uncomplicated F12.120
    cocaine F14.10
      with
        intoxication F14.129
          uncomplicated F14.120
    counseling and surveillance Z71.51
    hashish—*see* Abuse, drug, cannabis
    inhalant F18.10
    PCP (phencyclidine) (or related substance)—*see* Abuse, drug, hallucinogen
    psychoactive NEC F19.10
      with
        unspecified disorder F19.19
    solvent—*see* Abuse, drug, inhalant
    steroids F55.3
    stimulant NEC F15.10
      with
        intoxication F15.129
          uncomplicated F15.120
  hallucinogens—*see* Abuse, drug, hallucinogen
  hashish—*see* Abuse, drug, cannabis
  inhalant—*see* Abuse, drug, inhalant
  marihuana—*see* Abuse, drug, cannabis
  PCP (phencyclidine) (or related substance)—*see* Abuse, drug, hallucinogen
  physical (adult) (child)—*see* Maltreatment
  psychoactive substance—*see* Abuse, drug, psychoactive NEC
  psychological (adult) (child)—*see* Maltreatment
  sexual—*see* Maltreatment
  solvent—*see* Abuse, drug, inhalant
Acalculia R48.8
  developmental F81.2
Acanthosis (acquired) (nigricans) L83
  benign Q82.8
  congenital Q82.8
  seborrheic L82.1
    inflamed L82.0
  tongue K14.3
Acardia, acardius Q89.8
Acardiacus amorphus Q89.8
Acariasis B88.0
  scabies B86
Acarodermatitis (urticarioides) B88.0
Accelerated atrioventricular conduction I45.6
Accessory (congenital)
  atrioventricular conduction I45.6
  biliary duct or passage Q44.5
  carpal bones Q74.0
  cusp
    pulmonary Q22.3
  cystic duct Q44.5
  endocrine gland NEC Q89.2
  face bone (s) Q75.8
  finger (s) Q69.0
  foreskin N47.8
  frontonasal process Q75.8
  gallbladder Q44.1
  genital organ (s)
    female Q52.8
      external Q52.79
      internal NEC Q52.8
    male Q55.8
  genitourinary organs NEC Q89.8
    female Q52.8
    male Q55.8
  hallux Q69.2

Accessory, *continued*
heart Q24.8
valve, NEC Q24.8
pulmonary Q22.3
hepatic ducts Q44.5
liver Q44.7
duct Q44.5
navicular of carpus Q74.0
nipple Q83.3
parathyroid gland Q89.2
pituitary gland Q89.2
prepuce N47.8
sesamoid bones Q74.8
foot Q74.2
hand Q74.0
skin tags Q82.8
tarsal bones Q74.2
thumb Q69.1
thymus gland Q89.2
thyroid gland Q89.2
toes Q69.2
valve, heart
pulmonary Q22.3
Accident
birth—*see* Birth, injury
cerebrovascular (embolic) (ischemic) (thrombotic) I63.9
old (without sequelae) Z86.73
Accretio cordis (nonrheumatic) I31.0
Acculturation difficulty Z60.3
Acephalobrachia monster Q89.8
Acephalochirus monster Q89.8
Acephalogaster Q89.8
Acephalostomus monster Q89.8
Acephalothorax Q89.8
Acetonemia R79.89
in Type 1 diabetes E10.10
with coma E10.11
Achalasia (cardia) (esophagus) K22.0
congenital Q39.5
pylorus Q40.0
Achlorhydria, achlorhydric (neurogenic) K31.83
anemia D50.8
psychogenic F45.8
Achroma, cutis L80
Achromia parasitica B36.0
Achylia gastrica K31.89
psychogenic F45.8
Acid
peptic disease K30
stomach K30
psychogenic F45.8
Acidemia E87.2
metabolic (newborn) P19.9
first noted before onset of labor P19.0
first noted during labor P19.1
noted at birth P19.2
Acidity, gastric (high) K30
psychogenic F45.8
Acidocytopenia—*see* Agranulocytosis
Acidocytosis D72.1
Acidosis (lactic) (respiratory) E87.2
in Type 1 diabetes E10.10
with coma E10.11
mixed metabolic and respiratory, newborn P84
newborn P84
Aciduria
glutaric (type I) E72.3
type II E71.313
type III E71.5-
Acladiosis (skin) B36.0
Acleistocardia Q21.1
Acne L70.9
artificialis L70.8
atrophica L70.2
cachecticorum (Hebra) L70.8
conglobata L70.1
cystic L70.0
excoriée des jeunes filles L70.5
frontalis L70.2
indurata L70.0
infantile L70.4
lupoid L70.2
necrotic, necrotica (miliaris) L70.2

Acne, *continued*
neonatal L70.4
nodular L70.0
occupational L70.8
picker's L70.5
pustular L70.0
rodens L70.2
specified NEC L70.8
tropica L70.3
varioliformis L70.2
vulgaris L70.0
Acquired—*see also* condition
immunodeficiency syndrome (AIDS) B20
Acroasphyxia, chronic I73.89
Acrocephalopolysyndactyly Q87.0
Acrocephalosyndactyly Q87.0
Acrochondrohyperplasia—*see* Syndrome, Marfan's
Acrocyanosis I73.8
newborn P28.2
meaning transient blue hands and feet—omit code
Acrodermatitis L30.8
infantile papular L44.4
Acromegaly, acromegalia E22.0
Acronyx L60.0
Acroparesthesia (simple) (vasomotor) I73.89
Action, heart
disorder I49.9
irregular I49.9
psychogenic F45.8
Activation
mast cell (disorder) (syndrome) D89.40
idiopathic D89.42
monoclonal D89.41
secondary D89.43
specified type NEC D89.49
Active—*see* condition
Acute—*see also* condition
abdomen R10.0
gallbladder—*see* Cholecystitis, acute
Acyanotic heart disease (congenital) Q24.9
Adair-Dighton syndrome (brittle bones and blue sclera, deafness) Q78.0
Adamantinoma—*see also* Cyst, calcifying odontogenic
long bones C40.90
lower limb C40.2-
upper limb C40.0-
malignant C41.1
jaw (bone) (lower) C41.1
upper C41.0
tibial C40.2-
Adams-Stokes (-Morgagni) disease or syndrome I45.9
Adaption reaction—*see* Disorder, adjustment
Addiction (*see also* Dependence) F19.20
alcohol, alcoholic (ethyl) (methyl) (wood) (without remission) F10.20
with remission F10.21
drug—*see* Dependence, drug
ethyl alcohol (without remission) F10.20
with remission F10.21
ethyl alcohol (without remission) F10.20
with remission F10.21
methylated spirit (without remission) F10.20
with remission F10.21
tobacco—*see* Dependence, drug, nicotine
Addisonian crisis E27.2
Addison's
anemia (pernicious) D51.0
disease (bronze) or syndrome E27.1
Addison-Schilder complex E71.528
Additional—*see also* Accessory
chromosome (s) Q99.8
sex—*see* Abnormal, chromosome, sex
21—*see* Trisomy, 21
Adduction contracture, hip or other joint—*see* Contraction, joint
Adenitis—*see also* lymphadenitis
acute, unspecified site L04.9
axillary I88.9
acute L04.2
chronic or subacute I88.1
cervical I88.9
acute L04.0
chronic or subacute I88.1

Adenitis, *continued*
chronic, unspecified site I88.1
due to Pasteurella multocida (p. septica) A28.0
gangrenous L04.9
groin I88.9
acute L04.1
chronic or subacute I88.1
inguinal I88.9
acute L04.1
chronic or subacute I88.1
lymph gland or node, except mesenteric I88.9
acute—*see* Lymphadenitis, acute
chronic or subacute I88.1
mesenteric (acute) (chronic) (nonspecific) (subacute) I88.0
scrofulous (tuberculous) A18.2
strumous, tuberculous A18.2
subacute, unspecified site I88.1
Adenocarcinoma—*see also* Neoplasm, malignant, by site
renal cell C64-
Adenoiditis (chronic) J35.02
with tonsillitis J35.03
acute J03.90
recurrent J03.91
specified organism NEC J03.80
recurrent J03.81
staphylococcal J03.80
recurrent J03.81
streptococcal J03.00
recurrent J03.01
Adenoma—*see also* Neoplasm, benign, by site
apocrine
breast D24-
specified site NEC—*see* Neoplasm, skin, benign, by site
unspecified site D23.9
ceruminous D23.2-
Adenomatosis
endocrine (multiple) E31.20
single specified site—*see* Neoplasm, uncertain behavior, by site
specified site—*see* Neoplasm, benign, by site
unspecified site D12.6
Adenomatous
goiter (nontoxic) E04.9
with hyperthyroidism—*see* Hyperthyroidism, with, goiter, nodular
toxic—*see* Hyperthyroidism, with, goiter, nodular
Adenopathy (lymph gland) R59.9
generalized R59.1
Adenosclerosis I88.8
Adenovirus, as cause of disease classified elsewhere B97.0
Afibrinogenemia (*see also* Defect, coagulation) D68.8
acquired D65
congenital D68.2
Adherent—*see also* Adhesions
labia (minora) N90.89
pericardium (nonrheumatic) I31.0
rheumatic I09.2
scar (skin) L90.5
tendon in scar L90.5
Adhesions, adhesive (postinfective) K66.0
cardiac I31.0
rheumatic I09.2
cervicovaginal N88.1
congenital Q52.8
joint—*see* Ankylosis
temporomandibular M26.61-
labium (majus) (minus), congenital Q52.5
meninges (cerebral) (spinal) G96.12
congenital Q07.8
tuberculous (cerebral) (spinal) A17.0
nasal (septum) (to turbinates) J34.89
pericardium (nonrheumatic) I31.0
focal I31.8
rheumatic I09.2
preputial, prepuce N47.5
temporomandibular M26.61-
vagina (chronic) N89.5
Adiponecrosis neonatorum P83.8

Admission (for)—*see also* Encounter (for)
aftercare (*see also* Aftercare) Z51.89
radiation therapy (antineoplastic) Z51.0
attention to artificial opening (of) Z43.9
gastrostomy Z43.1
change of
dressing (nonsurgical) Z48.00
surgical dressing Z48.01
circumcision, ritual or routine (in absence of diagnosis) Z41.2
counseling—*see also* Counseling
dietary Z71.3
HIV Z71.7
human immunodeficiency virus Z71.7
non-attending third party Z71.0
procreative management NEC Z31.69
desensitization to allergens Z51.6
dietary surveillance and counseling Z71.3
examination at health care facility (adult) (*see also* Examination) Z00.00
with abnormal findings Z00.01
ear Z01.10
with abnormal findings NEC Z01.118
eye Z01.00
with abnormal findings Z01.01
hearing Z01.10
with abnormal findings NEC Z01.118
vision Z01.00
with abnormal findings Z01.01
followup examination Z09
intrauterine device management Z30.431
initial prescription Z30.014
prophylactic (measure)—*see also* Encounter, prophylactic measure
vaccination Z23
radiation therapy (antineoplastic) Z51.0
removal of
dressing (nonsurgical) Z48.00
implantable subdermal contraceptive Z30.46
intrauterine contraceptive device Z30.432
staples Z48.02
surgical dressing Z48.01
sutures Z48.02
sensitivity test—*see also* Test, skin
allergy NEC Z01.82
Mantoux Z11.1
vision examination Z01.00
with abnormal findings Z01.01
Adolescent X-linked adrenoleukodystrophy E71.521
Adrenal (gland)—*see* condition
Adrenalitis, adrenitis E27.8
autoimmune E27.1
Adrenogenital syndrome E25.9
congenital E25.0
salt loss E25.0
Adrenogenitalism, congenital E25.0
Adrenoleukodystrophy E71.529
neonatal E71.511
Xlinked E71.529
Addison only phenotype E71.528
Addison-Schilder E71.528
adolescent E71.521
adrenomyeloneuropathy E71.522
childhood cerebral E71.520
other specified E71.528
Adrenomyeloneuropathy E71.522
Adverse effect—*see* Table of Drugs and Chemicals, categories T36–T50, with 6th character 5
Aerodermectasia
subcutaneous (traumatic) T79.7
Aerophagy, aerophagia (psychogenic) F45.8
Aftercare (*see also* Care) Z51.89
following surgery (for) (on)
attention to
dressings (nonsurgical) Z48.00
surgical Z48.01
sutures Z48.02
specified NEC Z48.89
fracture *code to* fracture with seventh character D

Aftercare, *continued*
involving
removal of
dressings (nonsurgical) Z48.00
staples Z48.02
surgical dressings Z48.01
sutures Z48.02
Agammaglobulinemia (acquired) (secondary) (nonfamilial) D80.1
with
immunoglobulin-bearing B-lymphocytes D80.1
lymphopenia D81.9
common variable (CVAgamma) D80.1
lymphopenic D81.9
Aganglionosis (bowel) (colon) Q43.1
Agenesis
alimentary tract (complete) (partial) NEC Q45.8
upper Q40.8
anus, anal (canal) Q42.3
with fistula Q42.2
aorta Q25.41
appendix Q42.8
artery (peripheral) Q27.9
pulmonary Q25.79
umbilical Q27.0
bile duct or passage Q44.5
bone Q79.9
breast (with nipple present) Q83.8
with absent nipple Q83.0
cartilage Q79.9
cecum Q42.8
clavicle Q74.0
colon Q42.9
specified NEC Q42.8
corpus callosum Q04.0
digestive organ (s) or tract (complete) (partial)NEC Q45.8
upper Q40.8
endocrine (gland) NEC Q89.2
face
bones NEC Q75.8
gallbladder Q44.0
heart Q24.8
valve, NEC Q24.8
pulmonary Q22.0
intestine (small) Q41.9
large Q42.9
specified NEC Q42.8
genitalia, genital (organ(s))
female Q52.8
external Q52.71
internal NEC Q52.8
male Q55.8
parathyroid (gland) Q89.2
pelvic girdle (complete) (partial) Q74.2
pituitary (gland) Q89.2
rectum Q42.1
with fistula Q42.0
roof of orbit Q75.8
round ligament Q52.8
scapula Q74.0
scrotum Q55.29
septum
atrial Q21.1
shoulder girdle (complete) (partial) Q74.0
skull (bone) Q75.8
with
anencephaly Q00.0
encephalocele — *see* Encephalocele
hydrocephalus Q03.9
with spina bifida — *see* Spina bifida, by site, with hydrocephalus
microcephaly Q02
testicle Q55.0
thymus (gland) Q89.2
thyroid (gland) E03.1
cartilage Q31.8
Aglossia-adactylia syndrome Q87.0
Agnosia (body image) (other senses) (tactile) R48.1
developmental F88
verbal R48.1
auditory R48.1
developmental F80.2
developmental F80.2

Agranulocytosis (chronic) (cyclical) (genetic) (infantile) (periodic) (pernicious) (*see also* Neutropenia) D70.9
congenital D70.0
cytoreductive cancer chemotherapy sequela D70.1
drug-induced D70.2
due to cytoreductive cancer chemotherapy D70.1
due to infection D70.3
secondary D70.4
drug-induced D70.2
due to cytoreductive cancer chemotherapy D70.1
Agraphia (absolute) R48.8
with alexia R48.0
developmental F81.81
Ague (dumb)—*see* Malaria
AIDS (related complex) B20
AIPHI (acute idiopathic pulmonary hemorrhage in infants (over 28 days old)) R04.81
Air
anterior mediastinum J98.2
hunger, psychogenic F45.8
sickness T75.3
Airplane sickness T75.3
Alactasia, congenital E73.0
Albuminuria, albuminuric (acute) (chronic) (subacute) (*see also* Proteinuria) R80.9
orthostatic R80.2
postural R80.2
scarlatinal A38.8
Alcohol, alcoholic, alcohol-induced
addiction (without remission) F10.20
with remission F10.21
counseling and surveillance Z71.41
family member Z71.42
intoxication (acute) (without dependence) F10.129
with
delirium F10.121
dependence F10.229
with delirium F10.221
uncomplicated F10.220
uncomplicated F10.120
Alcoholism (chronic) (without remission) F10.20
with
psychosis—*see* Psychosis, alcoholic
remission F10.21
Aldrich (-Wiskott) syndrome (eczema-thrombocytopenia) D82.0
Aleukia
congenital D70.0
hemorrhagica D61.9
congenital D61.09
Alexia R48.0
developmental F81.0
secondary to organic lesion R48.0
Allergy, allergic (reaction) (to) T78.40
air-borne substance NEC (rhinitis) J30.89
anaphylactic reaction or shock T78.2
angioneurotic edema T78.3
animal (dander) (epidermal) (hair) (rhinitis) J30.81
bee sting (anaphylactic shock)—*see* Table of Drugs and Chemicals, by animal or substance, poisoning
biological—*see* Allergy, drug
colitis K52.29
food protein-induced K52.22
dander (animal) (rhinitis) J30.81
desensitization to allergens, encounter for Z51.6
dandruff (rhinitis) J30.81
drug, medicament & biological (any) (external) (internal) T78.40
correct substance properly administered—*see* Table of Drugs and Chemicals, by drug, adverse effect
wrong substance given or taken NEC (by accident) —*see* Table of Drugs and Chemicals, by drug, poisoning
due to pollen J30.1
dust (house) (stock) (rhinitis) J30.89
with asthma—*see* Asthma, allergic extrinsic
eczema—*see* Dermatitis, contact, allergic

ALLERGY, ALLERGIC–ANEMIA

Allergy, allergic, *continued*
  epidermal (animal) (rhinitis) J30.81
  feathers (rhinitis) J30.89
  food (any) (ingested) NEC T78.1
    anaphylactic shock—*see* Shock, anaphylactic, due to food
    dermatitis—*see* Dermatitis, due to, food
    dietary counseling and surveillance Z71.3
    in contact with skin L23.6
    rhinitis J30.5
    status (without reaction) Z91.018
      eggs Z91.012
      milk products Z91.011
      peanuts Z91.010
      seafood Z91.013
      specified NEC Z91.018
  gastrointestinal K52.29
    food protein-induced K52.22
    meaning colitis or gastroenteritis K52.59
    meaning other adverse food reaction NEC T78.1
  grain J30.1
  grass (hay fever) (pollen) J30.1
    asthma—*see* Asthma, allergic extrinsic
  hair (animal) (rhinitis) J30.81
  history (of)—*see* History, allergy
  horse serum—*see* Allergy, serum
  inhalant (rhinitis) J30.89
    pollen J30.1
  kapok (rhinitis) J30.89
  medicine—*see* Allergy, drug
  milk protein Z91.011
    anaphylactic reaction T78.07
    dermatitis L27.2
    enterocolitis syndrome K52.21
    enteropathy K52.22
    gastroenteritis K52.29
    gastroesophageal reflux (*see also* Reaction, adverse, food) K21.9
      with esophagitis K21.0
    proctocolitis K52.82
  nasal, seasonal due to pollen J30.1
  pneumonia J82
  pollen (any) (hay fever) J30.1
    asthma—*see* Asthma, allergic extrinsic
  primrose J30.1
  primula J30.1
  purpura D69.0
  ragweed (hay fever) (pollen) J30.1
    asthma—*see* Asthma, allergic extrinsic
  rose (pollen) J30.1
  seasonal NEC J30.2
  Senecio jacobae (pollen) J30.1
  serum (*see also* Reaction, serum) T80.69
    anaphylactic shock T80.59
  shock (anaphylactic) T78.2
    due to
      administration of blood and blood products T80.51
      immunization T80.52
      serum NEC T80.59
      vaccination T80.52
  specific NEC T78.49
  tree (any) (hay fever) (pollen) J30.1
    asthma—*see* Asthma, allergic extrinsic
  upper respiratory J30.9
  urticaria L50.0
  vaccine—*see* Allergy, serum
  wheat—*see* Allergy, food
Alopecia (hereditaria) (seborrheica) L65.9
  due to cytotoxic drugs NEC L65.8
  postinfective NEC L65.8
  specified NEC L65.8
Alport syndrome Q87.81
ALTE (apparent life threatening event) **in newborn and infant** R68.13
Alteration (of), Altered
  mental status R41.82
  pattern of family relationships affecting child Z62.898
Alymphocytosis D72.810
  thymic (with immunodeficiency) D82.1
Alymphoplasia, thymic D82.1
Amastia (with nipple present) Q83.8
  with absent nipple Q83.0

Amaurosis (acquired) (congenital)—*see also* Blindness
  hysterical F44.6
  Leber's congenital H35.50
Ambiguous genitalia Q56.4
Amblyopia (congenital) (ex anopsia) (partial) (suppression) H53.00-
  anisometropic—*see* Amblyopia, refractive
  hysterical F44.6
  suspect H53.04-
Amebiasis
  acute A06.0
  intestine A06.0
Ameloblastoma—*see also* Cyst, calcifying odontogenic
  long bones C40.9-
    lower limb C40.2-
    upper limb C40.0-
  malignant C41.1
    jaw (bone) (lower) C41.1
      upper C41.0
  tibial C40.2-
Amenorrhea N91.2
Amsterdam dwarfism Q87.1
Amygdalitis—*see* Tonsillitis
Amygdalolith J35.8
Amyotonia M62.89
  congenita G70.2
Anacidity, gastric K31.83
  psychogenic F45.8
Anaerosis of newborn P28.89
Analbuminemia E88.09
Anaphylactic
  purpura D69.0
  shock or reaction—*see* Shock, anaphylactic
Anaphylactoid shock or reaction—*see* Shock, anaphylactic
Anaphylaxis—*see* Shock, anaphylactic
Anarthria R47.1
Anasarca R60.1
  renal N04.9
Anastomosis
  arteriovenous ruptured brain I60.8
Android pelvis Q74.2
Anemia (essential) (general) (hemoglobin deficiency) (infantile) (primary) (profound) D64.9
  achlorhydric D50.8
  aplastic D61.9
    congenital D61.09
    drug-induced D61.1
    due to
      drugs D61.1
      external agents NEC D61.2
      infection D61.2
      radiation D61.2
    idiopathic D61.3
    red cell (pure) D60.9
      chronic D60.0
      congenital D61.01
    specified type NEC D61.89
    toxic D61.2
  aregenerative
    congenital D61.09
  atypical D64.9
  Baghdad spring D55.0
  blood loss (chronic) D50.0
    acute D62
  chlorotic D50.8
  chronica congenita aregenerativa D61.09
  congenital P61.4
    aplastic D61.09
    Heinz body D58.2
    spherocytic D58.0
  Cooley's (erythroblastic) D56.1
  deficiency D53.9
    enzyme D55.9
      glucose-6-phosphate dehydrogenase (G6PD) D55.0
    glucose-6-phosphate dehydrogenase D55.0
    G6PD D55.0
    nutritional D53.9
      with
        poor iron absorption D50.8
  Diamond-Blackfan (congenital hypoplastic) D61.01

Anemia, *continued*
  due to (in) (with)
    antineoplastic chemotherapy D64.81
    blood loss (chronic) D50.0
      acute D62
    chemotherapy, antineoplastic D64.81
    chronic disease classified elsewhere NEC D63.8
    hemorrhage (chronic) D50.0
      acute D62
    loss of blood (chronic) D50.0
      acute D62
    myxedema E03.9 [D63.8]
    Necator americanus B76.1 [D63.8]
    prematurity P61.2
  erythroblastic
    familial D56.1
    newborn (*see also* Disease, hemolytic) P55.9
    of childhood D56.1
  familial erythroblastic D56.1
  Fanconi's (congenital pancytopenia) D61.09
  favism D55.0
  glucose-6-phosphate dehydrogenase (G6PD) deficiency D55.0
  Heinz body, congenital D58.2
  hemolytic D58.9
    nonspherocytic
      congenital or hereditary NEC D55.8
        glucose-6-phosphate dehydrogenase deficiency D55.0
  hemorrhagic (chronic) D50.0
    acute D62
  Herrick's D57.1
  hookworm B76.9 [D63.8]
  hypochromic (idiopathic) (microcytic) (normoblastic) D50.9
    due to blood loss (chronic) D50.0
      acute D62
  hypoplasia, red blood cells D61.9
    congenital or familial D61.01
  hypoplastic (idiopathic) D61.9
    congenital or familial (of childhood) D61.01
  hypoproliferative (refractive) D61.9
  idiopathic D64.9
  iron deficiency D50.9
    secondary to blood loss (chronic) D50.0
      acute D62
    specified type NEC D50.8
  Joseph-Diamond-Blackfan (congenital hypoplastic) D61.01
  leukoerythroblastic D61.82
  malarial (*see also* Malaria) B54 [D63.8]
  marsh (*see also* Malaria) B54 [D63.8]
  Mediterranean (with other hemoglobinopathy) D56.9
  microcytic (hypochromic) D50.9
    due to blood loss (chronic) D50.0
      acute D62
    familial D56.8
  microdrepanocytosis D57.40
  microelliptopoikilocytic (RiettiGreppi Micheli) D56.9
  myelophthisic D61.82
  myeloproliferative D47.Z9
  newborn P61.4
    due to
      ABO (antibodies, isoimmunization, maternal/fetal incompatibility) P55.1
      Rh (antibodies, isoimmunization, maternal/fetal incompatibility) P55.0
    following fetal blood loss P61.3
    posthemorrhagic (fetal) P61.3
  normocytic (infectional) D64.9
    due to blood loss (chronic) D50.0
      acute D62
    myelophthisic D61.82
  nutritional (deficiency) D53.9
    with
      poor iron absorption D50.8
  of prematurity P61.2
  paludal (*see also* Malaria) B54 [D63.8]
  posthemorrhagic (chronic) D50.0
    acute D62
    newborn P61.3

Anemia, continued
  postoperative (postprocedural)
    due to (acute) blood loss D62
      chronic blood loss D50.0
    specified NEC D64.9
  progressive D64.9
    malignant D51.0
    pernicious D51.0
  pure red cell D60.9
    congenital D61.01
  Rietti-Greppi-Micheli D56.9
  secondary to
    blood loss (chronic) D50.0
      acute D62
    hemorrhage (chronic) D50.0
      acute D62
  semiplastic D61.89
  sickle-cell—see Disease, sicklecell
  sideropenic (refractory) D50.9
    due to blood loss (chronic) D50.0
      acute D62
  syphilitic (acquired) (late) A52.79 [D63.8]
  thalassemia D56.9
  thrombocytopenic—see Thrombocytopenia
  toxic D61.2
  tuberculous A18.89 [D63.8]
  Witts' (achlorhydric anemia) D50.8
Anesthesia, anesthetic R20.0
  dissociative F44.6
  functional (hysterical) F44.6
  hysterical F44.6
  testicular N50.9
Aneurysm (anastomotic) (artery) (cirsoid) (diffuse) (false)
               (fusiform) (multiple)
               (saccular) I72.9
  aorta, aortic (nonsyphilitic) I71.9
    congenital Q25.4
    root Q25.43
    sinus Q25.43
    valve (heart) (see also Endocarditis, aortic) I35.8
  arteriovenous (congenital)—see also Malformation,
               arteriovenous
    brain Q28.2
      ruptured I60.8
    berry (congenital) (nonruptured) I67.1
      ruptured I60.7
  brain I67.1
    arteriovenous (congenital) (nonruptured) Q28.2
      acquired I67.1
        ruptured I60.8
      ruptured I60.8
    berry (congenital) (nonruptured) I67.1
      ruptured (see also Hemorrhage, intracranial,
              subarachnoid) I60.7
    congenital Q28.3
      ruptured I60.7
    meninges I67.1
      ruptured I60.8
    miliary (congenital) (nonruptured) I67.1
      ruptured (see also Hemorrhage, intracranial,
              subarachnoid) I60.7
    mycotic I33.0-carotid artery (common) (external) I72.0
    ruptured into brain I60.0-
  cavernous sinus I67.1
    arteriovenous (congenital) (nonruptured) Q28.3
      ruptured I60.8
  circle of Willis I67.1
    congenital Q28.3
      ruptured I60.6
    ruptured I60.6
  congenital (peripheral) Q27.8
    brain Q28.3
      ruptured I60.7
    pulmonary Q25.79
  ductus arteriosus Q25.0
  endocardial, infective (any valve) I33.0
  infective I72.9
    endocardial (any valve) I33.0
  mycotic I72.9
    endocardial (any valve) I33.0
    ruptured, brain—see Hemorrhage, intracerebral,
              subarachnoid

Aneurysm, continued
  patent ductus arteriosus Q25.0
  pulmonary I28.1
    arteriovenous Q25.72
  tricuspid (heart) (valve) I07.8
Anger R45.4
Angina (attack) (cardiac) (chest) (heart) (pectoris) (syndrome)
               (vasomotor) I20.9
  aphthous B08.5
  croupous J05.0
  exudative, chronic J37.0
  Ludovici K12.2
  Ludwig's K12.2
  membranous J05.0
  monocytic—see Mononucleosis, infectious
  phlegmonous J36
  tonsil J36
  trachealis J05.0
Angioedema (allergic) (any site) (with urticaria) T78.3
Angioendothelioma—see Neoplasm, uncertain behavior,
               by site
  benign D18.00
    skin D18.01
    specified site NEC D18.09
  bone—see Neoplasm, bone, malignant
  Ewing's—see Neoplasm, bone, malignant
Angioma—see also Hemangioma, by site
  capillary I78.1
  hemorrhagicum hereditaria I78.0
  malignant—see Neoplasm, connective tissue, malignant
  plexiform D18.00
    skin D18.01
    specified site NEC D18.09
  senile I78.1
  skin D18.01
  specified site NEC D18.09
  spider I78.1
  stellate I78.1
Angiomatosis Q82.8
  encephalotrigeminal Q85.8
  hemorrhagic familial I78.0
  hereditary familial I78.0
Angioneurosis F45.8
Angioneurotic edema (allergic) (any site) (with urticaria)
               T78.3
Angiopathia, angiopathy I99.9
  peripheral I73.9
    specified type NEC I73.89
Angiospasm (peripheral) (traumatic) (vessel) I73.9
  cerebral G45.9
Angulation
  femur (acquired)—see also Deformity, limb, specified type
               NEC, thigh
    congenital Q74.2
  tibia (acquired)—see also Deformity, limb, specified type
               NEC, lower leg
    congenital Q74.2
  wrist (acquired)—see also Deformity, limb, specified type
               NEC, forearm
    congenital Q74.0
Angulus infectiosus (lips) K13.0
Anhydration, anhydremia E86.0
  with
    hypernatremia E87.0
    hyponatremia E87.1
Anhydremia E86.0
  with
    hypernatremia E87.0
    hyponatremia E87.1
Ankyloglossia Q38.1
Ankylosis (fibrous) (osseous) (joint) M24.60
  jaw (temporomandibular) M26.61-
  temporomandibular M26.61-
Anodontia (complete) (partial) (vera) K00.0
  acquired K08.10
Anomaly, anomalous (congenital) (unspecified type) Q89.9
  alimentary tract Q45.9
    upper Q40.9
  ankle (joint) Q74.2

Anomaly, continued
  aorta (arch) NEC Q25.40
    absence and aplasia Q25.41
    aneurysm (congenital) Q25.43
    coarctation (preductal) (postductal) Q25.1
    dilation (congenital) Q25.44
    double arch Q25.45
    hypoplasia Q25.42
    right aortic arch Q25.47
    tortuous arch Q25.46
  aqueduct of Sylvius Q03.0
    with spina bifida—see Spina bifida, with
               hydrocephalus
  arm Q74.0
  artery (peripheral) Q27.9
    pulmonary NEC Q25.79
    subclavian Q27.8
      origin Q25.48
    umbilical Q27.0
  atrial
    septa Q21.1
  atrioventricular
    excitation I45.6
    septum Q21.0
  Axenfeld's Q15.0
  biliary duct or passage Q44.5
  bladder Q64.70
    absence Q64.5
    diverticulum Q64.6
    exstrophy Q64.10
      cloacal Q64.12
      extroversion Q64.19
      specified type NEC Q64.19
      supravesical fissure Q64.11
    neck obstruction Q64.31
    specified type NEC Q64.79
  bone Q79.9
    arm Q74.0
    leg Q74.2
    pelvic girdle Q74.2
    shoulder girdle Q74.0
    skull Q75.9
      with
        anencephaly Q00.0
        encephalocele—see Encephalocele
        hydrocephalus Q03.9
          with spina bifida—see Spina bifida, by site,
               with hydrocephalus
        microcephaly Q02
  bursa Q79.9
  cardiac Q24.9
  carpus Q74.0
  cheek Q18.9
  chin Q18.9
  chromosomes, chromosomal Q99.9
    D (1)—see condition, chromosome 13
    E (3)—see condition, chromosome 18
    G—see condition, chromosome 21
    sex
      female phenotype Q97.8
      gonadal dysgenesis (pure) Q99.1
      Klinefelter's Q98.4
      male phenotype Q98.9
      Turner's Q96.9
    specified NEC Q99.8
  clavicle Q74.0
  common duct Q44.5
  communication
    left ventricle with right atrium Q21.0
  connection
    pulmonary venous Q26.4
      partial Q26.3
      total Q26.2
  cystic duct Q44.5
  dental
    arch relationship M26.20
    specified NEC M26.29
  dentofacial M26.9
    dental arch relationship M26.20
      specified NEC M26.29
    jaw size M26.00
      mandibular
        hypoplasia M26.04

ANOMALY–AORTA (AORTIC ARCH) ANOMALY

Anomaly, *continued*
malocclusion M26.4
dental arch relationship NEC M26.29
specified type NEC M26.89
temporomandibular joint M26.60-
adhesions M26.61-
ankylosis M26.61-
arthralgia M26.62-
articular disc M26.63-
specified type NEC M26.69
dermatoglyphic Q82.8
digestive organ (s) or tract Q45.9
lower Q43.9
upper Q40.9
ductus
arteriosus Q25.0
botalli Q25.0
ear (external) Q17.9
elbow Q74.0
endocrine gland NEC Q89.2
eye Q15.9
anterior segment Q13.9
specified NEC Q13.89
posterior segment Q14.9
specified NEC Q14.8
ptosis (eyelid) Q10.0
specified NEC Q15.8
eyelid Q10.3
ptosis Q10.0
face Q18.9
fascia Q79.9
femur NEC Q74.2
fibula NEC Q74.2
finger Q74.0
flexion (joint) NOS Q74.9
hip or thigh Q65.89
foot NEC Q74.2
varus (congenital) Q66.3
foramen
Botalli Q21.1
ovale Q21.1
forearm Q74.0
forehead Q75.8
gastrointestinal tract Q45.9
gallbladder (position) (shape) (size) Q44.1
genitalia, genital organ (s) or system
female Q52.9
external Q52.70
internal Q52.9
male Q55.9
hydrocele P83.5
specified NEC Q55.8
genitourinary NEC
female Q52.9
male Q55.9
Gerbode Q21.0
gyri Q07.9
hand Q74.0
heart Q24.9
patent ductus arteriosus (Botalli) Q25.0
septum Q21.9
auricular Q21.1
interatrial Q21.1
interventricular Q21.0
with pulmonary stenosis or atresia,
dextraposition of aorta
and hypertrophy of
right ventricle Q21.3
specified NEC Q21.8
ventricular Q21.0
with pulmonary stenosis or atresia,
dextraposition of aorta
and hypertrophy of
right ventricle Q21.3
tetralogy of Fallot Q21.3
valve NEC Q24.8
aortic
stenosis Q23.0
pulmonary Q22.3
stenosis Q22.1
heel NEC Q74.2
hepatic duct Q44.5
hip NEC Q74.2

Anomaly, *continued*
humerus Q74.0
hydatid of Morgagni
female Q50.5
male (epididymal) Q55.4
testicular Q55.29
hypophyseal Q89.2
ilium NEC Q74.2
integument Q84.9
ischium NEC Q74.2
joint Q74.9
ligament Q79.9
round Q52.8
limb Q74.9
lower NEC Q74.2
reduction deformity—*see* Defect, reduction, lower
limb
upper Q74.0
liver Q44.7
duct Q44.5
lower limb NEC Q74.2
meningeal bands or folds Q07.9
constriction of Q07.8
spinal Q06.9
meninges Q07.9
cerebral Q04.8
spinal Q06.9
meningocele Q05.9
mesentery Q45.9
metacarpus Q74.0
metatarsus NEC Q74.2
multiple NEC Q89.7
muscle Q79.9
musculoskeletal system, except limbs Q79.9
neck (any part) Q18.9
nerve Q07.9
acoustic Q07.8
optic Q07.8
nervous system (central) Q07.9
omphalomesenteric duct Q43.0
origin
artery
pulmonary Q25.79
parathyroid gland Q89.2
pelvic girdle NEC Q74.2
pelvis (bony) NEC Q74.2
penis (glans) Q55.69
pigmentation L81.9
congenital Q82.8
pituitary (gland) Q89.2
prepuce Q55.69
pulmonary Q33.9
artery NEC Q25.79
valve Q22.3
stenosis Q22.1
venous connection Q26.4
partial Q26.3
total Q26.2
radius Q74.0
respiratory system Q34.9
specified NEC Q34.8
rotation—*see* Malrotation
hip or thigh Q65.89
round ligament Q52.8
sacroiliac (joint) NEC Q74.2
scapula Q74.0
sex chromosomes NEC—*see also* Anomaly, chromosomes
female phenotype Q97.8
male phenotype Q98.9
shoulder Q74.0
simian crease Q82.8
sinus of Valsalva Q25.49
skull Q75.9
with
anencephaly Q00.0
encephalocele—*see* Encephalocele
hydrocephalus Q03.9
with spina bifida—*see* Spina bifida, by site,
with hydrocephalus
microcephaly Q02
specified organ or site NEC Q89.8
tarsus NEC Q74.2
tendon Q79.9

Anomaly, *continued*
thigh NEC Q74.2
thumb Q74.0
thymus gland Q89.2
thyroid (gland) Q89.2
cartilage Q31.8
tibia NEC Q74.2
toe NEC Q74.2
tooth, teeth K00.9
eruption K00.6
tragus Q17.9
ulna Q74.0
umbilical artery Q27.0
upper limb Q74.0
ureter Q62.8
obstructive NEC Q62.39
orthotopic ureterocele Q62.31
urinary tract Q64.9
ventricular
septa Q21.0
vitelline duct Q43.0
wrist Q74.0
Anonychia (congenital) Q84.3
acquired L60.8
Anorchia, anorchism, anorchidism Q55.0
Anorexia R63.0
nervosa F50.00
atypical F50.9
binge-eating type with purging F50.02
restricting type F50.01
Anosmia R43.0
hysterical F44.6
Anovulatory cycle N97.0
Anoxemia R09.02
newborn P84
Anoxia (pathological) R09.02
cerebral G93.1
newborn P84
due to
drowning T75.1
high altitude T70.29
intrauterine P84
newborn P84
Anteversion
femur (neck), congenital Q65.89
Anthrax
with pneumonia A22.1
cutaneous A22.0
colitis A22.2
gastrointestinal A22.2
inhalation A22.1
intestinal A22.2
pulmonary A22.1
respiratory A22.1
Anthropoid pelvis Q74.2
Antidiuretic hormone syndrome E22.2
Antibody
antiphospholipid R76.0
with
hemorrhagic disorder D68.312
hypercoagulable state D68.61
Anticardiolipin syndrome D68.61
Antiphospholipid
antibody
with hemorrhagic disorder D68.312
syndrome D68.61
Antritis J32.0
maxilla J32.0
acute J01.00
recurrent J01.01
Anuria R34
postrenal N13.8
Anusitis K62.89
Anxiety F41.9
depression F41.8
episodic paroxysmal F41.0
hysteria F41.8
panic type F41.0
separation, abnormal (of childhood) F93.0
specified NEC F41.8
Aorta (aortic arch) anomaly Q25.4-

Apepsia K30
  psychogenic F45.8
Apertognathia M26.09
Apert's syndrome Q87.0
Aphagia R13.0
  psychogenic F50.9
Aphasia (amnestic) (global) (nominal) (semantic) (syntactic)
        R47.01
  developmental (receptive type) F80.2
    expressive type F80.1
    Wernicke's F80.2
  sensory F80.2
  Wernicke's F80.2
Aphonia (organic) R49.1
  hysterical F44.4
  psychogenic F44.4
Aphthae, aphthous—*see also* condition
  Bednar's K12.0
  cachectic K14.0
  oral (recurrent) K12.0
  stomatitis (major) (minor) K12.0
  thrush B37.0
  ulcer (oral) (recurrent) K12.0
Aplasia—*see also* Agenesis
  abdominal muscle syndrome Q79.4
  aorta (congenital) Q25.41
  bone marrow (myeloid) D61.9
    congenital D61.01
  congenital pure red cell D61.01
  corpus callosum Q04.0
  erythrocyte congenital D61.01
  gallbladder, congenital Q44.0
  parathyroid-thymic D82.1
  red cell (with thymoma) D60.9
    acquired D60.9
      due to drugs D60.9
    congenital D61.01
    constitutional D61.01
    due to drugs D60.9
    hereditary D61.01
    of infants D61.01
    primary D61.01
    pure D61.01
      due to drugs D60.9
  round ligament Q52.8
  testicle Q55.0
  thymic, with immunodeficiency D82.1
  thyroid (congenital) (with myxedema) E03.1
Apnea, apneic (of) (spells) R06.81
  newborn NEC P28.4
    obstructive P28.4
    sleep (central) (obstructive) (primary) P28.3
  prematurity P28.4
  sleep G47.30
    central (primary) G47.31
      in conditions classified elsewhere G47.37
    obstructive (adult) (pediatric) G47.33
    primary central G47.31
    specified NEC G47.39
Apneumatosis, newborn P28.0
Apophysitis (bone)—*see also* Osteochondropathy
  juvenile M92.9
Apoplexia, apoplexy, apoplectic
  heat T67.0
Appendage
  testicular (organ of Morgagni) Q55.29
Appendicitis (pneumococcal) (retrocecal) K37
  with
    perforation or rupture K35.2
    peritoneal abscess K35.3
    peritonitis NEC K35.3
      generalized (with perforation or rupture) K35.2
      localized (with perforation or rupture) K35.3
  acute (catarrhal) (fulminating) (gangrenous) (obstructive)
                (retrocecal)
                (suppurative) K35.80
    with
      peritoneal abscess K35.3
      peritonitis NEC K35.3
        generalized (with perforation or rupture) K35.2
        localized (with perforation or rupture) K35.3
    specified NEC K35.89

Appendicopathia oxyurica B80
Appendix, appendicular—*see also* condition
  Morgagni
    male (epididymal) Q55.4
      testicular Q55.29
  testis Q55.29
Appetite
  depraved—*see* Pica
  excessive R63.2
  lack or loss (*see also* Anorexia) R63.0
    nonorganic origin F50.89
    psychogenic F50.89
  perverted (hysterical)—*see* Pica
Apprehensiveness, abnormal F41.9
ARC (AIDS-related complex) B20
Arnold-Chiari disease, obstruction or syndrome (type II)
        Q07.00
  with
    hydrocephalus Q07.02
      with spina bifida Q07.03
    spina bifida Q07.01
      with hydrocephalus Q07.03
  type III—*see* Encephalocele
  type IV Q04.8
Arrest, arrested
  cardiac I46.9
    due to
      cardiac condition I46.2
      specified condition NEC I46.8
    newborn P29.81
    postprocedural I97.12-
  development or growth
    bone—*see* Disorder, bone, development or growth
    child R62.50
  epiphyseal
    complete
      femur M89.15-
      humerus M89.12-
      tibia M89.16-
      ulna M89.13-
    forearm M89.13-
      specified NEC M89.13-
      ulna—*see* Arrest, epiphyseal, by type, ulna
    lower leg M89.16-
      specified NEC M89.168
      tibia—*see* Arrest, epiphyseal, by type, tibia
    partial
      femur M89.15-
      humerus M89.12-
      tibia M89.16-
      ulna M89.13-
      specified NEC M89.18
  growth plate—*see* Arrest, epiphyseal
  physeal—*see* Arrest, epiphyseal
  respiratory R09.2
    newborn P28.81
Arrhythmia (auricle) (cardiac) (juvenile) (nodal) (reflex) (sinus)
             (supraventricular)
             (transitory) (ventricle)
             I49.9
  block I45.9
  newborn
    bradycardia P29.12
    occurring before birth P03.819
      before onset of labor P03.810
      during labor P03.811
    tachycardia P29.11
  psychogenic F45.8
  vagal R55
Arrillaga-Ayerza syndrome (pulmonary sclerosis
                with pulmonary
                hypertension) I27.0
Arsenical pigmentation L81.8
  from drug or medicament—*see* Table of Drugs and
              Chemicals
Arteriosclerosis, arteriosclerotic (diffuse) (obliterans)
              (of) (senile) (with
              calcification) I70.90
  pulmonary (idiopathic) I27.0
Arteritis I77.6
  cerebral I67.7
    in
      systemic lupus erythematosus M32.19

Arteritis, *continued*
  coronary (artery) I25.89
    rheumatic I01.8
      chronic I09.89
Artery, arterial—*see also* condition
  single umbilical Q27.0
Arthralgia (allergic)—*see also* Pain, joint
  temporomandibular M26.62-
Arthritis, arthritic (acute) (chronic) (nonpyogenic) (subacute)
        M19.90
  due to or associated with
    acromegaly (*see also* subcategory M14.8-) E22.0
    bacterial disease (*see also* subcategory M01) A49.9
    erysipelas (*see also* category M01) A46
    erythema
      nodosum L52
    hemophilia D66 *[M36.2]*
    Henoch- (Schönlein) purpura D69.0 *[M36.4]*
    human parvovirus (*see also* category M01) B97.6
    Lyme disease A69.23
    serum sickness (*see also* Reaction, serum) T80.69
  in (due to)
    acromegaly (*see also* subcategory M14.8-) E22.0
    endocrine disorder NEC (*see also* subcategory M14.8-)
        E34.9
    enteritis, infectious NEC (*see also* category M01) A09
    erythema
      multiforme (*see also* subcategory M14.8-) L51.9
      nodosum (*see also* subcategory M14.8-) L52
    hemochromatosis (*see also* subcategory M14.8-)
        E83.118
    hemoglobinopathy NEC D58.2 *[M36.3]*
    hemophilia NEC D66 *[M36.2]*
    Hemophilus influenzae M00.8- *[B96.3]*
    Henoch (-Schönlein)purpura D69.0 *[M36.4]*
    hypogammaglobulinemia (*see also* subcategory
        M14.8-) D80.1
    hypothyroidism NEC (*see also* subcategory M14.8-)
        E03.9
    infection—*see* Arthritis, pyogenic or pyemic
      spine—*see* Spondylopathy, infective
    infectious disease NEC—*see* category M01
    Lyme disease A69.23
    metabolic disorder NEC (*see also* subcategory M14.8-)
        E88.9
    respiratory disorder NEC (*see also* subcategory M14.8-
) J98.9
    sarcoidosis D86.86
    Salmonella (arizonae) (choleraesuis) (typhimurium)
        A02.23
      specified organism NEC (*see also* category M01)
        A08.8
    thalassemia NEC D56.9 [M36.3]
  juvenile M08.90
    with systemic onset—*see* Still's disease
    ankle M08.97-
    elbow M08.92-
    foot joint M08.97-
    hand joint M08.94-
    hip M08.95-
    knee M08.96-
    multiple site M08.99
    pauciarticular M08.40
      ankle M08.47-
      elbow M08.42-
      foot joint M08.47-
      hand joint M08.44-
      hip M08.45-
      knee M08.46-
      shoulder M08.41-
      vertebrae M08.48
      wrist M08.43-
    rheumatoid—*see* Arthritis, rheumatoid, juvenile
    shoulder M08.91-
    vertebra M08.98
    specified type NEC M08.80
      ankle M08.87-
      elbow M08.82-
      foot joint M08.87-
      hand joint M08.84-
      hip M08.85-
      knee M08.86-
      multiple site M08.89

Arthritis, arthritic, *continued*
  shoulder M08.81-
  specified joint NEC M08.88
  vertebrae M08.88
  wrist M08.83-
  wrist M08.93-
 pneumococcal M00.10
  ankle M00.17-
  elbow M00.12-
  foot joint M00.17-
  hand joint M00.14-
  hip M00.15-
  knee M00.16-
  multiple site M00.19
  shoulder M00.11-
  vertebra M00.18
  wrist M00.13-
 pyogenic or pyemic (any site except spine) M00.9
  bacterial NEC M00.80
   ankle M00.87-
   elbow M00.82-
   foot joint M00.87-
   hand joint M00.84-
   hip M00.85-
   knee M00.86-
   multiple site M00.89
   shoulder M00.81-
   vertebra M00.88
   wrist M00.83-
  pneumococcal—*see* Arthritis, pneumococcal
  spine—*see* Spondylopathy, infective
  staphylococcal—*see* Arthritis, staphylococcal
  streptococcal—*see* Arthritis, streptococcal NEC
   pneumococcal—*see* Arthritis, pneumococcal
 rheumatoid M06.9
  juvenile (with or without rheumatoid factor) M08.00
   ankle M08.07-
   elbow M08.02-
   foot joint M08.07-
   hand joint M08.04-
   hip M08.05-
   knee M08.06-
   multiple site M08.09
   shoulder M08.01-
   vertebra M08.08
   wrist M08.03-
 septic (any site except spine)—*see* Arthritis, pyogenic or
          pyemic
  spine—*see* Spondylopathy, infective
 serum (nontherapeutic) (therapeutic)—*see* Arthropathy,
          postimmunization
 staphylococcal M00.00
  ankle M00.07-
  elbow M00.02-
  foot joint M00.07-
  hand joint M00.04-
  hip M00.05-
  knee M00.06-
  multiple site M00.09
  shoulder M00.01-
  vertebra M00.08
  wrist M00.03-
 streptococcal NEC M00.20
  ankle M00.27-
  elbow M00.22-
  foot joint M00.07-
  hand joint M00.24-
  hip M00.25-
  knee M00.26-
  multiple site M00.29
  shoulder M00.21-
  vertebra M00.28
  wrist M00.23-
 suppurative—*see* Arthritis, pyogenic or pyemic
 temporomandibular M26.69
Arthrodysplasia Q74.9
Arthrogryposis (congenital) Q68.8
 multiplex congenita Q74.3
Arthropathy (*see also* Arthritis) M12.9
 hemophilic NEC D66 *[M36.2]*
 in (due to)
  acromegaly E22.0 *[M14.8-]*
  endocrine disease NOS E34.9 [M14.8-]

Arthropathy, *continued*
 erythema
  multiforme L51.9 [M14.8-]
  nodosum L52 [M14.8-]
 hemochromatosis E83.118 [M14.8-]
 hemoglobinopathy NEC D58.2 *[M36.3]*
 hemophilia NEC D66 *[M36.2]*
 Henoch-Schönlein purpura D69.0 *[M36.4]*
 hypothyroidism E03.9 *[M14.8-]*
 infective endocarditis I33.0 *[M12.80]*
 metabolic disease NOS E88.9 *[M14.8-]*
 neoplastic disease NOS (*see also* Neoplasm) D49.9
         [M36.1]
 nutritional deficiency (*see also* subcategory M14.8-)
         E63.9
 sarcoidosis D86.86
 thyrotoxicosis (*see also* subcategory M14.8-) E05.90
 ulcerative colitis K51.90 *[M07.60]*
 viral hepatitis (postinfectious) NEC B19.9 *[M12.80]*
 Whipple's disease (*see also* subcategory M14.8-)
         K90.81
 postinfectious NEC B99 *[M12.80]*
  in (due to)
   viral hepatitis NEC B19.9 *[M12.80]*
 reactive M02.9
  in (due to)
   infective endocarditis I33.0 *[M02.9]*
 traumatic M12.50
  ankle M12.57-
  elbow M12.52-
  foot joint M12.57-
  hand joint M12.54-
  hip M12.55-
  knee M12.56-
  multiple site M12.59
  shoulder M12.51-
  specified joint NEC M12.58
  vertebrae M12.58
  wrist M12.53-
Arthus' phenomenon or reaction T78.41
 due to
  drug—*see* Table of Drugs and Chemicals, by drug
Artificial
 opening status (functioning) (without complication) Z93.9
  gastrostomy Z93.1
Ascariasis B77.9
 with
  complications NEC B77.89
  intestinal complications B77.0
  pneumonia, pneumonitis B77.81
Ascites (abdominal) R18.8
 cardiac I50.9
 heart I50.9
 malignant R18.0
 pseudochylous R18.8
Asperger's disease or syndrome F84.5
Asphyxia, asphyxiation (by) R09.01
 antenatal P84
 birth P84
 bunny bag—*see* Asphyxia, due to, mechanical threat to
         breathing, trapped in
         bed clothes
 drowning T75.1
 gas, fumes, or vapor—*see* Table of Drugs and Chemicals
 inhalation—*see* Inhalation
 intrauterine P84
 newborn P84
 pathological R09.01
 postnatal P84
  mechanical—*see* Asphyxia, due to, mechanical threat
         to breathing
 prenatal P84
 reticularis R23.1
 strangulation—*see* Asphyxia, due to, mechanical threat to
         breathing
 submersion T75.1
 traumatic T71.9
  due to
   foreign body (in)—*see* Foreign body, respiratory
         tract, causing asphyxia
   low oxygen content of ambient air T71.20

Asphyxia, asphyxiation, *continued*
 due to
  being trapped in
   low oxygen environment T71.29
    in car trunk T71.221
     circumstances undetermined
       T71.224
     done with intent to harm by
      another person T71.223
      self T71.222
    in refrigerator T71.231
     circumstances undetermined
       T71.234
     done with intent to harm by
      another person T71.233
      self T71.232
  cave-in T71.21
  mechanical threat to breathing (accidental)
       T71.191
   circumstances undetermined T71.194
   done with intent to harm by
    another person T71.193
    self T71.192
   hanging T71.161
    circumstances undetermined T71.164
    done with intent to harm by
     another person T71.163
     self T71.162
   plastic bag T71.121
    circumstances undetermined T71.124
    done with intent to harm by
     another person T71.123
     self T71.122
   smothering
    in furniture T71.151
     circumstances undetermined T71.154
     done with intent to harm by
      another person T71.153
      self T71.152
    under
     another person's body T71.141
      circumstances undetermined
       T71.144
      done with intent to harm T71.143
     pillow T71.111
      circumstances undetermined
       T71.114
      done with intent to harm by
       another person T71.113
       self T71.112
    trapped in bed clothes T71.131
     circumstances undetermined T71.134
     done with intent to harm by
      another person T71.133
      self T71.132
 vomiting, vomitus—*see* Foreign body, respiratory tract,
         causing asphyxia
Aspiration
 amniotic (clear) fluid (newborn) P24.10
  with
   pneumonia (pneumonitis) P24.11
   respiratory symptoms P24.11
 blood
  newborn (without respiratory symptoms) P24.20
   with
    pneumonia (pneumonitis) P24.21
    respiratory symptoms P24.21
  specified age NEC—*see* Foreign body, respiratory tract
 bronchitis J69.0
 food or foreign body (with asphyxiation)—*see* Asphyxia,
         food
 liquor (amnii) (newborn) P24.10
  with
   pneumonia (pneumonitis) P24.11
   respiratory symptoms P24.11
 meconium (newborn) (without respiratory symptoms)
         P24.00
  with
   pneumonitis (pneumonitis) P24.01
   respiratory symptoms P24.01
 milk (newborn) (without respiratory symptoms) P24.30

Aspiration, *continued*
    with
        pneumonia (pneumonitis) P24.31
        respiratory symptoms P24.31
        specified age NEC—*see* Foreign body, respiratory tract
    mucus—*see also* Foreign body, by site, causing asphyxia
        newborn P24.10
        with
            pneumonia (pneumonitis) P24.11
            respiratory symptoms P24.11
    neonatal P24.9
        specific NEC (without respiratory symptoms) P24.80
        with
            pneumonia (pneumonitis) P24.81
            respiratory symptoms P24.81
    newborn P24.9
        specific NEC (without respiratory symptoms) P24.80
        with
            pneumonia (pneumonitis) P24.81
            respiratory symptoms P24.81
    pneumonia J69.0
    pneumonitis J69.0
    syndrome of newborn—*see* Aspiration, by substance, with pneumonia
    vernix caseosa (newborn) P24.80
        with
            pneumonia (pneumonitis) P24.81
            respiratory symptoms P24.81
    vomitus—*see also* Foreign body, respiratory tract
        newborn (without respiratory symptoms) P24.30
        with
            pneumonia (pneumonitis) P24.31
            respiratory symptoms P24.31
Asplenia (congenital) Q89.01
Astasia (-abasia) (hysterical) F44.4
Asthenia, asthenic R53.1
    cardiac (*see also* Failure, heart) I50.9
        psychogenic F45.8
    cardiovascular (*see also* Failure, heart) I50.9
        psychogenic F45.8
    heart (*see also* Failure, heart) I50.9
        psychogenic F45.8
    hysterical F44.4
    myocardial (*see also* Failure, heart) I50.9
        psychogenic F45.8
    nervous F48.8
    neurocirculatory F45.8
Asthenopia—*see also* Discomfort, visual
    hysterical F44.6
    psychogenic F44.6
Asthma, asthmatic (bronchial) (catarrh) (spasmodic) J45.909
    with
        exacerbation (acute) J45.901
        hay fever—*see* Asthma, allergic extrinsic
        rhinitis, allergic—*see* Asthma, allergic extrinsic
        status asthmaticus J45.902
    allergic extrinsic J45.909
        with
            exacerbation (acute) J45.901
            status asthmaticus J45.902
    atopic—*see* Asthma, allergic extrinsic
    childhood J45.909
        with
            exacerbation (acute) J45.901
            status asthmaticus J45.902
    cough variant J45.991
    detergent J69.8
    due to
        detergent J69.8
    extrinsic, allergic—*see* Asthma, allergic extrinsic
    hay—*see* Asthma, allergic extrinsic
    idiosyncratic—*see* Asthma, nonallergic
    intermittent (mild) J45.20
        with
            exacerbation (acute) J45.21
            status asthmaticus J45.22
    intrinsic, nonallergic—*see* Asthma, nonallergic
    lateonset J45.909
        with
            exacerbation (acute) J45.901
            status asthmaticus J45.902

Asthma, asthmatic, *continued*
    mild intermittent J45.20
        with
            exacerbation (acute) J45.21
            status asthmaticus J45.22
    mild persistent J45.30
        with
            exacerbation (acute) J45.31
            status asthmaticus J45.32
    mixed J45.909
        with
            exacerbation (acute) J45.901
            status asthmaticus J45.902
    moderate persistent J45.40
        with
            exacerbation (acute) J45.41
            status asthmaticus J45.42
    nervous—*see* Asthma, nonallergic
    nonallergic (intrinsic) J45.909
        with
            exacerbation (acute) J45.901
            status asthmaticus J45.902
    persistent
        mild J45.30
        with
            exacerbation (acute) J45.31
            status asthmaticus J45.32
        moderate J45.40
        with
            exacerbation (acute) J45.41
            status asthmaticus J45.42
        severe J45.50
        with
            exacerbation (acute) J45.51
            status asthmaticus J45.52
    predominantly allergic J45.909
    severe persistent J45.50
        with
            exacerbation (acute) J45.51
            status asthmaticus J45.52
    specified NEC J45.998
Astroblastoma
    specified site—*see* Neoplasm, malignant, by site
    unspecified site C71.9
Astrocytoma (cystic)
    anaplastic
        specified site—*see* Neoplasm, malignant, by site
        unspecified site C71.9
    fibrillary
        specified site—*see* Neoplasm, malignant, by site
        unspecified site C71.9
    fibrous
        specified site—*see* Neoplasm, malignant, by site
        unspecified site C71.9
    gemistocytic
        specified site—*see* Neoplasm, malignant, by site
        unspecified site C71.9
    juvenile
        specified site—*see* Neoplasm, malignant, by site
        unspecified site C71.9
    pilocytic
        specified site—*see* Neoplasm, malignant, by site
        unspecified site C71.9
    piloid
        specified site—*see* Neoplasm, malignant, by site
        unspecified site C71.9
    protoplasmic
        specified site—*see* Neoplasm, malignant, by site
        unspecified site C71.9
    unspecified site C71.9
Astroglioma
    specified site—*see* Neoplasm, malignant, by site
    unspecified site C71.9
Asymmetrical face Q67.0
At risk
    for falling Z91.81
Ataxia, ataxy, ataxic R27.0
    cerebellar (hereditary) G11.9
        with defective DNA repair G11.3
        early-onset G11.1

Ataxia, ataxy, ataxic, *continued*
    in
        myxedema E03.9 *[G13.2]*
        neoplastic disease (*see also* Neoplasm) D49.9 *[G32.81]*
        specified disease NEC G32.81
    late-onset (Marie's) G11.2
    Friedreich's (heredofamilial) (cerebellar) (spinal) G11.1
    gait R26.0
        hysterical F44.4
    gluten M35.9 *[G32.81]*
        with celiac disease K90.0 *[G32.81]*
    hereditary G11.9
        cerebellar—*see* Ataxia, cerebellar
        spinal (Friedreich's) G11.1
    heredofamilial—*see* Ataxia, hereditary
    Hunt's G11.1
    hysterical F44.4
    Marie's (cerebellar) (heredofamilial) (late- onset) G11.2
    nonorganic origin F44.4
    nonprogressive, congenital G11.0
    psychogenic F44.4
    SangerBrown's (hereditary) G11.2
    spinal
        hereditary (Friedreich's) G11.1
    spinocerebellar, Xlinked recessive G11.1
    telangiectasia (LouisBar) G11.3
Ataxia-telangiectasia (Louis-Bar) G11.3
Atelectasis (massive) (partial) (pressure) (pulmonary) J98.11
    newborn P28.10
        due to resorption P28.11
        partial P28.19
        primary P28.0
        secondary P28.19
    primary (newborn) P28.0
Atelocardia Q24.9
Atheroma, atheromatous (*see also* Arteriosclerosis) I70.90
    aorta, aortic I70.0
        valve (*see also* Endocarditis, aortic) I35.8
    pulmonary valve (heart) (*see also* Endocarditis, pulmonary) I37.8
    tricuspid (heart) (valve) I36.8
    valve, valvular—*see* Endocarditis
Athlete's
    foot B35.3
    heart I51.7
Athyrea (acquired)—*see also* Hypothyroidism
    congenital E03.1
Atonia, atony, atonic
    capillary I78.8
    congenital P94.2
    intestine K59.8
        psychogenic F45.8
    stomach K31.89
        neurotic or psychogenic F45.8
    uterus (during labor) O62.2
        with hemorrhage (postpartum) O72.1
        postpartum (with hemorrhage) O72.1
        without hemorrhage O75.89
Atransferrinemia, congenital E88.09
Atresia, atretic
    alimentary organ or tract NEC Q45.8
        upper Q40.8
    ani, anus, anal (canal) Q42.3
        with fistula Q42.2
    aortic (orifice) (valve) Q23.0
        congenital with hypoplasia of ascending aorta and defective development of left ventricle (with mitral stenosis) Q23.4
        in hypoplastic left heart syndrome Q23.4
    aqueduct of Sylvius Q03.0
        with spina bifida—*see* Spina bifida, with hydrocephalus
    artery NEC Q27.8
        umbilical Q27.0
    bile duct (common) (congenital) (hepatic) Q44.2
        acquired—*see* Obstruction, bile duct
    cecum Q42.8
    choana Q30.0
    colon Q42.9
        specified NEC Q42.8

Atresia, atretic, *continued*
  common duct Q44.2
  cystic duct Q44.2
    acquired K82.8
      with obstruction K82.0
  digestive organs NEC Q45.8
  esophagus Q39.0
    with tracheoesophageal fistula Q39.1
  follicular cyst N83.0-
  foramen of
    Luschka Q03.1
      with spina bifida—*see* Spina bifida, with
             hydrocephalus
    Magendie Q03.1
      with spina bifida—*see* Spina bifida, with
             hydrocephalus
  gallbladder Q44.1
  genital organ
    external
      female Q52.79
      male Q55.8
    internal
      female Q52.8
      male Q55.8
  gullet Q39.0
    with tracheoesophageal fistula Q39.1
  hymen Q52.3
    acquired (postinfective) N89.6
  intestine (small) Q41.9
    large Q42.9
      specified NEC Q42.8
  iris, filtration angle Q15.0
  mitral valve Q23.2
    in hypoplastic left heart syndrome Q23.4
  nares (anterior) (posterior) Q30.0
  nose, nostril Q30.0
    acquired J34.89
  organ or site NEC Q89.8
  rectum Q42.1
    with fistula Q42.0
  ureter Q62.10
    pelvic junction Q62.11
    vesical orifice Q62.12
  ureteropelvic junction Q62.11
  ureterovesical orifice Q62.12
  vagina (congenital) Q52.4
    acquired (postinfectional) (senile) N89.5
Atrophy, atrophic (of)
  adrenal (capsule) (gland) E27.49
    primary (autoimmune) E27.1
  buccal cavity K13.79
  facioscapulohumeral (Landouzy-Déjérine) G71.0
  hemifacial Q67.4
    Romberg G51.8
  Landouzy-Déjérine G71.0
  laryngitis, infective J37.0
  lip K13.0
  muscle, muscular (diffuse) (general) (idiopathic) (primary)
             M62.50
    infantile spinal G12.0
    progressive (bulbar) G12.21
      infantile (spinal) G12.0
      spinal G12.9
        infantile G12.0
    pseudohypertrophic G71.0
    spinal G12.9
      infantile, type I (Werdnig-Hoffmann) G12.0
  pseudohypertrophic (muscle) G71.0
  rhinitis J31.0
  scar L90.5
  suprarenal (capsule) (gland) E27.49
    primary E27.1
  systemic affecting central nervous system
    in
      myxedema E03.9 *[G13.2]*
      neoplastic disease (*see also* Neoplasm) D49.9
           [G13.1]
      specified disease NEC G13.8
  testes N50.0
  thyroid (gland) (acquired) E03.4
    with cretinism E03.1
    congenital (with myxedema) E03.1

Atrophy, atrophic, *continued*
  turbinate J34.89
  WerdnigHoffmann G12.0
Attack, attacks
  AdamsStokes I45.9
  cyanotic, newborn P28.2
  drop NEC R55
  epileptic—*see* Epilepsy
  hysterical F44.9
  panic F41.0
  StokesAdams I45.9
  syncope R55
  transient ischemic (TIA) G45.9
    specified NEC G45.8
  unconsciousness R55
    hysterical F44.89
  vasomotor R55
  vasovagal (paroxysmal) (idiopathic) R55
  without alteration of consciousness—*see* Epilepsy,
             localizationrelated,
             symptomatic, with
             simple partial seizures
Attention (to)
  artificial
    opening (of) Z43.9
      digestive tract NEC Z43.4
        stomach Z43.1
  deficit disorder or syndrome F98.8
    with hyperactivity—*see* Disorder, attention-deficit
             hyperactivity
  gastrostomy Z43.1
  surgical dressings Z48.01
  sutures Z48.02
Austin Flint murmur (aortic insufficiency) I35.1
Autism, autistic (childhood) (infantile) F84.0
  atypical F84.9
  spectrum disorder F84.0
Autoerythrocyte sensitization (syndrome) D69.2
Autoimmune
  disease (systemic) M35.9
  lymphoproliferative syndrome *[ALPS]* D89.82
Avitaminosis (multiple) (*see also* Deficiency, vitamin) E56.9
  D E55.9
    with rickets E55.0
Automatism G93.89
  with temporal sclerosis G93.81
  epileptic—*see* Epilepsy, localizationrelated, symptomatic,
             with complex partial
             seizures
  paroxysmal, idiopathic—*see* Epilepsy, localizationrelated,
             symptomatic, with
             complex partial
             seizures
Autosensitivity, erythrocyte D69.2
Aversion
  oral R63.3
    newborn P92.-
      nonorganic origin F98.2
AVNRT (atrioventricular nodal re-entrant tachycardia) I47.1
AVRT (atrioventricular nodal re-entrant tachycardia) I47.1
Avulsion (traumatic)
  head (intracranial)
    scalp S08.0
  kidney S37.06
  scalp S08.0
  spleen S36.032
Awareness of heart beat R00.2
Axenfeld's
  anomaly or syndrome Q15.0
Ayerza's disease or syndrome (pulmonary artery sclerosis
             with pulmonary
             hypertension) I27.0

B

Babington's disease (familial hemorrhagic telangiectasia)
             I78.0
Baby
  crying constantly R68.11
  floppy (syndrome) P94.2
Bacilluria R82.71

Bacillus—*see also* Infection, bacillus
  coli infection (*see also* Escherichia coli) B96.20
  Shiga's A03.0
  suipestifer infection—*see* Infection, salmonella
Backache (postural) M54.9
  sacroiliac M53.3
Backward reading (dyslexia) F81.0
Bacteremia R78.81
  with sepsis—*see* Sepsis
Bacterium, bacteria, bacterial
  agent NEC, as cause of disease classified elsewhere
             B96.89
  in blood—*see* Bacteremia
  in urine R82.71
Bacteriuria, bacteruria R82.71
  asymptomatic R82.71
  urinary tract infection N39.0
Baelz's disease (cheilitis glandularis apostematosa) K13.0
Baerensprung's disease (eczema marginatum) B35.6
Balanitis (circinata) (erosiva) (gangrenosa) (phagedenic)
             (vulgaris) N48.1
  candidal B37.42
Balanoposthitis N47.6
Band (s)
  gallbladder (congenital) Q44.1
  vagina N89.5
Bandemia D72.825
Bannister's disease T78.3
Barton's fracture S52.56-
Basophilia D72.824
Basophilism (cortico-adrenal) (Cushing's) (pituitary) E24.0
Bateman's
  disease B08.1
  purpura (senile) D69.2
Bathing cramp T75.1
Battle exhaustion F43.0
Beach ear—*see* Swimmer's, ear
Beat (s)
  atrial, premature I49.1
  premature I49.40
    atrial I49.1
    auricular I49.1
    supraventricular I49.1
Becker's
  disease
    myotonia congenita, recessive form G71.12
  dystrophy G71.0
Beckwith-Wiedemann syndrome Q87.3
Bedbug bite (s)—*see* Bite(s), by site, superficial, insect
Bedclothes, asphyxiation or suffocation by—*see* Asphyxia,
             traumatic, due to,
             mechanical, trapped
Bednar's
  aphthae K12.0
Bedwetting—*see* Enuresis
Bee sting (with allergic or anaphylactic shock)—*see* Table of
             Drugs and Chemicals,
             by animal or substance,
             poisoning
Behavior
  drug seeking Z76.5
  self-damaging (lifestyle) Z72.89
Bell's
  palsy, paralysis G51.0
    infant or newborn P11.3
Bennett's fracture (displaced) S62.21-
Bent
  back (hysterical) F44.4
  nose M95.0
    congenital Q67.4
Bereavement (uncomplicated) Z63.4
Bergeron's disease (hysterical chorea) F44.4
Besnier's
  lupus pernio D86.3
  prurigo L20.0
Best's disease H35.50
Betalipoproteinemia, broad or floating E78.2
Betting and gambling Z72.6
Bifid (congenital)
  scrotum Q55.29
  toe NEC Q74.2
  uvula Q35.7

BITE(S)–BLISTER

Bite(s), *continued*
neck (*code to* Bite by specific site for esophagus, larynx,
pharynx, or trachea)
S11.95
involving
thyroid gland S11.15
specified site NEC S11.85
superficial NEC S10.87
insect S10.86
superficial NEC S10.97
insect S10.96
throat S11.85
superficial NEC S10.17
insect S10.16
nose (septum) (sinus) S01.25
superficial NEC S00.37
insect S00.36
occipital region—*see* Bite, scalp
oral cavity S01.552
superficial NEC S00.572
insect S00.562
orbital region—*see* Bite, eyelid
palate—*see* Bite, oral cavity
palm—*see* Bite, hand
parietal region—*see* Bite, scalp
pelvis S31.050
superficial NEC S30.870
insect S30.860
penis S31.25
superficial NEC S30.872
insect S30.862
perineum
female—*see* Bite, vulva
male—*see* Bite, pelvis
periocular area (with or without lacrimal passages)—*see*
Bite, eyelid
phalanges
finger—*see* Bite, finger
toe—*see* Bite, toe
pharynx S11.25
superficial NEC S10.17
insect S10.16
pinna—*see* Bite, ear
poisonous — *see* Table of Drugs and Chemicals, by
animal or substance,
poisoning
popliteal space—*see* Bite, knee
prepuce—*see* Bite, penis
pubic region—*see* Bite, abdomen, wall
rectovaginal septum—*see* Bite, vulva
red bug B88.0
reptile NEC—*see* Table of Drugs and Chemicals, by
animal or substance,
poisoning
nonvenomous—*see* Bite, by site
snake — *see* Table of Drugs and Chemicals, by animal
or substance, poisoning
sacral region—*see* Bite, back, lower
sacroiliac region—*see* Bite, back, lower
salivary gland—*see* Bite, oral cavity
scalp S01.05
superficial NEC S00.07
insect S00.06
scapular region—*see* Bite, shoulder
scrotum S31.35
superficial NEC S30.873
insect S30.863
sea-snake (venomous)—*see* Table of Drugs and
Chemicals, by animal
or substance, poisoning
shin—*see* Bite, leg
shoulder S41.05-
superficial NEC S40.27-
insect S40.26-
snake — *see* Table of Drugs and Chemicals, by animal or
substance, poisoning
nonvenomous—*see* Bite, by site
spermatic cord—*see* Bite, testis
spider (venomous) — *see* Table of Drugs and Chemicals,
by animal or substance,
poisoning
nonvenomous—*see* Bite, by site, superficial, insect

Bite(s), *continued*
sternal region—*see* Bite, thorax, front
submaxillary region—*see* Bite, head, specified site NEC
submental region—*see* Bite, head, specified site NEC
subungual
finger (s)—*see* Bite, finger
toe—*see* Bite, toe
superficial—*see* Bite, by site, superficial
supraclavicular fossa S11.85
supraorbital—*see* Bite, head, specified site NEC
temple, temporal region—*see* Bite, head, specified site
NEC
temporomandibular area—*see* Bite, cheek
testis S31.35
superficial NEC S30.873
insect S30.863
thigh S71.15-
superficial NEC S70.37-
insect S70.36-
thorax, thoracic (wall) S21.95
back S21.25-
with penetration into thoracic cavity S21.45-
breast—*see* Bite, breast
front S21.15-
with penetration into thoracic cavity S21.35-
superficial NEC S20.97
back S20.47-
front S20.37-
insect S20.96
back S20.46-
front S20.36-
throat—*see* Bite, neck, throat
thumb S61.05-
with
damage to nail S61.15-
superficial NEC S60.37-
insect S60.36-
thyroid S11.15
superficial NEC S10.87
insect S10.86
toe (s) S91.15-
with
damage to nail S91.25-
great S91.15-
with
damage to nail S91.25-
lesser S91.15-
with
damage to nail S91.25-
superficial NEC S90.47-
great S90.47-
insect S90.46-
great S90.46-
tongue S01.552
trachea S11.025
superficial NEC S10.17
insect S10.16
tunica vaginalis—*see* Bite, testis
tympanum, tympanic membrane—*see* Bite, ear
umbilical region S31.155
uvula—*see* Bite, oral cavity
vagina—*see* Bite, vulva
venomous—*see* Table of Drugs and Chemicals, by animal
or substance, poisoning
vulva S31.45
superficial NEC S30.874
insect S30.864
wrist S61.55-
superficial NEC S60.87-
insect S60.86-
Biting, cheek or lip K13.1
Biventricular failure (heart) I50.9
Blackfan-Diamond anemia or syndrome (congenital
hypoplastic anemia)
D61.01

Blackhead L70.0
Blackout R55
Bleeding—*see also* Hemorrhage
anal K62.5
anovulatory N97.0
gastrointestinal K92.2
intermenstrual (regular) N92.3
irregular N92.1

Bleeding, *continued*
irregular N92.6
nipple N64.59
nose R04.0
ovulation N92.3
pre-pubertal vaginal N93.1
puberty (excessive, with onset of menstrual periods)
N92.2
rectum, rectal K62.5
newborn P54.2
tendencies—*see* Defect, coagulation
uterus, uterine NEC N93.9
dysfunctional of functional N93.8
vagina, vaginal (abnormal) N93.9
dysfunctional or functional N93.8
newborn P54.6
pre-pubertal N93.1
vicarious N94.89
Blennorrhea (acute) (chronic)—*see also* Gonorrhea
inclusion (neonatal) (newborn) P39.1
lower genitourinary tract (gonococcal) A54.00
neonatorum (gonococcal ophthalmia) A54.31
Blepharitis (angularis) (ciliaris) (eyelid) (marginal)
(nonulcerative)
H01.009
left H01.006
lower H01.005
upper H01.004
right H01.003
lower H01.002
upper H01.001
Blepharochalasis H02.30
congenital Q10.0
Blepharoconjunctivitis H10.50-
Blepharoptosis H02.40-
congenital Q10.0
Blindness (acquired) (congenital) (both eyes) H54.0
color—*see* Deficiency, color vision
emotional (hysterical) F44.6
hysterical F44.6
word (developmental) F81.0
acquired R48.0
secondary to organic lesion R48.0
Blister (nonthermal)
abdominal wall S30.821
alveolar process S00.522
ankle S90.52-
antecubital space—*see* Blister, elbow
anus S30.827
arm (upper) S40.82-
auditory canal—*see* Blister, ear
auricle—*see* Blister, ear
axilla—*see* Blister, arm
back, lower S30.820
beetle dermatitis L24.89
breast S20.12-
brow S00.82
calf—*see* Blister, leg
canthus—*see* Blister, eyelid
cheek S00.82
internal S00.522
chest wall—*see* Blister, thorax
chin S00.82
costal region—*see* Blister, thorax
digit (s)
foot—*see* Blister, toe
hand—*see* Blister, finger
due to burn—*see* Burn, by site, second degree
ear S00.42-
elbow S50.32-
epiglottis S10.12
esophagus, cervical S10.12
eyebrow—*see* Blister, eyelid
eyelid S00.22-
face S00.82
fever B00.1
finger (s) S60.429
index S60.42-
little S60.42-
middle S60.42-
ring S60.42-
foot (except toe(s) alone) S90.82-
toe—*see* Blister, toe

Blister, *continued*
forearm S50.82-
elbow only—*see* Blister, elbow
forehead S00.82
fracture omit code
genital organ
female S30.826
male S30.825
gum S00.522
hand S60.52-
head S00.92
ear—*see* Blister, ear
eyelid—*see* Blister, eyelid
lip S00.521
nose S00.32
oral cavity S00.522
scalp S00.02
specified site NEC S00.82
heel—*see* Blister, foot
hip S70.22-
interscapular region S20.429
jaw S00.82
knee S80.22-
larynx S10.12
leg (lower) S80.82-
knee—*see* Blister, knee
upper—*see* Blister, thigh
lip S00.521
malar region S00.82
mammary—*see* Blister, breast
mastoid region S00.82
mouth S00.522
multiple, skin, nontraumatic R23.8
nail
finger—*see* Blister, finger
toe—*see* Blister, toe
nasal S00.32
neck S10.92
specified site NEC S10.82
throat S10.12
nose S00.32
occipital region S00.02
oral cavity S00.522
orbital region—*see* Blister, eyelid
palate S00.522
palm—*see* Blister, hand
parietal region S00.02
pelvis S30.820
penis S30.822
periocular area—*see* Blister, eyelid
phalanges
finger—*see* Blister, finger
toe—*see* Blister, toe
pharynx S10.12
pinna—*see* Blister, ear
popliteal space—*see* Blister, knee
scalp S00.02
scapular region—*see* Blister, shoulder
scrotum S30.823
shin—*see* Blister, leg
shoulder S40.22-
sternal region S20.329
submaxillary region S00.82
submental region S00.82
subungual
finger (s)—*see* Blister, finger
toe (s)—*see* Blister, toe
supraclavicular fossa S10.82
supraorbital S00.82
temple S00.82
temporal region S00.82
testis S30.823
thermal—*see* Burn, second degree, by site
thigh S70.32-
thorax, thoracic (wall) S20.92
back S20.42-
front S20.32-
throat S10.12
thumb S60.32-
toe (s) S90.42-
great S90.42-
tongue S00.522
trachea S10.12

Blister, *continued*
tympanum, tympanic membrane—*see* Blister, ear
upper arm—*see* Blister, arm (upper)
uvula S00.522
vagina S30.824
vocal cords S10.12
vulva S30.824
wrist S60.82-
Bloating R14.0
Block, blocked
arrhythmic I45.9
atrioventricular (incomplete) (partial) I44.30
with atrioventricular dissociation I44.2
complete I44.2
congenital Q24.6
congenital Q24.6
first degree I44.0
second degree (types I and II) I44.1
specified NEC I44.39
third degree I44.2
types I and II I44.1
cardiac I45.9
conduction I45.9
complete I44.2
foramen Magendie (acquired) G91.1
congenital Q03.1
with spina bifida—*see* Spina bifida, by site, with hydrocephalus
heart I45.9
complete (atrioventricular) I44.2
congenital Q24.6
first degree (atrioventricular) I44.0
second degree (atrioventricular) I44.1
third degree (atrioventricular) I44.2
Mobitz (types I and II) I44.1
portal (vein) I81
second degree (types I and II) I44.1
third degree I44.2
Wenckebach (types I and II) I44.1
Blocq's disease F44.4
Blood
in
feces K92.1
occult R19.5
urine—*see* Hematuria
occult in feces R19.5
pressure
decreased, due to shock following injury T79.4
examination only Z01.30
high—*see* Hypertension
borderline R03.0
incidental reading, without diagnosis of hypertension R03.0
transfusion
reaction or complication—*see* Complications, transfusion
Bloom (-Machacek) (-Torre) syndrome Q82.8
Blue
baby Q24.9
Blurring, visual H53.8
Blushing (abnormal) (excessive) R23.2
BMI—*see* Body, mass index
Boarder, hospital NEC Z76.4
accompanying sick person Z76.3
healthy infant or child Z76.2
foundling Z76.1
Blue
baby Q24.9
dot cataract Q12.0
sclera Q13.5
with fragility of bone and deafness Q78.0
Boder-Sedgwick syndrome (ataxia-telangiectasia) G11.3
Body, bodies
mass index (BMI)
pediatric
5th percentile to less than 85th percentile for age Z68.52
85th percentile to less than 95th percentile for age Z68.53
greater than or equal to ninety-fifth percentile for age Z68.54
less than fifth percentile for age Z68.51
rocking F98.4

Boeck's
disease or sarcoid—*see* Sarcoidosis
lupoid (miliary) D86.3
Bonnevie-Ullrich syndrome (*See also* Turner's Syndrome) Q87.1
Borderline
diabetes mellitus (prediabetes) R73.03
hypertension R03.0
Botalli, ductus (patent) (persistent) Q25.0
Botulism (foodborne intoxication) A05.1
infant A48.51
non-foodborne A48.52
wound A48.52
Bouillaud's disease or syndrome (rheumatic heart disease) I01.9
Bourneville's disease Q85.1
Boutonniere deformity (finger)—*see* Deformity, finger, boutonniere
Bowleg (s) (acquired) M21.16-
congenital Q68.5
Brachycardia R00.1
Bradycardia (sinoatrial) (sinus) (vagal) R00.1
neonatal P29.12
tachycardia syndrome I49.5
Bradypnea R06.89
Bradytachycardia I49.5
Brailsford's disease or osteochondrosis—*see* Osteochondrosis, juvenile, radius
Brain—*see also* condition
death G93.82
syndrome—*see* Syndrome, brain
Brash (water) R12
BRBPR K62.5
Breast—*see also* condition
buds E30.1
in newborn P96.89
dense R92.2
nodule N63
Breath
foul R19.6
holder, child R06.89
holding spell R06.89
shortness R06.02
Breathing
labored—*see* Hyperventilation
mouth R06.5
causing malocclusion M26.5
periodic R06.3
high altitude G47.32
Breathlessness R06.81
Brennemann's syndrome I88.0
Bright red blood per rectum (BRBPR) K62.5
Briquet's disorder or syndrome F45.0
Brissaud's
motor-verbal tic F95.2
Brittle
bones disease Q78.0
Broad—*see also* condition
beta disease E78.2
Broad- or floating-betalipoproteinemia E78.2
Broken
arm (meaning upper limb)—*see* Fracture, arm
bone—*see* Fracture
leg (meaning lower limb)—*see* Fracture, leg
nose S02.2-
tooth, teeth—*see* Fracture, tooth
Bromidism, bromism G92
due to
correct substance properly administered—*see* Table of Drugs and Chemicals, by drug, adverse effect
overdose or wrong substance given or taken—*see* Table of Drugs and Chemicals, by drug, poisoning
Bronchiolitis (acute) (infective) (subacute) J21.9
with
bronchospasm or obstruction J21.9
influenza, flu or grippe—*see* Influenza, with, respiratory manifestations NEC

BRONCHIOLITIS–BURN

Bronchiolitis, *continued*
    due to
        external agent—*see* Bronchitis, acute, due to
        human metapneumovirus J21.1
        respiratory syncytial virus J21.0
        specified organism NEC J21.8
    influenzal—*see* Influenza, with, respiratory manifestations
                           NEC
Bronchitis (diffuse) (fibrinous) (hypostatic) (infective)
                        (membranous) J40
    with
        influenza, flu or grippe—*see* Influenza, with,
                respiratory
                manifestations NEC
        tracheitis (I5 years of age and above) J40
            acute or subacute J20.9
            under I5 years of age J20.9
    acute or subacute (with bronchospasm or obstruction)
                      J20.9
        due to
            Haemophilus influenzae J20.1
            Mycoplasma pneumoniae J20.0
            radiation J70.0
            specified organism NEC J20.8
            Streptococcus J20.2
            virus
                coxsackie J20.3
                echovirus J20.7
                parainfluenza J20.4
                respiratory syncytial J20.5
                rhinovirus J20.6
        viral NEC J20.8
    allergic (acute) J45.909
        with
            exacerbation (acute) J45.901
            status asthmaticus J45.902
    asthmatic J45.9
    catarrhal (I5 years of age and above) J40
        acute—*see* Bronchitis, acute
        under I5 years of age J20.9
    mucopurulent (chronic) (recurrent) J41.1
        acute or subacute J20.9
    pneumococcal, acute or subacute J20.2
    viral NEC, acute or subacute (*see also* Bronchitis, acute)
                      J20.8
Bronchoalveolitis J18.0
Bronchocele meaning goiter E04.0
Bronchomycosis NOS B49 *[J99]*
    candidal B37.1
Bronchorrhea J98.09
    acute J20.9
Bronchospasm (acute) J98.01
    with
        bronchiolitis, acute J21.9
        bronchitis, acute (conditions in J20)—*see* Bronchitis,
                acute
    due to external agent—*see* condition, respiratory, acute,
                due to
    exercise induced J45.990
Bronze baby syndrome P83.8
Bruck-de Lange disease Q87.1
Brugsch's syndrome Q82.8
Bruise (skin surface intact)—*see also* Contusion
    with
        open wound—*see* Wound, open
        internal organ—*see* Injury, by site
    newborn P54.5
    scalp, due to birth injury, newborn P12.3
Bruit (arterial) R09.89
    cardiac R01.1
Bruxism
    psychogenic F45.8
Bubo I88.8
    indolent (nonspecific) I88.8
    inguinal (nonspecific) I88.8
        infective I88.8
    scrofulous (tuberculous) A18.2
    syphilitic (primary) A51.0
Buds
    breast E30.1
        in newborn P96.89

Bulimia (nervosa) F50.2
    atypical F50.9
    normal weight F50.9
Bulky
    stools R19.5
Buphthalmia, buphthalmos (congenital) Q15.0
Buried
    penis (congenital) Q55.64
Burkitt
    cell leukemia C91.0-
    lymphoma (malignant) C83.7-
        small noncleaved, diffuse C83.7-
        spleen C83.77
        undifferentiated C83.7-
    tumor C83.7-
    type
        acute lymphoblastic leukemia C91.0-
        undifferentiated C83.7-
Burn (electricity) (flame) (hot gas, liquid or hot object)
                      (radiation) (steam)
                      (thermal) T30.0
    abdomen, abdominal (muscle) (wall) T21.02
        first degree T21.12
        second degree T21.22
        third degree T21.32
    above elbow T22.039
        first degree T22.139
        left T22.032
            first degree T22.132
            second degree T22.232
            third degree T22.332
        right T22.031
            first degree T22.131
            second degree T22.231
            third degree T22.331
        second degree T22.239
        third degree T22.339
    acid (caustic) (external) (internal)—*see* Corrosion, by site
    alimentary tract NEC T28.2
        esophagus T28.1
        mouth T28.0
        pharynx T28.0
    alkaline (caustic) (external) (internal)—*see* Corrosion,
                by site
    ankle T25.019
        first degree T25.119
        left T25.012
            first degree T25.112
            second degree T25.212
            third degree T25.312
            multiple with foot—*see* Burn, lower, limb, multiple,
                  ankle and foot
        right T25.011
            first degree T25.111
            second degree T25.211
            third degree T25.311
        second degree T25.219
        third degree T25.319
    anus—*see* Burn, buttock
    arm (lower) (upper)—*see* Burn, upper, limb
    axilla T22.049
        first degree T22.149
        left T22.042
            first degree T22.142
            second degree T22.242
            third degree T22.342
        right T22.041
            first degree T22.141
            second degree T22.241
            third degree T22.341
        second degree T22.249
        third degree T22.349
    back (lower) T21.04
        first degree T21.14
        second degree T21.24
        third degree T21.34
        upper T21.03
            first degree T21.13
            second degree T21.23
            third degree T21.33
    blisters *code as* Burn, second degree, by site
    breast (s)—*see* Burn, chest wall

Burn, *continued*
    buttock (s) T21.05
        first degree T21.15
        second degree T21.25
        third degree T21.35
    calf T24.039
        first degree T24.139
        left T24.032
            first degree T24.132
            second degree T24.232
            third degree T24.332
        right T24.031
            first degree T24.131
            second degree T24.231
            third degree T24.331
        second degree T24.239
        third degree T24.339
    canthus (eye)—*see* Burn, eyelid
    caustic acid or alkaline—*see* Corrosion, by site
    cervix T28.3
    cheek T20.06
        first degree T20.16
        second degree T20.26
        third degree T20.36
    chemical (acids) (alkalines) (caustics) (external)
                      (internal)—*see*
                      Corrosion, by site
    chest wall T21.01
        first degree T21.11
        second degree T21.21
        third degree T21.31
    chin T20.03
        first degree T20.13
        second degree T20.23
        third degree T20.33
    colon T28.2
    conjunctiva (and cornea)—*see* Burn, cornea
    cornea (and conjunctiva) T26.1
        chemical—*see* Corrosion, cornea
    corrosion (external) (internal)—*see* Corrosion, by site
    deep necrosis of underlying tissue *code as* Burn, third
                      degree, by site
    dorsum of hand T23.069
        first degree T23.169
        left T23.062
            first degree T23.162
            second degree T23.262
            third degree T23.362
        right T23.061
            first degree T23.161
            second degree T23.261
            third degree T23.361
        second degree T23.269
        third degree T23.369
    due to ingested chemical agent—*see* Corrosion, by site
    ear (auricle) (external) (canal) T20.01
        first degree T20.11
        second degree T20.21
        third degree T20.31
    elbow T22.029
        first degree T22.129
        left T22.022
            first degree T22.122
            second degree T22.222
            third degree T22.322
        right T22.021
            first degree T22.121
            second degree T22.221
            third degree T22.321
        second degree T22.229
        third degree T22.329
    epidermal loss *code as* Burn, second degree, by site
    erythema, erythematous *code as* Burn, first degree, by site
    esophagus T28.1
    extent (percentage of body surface)
        less than 10 percent T31.0
        10–19 percent T31.10
            with 0–9 percent third degree burns T31.10
            with 10–19 percent third degree burns T31.11
    extremity—*see* Burn, limb

Burn, *continued*

eye (s) and adnexa T26.4-
  with resulting rupture and destruction of eyeball T26.2-
  conjunctival sac—*see* Burn, cornea
  cornea—*see* Burn, cornea
  lid—*see* Burn, eyelid
  periocular area—*see* Burn, eyelid
  specified site NEC T26.3-
eyeball—*see* Burn, eye
eyelid (s) T26.0-
  chemical—*see* Corrosion, eyelid
face—*see* Burn, head
finger T23.029
  first degree T23.129
  left T23.022
    first degree T23.122
    second degree T23.222
    third degree T23.322
  multiple sites (without thumb) T23.039
    with thumb T23.049
      first degree T23.149
      left T23.042
        first degree T23.142
        second degree T23.242
        third degree T23.342
      right T23.041
        first degree T23.141
        second degree T23.241
        third degree T23.341
      second degree T23.249
      third degree T23.349
    first degree T23.139
    left T23.032
      first degree T23.132
      second degree T23.232
      third degree T23.332
    right T23.031
      first degree T23.131
      second degree T23.231
      third degree T23.331
    second degree T23.239
    third degree T23.339
  right T23.021
    first degree T23.121
    second degree T23.221
    third degree T23.321
  second degree T23.229
  third degree T23.329
flank—*see* Burn, abdominal wall
foot T25.029
  first degree T25.129
  left T25.022
    first degree T25.122
    second degree T25.222
    third degree T25.322
  multiple with ankle—*see* Burn, lower, limb, multiple, ankle and foot
  right T25.021
    first degree T25.121
    second degree T25.221
    third degree T25.321
  second degree T25.229
  third degree T25.329
forearm T22.019
  first degree T22.119
  left T22.012
    first degree T22.112
    second degree T22.212
    third degree T22.312
  right T22.011
    first degree T22.111
    second degree T22.211
    third degree T22.311
  second degree T22.219
  third degree T22.319
forehead T20.06
  first degree T20.16
  second degree T20.26
  third degree T20.36
fourth degree *code as* Burn, third degree, by site
friction—*see* Burn, by site
from swallowing caustic or corrosive substance NEC—
        see Corrosion, by site

Burn, *continued*

full thickness skin loss *code as* Burn, third degree, by site
gastrointestinal tract NEC T28.2
  from swallowing caustic or corrosive substance T28.7
genital organs
  external
    female T21.07
      first degree T21.17
      second degree T21.27
      third degree T21.37
    male T21.06
      first degree T21.16
      second degree T21.26
      third degree T21.36
  internal T28.3
    from caustic or corrosive substance T28.8
groin—*see* Burn, abdominal wall
hand (s) T23.009
  back—*see* Burn, dorsum of hand
  finger—*see* Burn, finger
  first degree T23.109
  left T23.002
    first degree T23.102
    second degree T23.202
    third degree T23.302
  multiple sites with wrist T23.099
    first degree T23.199
    left T23.092
      first degree T23.192
      second degree T23.292
      third degree T23.392
    right T23.091
      first degree T23.191
      second degree T23.291
      third degree T23.391
    second degree T23.299
    third degree T23.399
  palm—*see* Burn, palm
  right T23.001
    first degree T23.101
    second degree T23.201
    third degree T23.301
  second degree T23.209
  third degree T23.309
  thumb—*see* Burn, thumb
head (and face) (and neck) (*Code by* Burn to specific site for cheek, chin, ear, eye, forehead, lip, neck, nose, or scalp) T20.00
  first degree T20.10
  multiple sites T20.09
    first degree T20.19
    second degree T20.29
    third degree T20.39
  second degree T20.20
  third degree T20.30
hip (s)—*see* Burn, thigh
inhalation—*see* Burn, respiratory tract
  caustic or corrosive substance (fumes)—*see* Corrosion, respiratory tract
internal organ (s) T28.40
  alimentary tract T28.2
    esophagus T28.1
  eardrum T28.41
  esophagus T28.1
  from caustic or corrosive substance (swallowing) NEC—*see* Corrosion, by site
  genitourinary T28.3
  mouth T28.0
  pharynx T28.0
  respiratory tract—*see* Burn, respiratory tract
  specified organ NEC T28.49
interscapular region—*see* Burn, back, upper
intestine (large) (small) T28.2
knee T24.029
  first degree T24.129
  left T24.022
    first degree T24.122
    second degree T24.222
    third degree T24.322

Burn, *continued*

  right T24.021
    first degree T24.121
    second degree T24.221
    third degree T24.321
  second degree T24.229
  third degree T24.329
labium (majus) (minus)—*see* Burn, genital organs, external, female
lacrimal apparatus, duct, gland or sac—*see* Burn, eye, specified site NEC
larynx T27.0
  with lung T27.1
leg (s) (lower) (upper)—*see* Burn, lower, limb
lightning—*see* Burn, by site
limb (s)
  lower (except ankle or foot alone)—*see* Burn, lower, limb
  upper—*see* Burn, upper limb
lip (s) T20.02
  first degree T20.12
  second degree T20.22
  third degree T20.32
lower
  back—*see* Burn, back
  limb T24.009 (*Code to* Burn by specific site for ankle, calf, foot, thigh, knee)
    first degree T24.109
    left T24.002
      first degree T24.102
      second degree T24.202
      third degree T24.302
    multiple sites, except ankle and foot T24.099
      ankle and foot T25.099
        first degree T25.199
        left T25.092
          first degree T25.192
          second degree T25.292
          third degree T25.392
        right T25.091
          first degree T25.191
          second degree T25.291
          third degree T25.391
        second degree T25.299
        third degree T25.399
      first degree T24.199
      left T24.092
        first degree T24.192
        second degree T24.292
        third degree T24.392
      right T24.091
        first degree T24.191
        second degree T24.291
        third degree T24.391
      second degree T24.299
      third degree T24.399
    right T24.001
      first degree T24.101
      second degree T24.201
      third degree T24.301
    second degree T24.209
    thigh—*see* Burn, thigh
    third degree T24.309
    toe—*see* Burn, toe
lung (with larynx and trachea) T27.1
mouth T28.0
neck T20.07
  first degree T20.17
  second degree T20.27
  third degree T20.37
nose (septum) T20.04
  first degree T20.14
  second degree T20.24
  third degree T20.34
ocular adnexa—*see* Burn, eye
orbit region—*see* Burn, eyelid
palm T23.059
  first degree T23.159
  left T23.052
    first degree T23.152
    second degree T23.252
    third degree T23.352

Burn, *continued*
    right T23.051
        first degree T23.151
        second degree T23.251
        third degree T23.351
      second degree T23.259
      third degree T23.359
    partial thickness *code as* Burn, unspecified degree, by site
    pelvis—*see* Burn, trunk
    penis—*see* Burn, genital organs, external, male
    perineum
      female—*see* Burn, genital organs, external, female
      male—*see* Burn, genital organs, external, male
    periocular area—*see* Burn, eyelid
    pharynx T28.0
    rectum T28.2
    respiratory tract T27.3
      larynx—*see* Burn, larynx
      specified part NEC T27.2
      trachea—*see* Burn, trachea
    sac, lacrimal—*see* Burn, eye, specified site NEC
    scalp T20.05
      first degree T20.15
      second degree T20.25
      third degree T20.35
    scapular region T22.069
      first degree T22.169
      left T22.062
        first degree T22.162
        second degree T22.262
        third degree T22.362
      right T22.061
        first degree T22.161
        second degree T22.261
        third degree T22.361
      second degree T22.269
      third degree T22.369
    sclera—*see* Burn, eye, specified site NEC
    scrotum—*see* Burn, genital organs, external, male
    shoulder T22.059
      first degree T22.159
      left T22.052
        first degree T22.152
        second degree T22.252
        third degree T22.352
      right T22.051
        first degree T22.151
        second degree T22.251
        third degree T22.351
      second degree T22.259
      third degree T22.359
    stomach T28.2
    temple—*see* Burn, head
    testis—*see* Burn, genital organs, external, male
    thigh T24.019
      first degree T24.119
      left T24.012
        first degree T24.112
        second degree T24.212
        third degree T24.312
      right T24.011
        first degree T24.111
        second degree T24.211
        third degree T24.311
      second degree T24.219
      third degree T24.319
    thorax (external)—*see* Burn, trunk
    throat (meaning pharynx) T28.0
    thumb (s) T23.019
      first degree T23.119
      left T23.012
        first degree T23.112
        second degree T23.212
        third degree T23.312
      multiple sites with fingers T23.049
        first degree T23.149
        left T23.042
          first degree T23.142
          second degree T23.242
          third degree T23.342

Burn, *continued*
    right T23.041
      first degree T23.141
      second degree T23.241
      third degree T23.341
    second degree T23.249
    third degree T23.349
    right T23.011
      first degree T23.111
      second degree T23.211
      third degree T23.311
    second degree T23.219
    third degree T23.319
    toe T25.039
      first degree T25.139
      left T25.032
        first degree T25.132
        second degree T25.232
        third degree T25.332
      right T25.031
        first degree T25.131
        second degree T25.231
        third degree T25.331
      second degree T25.239
      third degree T25.339
    tongue T28.0
    tonsil (s) T28.0
    trachea T27.0
      with lung T27.1
    trunk T21.00 *(Code to Burn by specific site for abdominal wall, buttock, upper limb, back, chest wall, genital organs, or scapular region)*
      first degree T21.10
      second degree T21.20
      specified site NEC T21.09
        first degree T21.19
        second degree T21.29
        third degree T21.39
      third degree T21.30
    unspecified site with extent of body surface involved specified
      less than 10 percent T31.0
      10−19 percent (0−9 percent third degree) T31.10
        with 10−19 percent third degree T31.11
    upper limb *(Code to Burn by specific site for above elbow, axilla, elbow, forearm, hand, scapular region, shoulder, upper back, or wrist)* T22.00
      first degree T22.10
      multiple sites T22.099
        first degree T22.199
        left T22.092
          first degree T22.192
          second degree T22.292
          third degree T22.392
        right T22.091
          first degree T22.191
          second degree T22.291
          third degree T22.391
        second degree T22.299
        third degree T22.399
      second degree T22.20
      third degree T22.30
    uterus T28.3
    vagina T28.3
    vulva—*see* Burn, genital organs, external, female
    wrist T23.079
      first degree T23.179
      left T23.072
        first degree T23.172
        second degree T23.272
        third degree T23.372
      multiple sites with hand T23.099
        first degree T23.199
        left T23.092
          first degree T23.192
          second degree T23.292
          third degree T23.392

Burn, *continued*
    right T23.091
      first degree T23.191
      second degree T23.291
      third degree T23.391
    second degree T23.299
    third degree T23.399
    right T23.071
      first degree T23.171
      second degree T23.271
      third degree T23.371
    second degree T23.279
    third degree T23.379
Burnett's syndrome E83.52
Bursitis M71.9
    specified NEC M71.50
      ankle M71.57-
      due to use, overuse or pressure—*see* Disorder, soft tissue, due to, use
      elbow M71.52-
      foot M71.57-
      hand M71.54-
      hip M71.55-
      knee M71.56-
      shoulder—*see* Bursitis, shoulder
      specified site NEC M71.58
      tibial collateral M76.4-
      wrist M71.53-

C

Cachexia R64
    dehydration E86.0
      with
        hypernatremia E87.0
        hyponatremia E87.1
Café au lait spots L81.3
Calciferol (vitamin D) deficiency E55.9
    with rickets E55.0
Calcification
    adrenal (capsule) (gland) E27.49
    cerebral (cortex) G93.89
    choroid plexus G93.89
    pericardium (*see also* Pericarditis) I31.1
    subcutaneous L94.2
    suprarenal (capsule) (gland) E27.49
Calcinosis (interstitial) (tumoral) (universalis) E83.59
    circumscripta (skin) L94.2
    cutis L94.2
Calculus, calculi, calculous
    biliary—*see also* Calculus, gallbladder
      specified NEC K80.80
        with obstruction K80.81
    bilirubin, multiple—*see* Calculus, gallbladder
    gallbladder K80.20
      with
        bile duct calculus—*see* Calculus, gallbladder and bile duct
        cholecystitis K80.10
          with obstruction K80.11
          acute K80.00
            with
              chronic cholecystitis K80.12
                with obstruction K80.13
              obstruction K80.01
          chronic K80.10
            with
              acute cholecystitis K80.12
                with obstruction K80.13
              obstruction K80.11
        specified NEC K80.18
          with obstruction K80.19
      obstruction K80.21
    intestinal (impaction) (obstruction) K56.49
    kidney (impacted) (multiple) (pelvis) (recurrent) (staghorn) N20.0
      with calculus, ureter N20.2
      congenital Q63.8
    nose J34.89
    pyelitis (impacted) (recurrent) N20.0
      with hydronephrosis N13.2
    pyelonephritis (impacted) (recurrent)—*see* category N20
      with hydronephrosis N13.2

Calculus, calculi, calculous, *continued*
    tonsil J35.8
    ureter (impacted) (recurrent) N20.1
        with calculus, kidney N20.2
            with hydronephrosis N13.2
                with infection N13.6
    urinary (duct) (impacted) (passage) (tract) N20.9
        with hydronephrosis N13.2
            with infection N13.6
    vagina N89.8
California
    encephalitis A83.5
Callositas, callosity (infected) L84
Callus (infected) L84
**CALME (Childhood asymmetric labium majus
                            enlargement) N90.61**
Calorie deficiency or malnutrition (*see also* Malnutrition)
                                                    E46
Calvé-Perthes disease M91.1-
Camptocormia (hysterical) F44.4
Canal—*see also* condition
    atrioventricular common Q21.2
Candidiasis, candidal B37.9
    balanitis B37.42
    bronchitis B37.1
    cheilitis B37.83
    congenital P37.5
    cystitis B37.41
    disseminated B37.7
    endocarditis B37.6
    enteritis B37.82
    esophagitis B37.81
    intertrigo B37.2
    lung B37.1
    meningitis B37.5
    mouth B37.0
    nails B37.2
    neonatal P37.5
    onychia B37.2
    oral B37.0
    osteomyelitis B37.89
    otitis externa B37.84
    paronychia B37.2
    perionyxis B37.2
    pneumonia B37.1
    proctitis B37.82
    pulmonary B37.1
    pyelonephritis B37.49
    sepsis B37.7
    skin B37.2
    specified site NEC B37.89
    stomatitis B37.0
    systemic B37.7
    urethritis B37.41
    urogenital site NEC B37.49
    vagina B37.3
    vulva B37.3
    vulvovaginitis B37.3
Canker (mouth) (sore) K12.0
    rash A38.9
Caput
    crepitus Q75.8
Carbuncle L02.93
    abdominal wall L02.231
    anus K61.0
    axilla L02.43-
    back (any part) L02.232
    breast N61.1
    buttock L02.33
    cheek (external) L02.03
    chest wall L02.233
    chin L02.03
    face NEC L02.03
    finger L02.53-
    flank L02.231
    foot L02.63-
    forehead L02.03
    genital—*see* Abscess, genital
    gluteal (region) L02.33
    groin L02.234
    hand L02.53-
    head NEC L02.831

Carbuncle, *continued*
    heel L02.63-
    hip L02.43-
    kidney—*see* Abscess, kidney
    knee L02.43-
    lower limb L02.43-
    navel L02.236
    neck L02.13
    nose (external) (septum) J34.0
    partes posteriores L02.33
    pectoral region L02.233
    perineum L02.235
    pinna—*see* Abscess, ear, external
    scalp L02.831
    specified site NEC L02.838
    temple (region) L02.03
    thumb L02.53-
    toe L02.63-
    trunk L02.239
        abdominal wall L02.231
        back L02.232
        chest wall L02.233
        groin L02.234
        perineum L02.235
        umbilicus L02.236
    umbilicus L02.236
    upper limb L02.43-
    urethra N34.0
    vulva N76.4
Carcinoma (malignant)—*see also* Neoplasm, by site,
                                                    malignant
    renal cell C64-
Cardiac—*see also* condition
    death, sudden—*see* Arrest, cardiac
    pacemaker
        in situ Z95.0
        management or adjustment Z45.018
    tamponade I31.4
Cardiochalasia K21.9
Cardiomegaly—*see also* Hypertrophy, cardiac
    congenital Q24.8
    idiopathic I51.7
Cardiomyopathy (familial) (idiopathic) I42.9
    constrictive NOS I42.5
    due to
        Friedreich's ataxia G11.1
        progressive muscular dystrophy G71.0
    hypertrophic (nonobstructive) I42.2
        obstructive I42.1
            congenital Q24.8
    in
        sarcoidosis D86.85
    metabolic E88.9 *[I43]*
        thyrotoxic E05.90 *[I43]*
            with thyroid storm E05.91 *[I43]*
    restrictive NEC I42.5
    secondary I42.9
    thyrotoxic E05.90 *[I43]*
        with thyroid storm E05.91 *[I43]*
Cardiopathy
    idiopathic I42.9
    mucopolysaccharidosis E76.3 *[I52]*
Cardiopathia nigra I27.0
Cardiosymphysis I31.0
Care (of) (for) (following)
    family member (handicapped) (sick)
        unavailable, due to
            absence (person rendering care) (sufferer) Z74.2
            inability (any reason) of person rendering care
                                                            Z74.2
    foundling Z76.1
    palliative Z51.5
    unavailable, due to
        absence of person rendering care Z74.2
        inability (any reason) of person rendering care Z74.2
    wellbaby Z76.2
Caries
    dental K02.9
Carnitine insufficiency E71.40
Carpenter's syndrome Q87.0

Carrier (suspected) **of**
    bacterial disease NEC Z22.39
        diphtheria Z22.2
        intestinal infectious NEC Z22.1
            typhoid Z22.0
        meningococcal Z22.31
        sexually transmitted Z22.4
        specified NEC Z22.39
        staphylococcal (Methicillin susceptible) Z22.321
            Methicillin resistant Z22.322
        streptococcal Z22.338
            group B Z22.330
    genetic Z14.8
        cystic fibrosis Z14.1
        hemophilia A (asymptomatic) Z14.01
            symptomatic Z14.02
    gonorrhea Z22.4
    HAA (hepatitis Australian-antigen) Z22.5
    HB (c) (s)-AG Z22.5
    hepatitis (viral) Z22.5
        Australia-antigen (HAA) Z22.5
        B surface antigen (HBsAg) Z22.5
            with acute delta- (super) infection B17.0
        C Z22.5
        specified NEC Z22.5
    infectious organism Z22.9
        specified NEC Z22.8
    meningococci Z22.31
    serum hepatitis—*see* Carrier, hepatitis
    staphylococci (Methicillin susceptible) Z22.321
        Methicillin resistant Z22.322
    streptococci Z22.338
        group B Z22.330
    syphilis Z22.4
    venereal disease Z22.4
Car sickness T75.3
Caruncle (inflamed)
    myrtiform N89.8
Caseation lymphatic gland (tuberculous) A18.2
Cat
    cry syndrome Q93.4
Cataract (cortical) (immature) (incipient) H26.9
    anterior
        and posterior axial embryonal Q12.0
            pyramidal Q12.0
    blue Q12.0
    central Q12.0
    cerulean Q12.0
    congenital Q12.0
    coraliform Q12.0
    coronary Q12.0
    crystalline Q12.0
    infantile—*see* Cataract, presenile
    juvenile—*see* Cataract, presenile
    nuclear
        embryonal Q12.0
    presenile H26.00-
    zonular (perinuclear) Q12.0
Cataracta—*see also* Cataract
    centralis pulverulenta Q12.0
    cerulea Q12.0
    congenita Q12.0
    coralliformis Q12.0
    coronaria Q12.0
    membranacea
        congenita Q12.0
Catarrh, catarrhal (acute) (febrile) (infectious) (inflammation)
                                            (*see also* condition) J00
    chronic J31.0
    gingivitis K05.00
        plaque induced K05.00
    larynx, chronic J37.0
    liver B15.9
    middle ear, chronic H65.2-
    mouth K12.1
    nasal (chronic)—*see* Rhinitis
    nasopharyngeal (chronic) J31.1
        acute J00
    pulmonary—*see* Bronchitis
    spring (eye) (vernal)—*see* Conjunctivitis, acute, atopic
    summer (hay)—*see* Fever, hay
    throat J31.2

Catarrh, catarrhal, *continued*
  tubotympanal—*see also* Otitis, media, nonsuppurative
      chronic H65.2-
Catatonic
  stupor R40.1
Cecitis K52.9
  with perforation, peritonitis, or rupture K65.8
Celiac
  disease (with steatorrhea) K90.0
  infantilism K90.0
Cellulitis (diffuse) (phlegmonous) (septic) (suppurative) L03.90
  abdominal wall L03.311
  ankle L03.11-
  anus K61.0
  axilla L03.11-
  back (any part) L03.312
  breast (acute) (nonpuerperal) N61.0
      nipple N61.0
  buttock L03.317
  cervical (meaning neck) L03.221
  cheek (external) L03.211
      internal K12.2
  chest wall L03.313
  chronic L03.90
  ear (external) H60.1-
  erysipelatous—*see* Erysipelas
  face NEC L03.211
  finger (intrathecal) (periosteal) (subcutaneous)
                                    (subcuticular) L03.01-
  foot L03.11-
  gangrenous—*see* Gangrene
  gluteal (region) L03.317
  groin L03.314
  head NEC L03.811
      face (any part, except ear, eye and nose) L03.211
  jaw (region) L03.211
  knee L03.11-
  lip K13.0
  lower limb L03.11-
      toe—*see* Cellulitis, toe
  mouth (floor) K12.2
  multiple sites, so stated L03.90
  navel L03.316
      newborn P38.9
          with mild hemorrhage P38.1
          without hemorrhage P38.9
  neck (region) L03.221
  nose (septum) (external) J34.0
  orbit, orbital H05.01-
      periorbital L03.213
  palate (soft) K12.2
  pectoral (region) L03.313
  pelvis, pelvic (chronic)
      female (*see also* Disease, pelvis, inflammatory) N73.2
          acute N73.0
      male K65.0
  perineal, perineum L03.315
  periorbital L03.213
  peritonsillar J36
  preseptal L03.213
  scalp (any part) L03.811
  specified site NEC L03.818
  submandibular (region) (space) (triangle) K12.2
      gland K11.3
  submaxillary (region) K12.2
      gland K11.3
  toe (intrathecal) (periosteal) (subcutaneous) (subcuticular)
                                    L03.03
  tonsil J36
  trunk L03.319
      abdominal wall L03.311
      back (any part) L03.312
      buttock L03.317
      chest wall L03.313
      groin L03.314
      perineal, perineum L03.315
      umbilicus L03.316
  umbilicus L03.316
  upper limb L03.11-
      axilla L03.11-
      finger L03.01-
      thumb L03.01-
  vaccinal T88.0

Central auditory processing disorder H93.25
Cephalematoma, cephalhematoma (calcified)
  newborn (birth injury) P12.0
Cephalgia, cephalalgia—*see also* Headache
  histamine G44.009
      intractable G44.001
      not intractable G44.009
Cerumen (accumulation) (impacted) H61.2-
Cervicalgia M54.2
Cervicitis (acute) (chronic) (nonvenereal) (senile (atrophic))
                                    (subacute) (with
                                    ulceration) N72
  chlamydial A56.09
  gonococcal A54.03
  trichomonal A59.09
Cervicocolpitis (emphysematosa) (*see also* Cervicitis) N72
Cestode infestation B71.9
  specified type NEC B71.8
Cestodiasis B71.9
Chafing L30.4
Chalasia (cardiac sphincter) K21.9
Chalazion H00.19
  left H00.16
      lower H00.15
      upper H00.14
  right H00.13
      lower H00.12
      upper H00.11
Chancre (any genital site) (hard) (hunterian) (mixed) (primary)
                                    (seronegative)
                                    (seropositive)
                                    (syphilitic) A51.0
  conjunctiva NEC A51.2
  extragenital A51.2
  eyelid A51.2
  lip A51.2
  nipple A51.2
  palate, soft A51.2
  soft A57
      bubo A57
      palate A51.2
  urethra A51.0
Change(s) (in) (of)—*see also* Removal
  circulatory I99.9
  contraceptive device Z30.433
  dressing (nonsurgical) Z48.00
      surgical Z48.01
  hypertrophic
      nasal sinus J34.89
      turbinate, nasal J34.3
      upper respiratory tract J39.8
  mental status R41.82
  sacroiliac joint M53.3
  skin R23.9
      acute, due to ultraviolet radiation L56.9
          specified NEC L56.8
      cyanosis R23.0
      flushing R23.2
      pallor R23.1
      petechiae R23.3
      specified change NEC R23.8
      swelling—*see* Mass, localized
  vascular I99.9
  voice R49.9
      psychogenic F44.4
CHARGE association Q89.8
Charley-horse (quadriceps) M62.831
  traumatic (quadriceps) S76.11-
Checking (of)
  implantable subdermal contraceptive Z30.46
  intrauterine contraceptive device Z30.431
Cheese itch B88.0
Cheilitis (acute) (angular) (catarrhal) (chronic) (exfoliative)
                                    (gangrenous)
                                    (glandular) (infectional)
                                    (suppurative)
                                    (ulcerative)(vesicular)
                                    K13.0
  actinic (due to sun) L56.8
      other than from sun L56.9
  candidal B37.83
Cheilodynia K13.0

Cheiloschisis—*see* Cleft, lip
Cheilosis (angular) K13.0
Cheiropompholyx L30.1
Chemotherapy (session) (for)
  cancer Z51.11
  neoplasm Z51.11
Cheyne-Stokes breathing (respiration) R06.3
Chickenpox—*see* Varicella
Chigger (infestation) B88.0
Child
  custody dispute Z65.3
Childhood
  cerebral X-linked adrenoleukodystrophy E71.520
  period of rapid growth Z00.2
Chill (s) R68.83
  with fever R50.9
  congestive in malarial regions B54
  without fever R68.83
Chinese dysentery A03.9
Chlamydia, chlamydial A74.9
  cervicitis A56.09
  conjunctivitis A74.0
  cystitis A56.01
  endometritis A56.11
  epididymitis A56.19
  female
      pelvic inflammatory disease A56.11
      pelviperitonitis A56.11
  orchitis A56.19
  peritonitis A74.81
  pharyngitis A56.4
  proctitis A56.3
  psittaci (infection) A70
  salpingitis A56.11
  sexually-transmitted infection NEC A56.8
  specified NEC A74.89
  urethritis A56.01
  vulvovaginitis A56.02
Chlamydiosis—*see* Chlamydia
Chlorotic anemia D50.8
Cholecystitis K81.9
  acute (emphysematous) (gangrenous) (suppurative) K81.0
  with
      calculus, stones in
          cystic duct—*see* Calculus, gallbladder, with
                                    cholecystitis, acute
          gallbladder—*see* Calculus, gallbladder, with
                                    cholecystitis, acute
          choledocholithiasis—*see* Calculus, bile duct, with
                                    cholecystitis, acute
          cholelithiasis—*see* Calculus, gallbladder, with
                                    cholecystitis, acute
      chronic cholecystitis K81.2
          with gallbladder calculus K80.12
              with obstruction K80.13
  chronic K81.1
      with acute cholecystitis K81.2
          with gallbladder calculus K80.12
              with obstruction K80.13
  emphysematous (acute)—*see* Cholecystitis, acute
  gangrenous—*see* Cholecystitis, acute
  suppurative—*see* Cholecystitis, acute
Choking sensation R09.89
Cholesteremia E78.0
Cholesterol
  elevated (high) E78.00
      with elevated (high) triglycerides E78.2
      screening for Z13.220
Cholesterolemia (essential) (pure) E78.00
  familial E78.01
  hereditary E78.01
Chondritis M94.8X9
  costal (Tietze's) M94.0
  patella, posttraumatic M22.4-
Chondromalacia (systemic) M94.20
  knee M94.26-
      patella M22.4-
Chondro-osteodysplasia (Morquio-Brailsford type) E76.219
Chondro-osteodystrophy E76.29
Chondropathia tuberosa M94.0
Chordee (nonvenereal) N48.89
  congenital Q54.4

Chorea (chronic) (gravis) (posthemiplegic) (senile) (spasmodic) G25.5
  with
    heart involvement I02.0
      active or acute (conditions in I01-) I02.0
      rheumatic I02.9
        with valvular disorder I02.0
      rheumatic heart disease (chronic) (inactive) (quiescent)—*code to* rheumatic heart condition involved
    hysterical F44.4
Chorioretinitis—*see also* Inflammation, chorioretinal
  in (due to)
    toxoplasmosis (acquired) B58.01
      congenital (active) P37.1 *[H32]*
Chromophytosis B36.0
Chylopericardium I31.3
  acute I30.9
Cicatricial (deformity)—*see* Cicatrix
Cicatrix (adherent) (contracted) (painful) (vicious) (*see also* Scar) L90.5
  adenoid (and tonsil) J35.8
  anus K62.89
  brain G93.89
  mouth K13.79
  muscle M62.89
    with contracture—*see* Contraction, muscle NEC
  palate (soft) K13.79
  rectum K62.89
  skin L90.5
    postinfective L90.5
    specified site NEC L90.5
  tonsil (and adenoid) J35.8
  vagina N89.8
    postoperative N99.2
  wrist, constricting (annular) L90.5
CINCA (chronic infantile neurological, cutaneous and articular syndrome) M04.2
Circulation
  failure (peripheral) R57.9
    newborn P29.89
  fetal, persistent P29.3
Circumcision (in absence of medical indication) (ritual) (routine) Z41.2
Cirrhosis, cirrhotic (hepatic) (liver) K74.60
  due to
    xanthomatosis E78.2
  pigmentary E83.110
  xanthomatous (biliary) K74.5
    due to xanthomatosis (familial) (metabolic) (primary) E78.2
Clam digger's itch B65.3
Clammy skin R23.1
Clark's paralysis G80.9
Claudication, intermittent I73.9
  cerebral (artery) G45.9
Clavus (infected) L84
Clawfoot (congenital) Q66.89
  acquired M21.53-
Clawtoe (congenital) Q66.89
  acquired M20.5X-
Cleft (congenital)—*see also* Imperfect, closure
  foot Q72.7
  hand Q71.6
  lip (unilateral) Q36.9
    with cleft palate Q37.9
      hard Q37.1
        with soft Q37.5
      soft Q37.3
        with hard Q37.5
    bilateral Q36.0
      with cleft palate Q37.8
        hard Q37.0
          with soft Q37.4
        soft Q37.2
          with hard Q37.4
    median Q36.1
  palate Q35.9
    with cleft lip (unilateral) Q37.9
      bilateral Q37.8

Cleft, *continued*
  hard Q35.1
    with
      cleft lip (unilateral) Q37.1
        bilateral Q37.0
      soft Q35.5
        with cleft lip (unilateral) Q37.5
          bilateral Q37.4
  medial Q35.5
  soft Q35.3
    with
      cleft lip (unilateral) Q37.3
        bilateral Q37.2
      hard Q35.5
        with cleft lip (unilateral) Q37.5
          bilateral Q37.4
  penis Q55.69
  scrotum Q55.29
  uvula Q35.7
Cleidocranial dysostosis Q74.0
Clicking hip (newborn) R29.4
Closed bite M26.29
Closure
  congenital, nose Q30.0
  foramen ovale, imperfect Q21.1
  hymen N89.6
  interauricular septum, defective Q21.1
  interventricular septum, defective Q21.0
  lacrimal duct—*see* Stenosis, lacrimal, duct
    congenital Q10.5
  nose (congenital) Q30.0
    acquired M95.0
  vagina N89.5
Clot (blood)—*see also* Embolism
  artery (obstruction) (occlusion)—*see* Embolism
  brain (intradural or extradural)—*see* Occlusion, artery, cerebral
  circulation I74.9
Clouded state R40.1
  epileptic—*see* Epilepsy, specified NEC
  paroxysmal—*see* Epilepsy, specified NEC
Cloudy antrum, antra J32.0
Clubfoot (congenital) Q66.89
  acquired M21.54-
  equinovarus Q66.0
  paralytic M21.54-
Clubhand (congenital) (radial) Q71.4-
  acquired M21.51-
Clumsiness, clumsy child syndrome F82
Cluttering F80.81
Coagulopathy—*see also* Defect, coagulation
  consumption D65
  intravascular D65
    newborn P60
Coalition
  calcaneo-scaphoid Q66.89
  tarsal Q66.89
Coarctation
  aorta (preductal) (postductal) Q25.1
  pulmonary artery Q25.71
Coccydynia, coccygodynia M53.3
Cockayne's syndrome Q87.1
Cock's peculiar tumor L72.3
Cold J00
  with influenza, flu, or grippe—*see* Influenza, with, respiratory manifestations NEC
  bronchial—*see* Bronchitis
  chest—*see* Bronchitis
  common (head) J00
  head J00
  on lung—*see* Bronchitis
  rose J30.1
  virus J00
Colibacillosis A49.8
  as the cause of other disease (*see also* Escherichia coli) B96.20
  generalized A41.50

Colic (bilious) (infantile) (intestinal) (recurrent) (spasmodic) R10.83
  abdomen R10.83
    psychogenic F45.8
  hysterical F45.8
  kidney N23
  mucous K58.9
    with constipation K58.1
    with diarrhea K58.0
    mixed K58.2
    other K58.8
    psychogenic F54
  nephritic N23
  psychogenic F45.8
  renal N23
  ureter N23
  uterus NEC N94.89
    menstrual—*see* Dysmenorrhea
Colitis (acute) (catarrhal) (chronic) (noninfective) (hemorrhagic) (*see also* Enteritis) K52.9
  allergic K52.29
    with
      food protein-induced enterocolitis syndrome K52.21
      proctocolitis K52.82
  amebic (acute) (*see also* Amebiasis) A06.0
  anthrax A22.2
  collagenous K52.831
  cystica superficialis K52.89
  dietary counseling and surveillance (for) Z71.3
  dietetic K52.29
  eosinophilic K52.82
  food hypersensitivity K52.29
  giardial A07.1
  granulomatous—*see* Enteritis, regional, large intestine
  infectious—*see* Enteritis, infectious
  indeterminate, so stated K52.3
  left sided K51.50
    with
      abscess K51.514
      complication K51.519
        specified NEC K51.518
      fistula K51.513
      obstruction K51.512
      rectal bleeding K51.511
  lymphocytic K52.832
  microscopic, other K52.838
    unspecified K52.839
  noninfective K52.9
    specified NEC K52.89
  septic—*see* Enteritis, infectious
  spastic K58.9
    with constipation K58.1
    with diarrhea K58.0
    mixed K58.2
    other K58.8
    psychogenic F54
  staphylococcal A04.8
    foodborne A05.0
  ulcerative (chronic) K51.90
    with
      complication K51.919
        abscess K51.914
        fistula K51.913
        obstruction K51.912
        rectal bleeding K51.911
        specified complication NEC K51.918
    enterocolitis—*see* Enterocolitis, ulcerative
    ileocolitis—*see* Ileocolitis, ulcerative
    mucosal proctocolitis—*see* Proctocolitis, mucosal
    proctitis—*see* Proctitis, ulcerative
    pseudopolyposis—*see* Polyp, colon, inflammatory
    psychogenic F54
    rectosigmoiditis—*see* Rectosigmoiditis, ulcerative
    specified type NEC K51.80
      with
        complication K51.819
          abscess K51.814
          fistula K51.813
          obstruction K51.812
          rectal bleeding K51.811
          specified complication NEC K51.818

Collagenosis, collagen disease (nonvascular) (vascular) M35.9
  specified NEC M35.8
Collapse R55
  adrenal E27.2
  cardiorespiratory R57.0
  cardiovascular R57.0
    newborn P29.89
  circulatory (peripheral) R57.9
  during or
    resulting from a procedure, not elsewhere classified
        T81.10
  general R55
  neurocirculatory F45.8
  postoperative T81.10
  valvular—*see* Endocarditis
  vascular (peripheral) R57.9
    newborn P29.89
Colles' fracture S52.53-
Collet (-Sicard) syndrome G52.7
Coloboma (iris) Q13.0
Colonization
  MRSA (Methicillin resistant Staphylococcus aureus)
    Z22.322
  MSSA (Methicillin susceptible Staphylococcus aureus)
    Z22.321
  status—*see* Carrier (suspected) of
Coma R40.20
  with
    motor response (none) R40.231
      abnormal R40.233
      extension R40.232
      flexion withdrawal R40.234
      localizes pain R40.235
      obeys commands R40.236
    opening of eyes (never) R40.211
      in response to
        pain R40.212
        sound R40.213
      spontaneous R40.214
    verbal response (none) R40.221
      confused conversation R40.224
      inappropriate words R40.223
      incomprehensible words R40.222
      oriented R40.225
  hyperosmolar (diabetic)—*see* Diabetes, coma
  hypoglycemic (diabetic)—*see* Diabetes, coma,
        hypoglycemic
    nondiabetic E15
  in diabetes—*see* Diabetes, coma
  insulin-induced—*see* Coma, hypoglycemic
  newborn P91.5
  persistent vegetative state R40.3
  specified NEC, without documented Glasgow coma scale
        score, or with partial
        Glasgow coma scale
        score reported R40.244
Comatose—*see* Coma
Comedo, comedones (giant) L70.0
Common
  arterial trunk Q20.0
  atrioventricular canal Q21.2
  atrium Q21.1
  cold (head) J00
  truncus (arteriosus) Q20.0
Communication
  between
    pulmonary artery and pulmonary vein, congenital
      Q25.72
  disorder
    social pragmatic F80.82
Complaint—*see also* Disease
  bowel, functional K59.9
    psychogenic F45.8
  intestine, functional K59.9
    psychogenic F45.8
  kidney—*see* Disease, renal
Complex
  Addison-Schilder E71.528
  Costen's M26.69
  Eisenmenger's (ventricular septal defect) I27.89
  Schilder-Addison E71.528

Complication(s) (from) (of)
  arteriovenous
    fistula, surgically created T82.9
      infection or inflammation T82.7
    shunt, surgically created T82.9
      infection or inflammation T82.7
    vascular (counterpulsation) T82.9
      infection or inflammation T82.7
  cardiac—*see also* Disease, heart
    device, implant or graft T82.9
      infection or inflammation T82.7
  cardiovascular device, graft or implant T82.9
    infection or inflammation T82.7
  catheter (device) NEC—*see also* Complications, prosthetic
        device or implant
    dialysis (vascular) T82.9
      infection and inflammation T82.7
    intravenous infusion T82.9
      infection or inflammation T82.7
  circulatory system I99.8
    postprocedural I97.89
      following cardiac surgery I97.19-
        postcardiotomy syndrome I97.0
      postcardiotomy syndrome I97.0
  delivery (*see also* Complications, obstetric) O75.9
    specified NEC O75.89
  extracorporeal circulation T80.90
  gastrointestinal K92.9
    postoperative
      malabsorption NEC K91.2
  gastrostomy (stoma) K94.20
    hemorrhage K94.21
    infection K94.22
    malfunction K94.23
    mechanical K94.23
    specified complication NEC K94.29
  infusion (procedure) T80.90
    infection T80.29
    sepsis T80.29
    serum reaction (*see also* Reaction, serum) T80.69
      anaphylactic shock (*see also* Shock, anaphylactic)
        T80.59
  injection (procedure) T80.90
    drug reaction—*see* Reaction, drug
    infection T80.29
    sepsis T80.29
  labor O75.9
    specified NEC O75.89
  metabolic E88.9
    postoperative E89.89
      specified NEC E89.89
  obstetric O75.9
    specified NEC O75.89
  perfusion NEC T80.90
  postprocedural—*see also* Complications, surgical
        procedure
    cardiac arrest
      following cardiac surgery I97.120
      following other surgery I97.121
    cardiac functional disturbance NEC
      following cardiac surgery I97.190
      following other surgery I97.191
    cardiac insufficiency
      following cardiac surgery I97.110
      following other surgery I97.111
    heart failure
      following cardiac surgery I97.130
      following other surgery I97.131
    hemorrhage (hematoma) (of)
      genitourinary organ or structure
        following procedure on genitourinary organ or
          structure N99.820
    specified NEC
      respiratory system J95.89
  prosthetic device or implant T85.9
    mechanical NEC T85.698
      ventricular shunt
        breakdown T85.01
        displacement T85.02
        leakage T85.03
        malposition T85.02
        obstruction T85.09
        perforation T85.09

Complication(s), *continued*
      protrusion T85.09
        specified NEC T85.09
  respiratory system J98.9
    postoperative J95.89
      air leak J95.812
      specified NEC J95.89
  surgical procedure (on) T81.9
    malabsorption (postsurgical)NEC K91.2
    postcardiotomy syndrome I97.0
    postcommissurotomy syndrome I97.0
    postvalvulotomy syndrome I97.0
    shock (hypovolemic) T81.19
  transfusion (blood) (lymphocytes) (plasma) T80.92
    circulatory overload E87.71
    febrile nonhemolytic transfusion reaction R50.84
    hemochromatosis E83.111
    hemolytic reaction (antigen unspecified) T80.919
    incompatibility reaction (antigen unspecified) T80.919
      acute (antigen unspecified) T80.910
      delayed (antigen unspecified) T80.911
      delayed serologic (DSTR) T80.89
    infection T80.29
      acute T80.22
    reaction NEC T80.89
    sepsis T80.29
    shock T80.89
  transplant T86.90
    bone marrow T86.00
      failure T86.02
      rejection T86.01
    failure T86.92
    heart T86.20
      with lung T86.30
        cardiac allograft vasculopathy T86.290
        failure T86.32
        rejection T86.31
      failure T86.22
      rejection T86.21
    infection T86.93
    kidney T86.10
      failure T86.12
      rejection T86.11
    liver T86.40
      failure T86.42
      rejection T86.41
    lung T86.819
      with heart T86.30
        failure T86.32
        rejection T86.31
      failure T86.811
      rejection T86.810
    malignant neoplasm C80.2
    peripheral blood stem cells T86.5
    post-transplant lymphoproliferative disorder (PTLD)
        D47.Z1
    rejection T86.91
    specified
      type NEC T86.99
    stem cell (from peripheral blood) (from umbilical cord)
        T86.5
    umbilical cord stem cells T86.5
  vaccination T88.1-
    anaphylaxis NEC T80.52-
    arthropathy—*see* Arthropathy, postimmunization
    cellulitis T88.0-
    encephalitis or encephalomyelitis G04.02
    infection (general) (local) NEC T88.0-
      meningitis G03.8
    myelitis G04.89
    protein sickness T80.62-
    rash T88.1-
    reaction (allergic) T88.1-
      serum T80.62-
    sepsis T88.0-
    serum intoxication, sickness, rash, or other serum
        reaction NEC T80.62-
      anaphylactic shock T80.52-
    shock (allergic) (anaphylactic) T80.52-
    vaccinia (generalized) (localized) T88.1-
  vascular I99.9
    device or implant T82.9
      infection or inflammation T82.7

Complication(s), *continued*
    ventricular (communicating) shunt (device) T85.9
        mechanical
            breakdown T85.01
            displacement T85.02
            leakage T85.03
            malposition T85.02
            obstruction T85.09
            perforation T85.09
            protrusion T85.09
            specified NEC T85.09

Compression
    facies Q67.1
    with injury *code by* Nature of injury
    laryngeal nerve, recurrent G52.2
        with paralysis of vocal cords and larynx J38.00
            bilateral J38.02
            unilateral J38.01
    nerve (*see also* Disorder, nerve) G58.9
        root or plexus NOS (in) G54.9
            neoplastic disease (*see also* Neoplasm) D49.9
                [G55]

Compulsion, compulsive
    neurosis F42.8
    states F42.9
    swearing F42.8
        in Gilles de la Tourette's syndrome F95.2
    tics and spasms F95.9

Concato's disease (pericardial polyserositis) A19.9
    nontubercular I31.1
    pleural—*see* Pleurisy, with effusion

Concealed penis Q55.69

Concretio cordis I31.1
    rheumatic I09.2

Concretion—*see also* Calculus
    prepuce (male) N47.8
    tonsil J35.8

Concussion (brain) (cerebral) (current) S06.0X-
    syndrome F07.81
    with
        loss of consciousness of 30 minutes or less S06.0X1
        loss of consciousness of unspecified duration S06.0X9

Condition—*see* Disease

Conditions arising in the perinatal period—*see* Newborn,
                affected by

Conduct disorder—*see* Disorder, conduct

Condyloma A63.0
    acuminatum A63.0
    gonorrheal A54.09
    latum A51.31
    syphilitic A51.31
        congenital A50.07
    venereal, syphilitic A51.31

Conflagration—*see also* Burn
    asphyxia (by inhalation of gases, fumes or vapors) (*see*
                also Table of Drugs and
                Chemicals) T59.9

Conflict (with)—*see also* Discord
    family Z73.9
    marital Z63.0
        involving divorce or estrangement Z63.5
    parentchild Z62.820
        parent-adopted child Z62.821
        parent-biological child Z62.820
        parent-foster child Z62.822

Congestion, congestive
    brain G93.89
    breast N64.59
    catarrhal J31.0
    chest R09.89
    glottis J37.0
    larynx J37.0
    lung R09.89
        active or acute—*see* Pneumonia

Conjunctivitis (staphylococcal) (streptococcal) NOS H10.9
    acute H10.3-
        atopic H10.1-
        chemical (*see also* Corrosion, cornea) H10.21-
        mucopurulent H10.02-
            viral—*see* Conjunctivitis, viral
        toxic H10.21-
    blennorrhagic (gonococcal) (neonatorum) A54.31
    chemical (acute) (*see also* Corrosion, cornea) H10.21-

Conjunctivitis, *continued*
    chlamydial A74.0
        neonatal P39.1
    epidemic (viral) B30.9
    gonococcal (neonatorum) A54.31
    in
        Chlamydia A74.0
        gonococci A54.31
    inclusion A74.0
    infantile P39.1
        gonococcal A54.31
    neonatal P39.1
        gonococcal A54.31
    viral B30.9

Conscious simulation (of illness) Z76.5

Consecutive—*see* condition

Consolidation lung (base)—*see* Pneumonia, lobar

Constipation (atonic) (neurogenic) (simple) (spastic) K59.00
    chronic K59.09
        idiopathic K59.04
    drug-induced K59.03
    functional K59.04
    outlet dysfunction K59.02
    psychogenic F45.8
    slow transit K59.01
    specified NEC K59.09

Constriction—*see also* Stricture
    external
        abdomen, abdominal (wall) S30.841
        alveolar process S00.542
        ankle S90.54-
        antecubital space S50.84-
        arm (upper) S40.84-
        auricle S00.44-
        axilla S40.84-
        back, lower S30.840
        breast S20.14-
        brow S00.84
        buttock S30.840
        calf S80.84-
        canthus S00.24-
        cheek S00.84
            internal S00.542
        chest wall—*see* Constriction, external, thorax
        chin S00.84
        clitoris S30.844
        costal region—*see* Constriction, external, thorax
        digit (s)
            foot—*see* Constriction, external, toe
            hand—*see* Constriction, external, finger
        ear S00.44-
        elbow S50.34-
        epididymis S30.843
        epigastric region S30.841
        esophagus, cervical S10.14
        eyebrow S00.24-
        eyelid S00.24-
        face S00.84
        finger (s) S60.44-
            index S60.44-
            little S60.44-
            middle S60.44-
            ring S60.44-
        flank S30.841
        foot (except toe(s) alone) S90.84-
            toe—*see* Constriction, external, toe
        forearm S50.84-
            elbow only S50.34-
        forehead S00.84
        genital organs, external
            female S30.846
            male S30.845
        groin S30.841
        gum S00.542
        hand S60.54-
        head S00.94
            ear S00.44-
            eyelid S00.24-
            lip S00.541
            nose S00.34
            oral cavity S00.542
            scalp S00.04
            specified site NEC S00.84

Constriction, *continued*
    heel S90.84-
    hip S70.24-
    inguinal region S30.841
    interscapular region S20.449
    jaw S00.84
    knee S80.24-
    labium (majus) (minus) S30.844
    larynx S10.14
    leg (lower) S80.84-
        knee S80.24-
        upper S70.34-
    lip S00.541
    lower back S30.840
    lumbar region S30.840
    malar region S00.84
    mammary S20.14-
    mastoid region S00.84
    mouth S00.542
    nail
        finger—*see* Constriction, external, finger
        toe—*see* Constriction, external, toe
    nasal S00.34
    neck S10.94
        specified site NEC S10.84
        throat S10.14
    nose S00.34
    occipital region S00.04
    oral cavity S00.542
    orbital region S00.24-
    palate S00.542
    palm S60.54-
    parietal region S00.04
    pelvis S30.840
    penis S30.842
    perineum
        female S30.844
        male S30.840
    periocular area S00.24-
    phalanges
        finger—*see* Constriction, external, finger
        toe—*see* Constriction, external, toe
    pharynx S10.14
    pinna S00.44-
    popliteal space S80.24-
    prepuce S30.842
    pubic region S30.840
    pudendum
        female S30.846
        male S30.845
    sacral region S30.840
    scalp S00.04
    scapular region S40.24-
    scrotum S30.843
    shin S80.84-
    shoulder S40.24-
    sternal region S20.349
    submaxillary region S00.84
    submental region S00.84
    subungual
        finger (s)—*see* Constriction, external, finger
        toe (s)—*see* Constriction, external, toe
    supraclavicular fossa S10.84
    supraorbital S00.84
    temple S00.84
    temporal region S00.84
    testis S30.843
    thigh S70.34-
    thorax, thoracic (wall) S20.94
        back S20.44-
        front S20.34-
    throat S10.14
    thumb S60.34-
    toe (s) (lesser) S90.44-
        great S90.44-
    tongue S00.542
    trachea S10.14
    tunica vaginalis S30.843
    uvula S00.542
    vagina S30.844
    vulva S30.844
    wrist S60.84-

Constriction, *continued*
  prepuce (acquired) (congenital) N47.1
  pylorus (adult hypertrophic) K31.1
    congenital or infantile Q40.0
    newborn Q40.0
Constrictive—*see* condition
Consultation
  medical—*see* Counseling, medical
  specified reason NEC Z71.89
  without complaint or sickness Z71.9
    feared complaint unfounded Z71.1
    specified reason NEC Z71.89
Consumption—*see* Tuberculosis
Contact (with)—*see also* Exposure (to)
  AIDS virus Z20.6
  anthrax Z20.810
  aromatic amines Z77.020
  arsenic Z77.010
  asbestos Z77.090
  bacterial disease NEC Z20.818
  body fluids (potentially hazardous) Z77.21
  benzene Z77.021
  chemicals (chiefly nonmedicinal) (hazardous) NEC
                  Z77.098
  chromium compounds Z77.018
  communicable disease Z20.9
    bacterial NEC Z20.818
    specified NEC Z20.89
    viral NEC Z20.828
  dyes Z77.098
  Escherichia coli (E. coli) Z20.01
  German measles Z20.4
  gonorrhea Z20.2
  hazardous metals NEC Z77.018
  hazardous substances NEC Z77.29
  hazards in the physical environment NEC Z77.128
  hazards to health NEC Z77.9
  HIV Z20.6
  HTLV-III/LAV Z20.6
  human immunodeficiency virus Z20.6
  infection Z20.9
    specified NEC Z20.89
  intestinal infectious disease NEC Z20.09
    Escherichia Coli (E. coli) Z20.01
  lead Z77.011
  meningococcus Z20.811
  mold (toxic) Z77.120
  nickel dust Z77.018
  poliomyelitis Z20.89
  rabies Z20.3
  rubella Z20.4
  sexually-transmitted disease Z20.2
  smallpox (laboratory) Z20.89
  syphilis Z20.2
  tuberculosis Z20.1
  varicella Z20.820
  venereal disease Z20.2
  viral disease NEC Z20.828
  viral hepatitis Z20.5
Contamination, food—*see* Intoxication, foodborne
Contraception, contraceptive
  advice Z30.09
  counseling Z30.09
  device (intrauterine) (in situ) Z97.5
    checking Z30.431
    complications—*see* Complications, intrauterine,
              contraceptive device
    in place Z97.5
    initial prescription Z30.014
      barrier Z30.018
      diaphragm Z30.018
      subdermal implantable Z30.017
      transdermal patch hormonal Z30.016
      vaginal ring hormonal Z30.015
    maintenance Z30.40
      barrier Z30.49
      diaphragm Z30.49
      subdermal implantable Z30.46
      transdermal patch hormonal Z30.45
      vaginal ring hormonal Z30.44
    reinsertion Z30.433
    removal Z30.432
    replacement Z30.433

Contraception, contraceptive, *continued*
  emergency (postcoital) Z30.012
  initial prescription Z30.019
    injectable Z30.013
    intrauterine device Z30.014
    pills Z30.011
    postcoital (emergency) Z30.012
    specified type NEC Z30.018
    subdermal implantable Z30.019
  maintenance Z30.40
    examination Z30.8
    injectable Z30.42
    intrauterine device Z30.431
    pills Z30.41
    specified type NEC Z30.49
    subdermal implantable Z30.46
    transdermal patch Z30.45
    vaginal ring Z30.44
  management Z30.9
    specified NEC Z30.8
  postcoital (emergency) Z30.012
  prescription Z30.019
    repeat Z30.40
  sterilization Z30.2
  surveillance (drug)—*see* Contraception, maintenance
Contraction (s), contracture, contracted
  Achilles tendon—*see also* Short, tendon, Achilles
    congenital Q66.89
  bladder N32.89
    neck or sphincter N32.0
  hourglass
    bladder N32.89
      congenital Q64.79
    gallbladder K82.0
      congenital Q44.1
    stomach K31.89
      congenital Q40.2
      psychogenic F45.8
  hysterical F44.4
  joint (abduction) (acquired) (adduction) (flexion) (rotation)
                  M24.50
    congenital NEC Q68.8
      hip Q65.89
    hip M24.55-
      congenital Q65.89
  muscle (postinfective) (postural) NEC M62.40
    with contracture of joint—*see* Contraction, joint
    congenital Q79.8
      sternocleidomastoid Q68.0
    hysterical F44.4
    posttraumatic—*see* Strabismus, paralytic
    psychogenic F45.8
      conversion reaction F44.4
    psychogenic F45.8
      conversion reaction F44.4
  premature
    atrium I49.1
    supraventricular I49.1
  pylorus NEC—*see also* Pylorospasm
    psychogenic F45.8
  sternocleidomastoid (muscle), congenital Q68.0
  stomach K31.89
    hourglass K31.89
      congenital Q40.2
      psychogenic F45.8
    psychogenic F45.8
  urethra—*see also* Stricture, urethra
    orifice N32.0
  vagina (outlet) N89.5
  vesical N32.89
    neck or urethral orifice N32.0
Contusion (skin surface intact) T14.8
  abdomen, abdominal (muscle) (wall) S30.1
  adnexa, eye NEC S05.8X-
  adrenal gland S37.812
  alveolar process S00.532
  ankle S90.0-
  antecubital space S50.1-
  anus S30.3
  arm (upper) S40.02-
    lower (with elbow) S50.1-
  auditory canal S00.43-
  auricle S00.43-

Contusion, *continued*
  axilla S40.02-
  back S20.22-
    lower S30.0
  bile duct S36.13
  bladder S37.22
  bone NEC T14.8
  brain (diffuse)—*see* Injury, intracranial, diffuse
    focal—*see* Injury, intracranial, focal
  brainstem S06.38-
  breast S20.0-
  broad ligament S37.892
  brow S00.83
  buttock S30.0
  canthus, eye S00.1-
  cauda equina S34.3
  cerebellar, traumatic S06.37-
  cerebral S06.33-
    left side S06.32-
    right side S06.31-
  cheek S00.83
    internal S00.532
  chest (wall)—*see* Contusion, thorax
  chin S00.83
  clitoris S30.23
  colon—*see* Injury, intestine, large, contusion
  common bile duct S36.13
  conjunctiva S05.1-
    with foreign body (in conjunctival sac)—*see* Foreign
                  body, conjunctival sac
  conus medullaris (spine) S34.139
  cornea S05.1-
    with foreign body—*see* Foreign body, cornea
  corpus cavernosum S30.21
  cortex (brain) (cerebral)—*see* Injury, intracranial, diffuse
    focal—*see* Injury, intracranial, focal
  costal region—*see* Contusion, thorax
  cystic duct S36.13
  diaphragm S27.802
  duodenum S36.420
  ear S00.43-
  elbow S50.0-
    with forearm S50.1-
  epididymis S30.22
  epigastric region S30.1
  epiglottis S10.0
  esophagus (thoracic) S27.812
    cervical S10.0
  eyeball S05.1-
  eyebrow S00.1-
  eyelid (and periocular area) S00.1-
  face NEC S00.83
  fallopian tube S37.529
    bilateral S37.522
    unilateral S37.521
  femoral triangle S30.1
  finger (s) S60.00
    with damage to nail (matrix) S60.10
    index S60.02-
      with damage to nail S60.12-
    little S60.05-
      with damage to nail S60.15-
    middle S60.03-
      with damage to nail S60.13-
    ring S60.04-
      with damage to nail S60.14-
    thumb—*see* Contusion, thumb
  flank S30.1
  foot (except toe(s) alone) S90.3-
    toe—*see* Contusion, toe
  forearm S50.1-
    elbow only S50.0-
  forehead S00.83
  gallbladder S36.122
  genital organs, external
    female S30.202
    male S30.201
  globe (eye) S05.1-
  groin S30.1
  gum S00.532
  hand S60.22-
    finger (s)—*see* Contusion, finger
    wrist S60.21-

Contusion, *continued*
head S00.93
ear S00.43-
eyelid S00.1-
lip S00.531
nose S00.33
oral cavity S00.532
scalp S00.03
specified part NEC S00.83
heel S90.3-
hepatic duct S36.13
hip S70.0-
ileum S36.428
iliac region S30.1
inguinal region S30.1
interscapular region S20.229
intra-abdominal organ S36.92
refer to specific organ under contusion
colon—*see* Injury, intestine, large, contusion
small intestine—*see* Injury, intestine, small, contusion
specified organ NEC S36.892
iris (eye) S05.1-
jaw S00.83
jejunum S36.428
kidney S37.01-
major (greater than 2 cm) S37.02-
minor (less than 2 cm) S37.01-
knee S80.0-
labium (majus) (minus) S30.23
lacrimal apparatus, gland or sac S05.8X-
larynx S10.0
leg (lower) S80.1-
knee S80.0-
lens S05.1-
lip S00.531
liver S36.112
lower back S30.0
lumbar region S30.0
lung S27.329
bilateral S27.322
unilateral S27.321
malar region S00.83
mastoid region S00.83
membrane, brain—*see* Injury, intracranial, diffuse
focal—*see* Injury, intracranial, focal
mesentery S36.892
mesosalpinx S37.892
mouth S00.532
muscle—*see* Contusion, by site
nail
finger—*see* Contusion, finger, with damage to nail
toe—*see* Contusion, toe, with damage to nail
nasal S00.33
neck S10.93
specified site NEC S10.83
throat S10.0
nerve—*see* Injury, nerve
newborn P54.5
nose S00.33
occipital
lobe (brain)—*see* Injury, intracranial, diffuse
focal—*see* Injury, intracranial, focal
region (scalp) S00.03
orbit (region) (tissues) S05.1-
ovary S37.429
bilateral S37.422
unilateral S37.421
palate S00.532
pancreas S36.229
body S36.221
head S36.220
tail S36.222
parietal
lobe (brain)—*see* Injury, intracranial, diffuse
focal—*see* Injury, intracranial, focal
region (scalp) S00.03
pelvic organ S37.92
adrenal gland S37.812
bladder S37.22
fallopian tube—*see* Contusion, fallopian tube
kidney—*see* Contusion, kidney
ovary—*see* Contusion, ovary
prostate S37.822

Contusion, *continued*
specified organ NEC S37.892
ureter S37.12
urethra S37.32
uterus S37.62
pelvis S30.0
penis S30.21
perineum
female S30.23
male S30.0
periocular area S00.1-
peritoneum S36.81
periurethral tissue S37.32
pharynx S10.0
pinna S00.43-
popliteal space S80.0-
prepuce S30.21
prostate S37.822
pubic region S30.1
pudendum
female S30.202
male S30.201
quadriceps femoris S70.1-
rectum S36.62
retroperitoneum S36.892
round ligament S37.892
sacral region S30.0
scalp S00.03
due to birth injury P12.3
scapular region S40.01-
sclera S05.1-
scrotum S30.22
seminal vesicle S37.892
shoulder S40.01-
skin NEC T14.8
small intestine—*see* Injury, intestine, small, contusion
spermatic cord S37.892
spinal cord—*see* Injury, spinal cord, by region
cauda equina S34.3
conus medullaris S34.139
spleen S36.029
major S36.021
minor S36.020
sternal region S20.219
stomach S36.32
subconjunctival S05.1-
subcutaneous NEC T14.8
submaxillary region S00.83
submental region S00.83
subperiosteal NEC T14.8
subungual
finger—*see* Contusion, finger, with damage to nail
toe—*see* Contusion, toe, with damage to nail
supraclavicular fossa S10.83
supraorbital S00.83
suprarenal gland S37.812
temple (region) S00.83
temporal
lobe (brain)—*see* Injury, intracranial, diffuse
focal—*see* Injury, intracranial, focal
region S00.83
testis S30.22
thigh S70.1-
thorax (wall) S20.20
back S20.22-
front S20.21-
throat S10.0
thumb S60.01-
with damage to nail S60.11-
toe (s) (lesser) S90.12-
with damage to nail S90.22-
great S90.11-
with damage to nail S90.21-
specified type NEC S90.221
tongue S00.532
trachea (cervical) S10.0
thoracic S27.52
tunica vaginalis S30.22
tympanum, tympanic membrane S00.43-
ureter S37.12
urethra S37.32
urinary organ NEC S37.892
uterus S37.62

Contusion, *continued*
uvula S00.532
vagina S30.23
vas deferens S37.892
vesical S37.22
vocal cord (s) S10.0
vulva S30.23
wrist S60.21-
Conversion hysteria, neurosis or reaction F44.9
Converter, tuberculosis (test reaction) R76.11
Convulsions (idiopathic) (*see also* Seizure (s)) R56.9
febrile R56.00
with status epilepticus G40.901
complex R56.01
with status epilepticus G40.901
simple R56.00
infantile P90
epilepsy—*see* Epilepsy
myoclonic G25.3
neonatal, benign (familial)—*see* Epilepsy, generalized,
idiopathic
newborn P90
post traumatic R56.1
recurrent R56.9
scarlatinal A38.8
Convulsive—*see also* Convulsions
Cooley's anemia D56.1
Copra itch B88.0
Creotoxism A05.9
Coprophagy F50.89
Cor
pulmonale (chronic) I27.81
triloculare Q20.8
biventriculare Q21.1
Corbus' disease (gangrenous balanitis) N48.1
Corn (infected) L84
Cornelia de Lange syndrome Q87.1
Cornual gestation or pregnancy O00.8-
Coryza (acute) J00
with grippe or influenza—*see* Influenza, with, respiratory
manifestations NEC
Costen's syndrome or complex M26.69
Costochondritis M94.0
Cot death R99
Cough (affected) (chronic) (epidemic) (nervous) R05
with hemorrhage—*see* Hemoptysis
bronchial R05
with grippe or influenza—*see* Influenza, with,
respiratory
manifestations NEC
functional F45.8
hysterical F45.8
laryngeal, spasmodic R05
psychogenic F45.8
Counseling (for) Z71.9
abuse NEC
perpetrator Z69.82
victim Z69.81
alcohol abuser Z71.41
family Z71.42
child abuse
non-parental
perpetrator Z69.021
victim Z69.020
parental
perpetrator Z69.011
victim Z69.010
contraceptive Z30.09
dietary Z71.3
drug abuser Z71.51
family member Z71.52
family Z71.89
for non-attending third party Z71.0
related to sexual behavior or orientation Z70.2
genetic NEC Z31.5
health (advice) (education) (instruction)—*see* Counseling,
medical
human immunodeficiency virus (HIV) Z71.7
insulin pump use Z46.81
medical (for) Z71.9
human immunodeficiency virus (HIV) Z71.7
on behalf of another Z71.0
specified reason NEC Z71.89

Counseling, *continued*
  natural family planning
    to avoid pregnancy Z30.02
  perpetrator (of)
    abuse NEC Z69.82
    child abuse
      non-parental Z69.021
      parental Z69.011
    rape NEC Z69.82
    spousal abuse Z69.12
  procreative NEC Z31.69
    using natural family planning Z31.61
  rape victim Z69.81
  specified reason NEC Z71.89
  spousal abuse (perpetrator) Z69.12
    victim Z69.11
  substance abuse Z71.89
    alcohol Z71.41
    drug Z71.51
    tobacco Z71.6
  tobacco use Z71.6
  use (of)
    insulin pump Z46.81
  victim (of)
    abuse Z69.81
    child abuse
      by parent Z69.010
      non-parental Z69.020
    rape NEC Z69.81
Coxsackie (virus) (infection) B34.1
  as cause of disease classified elsewhere B97.11
  enteritis A08.3
  meningitis (aseptic) A87.0
  pharyngitis B08.5
Crabs, meaning pubic lice B85.3
Crack baby P04.41
Cracked tooth K03.81
Cradle cap L21.0
Cramp (s) R25.2
  abdominal—*see* Pain, abdominal
  bathing T75.1
  colic R10.83
    psychogenic F45.8
  due to immersion T75.1
  fireman T67.2
  heat T67.2
  immersion T75.1
  intestinal—*see* Pain, abdominal
    psychogenic F45.8
  limb (lower) (upper)NEC R25.2
    sleep related G47.62
  muscle (limb) (general) R25.2
    due to immersion T75.1
    psychogenic F45.8
  salt-depletion E87.1
  stoker's T67.2
  swimmer's T75.1
Craniocleidodysostosis Q74.0
Craniofenestria (skull) Q75.8
Craniolacunia (skull) Q75.8
Cranioschisis Q75.8
Creotoxism A05.9
Crepitus
  caput Q75.8
  joint—*see* Derangement, joint, specified type NEC
Crib death R99
Cribriform hymen Q52.3
Cri-du-chat syndrome Q93.4
Crigler-Najjar disease or syndrome E80.5
Crisis
  abdomen R10.0
  acute reaction F43.0
  addisonian E27.2
  adrenal (cortical) E27.2
  celiac K90.0
  Dietl's N13.8
  emotional—*see also* Disorder, adjustment
    acute reaction to stress F43.0
    specific to childhood and adolescence F93.8
  oculogyric H51.8
    psychogenic F45.8
  psychosexual identity F64.2

Crisis, *continued*
  sickle-cell D57.00
    with
      acute chest syndrome D57.01
      splenic sequestration D57.02
  state (acute reaction) F43.0
Crocq's disease (acrocyanosis) I73.89
Crohn's disease— *see* Enteritis, regional
Crooked septum, nasal J34.2
Croup, croupous (catarrhal) (infectious) (inflammatory)
                        (nondiphtheritic) J05.0
  bronchial J20.9
Crush, crushed, crushing T14.8
  ankle S97.0-
  arm (upper) (and shoulder) S47.-
  finger (s) S67.1-
    with hand (and wrist) S67.2-
    index S67.19-
    little S67.19-
    middle S67.19-
    ring S67.19-
    thumb—*see* Crush, thumb
  foot S97.8-
    toe—*see* Crush, toe
  hand (except fingers alone) S67.2-
    with wrist S67.4-
  thumb S67.0-
    with hand (and wrist) S00.44-
  toe (s) S97.10-
    great S97.11-
    lesser S97.12-
  wrist S67.3-
    with hand S67.4-
Crusta lactea L21.0
Crying (constant) (continuous) (excessive)
  child, adolescent, or adult R45.83
  infant (baby) (newborn) R68.11
Cryptitis (anal) (rectal) K62.89
Cryptopapillitis (anus) K62.89
Cryptophthalmos Q11.2
  syndrome Q87.0
Cryptorchid, cryptorchism, cryptorchidism Q53.9
  bilateral Q53.20
    abdominal Q53.21
    perineal Q53.22
  unilateral Q53.10
    abdominal Q53.11
    perineal Q53.12
Cryptosporidiosis A07.2
  hepatobiliary B88.8
  respiratory B88.8
Cubitus
  congenital Q68.8
  valgus (acquired) M21.0-
    congenital Q68.8
  varus (acquired) M21.1-
    congenital Q68.8
Cultural deprivation or shock Z60.3
Curvature
  organ or site, congenital NEC—*see* Distortion
  penis (lateral) Q55.61
  Pott's (spinal) A18.01
  radius, idiopathic, progressive (congenital) Q74.0
  spine (acquired) (angular) (idiopathic) (incorrect)
                        (postural)— *see*
                        Dorsopathy, deforming
    congenital Q67.5
    due to or associated with
      osteitis
        deformans M88.88
        tuberculosis (Pott's curvature) A18.01
    tuberculous A18.01
Cushingoid due to steroid therapy E24.2
  correct substance properly administered—*see* Table of
                        Drugs and Chemicals,
                        by drug, adverse effect
  overdose or wrong substance given or taken—*see*
                        Table of Drugs and
                        Chemicals, by drug,
                        poisoning

Cushing's
  syndrome or disease E24.9
    drug-induced E24.2
    iatrogenic E24.2
    pituitary-dependent E24.0
    specified NEC E24.8
  ulcer—*see* Ulcer, peptic, acute
Cutaneous—*see also* condition
  hemorrhage R23.3
Cutis—*see also* condition
  hyperelastica Q82.8
  osteosis L94.2
  verticis gyrata Q82.8
    acquired L91.8
Cyanosis R23.0
  due to
    patent foramen botalli Q21.1
    persistent foramen ovale Q21.1
  enterogenous D74.8
Cyanotic heart disease I24.9
  congenital Q24.9
Cycle
  anovulatory N97.0
  menstrual, irregular N92.6
Cyclical vomiting (*see also* Vomiting, cyclical) G43.A0
  psychogenic F50.89
Cyclopia, cyclops Q87.0
Cyclopism Q87.0
Cynanche
  tonsillaris J36
Cyst (colloid) (mucous) (simple) (retention)
  adenoid (infected) J35.8
  antrum J34.1
  anus K62.89
  arachnoid, brain (acquired) G93.0
    congenital Q04.6
  Baker's M71.2-
    ruptured M66.0
  Bartholin's gland N75.0
  bone (local) NEC M85.60
    specified type NEC M85.60
      ankle M85.67-
      foot M85.67-
      forearm M85.63-
      hand M85.64-
      jaw M27.40
        developmental (nonodontogenic) K09.1
        odontogenic K09.0
      lower leg M85.66-
      multiple site M85.69
      neck M85.68
      rib M85.68
      shoulder M85.61-
      skull M85.68
      specified site NEC M85.68
      thigh M85.65-
      toe M85.67-
      upper arm M85.62-
      vertebra M85.68
  brain (acquired) G93.0
    congenital Q04.6
    third ventricle (colloid), congenital Q04.6
  canal of Nuck (female) N94.89
    congenital Q52.4
  canthus—*see* Cyst, conjunctiva
  choledochus, congenital Q44.4
  congenital NEC Q89.8
    kidney Q61.00
      more than one (multiple) Q61.02
        specified as polycystic Q61.3
          infantile type NEC Q61.19
            collecting duct dilation Q61.11
      solitary Q61.01
    prepuce Q55.69
    thymus (gland) Q89.2
  corpus
    albicans N83.29-
    luteum (hemorrhagic) (ruptured) N83.1-
  Dandy-Walker Q03.1
    with spina bifida—*see* Spina bifida

COUNSELING–CYST

Cyst, *continued*
  dental (root) K04.8
    developmental K09.0
    eruption K09.0
    primordial K09.0
  dentigerous (mandible) (maxilla) K09.0
  dermoid—*see* Neoplasm, benign, by site
    implantation
      vagina N89.8
  developmental K09.1
    odontogenic K09.0
  eruption K09.0
  ethmoid sinus J34.1
  eyelid (sebaceous) H02.829
    infected—*see* Hordeolum
    left H02.826
      lower H02.825
      upper H02.824
    right H02.823
      lower H02.822
      upper H02.821
  fallopian tube N83.8
    congenital Q50.4
  follicle (graafian) (hemorrhagic) N83.0-
  follicular (atretic) (hemorrhagic) (ovarian) N83.0-
    dentigerous K09.0
    odontogenic K09.0
  frontal sinus J34.1
  gingiva K09.0
  graafian follicle (hemorrhagic) N83.0-
  granulosal lutein (hemorrhagic) N83.1-
  hemangiomatous D18.00
    skin D18.01
    specified site NEC D18.09
  hydatid (*see also* Echinococcus) B67.90
    Morgagni
      male (epididymal) Q55.4
        testicular Q55.29
  hymen N89.8
    embryonic Q52.4
  implantation (dermoid)
    vagina N89.8
  jaw (bone) M27.40
    developmental (odontogenic) K09.0
  kidney (acquired) N28.1
    congenital Q61.00
    more than one (multiple) Q61.02
      specified as polycystic Q61.3
        infantile type (autosomal recessive) NEC Q61.19
          collecting duct dilation Q61.11
    simple N28.1
    solitary (single) Q61.01
      acquired N28.1
  lateral periodontal K09.0
  lip (gland) K13.0
  lutein N83.1-
  mandible M27.40
    dentigerous K09.0
  maxilla M27.40
    dentigerous K09.0
  Morgagni (hydatid)
    male (epididymal) Q55.4
      testicular Q55.29
  Müllerian duct Q50.4
    appendix testis Q55.29
    male Q55.29
  nose (turbinates) J34.1
    sinus J34.1
  odontogenic, developmental K09.0
  omentum (lesser) K66.8
    congenital Q45.8
  ovary, ovarian (twisted) N83.20-
    adherent N83.20-
    corpus
      albicans N83.29-
      luteum (hemorrhagic) N83.1-
    developmental Q50.1
    due to failure of involution NEC N83.20-
    follicular (graafian) (hemorrhagic) N83.0-
    hemorrhagic N83.20-

Cyst, *continued*
    retention N83.29-
    serous N83.20-
    specified NEC N83.29-
    theca lutein (hemorrhagic) N83.1-
  paramesonephric duct Q50.4
    male Q55.29
  paranephric N28.1
  paraphysis, cerebri, congenital Q04.6
  pericardial (congenital) Q24.8
    acquired (secondary) I31.8
  pericoronal K09.0
  periodontal K04.8
    lateral K09.0
  peripelvic (lymphatic) N28.1
  pilar L72.11
  pilonidal (infected) (rectum) L05.91
    with abscess L05.01
  porencephalic Q04.6
    acquired G93.0
  prepuce N47.4
    congenital Q55.69
  primordial (jaw) K09.0
  rectum (epithelium) (mucous) K62.89
  renal—*see* Cyst, kidney
  retention (ovary) N83.29-
  sebaceous (duct) (gland) L72.3
    breast—*see* Dysplasia, mammary, specified type NEC
    eyelid—*see* Cyst, eyelid
    genital organ NEC
      female N94.89
      male N50.89
    scrotum L72.3
  serous (ovary) N83.20-
  sinus (accessory) (nasal) J34.1
  skin L72.9
    sebaceous L72.3
  solitary
    bone—*see* Cyst, bone, solitary
    jaw M27.40
    kidney N28.1
  sphenoid sinus J34.1
  testis N44.2
    tunica albuginea N44.1
  theca lutein (ovary) N83.1-
  thyroglossal duct (infected) (persistent) Q89.2
  thyrolingual duct (infected) (persistent) Q89.2
  tonsil J35.8
  trichilemmal (proliferating) L72.12
  trichodermal L72.12
  turbinate (nose) J34.1
  vagina, vaginal (implantation) (inclusion) (squamous cell) (wall) N89.8
    embryonic Q52.4
Cystic—*see also* condition
  corpora lutea (hemorrhagic) N83.1-
  kidney (congenital) Q61.9
    infantile type NEC Q61.19
      collecting duct dilatation Q61.11
    medullary Q61.5
  ovary N83.20-
Cystitis (exudative) (hemorrhagic) (septic) (suppurative) N30.90
  acute N30.00
    with hematuria N30.01
    of trigone N30.00
      with hematuria N30.31
  blennorrhagic (gonococcal) A54.01
  chlamydial A56.01
  gonococcal A54.01
  trichomonal A59.03
Cystoma—*see also* Neoplasm, benign, by site
  simple (ovary) N83.29-
Cytomegalic inclusion disease
  congenital P35.1
Cytomegalovirus infection B25.9

D

Da Costa's syndrome F45.8
Dacryocystitis H04.30-
  neonatal P39.1
Dactylitis
  bone—*see* Osteomyelitis
  sickle-cell D57.00
    Hb C D57.219
    Hb SS D57.00
    specified NEC D57.819
  skin L08.9
  syphilitic A52.77
  tuberculous A18.03
Dactylosymphysis Q70.9
  fingers—*see* Syndactylism, complex, fingers
  toes—*see* Syndactylism, complex, toes
Damage
  brain (nontraumatic) G93.9
    anoxic, hypoxic G93.1
      child NEC G80.9
    due to birth injury P11.2
  cerebral NEC—*see* Damage, brain
  eye, birth injury P15.3
  vascular I99.9
Dandruff L21.0
Dandy-Walker syndrome Q03.1
  with spina bifida—*see* Spina bifida
Danlos' syndrome Q79.6
Darier (-White) disease (congenital) Q82.8
  meaning erythema annulare centrifugum L53.1
Darier-Roussy sarcoid D86.3
De la Tourette's syndrome F95.2
De Lange's syndrome Q87.1
De Morgan's spots (senile angiomas) I78.1
Dead
  fetus, retained (mother) O36.4
    early pregnancy O02.1
Deafmutism (acquired) (congenital) NEC H91.3
  hysterical F44.6
Deafness (acquired) (complete) (hereditary) (partial) H91.9-
  with blue sclera and fragility of bone Q78.0
  central—*see* Deafness, sensorineural
  conductive H90.2
    and sensorineural, mixed H90.8
      bilateral H90.6
    bilateral H90.0
    unilateral H90.1-
      with restrictive hearing on contralateral side H90.A-
  congenital H90.5
    with blue sclera and fragility of bone Q78.0
  due to toxic agents—*see* Deafness, ototoxic
  emotional (hysterical) F44.6
  functional (hysterical) F44.6
  high frequency H91.9-
  hysterical F44.6
  low frequency H91.9-
  mixed conductive and sensorineural H90.8
    bilateral H90.6
    unilateral H90.7-
  nerve—*see* Deafness, sensorineural
  neural—*see* Deafness, sensorineural
  psychogenic (hysterical) F44.6
  sensorineural H90.5
    and conductive, mixed H90.8
      bilateral H90.6
    bilateral H90.3
    unilateral H90.4-
  sensory—*see* Deafness, sensorineural
  word (developmental) H93.25
Death (cause unknown) (of) (unexplained) (unspecified cause) R99
  brain G93.82
  cardiac (sudden) (with successful resuscitation)—*code to* underlying disease
    family history of Z82.41
    personal history of Z86.74
  family member (assumed) Z63.4
Debility (chronic) (general) (nervous) R53.81
  congenital or neonatal NOS P96.9
  nervous R53.81

Débove's disease (splenomegaly) R16.1
Decalcification
  teeth K03.89
Decrease (d)
  absolute neutrophil count—*see* Neutropenia
  blood
    platelets—*see* Thrombocytopenia
    pressure R03.1
      due to shock following
        injury T79.4
        operation T81.19
  leukocytes D72.819
    specified NEC D72.818
  lymphocytes D72.810
  respiration, due to shock following injury T79.4
  tolerance
    fat K90.49
    glucose R73.09
    salt and water E87.8
  vision NEC H54.7
  white blood cell count D72.819
    specified NEC D72.818
Defect, defective Q89.9
  3-beta-hydroxysterioid dehydrogenase E25.0
  11-hydroxylase E25.0
  21-hydroxylase E25.0
  atrial septal (ostium secundum type) Q21.1
    ostium primum type Q21.2
  atrioventricular
    canal Q21.2
    septum Q21.2
  auricular septal Q21.1
  bilirubin excretion NEC E80.6
  bulbar septum Q21.0
  cell membrane receptor complex (CR3) D71
  circulation I99.9
    congenital Q28.9
    newborn Q28.9
  coagulation (factor) (*see also* Deficiency, factor) D68.9
    newborn, transient P61.6
  conduction (heart) I45.9
    bone—*see* Deafness, conductive
  coronary sinus Q21.1
  cushion, endocardial Q21.2
  diaphragm
    with elevation, eventration or hernia—*see* Hernia,
          diaphragm
    congenital Q79.1
      with hernia Q79.0
      gross (with hernia) Q79.0
  extensor retinaculum M62.89
  filling
    bladder R93.41
    kidney R93.42-
    renal pelvis R93.41
    ureter R93.41
    urinary organs, specified NEC R93.49
  Gerbode Q21.0
  interatrial septal Q21.1
  interauricular septal Q21.1
  interventricular septal Q21.0
    with dextroposition of aorta, pulmonary stenosis and
          hypertrophy of right
          ventricle Q21.3
    in tetralogy of Fallot Q21.3
  learning (specific)—*see* Disorder, learning
  obstructive, congenital
    ureter Q62.39
      orthotopic ureterocele Q62.31
  ostium
    primum Q21.2
    secundum Q21.1
  reduction
    limb Q73.8
      lower Q72.9-
        longitudinal
          femur Q72.4-
          fibula Q72.6-
          tibia Q72.5-
        specified type NEC Q72.89-
      upper Q71.9-
        longitudinal

Defect, defective, *continued*
        radius Q71.4-
        ulna Q71.5-
        specified type NEC Q71.89-
  respiratory system, congenital Q34.9
  septal (heart) NOS Q21.9
    atrial Q21.1
    ventricular (*see also* Defect, ventricular septal) Q21.0
  sinus venosus Q21.1
  speech R47.9
    developmental F80.9
    specified NEC R47.89
  vascular (local) I99.9
    congenital Q27.9
  ventricular septal Q21.0
    in tetralogy of Fallot Q21.3
  vision NEC H54.7
Defibrination (syndrome) D65
  newborn P60
Deficiency, deficient
  3-beta-hydroxysterioid dehydrogenase E25.0
  11-hydroxylase E25.0
  21-hydroxylase E25.0
  abdominal muscle syndrome Q79.4
  anti-hemophilic
    factor (A) D66
      B D67
    globulin (AHG) NEC D66
  attention (disorder) (syndrome) F98.8
    with hyperactivity—*see* Disorder, attention-deficit
          hyperactivity
  beta-glucuronidase E76.29
  calcium (dietary) E58
  carnitine E71.40
    due to
      hemodialysis E71.43
      inborn errors of metabolism E71.42
      Valproic acid therapy E71.43
    iatrogenic E71.43
    muscle palmityltransferase E71.314
    primary E71.41
    secondary E71.448
  cell membrane receptor complex (CR3) D71
  clotting (blood) (*see also* Deficiency, coagulation factor)
          D68.9
  coagulation NOS D68.9
  combined glucocorticoid and mineralocorticoid E27.49
  corticoadrenal E27.40
    primary E27.1
  dehydrogenase
    long chain/very long chain acyl CoA E71.310
    medium chain acyl CoA E71.311
    short chain acyl CoA E71.312
  diet E63.9
  disaccharidase E73.9
  edema—*see* Malnutrition, severe
  enzymes, circulating NEC E88.09
  factor—*see also* Deficiency, coagulation
    IX (congenital) (functional) (hereditary) (with functional
          defect) D67
    VIII (congenital) (functional) (hereditary) (with functional
          defect) D66
  fibrinogen (congenital) (hereditary) D68.2
    acquired D65
  gammaglobulin in blood D80.1
    hereditary D80.0
  glucocorticoid E27.49
    mineralocorticoid E27.49
  glucose-6-phosphate dehydrogenase anemia D55.0
  glucuronyl transferase E80.5
  hearing—*see* Deafness
  high grade F70
  hemoglobin D64.9
  immunity D84.9
    cell-mediated D84.8
      with thrombocytopenia and eczema D82.0
    combined D81.9
  lactase
    congenital E73.0
    secondary E73.1
  menadione (vitamin K) E56.1
    newborn P53
  mineralocorticoid E27.49

Deficiency, deficient, *continued*
    with glucocorticoid E27.49
  muscle
    carnitine (palmityltransferase) E71.314
    NADH diaphorase or reductase (congenital) D74.0
    NADH-methemoglobin reductase (congenital) D74.0
  natrium E87.1
  phosphoenolpyruvate carboxykinase E74.4
  protein (*see also* Malnutrition) E46
  pseudocholinesterase E88.09
  pyruvate
    carboxylase E74.4
    dehydrogenase E74.4
  salt E87.1
  secretion
    urine R34
  short stature homeobox gene (SHOX)
    with
      dyschondrosteosis Q78.8
      short stature (idiopathic) E34.3
      Turner's syndrome Q96.9
  sodium (Na) E87.1
  thrombokinase D68.2
    newborn P53
  vascular I99.9
  vitamin (multiple)NOS E56.9
    K E56.1
      of newborn P53
Deficit—*see also* Deficiency
  attention and concentration R41.840
    disorder—*see* Attention, deficit
  concentration R41.840
  oxygen R09.02
Deflection
  radius M21.83-
  septum (acquired) (nasal) (nose) J34.2
  spine—*see* Curvature, spine
  turbinate (nose) J34.2
Defluvium
  capillorum—*see* Alopecia
  unguium L60.8
Deformity Q89.9
  alimentary tract, congenital Q45.9
    upper Q40.9
  anus (acquired) K62.89
    congenital Q43.9
  aorta (arch) (congenital) Q25.40
  aortic
    cusp or valve (congenital) Q23.8
      acquired (*see also* Endocarditis, aortic) I35.8
  artery (congenital) (peripheral) NOS Q27.9
    umbilical Q27.0
  atrial septal Q21.1
  bile duct (common) (congenital) (hepatic) Q44.5
    acquired K83.8
  biliary duct or passage (congenital) Q44.5
    acquired K83.8
  bladder (neck) (trigone) (sphincter) (acquired) N32.89
    congenital Q64.79
  bone (acquired) NOS M95.9
    congenital Q79.9
  brain (congenital) Q04.9
    acquired G93.89
  bursa, congenital Q79.9
  cerebral, acquired G93.89
    congenital Q04.9
  cheek (acquired) M95.2
    congenital Q18.9
  chin (acquired) M95.2
    congenital Q18.9
  cystic duct (congenital) Q44.5
    acquired K82.8
  Dandy-Walker Q03.1
    with spina bifida—*see* Spina bifida
  diaphragm (congenital) Q79.1
    acquired J98.6
  digestive organ NOS Q45.9
  ductus arteriosus Q25.0
  ear (acquired)—*see also* Disorder, pinna, deformity
    congenital (external) Q17.9
  ectodermal (congenital) NEC Q84.9
  endocrine gland NEC Q89.2

Deformity, *continued*
eye, congenital Q15.9
face (acquired) M95.2
congenital Q18.9
flexion (joint) (acquired) (*see also* Deformity, limb, flexion) M21.20
congenital NOS Q74.9
hip Q65.89
foot (acquired)—*see also* Deformity, limb, lower leg
cavovarus (congenital) Q66.1
congenital NOS Q66.9
specified type NEC Q66.89
specified type NEC M21.6X-
valgus (congenital) Q66.6
acquired M21.07-
varus (congenital) NEC Q66.3
acquired M21.17-
forehead (acquired) M95.2
congenital Q75.8
frontal bone (acquired) M95.2
congenital Q75.8
gallbladder (congenital) Q44.1
acquired K82.8
gastrointestinal tract (congenital) NOS Q45.9
acquired K63.89
genitalia, genital organ (s) or system NEC
female (congenital) Q52.9
acquired N94.89
external Q52.70
male (congenital) Q55.9
acquired N50.89
head (acquired) M95.2
congenital Q75.8
heart (congenital) Q24.9
septum Q21.9
auricular Q21.1
ventricular Q21.0
hepatic duct (congenital) Q44.5
acquired K83.8
humerus (acquired) M21.82-
congenital Q74.0
hypophyseal (congenital) Q89.2
ilium (acquired) M95.5
congenital Q74.2
integument (congenital) Q84.9
ischium (acquired) M95.5
congenital Q74.2
ligament (acquired)—*see* Disorder, ligament
congenital Q79.9
limb (acquired) M21.90
congenital, except reduction deformity Q74.9
flat foot M21.4-
specified type NEC M21.80
lower leg M21.86-
lip (acquired) NEC K13.0
congenital Q38.0
liver (congenital) Q44.7
acquired K76.89
Madelung's (radius) Q74.0
meninges or membrane (congenital) Q07.9
cerebral Q04.8
metacarpus (acquired)—*see* Deformity, limb, forearm
congenital Q74.0
mitral (leaflets) (valve) I05.8
parachute Q23.2
stenosis, congenital Q23.2
mouth (acquired) K13.79
congenital Q38.6
multiple, congenital NEC Q89.7
muscle (acquired) M62.89
congenital Q79.9
sternocleidomastoid Q68.0
musculoskeletal system (acquired) M95.9
congenital Q79.9
nail (acquired) L60.8
congenital Q84.6
nasal—*see* Deformity, nose
neck (acquired) M95.3
congenital Q18.9
sternocleidomastoid Q68.0
nervous system (congenital) Q07.9
nose (acquired) (cartilage) M95.0

Deformity, *continued*
bone (turbinate) M95.0
congenital Q30.9
bent or squashed Q67.4
septum (acquired) J34.2
congenital Q30.8
parathyroid (gland) Q89.2
pelvis, pelvic (acquired) (bony) M95.5
congenital Q74.2
penis (glans) (congenital) Q55.69
acquired N48.89
pinna, acquired—*see also* Disorder, pinna, deformity
congenital Q17.9
pituitary (congenital) Q89.2
posture—*see* Dorsopathy, deforming
prepuce (congenital) Q55.69
acquired N47.8
rectum (congenital) Q43.9
acquired K62.89
respiratory system (congenital) Q34.9
rotation (joint) (acquired)—*see* Deformity, limb, specified site NEC
congenital Q74.9
hip M21.85-
congenital Q65.89
sacroiliac joint (congenital) Q74.2
acquired—*see* subcategory M43.8
septum, nasal (acquired) J34.2
shoulder (joint) (acquired) M21.92-
congenital Q74.0
skull (acquired) M95.2
congenital Q75.8
with
anencephaly Q00.0
encephalocele—*see* Encephalocele
hydrocephalus Q03.9
with spina bifida—*see* Spina bifida, by site, with hydrocephalus
microcephaly Q02
spinal—*see* Dorsopathy, deforming
nerve root (congenital) Q07.9
Sprengel's (congenital) Q74.0
sternocleidomastoid (muscle), congenital Q68.0
thymus (tissue) (congenital) Q89.2
thyroid (gland) (congenital) Q89.2
toe (acquired) M20.6-
congenital Q66.9
hallux valgus M20.1-
tricuspid (leaflets) (valve) I07.8
atresia or stenosis Q22.4
Ebstein's Q22.5
urachus (congenital) Q64.4
urinary tract (congenital) Q64.9
urachus Q64.4
vagina (acquired) N89.8
congenital Q52.4
valgus NEC M21.00
knee M21.06-
varus NEC M21.10
knee M21.16-
vesicourethral orifice (acquired) N32.89
congenital NEC Q64.79

Degeneration, degenerative
brain (cortical) (progressive) G31.9
childhood G31.9
specified NEC G31.89
cystic G31.89
congenital Q04.6
in
congenital hydrocephalus Q03.9
with spina bifida—*see also* Spina bifida
Hunter's syndrome E76.1
cerebrovascular I67.9
due to hypertension I67.4
cortical (cerebellar) (parenchymatous) G31.89
cutis L98.8
intervertebral disc NOS
sacrococcygeal region M53.3
kidney N28.89
amyloid E85.4 [N29]
cystic, congenital Q61.9
fatty N28.89

Degeneration, degenerative, *continued*
polycystic Q61.3
infantile type (autosomal recessive) NEC Q61.19
collecting duct dilatation Q61.11
muscle (fatty) (fibrous) (hyaline) (progressive) M62.89
heart—*see* Degeneration, myocardial
myocardial, myocardium (fatty) (hyaline) (senile) I51.5
with rheumatic fever (conditions in I00) I09.0
active, acute or subacute I01.2
with chorea I02.0
inactive or quiescent (with chorea) I09.0
nasal sinus (mucosa) J32.9
frontal J32.1
maxillary J32.0
nervous system G31.9
fatty G31.89
specified NEC G31.89
ovary N83.8
cystic N83.20-
microcystic N83.20-
pulmonary valve (heart) I37.8
sinus (cystic)—*see also* Sinusitis
polypoid J33.1
skin L98.8
colloid L98.8
spinal (cord) G31.89
familial NEC G31.89
fatty G31.89
tricuspid (heart) (valve) I07.9
turbinate J34.89
Deglutition
paralysis R13.0
hysterical F44.4
pneumonia J69.0
Dehiscence (of)
closure
laceration (internal) (external) T81.33
traumatic laceration (external) (internal) T81.33
traumatic injury wound repair T81.33
wound T81.30
traumatic repair T81.33
Dehydration E86.0
hypertonic E87.0
hypotonic E87.1
newborn P74.1
Delay, delayed
closure, ductus arteriosus (Botalli) P29.3
conduction (cardiac) (ventricular) I45.9
development R62.50
intellectual (specific) F81.9
language F80.9
due to hearing loss F80.4
learning F81.9
pervasive F84.9
physiological R62.50
specified stage NEC R62.0
reading F81.0
sexual E30.0
speech F80.9
due to hearing loss F80.4
spelling F81.81
gastric emptying K30
menarche E30.0
milestone R62.0
passage of meconium (newborn) P76.0
primary respiration P28.9
puberty (constitutional) E30.0
separation of umbilical cord P96.82
sexual maturation, female E30.0
vaccination Z28.9
Deletion(s)
autosome Q93.9
identified by fluorescence in situ hybridization (FISH) Q93.89
identified by in situ hybridization (ISH) Q93.89
chromosome
seen only at prometaphase Q93.89
short arm
5p Q93.4
22q11.2 Q93.81
specified NEC Q93.89
microdeletions NEC Q93.88

Delinquency (juvenile) (neurotic) F91.8
   group Z72.810
Delinquent immunization status Z28.3
Delirium, delirious (acute or subacute) (not alcohol- or
                       drug-induced) (with
                       dementia) R41.0
   exhaustion F43.0
Delivery (childbirth) (labor)
   cesarean (for)
      fetal-maternal hemorrhage O43.01-
      placental insufficiency O36.51-
      placental transfusion syndromes
         fetomaternal O43.01-
         fetus to fetus O43.02-
         maternofetal O43.01-
      pre-eclampsia O14.9-
         mild O14.0-
         moderate O14.0-
         severe
            with hemolysis, elevated liver enzymes and low
                  platelet count (HELLP)
                  O14.2-
   complicated O75.9
      by
         premature rupture, membranes (see also
            Pregnancy, complicated
            by, premature rupture
            of membranes) O42.90
   missed (at or near term) O36.4
Dementia (degenerative (primary)) (old age) (persisting)
                     F03.90
   in (due to)
      hypercalcemia E83.52 [F02.80]
         with behavioral disturbance E83.52 [F02.81]
      hypothyroidism, acquired E03.9 [F02.80]
         with behavioral disturbance E03.9 [F02.81]
         due to iodine deficiency E01.8 [F02.80]
            with behavioral disturbance E01.8 [F02.81]
Demodex folliculorum (infestation) B88.0
Dentia praecox K00.6
Dentigerous cyst K09.0
Dentin
   sensitive K03.89
Dentition (syndrome) K00.7
   delayed K00.6
   difficult K00.7
   precocious K00.6
   premature K00.6
   retarded K00.6
Dependence (on) (syndrome) F19.20
   with remission F19.21
   alcohol (ethyl) (methyl) (without remission) F10.20
      with
         amnestic disorder, persisting F10.26
         anxiety disorder F10.280
         dementia, persisting F10.27
         intoxication F10.229
           with delirium F10.221
           uncomplicated F10.220
         mood disorder F10.24
      counseling and surveillance Z71.41
   amphetamine (s) (type)—see Dependence, drug,
            stimulant NEC
   benzedrine—see Dependence, drug, stimulant NEC
   bhang—see Dependence, drug, cannabis
   caffeine—see Dependence, drug, stimulant NEC
   cannabis (sativa) (indica) (resin) (derivatives) (type)— see
            Dependence, drug,
            cannabis
   coca (leaf) (derivatives)—see Dependence, drug, cocaine
   cocaine—see Dependence, drug, cocaine
   combinations of drugs F19.20
   dagga—see Dependence, drug, cannabis
   dexamphetamine—see Dependence, drug, stimulant NEC
   dexedrine—see Dependence, drug, stimulant NEC
   dextro-nor-pseudo-ephedrine—see Dependence, drug,
            stimulant NEC
   diazepam—see Dependence, drug, sedative
   drug NEC F19.20
      cannabis F12.20
         with
           intoxication F12.229
             uncomplicated F12.220

Dependence, *continued*
     in remission F12.21
     cocaine F14.20
       with
          intoxication F14.229
            uncomplicated F14.220
          withdrawal F14.23
       in remission F14.21
       withdrawal symptoms in newborn P96.1
     counseling and surveillance Z71.51
     inhalant F18.20
       with
          intoxication F18.229
            uncomplicated F18.220
       in remission F18.21
     nicotine F17.200
       with disorder F17.209
         remission F17.201
         specified disorder NEC F17.208
         withdrawal F17.203
       chewing tobacco F17.220
         with disorder F17.229
           remission F17.221
           specified disorder NEC F17.228
           withdrawal F17.223
       cigarettes F17.210
         with disorder F17.219
           remission F17.211
           specified disorder NEC F17.218
       specified product NEC F17.290
         with disorder F17.299
           remission F17.291
           specified disorder NEC F17.298
           withdrawal F17.293
     psychoactive NEC F19.20
       with
          unspecified disorder F19.29
     stimulant NEC F15.20
       with
          intoxication F15.229
            uncomplicated F15.220
          withdrawal F15.23
       in remission F15.21
   ethyl
      alcohol (without remission) F10.20
         with remission F10.21
   ganja—see Dependence, drug, cannabis
   glue (airplane) (sniffing)—see Dependence, drug, inhalant
   hashish—see Dependence, drug, cannabis
   hemp—see Dependence, drug, cannabis
   Indian hemp—see Dependence, drug, cannabis
   inhalants—see Dependence, drug, inhalant
   maconha—see Dependence, drug, cannabis
   marihuana—see Dependence, drug, cannabis
   methyl
      alcohol (without remission) F10.20
         with remission F10.21
   nicotine—see Dependence, drug, nicotine
   on
      care provider (because of) Z74.9
         no other household member able to render care
            Z74.2
      renal dialysis (hemodialysis) (peritoneal) Z99.2
      respirator Z99.11
      ventilator Z99.11
      wheelchair Z99.3
   PCP (phencyclidine) (see also Abuse, drug, hallucinogen)
            F16.20
   phencyclidine (PCP) (and related substances) (see
            also Abuse, drug,
            hallucinogen) F16.20
   phenmetrazine—see Dependence, drug, stimulant NEC
   polysubstance F19.20
   psychostimulant NEC—see Dependence, drug, stimulant
            NEC
   specified drug NEC—see Dependence, drug
   stimulant NEC—see Dependence, drug, stimulant NEC
   substance NEC—see Dependence, drug
   tobacco—see Dependence, drug, nicotine
      counseling and surveillance Z71.6
   volatile solvents—see Dependence, drug, inhalant

Depletion
   extracellular fluid E86.9
   plasma E86.1
   salt or sodium E87.1
      causing heat exhaustion or prostration T67.4
      nephropathy N28.9
   volume NOS E86.9
Depolarization, premature I49.40
   atrial I49.1
   specified NEC I49.49
Deposit
   bone in Boeck's sarcoid D86.89
Depression (acute) (mental) F32.9
   anaclitic—see Disorder, adjustment
   anxiety F41.8
   atypical (single episode) F32.89
   central nervous system R09.2
   cerebral R29.818
      newborn P91.4
   major F32.9
   medullary G93.89
   psychogenic (reactive) (single episode) F32.9
   reactive (psychogenic) (single episode) F32.9
      psychotic (single episode) F32.3
   recurrent—see Disorder, depressive, recurrent
   respiratory center G93.89
   situational F43.21
   skull Q67.4
   specified NEC (single episode) F32.89
Deprivation
   cultural Z60.3
   emotional NEC Z65.8
      affecting infant or child—see Maltreatment, child,
            psychological
   social Z60.4
      affecting infant or child—see Maltreatment, child,
            psychological
De Quervain's
   syndrome E34.51
Derangement
   joint (internal) M24.9
      ankylosis—see Ankylosis
      temporomandibular M26.69
Dermatitis (eczematous) L30.9
   acarine B88.0
   ammonia L22
   arsenical (ingested) L27.8
   artefacta L98.1
      psychogenic F54
   atopic L20.9
      psychogenic F54
      specified NEC L20.89
   cercarial B65.3
   contact (occupational) L25.9
      allergic L23.9
         due to
           adhesives L23.1
           cement L24.5
           chemical products NEC L23.5
           chromium L23.0
           cosmetics L23.2
           dander (cat) (dog) L23.81
           drugs in contact with skin L23.3
           dyes L23.4
           food in contact with skin L23.6
           hair (cat) (dog) L23.81
           insecticide L23.5
           metals L23.0
           nickel L23.0
           plants, non-food L23.7
           plastic L23.5
           rubber L23.5
           specified agent NEC L23.89
      due to
         dander (cat) (dog) L23.81
         hair (cat) (dog) L23.81
   contusiformis L52
   diabetic—see E08-E13 with .620
   diaper L22

Dermatitis, *continued*
due to
adhesive (s) (allergic) (contact) (plaster) L23.1
alcohol (irritant) (skin contact) (substances in category T51) L24.2
taken internally L27.8
alkalis (contact) (irritant) L24.5
arsenic (ingested) L27.8
cereal (ingested) L27.2
chemical (s) NEC L25.3
taken internally L27.8
coffee (ingested) L27.2
cosmetics (contact) L25.0
allergic L23.2
dander (cat) (dog) L23.81
Demodex species B88.0
Dermanyssus gallinae B88.0
drugs and medicaments (generalized) (internal use) L27.0
in contact with skin L25.1
allergic L23.3
localized skin eruption L27.1
specified substance—*see* Table of Drugs and Chemicals
dyes (contact) L25.2
allergic L23.4
fish (ingested) L27.2
flour (ingested) L27.2
food (ingested) L27.2
in contact with skin L25.4
fruit (ingested) L27.2
furs (allergic) (contact) L23.81
hair (cat) (dog) L23.81
infrared rays L59.8
ingestion, ingested substance L27.9
chemical NEC L27.8
drugs and medicaments—*see* Dermatitis, due to, drugs
food L27.2
specified NEC L27.8
insecticide in contact with skin L24.5
internal agent L27.9
drugs and medicaments (generalized)—*see* Dermatitis, due to, drugs
food L27.2
irradiation—*see* Dermatitis, due to, radioactive substance
lacquer tree (allergic) (contact) L23.7
light (sun) NEC L57.8
acute L56.8
other L59.8
Lyponyssoides sanguineus B88.0
milk (ingested) L27.2
plants NEC (contact) L25.5
allergic L23.7
plasters (adhesive) (any) (allergic) (contact) L23.1
primrose (allergic) (contact) L23.7
primula (allergic) (contact) L23.7
radiation L59.8
nonionizing (chronic exposure) L57.8
sun NEC L57.8
acute L56.8
ragweed (allergic) (contact) L23.7
Rhus (allergic) (contact) (diversiloba) (radicans) (toxicodendron) (venenata) (verniciflua) L23.7
Senecio jacobaea (allergic) (contact) L23.7
specified agent NEC (contact) L25.8
allergic L23.89
sunshine NEC L57.8
acute L56.8
ultraviolet rays (sun NEC) (chronic exposure) L57.8
acute L56.8
vaccine or vaccination L27.0
specified substance—*see* Table of Drugs and Chemicals
dyshydrotic L30.1
dysmenorrheica N94.6
exfoliative, exfoliativa (generalized) L26
neonatorum L00
eyelid
due to
Demodex species B88.0

Dermatitis, *continued*
facta, factitia, factitial L98.1
psychogenic F54
flexural NEC L20.82
friction L30.4
gangrenosa, gangrenous infantum L08.0
harvest mite B88.0
irritant—*see* Dermatitis, contact, irritant
Jacquet's (diaper dermatitis) L22
Leptus B88.0
mite B88.0
napkin L22
purulent L08.0
pyococcal L08.0
pyogenica L08.0
Ritter's (exfoliativa) L00
schistosome B65.3
seborrheic L21.9
infantile L21.1
specified NEC L21.8
sensitization NOS L23.9
septic L08.0
suppurative L08.0
traumatic NEC L30.4
ultraviolet (sun) (chronic exposure) L57.8
acute L56.8
Dermatolysis (exfoliativa) (congenital) Q82.8
Dermatomegaly NEC Q82.8
Dermatomycosis B36.9
furfuracea B36.0
specified type NEC B36.8
Dermatomyositis (acute) (chronic)—*see also* Dermatopolymyositis
in (due to) neoplastic disease (*see also* Neoplasm) D49.9 [M36.0]
Dermatoneuritis of children—*see* Poisoning, mercury
Dermatophytosis (epidermophyton) (infection) (Microsporum) (tinea) (Trichophyton) B35.9
beard B35.0
body B35.4
capitis B35.0
corporis B35.4
deep-seated B35.8
disseminated B35.8
foot B35.3
granulomatous B35.8
groin B35.6
hand B35.2
nail B35.1
perianal (area) B35.6
scalp B35.0
specified NEC B35.8
Dermatopolymyositis M33.90
with
myopathy M33.92
respiratory involvement M33.91
specified organ involvement NEC M33.99
juvenile M33.00
with
myopathy M33.02
respiratory involvement M33.01
specified organ involvement NEC M33.09
Dermatopolyneuritis—*see* Poisoning, mercury
Dermatorrhexis Q79.6
acquired L57.4
Dermatosis L98.9
factitial L98.1
menstrual NEC L98.8
Dermophytosis—*see* Dermatophytosis
Despondency F32.9
Destruction, destructive—*see also* Damage
joint—*see also* Derangement, joint, specified type NEC
sacroiliac M53.3
rectal sphincter K62.89
septum (nasal) J34.89
Detergent asthma J69.8
Deterioration
general physical R53.81

Development
abnormal, bone Q79.9
arrested R62.50
bone—*see* Arrest, development or growth, bone
child R62.50
due to malnutrition E45
defective, congenital—*see also* Anomaly, by site
left ventricle Q24.8
in hypoplastic left heart syndrome Q23.4
delayed (*see also* Delay, development) R62.50
arithmetical skills F81.2
language (skills) (expressive) F80.1
learning skill F81.9
mixed skills F88
motor coordination F82
reading F81.0
specified learning skill NEC F81.89
speech F80.9
spelling F81.81
written expression F81.81
imperfect, congenital—*see also* Anomaly, by site
heart Q24.9
lungs Q33.6
incomplete
bronchial tree Q32.4
organ or site not listed—*see* Hypoplasia, by site
respiratory system Q34.9
sexual, precocious NEC E30.1
tardy, mental (*see also* Disability, intellectual) F79
Developmental—*see* condition
testing, infant or child—*see* Examination, child
Deviation (in)
midline (jaw) (teeth) (dental arch) M26.29
specified site NEC—*see* Malposition
nasal septum J34.2
congenital Q67.4
septum (nasal) (acquired) J34.2
congenital Q67.4
sexual F65.9
transvestism F64.1
teeth, midline M26.29
Device
cerebral ventricle (communicating) in situ Z98.2
drainage, cerebrospinal fluid, in situ Z98.2
Devil's
pinches (purpura simplex) D69.2
Dextraposition, aorta Q20.3
in tetralogy of Fallot Q21.3
Dextrocardia (true) Q24.0
with
complete transposition of viscera Q89.3
situs inversus Q89.3
Dextrotransposition, aorta Q20.3
Dhobi itch B35.6
Di George's syndrome D82.1
Diabetes, diabetic (mellitus) (sugar) E11.9
bronzed E83.110
dietary counseling and surveillance Z71.3
due to drug or chemical E09.9
with
amyotrophy E09.44
arthropathy NEC E09.618
autonomic (poly)neuropathy E09.43
cataract E09.36
Charcot's joints E09.610
chronic kidney disease E09.22
circulatory complication NEC E09.59
complication E09.8
specified NEC E09.69
dermatitis E09.620
foot ulcer E09.621
gangrene E09.52
gastroparesis E09.43
glomerulonephrosis, intracapillary E09.21
glomerulosclerosis, intercapillary E09.21
hyperglycemia E09.65
hyperosmolarity E09.00
with coma E09.01
hypoglycemia E09.649
with coma E09.641
ketoacidosis E09.10
with coma E09.11
kidney complications NEC E09.29

Diabetes, diabetic (mellitus) (sugar), *continued*
  Kimmelsteil-Wilson disease E09.21
  mononeuropathy E09.41
  myasthenia E09.44
  necrobiosis lipoidica E09.620
  nephropathy E09.21
  neuralgia E09.42
  neurologic complication NEC E09.49
  neuropathic arthropathy E09.610
  neuropathy E09.40
  ophthalmic complication NEC E09.39
  oral complication NEC E09.638
  periodontal disease E09.630
  peripheral angiopathy E09.51
    with gangrene E09.52
  polyneuropathy E09.42
  renal complication NEC E09.29
  renal tubular degeneration E09.29
  retinopathy E09.319
    with macular edema E09.311
    nonproliferative E09.329
      with macular edema E09.321
      mild E09.329
        with macular edema E09.321
      moderate E09.339
        with macular edema E09.331
      severe E09.349
        with macular edema E09.341
    proliferative E09.359
      with macular edema E09.351
  skin complication NEC E09.628
  skin ulcer NEC E09.622
due to underlying condition E08.9
  with
    amyotrophy E08.44
    arthropathy NEC E08.618
    autonomic (poly)neuropathy E08.43
    cataract E08.36
    Charcot's joints E08.610
    chronic kidney disease E08.22
    circulatory complication NEC E08.59
    complication E08.8
      specified NEC E08.69
    dermatitis E08.620
    foot ulcer E08.621
    gangrene E08.52
    gastroparesis E08.43
    glomerulonephrosis, intracapillary E08.21
    glomerulosclerosis, intercapillary E08.21
    hyperglycemia E08.65
    hyperosmolarity E08.00
      with coma E08.01
    hypoglycemia E08.649
      with coma E08.641
    ketoacidosis E08.10
      with coma E08.11
    kidney complications NEC E08.29
    Kimmelsteil-Wilson disease E08.21
    mononeuropathy E08.41
    myasthenia E08.44
    necrobiosis lipoidica E08.620
    nephropathy E08.21
    neuralgia E08.42
    neurologic complication NEC E08.49
    neuropathic arthropathy E08.610
    neuropathy E08.40
    ophthalmic complication NEC E08.39
    oral complication NEC E08.638
    periodontal disease E08.630
    peripheral angiopathy E08.51
      with gangrene E08.52
    polyneuropathy E08.42
    renal complication NEC E08.29
    renal tubular degeneration E08.29
    retinopathy E08.319
      with macular edema E08.311
      nonproliferative E08.329
        with macular edema E08.321
        mild E08.329
          with macular edema E08.321
        moderate E08.339
          with macular edema E08.331

Diabetes, diabetic (mellitus) (sugar), *continued*
    severe E08.349
      with macular edema E08.341
    proliferative E08.359
      with macular edema E08.351
  skin complication NEC E08.628
  skin ulcer NEC E08.622
gestational (in pregnancy) O24.419
  affecting newborn P70.0
  diet controlled O24.410
  insulin (and diet)controlled O24.414
  oral hypoglycemic drug controlled O24.415
inadequately controlled—*code to* Diabetes, by type, with
                                    hyperglycemia
insulin dependent—*code to* type of diabetes
juvenile-onset—*see* Diabetes, type 1
ketosis-prone—*see* Diabetes, type 1
latent R73.09
neonatal (transient) P70.2
non-insulin dependent—*code to* type of diabetes
out of control—*code to* Diabetes, by type, with
                          hyperglycemia
poorly controlled—*code to* Diabetes, by type, with
                             hyperglycemia
postpancreatectomy—*see* Diabetes, specified type NEC
postprocedural—*see* Diabetes, specified type NEC
prediabetes R73.03
secondary diabetes mellitus NEC—*see* Diabetes, specified
                                    type NEC
steroid-induced—*see* Diabetes, due to, drug or chemical
type 1 E10.9
  with
    amyotrophy E10.44
    arthropathy NEC E10.618
    autonomic (poly)neuropathy E10.43
    cataract E10.36
    Charcot's joints E10.610
    chronic kidney disease E10.22
    circulatory complication NEC E10.59
    complication E10.8
      specified NEC E10.69
    dermatitis E10.620
    foot ulcer E10.621
    gangrene E10.52
    gastroparesis E10.43
    glomerulonephrosis, intracapillary E10.21
    glomerulosclerosis, intercapillary E10.21
    hyperglycemia E10.65
    hypoglycemia E10.649
      with coma E10.641
    ketoacidosis E10.10
      with coma E10.11
    kidney complications NEC E10.29
    Kimmelsteil-Wilson disease E10.21
    mononeuropathy E10.41
    myasthenia E10.44
    necrobiosis lipoidica E10.620
    nephropathy E10.21
    neuralgia E10.42
    neurologic complication NEC E10.49
    neuropathic arthropathy E10.610
    neuropathy E10.40
    ophthalmic complication NEC E10.39
    oral complication NEC E10.638
    periodontal disease E10.630
    peripheral angiopathy E10.51
      with gangrene E10.52
    polyneuropathy E10.42
    renal complication NEC E10.29
    renal tubular degeneration E10.29
    retinopathy E10.319
      with macular edema E10.311
      nonproliferative E10.329
        with macular edema E10.321
        mild E10.329
          with macular edema E10.321
        moderate E10.339
          with macular edema E10.331
        severe E10.349
          with macular edema E10.341
      proliferative E10.359
        with macular edema E10.351

Diabetes, diabetic (mellitus) (sugar), *continued*
    skin complication NEC E10.628
    skin ulcer NEC E10.622
  type 2 E11.9
    with
      amyotrophy E11.44
      arthropathy NEC E11.618
      autonomic (poly)neuropathy E11.43
      cataract E11.36
      Charcot's joints E11.610
      chronic kidney disease E11.22
      circulatory complication NEC E11.59
      complication E11.8
        specified NEC E11.69
      dermatitis E11.620
      foot ulcer E11.621
      gangrene E11.52
      gastroparesis E11.43
      glomerulonephrosis, intracapillary E11.21
      glomerulosclerosis, intercapillary E11.21
      hyperglycemia E11.65
      hyperosmolarity E11.00
        with coma E11.01
      hypoglycemia E11.649
        with coma E11.641
      kidney complications NEC E11.29
      Kimmelsteil-Wilson disease E11.21
      mononeuropathy E11.41
      myasthenia E11.44
      necrobiosis lipoidica E11.620
      nephropathy E11.21
      neuralgia E11.42
      neurologic complication NEC E11.49
      neuropathic arthropathy E11.610
      neuropathy E11.40
      ophthalmic complication NEC E11.39
      oral complication NEC E11.638
      periodontal disease E11.630
      peripheral angiopathy E11.51
        with gangrene E11.52
      polyneuropathy E11.42
      renal complication NEC E11.29
      renal tubular degeneration E11.29
      retinopathy E11.319
        with macular edema E11.311
        nonproliferative E11.329
          with macular edema E11.321
          mild E11.329
            with macular edema E11.321
          moderate E11.339
            with macular edema E11.331
          severe E11.349
            with macular edema E11.341
        proliferative E11.359
          with macular edema E11.351
      skin complication NEC E11.628
      skin ulcer NEC E11.622
Diagnosis deferred R69
Dialysis (intermittent) (treatment)
  noncompliance (with) Z91.15
  renal (hemodialysis) (peritoneal), status Z99.2
Diamond-Blackfan anemia (congenital hypoplastic) D61.01
Diamond-Gardener syndrome (autoerythrocyte
                                  sensitization) D69.2
Diaper rash L22
Diaphoresis (excessive) R61
Diaphragmatitis, diaphragmitis J98.6
Diarrhea, diarrheal (disease) (infantile) (inflammatory) R19.7
  allergic K52.29
  amebic (*see also* Amebiasis) A06.0
    acute A06.0
  cachectic NEC K52.89
  chronic (noninfectious) K52.9
  dietetic K52.29
  due to
    Campylobacter A04.5
    Escherichia coli A04.4
      enteroaggregative A04.4
      enterohemorrhagic A04.3
      enteropathogenic A04.0
      enterotoxigenic A04.1
      specified NEC A04.4
    food hypersensitivity K52.29

Diarrhea, *continued*
    specified organism NEC A08.8
        bacterial A04.8
        viral A08.39
    dysenteric A09
    endemic A09
    epidemic A09
    functional K59.1
        following gastrointestinal surgery K91.89
        psychogenic F45.8
    Giardia lamblia A07.1
    giardial A07.1
    infectious A09
    mite B88.0
    nervous F45.8
    noninfectious K52.9
    psychogenic F45.8
    specified
        bacterial A04.8
        virus NEC A08.39

Diastasis
    cranial bones M84.88
        congenital NEC Q75.8
    joint (traumatic)—*see* Dislocation

Diathesis
    hemorrhagic (familial) D69.9
        newborn NEC P53

Didymytis N45.1
    with orchitis N45.3

Dietary
    surveillance and counseling Z71.3

Dietl's crisis N13.8

Difficult, difficulty (in)
    acculturation Z60.3
    feeding R63.3
        newborn P92.9
            breast P92.5
            specified NEC P92.8
        nonorganic (infant or child) F98.29
    reading (developmental) F81.0
        secondary to emotional disorders F93.9
    spelling (specific) F81.81
        with reading disorder F81.89
        due to inadequate teaching Z55.8
    swallowing—*see* Dysphagia
    walking R26.2

DiGeorge's syndrome (thymic hypoplasia) D82.1

Dilatation
    aorta (congenital) Q25.44
    bladder (sphincter) N32.89
        congenital Q64.79
    colon K59.39
        congenital Q43.1
        psychogenic F45.8
        toxic K59.31
    common duct (acquired) K83.8
        congenital Q44.5
    cystic duct (acquired) K82.8
        congenital Q44.5
    ileum K59.8
        psychogenic F45.8
    jejunum K59.8
        psychogenic F45.8
    Meckel's diverticulum (congenital) Q43.0
    rectum K59.39
    sphincter ani K62.89
    stomach K31.89
        acute K31.0
        psychogenic F45.8
    vesical orifice N32.89

Dilated, dilation—*see* Dilatation

Diminished, diminution
    hearing (acuity)—*see* Deafness
    sense or sensation (cold) (heat) (tactile) (vibratory) R20.8
    vision NEC H54.7

Dimitri-Sturge-Weber disease Q85.8

Dimple
    congenital, sacral Q82.6
        parasacral Q82.6
    parasacral, pilonidal or postanal—*see* Cyst, pilonidal

Diphallus Q55.69

Diplegia (upper limbs) G83.0
    lower limbs G82.20

Dipsomania F10.20
    with
        psychosis—*see* Psychosis, alcoholic
        remission F10.21

Dirt-eating child F98.3

Disability, disabilities
    intellectual F79
        with
            autistic features F84.9
        mild (I.Q.50–69) F70
        moderate (I.Q.35–49) F71
        profound (I.Q. under 20) F73
        severe (I.Q.20–34) F72
        specified level NEC F78
    knowledge acquisition F81.9
    learning F81.9
    limiting activities Z73.6
    spelling, specific F81.81

Disappearance of family member Z63.4

Discharge (from)
    abnormal finding in—*see* Abnormal, specimen
    breast (female) (male) N64.52
    diencephalic autonomic idiopathic—*see* Epilepsy,
                        specified NEC
    ear—*see also* Otorrhea
        blood—*see* Otorrhagia
    excessive urine R35.8
    nipple N64.52
    penile R36.9
    postnasal R09.82
    prison, anxiety concerning Z65.2
    urethral R36.9
        without blood R36.0
    vaginal N89.8

Discoloration
    nails L60.8

Discord (with)
    family Z63.8

Discordant connection
    ventriculoarterial Q20.3

Discrepancy
    leg length (acquired)—*see* Deformity, limb, unequal length
        congenital—*see* Defect, reduction, lower limb

Disease, diseased—*see also* Syndrome
    acid-peptic K30
    Adams-Stokes (-Morgagni) (syncope with heart block)
                        I45.9
    adenoids (and tonsils) J35.9
    airway
        reactive—*see* Asthma
    angiospastic I73.9
        cerebral G45.9
    anus K62.9
        specified NEC K62.89
    aortic (heart) (valve) I35.9
        rheumatic I06.9
    Ayerza's (pulmonary artery sclerosis with pulmonary
            hypertension) I27.0
    Babington's (familial hemorrhagic telangiectasia) I78.0
    Baelz's (cheilitis glandularis apostematosa) K13.0
    Bannister's T78.3
    Bateman's B08.1
    Becker
        myotonia congenita G71.12
    bladder N32.9
        specified NEC N32.89
    bleeder's D66
    blood D75.9
        vessel I99.9
    Bouillaud's (rheumatic heart disease) I01.9
    Bourneville (-Brissaud) (tuberous sclerosis) Q85.1
    bowel K63.9
        functional K59.9
            psychogenic F45.8
    brain G93.9
        parasitic NEC B71.9 *[G94]*
        specified NEC G93.89
    broad
        beta E78.2
    bronze Addison's E27.1
    cardiopulmonary, chronic I27.9
    cardiovascular (atherosclerotic) I25.10
    celiac (adult) (infantile) K90.0

Disease, diseased, *continued*
    chigo, chigoe B88.1
    childhood granulomatous D71
    chlamydial A74.9
        specified NEC A74.89
    collagen NOS (nonvascular) (vascular) M35.9
        specified NEC M35.8
    colon K63.9
        functional K59.9
            congenital Q43.2
    Concato's (pericardial polyserositis) A19.9
        nontubercular I31.1
        pleural—*see* Pleurisy, with effusion
    conjunctiva H11.9
        chlamydial A74.0
        viral B30.9
    connective tissue, systemic (diffuse) M35.9
        in (due to)
            hypogammaglobulinemia D80.1 *[M36.8]*
        specified NEC M35.8
    Crocq's (acrocyanosis) I73.89
    cystic
        kidney, congenital Q61.9
    cytomegalic inclusion (generalized) B25.9
        congenital P35.1
    cytomegaloviral B25.9
    Débove's (splenomegaly) R16.1
    diaphorase deficiency D74.0
    diaphragm J98.6
    diarrheal, infectious NEC A09
    disruptive F91.9
        mood dysregulation F34.81
        specified NEC F91.8
    disruptive behavior F91.9
    Duchenne-Griesinger G71.0
    Duchenne's
        muscular dystrophy G71.0
        pseudohypertrophy, muscles G71.0
    Dupré's (meningism) R29.1
    dysmorphic body F45.22
    Eddowes' (brittle bones and blue sclera) Q78.0
    Edsall's T67.2
    Eichstedt's (pityriasis versicolor) B36.0
    end stage renal (ESRD) N18.6
    English (rickets) E55.0
    Erb (-Landouzy) G71.0
    esophagus K22.9
        functional K22.4
        psychogenic F45.8
    eustachian tube—*see* Disorder, eustachian tube
    external
        auditory canal—*see* Disorder, ear, external
        ear—*see* Disorder, ear, external
    facial nerve (seventh) G51.9
        newborn (birth injury) P11.3
    Fanconi's (congenital pancytopenia) D61.09
    fascia NEC—*see also* Disorder, muscle
        inflammatory—*see* Myositis
        specified NEC M62.89
    Fede's K14.0
    female pelvic inflammatory (*see also* Disease, pelvis,
                 inflammatory) N73.9
    fifth B08.3
    Fothergill's
        scarlatina anginosa A38.9
    Friedreich's
        combined systemic or ataxia G11.1
        myoclonia G25.3
    frontal sinus—*see* Sinusitis, frontal
    fungus NEC B49
    Gaisböck's (polycythemia hypertonica) D75.1
    gastroesophageal reflux (GERD) K21.9
        with esophagitis K21.0
    gastrointestinal (tract) K92.9
        functional K59.9
            psychogenic F45.8
        specified NEC K92.89
    Gee (-Herter) (-Heubner) (-Thaysen) (nontropical sprue)
                 K90.0
    genital organs
        female N94.9
        male N50.9

Disease, diseased, *continued*
Gibert's (pityriasis rosea) L42
Gilles de la Tourette's (motor-verbal tic) F95.2
Goldstein's (familial hemorrhagic telangiectasia) I78.0
graft-versus-host (GVH) D89.813
   acute D89.810
   acute on chronic D89.812
   chronic D89.811
granulomatous (childhood) (chronic) D71
Grisel's M43.6
Gruby's (tinea tonsurans) B35.0
Guinon's (motor-verbal tic) F95.2
hair (color) (shaft) L67.9
   follicles L73.9
      specified NEC L73.8
Hamman's (spontaneous mediastinal emphysema) J98.2
hand, foot, and mouth B08.4
heart (organic) I51.9
   with
      pulmonary edema (acute) (*see also* Failure,
               ventricular, left) I50.1
      rheumatic fever (conditions in I00)
         active I01.9
            with chorea I02.0
            specified NEC I01.8
         inactive or quiescent (with chorea) I09.9
            specified NEC I09.89
   aortic (valve) I35.9
   black I27.0
   congenital Q24.9
      cyanotic Q24.9
      specified NEC Q24.8
   fibroid—*see* Myocarditis
   functional I51.89
      psychogenic F45.8
   hyperthyroid (*see also* Hyperthyroidism) E05.90 [I43]
      with thyroid storm E05.91 [I43]
   kyphoscoliotic I27.1
   mitral I05.9
      specified NEC I0
   psychogenic (functional) F45.8
   pulmonary (chronic) I27.9
      in schistosomiasis B65.9 *[I52]*
      specified NEC I27.89
   rheumatic (chronic) (inactive) (old) (quiescent) (with
               chorea) I09.9
      active or acute I01.9
         with chorea (acute) (rheumatic) (Sydenham's)
               I02.0
   thyrotoxic (*see also* Thyrotoxicosis) E05.90 [I43]
      with thyroid storm E05.91 [I43]
Hebra's
   pityriasis
      maculata et circinata L42
hemoglobin or Hb
   abnormal (mixed) NEC D58.2
      with thalassemia D56.9
   AS genotype D57.3
   Bart's D56.0
   C (Hb-C) D58.2
      with other abnormal hemoglobin NEC D58.2
      elliptocytosis D58.1
      Hb-S D57.2-
      sickle-cell D57.2-
      thalassemia D56.8
   Constant Spring D58.2
   D (Hb-D) D58.2
   E (Hb-E) D58.2
   E-beta thalassemia D56.5
   elliptocytosis D58.1
   H (Hb-H) (thalassemia) D56.0
      with other abnormal hemoglobin NEC D56.9
      Constant Spring D56.0
   I thalassemia D56.9
   M D74.0
   S or SS D57.1
   SC D57.2-
   SD D57.8-
   SE D57.8-
   spherocytosis D58.0
   unstable, hemolytic D58.2

Disease, diseased, *continued*
hemolytic (newborn) P55.9
   due to or with
      incompatibility
         ABO (blood group) P55.1
hemorrhagic D69.9
   newborn P53
Henoch (-Schönlein) (purpura nervosa) D69.0
hepatic—*see* Disease, liver
Herter (-Gee) (-Heubner) (nontropical sprue) K90.0
Heubner-Herter (nontropical sprue) K90.0
high fetal gene or hemoglobin thalassemia D56.9
hip (joint) M25.9
   congenital Q65.89
   suppurative M00.9
host-versus-graft D89.813
   acute D89.810
   acute on chronic D89.812
   chronic D89.811
human immunodeficiency virus (HIV) B20
hyaline (diffuse) (generalized)
   membrane (lung) (newborn) P22.0
immune D89.9
inclusion B25.9
   salivary gland B25.9
infectious, infective B99.9
   congenital P37.9
      specified NEC P37.8
      viral P35.9
         specified type NEC P35.8
   specified NEC B99.8
inflammatory
   prepuce
      balanoposthitis N47.6
intestine K63.9
   functional K59.9
      psychogenic F45.8
      specified NEC K59.8
jigger B88.1
joint—*see also* Disorder, joint
   sacroiliac M53.3
Jourdain's (acute gingivitis) K05.00
   plaque induced K05.00
kidney (functional) (pelvis) N28.9
   chronic N18.9
      hypertensive—*see* Hypertension, kidney
      stage 1 N18.1
      stage 2 (mild) N18.2
      stage 3 (moderate) N18.3
      stage 4 (severe) N18.4
      stage 5 N18.5
   cystic (congenital) Q61.9
   in (due to)
      multicystic Q61.4
      polycystic Q61.3
         childhood type NEC Q61.19
            collecting duct dilatation Q61.11
Kimmelstiel (-Wilson) (intercapillary polycystic (congenital)
               glomerulosclerosis)—
               see E08-E13 with .21
kissing—*see* Mononucleosis, infectious
Kok Q89.8
Kostmann's (infantile genetic agranulocytosis) D70.0
Lenegre's I44.2
Lev's (acquired complete heart block) I44.2
lip K13.0
Lobstein's (brittle bones and blue sclera) Q78.0
Ludwig's (submaxillary cellulitis) K12.2
lung J98.4
   in
      sarcoidosis D86.0
      systemic
         lupus erythematosus M32.13
      interstitial J84.9
         of childhood, specified NEC J84.848
         specified NEC J84.89
Lutembacher's (atrial septal defect with mitral stenosis)
               Q21.1
Lyme A69.20
lymphoproliferative D47.9
   specified NEC D47.Z9
   T-gamma D47.Z9

Disease, diseased, *continued*
maple-syrup-urine E71.0
Marion's (bladder neck obstruction) N32.0
medullary center (idiopathic) (respiratory) G93.89
metabolic, metabolism E88.9
   bilirubin E80.7
Minot's (hemorrhagic disease, newborn) P53
mitral (valve) I05.9
Morgagni-Adams-Stokes (syncope with heart block) I45.9
Morvan's G60.8
muscle M62.9
   specified type NEC M62.89
   tone, newborn P94.9
      specified NEC P94.8
myocardium, myocardial (*see also* Degeneration,
               myocardial) I51.5
   primary (idiopathic) I42.9
myoneural G70.9
nails L60.9
   specified NEC L60.8
nasal J34.9
neuromuscular system G70.9
neutropenic D70.9
nerve—*see* Disorder, nerve
nervous system G98.8
   congenital Q07.9
nose J34.9
Osler-Rendu (familial hemorrhagic telangiectasia) I78.0
ovary (noninflammatory) N83.9
   cystic N83.20-
   inflammatory—*see* Salpingo-oophoritis
   polycystic E28.2
   specified NEC N83.8
pancreas K86.9
   cystic K86.2
   fibrocystic E84.9
   specified NEC K86.8
parasitic B89
   cerebral NEC B71.9 *[G94]*
   intestinal NOS B82.9
   mouth B37.0
   skin NOS B88.9
   specified type—see Infestation
   tongue B37.0
pelvis, pelvic
   gonococcal (acute) (chronic) A54.24
   inflammatory (female) N73.9
      acute N73.0
      chronic N73.1
      specified NEC N73.8
Pick's I31.1
pinworm B80
Pollitzer's (hidradenitis suppurativa) L73.2
polycystic
   kidney or renal Q61.3
      childhood type NEC Q61.19
         collecting duct dilatation Q61.11
   ovary, ovaries E28.2
prepuce N47.8
   inflammatory N47.7
      balanoposthitis N47.6
Pringle's (tuberous sclerosis) Q85.1
Puente's (simple glandular cheilitis) K13.0
pulmonary—*see also* Disease, lung
   heart I27.9
      specified NEC I27.89
   hypertensive (vascular) I27.0
   valve I37.9
      rheumatic I09.89
rag picker's or rag sorter's A22.1
rectum K62.9
   specified NEC K62.89
renal (functional) (pelvis) (*see also* Disease, kidney) N28.9
   with
      edema—*see* Nephrosis
      glomerular lesion—*see* Glomerulonephritis
         with edema—*see* Nephrosis
      interstitial nephritis N12
   acute N28.9
   chronic (*see also* Disease, kidney, chronic) N18.9
   cystic, congenital Q61.9
   diabetic—*see* E08-E13 with .22
   end-stage (failure) N18.6

DISEASE, DISEASED—DISORDER

DISORDER-DISORDER

Disorder, *continued*
  amino-acid
    homocystinuria E72.11
    metabolism—*see* Disturbance, metabolism, amino-
          acid
      specified NEC E72.8
    neonatal, transitory P74.8
  anxiety F41.9
    illness F45.21
    mixed
      with depression (mild) F41.8
    phobic F40.9
      of childhood F40.8
    specified NEC F41.8
  attention-deficit hyperactivity (adolescent) (adult) (child)
          F90.9
    combined type F90.2
    hyperactive type F90.1
    inattentive type F90.0
    specified type NEC F90.8
  attention-deficit without hyperactivity (adolescent) (adult)
          (child) F90.0
  auditory processing (central) H93.25
  autistic F84.0
  balance
    acid-base E87.8
      mixed E87.4
    electrolyte E87.8
    fluid NEC E87.8
  beta-amino-acid metabolism E72.8
  bilirubin excretion E80.6
  binge-eating F50.81
  bladder N32.9
    specified NEC N32.89
  bleeding D68.9
  body dysmorphic F45.22
  Briquet's F45.0
  cannabis use
    due to drug abuse—*see* Abuse, drug, cannabis
    due to drug dependence—*see* Dependence, drug,
          cannabis
  carnitine metabolism E71.40
  central auditory processing H93.25
  character NOS F60.9
  coagulation (factor) (*see also* Defect, coagulation) D68.9
    newborn, transient P61.6
  coccyx NEC M53.3
  conduct (childhood) F91.9
    adjustment reaction—*see* Disorder, adjustment
    adolescent onset type F91.2
    childhood onset type F91.1
    depressive F91.8
    group type F91.2
    hyperkinetic—*see* Disorder, attention-deficit
          hyperactivity
    oppositional defiance F91.3
    socialized F91.2
    solitary aggressive type F91.1
    specified NEC F91.8
    unsocialized (aggressive) F91.1
  conduction, heart I45.9
  cornea H18.9
    deformity—*see* Deformity, cornea
    degeneration—*see* Degeneration, cornea
    due to contact lens H18.82-
  defiant oppositional F91.3
  depressive F32.9
    major F32.9
      with psychotic symptoms F32.3
      in remission (full) F32.5
        partial F32.4
      recurrent F33.9
      single episode F32.9
        mild F32.0
        moderate F32.1
        severe (without psychotic symptoms) F32.2
          with psychotic symptoms F32.3
  developmental F89
    arithmetical skills F81.2
    coordination (motor) F82
    expressive writing F81.81
    language F80.9
      expressive F80.1

Disorder, *continued*
  language F80.9
    expressive F80.1
    mixed receptive and expressive F80.2
    receptive type F80.2
    specified NEC F80.89
  learning F81.9
    arithmetical F81.2
    reading F81.0
  mixed F88
  motor coordination or function F82
  pervasive F84.9
    specified NEC F84.8
  phonological F80.0
  reading F81.0
  scholastic skills—*see also* Disorder, learning
    mixed F81.89
  specified NEC F88
  speech F80.9
    articulation F80.0
    specified NEC F80.89
  written expression F81.81
  diaphragm J98.6
  digestive (system) K92.9
    newborn P78.9
      specified NEC P78.89
    postprocedural—*see* Complication, gastrointestinal
    psychogenic F45.8
  disc (intervertebral) M51.9
    with
      myelopathy
        sacroiliac region M53.3
        sacrococcygeal region M53.3
      specified NEC
        sacrococcygeal region M53.3
  dissociative F44.9
    affecting
      motor function F44.4
        and sensation F44.7
      sensation F44.6
        and motor function F44.7
    brief reactive F43.0
  drug related F19.99
    abuse—*see* Abuse, drug
    dependence—*see* Dependence, drug
  eating (adult) (psychogenic) F50.9
    anorexia—*see* Anorexia
    binge F50.81
    bulimia F50.2
    child F98.29
      pica F98.3
      rumination disorder F98.21
    other F50.89
    pica F50.89
      childhood F98.3
  electrolyte (balance) NEC E87.8
    acidosis (metabolic) (respiratory) E87.2
    alkalosis (metabolic) (respiratory) E87.3
  emotional (persistent) F34.9
    of childhood F93.9
      specified NEC F93.8
  esophagus K22.9
    functional K22.4
    psychogenic F45.8
  eustachian tube H69.9-
    infection—*see* Salpingitis, eustachian
    obstruction—*see* Obstruction, eustachian tube
    patulous—*see* Patulous, eustachian tube
    specified NEC H69.8-
  factitious F68.10
    with predominantly
      psychological symptoms F68.11
        with physical symptoms F68.13
      physical symptoms F68.12
        with psychological symptoms F68.13
  factor, coagulation—*see* Defect, coagulation
  fatty acid
    metabolism E71.30
      specified NEC E71.39

Disorder, *continued*
  oxidation
    LCAD E71.310
    MCAD E71.311
    SCAD E71.312
    specified deficiency NEC E71.318
  feeding (infant or child) (*see also* Disorder, eating) R63.3
  feigned (with obvious motivation) Z76.5
    without obvious motivation—*see* Disorder, factitious
  fibroblastic M72.9
  fluency
    childhood onset F80.81
    in conditions classified elsewhere R47.82
  fluid balance E87.8
  follicular (skin) L73.9
    specified NEC L73.8
  functional polymorphonuclear neutrophils D71
  gamma-glutamyl cycle E72.8
  gastric (functional) K31.9
    motility K30
    psychogenic F45.8
    secretion K30
  gastrointestinal (functional) NOS K92.9
    newborn P78.9
    psychogenic F45.8
  gender-identity or -role F64.9
    childhood F64.2
    effect on relationship F66
    of adolescence or adulthood (nontranssexual) F64.0
    specified NEC F64.8
    uncertainty F66
  genitourinary system
    female N94.9
    male N50.9
    psychogenic F45.8
  glomerular (in) N05.9
    disseminated intravascular coagulation D65 [N08]
    Henoch (-Schönlein) purpura D69.0 [N08]
    sepsis NEC A41. - [N08]
    subacute bacterial endocarditis I33.0 [N08]
    systemic lupus erythematosus M32.14
  gluconeogenesis E74.4
  habit (and impulse) F63.9
    involving sexual behavior NEC F65.9
    specified NEC F63.89
  heart action I49.9
  hoarding F42.3
  hypochondriacal F45.20
    body dysmorphic F45.22
  identity
    dissociative F44.81
    of childhood F93.8
  immune mechanism (immunity) D89.9
    specified type NEC D89.89
  integument, newborn P83.9
    specified NEC P83.8
  intestine, intestinal
    carbohydrate absorption NEC E74.39
      postoperative K91.2
    functional NEC K59.9
    psychogenic F45.8
  joint M25.9
    psychogenic F45.8
  language (developmental) F80.9
    expressive F80.1
    mixed receptive and expressive F80.2
    receptive F80.2
  learning (specific) F81.9
    acalculia R48.8
    alexia R48.0
    mathematics F81.2
    reading F81.0
    specified NEC F81.89
    spelling F81.81
    written expression F81.81
  liver K76.9
    malarial B54 [K77]
  lymphoproliferative, post-transplant (PTLD) D47.Z1
  menstrual N92.6
    psychogenic F45.8
    specified NEC N92.5

Disorder, *continued*
  mental (or behavioral) (nonpsychotic) F99
    following organic brain damage F07.9
      postconcussional syndrome F07.81
      specified NEC F07.89
    infancy, childhood or adolescence F98.9
    neurotic—*see* Neurosis
  metabolic, amino acid, transitory, newborn P74.8
  metabolism NOS E88.9
    amino-acid E72.9
      aromatic
        hyperphenylalaninemia E70.1
          classical phenylketonuria E70.0
      branched chain E71.2
        maple syrup urine disease E71.0
      glycine E72.50
      other specified E72.8
        beta-amino acid E72.8
        gamma-glutamyl cycle E72.8
      straight-chain E72.8
    bilirubin E80.7
      specified NEC E80.6
    calcium E83.50
      hypercalcemia E83.52
      hypocalcemia E83.51
      other specified E83.59
    congenital E88.9
    glutamine E72.8
    mitochondrial E88.40
      MELAS syndrome E88.41
      MERRF syndrome (myoclonic epilepsy associated
             with ragged-red fibers)
             E88.42
      other specified E88.49
    plasma protein NEC E88.09
    pyruvate E74.4
    serine E72.8
    sodium E87.8
    threonine E72.8
  micturition NEC R39.198
    feeling of incomplete emptying R39.14
    hesitancy R39.11
    need to immediately re-void R39.191
    poor stream R39.12
    position dependent R39.192
    psychogenic F45.8
    split stream R39.13
    straining R39.16
    urgency R39.15
  mitochondrial metabolism E88.40
  mixed
    anxiety and depressive F41.8
    of scholastic skills (developmental) F81.89
    receptive expressive language F80.2
  mood (affective), unspecified F39
  movement G25.9
    hysterical F44.4
    in diseases classified elsewhere—*see* category G26
    stereotyped F98.4
  muscle M62.9
    attachment, spine—*see* Enthesopathy, spinal
    psychogenic F45.8
    specified type NEC M62.89
    tone, newborn P94.9
      specified NEC P94.8
  musculoskeletal system, soft tissue—*see* Disorder, soft
             tissue
    psychogenic F45.8
  myoneural G70.9
    due to lead G70.1
    specified NEC G70.89
    toxic G70.1
  nerve G58.9
    cranial G52.9
      multiple G52.7
      seventh NEC G51.8
      sixth NEC—*see* Strabismus, paralytic, sixth nerve
    facial G51.9
      specified NEC G51.8
  neuromuscular G70.9
    hereditary NEC G71.9
    specified NEC G70.89
    toxic G70.1

Disorder, *continued*
  neurotic F48.9
    specified NEC F48.8
  neutrophil, polymorphonuclear D71
  nose J34.9
    specified NEC J34.89
  obsessive-compulsive F42.9
    excoriation (skin picking) disorder F42.4
    hoarding disorder F42.3
    mixed obsessional thoughts and acts F42.2
    other F42.8
  oppositional defiant F91.3
  overanxious F41.1
    of childhood F93.8
  panic F41.0
  parietoalveolar NEC J84.09
  paroxysmal, mixed R56.9
  peroxisomal E71.50
    biogenesis
      neonatal adrenoleukodystrophy E71.511
      specified disorder NEC E71.518
      Zellweger syndrome E71.510
    rhizomelic chondrodysplasia punctata E71.540
    specified form NEC E71.548
      group 1 E71.518
      group 2 E71.53
      group 3 E71.542
    X-linked adrenoleukodystrophy E71.529
      adolescent E71.521
      adrenomyeloneuropathy E71.522
      childhood E71.520
      specified form NEC E71.528
    Zellweger-like syndrome E71.54
  personality (*see also* Personality) F60.9
    pathological NEC F60.9
  pervasive, developmental F84.9
  pigmentation L81.9
    choroid, congenital Q14.3
    diminished melanin formation L81.6
    iron L81.8
    specified NEC L81.8
  polymorphonuclear neutrophils D71
  postconcussional F07.81
  postprocedural (postoperative)—*see* Complications,
             postprocedural
  post-traumatic stress (PTSD) F43.10
    acute F43.11
    chronic F43.12
  premenstrual dysphoric (PMDD) F32.81
  prepuce N47.8
  psychogenic NOS (*see also* condition) F45.9
    anxiety F41.8
    appetite F50.9
    asthenic F48.8
    cardiovascular (system) F45.8
    compulsive F42.8
    cutaneous F54
    depressive F32.9
    digestive (system) F45.8
    dysmenorrheic F45.8
    dyspnelc F45.8
    endocrine (system) F54
    eye NEC F45.8
    feeding—*see* Disorder, eating
    functional NEC F45.8
    gastric F45.8
    gastrointestinal (system) F45.8
    genitourinary (system) F45.8
    heart (function) (rhythm) F45.8
    hyperventilatory F45.8
    hypochondriacal—*see* Disorder, hypochondriacal
    intestinal F45.8
    joint F45.8
    learning F81.9
    limb F45.8
    lymphatic (system) F45.8
    menstrual F45.8
    micturition F45.8
    monoplegic NEC F44.4
    motor F44.4
    muscle F45.8
    musculoskeletal F45.8

Disorder, *continued*
    neurocirculatory F45.8
    obsessive F42.8
    organ or part of body NEC F45.8
    paralytic NEC F44.4
    phobic F40.9
    physical NEC F45.8
    rectal F45.8
    respiratory (system) F45.8
    rheumatic F45.8
    specified part of body NEC F45.8
    stomach F45.8
  psychomotor NEC F44.4
    hysterical F44.4
  psychoneurotic—*see also* Neurosis
    mixed NEC F48.8
  psychophysiologic—*see* Disorder, somatoform
  psychosexual F65.9
    development F66
    identity of childhood F64.2
  psychosomatic NOS—*see* Disorder, somatoform
    multiple F45.0
    undifferentiated F45.1
  psychotic—*see* Psychosis
    transient (acute) F23
  puberty E30.9
    specified NEC E30.8
  pulmonary (valve)—*see* Endocarditis, pulmonary
  pyruvate metabolism E74.4
  reading R48.0
    developmental (specific) F81.0
  receptive language F80.2
  refraction H52.7
  respiratory function, impaired—*see also* Failure,
             respiration
    postprocedural—*see* Complication, postoperative,
             respiratory system
    psychogenic F45.8
  sacrum, sacrococcygeal NEC M53.3
  schizoid of childhood F84.5
  seizure (*see also* Epilepsy) G40.909
    intractable G40.919
      with status epilepticus G40.911
  semantic pragmatic F80.89
    with autism F84.0
  sense of smell R43.1
    psychogenic F45.8
  separation anxiety, of childhood F93.0
  sexual
    preference (*see also* Deviation, sexual) F65.9
  shyness, of childhood and adolescence F40.10
  sibling rivalry F93.8
  sickle-cell (sickling) (homozygous)—*see* Disease,
             sickle-cell
    heterozygous D57.3
    specified type NEC D57.8-
    trait D57.3
  sinus (nasal) J34.9
    specified NEC J34.89
  skin L98.9
    hypertrophic L91.9
      specified NEC L91.8
    newborn P83.9
      specified NEC P83.8
    picking F42.4
  sleep G47.9
    terrors F51.4
    walking F51.3
  sleep-wake pattern or schedule—*see* Disorder, sleep,
             circadian rhythm
  social
    anxiety of childhood F40.10
    functioning in childhood F94.9
      specified NEC F94.8
    pragmatic F80.82
  somatization F45.0
  somatoform F45.9
    pain (persistent) F45.41
    somatization (multiple) (long-lasting) F45.0
    specified NEC F45.8
    undifferentiated F45.1

DISORDER-DIURESIS

Disorder, *continued*
  specific
    arithmetical F81.2
    developmental, of motor F82
    reading F81.0
    speech and language F80.9
    spelling F81.81
    written expression F81.81
  speech R47.9
    articulation (functional) (specific) F80.0
    developmental F80.9
    specified NEC R47.89
  spelling (specific) F81.81
  stereotyped, habit or movement F98.4
  stomach (functional)—*see* Disorder, gastric
  stress F43.9
    acute F43.0
    post-traumatic F43.10
      acute F43.11
      chronic F43.12
  temperature regulation, newborn P81.9
  thyroid (gland) E07.9
    function NEC, neonatal, transitory P72.2
    iodine-deficiency related E01.8
    specified NEC E07.89
  tic—*see* Tic
  tobacco use
    mild Z72.0
    moderate or severe F17.200
  tooth K08.9
    eruption K00.6
  Tourette's F95.2
  trauma and stressor related F43.9
  tubulo-interstitial (in)
    lymphoma NEC C85.9- *[N16]*
    Salmonella infection A02.25
    sarcoidosis D86.84
    sepsis A41.9 *[N16]*
      streptococcal A40.9 *[N16]*
    systemic lupus erythematosus M32.15
    toxoplasmosis B58.83
    transplant rejection T86.91 *[N16]*
  unsocialized aggressive F91.1
  white blood cells D72.9
    specified NEC D72.89
Disorientation R41.0
Displacement, displaced
  acquired traumatic of bone, cartilage, joint, tendon
        NEC—*see* Dislocation
  bladder (acquired) N32.89
    congenital Q64.19
  gallbladder (congenital) Q44.1
  intervertebral disc NEC
    sacrococcygeal region M53.3
  Meckel's diverticulum Q43.0
  nail (congenital) Q84.6
    acquired L60.8
  sacro-iliac (joint) (congenital) Q74.2
    current injury S33.2
    old—*see* subcategory M53.2
  ventricular septum Q21.0
Disruption (of)
  closure of
    laceration (external) (internal) T81.33
    traumatic laceration (external) (internal) T81.33
  family Z63.8
    due to
      absence of family member due to military
        deployment Z63.31
      absence of family member NEC Z63.32
      alcoholism and drug addiction in family Z63.72
      bereavement Z63.4
      death (assumed) or disappearance of family
        member Z63.4
      divorce or separation Z63.5
      drug addiction in family Z63.72
      stressful life events NEC Z63.79
  wound T81.30
    traumatic injury repair T81.33
    traumatic injury wound repair T81.33

Dissociation
  auriculoventricular or atrioventricular (AV) (any degree)
        (isorhythmic) I45.89
    with heart block I44.2
Dissociative reaction, state F44.9
Distension, distention
  abdomen R14.0
  bladder N32.89
  stomach K31.89
    acute K31.0
    psychogenic F45.8
Distortion(s) (congenital)
  bile duct or passage Q44.5
  clavicle Q74.0
  common duct Q44.5
  cystic duct Q44.5
  endocrine NEC Q89.2
  face bone (s) NEC Q75.8
  genitalia, genital organ (s)
    female Q52.8
      external Q52.79
      internal NEC Q52.8
  hepatic duct Q44.5
  intrafamilial communications Z63.8
  jaw NEC M26.89
  parathyroid (gland) Q89.2
  pituitary (gland) Q89.2
  sacroiliac joint Q74.2
  scapula Q74.0
  shoulder girdle Q74.0
  skull bone (s) NEC Q75.8
    with
      anencephalus Q00.0
      encephalocele—*see* Encephalocele
      hydrocephalus Q03.9
        with spina bifida—*see* Spina bifida, with
            hydrocephalus
      microcephaly Q02
  thymus (gland) Q89.2
  thyroid (gland) Q89.2
Distress
  abdomen—*see* Pain, abdominal
  acute respiratory R06.00
    syndrome (adult) (child) J80
  epigastric R10.13
  fetal P84
  gastrointestinal (functional) K30
    psychogenic F45.8
  intestinal (functional) NOS K59.9
    psychogenic F45.8
  respiratory R06.00
    child J80
    newborn P22.9
      specified NEC P22.8
    orthopnea R06.01
    psychogenic F45.8
    shortness of breath R06.02
    specified type NEC R06.09
Disturbance(s)—*see also* Disease
  absorption K90.9
    calcium E58
    carbohydrate K90.49
    fat K90.49
      pancreatic K90.3
    protein K90.49
    starch K90.49
    vitamin—*see* Deficiency, vitamin
  acid-base equilibrium E87.8
    mixed E87.4
  activity and attention (with hyperkinesis)—*see* Disorder,
        attention-deficit
        hyperactivity
  assimilation, food K90.9
  blood clotting (mechanism) (*see also* Defect, coagulation)
        D68.9
  cerebral
    status, newborn P91.9
      specified NEC P91.8
  circulatory I99.9
  conduct (*see also* Disorder, conduct) F91.9
    adjustment reaction—*see* Disorder, adjustment
    disruptive F91.9

Disturbance(s), *continued*
  hyperkinetic—*see* Disorder, attention-deficit
        hyperactivity
    socialized F91.2
    specified NEC F91.8
    unsocialized F91.1
  digestive K30
    psychogenic F45.8
  electrolyte—*see also* Imbalance, electrolyte
    newborn, transitory P74.4
      specified type NEC P74.4
  emotions specific to childhood and adolescence F93.9
    with
      anxiety and fearfulness NEC F93.8
      oppositional disorder F91.3
      sensitivity (withdrawal) F40.10
      shyness F40.10
      social withdrawal F40.10
    involving relationship problems F93.8
    mixed F93.8
    specified NEC F93.8
  equilibrium R42
  gait—*see* Gait
    hysterical F44.4
    psychogenic F44.4
  gastrointestinal (functional) K30
    psychogenic F45.8
  heart, functional (conditions in I44-I50)
    due to presence of (cardiac) prosthesis I97.19-
    postoperative I97.89
      cardiac surgery I97.19-
  keratinization NEC
    lip K13.0
  metabolism E88.9
    amino-acid E72.9
      straight-chain E72.8
    general E88.9
    glutamine E72.8
    neonatal, transitory P74.9
      calcium and magnesium P71.9
        specified type NEC P71.8
      specified NEC P74.8
    threonine E72.8
  nervous, functional R45.0
  ocular motion H51.9
    psychogenic F45.8
  oculogyric H51.8
    psychogenic F45.8
  oculomotor H51.9
    psychogenic F45.8
  personality (pattern) (trait) (*see also* Disorder, personality)
        F60.9
  psychomotor F44.4
  rhythm, heart I49.9
  sensation (cold) (heat) (localization) (tactile discrimination)
        (texture) (vibratory) NEC
        R20.9
    hysterical F44.6
  sensory—*see* Disturbance, sensation
  situational (transient)—*see also* Disorder, adjustment
    acute F43.0
  sleep G47.9
    nonorganic origin F51.9
  smell—*see* Disturbance, sensation, smell
  speech R47.9
    developmental F80.9
    specified NEC R47.89
  taste—*see* Disturbance, sensation, taste
  temperature
    regulation, newborn P81.9
      specified NEC P81.8
    sense R20.8
      hysterical F44.6
  tooth
    eruption K00.6
  vascular I99.9
  vision, visual H53.9
    specified NEC H53.8
  voice R49.9
    psychogenic F44.4
    specified NEC R49.8
Diuresis R35.8

Diverticulum, diverticula (multiple) K57.90
    Meckel's (displaced) (hypertrophic) Q43.0
    pericardium (congenital) (cyst) Q24.8
        acquired I31.8
Division
    glans penis Q55.69
Divorce, causing family disruption Z63.5
Dizziness R42
    hysterical F44.89
    psychogenic F45.8
DNR (do not resuscitate) Z66
Dorsalgia M54.9
Double
    aortic arch Q25.45
    albumin E88.09
Down syndrome Q90.9
Drinking (alcohol)
    excessive, to excess NEC (without dependence) F10.10
        habitual (continual) (without remission) F10.20
            with remission F10.21
Drip, postnasal (chronic) R09.82
    due to
        allergic rhinitis—*see* Rhinitis, allergic
        common cold J00
        nasopharyngitis—*see* Nasopharyngitis
        other know condition—*code to* condition
        sinusitis—*see* Sinusitis
Drop (in)
    attack NEC R55
Dropped heart beats I45.9
Dropsy, dropsical—*see also* Hydrops
    abdomen R18.8
    brain—*see* Hydrocephalus
    newborn due to isoimmunization P56.0
Drowned, drowning (near) T75.1
Drowsiness R40.0
Drug
    abuse counseling and surveillance Z71.51
    addiction—*see* Dependence
    dependence—*see* Dependence
    habit—*see* Dependence
    harmful use—*see* Abuse, drug
    induced fever R50.2
    overdose—*see* Table of Drugs and Chemicals, by drug,
                poisoning
    poisoning—*see* Table of Drugs and Chemicals, by drug,
                poisoning
    resistant organism infection (*see also* Resistant, organism,
                to, drug) Z16.30
    therapy
        long term (current) (prophylactic)—*see* Therapy, drug
            long-term (current)
            (prophylactic)
        short term—omit code
    wrong substance given or taken in error—*see* Table of
              Drugs and Chemicals,
              by drug, poisoning
Drunkenness (without dependence) F10.129
    acute in alcoholism F10.229
    chronic (without remission) F10.20
        with remission F10.21
    pathological (without dependence) F10.129
        with dependence F10.229
Dry, dryness—*see also* condition
    mouth R68.2
        due to dehydration E86.0
    nose J34.89
Dubin-Johnson disease or syndrome E80.6
Dubowitz' syndrome Q87.1
Duchenne-Griesinger disease G71.0
Duchenne's
    disease or syndrome
        muscular dystrophy G71.0
    paralysis
        birth injury P14.0
        due to or associated with
            muscular dystrophy G71.0
Duodenitis (nonspecific) (peptic) K29.80
    with bleeding K29.81

Duplication, duplex—*see also* Accessory
    alimentary tract Q45.8
    biliary duct (any) Q44.5
    cystic duct Q44.5
    digestive organs Q45.8
    frontonasal process Q75.8
Dupré's disease (meningism) R29.1
Dwarfism E34.3
    achondroplastic Q77.4
    congenital E34.3
    constitutional E34.3
    hypochondroplastic Q77.4
    hypophyseal E23.0
    infantile E34.3
    Laron-type E34.3
    Lorain (-Levi) type E23.0
    metatropic Q77.8
    nephrotic-glycosuric (with hypophosphatemic rickets)
                E72.09
    nutritional E45
    penis Q55.69
    pituitary E23.0
    renal N25.0
    thanatophoric Q77.1
Dysarthria R47.1
Dysbasia R26.2
    hysterical F44.4
    nonorganic origin F44.4
    psychogenic F44.4
Dysbetalipoproteinemia (familial) E78.2
Dyscalculia R48.8
    developmental F81.2
Dyschezia K59.00
Dyscranio-pygo-phalangy Q87.0
    stomach K31.89
        psychogenic F45.8
Dysentery, dysenteric (catarrhal) (diarrhea) (epidemic)
                (hemorrhagic)
                (infectious) (sporadic)
                (tropical) A09
    amebic (*see also* Amebiasis) A06.0
        acute A06.0
        chronic A06.1
    arthritis (*see also* category M01) A09
        bacillary (*see also* category M01) A03.9
    bacillary A03.9
        arthritis (*see also* category M01)
        Shigella A03.9
            boydii A03.2
            dysenteriae A03.0
            flexneri A03.1
            group A A03.0
            group B A03.1
            group C A03.2
            group D A03.3
            sonnei A03.3
            specified type NEC A03.8
    candidal B37.82
    Chinese A03.9
    Giardia lamblia A07.1
    Lamblia A07.1
    monilial B37.82
    Salmonella A02.0
    viral (*see also* Enteritis, viral) A08.4
Dysequilibrium R42
Dysesthesia R20.8
    hysterical F44.6
Dysfunction
    autonomic
        somatoform F45.8
    bleeding, uterus N93.8
    cerebral G93.89
    colon K59.9
        psychogenic F45.8
    rectum K59.9
        psychogenic F45.8
    sexual (due to) R37
    sinoatrial node I49.5
    somatoform autonomic F45.8
    temporomandibular (joint) M26.69
        joint-pain syndrome M26.62-

Dysfunction, *continued*
    ventricular I51.9
        with congestive heart failure I50.9—left, reversible,
                following sudden
                emotional stress I51.81
Dysgenesis
    gonadal (due to chromosomal anomaly) Q96.9
    tidal platelet D69.3
Dyshidrosis, dysidrosis L30.1
Dyskeratosis L85.8
    congenital Q82.8
Dyskinesia G24.9
    hysterical F44.4
    nonorganic origin F44.4
    psychogenic F44.4
Dyslalia (developmental) F80.0
Dyslexia R48.0
    developmental F81.0
Dyslipidemia E78.5
Dysmenorrhea (essential) (exfoliative) N94.6
    congestive (syndrome) N94.6
    primary N94.4
    psychogenic F45.8
    secondary N94.5
Dysmetabolic syndrome X E88.81
Dysmorphism (due to)
    alcohol Q86.0
Dysmorphophobia (non-delusional) F45.22
    delusional F22
Dysorexia R63.0
    psychogenic F50.89
Dysostosis
    cleidocranial, cleidocranialis Q74.0
    multiplex E76.01
Dyspareunia N94.10
    deep N94.12
    other specified N94.19
    superficial (introital) N94.11
Dyspepsia R10.13
    atonic K30
    functional (allergic) (congenital) (gastrointestinal)
                (occupational) (reflex)
                K30
    nervous F45.8
    neurotic F45.8
    psychogenic F45.8
Dysphagia R13.10
    cervical R13.19
    functional (hysterical) F45.8
    hysterical F45.8
    nervous (hysterical) F45.8
    neurogenic R13.19
    oral phase R13.11
    oropharyngeal phase R13.12
    pharyngeal phase R13.13
    pharyngoesophageal phase R13.14
    psychogenic F45.8
    specified NEC R13.19
Dysphagocytosis, congenital D71
Dysphasia R47.02
    developmental
        expressive type F80.1
        receptive type F80.2
Dysphonia R49.0
    functional F44.4
    hysterical F44.4
    psychogenic F44.4
Dysplasia—*see also* Anomaly
    acetabular, congenital Q65.89
    alveolar capillary, with vein misalignment J84.843
    anus (histologically confirmed) (mild) (moderate) K62.82
        severe D01.3
    brain Q07.9
    bronchopulmonary, perinatal P27.1
    colon D12.6
    ectodermal (anhidrotic) (congenital) (hereditary) Q82.4
        hydrotic Q82.8
    high grade, focal D12.6
    hip, congenital Q65.89
    joint, congenital Q74.8
    kidney Q61.4
        multicystic Q61.4
    leg Q74.2

Dysplasia, *continued*
   lung, congenital (not associated with short gestation)
          Q33.6
   oculodentodigital Q87.0
   renal Q61.4
      multicystic Q61.4
   skin L98.8
   thymic, with immunodeficiency D82.1
Dyspnea (nocturnal) (paroxysmal) R06.00
   asthmatic (bronchial) J45.909
      with
         exacerbation (acute) J45.901
         bronchitis J45.909
            with
               exacerbation (acute) J45.901
               status asthmaticus J45.902
            chronic J44.9
         status asthmaticus J45.902
   functional F45.8
   hyperventilation R06.4
   hysterical F45.8
   newborn P28.89
   orthopnea R06.01
   psychogenic F45.8
   shortness of breath R06.02
   specified type NEC R06.09
Dyspraxia R27.8
   developmental (syndrome) F82
Dysproteinemia E88.09
Dysrhythmia
   cardiac I49.9
      newborn
         bradycardia P29.12
         occurring before birth P03.819
            before onset of labor P03.810
            during labor P03.811
         tachycardia P29.11
      postoperative I97.89
   cerebral or cortical—*see* Epilepsy
Dyssomnia—*see* Disorder, sleep
Dyssynergia
   cerebellaris myoclonica (Hunt's ataxia) G11.1
Dystocia O66.9
   affecting newborn P03.1
Dystrophy, dystrophia
   Becker's type G71.0
   Duchenne's type G71.0
   Erb's G71.0
   Gower's muscular G71.0
   infantile neuraxonal G31.89
   Landouzy-Déjérine G71.0
   Leyden-Möbius G71.0
   muscular G71.0
      benign (Becker type) G71.0
      congenital (hereditary) (progressive) (with specific
            morphological
            abnormalities of the
            muscle fiber) G71.0
      distal G71.0
      Duchenne type G71.0
      Emery-Dreifuss G71.0
      Erb type G71.0
      facioscapulohumeral G71.0
      Gower's G71.0
      hereditary (progressive) G71.0
      Landouzy-Déjérine type G71.0
      limb-girdle G71.0
      progressive (hereditary) G71.0
      pseudohypertrophic (infantile) G71.0
      severe (Duchenne type) G71.0
   ocular G71.0
   oculocerebrorenal E72.03
   oculopharyngeal G71.0
   retinal (hereditary) H35.50
      involving
         sensory area H35.53
   scapuloperoneal G71.0
   skin NEC L98.8
Dysuria R30.0
   psychogenic F45.8

E

Ear—*see also* condition
   wax (impacted) H61.20
      left H61.22
         with right H61.23
      right H61.21
         with left H61.23
Earache—*see* subcategory H92.0
Eccentro-osteochondrodysplasia E76.29
Ecchymosis R58
   newborn P54.5
   spontaneous R23.3
   traumatic—*see* Contusion
Echovirus, as cause of disease classified elsewhere
          B97.12
Ectasia, ectasis
   annuloaortic I35.8
Ecthyma L08.0
   gangrenosum L08.0
Ectodermosis erosiva pluriorificialis L51.1
Ectopic, ectopia (congenital)
   abdominal viscera Q45.8
      due to defect in anterior abdominal wall Q79.59
   atrial beats I49.1
   beats I49.49
      atrial I49.1
   bladder Q64.10
   testis Q53.00
      bilateral Q53.02
      unilateral Q53.01
   thyroid Q89.2
   vesicae Q64.10
Ectropion H02.109
   cervix N86
      with cervicitis N72
   lip (acquired) K13.0
      congenital Q38.0
Eczema (acute) (chronic) (erythematous) (fissum) (rubrum)
         (squamous) (*see also*
         Dermatitis) L30.9
   contact—*see* Dermatitis, contact
   dyshydrotic L30.1
   flexural L20.82
   infantile L20.83
      intertriginous L21.1
      seborrheic L21.1
   intertriginous NEC L30.4
      infantile L21.1
   intrinsic (allergic) L20.84
   marginatum (hebrae) B35.6
   vaccination, vaccinatum T88.1
Eddowes (-Spurway) syndrome Q78.0
Edema, edematous (infectious) (pitting) (toxic) R60.9
   with nephritis—*see* Nephrosis
   allergic T78.3
   angioneurotic (allergic) (any site) (with urticaria) T78.3
   brain (cytotoxic) (vasogenic) G93.6
      due to birth injury P11.0
      newborn (anoxia or hypoxia) P52.4
         birth injury P11.0
      traumatic—*see* Injury, intracranial, cerebral edema
   circumscribed, acute T78.3
   conjunctiva H11.42-
   due to
      salt retention E87.0
   epiglottis—*see* Edema, glottis
   essential, acute T78.3
   generalized R60.1
   glottis, glottic, glottidis (obstructive) (passive) J38.4
      allergic T78.3
   intracranial G93.6
   legs R60.0
   localized R60.0
   lower limbs R60.0
   lung J81.1
      acute J81.0
      due to
         high altitude T70.29
         near drowning T75.1
   penis N48.89
   periodic T78.3
   Quincke's T78.3
   salt E87.0

Edentulism—*see* Absence, teeth, acquired
Edsall's disease T67.2
Educational handicap Z55.9
   specified NEC Z55.8
Edward's syndrome—*see* Trisomy, 18
Effect, adverse
   abuse—*see* Maltreatment
   altitude (high)—*see* Effect, adverse, high altitude
   biological, correct substance properly administered—*see*
         Effect, adverse, drug
   blood (derivatives) (serum) (transfusion)—*see*
         Complications,
         transfusion
   chemical substance—*see* Table of Drugs and Chemicals
   cold (temperature) (weather) T69.9
      chilblains T69.1
      frostbite—*see* Frostbite
      specified effect NEC T69.8
   drugs and medicaments T88.7
      specified drug—*see* Table of Drugs and Chemicals, by
         drug, adverse effect
      specified effect—*code to* condition
   electric current, electricity (shock) T75.4
      burn—*see* Burn
   exposure—*see* Exposure
   external cause NEC T75.89
   foodstuffs T78.1
      allergic reaction—*see* Allergy, food
      causing anaphylaxis—*see* Shock, anaphylactic,
         due to food
      noxious—*see* Poisoning, food, noxious
   gases, fumes, or vapors T59.9-
      specified agent—*see* Table of Drugs and Chemicals
   glue (airplane) sniffing
      due to drug abuse—*see* Abuse, drug, inhalant
      due to drug dependence—*see* Dependence, drug,
         inhalant
   heat—*see* Heat
   high altitude NEC T70.29
      anoxia T70.29
      on
         ears T70.0
         sinuses T70.1
      polycythemia D75.1
   hot weather—*see* Heat
   hunger T73.0
   immersion, foot—*see* Immersion
   immunization—*see* Complications, vaccination
   immunological agents—*see* Complications, vaccination
   infusion—*see* Complications, infusion
   lack of care of infants—*see* Maltreatment, child
   medical care T88.9
      specified NEC T88.8
   medicinal substance, correct, properly administered—*see*
         Effect, adverse, drug
   motion T75.3
   serum NEC (*see also* Reaction, serum) T80.69
   specified NEC T78.8
   strangulation—*see* Asphyxia, traumatic
   submersion T75.1
   toxic—*see* Table of Drugs and Chemicals, by animal or
         substance, poisoning
   transfusion—*see* Complications, transfusion
   ultraviolet (radiation) (rays) NOS T66
      burn—*see* Burn
      dermatitis or eczema—*see* Dermatitis, due to,
         ultraviolet rays
      acute L56.8
   vaccine (any)—*see* Complications, vaccination
   whole blood—*see* Complications, transfusion
Effect (s) (of) (from)—*see* Effect, adverse NEC
Effects, late—*see* Sequelae
Effort syndrome (psychogenic) F45.8
Effusion
   brain (serous) G93.6
   bronchial—*see* Bronchitis
   cerebral G93.6
   cerebrospinal—*see also* Meningitis
      vessel G93.6
   chest—*see* Effusion, pleura
   intracranial G93.6

DYSPLASIA-EFFUSION

Effusion, *continued*
  joint M25.40
    ankle M25.47-
    elbow M25.42-
    foot joint M25.47-
    hand joint M25.44-
    hip M25.45-
    knee M25.46-
    shoulder M25.41-
    specified joint NEC M25.48
    wrist M25.43-
  malignant pleural J91.0
  pericardium, pericardial (noninflammatory) I31.3
    acute—*see* Pericarditis, acute
  peritoneal (chronic) R18.8
  pleura, pleurisy, pleuritic, pleuropericardial J90
    due to systemic lupus erythematosus M32.13
    malignant J91.0
    newborn P28.89
  spinal—*see* Meningitis
  thorax, thoracic—*see* Effusion, pleura
Ehlers-Danlos syndrome Q79.6
Ehrlichiosis A77.40
Eichstedt's disease B36.0
Eisenmenger's
  complex or syndrome I27.89
  defect Q21.8
Ekman's syndrome (brittle bones and blue sclera) Q78.0
Elastic skin Q82.8
  acquired L57.4
Elastoma (juvenile) Q82.8
  Miescher's L87.2
Electric current, electricity, effects (concussion) (fatal)
           (nonfatal) (shock) T75.4
  burn—*see* Burn
Electrocution T75.4
  from electroshock gun (taser) T75.4
Electrolyte imbalance E87.8
Elevated, elevation
  blood pressure—*see also* Hypertension
    reading (incidental) (isolated) (nonspecific), no
        diagnosis of
        hypertension R03.0
  blood sugar R73.9
  body temperature (of unknown origin) R50.9
  C-reactive protein (CRP) R79.82
  cholesterol E78.00
    with high triglycerides E78.2
  erythrocyte sedimentation rate R70.0
  fasting glucose R73.01
  finding on laboratory examination—*see* Findings,
        abnormal, inconclusive,
        without diagnosis, by
        type of exam
  glucose tolerance (oral) R73.02
  leukocytes D72.829
  liver function
    test R79.89
      bilirubin R17
  lymphocytes D72.820
  scapula, congenital Q74.0
  sedimentation rate R70.0
  triglycerides E78.1
    with high cholesterol E78.2
  white blood cell count D72.829
    specified NEC D72.828
Elliptocytosis (congenital) (hereditary) D58.1
  Hb C (disease) D58.1
  hemoglobin disease D58.1
  sickle-cell (disease) D57.8-
    trait D57.3
Elongated, elongation (congenital)—*see also* Distortion
  bone Q79.9
  cystic duct Q44.5
  frenulum, penis Q55.69
  labia minora (acquired) N90.69
Embolism (multiple) (paradoxical) I74.9
  artery I74.9
  portal (vein) I81
  pulmonary (acute) (artery) (vein) I26.99
    with acute cor pulmonale I26.09
    chronic I27.82
      personal history of Z86.71

Embolism, *continued*
  pyemic (multiple) I76
    following
      Hemophilus influenzae A41.3
      pneumococcal A40.3
        with pneumonia J13
      specified organism NEC A41.89
      staphylococcal A41.2
      streptococcal A40.9
  renal (artery) N28.0
    vein I82.3
  vein (acute) I82.90
    renal I82.3
Embryoma—*see also* Neoplasm, uncertain behavior, by site
  kidney C64.-
  malignant—*see also* Neoplasm, malignant, by site
    kidney C64.-
Emesis—*see* vomiting
Emotional lability R45.86
Emphysema (atrophic) (bullous) (chronic) (interlobular)
             (lung) (obstructive)
             (pulmonary) (senile)
             (vesicular) J43.9
  cellular tissue (traumatic) T79.7
  connective tissue (traumatic) T79.7
  eyelid (s) H02.89
    traumatic T79.7
  interstitial J98.2
    congenital P25.0
    perinatal period P25.0
  laminated tissue T79.7
  mediastinal J98.2
    newborn P25.2
  subcutaneous (traumatic) T79.7
    nontraumatic J98.2
  traumatic T79.7
Empyema (acute) (chest) (double) (pleura)
             (supradiaphragmatic)
             (thorax) J86.9
  with fistula J86.0
  gallbladder K81.0
Enanthema, viral B09
Encephalitis (chronic) (hemorrhagic) (idiopathic)(spurious)
             (subacute) G04.90
  acute (*see also* Encephalitis, viral) A86
    disseminated G04.00
      infectious G04.01
      noninfectious G04.81
      postimmunization (postvaccination) G04.02
      postinfectious G04.01
  California (virus) A83.5
  disseminated, acute G04.00
    necrotizing hemorrhagic G04.30
      postimmunization G04.32
      postinfectious G04.31
      specified NEC G04.39
  due to
    cat scratch disease A28.1
    human immunodeficiency virus (HIV) disease B20
        [G05.3]
    malaria—*see* Malaria
    smallpox inoculation G04.02
  Eastern equine A83.2
  endemic (viral) A86
  epidemic NEC (viral) A86
  equine (acute) (infectious) (viral) A83.9
    Eastern A83.2
  following vaccination or other immunization procedure
        G04.02
  herpes zoster B02.0
  herpesviral B00.4
    due to herpesvirus 7 B10.09
    specified NEC B10.09
  in (due to)
    herpes (simplex) virus B00.4
      due to herpesvirus 7 B10.09
      specified NEC B10.09
    infectious disease NEC B99 [G05.3]
    influenza—*see* Influenza, with, encephalopathy
      congenital P37.1
    listeriosis A32.12
    measles B05.0
    parasitic disease NEC B89 [G05.3]

Encephalitis, *continued*
    systemic lupus erythematosus M32.19
    toxoplasmosis (acquired) B58.2
  infectious (acute) (virus) NEC A86
  La Crosse A83.5
  lupus erythematosus, systemic M32.19
  otitic NEC H66.40 [G05.3]
  parasitic NOS B71.9
  postchickenpox B01.11
  postexanthematous NEC B09
  postimmunization G04.02
  postinfectious NEC G04.01
  postmeasles B05.0
  postvaccinal G04.02
  postvaricella B01.11
  postviral NEC A86
  St. Louis A83.3
  toxic NEC G92
  type
    C A83.3
  viral, virus A86
    arthropod-borne NEC A85.2
      mosquito-borne A83.9
        California virus A83.5
        Eastern equine A83.2
        St. Louis A83.3
        type C A83.3
Encephalomalacia (brain) (cerebellar) (cerebral)—*see*
        Softening, brain
Encephalomyelitis (*see also* Encephalitis) G04.90
  acute disseminated G04.00
    infectious G04.01
    noninfectious G04.81
    postimmunization G04.02
    postinfectious G04.01
  acute necrotizing hemorrhagic G04.30
    postimmunization G04.32
    postinfectious G04.31
    specified NEC G04.39
  equine A83.9
    Eastern A83.2
  in diseases classified elsewhere G05.3
  postchickenpox B01.11
  postinfectious NEC G04.01
  postmeasles B05.0
  postvaccinal G04.02
  postvaricella B01.11
Encephalopathy (acute) G93.40
  acute necrotizing hemorrhagic G04.30
    postimmunization G04.32
    postinfectious G04.31
    specified NEC G04.39
  congenital Q07.9
  due to
    drugs (*see also* Table of Drugs and Chemicals) G92
  hyperbilirubinemic, newborn P57.9
    due to isoimmunization (conditions in P55) P57.0
  hypertensive I67.4
  hypoglycemic E16.2
  hypoxic—*see* Damage, brain, anoxic
  hypoxic ischemic P91.60
    mild P91.61
    moderate P91.62
    severe P91.63
  in (due to) (with)
    birth injury P11.1
    hyperinsulinism E16.1 [G94]
    influenza—*see* Influenza, with, encephalopathy
    lack of vitamin (*see also* Deficiency, vitamin) E56.9
        [G32.89]
    neoplastic disease (*see also* Neoplasm) D49.9 [G13.1]
    serum (*see also* Reaction, serum) T80.69
    syphilis A52.17
    trauma (postconcussional) F07.81
      current injury—*see* Injury, intracranial
    vaccination G04.02
  lead—*see* Poisoning, lead
  metabolic G93.41
    drug induced G92
    toxic G92
  postcontusional F07.81
    current injury—*see* Injury, intracranial, diffuse
  postradiation G93.89

Encephalopathy, *continued*
  toxic G92
    metabolic G92
  traumatic (postconcussional) F07.81
    current injury—*see* Injury, intracranial
Encephalorrhagia—*see* Hemorrhage, intracranial,
                  intracerebral
Encephalosis, posttraumatic F07.81
Encopresis R15.9
  functional F98.1
  nonorganic origin F98.1
  psychogenic F98.1
Encounter (with health service) (for) Z76.89
  administrative purpose only Z02.9
    examination for
      adoption Z02.82
      armed forces Z02.3
      disability determination Z02.71
      driving license Z02.4
      employment Z02.1
      insurance Z02.6
      medical certificate NEC Z02.79
      paternity testing Z02.81
      residential institution admission Z02.2
      school admission Z02.0
      sports Z02.5
      specified reason NEC Z02.89
  aftercare—*see* Aftercare
  check-up—*see* Examination
  chemotherapy for neoplasm Z51.11
  counseling—*see* Counseling
  desensitization to allergens Z51.6
  examination—*see* Examination
  expectant parent (s) (adoptive) pre-birth pediatrician visit
                Z76.81
  fluoride varnish application Z29.3
  genetic
    counseling Z31.5
    testing—*see* Test, genetic
  hearing conservation and treatment Z01.12
  instruction (in)
    child care (postpartal) (prenatal) Z32.3
    natural family planning
      procreative Z31.61
      to avoid pregnancy Z30.02
  laboratory (as part of a general medical examination)
                Z00.00
    with abnormal findings Z00.01
  mental health services (for)
    abuse NEC
      perpetrator Z69.82
      victim Z69.81
    child abuse
      non-parental
        perpetrator Z69.021
        victim Z69.020
      parental
        perpetrator Z69.011
        victim Z69.010
    spousal or partner abuse
      perpetrator Z69.12
      victim Z69.11
  observation (for) (ruled out)
    exposure to (suspected)
      anthrax Z03.810
      biological agent NEC Z03.818
  pediatrician visit, by expectant parent (s) (adoptive) Z76.81
  pregnancy
    supervision of—*see* Pregnancy, supervision of
    test Z32.00
      result negative Z32.02
      result positive Z32.01
  prophylactic measures
    antivenin Z29.12
    fluoride administration Z29.3
    other specified Z29.8
    rabies immune globulin Z29.14
    respiratory syncytial virus (RSV) immune globulin
                Z29.11
    Rho(D) immune globulin Z29.13
    unspecified Z29.9
  radiation therapy (antineoplastic) Z51.0

Encounter, *continued*
  radiological (as part of a general medical examination)
                Z00.00
    with abnormal findings Z00.01
  repeat cervical smear to confirm findings of recent normal
              smear following initial
              abnormal smear
              Z01.42
  respiratory syncytial virus immune globulin administration
              Z29.11
  suspected condition, ruled out
    fetal anomaly Z03.73
    fetal growth Z03.74
  suspected exposure (to), ruled out
    anthrax Z03.810
    biological agents NEC Z03.818
  therapeutic drug level monitoring Z51.81
  to determine fetal viability of pregnancy O36.80
  training
    insulin pump Z46.81
  X-ray of chest (as part of a general medical examination)
                Z00.00
    with abnormal findings Z00.01
Endocarditis (chronic) (marantic) (nonbacterial) (thrombotic)
              (valvular) I38
  with rheumatic fever (conditions in I00)
    active—*see* Endocarditis, acute, rheumatic
    inactive or quiescent (with chorea) I09.1
  acute or subacute I33.9
    infective I33.0
    rheumatic (aortic) (mitral) (pulmonary) (tricuspid) I01.1
      with chorea (acute) (rheumatic) (Sydenham's) I02.0
  aortic (heart) (nonrheumatic) (valve) I35.8
    with
      mitral disease I08.0
        with tricuspid (valve) disease I08.3
        active or acute I01.1
          with chorea (acute) (rheumatic)
              (Sydenham's) I02.0
      rheumatic fever (conditions in I00)
        active—*see* Endocarditis, acute, rheumatic
        inactive or quiescent (with chorea) I06.9
      tricuspid (valve) disease I08.2
        with mitral (valve) disease I08.3
    acute or subacute I33.9
    arteriosclerotic I35.8
    rheumatic I06.9
      with mitral disease I08.0
        with tricuspid (valve) disease I08.3
        active or acute I01.1
          with chorea (acute) (rheumatic)
              (Sydenham's) I02.0
      active or acute I01.1
        with chorea (acute) (rheumatic) (Sydenham's)
              I02.0
    specified NEC I06.8
    specified cause NEC I35.8
  atypical verrucous (Libman-Sacks) M32.11
  bacterial (acute) (any valve) (subacute) I33.0
  candidal B37.6
  constrictive I33.0
  due to
    Serratia marcescens I33.0
  infectious or infective (acute) (any valve) (subacute) I33.0
  lenta (acute) (any valve) (subacute) I33.0
  Libman-Sacks M32.11
  malignant (acute) (any valve) (subacute) I33.0
  mitral (chronic) (double) (fibroid) (heart) (inactive) (valve)
              (with chorea) I05.9
    with
      aortic (valve) disease I08.0
        with tricuspid (valve) disease I08.3
        active or acute I01.1
          with chorea (acute) (rheumatic)
              (Sydenham's) I02.0
      rheumatic fever (conditions in I00)
        active—*see* Endocarditis, acute, rheumatic
        inactive or quiescent (with chorea) I05.9
    active or acute I01.1
      with chorea (acute) (rheumatic) (Sydenham's) I02.0
    bacterial I33.0

Endocarditis, *continued*
  nonrheumatic I34.8
    acute or subacute I33.9
    specified NEC I05.8
  monilial B37.6
  mycotic (acute) (any valve) (subacute) I33.0
  pneumococcal (acute) (any valve) (subacute) I33.0
  pulmonary (chronic) (heart) (valve) I37.8
    with rheumatic fever (conditions in I00)
      active—*see* Endocarditis, acute, rheumatic
      inactive or quiescent (with chorea) I09.89
        with aortic, mitral or tricuspid disease I08.8
    acute or subacute I33.9
      rheumatic I01.1
        with chorea (acute) (rheumatic) (Sydenham's)
              I02.0
    arteriosclerotic I37.8
    congenital Q22.2
  purulent (acute) (any valve) (subacute) I33.0
  rheumatic (chronic) (inactive) (with chorea) I09.1
    active or acute (aortic) (mitral) (pulmonary) (tricuspid)
              I01.1
      with chorea (acute) (rheumatic) (Sydenham's) I02.0
  septic (acute) (any valve) (subacute) I33.0
  streptococcal (acute) (any valve) (subacute) I33.0
  subacute—*see* Endocarditis, acute
  suppurative (acute) (any valve) (subacute) I33.0
  toxic I33.9
  tricuspid (chronic) (heart) (inactive) (rheumatic) (valve)
              (with chorea) I07.9
    with
      aortic (valve) disease I08.2
        mitral (valve) disease I08.3
      mitral (valve) disease I08.1
        aortic (valve) disease I08.3
      rheumatic fever (conditions in I00)
        active—*see* Endocarditis, acute, rheumatic
        inactive or quiescent (with chorea) I07.8
    active or acute I01.1
      with chorea (acute) (rheumatic) (Sydenham's) I02.0
    arteriosclerotic I36.8
    nonrheumatic I36.8
      acute or subacute I33.9
    specified cause, except rheumatic I36.8
  ulcerative (acute) (any valve) (subacute) I33.0
  vegetative (acute) (any valve) (subacute) I33.0
  verrucous (atypical) (nonbacterial) (nonrheumatic) M32.11
Endocardium, endocardial—*see also* condition
  cushion defect Q21.2
Endocervicitis—*see also* Cervicitis
  hyperplastic N72
Endometritis (decidual) (nonspecific) (purulent) (senile)
             (atrophic) (suppurative)
             N71.9
  acute N71.0
  blennorrhagic (gonococcal) (acute) (chronic) A54.24
  cervix, cervical (with erosion or ectropion)—*see also*
             Cervicitis
    hyperplastic N72
  chlamydial A56.11
  gonococcal, gonorrheal (acute) (chronic) A54.24
  hyperplastic (*see also* Hyperplasia, endometrial) N85.00-
    cervix N72
Engorgement
  breast N64.59
    newborn P83.4
Enlargement, enlarged—*see also* Hypertrophy
  adenoids J35.2
    with tonsils J35.3
  gingival K06.1
  labium majus (childhood asymmetric) CALME N90.61
  lymph gland or node R59.9
    generalized R59.1
    localized R59.0
  tonsils J35.1
    with adenoids J35.3
Enteritis (acute) (diarrheal) (hemorrhagic) (noninfective) K52.9
  aertrycke infection A02.0
  allergic K52.29
    with
      eosinophilic gastritis or gastroenteritis K52.81
      food protein-induced enterocolitis syndrome K52.21
      food protein-induced enteropathy K52.22

Enteritis, *continued*
  amebic (acute) A06.0
  bacillary NOS A03.9
  candidal B37.82
  chronic (noninfectious) K52.9
    ulcerative—*see* Colitis, ulcerative
  Clostridium
    botulinum (food poisoning) A05.1
  coxsackie virus A08.39
  dietetic K52.29
  due to
    coxsackie virus A08.39
    echovirus A08.39
    enterovirus NEC A08.39
    food hypersensitivity K52.29
    torovirus A08.39
  echovirus A08.39
  enterovirus NEC A08.39
  eosinophilic K52.81
  epidemic (infectious) A09
  fulminant (*see also* Ischemia, intestine, acute) K55.019
    ischemic K55.9
      acute (*see also* Ischemia, intestine, acute) K55.019
  giardial A07.1
  infectious NOS A09
    due to
      Arizona (bacillus) A02.0
      Campylobacter A04.5
      Escherichia coli A04.4
        enteroaggregative A04.4
        enterohemorrhagic A04.3
        enteropathogenic A04.0
        enterotoxigenic A04.1
        specified NEC A04.4
      enterovirus A08.39
      specified
        bacteria NEC A04.8
        virus NEC A08.39
      virus NEC A08.4
        specified type NEC A08.39
  necroticans A05.2
  noninfectious K52.9
  parasitic NEC B82.9
  regional (of) K50.90
    with
      complication K50.919
        abscess K50.914
        fistula K50.913
        intestinal obstruction K50.912
        rectal bleeding K50.911
        specified complication NEC K50.918
    large intestine (colon) (rectum) K50.10
      with
        complication K50.119
          abscess K50.114
          fistula K50.113
          intestinal obstruction K50.112
          rectal bleeding K50.111
          small intestine (duodenum) (ileum) (jejunum) involvement K50.80
          with
            complication K50.819
              abscess K50.814
              fistula K50.813
              intestinal obstruction K50.812
              rectal bleeding K50.811
              specified complication NEC K50.818
        specified complication NEC K50.118
    rectum—*see* Enteritis, regional, large intestine
    small intestine (duodenum) (ileum) (jejunum) K50.00
      with
        complication K50.019
          abscess K50.014
          fistula K50.013
          intestinal obstruction K50.012
          large intestine (colon) (rectum) involvement K50.80

Enteritis, *continued*
  with
    complication K50.819
      abscess K50.814
      fistula K50.813
      intestinal obstruction K50.812
      rectal bleeding K50.811
      specified complication NEC K50.818
    rectal bleeding K50.011
    specified complication NEC K50.018
  rotaviral A08.0
  Salmonella, salmonellosis (arizonae) (choleraesuis) (enteritidis) (typhimurium) A02.0
  septic A09
  staphylococcal A04.8
    due to food A05.0
  torovirus A08.39
  viral A08.4
    enterovirus A08.39
    Rotavirus A08.0
    specified NEC A08.39
    virus specified NEC A08.39
Enterobiasis B80
Enterobius vermicularis (infection) (infestation) B80
Enterocolitis (*see also* Enteritis) K52.9
  fulminant ischemic (*see also* Ischemia, intestine, acute) K55.059
  hemorrhagic (acute) (*see also* Ischemia, intestine, acute) K55.059
  infectious NEC A09
  necrotizing
    due to Clostridium difficile A04.7
    in newborn P77.9
      stage 1 (without pneumatosis, without perforation) P77.1
      stage 2 (with pneumatosis, without perforation) P77.2
      stage 3 (with pneumatosis, with perforation) P77.3
    stage 1 (excluding newborns) K55.31
    stage 2 (excluding newborns) K55.32
    stage 3 (excluding newborns) K55.33
    unspecified K55.30
  noninfectious K52.9
    newborn—*see* Enterocolitis, necrotizing in newborn
  protein-induced syndrome K52.21
Enteropathy K63.9
  food protein-induced K52.22
  gluten-sensitive
    celiac K90.0
    non-celiac K90.41
  protein-losing K90.49
Enterorrhagia K92.2
Enterospasm—*see also* Syndrome, irritable, bowel
  psychogenic F45.8
Enterovirus, as cause of disease classified elsewhere B97.10
  coxsackievirus B97.11
  echovirus B97.12
  other specified B97.19
Enuresis R32
  functional F98.0
  habit disturbance F98.0
  nocturnal N39.44
    psychogenic F98.0
  nonorganic origin F98.0
  psychogenic F98.0
Eosinophilia (allergic) (hereditary) (idiopathic) (secondary) D72.1
  with
    angiolymphoid hyperplasia (ALHE) D18.01
Eosinophilia-myalgia syndrome M35.8
Ependymoblastoma
  specified site—*see* Neoplasm, malignant, by site
  unspecified site C71.9
Ependymoma (epithelial) (malignant)
  anaplastic
    specified site—*see* Neoplasm, malignant, by site
    unspecified site C71.9
  benign
    specified site—*see* Neoplasm, benign, by site
    unspecified site D33.2

Ependymoma, *continued*
  specified site—*see* Neoplasm, malignant, by site
  unspecified site C71.9
Ependymopathy G93.89
Epidermodysplasia verruciformis B07.8
Epidermolysis
  bullosa (congenital) Q81.9
    dystrophica Q81.2
    letalis Q81.1
    simplex Q81.0
    specified NEC Q81.8
  necroticans combustiformis L51.2
    due to drug—*see* Table of Drugs and Chemicals, by drug
Epididymitis (acute) (nonvenereal) (recurrent) (residual) N45.1
  with orchitis N45.3
  blennorrhagic (gonococcal) A54.23
  chlamydial A56.19
  gonococcal A54.23
  syphilitic A52.76
Epididymo-orchitis (*see also* Epididymitis) N45.3
Epiglottitis, epiglottiditis (acute) J05.10
  with obstruction J05.11
  chronic J37.0
Epilepsia partialis continua (*see also* Kozhevnikof's epilepsy) G40.1-
Epilepsy, epileptic, epilepsia (attack) (cerebral) (convulsion) (fit) (seizure) G40.909
  Note: the following terms are to be considered equivalent to intractable: pharmacoresistant (pharmacologically resistant), treatment resistant, refractory (medically) and poorly controlled
  benign childhood with centrotemporal EEG spikes—*see* Epilepsy, localization-related, idiopathic
  benign myoclonic in infancy G40.80-
  childhood
    with occipital EEG paroxysms—*see* Epilepsy, localization-related, idiopathic
    absence G40.A09
      intractable G40.A19
        with status epilepticus G40.A11
        without status epilepticus G40.A19
      not intractable G40.A09
        with status epilepticus G40.A01
        without status epilepticus G40.A09
  generalized
    idiopathic G40.309
      intractable G40.319
        with status epilepticus G40.311
        without status epilepticus G40.319
      not intractable G40.309
        with status epilepticus G40.301
        without status epilepticus G40.309
    specified NEC G40.409
      intractable G40.419
        with status epilepticus G40.411
        without status epilepticus G40.419
      not intractable G40.409
        with status epilepticus G40.401
        without status epilepticus G40.409
  impulsive petit mal—*see* Epilepsy, juvenile myoclonic
  intractable G40.919
    with status epilepticus G40.911
    without status epilepticus G40.919
  juvenile absence G40.A09
    intractable G40.A19
      with status epilepticus G40.A11
      without status epilepticus G40.A19
    not intractable G40.A09
      with status epilepticus G40.A01
      without status epilepticus G40.A09
  juvenile myoclonic G40.B09
    intractable G40.B19
      with status epilepticus G40.B11
      without status epilepticus G40.B19

EPILEPSY, EPILEPTIC, EPILEPSIA-EVISCERATION

Examination (for) (following) (general) (of) (routine) Z00.00
  with abnormal findings Z00.01
  abuse, physical (alleged), ruled out
    child Z04.72
  adolescent (development state) Z00.3
  alleged rape or sexual assault (victim), ruled out
    child Z04.42
  annual (adult) (periodic) (physical) Z00.00
    with abnormal findings Z00.01
    gynecological Z01.419
      with abnormal findings Z01.411
  blood—see Examination, laboratory
  blood pressure Z01.30
    with abnormal findings Z01.31
  cervical Papanicolaou smear Z12.4
    as part of routine gynecological examination Z01.419
      with abnormal findings Z01.411
  child (over 28 days old) Z00.129
    with abnormal findings Z00.121
    under 28 days old—see Newborn, examination
  contraceptive (drug) maintenance (routine) Z30.8
    device (intrauterine) Z30.431
  ear Z01.10
    with abnormal findings NEC Z01.118
  eye Z01.00
    with abnormal findings Z01.01
  developmental—see Examination, child
  following
    accident NEC Z04.3
      transport Z04.1
      work Z04.2
    assault, alleged, ruled out
      child Z04.72
    motor vehicle accident Z04.1
    treatment (for) Z09
      combined NEC Z09
        fracture Z09
        malignant neoplasm Z08
      malignant neoplasm Z08
      mental disorder Z09
      specified condition NEC Z09
  follow-up (routine) (following) Z09
    chemotherapy NEC Z09
      malignant neoplasm Z08
    fracture Z09
    malignant neoplasm Z08
    radiotherapy NEC Z09
      malignant neoplasm Z08
    surgery NEC Z09
      malignant neoplasm Z08
  gynecological Z01.419
    with abnormal findings Z01.411
    for contraceptive maintenance Z30.8
  health—see Examination, medical
  hearing Z01.10
    with abnormal findings NEC Z01.118
    following failed hearing screening Z01.110
  immunity status testing Z01.84
  laboratory (as part of a general medical examination) Z00.00
    with abnormal findings Z00.01
    preprocedural Z01.812
  lactating mother Z39.1
  medical (adult) (for) (of) Z00.00
    with abnormal findings Z00.01
    administrative purpose only Z02.9
      specified NEC Z02.89
    admission to
      school Z02.0
        following illness or medical treatment Z02.0
      summer camp Z02.89
    adoption Z02.82
    blood alcohol or drug level Z02.83
    camp (summer) Z02.89
    general (adult) Z00.00
      with abnormal findings Z00.01
    medicolegal reasons NEC Z04.8
    participation in sport Z02.5
    pre-operative—see Examination, pre-procedural
    pre-procedural
      cardiovascular Z01.810
      respiratory Z01.811
      specified NEC Z01.818

Examination, *continued*
  preschool children
    for admission to school Z02.0
    sport competition Z02.5
  medicolegal reason NEC Z04.8
  newborn—see Newborn, examination
  pelvic (annual) (periodic) Z01.419
    with abnormal findings Z01.411
  period of rapid growth in childhood Z00.2
  periodic (adult) (annual) (routine) Z00.00
    with abnormal findings Z00.01
  physical (adult)—see also Examination, medical Z00.00
    sports Z02.5
  pre-chemotherapy (antineoplastic) Z01.818
  pre-procedural (pre-operative)
    cardiovascular Z01.810
    laboratory Z01.812
    respiratory Z01.811
    specified NEC Z01.818
  prior to chemotherapy (antineoplastic) Z01.818
  radiological (as part of a general medical examination) Z00.00
    with abnormal findings Z00.01
  repeat cervical smear to confirm findings of recent normal smear following initial abnormal smear Z01.42
  skin (hypersensitivity) Z01.82
  special (see also Examination, by type) Z01.89
    specified type NEC Z01.89
  specified type or reason NEC Z04.8
  teeth Z01.20
    with abnormal findings Z01.21
  urine—see Examination, laboratory
  vision Z01.00
    with abnormal findings Z01.01
Exanthem, exanthema—see also Rash
  with enteroviral vesicular stomatitis B08.4
  subitum B08.20
    due to human herpesvirus 6 B08.21
    due to human herpesvirus 7 B08.22
  viral, virus B09
    specified type NEC B08.8
Excess, excessive, excessively
  alcohol level in blood R78.0
  crying
    in child, adolescent, or adult R45.83
    in infant R68.11
  development, breast N62
  drinking (alcohol) NEC (without dependence) F10.10
    habitual (continual) (without remission) F10.20
  eating R63.2
  foreskin N47.8
  gas R14.0
  large
    colon K59.39
      congenital Q43.8
      toxic K59.31
    infant P08.0
    organ or site, congenital NEC—see Anomaly, by site
  long
    organ or site, congenital NEC—see Anomaly, by site
  menstruation (with regular cycle) N92.0
    with irregular cycle N92.1
  napping Z72.821
  natrium E87.0
  secretion—see also Hypersecretion
    sweat R61
  skin and subcutaneous tissue L98.7
  sodium (Na) E87.0
  sweating R61
  thirst R63.1
    due to deprivation of water T73.1
  weight
    gain R63.5
    loss R63.4
Excitation
  anomalous atrioventricular I45.6
Excoriation (traumatic)—see also Abrasion
  neurotic L98.1
  skin picking disorder F42.4

Exhaustion, exhaustive (physical NEC) R53.83
  battle F43.0
  cardiac—see Failure, heart
  delirium F43.0
  heat (see also Heat, exhaustion) T67.5
    due to
      salt depletion T67.4
      water depletion T67.3
  psychosis F43.0
Exomphalos Q79.2
  meaning hernia—see Hernia, umbilicus
Exotropia—see Strabismus, divergent concomitant
Explanation of
  investigation finding Z71.2
  medication Z71.89
Exposure (to) (also Contact, with) T75.89
  AIDS virus Z20.6
  anthrax Z20.810
  aromatic amines Z77.020
  aromatic (hazardous) compounds NEC Z77.028
  aromatic dyes NOS Z77.028
  arsenic Z77.010
  asbestos Z77.090
  bacterial disease NEC Z20.818
  benzene Z77.021
  body fluids (potentially hazardous) Z77.21
  chemicals (chiefly nonmedicinal) (hazardous) NEC Z77.098
  chromium compounds Z77.018
  communicable disease Z20.9
    bacterial NEC Z20.818
    specified NEC Z20.89
    viral NEC Z20.828
  disaster Z65.5
  dyes Z77.098
  environmental tobacco smoke (acute) (chronic) Z77.22
  Escherichia coli (E. coli) Z20.01
  German measles Z20.4
  gonorrhea Z20.2
  hazardous metals NEC Z77.018
  hazardous substances NEC Z77.29
  hazards in the physical environment NEC Z77.128
  hazards to health NEC Z77.9
  human immunodeficiency virus (HIV) Z20.6
  human T-lymphotropic virus type-1 (HTLV-1) Z20.89
  infestation (parasitic) NEC Z20.7
  intestinal infectious disease NEC Z20.09
    Escherichia coli (E. coli) Z20.01
  lead Z77.011
  meningococcus Z20.811
  mold (toxic) Z77.120
  nickel dust Z77.018
  poliomyelitis Z20.89
  polycyclic aromatic hydrocarbons Z77.028
  prenatal (drugs) (toxic chemicals)—see Newborn, affected by noxious substances transmitted via placenta or breast milk
  rabies Z20.3
  rubella Z20.4
  second hand tobacco smoke (acute) (chronic) Z77.22
    in the perinatal period P96.81
  sexually-transmitted disease Z20.2
  smallpox (laboratory) Z20.89
  syphilis Z20.2
  tuberculosis Z20.1
  varicella Z20.820
  venereal disease Z20.2
  viral disease NEC Z20.828
Exstrophy
  abdominal contents Q45.8
  bladder Q64.10
    cloacal Q64.12
    specified type NEC Q64.19
    supravesical fissure Q64.11
Extrasystoles (supraventricular) I49.49
  atrial I49.1
  auricular I49.1
Extravasation
  pelvicalyceal N13.8
  pyelosinus N13.8
  vesicant agent
    antineoplastic chemotherapy T80.810
    other agent NEC T80.818

F

Failure, failed
aortic (valve) I35.8
  rheumatic I06.8
biventricular I50.9
cardiorenal (chronic) I50.9
cardiorespiratory (*see also* Failure, heart) R09.2
circulation, circulatory (peripheral) R57.9
  newborn P29.89
compensation—*see* Disease, heart
compliance with medical treatment or regimen—*see*
              Noncompliance
expansion terminal respiratory units (newborn) (primary)
              P28.0
gain weight (child over 28 days old) R62.51
  newborn P92.6
heart (acute) (senile) (sudden) I50.9
  biventricular I50.9
  combined left-right sided I50.9
  compensated I50.9
  congestive (compensated) (decompensated) I50.9
    with rheumatic fever (conditions in I00)
      active I01.8
      inactive or quiescent (with chorea) I09.81
    newborn P29.0
    rheumatic (chronic) (inactive) (with chorea) I09.81
      active or acute I01.8
        with chorea I02.0
  decompensated I50.9
    newborn P29.0
  diastolic (congestive) I50.30
    combined with systolic (congestive) I50.40
      acute (congestive) I50.41
        and (on) chronic (congestive) I50.43
      chronic (congestive) I50.42
        and (on) acute (congestive) I50.43
  due to presence of cardiac prosthesis I97.13-
  following cardiac surgery I97.13-
  high output NOS I50.9
  low output (syndrome)NOS I50.9
  systolic (congestive) I50.20
    combined with diastolic (congestive) I50.40
      acute (congestive) I50.41
        and (on) chronic (congestive) I50.43
      chronic (congestive) I50.42
        and (on) acute (congestive) I50.43
  postprocedural I97.13-
kidney (*see also* Disease, kidney, chronic) N19
  acute (*see also* Failure, renal, acute) N17.9-
  diabetic—*see* E08-E13 with .22
mitral I05.8
myocardial, myocardium (*see also* Failure, heart) I50.9
  chronic (*see also* Failure, heart, congestive) I50.9
  congestive (*see also* Failure, heart, congestive) I50.9
ovulation causing infertility N97.0
renal N19
  with
    tubular necrosis (acute) N17.0
  acute N17.9
    with
      cortical necrosis N17.1
      medullary necrosis N17.2
      tubular necrosis N17.0
    specified NEC N17.8
  chronic N18.9
  congenital P96.0
  end stage N18.6
respiration, respiratory J96.90
  with
    hypercapnia J96.92
    hypoxia J96.91
  acute J96.00
    with
      hypercapnia J96.02
      hypoxia J96.01
  center G93.89
  chronic J96.10
    with
      hypercapnia J96.12
      hypoxia J96.11
  newborn P28.5

Failure, failed, *continued*
  postprocedural (acute) J95.821
    acute and chronic J95.822
to thrive (child over 28 days old) R62.51
  newborn P92.6
transplant T86.92
  bone T86.831
    marrow T86.02
  heart T86.22
    with lung (s) T86.32
  kidney T86.12
  liver T86.42
  lung (s) T86.811
    with heart T86.32
  stem cell (peripheral blood) (umbilical cord) T86.5
ventricular (*see also* Failure, heart) I50.9
  left I50.1
    with rheumatic fever (conditions in I00)
      active I01.8
        with chorea I02.0
      inactive or quiescent (with chorea) I09.81
    rheumatic (chronic) (inactive) (with chorea) I09.81
      active or acute I01.8
        with chorea I02.0
  right (*see also* Failure, heart, congestive) I50.9
vital centers, newborn P91.8
Fainting (fit) R55
Fallot's
tetrad or tetralogy Q21.3
Family, familial—*see also* condition
disruption Z63.8
  involving divorce or separation Z63.5
planning advice Z30.09
problem Z63.9
  specified NEC Z63.8
retinoblastoma C69.2-
Fanconi's anemia (congenital pancytopenia) D61.09
Fasciitis M72.9
infective M72.8
  necrotizing M72.6
necrotizing M72.6
Fascioscapulohumeral myopathy G71.0
Fast pulse R00.0
Fat
in stool R19.5
Fatigue R53.83
auditory deafness—*see* Deafness
chronic R53.82
combat F43.0
general R53.83
heat (transient) T67.6
muscle M62.89
Faucitis J02.9
Favism (anemia) D55.0
Favus—*see* Dermatophytosis
Fear complex or reaction F40.9
Fear of—*see* Phobia
Feared complaint unfounded Z71.1
Febris, febrile—*see also* Fever
rubra A38.9
Fecal
incontinence R15.9
smearing R15.1
soiling R15.1
urgency R15.2
Fecalith (impaction) K56.41
Fede's disease K14.0
Feeble rapid pulse due to shock following injury T79.4
Feeble-minded F70
Feeding
difficulties R63.3
problem R63.3
  newborn P92.9
    specified NEC P92.8
  nonorganic (adult)—*see* Disorder, eating
Feeling (of)
foreign body in throat R09.89
Feet—*see* condition
Feigned illness Z76.5
Fetid
breath R19.6

Fetus, fetal—*see also* condition
alcohol syndrome (dysmorphic) Q86.0
lung tissue P28.0
Fever (inanition) (of unknown origin) (persistent) (with chills)
            (with rigor) R50.9
American
  spotted A77.0
Bullis A77.0
catarrhal (acute) J00
  chronic J31.0
cerebrospinal meningococcal A39.0
due to
  conditions classified elsewhere R50.81
  heat T67.0
ephemeral (of unknown origin) R50.9
erysipelatous—*see* Erysipelas
glandular—*see* Mononucleosis, infectious
hay (allergic) J30.1
  with asthma (bronchial) J45.909
    with
      exacerbation (acute) J45.901
      status asthmaticus J45.902
  due to
    allergen other than pollen J30.89
    pollen, any plant or tree J30.1
heat (effects) T67.0
intermittent (bilious)—*see also* Malaria
  of unknown origin R50.9
  pernicious B50.9
Lone Star A77.0
mountain—*see also* Brucellosis
  meaning Rocky Mountain spotted fever A77.0
newborn P81.9
  environmental P81.0
persistent (of unknown origin) R50.9
petechial A39.0
postimmunization R50.83
postoperative R50.82
  due to infection T81.4
posttransfusion R50.84
postvaccination R50.83
presenting with conditions classified elsewhere R50.81
rheumatic (active) (acute) (chronic) (subacute) I00
  with central nervous system involvement I02.9
  active with heart involvement (*see category*) I01
  inactive or quiescent with
    cardiac hypertrophy I09.89
    carditis I09.9
    endocarditis I09.1
      aortic (valve) I06.9
        with mitral (valve) disease I08.0
      mitral (valve) I05.9
        with aortic (valve) disease I08.0
      pulmonary (valve) I09.89
      tricuspid (valve) I07.8
    heart disease NEC I09.89
    heart failure (congestive) (conditions in I50.9)
              I09.81
    left ventricular failure (conditions in I50.1) I09.81
    myocarditis, myocardial degeneration (conditions in
             I51.4) I09.0
    pancarditis I09.9
    pericarditis I09.2
Rocky Mountain spotted A77.0
rose J30.1
Sao Paulo A77.0
spotted A77.9
  American A77.0
  Brazilian A77.0
  cerebrospinal meningitis A39.0
  Columbian A77.0
  due to Rickettsia
    rickettsii A77.0
  Ehrlichiosis A77.40
  Rocky Mountain spotted A77.0
scarlet A38.9
swine A02.8
thermic T67.0
unknown origin R50.9
uveoparotid B86.69

Fever, *continued*
  West Nile (viral) A92.30
    with
      complications NEC A92.39
      cranial nerve disorders A92.32
      encephalitis A92.31
      encephalomyelitis A92.31
      neurologic manifestation NEC A92.32
      optic neuritis A92.32
      polyradiculitis A92.32
  Zika virus A92.5
Fibrillation
  muscular M62.89
Fibrinogenopenia D68.8
  acquired D65
  congenital D68.2
Fibrinolysis (hemorrhagic) (acquired) D65
  newborn, transient P60
Fibrocystic
  disease—*see also* Fibrosis, cystic
    pancreas E84.9
Fibromatosis M72.9
  gingival K06.1
Fibromyxolipoma D17.9
Fibrosis, fibrotic
  anal papillae K62.89
  cystic (of pancreas) E84.9
    with
      distal intestinal obstruction syndrome E84.19
      fecal impaction E84.19
      intestinal manifestations NEC E84.19
      pulmonary manifestations E84.0
      specified manifestations NEC E84.8
  pericardium I31.0
  rectal sphincter K62.89
  skin L90.5
Fibroplasia, retrolental H35.17-
Fiedler's
  myocarditis (acute) I40.1
Fifth disease B08.3
Filatov's disease—*see* Mononucleosis, infectious
Findings, abnormal, inconclusive, without diagnosis—
                              see also Abnormal
  alcohol in blood R78.0
  antenatal screening of mother O28.9
    biochemical O28.1
    chromosomal O28.5
    cytological O28.2
    genetic O28.5
    hematological O28.0
    radiological O28.4
    specified NEC O28.8
    ultrasonic O28.3
  bacteriuria R82.71
  bicarbonate E87.8
  blood sugar R73.09
    high R73.9
    low (transient) E16.2
  chloride E87.8
  cholesterol E78.9
    high E78.00
      with high triglycerides E78.2
  culture
    blood R78.81
    positive—*see* Positive, culture
  echocardiogram R93.1
  glycosuria R81
  heart
    shadow R93.1
    sounds R01.2
  hematinuria R82.3
  hemoglobinuria R82.3
  in blood (of substance not normally found in blood) R78.9
    alcohol (excessive level) R78.0
    lead R78.71
  neonatal screening P09
  PPD R76.11
  radiologic (X-ray) R93.8
    abdomen R93.5
    intrathoracic organs NEC R93.1
    retroperitoneum R93.5
  sodium (deficiency) E87.1
    excess E87.0

Findings, abnormal, inconclusive, without diagnosis,
continued
  sedimentation rate, elevated R70.0
  triglycerides E78.9
    high E78.1
      with high cholesterol E78.2
  tuberculin skin test (without active tuberculosis) R76.11
  urine
    bacteriuria R82.71
    culture positive R82.79
    glucose R81
    hemoglobin R82.3
    sugar R81
Fire, Saint Anthony's—*see* Erysipelas
Fissure, fissured
  anus, anal K60.2
    acute K60.0
    chronic K60.1
    congenital Q43.8
  lip K13.0
    congenital—*see* Cleft, lip
Fistula (cutaneous) L98.8
  abdominothoracic J86.0
  accessory sinuses—*see* Sinusitis
  anus, anal (recurrent) (infectional) K60.3
    congenital Q43.6
  arteriovenous (acquired) (nonruptured) I77.0
    brain I67.1
      congenital Q28.2
        ruptured I60.8
      ruptured I60.8
    cerebral—*see* Fistula, arteriovenous, brain
    congenital (peripheral)—*see also* Malformation,
                                arteriovenous
      brain Q28.2
        ruptured I60.8
      pulmonary Q25.72
    pulmonary I28.0
      congenital Q25.72
    surgically created (for dialysis) Z99.2
  brain G93.89
  breast N61.0
  bronchial J86.0
  bronchocutaneous, bronchomediastinal, bronchopleural,
                                bronchopleuro-
                                mediastinal (infective)
                                J86.0
  bronchoesophageal J86.0
    congenital Q39.2
      with atresia of esophagus Q39.1
  bronchovisceral J86.0
  buccal cavity (infective) K12.2
  chest (wall) J86.0
  costal region J86.0
  cystic duct—*see also* Fistula, gallbladder
    congenital Q44.5
  diaphragm J86.0
  esophagobronchial J86.0
    congenital Q39.2
      with atresia of esophagus Q39.1
  esophagocutaneous K22.8
  esophagopleural-cutaneous J86.0
  esophagotracheal J86.0
    congenital Q39.2
      with atresia of esophagus Q39.1
  esophagus K22.8
    congenital Q39.2
      with atresia of esophagus Q39.1
  ethmoid—*see* Sinusitis, ethmoidal
  hepatopleural J86.0
  hepatopulmonary J86.0
  lip K13.0
    congenital Q38.0
  lung J86.0
  mammary (gland) N61.0
  maxillary J32.0
  mediastinal J86.0
  mediastinobronchial J86.0
  mediastinocutaneous J86.0
  mouth K12.2
  nasal J34.89
    sinus—*see* Sinusitis

Fistula, *continued*
  nose J34.89
  oral (cutaneous) K12.2
    maxillary J32.0
  oroantral J32.0
  parotid (gland) K11.4
    region K12.2
  pleura, pleural, pleurocutaneous, pleuroperitoneal J86.0
  pleuropericardial I31.8
  pulmonary J86.0
    arteriovenous I28.0
      congenital Q25.72
  pulmonoperitoneal J86.0
  rectum (to skin) K60.4
    congenital Q43.6
      with absence, atresia and stenosis Q42.0
  skin L98.8
  submaxillary (gland) K11.4
    region K12.2
  thoracic J86.0
  thoracoabdominal J86.0
  thoracogastric J86.0
  thoracointestinal J86.0
  thorax J86.0
  thyroglossal duct Q89.2
  tracheoesophageal J86.0
    congenital Q39.2
      with atresia of esophagus Q39.1
Fit R56.9
  epileptic—*see* Epilepsy
  fainting R55
  newborn P90
Flat
  foot (acquired) (fixed type) (painful) (postural)—*see also*
                                Deformity, limb, flat foot
    congenital (rigid) (spastic (everted)) Q66.5-
  pelvis M95.5
    congenital Q74.2
Flattening
  nose (congenital) Q67.4
    acquired M95.0
Flatulence R14.3
  psychogenic F45.8
Flexion
  deformity, joint (*see also* Deformity, limb, flexion) M21.20
    hip, congenital Q65.89
Flint murmur (aortic insufficiency) I35.1
Floating
  gallbladder, congenital Q44.1
Flooding N92.0
Floppy
  baby syndrome (nonspecific) P94.2
Flu—*see also* Influenza
  avian (*see also* Influenza, due to, identified novel influenza
                                A virus) J09.X2
  bird (*see also* Influenza, due to, identified novel influenza A
                                virus) J09.X2
  intestinal NEC A08.4
  swine (viruses that normally cause infections in pigs)
                                (*see also* Influenza,
                                due to, identified novel
                                influenza A virus)
                                J09.X2
Fluid
  abdomen R18.8
  loss (acute) E86.9
  peritoneal cavity R18.8
  retention R60.9
Fluoride varnish application Z29.3
FNHTR (febrile nonhemolytic transfusion reaction) R50.84
Follicle
  graafian, ruptured, with hemorrhage N83.0-
Folliculitis (superficial) L73.9
  cyst N83.0-
  gonococcal (acute) (chronic) A54.01
Folling's disease E70.0
Follow-up—*see* Examination, follow-up
Food
  allergy L27.2
  asphyxia (from aspiration or inhalation)—*see* Foreign
                                body, by site
  choked on—*see* Foreign body, by site
  cyst N83.0-

Foreign body, *continued*

leg (lower) S80.85-
    knee S80.25-
    upper—*see* Foreign body, superficial, thigh
lip S00.551
lower back S30.850
lumbar region S30.850
malar region S00.85
mammary—*see* Foreign body, superficial, breast
mastoid region S00.85
mouth S00.552
nail
    finger—*see* Foreign body, superficial, finger
    toe—*see* Foreign body, superficial, toe
nape S10.85
nasal S00.35
neck S10.95
    specified site NEC S10.85
    throat S10.15
nose S00.35
occipital region S00.05
oral cavity S00.552
orbital region—*see* Foreign body, superficial, eyelid
palate S00.552
palm—*see* Foreign body, superficial, hand
parietal region S00.05
pelvis S30.850
penis S30.852
perineum
    female S30.854
    male S30.850
periocular area S00.25-
phalanges
    finger—*see* Foreign body, superficial, finger
    toe—*see* Foreign body, superficial, toe
pharynx S10.15
pinna S00.45-
popliteal space S80.25-
prepuce S30.852
pubic region S30.850
pudendum
    female S30.856
    male S30.855
sacral region S30.850
scalp S00.05
scapular region S40.25-
scrotum S30.853
shin S80.85-
shoulder S40.25-
sternal region S20.359
submaxillary region S00.85
submental region S00.85
subungual
    finger (s)—*see* Foreign body, superficial, finger
    toe (s)—*see* Foreign body, superficial, toe
supraclavicular fossa S10.85
supraorbital S00.85
temple S00.85
temporal region S00.85
testis S30.853
thigh S70.35-
thorax, thoracic (wall) S20.95
    back S20.45-
    front S20.35-
throat S10.15
thumb S60.35-
toe (s) (lesser) S90.456
    great S90.45-
tongue S00.552
trachea S10.15
tunica vaginalis S30.853
tympanum, tympanic membrane S00.45-
uvula S00.552
vagina S30.854
vocal cords S10.15
vulva S30.854
wrist S60.85-
swallowed T18.9
trachea T17.408
    causing
        asphyxiation T17.400
            food (bone) (seed) T17.420

Foreign body, *continued*

    gastric contents (vomitus) T17.410
    specified type NEC T17.490
    injury NEC T17.408
        food (bone) (seed) T17.428
        gastric contents (vomitus) T17.418
        specified type NEC T17.498
type of fragment—*see* Retained, foreign body fragments
            (type of)

Fothergill's

disease (trigeminal neuralgia)—*see also* Neuralgia,
            trigeminal
    scarlatina anginosa A38.9

Foul breath R19.6
Foundling Z76.1
Fracture (abduction) (adduction) (separation) T14.8

acetabulum S32.40-
    column
        anterior (displaced) (iliopubic) S32.43-
            nondisplaced S32.436
        posterior (displaced) (ilioischial) S32.443
            nondisplaced S32.44-
    dome (displaced) S32.48-
        nondisplaced S32.48
    specified NEC S32.49-
    transverse (displaced) S32.45-
        with associated posterior wall fracture (displaced)
            S32.46-
            nondisplaced S32.46-
        nondisplaced S32.45-
    wall
        anterior (displaced) S32.41-
            nondisplaced S32.41-
        medial (displaced) S32.47-
            nondisplaced S32.47-
        posterior (displaced) S32.42-
            with associated transverse fracture (displaced)
                S32.46-
                nondisplaced S32.46-
            nondisplaced S32.42-
ankle S82.899
    bimalleolar (displaced) S82.84-
        nondisplaced S82.84-
    lateral malleolus only (displaced) S82.6-
        nondisplaced S82.6-
    medial malleolus (displaced) S82.5-
        associated with Maisonneuve's fracture—*see*
                Fracture,
                Maisonneuve's
        nondisplaced S82.5-
    talus—*see* Fracture, tarsal, talus
    trimalleolar (displaced) S82.85-
        nondisplaced S82.85-
arm (upper)—*see also* Fracture, humerus, shaft
    humerus—*see* Fracture, humerus
    radius—*see* Fracture, radius
    ulna—*see* Fracture, ulna
astragalus—*see* Fracture, tarsal, talus
Barton's—*see* Barton's fracture
base of skull—*see* Fracture, skull, base
basicervical (basal) (femoral) S72.0
Bennett's—*see* Bennett's fracture
bimalleolar—*see* Fracture, ankle, bimalleolar
blowout S02.3-
bone NEC T14.8
    birth injury P13.9
    following insertion of orthopedic implant, joint
                prosthesis or bone
                plate—*see* Fracture,
                following insertion of
                orthopedic implant,
                joint prosthesis or bone
                plate
    in (due to) neoplastic disease NEC—*see* Fracture,
                pathological, due to,
                neoplastic disease
burst—*see* Fracture, traumatic, by site
calcaneus—*see* Fracture, tarsal, calcaneus
carpal bone (s) S62.10-
    capitate (displaced) S62.13-
        nondisplaced S62.13-
    cuneiform—*see* Fracture, carpal bone, triquetrum
    hamate (body) (displaced) S62.143

Fracture, *continued*

hook process (displaced) S62.15-
    nondisplaced S62.15-
    nondisplaced S62.14-
larger multangular—*see* Fracture, carpal bones,
              trapezium
lunate (displaced) S62.12-
    nondisplaced S62.12-
navicular S62.00-
    distal pole (displaced) S62.01-
        nondisplaced S62.01-
    middle third (displaced) S62.02-
        nondisplaced S62.02-
    proximal third (displaced) S62.03-
        nondisplaced S62.03-
    volar tuberosity—*see* Fracture, carpal bones,
              navicular, distal pole
os magnum—*see* Fracture, carpal bones, capitate
pisiform (displaced) S62.16-
    nondisplaced S62.16-
semilunar—*see* Fracture, carpal bones, lunate
smaller multangular—*see* Fracture, carpal bones,
              trapezoid
trapezium (displaced) S62.17-
    nondisplaced S62.17-
trapezoid (displaced) S62.18-
    nondisplaced S62.18-
triquetrum (displaced) S62.11-
    nondisplaced S62.11-
unciform—*see* Fracture, carpal bones, hamate
clavicle S42.00-
    acromial end (displaced) S42.03-
        nondisplaced S42.03-
    birth injury P13.4
    lateral end—*see* Fracture, clavicle, acromial end
    shaft (displaced) S42.02-
        nondisplaced S42.02-
    sternal end (anterior) (displaced) S42.01-
        nondisplaced S42.01-
        posterior S42.01-
coccyx S32.2
collar bone—*see* Fracture, clavicle
Colles'—*see* Colles' fracture
coronoid process—*see* Fracture, ulna, upper end,
              coronoid process
corpus cavernosum penis S39.840
costochondral, costosternal junction—*see* Fracture, rib
cranium—*see* Fracture, skull
cricoid cartilage S12.8
cuboid (ankle)—*see* Fracture, tarsal, cuboid
cuneiform
    foot—*see* Fracture, tarsal, cuneiform
    wrist—*see* Fracture, carpal, triquetrum
delayed union—*see* Delay, union, fracture
due to
    birth injury—*see* Birth, injury, fracture
Dupuytren's—*see* Fracture, ankle, lateral malleolus
elbow S42.40-
ethmoid (bone) (sinus)—*see* Fracture, skull, base
face bone S02.92-
fatigue—*see also* Fracture, stress
femur, femoral S72.9-
    basicervical (basal) S72.0
    birth injury P13.2
    capital epiphyseal S79.01-
    condyles, epicondyles—*see* Fracture, femur, lower end
    distal end—*see* Fracture, femur, lower end
    epiphysis
        head—*see* Fracture, femur, upper end, epiphysis
        lower—*see* Fracture, femur, lower end, epiphysis
        upper—*see* Fracture, femur, upper end, epiphysis
    head—*see* Fracture, femur, upper end, head
    intertrochanteric—*see* Fracture, femur, trochanteric
    intratrochanteric—*see* Fracture, femur, trochanteric
    lower end S72.40-
        condyle (displaced) S72.41-
            lateral (displaced) S72.42-
                nondisplaced S72.42-
            medial (displaced) S72.43-
                nondisplaced S72.43-
            nondisplaced S72.41-
        epiphysis (displaced) S72.44-
            nondisplaced S72.44-

Fracture, *continued*
  physeal S79.10-
    Salter-Harris
      Type I S79.11-
      Type II S79.12-
      Type III S79.13-
      Type IV S79.14-
      specified NEC S79.19-
  specified NEC S72.49-
  supracondylar (displaced) S72.45-
    with intracondylar extension (displaced)
      S72.46-
    nondisplaced S72.46-
  nondisplaced S72.45-
  torus S72.47-
  neck—*see* Fracture, femur, upper end, neck
  pertrochanteric—*see* Fracture, femur, trochanteric
  shaft (lower third) (middle third) (upper third) S72.30-
    comminuted (displaced) S72.35-
      nondisplaced S72.35-
    oblique (displaced) S72.33-
      nondisplaced S72.33-
    segmental (displaced) S72.36-
      nondisplaced S72.36-
    specified NEC S72.39-
    spiral (displaced) S72.34-
      nondisplaced S72.34-
    transverse (displaced) S72.32-
      nondisplaced S72.32-
  specified site NEC—*see* subcategory S72.8
  subcapital (displaced) S72.01-
  subtrochanteric (region) (section) (displaced) S72.2-
    nondisplaced S72.2-
  transcervical—*see* Fracture, femur, upper end, neck
  transtrochanteric—*see* Fracture, femur, trochanteric
  trochanteric S72.10-
    apophyseal (displaced) S72.13-
      nondisplaced S72.13-
    greater trochanter (displaced) S72.11-
      nondisplaced S72.11-
    intertrochanteric (displaced) S72.14-
      nondisplaced S72.14-
    lesser trochanter (displaced) S72.12-
      nondisplaced S72.12-
  upper end S72.00-
    apophyseal (displaced) S72.13-
      nondisplaced S72.13-
    cervicotrochanteric—*see* Fracture, femur, upper
      end, neck, base
    epiphysis (displaced) S72.02-
      nondisplaced S72.02-
    head S72.05-
      articular (displaced) S72.06-
        nondisplaced S72.06-
      specified NEC S72.09-
    intertrochanteric (displaced) S72.14-
      nondisplaced S72.14-
    intracapsular S72.01-
    midcervical (displaced) S72.03-
      nondisplaced S72.03-
    neck S72.00-
      base (displaced) S72.04-
        nondisplaced S72.04-
      specified NEC S72.09-
    pertrochanteric—*see* Fracture, femur, upper end,
      trochanteric
  physeal S79.00-
    Salter-Harris type I S79.01-
    specified NEC S79.09-
  subcapital (displaced) S72.01-
  subtrochanteric (displaced) S72.2-
    nondisplaced S72.2-
  transcervical—*see* Fracture, femur, upper end,
    midcervical
  trochanteric S72.10-
    greater (displaced) S72.11-
      nondisplaced S72.11-
    lesser (displaced) S72.12-
      nondisplaced S72.12-
fibula (shaft) (styloid) S82.40-
  comminuted (displaced) S82.45-
    nondisplaced S82.45-

Fracture, *continued*
  involving ankle or malleolus—*see* Fracture, fibula,
    lateral malleolus
  lateral malleolus (displaced) S82.6-
    nondisplaced S82.6-
  lower end
    physeal S89.30-
      Salter-Harris
        Type I S89.31-
        Type II S89.32-
        specified NEC S89.39-
    specified NEC S82.83-
    torus S82.82-
  oblique (displaced) S82.43-
    nondisplaced S82.43-
  segmental (displaced) S82.46-
    nondisplaced S82.46-
  specified NEC S82.49-
  spiral (displaced) S82.44-
    nondisplaced S82.44-
  transverse (displaced) S82.42-
    nondisplaced S82.42-
  upper end
    physeal S89.20-
      Salter-Harris
        Type I S89.21-
        Type II S89.22-
        specified NEC S89.29-
    specified NEC S82.83-
    torus S82.81-
  finger (except thumb) S62.60-
    distal phalanx (displaced) S62.63-
      nondisplaced S62.66-
    index S62.60-
      distal phalanx (displaced) S62.63-
        nondisplaced S62.66-
      medial phalanx (displaced) S62.62-
        nondisplaced S62.65-
      proximal phalanx (displaced) S62.61-
        nondisplaced S62.64-
    little S62.60-
      distal phalanx (displaced) S62.63-
        nondisplaced S62.66-
      medial phalanx (displaced) S62.62-
        nondisplaced S62.65-
      proximal phalanx (displaced) S62.61-
        nondisplaced S62.64-
    medial phalanx (displaced) S62.62-
      nondisplaced S62.65-
    middle S62.60-
      distal phalanx (displaced) S62.63-
        nondisplaced S62.66-
      medial phalanx (displaced) S62.62-
        nondisplaced S62.65-
      proximal phalanx (displaced) S62.61-
        nondisplaced S62.64-
    proximal phalanx (displaced) S62.61-
      nondisplaced S62.64-
    ring S62.60-
      distal phalanx (displaced) S62.63-
        nondisplaced S62.66-
      medial phalanx (displaced) S62.62-
        nondisplaced S62.65-
      proximal phalanx (displaced) S62.61-
        nondisplaced S62.64-
    thumb—*see* Fracture, thumb
  foot S92.90-
    astragalus—*see* Fracture, tarsal, talus
    calcaneus—*see* Fracture, tarsal, calcaneus
    cuboid—*see* Fracture, tarsal, cuboid
    cuneiform—*see* Fracture, tarsal, cuneiform
    metatarsal—*see* Fracture, metatarsal
    navicular—*see* Fracture, tarsal, navicular
    sesamoid S92.81-
    talus—*see* Fracture, tarsal, talus
    tarsal—*see* Fracture, tarsal
    toe—*see* Fracture, toe
  forearm S52.9-
    radius—*see* Fracture, radius
    ulna—*see* Fracture, ulna
  fossa (anterior) (middle) (posterior) S02.19-
  frontal (bone) (skull) S02.0-
    sinus S02.19-

Fracture, *continued*
  greenstick—*see* Fracture, by site
  hallux—*see* Fracture, toe, great
  hand S62.9-
    carpal—*see* Fracture, carpal bone
    finger (except thumb)—*see* Fracture, finger
    metacarpal—*see* Fracture, metacarpal
    navicular (scaphoid) (hand)—*see* Fracture, carpal
      bone, navicular
    thumb—*see* Fracture, thumb
  healed or old
    with complications—*code by* Nature of the
      complication
  heel bone—*see* Fracture, tarsal, calcaneus
  Hill-Sachs S42.29-
  hip—*see* Fracture, femur, neck
  humerus S42.30-
    anatomical neck—*see* Fracture, humerus, upper end
    articular process—*see* Fracture, humerus, lower end
    capitellum—*see* Fracture, humerus, lower end,
      condyle, lateral
    distal end—*see* Fracture, humerus, lower end
    epiphysis
      lower—*see* Fracture, humerus, lower end, physeal
      upper—*see* Fracture, humerus, upper end, physeal
    external condyle—*see* Fracture, humerus, lower end,
      condyle, lateral
    great tuberosity—*see* Fracture, humerus, upper end,
      greater tuberosity
    intercondylar—*see* Fracture, humerus, lower end
    internal epicondyle—*see* Fracture, humerus, lower
      end, epicondyle, medial
    lesser tuberosity—*see* Fracture, humerus, upper end,
      lesser tuberosity
    lower end S42.40-
      condyle
        lateral (displaced) S42.45-
          nondisplaced S42.45-
        medial (displaced) S42.46-
          nondisplaced S42.46-
      epicondyle
        lateral (displaced) S42.43-
          nondisplaced S42.43-
        medial (displaced) S42.44-
          incarcerated S42.44-
          nondisplaced S42.44-
      physeal S49.10-
        Salter-Harris
          Type I S49.11-
          Type II S49.12-
          Type III S49.13-
          Type IV S49.14-
          specified NEC S49.19-
      specified NEC (displaced) S42.49-
        nondisplaced S42.49-
      supracondylar (simple) (displaced) S42.41-
        comminuted (displaced) S42.42-
          nondisplaced S42.42-
        nondisplaced S42.41-
      torus S42.48-
      transcondylar (displaced) S42.47-
        nondisplaced S42.47-
    proximal end—*see* Fracture, humerus, upper end
    shaft S42.30-
      comminuted (displaced) S42.35-
        nondisplaced S42.35-
      greenstick S42.31-
      oblique (displaced) S42.33
        nondisplaced S42.33-
      segmental (displaced) S42.36-
        nondisplaced S42.36-
      specified NEC S42.39-
      spiral (displaced) S42.34-
        nondisplaced S42.34-
      transverse (displaced) S42.32-
        nondisplaced S42.32-
    supracondylar—*see* Fracture, humerus, lower end
    surgical neck—*see* Fracture, humerus, upper end,
      surgical neck
    trochlea—*see* Fracture, humerus, lower end, condyle,
      medial
    tuberosity—*see* Fracture, humerus, upper end
    upper end S42.20-

Fracture, *continued*

anatomical neck—*see* Fracture, humerus, upper end, specified NEC
articular head—*see* Fracture, humerus, upper end, specified NEC
epiphysis—*see* Fracture, humerus, upper end, physeal
greater tuberosity (displaced) S42.25-
   nondisplaced S42.25-
lesser tuberosity (displaced) S42.26-
   nondisplaced S42.26-
physeal S49.00-
   Salter-Harris
     Type I S49.01-
     Type II S49.02-
     Type III S49.03-
     Type IV S49.04-
   specified NEC S49.09-
specified NEC (displaced) S42.29-
   nondisplaced S42.29-
surgical neck (displaced) S42.21-
   four-part S42.24-
   nondisplaced S42.21-
   three-part S42.23-
   two-part (displaced) S42.22-
     nondisplaced S42.22-
torus S42.27-
transepiphyseal—*see* Fracture, humerus, upper end, physeal
hyoid bone S12.8
ilium S32.30-
   with disruption of pelvic ring—*see* Disruption, pelvic ring
   avulsion (displaced) S32.31-
     nondisplaced S32.31-
   specified NEC S32.39-
impaction, impacted—*code as* Fracture, by site
innominate bone—*see* Fracture, ilium
instep—*see* Fracture, foot
ischium S32.60-
   with disruption of pelvic ring—*see* Disruption, pelvic ring
   avulsion (displaced) S32.61-
     nondisplaced S32.61-
   specified NEC S32.69-
jaw (bone) (lower)—*see* Fracture, mandible
   upper—*see* Fracture, maxilla
knee cap—*see* Fracture, patella
larynx S12.8
late effects—*see* Sequelae, fracture
leg (lower) S82.9-
   ankle—*see* Fracture, ankle
   femur—*see* Fracture, femur
   fibula—*see* Fracture, fibula
   malleolus—*see* Fracture, ankle
   patella—*see* Fracture, patella
   specified site NEC S82.89-
   tibia—*see* Fracture, tibia
lumbosacral spine S32.9
Maisonneuve's (displaced) S82.86-
   nondisplaced S82.86-
malar bone (*see also* Fracture, maxilla) S02.40-
malleolus—*see* Fracture, ankle
malunion—*see* Fracture, by site
mandible (lower jaw (bone)) S02.609-
   alveolus S02.67-
   angle (of jaw) S02.65-
   body, unspecified S02.60-
   condylar process S02.61-
   coronoid process S02.63-
   ramus, unspecified S02.64-
   specified site NEC S02.69-
   subcondylar process S02.62-
   symphysis S02.66-
march—*see* Fracture, traumatic, stress, by site
metacarpal S62.309
   base (displaced) S62.319
     nondisplaced S62.349
   fifth S62.30-
     base (displaced) S62.31-
       nondisplaced S62.34-
     neck (displaced) S62.33-
       nondisplaced S62.36-

Fracture, *continued*

shaft (displaced) S62.32-
     nondisplaced S62.35-
   specified NEC S62.398
first S62.20-
   base NEC (displaced) S62.23-
     nondisplaced S62.23-
   Bennett's—*see* Bennett's fracture
   neck (displaced) S62.25-
     nondisplaced S62.25-
   shaft (displaced) S62.24-
     nondisplaced S62.24-
   specified NEC S62.29-
fourth S62.30-
   base (displaced) S62.31-
     nondisplaced S62.34-
   neck (displaced) S62.33-
     nondisplaced S62.36-
   shaft (displaced) S62.32-
     nondisplaced S62.35-
   specified NEC S62.39-
neck (displaced) S62.33-
   nondisplaced S62.36-
Rolando's—*see* Rolando's fracture
second S62.30-
   base (displaced) S62.31-
     nondisplaced S62.34-
   neck (displaced) S62.33-
     nondisplaced S62.36-
   shaft (displaced) S62.32-
     nondisplaced S62.35-
   specified NEC S62.39-
shaft (displaced) S62.32-
   nondisplaced S62.35-
third S62.30-
   base (displaced) S62.31-
     nondisplaced S62.34-
   neck (displaced) S62.33-
     nondisplaced S62.36-
   shaft (displaced) S62.32-
     nondisplaced S62.35-
   specified NEC S62.39-
specified NEC S62.399
metastatic—*see* Fracture, pathological, due to, neoplastic disease—*see also* Neoplasm
metatarsal bone S92.30-
   fifth (displaced) S92.35-
     nondisplaced S92.35-
   first (displaced) S92.31-
     nondisplaced S92.31-
   fourth (displaced) S92.34-
     nondisplaced S92.34-
   second (displaced) S92.32-
     nondisplaced S92.32-
   third (displaced) S92.33-
     nondisplaced S92.33-
   physeal S99.10-
     Salter-Harris
       Type I S99.11-
       Type II S99.12-
       Type III S99.13-
       Type IV S99.14-
     specified NEC S99.19-
Monteggia's—*see* Monteggia's fracture
multiple
   hand (and wrist) NEC—*see* Fracture, by site
   ribs—*see* Fracture, rib, multiple
nasal (bone(s)) S02.2-
navicular (scaphoid) (foot)—*see also* Fracture, tarsal, navicular
   hand—*see* Fracture, carpal, navicular
neck S12.9
   cervical vertebra S12.9
     fifth (displaced) S12.400
       nondisplaced S12.401
       specified type NEC (displaced) S12.490
         nondisplaced S12.491
     first (displaced) S12.000
       burst (stable) S12.01
         unstable S12.02
       lateral mass (displaced) S12.040
         nondisplaced S12.041

Fracture, *continued*

nondisplaced S12.001
posterior arch (displaced) S12.030
   nondisplaced S12.031
specified type NEC (displaced) S12.090
   nondisplaced S12.091
fourth (displaced) S12.300
   nondisplaced S12.301
   specified type NEC (displaced) S12.390
     nondisplaced S12.391
second (displaced) S12.100
   nondisplaced S12.101
   dens (anterior) (displaced) (type II) S12.110
     nondisplaced S12.112
     posterior S12.111
   specified type NEC (displaced) S12.120
     nondisplaced S12.121
   specified type NEC (displaced) S12.190
     nondisplaced S12.191
seventh (displaced) S12.600
   nondisplaced S12.601
   specified type NEC (displaced) S12.690
     displaced S12.691
sixth (displaced) S12.500
   nondisplaced S12.501
   specified type NEC (displaced) S12.590
     displaced S12.591
third (displaced) S12.200
   nondisplaced S12.201
   specified type NEC (displaced) S12.290
     displaced S12.291
hyoid bone S12.8
larynx S12.8
specified site NEC S12.8
thyroid cartilage S12.8
trachea S12.8
neoplastic NEC—*see* Fracture, pathological, due to, neoplastic disease
newborn—*see* Birth, injury, fracture
nontraumatic—*see* Fracture, pathological
nonunion—*see* Nonunion, fracture
nose, nasal (bone) (septum) S02.2-
occiput—*see* Fracture, skull, base, occiput
olecranon (process) (ulna)—*see* Fracture, ulna, upper end, olecranon process
orbit, orbital (bone) (region) S02.8-
   floor (blow-out) S02.3-
   roof S02.19-
   calcis—*see* Fracture, tarsal, calcaneus
   magnum—*see* Fracture, carpal, capitate
   pubis—*see* Fracture, pubis
palate S02.8-
parietal bone (skull) S02.0-
patella S82.00-
   comminuted (displaced) S82.04-
     nondisplaced S82.04-
   longitudinal (displaced) S82.02-
     nondisplaced S82.02-
   osteochondral (displaced) S82.01-
     nondisplaced S82.01-
   specified NEC S82.09-
   transverse (displaced) S82.03-
     nondisplaced S82.03-
pedicle (of vertebral arch)—*see* Fracture, vertebra
pelvis, pelvic (bone) S32.9
   acetabulum—*see* Fracture, acetabulum
   circle—*see* Disruption, pelvic ring
   ilium—*see* Fracture, ilium
   ischium—*see* Fracture, ischium
   multiple
     with disruption of pelvic ring (circle)—*see* Disruption, pelvic ring
     without disruption of pelvic ring (circle) S32.82
   pubis—*see* Fracture, pubis
   specified site NEC S32.89
   sacrum—*see* Fracture, sacrum
phalanx
   foot—*see* Fracture, toe
   hand—*see* Fracture, finger
pisiform—*see* Fracture, carpal, pisiform
pond—*see* Fracture, skull

Fracture, *continued*
- prosthetic device, internal—*see* Complications, prosthetic device, by site, mechanical
- pubis S32.50-
  - with disruption of pelvic ring—*see* Disruption, pelvic ring
  - specified site NEC S32.59-
  - superior rim S32.51-
- radius S52.9-
  - distal end—*see* Fracture, radius, lower end
  - head—*see* Fracture, radius, upper end, head
  - lower end S52.50-
    - Barton's—*see* Barton's fracture
    - Colles'—*see* Colles' fracture
    - extraarticular NEC S52.55-
    - intraarticular NEC S52.57-
    - physeal S59.20-
      - Salter-Harris
        - Type I S59.21-
        - Type II S59.22-
        - Type III S59.23-
        - Type IV S59.24-
        - specified NEC S59.29-
    - Smith's—*see* Smith's fracture
    - specified NEC S52.59-
    - styloid process (displaced) S52.51-
      - nondisplaced S52.51-
    - torus S52.52-
  - neck—*see* Fracture, radius, upper end
  - proximal end—*see* Fracture, radius, upper end
  - shaft S52.30-
    - bent bone S52.38-
    - comminuted (displaced) S52.35-
      - nondisplaced S52.35-
    - Galeazzi's—*see* Galeazzi's fracture
    - greenstick S52.31-
    - oblique (displaced) S52.33-
      - nondisplaced S52.33-
    - segmental (displaced) S52.36-
      - nondisplaced S52.36-
    - specified NEC S52.39-
    - spiral (displaced) S52.34-
      - nondisplaced S52.34-
    - transverse (displaced) S52.32-
      - nondisplaced S52.32-
  - upper end S52.10-
    - head (displaced) S52.12-
      - nondisplaced S52.12-
    - neck (displaced) S52.13-
      - nondisplaced S52.13-
    - specified NEC S52.18-
    - physeal S59.10-
      - Salter-Harris
        - Type I S59.11-
        - Type II S59.12-
        - Type III S59.13-
        - Type IV S59.14-
        - specified NEC S59.19-
    - torus S52.11-
- ramus
  - inferior or superior, pubis—*see* Fracture, pubis
  - mandible—*see* Fracture, mandible
- rib S22.3-
  - with flail chest—*see* Flail, chest
  - multiple S22.4-
    - with flail chest—*see* Flail, chest
- root, tooth—*see* Fracture, tooth
- sacrum S32.10
  - specified NEC S32.19
  - Type
    - 1 S32.14
    - 2 S32.15
    - 3 S32.16
    - 4 S32.17
  - Zone
    - I S32.119
      - displaced (minimally) S32.111
        - severely S32.112
      - nondisplaced S32.110

Fracture, *continued*
- II S32.129
  - displaced (minimally) S32.121
    - severely S32.122
  - nondisplaced S32.120
- III S32.139
  - displaced (minimally) S32.131
    - severely S32.132
  - nondisplaced S32.130
- scaphoid (hand)—*see also* Fracture, carpal, navicular
  - foot—*see* Fracture, tarsal, navicular
- semilunar bone, wrist—*see* Fracture, carpal, lunate
- sequelae—*see* Sequelae, fracture
- sesamoid bone
  - foot S92.81-
  - hand—*see* Fracture, carpal
  - other—*code by* site under Fracture
- shepherd's—*see* Fracture, tarsal, talus
- shoulder (girdle) S42.9-
- sinus (ethmoid) (frontal) S02.19-
- skull S02.91-
  - base S02.10-
    - occiput S02.119
      - condyle S02.11-
        - type I S02.11-
        - type II S02.11-
        - type III S02.11
    - specified NEC S02.118-
    - specified NEC S02.19-
  - birth injury P13.0
  - frontal bone S02.0-
  - parietal bone S02.0-
  - specified site NEC S02.8-
  - temporal bone S02.19-
  - vault S02.0-
- Smith's—*see* Smith's fracture
- sphenoid (bone) (sinus) S02.19-
- spontaneous (cause unknown)—*see* Fracture, pathological
- stave (of thumb)—*see* Fracture, metacarpal, first
- sternum S22.20
  - with flail chest—*see* Flail, chest
  - body S22.22
  - manubrium S22.21
  - xiphoid (process) S22.24
- stress M84.30
  - ankle M84.37-
  - carpus M84.34-
  - clavicle M84.31-
  - femoral neck M84.359
  - femur M84.35-
  - fibula M84.36-
  - finger M84.34-
  - hip M84.359
  - humerus M84.32-
  - ilium M84.350
  - ischium M84.350
  - metacarpus M84.34-
  - metatarsus M84.37-
  - pelvis M84.350
  - radius M84.33-
  - rib M84.38
  - scapula M84.31-
  - skull M84.38
  - tarsus M84.37-
  - tibia M84.36-
  - toe M84.37-
  - ulna M84.33-
- supracondylar, elbow—*see* Fracture, humerus, lower end, supracondylar
- symphysis pubis—*see* Fracture, pubis
- talus (ankle bone)—*see* Fracture, tarsal, talus
- tarsal bone (s) S92.20-
  - astragalus—*see* Fracture, tarsal, talus
  - calcaneus S92.00-
    - anterior process (displaced) S92.02-
      - nondisplaced S92.02-
    - body (displaced) S92.01-
      - nondisplaced S92.01-
    - extraarticular NEC (displaced) S92.05-
      - nondisplaced S92.05-

Fracture, *continued*
- intraarticular (displaced) S92.06-
  - nondisplaced S92.06-
- physeal S99.00-
  - Salter-Harris
    - Type I S99.01-
    - Type II S99.02-
    - Type III S99.03-
    - Type IV S99.04-
    - specified NEC S99.09-
- tuberosity (displaced) S92.04-
  - avulsion (displaced) S92.03-
    - nondisplaced S92.03-
  - nondisplaced S92.04-
- cuboid (displaced) S92.21-
  - nondisplaced S92.21-
- cuneiform
  - intermediate (displaced) S92.23-
    - nondisplaced S92.23-
  - lateral (displaced) S92.22-
    - nondisplaced S92.22-
  - medial (displaced) S92.24-
    - nondisplaced S92.24-
- navicular (displaced) S92.25-
  - nondisplaced S92.25-
- scaphoid—*see* Fracture, tarsal, navicular
- talus S92.10-
  - avulsion (displaced) S92.15-
    - nondisplaced S92.15-
  - body (displaced) S92.12-
    - nondisplaced S92.12-
  - dome (displaced) S92.14-
    - nondisplaced S92.14-
  - head (displaced) S92.12-
    - nondisplaced S92.12-
  - lateral process (displaced) S92.14-
    - nondisplaced S92.14-
  - neck (displaced) S92.11-
    - nondisplaced S92.11-
  - posterior process (displaced) S92.13-
    - nondisplaced S92.13-
  - specified NEC S92.19-
- temporal bone (styloid) S02.19-
- thorax (bony) S22.9
  - with flail chest—*see* Flail, chest
  - rib S22.3-
    - multiple S22.4-
      - with flail chest—*see* Flail, chest
- thumb S62.50-
  - distal phalanx (displaced) S62.52-
    - nondisplaced S62.52-
  - proximal phalanx (displaced) S62.51-
    - nondisplaced S62.51-
- thyroid cartilage S12.8
- tibia (shaft) S82.20-
  - comminuted (displaced) S82.25-
    - nondisplaced S82.25-
  - condyles—*see* Fracture, tibia, upper end
  - distal end—*see* Fracture, tibia, lower end
  - epiphysis
    - lower—*see* Fracture, tibia, lower end
    - upper—*see* Fracture, tibia, upper end
  - head (involving knee joint)—*see* Fracture, tibia, upper end
  - intercondyloid eminence—*see* Fracture, tibia, upper end
  - involving ankle or malleolus—*see* Fracture, ankle, medial malleolus
  - lower end S82.30-
    - physeal S89.10-
      - Salter-Harris
        - Type I S89.11-
        - Type II S89.12-
        - Type III S89.13-
        - Type IV S89.14-
        - specified NEC S89.19-
    - pilon (displaced) S82.87-
      - nondisplaced S82.87-
    - specified NEC S82.39-
    - torus S82.31-
  - malleolus—*see* Fracture, ankle, medial malleolus

FRACTURE-FRACTURE

Fracture, *continued*
  oblique (displaced) S82.23-
    nondisplaced S82.23-
  pilon—*see* Fracture, tibia, lower end, pilon
  proximal end—*see* Fracture, tibia, upper end
  segmental (displaced) S82.26-
    nondisplaced S82.26-
  specified NEC S82.29-
  spiral (displaced) S82.24-
    nondisplaced S82.24-
  transverse (displaced) S82.22-
    nondisplaced S82.22-
  tuberosity—*see* Fracture, tibia, upper end, tuberosity
  upper end S82.10-
    bicondylar (displaced) S82.14-
      nondisplaced S82.14-
    lateral condyle (displaced) S82.12-
      nondisplaced S82.12-
    medial condyle (displaced) S82.13-
      nondisplaced S82.13-
    physeal S89.00-
      Salter-Harris
        Type I S89.01-
        Type II S89.02-
        Type III S89.03-
        Type IV S89.04-
      specified NEC S89.09-
    plateau—*see* Fracture, tibia, upper end, bicondylar
    spine (displaced) S82.11-
      nondisplaced S82.11-
    torus S82.16-
    specified NEC S82.19-
    tuberosity (displaced) S82.15-
      nondisplaced S82.15-
  toe S92.91-
    great (displaced) S92.40-
      distal phalanx (displaced) S92.42-
        nondisplaced S92.42-
      nondisplaced S92.40-
      proximal phalanx (displaced) S92.41-
        nondisplaced S92.41-
      specified NEC S92.49-
    lesser (displaced) S92.50-
      distal phalanx (displaced) S92.53-
        nondisplaced S92.53-
      medial phalanx (displaced) S92.52-
        nondisplaced S92.52-
      nondisplaced S92.50-
      proximal phalanx (displaced) S92.51-
        nondisplaced S92.51-
      specified NEC S92.59-
  tooth (root) S02.5-
  trachea (cartilage) S12.8
  trapezium or trapezoid bone—*see* Fracture, carpal
  trimalleolar—*see* Fracture, ankle, trimalleolar
  triquetrum (cuneiform of carpus)—*see* Fracture, carpal, triquetrum
  trochanter—*see* Fracture, femur, trochanteric
  tuberosity (external)—*code by* site under Fracture
  ulna (shaft) S52.20-
    bent bone S52.28-
    coronoid process—*see* Fracture, ulna, upper end, coronoid process
    distal end—*see* Fracture, ulna, lower end
    head S52.00-
    lower end S52.60-
      physeal S59.00-
        Salter-Harris
          Type I S59.01-
          Type II S59.02-
          Type III S59.03-
          Type IV S59.04-
        specified NEC S59.09-
      specified NEC S52.69-
      styloid process (displaced) S52.61-
        nondisplaced S52.61-
      torus S52.62-
    proximal end—*see* Fracture, ulna, upper end
    shaft S52.20-
      comminuted (displaced) S52.25-
        nondisplaced S52.25-
      greenstick S52.21-

Fracture, *continued*
  Monteggia's—*see* Monteggia's fracture
  oblique (displaced) S52.23-
    nondisplaced S52.23-
  segmental (displaced) S52.26-
    nondisplaced S52.26-
  specified NEC S52.29-
  spiral (displaced) S52.24-
    nondisplaced S52.24-
  transverse (displaced) S52.22-
    nondisplaced S52.22-
  upper end S52.00-
    coronoid process (displaced) S52.04-
      nondisplaced S52.04-
    olecranon process (displaced) S52.02-
      with intraarticular extension S52.03-
      nondisplaced S52.02-
        with intraarticular extension S52.03-
    specified NEC S52.09-
    torus S52.01-
  unciform—*see* Fracture, carpal, hamate
  vault of skull S02.0-
  vertebra, vertebral (arch) (body) (column) (neural arch) (pedicle) (spinous process) (transverse process)
    atlas—*see* Fracture, neck, cervical vertebra, first
    axis—*see* Fracture, neck, cervical vertebra, second
    cervical (teardrop) S12.9
      axis—*see* Fracture, neck, cervical vertebra, second
      first (atlas)—*see* Fracture, neck, cervical vertebra, first
      second (axis)—*see* Fracture, neck, cervical vertebra, second
    vertex S02.0-
    vomer (bone) S02.2-
    wrist S62.10-
      carpal—*see* Fracture, carpal bone
      navicular (scaphoid) (hand)—*see* Fracture, carpal, navicular
  zygoma S02.402
    left side S02.40F
    right side S02.40E

Fragile, fragility
  bone, congenital (with blue sclera) Q78.0
  X chromosome Q99.2

Fragilitas
  ossium (with blue sclerae) (hereditary) Q78.0

Frank's essential thrombocytopenia D69.3

Fraser's syndrome Q87.0

Freckle (s) L81.2
  retinal D49.81

Frederickson's hyperlipoproteinemia, type
  IIA E78.0
  IIB and III E78.2

Freeman Sheldon syndrome Q87.0

Frenum, frenulum
  tongue (shortening) (congenital) Q38.1

Frequency micturition (nocturnal) R35.0
  psychogenic F45.8

Friction
  burn—*see* Burn, by site
  sounds, chest R09.89

Friedreich's
  ataxia G11.1
  combined systemic disease G11.1
  facial hemihypertrophy Q67.4
  sclerosis (cerebellum) (spinal cord) G11.1

Fugue R68.89
  reaction to exceptional stress (transient) F43.0

Fulminant, fulminating—*see* condition

Functional—*see also* condition
  bleeding (uterus) N93.8

Fungus, fungous
  cerebral G93.89
  disease NOS B49
  infection—*see* Infection, fungus

Funnel
  breast (acquired) M95.4
    congenital Q67.6
  chest (acquired) M95.4
    congenital Q67.6

Funnel, *continued*
  pelvis (acquired) M95.5
    congenital Q74.2

FUO (fever of unknown origin) R50.9

Furfur L21.0
  microsporon B36.0

Furuncle L02.92
  abdominal wall L02.221
  ankle L02.42-
  anus K61.0
  axilla (region) L02.42-
  back (any part) L02.222
  breast N61.1
  buttock L02.32
  cheek (external) L02.02
  chest wall L02.223
  chin L02.02
  face L02.02
  flank L02.221
  foot L02.62-
  forehead L02.02
  gluteal (region) L02.32
  groin L02.224
  hand L02.52-
  head L02.821
    face L02.02
  hip L02.42-
  kidney—*see* Abscess, kidney
  knee L02.42-
  leg (any part) L02.42-
  lower limb L02.42-
  malignant A22.0
  mouth K12.2
  navel L02.226
  neck L02.12
  nose J34.0
  orbit, orbital—*see* Abscess, orbit
  partes posteriores L02.32
  pectoral region L02.223
  perineum L02.225
  scalp L02.821
  specified site NEC L02.828
  submandibular K12.2
  temple (region) L02.02
  thumb L02.52-
  toe L02.62-
  trunk L02.229
    abdominal wall L02.221
    back L02.222
    chest wall L02.223
    groin L02.224
    perineum L02.225
    umbilicus L02.226
  umbilicus L02.226
  upper limb L02.42-
  vulva N76.4

Fusion, fused (congenital)
  astragaloscaphoid Q74.2
  atria Q21.1
  auricles, heart Q21.1
  choanal Q30.0
  cusps, heart valve NEC Q24.8
    pulmonary Q22.1
  fingers Q70.0-
  hymen Q52.3
  limb, congenital Q74.8
    lower Q74.2
    upper Q74.0
  nares, nose, nasal, nostril (s) Q30.0
  ossicles Q79.9
    auditory Q16.3
  pulmonic cusps Q22.1
  sacroiliac (joint) (acquired) M43.28
    congenital Q74.2
  toes Q70.2
  ventricles, heart Q21.0

Fussy baby R68.12

G

Gain in weight (abnormal) (excessive)—*see also* Weight, gain

Gaisböck's disease (polycythemia hypertonica) D75.1

Gait abnormality R26.9
- ataxic R26.0
- hysterical (ataxic) (staggering) F44.4
- paralytic R26.1
- spastic R26.1
- specified type NEC R26.89
- staggering R26.0
- unsteadiness R26.81
- walking difficulty NEC R26.2

Galactophoritis N61.0

Galactorrhea O92.6
- not associated with childbirth N64.3

Galeazzi's fracture S52.37-

Gallbladder—*see also* condition
- acute K81.0

Gambling Z72.6

Ganglion (compound) (diffuse) (joint) (tendon (sheath)) M67.40
- ankle M67.47-
- foot M67.47-
- forearm M67.43-
- hand M67.44-
- lower leg M67.46-
- multiple sites M67.49
- pelvic region M67.45-
- periosteal—*see* Periostitis
- shoulder region M67.41-
- specified site NEC M67.48
- thigh region M67.45-
- upper arm M67.42-
- wrist M67.43-

Ganglionitis
- geniculate G51.1
- newborn (birth injury) P11.3

Gangliosidosis E75.10
- Tay-Sachs disease E75.02

Gangrene, gangrenous (connective tissue) (dropsical) (dry) (moist) (skin) (ulcer) (*see also* Necrosis) I96
- appendix K35.80
  - with
    - perforation or rupture K35.2
    - peritoneal abscess K35.3
    - peritonitis NEC K35.3
      - generalized (with perforation or rupture) K35.2
      - localized (with perforation or rupture) K35.3
- epididymis (infectional) N45.1
- erysipelas—*see* Erysipelas
- glossitis K14.0
- laryngitis J04.0
- pancreas
  - infected K85.82
  - idiopathic
    - infected K85.02
    - uninfected K85.01
  - uninfected K85.81
- quinsy J36
- testis (infectional) N45.2
  - noninfective N44.8
- uvulitis K12.2

Gardner-Diamond syndrome (autoerythrocyte sensitization) D69.2

Gargoylism E76.01

Gas R14.3
- excessive R14.0
- on stomach R14.0
- pains R14.1

Gastrectasis K31.0
- psychogenic F45.8

Gastric—*see* condition

Gastritis (simple) K29.70
- with bleeding K29.71
- acute (erosive) K29.00
  - with bleeding K29.01
- dietary counseling and surveillance Z71.3
- eosinophilic K52.81
- viral NEC A08.4

Gastroduodenitis K29.90
- with bleeding K29.91
- virus, viral A08.4
  - specified type NEC A08.39

Gastroenteritis (acute) (chronic) (noninfectious) (*see also* Enteritis) K52.9
- allergic K52.29
  - with
    - eosinophilic gastritis or gastroenteritis K52.81
    - food protein-induced enterocolitis syndrome K52.21
    - food protein-induced enteropathy K52.22
- dietetic K52.29
- eosinophilic K52.81
- epidemic (infectious) A09
- food hypersensitivity K52.29
- infectious—*see* Enteritis, infectious
- noninfectious K52.9
  - specified NEC K52.89
- rotaviral A08.0
- Salmonella A02.0
- viral NEC A08.4
  - acute infectious A08.39
  - infantile (acute) A08.39
  - rotaviral A08.0
  - severe of infants A08.39
  - specified type NEC A08.39

Gastroenteropathy (*see also* Gastroenteritis) K52.9
- infectious A09

Gastrojejunitis (*see also* Enteritis) K52.9

Gastropathy K31.9
- erythematous K29.70
- exudative K90.89

Gastrorrhagia K92.2
- psychogenic F45.8

Gastroschisis (congenital) Q79.3

Gastrospasm (neurogenic) (reflex) K31.89
- neurotic F45.8
- psychogenic F45.8

Gastrostomy
- attention to Z43.1
- status Z93.1

Gee (-Herter)(-Thaysen) disease (nontropical sprue) K90.0

Gemistocytoma
- specified site—*see* Neoplasm, malignant, by site
- unspecified site C71.9

General, generalized—*see* condition

Genetic
- carrier (status)
  - cystic fibrosis Z14.1
  - hemophilia A (asymptomatic) Z14.01
    - symptomatic Z14.02
  - specified NEC Z14.8

Genu
- congenital Q74.1
- extrorsum (acquired) M21.16-
  - congenital Q74.1
- introrsum (acquired) M21.06-
  - congenital Q74.1
- recurvatum (acquired) M21.86-
  - congenital Q68.2
- valgum (acquired) (knock-knee) M21.06-
  - congenital Q74.1
- varum (acquired) (bowleg) M21.16-
  - congenital Q74.1

Geographic tongue K14.1

Geophagia—*see* Pica

Gerbode defect Q21.0

GERD (gastroesophageal reflux disease) K21.9

Gerhardt's
- syndrome (vocal cord paralysis) J38.00
  - bilateral J38.02
  - unilateral J38.01

German measles—*see also* Rubella
- exposure to Z20.4

Germinoblastoma (diffuse) C85.9-
- follicular C82.9-

Gerstmann's syndrome R48.8
- developmental F81.2

Gianotti-Crosti disease L44.4

Giant
- urticaria T78.3

Giardiasis A07.1

Gibert's disease or pityriasis L42

Giddiness R42
- hysterical F44.89
- psychogenic F45.8

Gigantism (cerebral) (hypophyseal) (pituitary) E22.0

Gilbert's disease or syndrome E80.4

Gilles de la Tourette's disease or syndrome (motor-verbal tic) F95.2

Gingivitis K05.10
- acute (catarrhal) K05.00
  - plaque induced K05.00

Gingivoglossitis K14.0

Gingivostomatitis K05.10
- herpesviral B00.2

Glaucoma H40.9
- childhood Q15.0
- congenital Q15.0
- in (due to)
  - endocrine disease NOS E34.9 *[H42]*
  - Lowe's syndrome E72.03 *[H42]*
  - metabolic disease NOS E88.9 *[H42]*
- infantile Q15.0
- newborn Q15.0
- secondary (to) H40.5-
  - trauma H40.3-
- traumatic—*see also* Glaucoma, secondary, trauma
  - newborn (birth injury) P15.3

Gleet (gonococcal) A54.01

Glioblastoma (multiforme)
- with sarcomatous component
  - specified site—*see* Neoplasm, malignant, by site
  - unspecified site C71.9
- giant cell
  - specified site—*see* Neoplasm, malignant, by site
  - unspecified site C71.9
- specified site—*see* Neoplasm, malignant, by site
- unspecified site C71.9

Glioma (malignant)
- astrocytic
  - specified site—*see* Neoplasm, malignant, by site
  - unspecified site C71.9
- mixed
  - specified site—*see* Neoplasm, malignant, by site
  - unspecified site C71.9
- nose Q30.8
- specified site NEC—*see* Neoplasm, malignant, by site
- subependymal D43.2
  - specified site—*see* Neoplasm, uncertain behavior, by site
  - unspecified site D43.2
- unspecified site C71.9

Gliosarcoma
- specified site—*see* Neoplasm, malignant, by site
- unspecified site C71.9

Gliosis (cerebral) G93.89

Globinuria R82.3

Globus (hystericus) F45.8

Glomangioma D18.00
- skin D18.01
- specified site NEC D18.09

Glomangiomyoma D18.00
- intra-abdominal D18.03
- intracranial D18.02
- skin D18.01
- specified site NEC D18.09

Glomerulonephritis (*see also* Nephritis) N05.9
- with
  - edema—*see* Nephrosis
  - minimal change N05.0
  - minor glomerular abnormality N05.0
- acute N00.9
- chronic N03.9
- in (due to)
  - defibrination syndrome D65 *[N08]*
  - disseminated intravascular coagulation D65 *[N08]*
  - Henoch (-Schönlein) purpura D69.0 *[N08]*
  - sepsis A41.9 *[N08]*
    - streptococcal A40- *[N08]*
  - subacute bacterial endocarditis I33.0 *[N08]*
  - systemic lupus erythematosus M32.14

Glomerulonephritis, *continued*
poststreptococcal NEC N05.9
acute N00.9
chronic N03.9
proliferative NEC (*see also* N00-N07 with fourth character
.8) N05.8
diffuse (lupus) M32.14
Glossitis (chronic superficial) (gangrenous) (Moeller's) K14.0
areata exfoliativa K14.1
benign migratory K14.1
cortical superficial, sclerotic K14.0
interstitial, sclerous K14.0
superficial, chronic K14.0
Glottitis (*see also* Laryngitis) J04.0
Glue
ear H65.3-
sniffing (airplane)—*see* Abuse, drug, inhalant
dependence—*see* Dependence, drug, inhalant
Glycogenosis (diffuse) (generalized)—*see also* Disease,
glycogen storage
pulmonary interstitial J84.842
Glycopenia E16.2
Glycosuria R81
renal E74.8
Goiter (plunging) (substernal) E04.9
with
hyperthyroidism (recurrent)—*see* Hyperthyroidism,
with, goiter
thyrotoxicosis—*see* Hyperthyroidism, with, goiter
adenomatous—*see* Goiter, nodular
due to
iodine-deficiency (endemic) E01.2
endemic (iodine-deficiency) E01.2
diffuse E01.0
multinodular E01.1
iodine-deficiency (endemic) E01.2
diffuse E01.0
multinodular E01.1
nodular E01.1
lingual Q89.2
nodular (nontoxic) (due to) E04.9
endemic E01.1
iodine-deficiency E01.1
sporadic E04.9
nontoxic E04.9
diffuse (colloid) E04.0
multinodular E04.2
simple E04.0
specified NEC E04.8
uninodular E04.1
simple E04.0
Goldberg syndrome Q89.8
Goldberg-Maxwell syndrome E34.51
Goldenhar (-Gorlin) syndrome Q87.0
Goldflam-Erb disease or syndrome G70.00
with exacerbation (acute) G70.01
in crisis G70.01
Goldscheider's disease Q81.8
Goldstein's disease (familial hemorrhagic telangiectasia)
I78.0
Gonococcus, gonococcal (disease) (infection) (*see also*
condition) A54.9
conjunctiva, conjunctivitis (neonatorum) A54.31
eye A54.30
conjunctivitis A54.31
newborn A54.31
fallopian tubes (acute) (chronic) A54.24
genitourinary (organ) (system) (tract) (acute)
lower A54.00
pelviperitonitis A54.24
pelvis (acute) (chronic) A54.24
pyosalpinx (acute) (chronic) A54.24
urethra (acute) (chronic) A54.01
with abscess (accessory gland) (periurethral) A54.1
vulva (acute) (chronic) A54.02
Gonorrhea (acute) (chronic) A54.9
Bartholin's gland (acute) (chronic)(purulent) A54.02
with abscess (accessory gland) (periurethral) A54.1
bladder A54.01
cervix A54.03
conjunctiva, conjunctivitis (neonatorum) A54.31
contact Z20.2
exposure to Z20.2

Gonorrhea, *continued*
fallopian tube A54.24
lower genitourinary tract A54.00
ovary (acute) (chronic) A54.24
pelvis (acute) (chronic) A54.24
female pelvic inflammatory disease A54.24
urethra A54.01
vagina A54.02
vulva A54.02
Gorlin-Chaudry-Moss syndrome Q87.0
Gougerot-Carteaud disease or syndrome (confluent
reticulate
papillomatosis) L83
Gouley's syndrome (constrictive pericarditis) I31.1
Gower's
muscular dystrophy G71.0
syndrome (vasovagal attack) R55
Graft-versus-host disease D89.813
acute D89.810
acute on chronic D89.812
chronic D89.811
Grain mite (itch) B88.0
Granular—*see also* condition
inflammation, pharynx J31.2
Granuloma L92.9
abdomen K66.8
from residual foreign body L92.3
pyogenicum L98.0
beryllium (skin) L92.3
brain (any site) G06.0
candidal (cutaneous) B37.2
cerebral (any site) G06.0
foreign body (in soft tissue) NEC M60.20
skin L92.3
subcutaneous tissue L92.3
gland (lymph) I88.8
hepatic NEC K75.3
in (due to)
sarcoidosis D86.89
Hodgkin C81.9-
intracranial (any site) G06.0
monilial (cutaneous) B37.2
operation wound T81.89
foreign body—*see* Foreign body, accidentally left
during a procedure
stitch T81.89
pyogenic, pyogenicum (of) (skin) L98.0
rectum K62.89
reticulohistiocytic D76.3
septic (skin) L98.0
silica (skin) L92.3
skin L92.9
from residual foreign body L92.3
pyogenicum L98.0
stitch (postoperative) T81.89
suppurative (skin) L98.0
telangiectaticum (skin) L98.0
Granulomatosis L92.9
progressive septic D71
Grawitz tumor C64.-
Green sickness D50.8
Grief F43.21
prolonged F43.29
reaction (*see also* Disorder, adjustment) F43.20
Grinding, teeth
psychogenic F45.8
sleep related G47.63
Grisel's disease M43.6
Growing pains, children R29.898
Growth (fungoid) (neoplastic) (new)—*see also* Neoplasm
adenoid (vegetative) J35.8
benign—*see* Neoplasm, benign, by site
malignant—*see* Neoplasm, malignant, by site
rapid, childhood Z00.2
secondary—*see* Neoplasm, secondary, by site
Gruby's disease B35.0
Guerin-Stern syndrome Q74.3
Guinon's disease (motor-verbal tic) F95.2
Gumboil K04.7
Gynecological examination (periodic) (routine) Z01.419
with abnormal findings Z01.411
Gynecomastia N62
Gyrate scalp Q82.8

H

**Haemophilus (H.) influenzae, as cause of disease
classified elsewhere**
B96.3
Hailey-Hailey disease Q82.8
Hair—*see also* condition
plucking F63.3
in stereotyped movement disorder F98.4
tourniquet syndrome—*see also* Constriction, external,
by site
finger S60.44-
penis S30.842
thumb S60.34-
toe S90.44-
Hairball in stomach T18.2
Hair-pulling, pathological (compulsive) F63.3
Halitosis R19.6
Hallerman-Streiff syndrome Q87.0
Hallucination R44.3
auditory R44.0
gustatory R44.2
olfactory R44.2
specified NEC R44.2
tactile R44.2
visual R44.1
Hallux
rigidus (acquired) M20.2-
congenital Q74.2
valgus (acquired) M20.1-
congenital Q66.6
Hamartoma, hamartoblastoma Q85.9
Hamartosis Q85.9
Hammer toe (acquired) NEC—*see also* Deformity, toe,
hammer toe
congenital Q66.89
Hand-foot syndrome L27.1
Handicap, handicapped
educational Z55.9
specified NEC Z55.8
Hangover (alcohol) F10.129
Hanhart's syndrome Q87.0
Hardening
brain G93.89
Harelip (complete) (incomplete)—*see* Cleft, lip
Harmful use (of)
alcohol F10.10
cannabinoids—*see* Abuse, drug, cannabis
cocaine—*see* Abuse, drug, cocaine
drug—*see* Abuse, drug
hallucinogens—*see* Abuse, drug, hallucinogen
PCP (phencyclidine)—*see* Abuse, drug, hallucinogen
Hay fever (*see also* Fever, hay) J30.1
Hb (abnormal)
Bart's disease D56.0
disease—*see* Disease, hemoglobin
trait—*see* Trait
Head—*see* condition
Headache R51
chronic daily R51
cluster G44.009
intractable G44.001
not intractable G44.009
daily chronic R51
histamine G44.009
intractable G44.001
not intractable G44.009
nasal septum R51
periodic syndromes in adults and children G43.C0
with refractory migraine G43.C1
intractable G43.C1
not intractable G43.C0
without refractory migraine G43.C0
tension (-type) G44.209
chronic G44.229
intractable G44.221
not intractable G44.229
episodic G44.219
intractable G44.211
not intractable G44.219
intractable G44.201
not intractable G44.209

Hearing examination Z01.10
  with abnormal findings NEC Z01.118
  following failed hearing screening Z01.110
  for hearing conservation and treatment Z01.12
Heart—*see* condition
Heart beat
  abnormality R00.9
    specified NEC R00.8
  awareness R00.2
  rapid R00.0
  slow R00.1
Heartburn R12
  psychogenic F45.8
Heat (effects) T67.9
  apoplexy T67.0
  burn (*see also* Burn) L55.9
  cramps T67.2
  exhaustion T67.5
    anhydrotic T67.3
    due to
      salt (and water) depletion T67.4
      water depletion T67.3
        with salt depletion T67.4
  fatigue (transient) T67.6
  fever T67.0
  hyperpyrexia T67.0
  prickly L74.0
  pyrexia T67.0
  rash L74.0
  stroke T67.0
  syncope T67.1
Heavy-for-dates NEC (infant) (4000g to 4499g) P08.1
  exceptionally (4500g or more) P08.0
Heerfordt's disease D86.89
Heinz body anemia, congenital D58.2
Heloma L84
Hemangioendothelioma—*see also* Neoplasm, uncertain
                behavior, by site
  benign D18.00
    skin D18.01
    specified site NEC D18.09
  bone (diffuse)—*see* Neoplasm, bone, malignant
  epithelioid—*see also* Neoplasm, uncertain behavior,
                by site
    malignant—*see* Neoplasm, malignant, by site
  malignant—*see* Neoplasm, connective tissue, malignant
Hemangiofibroma—*see* Neoplasm, benign, by site
Hemangiolipoma—*see* Lipoma
Hemangioma D18.00
  arteriovenous D18.00
    skin D18.01
    specified site NEC D18.09
  capillary D18.00
    skin D18.01
    specified site NEC D18.09
  cavernous D18.00
    skin D18.01
    specified site NEC D18.09
  epithelioid D18.00
    skin D18.01
    specified site NEC D18.09
  histiocytoid D18.00
    skin D18.01
    specified site NEC D18.09
  infantile D18.00
    skin D18.01
    specified site NEC D18.09
  intramuscular D18.00
    skin D18.01
    specified site NEC D18.09
  juvenile D18.00
  malignant—*see* Neoplasm, connective tissue, malignant
  plexiform D18.00
    skin D18.01
    specified site NEC D18.09
  racemose D18.00
    skin D18.01
    specified site NEC D18.09
  sclerosing—*see* Neoplasm, skin, benign
  simplex D18.00
    skin D18.01
    specified site NEC D18.09
  skin D18.01

Hemangioma, *continued*
  specified site NEC D18.09
  venous D18.00
    skin D18.01
    specified site NEC D18.09
  verrucous keratotic D18.00
    skin D18.01
    specified site NEC D18.09
Hemangiomatosis (systemic) I78.8
  involving single site—*see* Hemangioma
Hemarthrosis (nontraumatic) M25.00
  ankle M25.07-
  elbow M25.02-
  foot joint M25.07-
  hand joint M25.04-
  hip M25.05-
  in hemophilic arthropathy—*see* Arthropathy, hemophilic
  knee M25.06-
  shoulder M25.01-
  specified joint NEC M25.08
  traumatic—*see* Sprain, by site
  vertebrae M25.08
  wrist M25.03
Hematemesis K92.0
  with ulcer—*code by* site under Ulcer, with hemorrhage
                K27.4
  newborn, neonatal P54.0
    due to swallowed maternal blood P78.2
Hematocele
  female NEC N94.89
    with ectopic pregnancy O00.90
      with uterine pregnancy O00.91
Hematochezia (*see also* Melena) K92.1
Hematoma (traumatic) (skin surface intact)—*see also*
                Contusion
  with
    injury of internal organs—*see* Injury, by site
    open wound—*see* Wound, open
  auricle—*see* Contusion, ear
    nontraumatic—*see* Disorder, pinna, hematoma
  birth injury NEC P15.8
  brain (traumatic)
    with
      cerebral laceration or contusion (diffuse)—*see*
                Injury, intracranial,
                diffuse
      focal—*see* Injury, intracranial, focal
    cerebellar, traumatic S06.37-
    newborn NEC P52.4
      birth injury P10.1
    intracerebral, traumatic—*see* Injury, intracranial,
                intracerebral
                hemorrhage
    nontraumatic—*see* Hemorrhage, intracranial
    subarachnoid, arachnoid, traumatic—*see* Injury,
                intracranial,
                subarachnoid
                hemorrhage
    subdural, traumatic—*see* Injury, intracranial, subdural
                hemorrhage
  breast (nontraumatic) N64.89
  cerebral—*see* Hematoma, brain
  cerebrum S06.36-
    left S06.35-
    right S06.34-
  face, birth injury P15.4
  genital organ NEC (nontraumatic)
    female (nonobstetric) N94.89
      traumatic S30.202
  internal organs—*see* Injury, by site
  intracerebral, traumatic—*see* Injury, intracranial,
                intracerebral
                hemorrhage
  intraoperative—*see* Complications, intraoperative,
                hemorrhage
  labia (nontraumatic) (nonobstetric) N90.89
  pelvis (female) (nontraumatic) (nonobstetric) N94.89
    traumatic—*see* Injury, by site
  perianal (nontraumatic) K64.5
  superficial, newborn P54.5
  vagina (ruptured) (nontraumatic) N89.8
Hematomyelitis G04.90

Hematoperitoneum—*see* Hemoperitoneum
Hematopneumothorax (*see* Hemothorax)
Hematopoiesis, cyclic D70.4
Hematuria R31.9
  benign (familial) (of childhood)—*see also* Hematuria,
                idiopathic
    essential microscopic R31.1
  gross R31.0
  microscopic NEC (with symptoms) R31.29
    asymptomatic R31.21
    benign essential R31.1
Hemiatrophy R68.89
  face, facial, progressive (Romberg) G51.8
Hemiplegia G81.9-
  ascending NEC G81.90
    spinal G95.89
  flaccid G81.0-
  hysterical F44.4
  newborn NEC P91.8
    birth injury P11.9
  spastic G81.1-
    congenital G80.2
Hemispasm (facial) R25.2
Hemitremor R25.1
Hemochromatosis E83.119
  with refractory anemia D46.1
  due to repeated red blood cell transfusion E83.111
  hereditary (primary) E83.110
  primary E83.110
  specified NEC E83.118
Hemoglobin—*see also* condition
  abnormal (disease)—*see* Disease, hemoglobin
  AS genotype D57.3
  Constant Spring D58.2
  E-beta thalassemia D56.5
  fetal, hereditary persistence (HPFH) D56.4
  H Constant Spring D56.0
  low NOS D64.9
  S (Hb S), heterozygous D57.3
Hemoglobinopathy (mixed) D58.2
  with thalassemia D56.8
  sickle-cell D57.1
    with thalassemia D57.40
      with crisis (vaso-occlusive pain) D57.419
        with
          acute chest syndrome D57.411
          splenic sequestration D57.412
      without crisis D57.40
Hemoglobinuria R82.3
Hemopericardium I31.2
  newborn P54.8
  traumatic—*see* Injury, heart, with hemopericardium
Hemophilia (classical) (familial) (hereditary) D66
  A D66
  B D67
  acquired D68.311
  autoimmune D68.311
  secondary D68.311
Hemoptysis R04.2
  newborn P26.9
Hemorrhage, hemorrhagic (concealed) R58
  acute idiopathic pulmonary, in infants R04.81
  adenoid J35.8
  adrenal (capsule) (gland) E27.49
    medulla E27.8
    newborn P54.4
  alveolar
    lung, newborn P26.8
  anemia (chronic) D50.0
    acute D62
  antepartum (with) O46.90
    before 20 weeks gestation O20.9
      specified type NEC O20.8
      threatened abortion O20.0
  anus K62.5
  basilar (ganglion) I61.0
  brain (miliary) (nontraumatic)—*see* Hemorrhage,
              intracranial,
              intracerebral
    due to
      birth injury P10.1
    newborn P52.4
      birth injury P10.1

Hemorrhage, hemorrhagic, *continued*
  brainstem (nontraumatic) I61.3
    traumatic S06.38-
  breast N64.59
  bowel K92.2
    newborn P54.3
  bulbar I61.5
  cecum K92.2
  cerebellar, cerebellum (nontraumatic) I61.4
    newborn P52.6
    traumatic S06.37-
  cerebral, cerebrum—*see also* Hemorrhage, intracranial,
                     intracerebral
    newborn (anoxic) P52.4
      birth injury P10.1
    lobe I61.1
  cerebromeningeal I61.8
  cerebrospinal—*see* Hemorrhage, intracranial,
                    intracerebral
  colon K92.2
  conjunctiva H11.3-
    newborn P54.8
  corpus luteum (ruptured) cyst N83.1-
  cortical (brain) I61.1
  cranial—*see* Hemorrhage, intracranial
  cutaneous R23.3
    due to autosensitivity, erythrocyte D69.2
    newborn P54.5
  disease D69.9
    newborn P53
  duodenum, duodenal K92.2
    ulcer—*see* Ulcer, duodenum, with hemorrhage
  epicranial subaponeurotic (massive), birth injury P12.2
  epidural (traumatic)—*see also* Injury, intracranial, epidural
                    hemorrhage
    nontraumatic I62.1
  esophagus K22.8
    varix I85.01
  extradural (traumatic)—*see* Injury, intracranial, epidural
                    hemorrhage
    birth injury P10.8
    newborn (anoxic) (nontraumatic) P52.8
    nontraumatic I62.1
  gastric—*see* Hemorrhage, stomach
  gastroenteric K92.2
    newborn P54.3
  gastrointestinal (tract) K92.2
    newborn P54.3
  genitourinary (tract) NOS R31.9
  graafian follicle cyst (ruptured) N83.0-
  intermenstrual (regular) N92.3
    irregular N92.1
  internal (organs) EC R58
    capsule I61.0
    newborn P54.8
    intestine K92.2
    newborn P54.3
  intra-alveolar (lung), newborn P26.8
  intracerebral (nontraumatic)—*see* Hemorrhage,
                    intracranial,
                    intracerebral
  intracranial (nontraumatic) I62.9
    birth injury P10.9
    epidural, nontraumatic I62.1
    extradural, nontraumatic I62.1
    intracerebral (nontraumatic) (in) I61.9
      brain stem I61.3
      cerebellum I61.4
      newborn P52.4
        birth injury P10.1
      hemisphere I61.2
        cortical (superficial) I61.1
        subcortical (deep) I61.0
      intraventricular I61.5
      multiple localized I61.6
      specified NEC I61.8
      superficial I61.1
      traumatic (diffuse)—*see* Injury, intracranial, diffuse
      focal—*see* Injury, intracranial, focal
    subarachnoid (nontraumatic) (from) I60.9
      newborn P52.5
        birth injury P10.3

Hemorrhage, hemorrhagic, *continued*
  intracranial (cerebral)artery I60.7
    anterior communicating I60.2-
    basilar I60.4
    carotid siphon and bifurcation I60.0-
    communicating I60.7
      anterior I60.2-
      posterior I60.3-
    middle cerebral I60.1-
    posterior communicating I60.3-
    specified artery NEC I60.6
    vertebral I60.5-
    specified NEC I60.8
    traumatic S06.6X-
  subdural (nontraumatic) I62.00
    acute I62.01
    birth injury P10.0
    chronic I62.03
    newborn (anoxic) (hypoxic) P52.8
      birth injury P10.0
    spinal G95.19
    subacute I62.02
    traumatic—*see* Injury, intracranial, subdural
                    hemorrhage
    traumatic—*see* Injury, intracranial, focal brain injury
  intrapontine I61.3
  intraventricular I61.5
    newborn (nontraumatic) (*see also* Newborn, affected
                  by, hemorrhage) P52.3
      due to birth injury P10.2
      grade
        1 P52.0
        2 P52.1
        3 P52.21
        4 P52.22
  lenticular striate artery I61.0
  lung R04.89
    newborn P26.9
      massive P26.1
      specified NEC P26.8
  medulla I61.3
  membrane (brain) I60.8
    spinal cord—*see* Hemorrhage, spinal cord
  meninges, meningeal (brain) (middle) I60.8
    spinal cord—*see* Hemorrhage, spinal cord
  mouth K13.79
  mucous membrane NEC R58
    newborn P54.8
  nail (subungual) L60.8
  nasal turbinate R04.0
    newborn P54.8
  newborn P54.9
    specified NEC P54.8
  nipple N64.59
  nose R04.0
    newborn P54.8
  ovary NEC N83.8
  pericardium, pericarditis I31.2
  peritonsillar tissue J35.8
    due to infection J36
  petechial R23.3
    due to autosensitivity, erythrocyte D69.2
  pons, pontine I61.3
  posterior fossa (nontraumatic) I61.8
    newborn P52.6
  postnasal R04.0
  pulmonary R04.89
    newborn P26.9
      massive P26.1
      specified NEC P26.8
  purpura (primary) D69.3
  rectum (sphincter) K62.5
    newborn P54.2
  skin R23.3
    newborn P54.5
  slipped umbilical ligature P51.8
  stomach K92.2
    newborn P54.3
    ulcer—*see* Ulcer, stomach, with hemorrhage
  subconjunctival—*see also* Hemorrhage, conjunctiva
    birth injury P15.3
  subcortical (brain) I61.0
  subcutaneous R23.3

Hemorrhage, hemorrhagic, *continued*
  subependymal
    newborn P52.0
      with intraventricular extension P52.1
        and intracerebral extension P52.22
  subungual L60.8
  suprarenal (capsule) (gland) E27.49
    newborn P54.4
  tonsil J35.8
  ulcer—*code by* site under Ulcer, with hemorrhage K27.4
  umbilicus, umbilical
    cord
      after birth, newborn P51.9
      complicating delivery O69.5
    newborn P51.9
      massive P51.0
      slipped ligature P51.8
    stump P51.9
  uterus, uterine (abnormal) N93.9
    dysfunctional or functional N93.8
    intermenstrual (regular) N92.3
      irregular N92.1
    pubertal N92.2
  vagina (abnormal) N93.9
    newborn P54.6
  ventricular I61.5
  viscera NEC R58
    newborn P54.8
Hemorrhoids (bleeding) (without mention of degree) K64.9
  1st degree (grade/stage I) (without prolapse outside of
                    anal canal) K64.0
  2nd degree (grade/stage II) (that prolapse with
                    straining but retract
                    spontaneously) K64.1
  3rd degree (grade/stage III) (that prolapse with straining
                    and require manual
                    replacement back
                    inside anal canal)
                    K64.2
  4th degree (grade/stage IV) (with prolapsed tissue that
                    cannot be manually
                    replaced) K64.3
  external K64.4
    with
      thrombosis K64.5
  internal (without mention of degree) K64.8
  prolapsed K64.8
  skin tags
    anus K64.4
    residual K64.4
  specified NEC K64.8
  strangulated (*see also* Hemorrhoids, by degree) K64.8
  thrombosed (*see also* Hemorrhoids, by degree) K64.5
  ulcerated (*see also* Hemorrhoids, by degree) K64.8
Hemothorax (bacterial) (nontuberculous) J94.2
  newborn P54.8
Henoch (-Schönlein) disease or syndrome (purpura) D69.0
Hepatitis K75.9
  acute (infectious) (viral) B17.9
  B B19.10
    acute B16.9
  C (viral) B19.20
    acute B17.10
    chronic B18.2
  catarrhal (acute) B15.9
  chronic K73.9
    active NEC K73.2
  epidemic B15.9
  fulminant NEC K75.3
    neonatal giant cell P59.29
  history of
    B Z86.19
    C Z86.19
  homologous serum—*see* Hepatitis, viral, type B
  in (due to)
    toxoplasmosis (acquired) B58.1
      congenital (active) P37.1 *[K77]*
  infectious, infective (acute) (chronic) (subacute) B15.9
  neonatal (idiopathic) (toxic) P59.29
  newborn P59.29
  viral, virus B19.9
    acute B17.9
      C B18.2

Hepatitis, *continued*
    in remission, any type—*code to* Hepatitis, chronic,
          by type
    type
        A B15.9
        B 19.10
            acute B16.9
        C B19.20
            acute B17.10
            chronic B18.2
Hepatomegaly—*see also* Hypertrophy, liver
    in mononucleosis
        gammaherpesviral B27.09
        infectious specified NEC B27.89
Herlitz' syndrome Q81.1
Hernia, hernial (acquired) (recurrent) K46.9
    with
        gangrene—*see* Hernia, by site, with, gangrene
        incarceration—*see* Hernia, by site, with, obstruction
        irreducible—*see* Hernia, by site, with, obstruction
        obstruction—*see* Hernia, by site, with, obstruction
        strangulation—*see* Hernia, by site, with, obstruction
    diaphragm, diaphragmatic K44.9
        with
            gangrene (and obstruction) K44.1
            obstruction K44.0
        congenital Q79.0
    direct (inguinal)—*see* Hernia, inguinal
    diverticulum, intestine—*see* Hernia, abdomen
    double (inguinal)—*see* Hernia, inguinal, bilateral
    epigastric (*see also* Hernia, ventral) K43.9
    esophageal hiatus—*see* Hernia, hiatal
    external (inguinal)—*see* Hernia, inguinal
    hiatal (esophageal) (sliding) K44.9
        with
            gangrene (and obstruction) K44.1
            obstruction K44.0
        congenital Q40.1
    indirect (inguinal)—*see* Hernia, inguinal
    incisional K43.2
        with
            gangrene (and obstruction) K43.1
            obstruction K43.0
    inguinal (direct) (external) (funicular) (indirect) (internal)
            (oblique) (scrotal)
            (sliding) K40.90
        with
            gangrene (and obstruction) K40.40
                not specified as recurrent K40.40
                recurrent K40.41
            obstruction K40.30
                not specified as recurrent K40.30
                recurrent K40.31
        not specified as recurrent K40.90
        recurrent K40.91
        bilateral K40.20
            with
                gangrene (and obstruction) K40.10
                    not specified as recurrent K40.10
                    recurrent K40.11
                obstruction K40.00
                  not specified as recurrent K40.00
                  recurrent K40.01
            not specified as recurrent K40.20
            recurrent K40.21
        unilateral K40.90
            with
                gangrene (and obstruction) K40.40
                    not specified as recurrent K40.40
                    recurrent K40.41
                obstruction K40.30
                  not specified as recurrent K40.30
                  recurrent K40.31
            not specified as recurrent K40.90
            recurrent K40.91
    irreducible—*see also* Hernia, by site, with obstruction
        with gangrene—*see* Hernia, by site, with gangrene
    linea (alba) (semilunaris)—*see* Hernia, ventral
    midline—*see* Hernia, ventral
    oblique (inguinal)—*see* Hernia, inguinal
    obstructive—*see also* Hernia, by site, with obstruction
        with gangrene—*see* Hernia, by site, with gangrene

Hernia, hernial, *continued*
    scrotum, scrotal—*see* Hernia, inguinal
    sliding (inguinal)—*see also* Hernia, inguinal
        hiatus—*see* Hernia, hiatal
    spigelian—*see* Hernia, ventral
    spinal—*see* Spina bifida
    strangulated—*see also* Hernia, by site, with obstruction
        with gangrene—*see* Hernia, by site, with gangrene
    subxiphoid—*see* Hernia, ventral
    supra-umbilicus—*see* Hernia, ventral
    tendon—*see* Disorder, tendon, specified type NEC
    tunica vaginalis Q55.29
    umbilicus, umbilical K42.9
        with
            gangrene (and obstruction) K42.1
            obstruction K42.0
    ventral K43.9
        with
            gangrene (and obstruction) K43.7
            obstruction K43.6
        recurrent—*see* Hernia, incisional
        incisional K43.2
            with
                gangrene (and obstruction) K43.1
                obstruction K43.0
        specified NEC K43.9
            with
                gangrene (and obstruction) K43.7
                obstruction K43.6
Herpangina B08.5
Herpes, herpesvirus, herpetic B00.9
    anogenital A60.9
        urogenital tract A60.00
            cervix A60.03
            male genital organ NEC A60.02
            penis A60.01
            specified site NEC A60.09
            vagina A60.04
            vulva A60.04
    circinatus B35.4
        bullous L12.0
    encephalitis B00.4
        due to herpesvirus 7 B10.09
        specified NEC B10.09
    genital, genitalis A60.00
        female A60.09
        male A60.02
    gingivostomatitis B00.2
    human B00.9
        1—*see* Herpes, simplex
        2—*see* Herpes, simplex
        4—*see* Mononucleosis, Epstein-Barr (virus)
        7
            encephalitis B10.09
    meningitis (simplex) B00.3
        zoster B02.1
    pharyngitis, pharyngotonsillitis B00.2
    simplex B00.9
        complicated NEC B00.89
        congenital P35.2
        specified complication NEC B00.89
        visceral B00.89
    stomatitis B00.2
    tonsurans B35.0
    visceral B00.89
    whitlow B00.89
    zoster (*see also* condition) B02.9
        complicated NEC B02.8
Herter-Gee Syndrome K90.0
Hesitancy
    of micturition R39.11
    urinary R39.11
Heubner-Herter disease K90.0
Hiccup, hiccough R06.6
    epidemic B33.0
    psychogenic F45.8
Hidden penis (congenital) Q55.64
Hidradenitis (axillaris) (suppurative) L73.2
High
    altitude effects T70.20
        anoxia T70.29

High, *continued*
    on
        ears T70.0
        sinuses T70.1
    polycythemia D75.1
    blood pressure—*see also* Hypertension
        borderline R03.0
        reading (incidental) (isolated) (nonspecific), without
            diagnosis of
            hypertension R03.0
    cholesterol E78.00
        with high triglycerides E78.2
    expressed emotional level within family Z63.8
    palate, congenital Q38.5
    risk
        infant NEC Z76.2
        sexual behavior (heterosexual) Z72.51
            bisexual Z72.53
            homosexual Z72.52
    temperature (of unknown origin) R50.9
    triglycerides E78.1
        with high cholesterol E78.2
Hippel's disease Q85.8
Hirschsprung's disease or megacolon Q43.1
Hirsutism, hirsuties L68.0
Hirudiniasis
    external B88.3
Histiocytosis D76.3
    lipid, lipoid D76.3
    mononuclear phagocytes NEC D76.1
    non-Langerhans cell D76.3
    polyostotic sclerosing D76.3
    sinus, with massive lymphadenopathy D76.3
    syndrome NEC D76.3
History
    family (of)—*see also* History, personal (of)
        alcohol abuse Z81.1
        allergy NEC Z84.89
        anemia Z83.2
        arthritis Z82.61
        asthma Z82.5
        blindness Z82.1
        cardiac death (sudden) Z82.41
        carrier of genetic disease Z84.81
        chromosomal anomaly Z82.79
        chronic
            disabling disease NEC Z82.8
            lower respiratory disease Z82.5
        colonic polyps Z83.71
        congenital malformations and deformations Z82.79
            polycystic kidney Z82.71
        consanguinity Z84.3
        deafness Z82.2
        diabetes mellitus Z83.3
        disability NEC Z82.8
        disease or disorder (of)
            allergic NEC Z84.89
            behavioral NEC Z81.8
            blood and blood-forming organs Z83.2
            cardiovascular NEC Z82.49
            chronic disabling Z82.8
            digestive Z83.79
            ear NEC Z83.52
            endocrine NEC Z83.49
            eye NEC Z83.518
                glaucoma Z83.511
            familial hypercholesterolemia Z83.42
            genitourinary NEC Z84.2
            glaucoma Z83.511
            hematological Z83.2
            immune mechanism Z83.2
            infectious NEC Z83.1
            ischemic heart Z82.49
            kidney Z84.1
            mental NEC Z81.8
            metabolic Z83.49
            musculoskeletal NEC Z82.69
            neurological NEC Z82.0
            nutritional Z83.49
            parasitic NEC Z83.1
            psychiatric NEC Z81.8
            respiratory NEC Z83.6

History, *continued*

- skin and subcutaneous tissue NEC Z84.0
  - specified NEC Z84.89
- drug abuse NEC Z81.3
- epilepsy Z82.0
- familial hypercholesterolemia Z83.42
- genetic disease carrier Z84.81
- glaucoma Z83.511
- hearing loss Z82.2
- human immunodeficiency virus (HIV) infection Z83.0
- hypercholesterolemia (familial) Z83.42
- Huntington's chorea Z82.0
- intellectual disability Z81.0
- leukemia Z80.6
- malignant neoplasm (of) NOS Z80.9
  - bladder Z80.52
  - breast Z80.3
  - bronchus Z80.1
  - digestive organ Z80.0
  - gastrointestinal tract Z80.0
  - genital organ Z80.49
    - ovary Z80.41
    - prostate Z80.42
    - specified organ NEC Z80.49
    - testis Z80.43
  - hematopoietic NEC Z80.7
  - intrathoracic organ NEC Z80.2
  - kidney Z80.51
  - lung Z80.1
  - lymphatic NEC Z80.7
  - ovary Z80.41
  - prostate Z80.42
  - respiratory organ NEC Z80.2
  - specified site NEC Z80.8
  - testis Z80.43
  - trachea Z80.1
  - urinary organ or tract Z80.59
    - bladder Z80.52
    - kidney Z80.51
- mental
  - disorder NEC Z81.8
- multiple endocrine neoplasia (MEN) syndrome Z83.41
- osteoporosis Z82.62
- polycystic kidney Z82.71
- polyps (colon) Z83.71
- psychiatric disorder Z81.8
- psychoactive substance abuse NEC Z81.3
- respiratory condition NEC Z83.6
  - asthma and other lower respiratory conditions Z82.5
- self-harmful behavior Z81.8
- SIDS (sudden infant death syndrome) Z84.82
- skin condition Z84.0
- specified condition NEC Z84.89
- stroke (cerebrovascular) Z82.3
- substance abuse NEC Z81.4
  - alcohol Z81.1
  - drug NEC Z81.3
  - psychoactive NEC Z81.3
  - tobacco Z81.2
- sudden cardiac death Z82.41
- sudden infant death syndrome Z84.82
- tobacco abuse Z81.2
- violence, violent behavior Z81.8
- visual loss Z82.1
- **personal (of)**—*see also* History, family (of)
  - **abuse**
    - childhood Z62.819
      - physical Z62.810
      - psychological Z62.811
      - sexual Z62.810
  - alcohol dependence F10.21
  - allergy (to) Z88.9
    - antibiotic agent NEC Z88.1
    - drugs, medicaments and biological substances Z88.9
      - specified NEC Z88.8
    - food Z91.018
      - additives Z91.02
      - eggs Z91.012
      - milk products Z91.011
      - peanuts Z91.010
      - seafood Z91.013
      - specified food NEC Z91.018

History, *continued*

- insect Z91.038
  - bee Z91.030
- latex Z91.040
- medicinal agents Z88.9
  - specified NEC Z88.8
- narcotic agent Z88.5
- nonmedicinal agents Z91.048
- penicillin Z88.0
- serum Z88.7
- sulfonamides Z88.2
- vaccine Z88.7
- anaphylactic shock Z87.892
- anaphylaxis Z87.892
- behavioral disorders Z86.59
- brain injury (traumatic) Z87.820
- cancer—*see* History, personal (of), malignant neoplasm (of)
- cardiac arrest (death), successfully resuscitated Z86.74
- cerebral infarction without residual deficit Z86.73
- chemotherapy for neoplastic condition Z92.21
- cleft lip (corrected) Z87.730
- cleft palate (corrected) Z87.730
- congenital malformation (corrected) Z87.798
  - circulatory system (corrected) Z87.74
  - digestive system (corrected)NEC Z87.738
  - ear (corrected) Z87.720
  - eye (corrected) Z87.721
  - face and neck (corrected) Z87.790
  - genitourinary system (corrected) NEC Z87.718
  - heart (corrected) Z87.74
  - integument (corrected) Z87.76
  - limb (s) (corrected) Z87.76
  - musculoskeletal system (corrected) Z87.76
  - neck (corrected) Z87.790
  - nervous system (corrected)NEC Z87.728
  - respiratory system (corrected) Z87.75
  - sense organs (corrected)NEC Z87.728
  - specified NEC Z87.798
- disease or disorder (of) Z87.898
  - blood and blood-forming organs Z86.2
  - connective tissue NEC Z87.39
  - ear Z86.69
  - endocrine Z86.39
    - specified type NEC Z86.39
  - eye Z86.69
  - hematological Z86.2
  - Hodgkin Z85.71
  - immune mechanism Z86.2
  - infectious Z86.19
    - Methicillin resistant Staphylococcus aureus (MRSA) Z86.14
    - tuberculosis Z86.11
  - mental NEC Z86.59
  - metabolic Z86.39
    - specified type NEC Z86.39
  - musculoskeletal NEC Z87.39
  - nervous system Z86.69
  - nutritional Z86.39
  - respiratory system NEC Z87.09
  - sense organs Z86.69
  - specified site or type NEC Z87.898
  - urinary system NEC Z87.448
- drug therapy
  - antineoplastic chemotherapy Z92.21
  - immunosupression Z92.25
  - inhaled steroids Z92.240
  - monoclonal drug Z92.22
  - specified NEC Z92.29
  - steroid Z92.241
  - systemic steroids Z92.241
- encephalitis Z86.61
- extracorporeal membrane oxygenation (ECMO) Z92.81
- fall, falling Z91.81
- hepatitis
  - B Z86.19
  - C Z86.19
- Hodgkin disease Z85.71
- hypospadias (corrected) Z87.710
- immunosupression therapy Z92.25

History, *continued*

- infection NEC Z86.19
  - central nervous system Z86.61
  - Methicillin resistant Staphylococcus aureus (MRSA) Z86.14
- in utero procedure while a fetus Z98.871
- leukemia Z85.6
- lymphoma (non-Hodgkin) Z85.72
- malignant melanoma (skin) Z85.820
- malignant neoplasm (of) Z85.9
  - bone Z85.830
  - brain Z85.841
  - carcinoid—*see* History, personal (of), malignant neoplasm, by site, carcinoid
  - endocrine gland NEC Z85.858
  - eye Z85.840
  - hematopoietic NEC Z85.79
  - kidney NEC Z85.528
    - carcinoid Z85.520
- maltreatment Z91.89
- meningitis Z86.61
- mental disorder Z86.59
- Methicillin resistant Staphylococcus aureus (MRSA) Z86.14
- neglect (in)
  - childhood Z62.812
- neoplasm
  - malignant—*see* History of, malignant neoplasm
  - uncertain behavior Z86.03
- nephrotic syndrome Z87.441
- nicotine dependence Z87.891
- noncompliance with medical treatment or regimen—*see* Noncompliance
- nutritional deficiency Z86.39
- parasuicide (attempt) Z91.5
- physical trauma NEC Z87.828
  - self-harm or suicide attempt Z91.5
- pneumonia (recurrent) Z87.01
- poisoning NEC Z91.89
  - self-harm or suicide attempt Z91.5
- procedure while a fetus Z98.871
- prolonged reversible ischemic neurologic deficit (PRIND) Z86.73
- psychological
  - abuse
    - child Z62.811
  - trauma, specified NEC Z91.49
- respiratory condition NEC Z87.09
- retained foreign body fully removed Z87.821
- risk factors NEC Z91.89
- self-harm Z91.5
- self-poisoning attempt Z91.5
- specified NEC Z87.898
- steroid therapy (systemic) Z92.241
  - inhaled Z92.240
- stroke without residual deficits Z86.73
- substance abuse NEC F10-F19 with fifth character 1
- sudden cardiac arrest Z86.74
- sudden cardiac death successfully resuscitated Z86.74
- suicide attempt Z91.5
- surgery NEC Z98.890
- tobacco dependence Z87.891
- transient ischemic attack (TIA) without residual deficits Z86.73
- trauma (physical) NEC Z87.828
  - psychological NEC Z91.49
  - self-harm Z91.5
- traumatic brain injury Z87.820
- **HIV** (*see also* Human, immunodeficiency virus) B20
  - laboratory evidence (nonconclusive) R75
  - positive, seropositive Z21
  - nonconclusive test (in infants) R75
- **Hives** (bold)—*see* Urticaria
- **Hoarseness** R49.0
- **Hoffmann's syndrome** E03.9 *[G73.7]*
- **Homelessness** Z59.0
- **Hooded**
  - clitoris Q52.6
  - penis Q55.69

Hordeolum (eyelid) (externum) (recurrent) H00.019
  internum H00.029
    left H00.026
      lower H00.025
      upper H00.024
    right H00.023
      lower H00.022
      upper H00.021
  left H00.016
    lower H00.015
    upper H00.014
  right H00.013
    lower H00.012
    upper H00.011
Horseshoe kidney (congenital) Q63.1
Hospital hopper syndrome—*see* Disorder, factitious
Hospitalism in children—*see* Disorder, adjustment
Human
  bite (open wound)—*see also* Bite
    intact skin surface—*see* Bite, superficial
  herpesvirus—*see* Herpes
  immunodeficiency virus (HIV) disease (infection) B20
    asymptomatic status Z21
    contact Z20.6
    counseling Z71.7
    exposure to Z20.6
    laboratory evidence R75
  papillomavirus (HPV)
    screening for Z11.51
Hunger T73.0
  air, psychogenic F45.8
Hunter's
  syndrome E76.1
Hunt's
  dyssynergia cerebellaris myoclonica G11.1
Hutchinson's
  disease, meaning
    pompholyx (cheiropompholyx) L30.1
Hyaline membrane (disease) (lung) (pulmonary) (newborn) P22.0
Hydatid
  Morgagni
    male (epididymal) Q55.4
      testicular Q55.29
Hydradenitis (axillaris) (suppurative) L73.2
Hydramnios O40.-
Hydroadenitis (axillaris) (suppurative) L73.2
Hydrocele (spermatic cord) (testis) (tunica vaginalis) N43.3
  communicating N43.2
    congenital P83.5
  congenital P83.5
  encysted N43.0
  female NEC N94.89
  infected N43.1
  newborn P83.5
  round ligament N94.89
  specified NEC N43.2
  spinalis—*see* Spina bifida
  vulva N90.89
Hydrocephalus (acquired) (external) (internal) (malignant) (recurrent) G91.9
  aqueduct Sylvius stricture Q03.0
  communicating G91.0
  congenital (external) (internal) Q03.9
    with spina bifida Q05.4
      cervical Q05.0
      dorsal Q05.1
      lumbar Q05.2
      lumbosacral Q05.2
      sacral Q05.3
      thoracic Q05.1
      thoracolumbar Q05.1
    specified NEC Q03.8
  due to toxoplasmosis (congenital) P37.1
  foramen Magendie block (acquired) G91.1
    congenital (*see also* Hydrocephalus, congenital) Q03.1
  newborn Q03.9
    with spina bifida—*see* Spina bifida, with hydrocephalus
  noncommunicating G91.1

Hydrocephalus, *continued*
  normal pressure G91.2
    secondary G91.0
  obstructive G91.1
  otitic G93.2
Hydromicrocephaly Q02
Hydromphalos (since birth) Q45.8
Hydronephrosis (atrophic) (early) (functionless) (intermittent) (primary) (secondary) NEC N13.30
  with
    obstruction (by) (of)
      renal calculus N13.2
      ureteral NEC N13.1
        calculus N13.2
      ureteropelvic junction N13.0
        congenital Q62.0
      with infection N13.6
    ureteral stricture NEC N13.1
  congenital Q62.0
  specified type NEC N13.39
Hydroperitoneum R18.8
Hydrophthalmos Q15.0
Hydrops R60.9
  abdominis R18.8
  fetalis P83.2
    due to
      ABO isoimmunization P56.0
      alpha thalassemia D56.0
      hemolytic disease P56.90
        specified NEC P56.99
      isoimmunization (ABO) (Rh) P56.0
      other specified nonhemolytic disease NEC P83.2
      Rh incompatibility P56.0
    newborn (idiopathic) P83.2
      due to
        ABO isoimmunization P56.0
        alpha thalassemia D56.0
        hemolytic disease P56.90
          specified NEC P56.99
        isoimmunization (ABO) (Rh) P56.0
        Rh incompatibility P56.0
  nutritional—*see* Malnutrition, severe
  pericardium—*see* Pericarditis
  pleura—*see* Hydrothorax
  spermatic cord—*see* Hydrocele
Hydropyonephrosis N13.6
Hydrorrhea (nasal) J34.89
Hydrosadenitis (axillaris) (suppurative) L73.2
Hyperacidity (gastric) K31.89
  psychogenic F45.8
Hyperactive, hyperactivity F90.9
  bowel sounds R19.12
  child F90.9
    attention deficit—*see* Disorder, attention-deficit hyperactivity
  detrusor muscle N32.81
  gastrointestinal K31.89
    psychogenic F45.8
  nasal mucous membrane J34.3
Hyperadrenocorticism E24.9
  congenital E25.0
  iatrogenic E24.2
    correct substance properly administered—*see* Table of Drugs and Chemicals, by drug, adverse effect
    overdose or wrong substance given or taken—*see* Table of Drugs and Chemicals, by drug, poisoning
  not associated with Cushing's syndrome E27.0
  pituitary-dependent E24.0
Hyperbetalipoproteinemia (familial) E78.0
  with prebetalipoproteinemia E78.2
Hyperbilirubinemia
  constitutional E80.6
  familial conjugated E80.6
  neonatal (transient)—*see* Jaundice, newborn
Hypercalcemia, hypocalciuric, familial E83.52
Hypercalciuria, idiopathic E83.52
Hypercapnia R06.89
  newborn P84
Hyperchloremia E87.8

Hyperchlorhydria K31.89
  neurotic F45.8
  psychogenic F45.8
Hypercholesterolemia (essential) (primary) (pure) E78.00
  with hyperglyceridemia, endogenous E78.2
  dietary counseling and surveillance Z71.3
  familial E78.01
  family history of Z83.42
  hereditary E78.01
Hyperchylia gastrica, psychogenic F45.8
Hypercorticalism, pituitary-dependent E24.0
Hypercorticosolism—*see* Cushing's, syndrome
Hypercorticosteronism E24.2
  correct substance properly administered—*see* Table of Drugs and Chemicals, by drug, adverse effect
  overdose or wrong substance given or taken—*see* Table of Drugs and Chemicals, by drug, poisoning
Hypercortisonism E24.2
  correct substance properly administered—*see* Table of Drugs and Chemicals, by drug, adverse effect
  overdose or wrong substance given or taken—*see* Table of Drugs and Chemicals, by drug, poisoning
Hyperekplexia Q89.8
Hyperelectrolytemia E87.8
Hyperemia (acute) (passive) R68.89
  anal mucosa K62.89
  ear internal, acute—*see* subcategory H83.0
  labyrinth—*see* subcategory H83.0
Hyperemesis R11.10
  with nausea R11.2
  projectile R11.12
  psychogenic F45.8
Hyperexplexia Q89.8
Hyperfunction
  adrenal cortex, not associated with Cushing's syndrome E27.0
    virilism E25.9
      congenital E25.0
Hyperglycemia, hyperglycemic (transient) R73.9
  coma—*see* Diabetes, by type, with coma
  postpancreatectomy E89.1
Hyperhidrosis, hyperhidrosis R61
  generalized R61
  psychogenic F45.8
  secondary R61
    focal L74.52
Hyperkeratosis (*see also* Keratosis) L85.9
  follicularis Q82.8
Hyperlipemia, hyperlipidemia E78.5
  combined E78.2
  group
    A E78.00
    C E78.2
  mixed E78.2
Hyperlipoproteinemia E78.5
  Fredrickson's type
    IIa E78.00
    IIb E78.2
    III E78.2
  low-density-lipoprotein-type (LDL) E78.00
  very-low-density-lipoprotein-type (VLDL) E78.1
Hypermagnesemia E83.41
  neonatal P71.8
Hypermenorrhea N92.0
Hypermobility, hypermotility
  colon—*see* Syndrome, irritable bowel
    psychogenic F45.8
  intestine (*see also* Syndrome, irritable bowel) K58.9
    psychogenic F45.8
  stomach K31.89
    psychogenic F45.8
Hypernatremia E87.0
Hypernephroma C64.-
Hyperopia—*see* Hypermetropia
Hyperorexia nervosa F50.2
Hyperosmolality E87.0

Hyperostosis (monomelic)—*see also* Disorder, bone, density and structure, specified NEC
  skull M85.2
    congenital Q75.8
Hyperperistalsis R19.2
  psychogenic F45.8
Hyperpigmentation—*see also* Pigmentation
  melanin NEC L81.4
Hyperplasia, hyperplastic
  adenoids J35.2
  adrenal (capsule) (cortex) (gland) E27.8
    with
      sexual precocity (male) E25.9
        congenital E25.0
      virilism, adrenal E25.9
        congenital E25.0
      virilization (female) E25.9
        congenital E25.0
    congenital E25.0
    salt-losing E25.0
  adrenomedullary E27.5
  angiolymphoid, eosinophilia (ALHE) D18.01
  bone NOS Q79.9
    face Q75.8
    skull—*see* Hypoplasia, skull
  cervix (uteri) (basal cell) (endometrium) (polypoid)—*see also* Dysplasia, cervix
    congenital Q51.828
  endocervicitis N72
  epithelial L85.9
    focal, oral, including tongue K13.29
    nipple N62
    skin L85.9
    tongue K13.29
  face Q18.8
    bone (s) Q75.8
  genital
    female NEC N94.89
    male N50.89
  gingiva K06.1
  gum K06.1
  nose
    lymphoid J34.89
    polypoid J33.9
  tonsils (faucial) (infective) (lingual) (lymphoid) J35.1
    with adenoids J35.3
Hyperpnea—*see* Hyperventilation
Hyperproteinemia E88.09
Hyperpyrexia R50.9
  heat T67.0
    rheumatic—*see* Fever, rheumatic
  unknown origin R50.9
Hypersecretion
  ACTH (not associated with Cushing's syndrome) E27.0
    pituitary E24.0
  corticoadrenal E24.9
  cortisol E24.9
  gastric K31.89
    psychogenic F45.8
  hormone (s)
    ACTH (not associated with Cushing's syndrome) E27.0
      pituitary E24.0
    antidiuretic E22.2
    growth E22.0
Hypersensitive, hypersensitiveness, hypersensitivity—*see also* Allergy
  gastrointestinal K52.29
    psychogenic F45.8
  reaction T78.40
Hypertension, hypertensive (accelerated) (benign) (essential) (idiopathic) (malignant) (systemic) I10
  benign, intracranial G93.2
  borderline R03.0
  complicating
    pregnancy O16.-
      gestational (pregnancy induced) (transient) (without proteinuria) O13.-

Hypertension, hypertensive, *continued*
  with proteinuria O14.9-
    mild pre-eclampsia O14.0-
    moderate pre-eclampsia O14.0-
    severe pre-eclampsia O14.1-
      with hemolysis, elevated liver enzymes and low platelet count (HELLP) O14.2-
  pre-existing O10.91-
    with
      pre-eclampsia O11.-
    essential O10.01-
    secondary O10.41-
  encephalopathy I67.4
  lesser circulation I27.0
  newborn P29.2
    pulmonary (persistent) P29.3
  psychogenic F45.8
  pulmonary (artery) (secondary) NEC I27.2
    with
      cor pulmonale (chronic) I27.2
        acute I26.09
      right heart ventricular strain/failure I27.2
        acute I26.09
    of newborn (persistent) P29.3
    primary (idiopathic) I27.0
Hyperthermia (of unknown origin)—*see also* Hyperpyrexia
  newborn P81.9
    environmental P81.0
Hyperthyroidism (latent) (pre-adult) (recurrent) E05.90
  with
    goiter (diffuse) E05.00
      with thyroid storm E05.01
      nodular (multinodular) E05.20
        with thyroid storm E05.21
      uninodular E05.10
        with thyroid storm E05.11
    storm E05.91
  due to ectopic thyroid tissue E05.30
    with thyroid storm E05.31
  intracranial (benign) G93.2
  neonatal, transitory P72.1
  specified NEC E05.80
    with thyroid storm E05.81
Hypertony, hypertonia, hypertonicity
  stomach K31.89
    psychogenic F45.8
Hypertrophy, hypertrophic
  adenoids (infective) J35.2
    with tonsils J35.3
  anal papillae K62.89
  bladder (sphincter) (trigone) N32.89
  brain G93.89
  breast N62
    cystic—*see* Mastopathy, cystic
    newborn P83.4
    pubertal, massive N62
  cardiac (chronic) (idiopathic) I51.7
    with rheumatic fever (conditions in I00)
      active I01.8
      inactive or quiescent (with chorea) I09.89
    congenital NEC Q24.8
    rheumatic (with chorea) I09.89
      active or acute I01.8
        with chorea I02.0
  foot (congenital) Q74.2
  frenulum, frenum (tongue) K14.8
    lip K13.0
  gland, glandular R59.9
    generalized R59.1
    localized R59.0
  gum (mucous membrane) K06.1
  hemifacial 67.4
  lingual tonsil (infective) J35.1
    with adenoids J35.3
  lip K13.0
    congenital Q18.6
  liver R16.0
  lymph, lymphatic gland R59.9
    generalized R59.1
    localized R59.0
  Meckel's diverticulum (congenital) Q43.0

Hypertrophy, hypertrophic, *continued*
  mucous membrane
    gum K06.1
    nose (turbinate) J34.3
  myocardium—*see also* Hypertrophy, cardiac
    idiopathic I42.2
  nasal J34.89
    alae J34.89
    bone J34.89
    cartilage J34.89
    mucous membrane (septum) J34.3
    sinus J34.89
    turbinate J34.3
  nasopharynx, lymphoid (infectional) (tissue) (wall) J35.2
  nipple N62
  palate (hard) M27.8
    soft K13.79
  pharyngeal tonsil J35.2
  pharynx J39.2
    lymphoid (infectional) (tissue) (wall) J35.2
  prepuce (congenital) N47.8
    female N90.89
  pseudomuscular G71.0
  pylorus (adult) (muscle) (sphincter) K31.1
    congenital or infantile Q40.0
  rectal, rectum (sphincter) K62.89
  rhinitis (turbinate) J31.0
  scar L91.0
    specified NEC L91.8
  skin L91.9
  testis N44.8
    congenital Q55.29
  toe (congenital) Q74.2
    acquired—*see also* Deformity, toe, specified NEC
  tonsils (faucial) (infective) (lingual) (lymphoid) J35.1
    with adenoids J35.3
  uvula K13.79
  ventricle, ventricular (heart)—*see also* Hypertrophy, cardiac
    congenital Q24.8
    in tetralogy of Fallot Q21.3
  vulva N90.60
    childhood asymmetric labium majus enlargement (CALME) N90.61
    other specified N90.69
Hyperventilation (tetany) R06.4
  hysterical F45.8
  psychogenic F45.8
  syndrome F45.8
Hypoacidity, gastric K31.89
  psychogenic F45.8
Hypoadrenalism, hypoadrenia E27.40
  primary E27.1
Hypoadrenocorticism E27.40
  pituitary E23.0
  primary E27.1
Hypoalbuminemia E88.09
Hypoaldosteronism E27.40
Hypocalcemia E83.51
  dietary E58
  neonatal P71.1
    due to cow's milk P71.0
  phosphate-loading (newborn) P71.1
Hypochloremia E87.8
Hypochlorhydria K31.89
  neurotic F45.8
  psychogenic F45.8
Hypochromasia, blood cells D50.8
Hypoeosinophilia D72.89
Hypofibrinogenemia D68.8
  acquired D65
  congenital (hereditary) D68.2
Hypofunction
  adrenocortical E27.40
    primary E27.1
  corticoadrenal NEC E27.40
Hypogammaglobulinemia (*see also* Agammaglobulinemia) D80.1
  hereditary D80.0
  nonfamilial D80.1
  transient, of infancy D80.7

Hypoglycemia (spontaneous) E16.2
  coma E15
    diabetic—*see* Diabetes, coma
  diabetic—*see* Diabetes, hypoglycemia
  dietary counseling and surveillance Z71.3
  neonatal (transitory) P70.4
  transitory neonatal P70.4
Hypometabolism R63.8
Hypomotility
  gastrointestinal (tract) K31.89
    psychogenic F45.8
  intestine K59.8
    psychogenic F45.8
  stomach K31.89
    psychogenic F45.8
Hyponatremia E87.1
Hypo-osmolality E87.1
Hypoperfusion (in)
  newborn P96.89
Hypophyseal, hypophysis—*see also* condition
  gigantism E22.0
Hypoplasia, hypoplastic
  alimentary tract, congenital Q45.8
    upper Q40.8
  anus, anal (canal) Q42.3
    with fistula Q42.2
  aorta, aortic Q25.42
    ascending, in hypoplastic left heart syndrome Q23.4
    valve Q23.1
      in hypoplastic left heart syndrome Q23.4
  artery (peripheral) Q27.8
    pulmonary Q25.79
    umbilical Q27.0
  biliary duct or passage Q44.5
  bone NOS Q79.9
    marrow D61.9
      megakaryocytic D69.49
    skull—*see* Hypoplasia, skull
  brain Q02
  cecum Q42.8
  cephalic Q02
  clavicle (congenital) Q74.0
  colon Q42.9
    specified NEC Q42.8
  corpus callosum Q04.0
  digestive organ (s) or tract NEC Q45.8
    upper (congenital) Q40.8
  endocrine (gland) NEC Q89.2
  erythroid, congenital D61.01
  focal dermal Q82.8
  gallbladder Q44.0
  genitalia, genital organ (s)
    female, congenital Q52.8
      external Q52.79
      internal NEC Q52.8
    in adiposogenital dystrophy E23.6
  intestine (small) Q41.9
    large Q42.9
      specified NEC Q42.8
  jaw M26.09
    lower M26.04
  left heart syndrome Q23.4
  lung (lobe) (not associated with short gestation) Q33.6
    associated with immaturity, low birth weight, prematurity, or short gestation P28.0
  mandible, mandibular M26.04
  medullary D61.9
  megakaryocytic D69.49
  metacarpus—*see* Defect, reduction, upper limb, specified type NEC
  metatarsus—*see* Defect, reduction, lower limb, specified type NEC
  optic nerve H47.03-
  parathyroid (gland) Q89.2
  pelvis, pelvic girdle Q74.2
  penis (congenital) Q55.62
  pituitary (gland) (congenital) Q89.2
  pulmonary (not associated with short gestation) Q33.6
    associated with short gestation P28.0
  rectum Q42.1
    with fistula Q42.0
  scapula Q74.0

Hypoplasia, hypoplastic, *continued*
  shoulder girdle Q74.0
  skin Q82.8
  skull (bone) Q75.8
    with
      anencephaly Q00.0
      encephalocele—*see* Encephalocele
      hydrocephalus Q03.9
        with spina bifida—*see* Spina bifida, by site, with hydrocephalus
      microcephaly Q02
  thymic, with immunodeficiency D82.1
  thymus (gland) Q89.2
    with immunodeficiency D82.1
  thyroid (gland) E03.1
    cartilage Q31.2
  umbilical artery Q27.0
Hypopyrexia R68.0
Hypospadias Q54.9
  balanic Q54.0
  coronal Q54.0
  glandular Q54.0
  penile Q54.1
  penoscrotal Q54.2
  perineal Q54.3
  specified NEC Q54.8
Hypotension (arterial) (constitutional) I95.9
  orthostatic (chronic) I95.1
  postural I95.1
Hypothermia (accidental) T68
  low environmental temperature T68
  neonatal P80.9
    environmental (mild) NEC P80.8
    mild P80.8
    severe (chronic) (cold injury syndrome) P80.0
    specified NEC P80.8
  not associated with low environmental temperature R68.0
Hypothyroidism (acquired) E03.9
  congenital (without goiter) E03.1
    with goiter (diffuse) E03.0
  due to
    iodine-deficiency, acquired E01.8
      subclinical E02
  iodine-deficiency (acquired) E01.8
    congenital—*see* Syndrome, iodine- deficiency, congenital
    subclinical E02
  neonatal, transitory P72.2
  specified NEC E03.8
Hypotonia, hypotonicity, hypotony
  congenital (benign) P94.2
Hypoventilation R06.89
Hypovolemia E86.1
  surgical shock T81.19
  traumatic (shock) T79.4
Hypoxemia R09.02
  newborn P84
Hypoxia (*see also* Anoxia) R09.02
  intrauterine P84
  newborn P84
Hysteria, hysterical (conversion) (dissociative state) F44.9
  anxiety F41.8
  psychosis, acute F44.9

I

Ichthyoparasitism due to Vandellia cirrhosa B88.8
Ichthyosis (congenital) Q80.9
  palmaris and plantaris Q82.8
Icterus—*see also* Jaundice
  conjunctiva R17
    newborn P59.9
  hemorrhagic (acute) (leptospiral) (spirochetal) A27.0
    newborn P53
  infectious B15.9
Ictus solaris, solis T67.0
Ideation
  homicidal R45.850
  suicidal R45.851
Identity disorder (child) F64.9
  gender role F64.2
  psychosexual F64.2
Idioglossia F80.0

Idiopathic—*see* condition
Idiopathic—*see* condition
Idiot, idiocy (congenital) F73
  microcephalic Q02
IgE asthma J45.909
IIAC (idiopathic infantile arterial calcification) Q28.8
Ileitis (chronic) (noninfectious) (*see also* Enteritis) K52.9
  infectious A09
  regional (ulcerative)—*see* Enteritis, regional, small intestine
  segmental—*see* Enteritis, regional
  terminal (ulcerative)—*see* Enteritis, regional, small intestine
Ileocolitis (*see also* Enteritis) K52.9
  regional—*see* Enteritis, regional
  infectious A09
Ileus (bowel) (colon) (inhibitory) (intestine) K56.7
  adynamic K56.0
  meconium P76.0
    in cystic fibrosis E84.11
    meaning meconium plug (without cystic fibrosis) P76.0
  neurogenic K56.0
    Hirschsprung's disease or megacolon Q43.1
  newborn
    due to meconium P76.0
      in cystic fibrosis E84.11
      meaning meconium plug (without cystic fibrosis) P76.0
    transitory P76.1
  obstructive K56.69
  paralytic K56.0
Illness (*see also* Disease) R69
Imbalance R26.89
  electrolyte E87.8
    neonatal, transitory NEC P74.4
  endocrine E34.9
  eye muscle NOS H50.9
  hysterical F44.4
  posture R29.3
  protein-energy—*see* Malnutrition
Immaturity (less than 37 completed weeks)—*see also* Preterm, newborn
  extreme of newborn (less than 28 completed weeks of gestation) (less than 196 completed days of gestation) (unspecified weeks of gestation) P07.20
    gestational age
      23 completed weeks (23 weeks, 0 days through 23 weeks, 6 days) P07.22
      24 completed weeks (24 weeks, 0 days through 24 weeks, 6 days) P07.23
      25 completed weeks (25 weeks, 0 days through 25 weeks, 6 days) P07.24
      26 completed weeks (26 weeks, 0 days through 26 weeks, 6 days) P07.25
      27 completed weeks (27 weeks, 0 days through 27 weeks, 6 days) P07.26
      less than 23 completed weeks P07.21
  fetus or infant light-for-dates—*see* Light-for-dates
  lung, newborn P28.0
  organ or site NEC—*See* Hypoplasia
  pulmonary, newborn P28.0
  sexual (female) (male), after puberty E30.0
Immersion T75.1
  hand T69.01-
  foot T69.02-
Immunization—*see also* Vaccination
  ABO—*see* Incompatibility, ABO
    in newborn P55.1
  complication—*see* Complications, vaccination
  encounter for Z23
  not done (not carried out) Z28.9
    because (of)
      acute illness of patient Z28.01
      allergy to vaccine (or component) Z28.04
      caregiver refusal Z28.82
      chronic illness of patient Z28.02
      contraindication NEC Z28.09
      group pressure Z28.1
      guardian refusal Z28.82
      immune compromised state of patient Z28.03

Immunization, *continued*
    parent refusal Z28.82
    patient's belief Z28.1
    patient had disease being vaccinated against
        Z28.81
    patient refusal Z28.21
    religious beliefs of patient Z28.1
    specified reason NEC Z28.89
       of patient Z28.29
    unspecified patient reason Z28.20
  Rh factor
    affecting management of pregnancy NEC O36.09-
      anti-D antibody O36.01-
    from transfusion—*see* Complication(s), transfusion,
            incompatibility reaction,
            Rh (factor)
Immunodeficiency D84.9
  with
    thrombocytopenia and eczema D82.0
  combined D81.9
    severe D81.9
  severe combined (SCID) D81.9
Impaction, impacted
  bowel, colon, rectum (*see also* Impaction, fecal) K56.49
  cerumen (ear) (external) H61.2-
  fecal, feces K56.41
  intestine (calculous) NEC (*see also* Impaction, fecal)
           K56.49
  turbinate J34.89
Impaired, impairment (function)
  auditory discrimination—*see* Abnormal, auditory
          perception
  dual sensory Z73.82
  fasting glucose R73.01
  glucose tolerance (oral) R73.02
  hearing—*see* Deafness
  heart—*see* Disease, heart
  rectal sphincter R19.8
  vision NEC H54.7
    both eyes H54.3
Impediment, speech R47.9
  psychogenic (childhood) F98.8
  slurring R47.81
  specified NEC R47.89
Imperception auditory (acquired)—*see also* Deafness
  congenital H93.25
Imperfect
  aeration, lung (newborn)NEC—*see* Atelectasis
  closure (congenital)
    alimentary tract NEC Q45.8
      lower Q43.8
      upper Q40.8
    atrioventricular ostium Q21.2
    atrium (secundum) Q21.1
    ductus
      arteriosus Q25.0
      Botalli Q25.0
    esophagus with communication to bronchus or trachea
         Q39.1
    foramen
      botalli Q21.1
      ovale Q21.1
    genitalia, genital organ (s)or system
      female Q52.8
        external Q52.79
        internal NEC Q52.8
      male Q55.8
    interatrial ostium or septum Q21.1
    interauricular ostium or septum Q21.1
    interventricular ostium or septum Q21.0
    omphalomesenteric duct Q43.0
    ostium
      interatrial Q21.1
      interauricular Q21.1
      interventricular Q21.0
    roof of orbit Q75.8
    septum
      atrial (secundum) Q21.1
      interatrial (secundum) Q21.1
      interauricular (secundum) Q21.1
      interventricular Q21.0
        in tetralogy of Fallot Q21.3

Imperfect, *continued*
    ventricular Q21.0
      with pulmonary stenosis or atresia,
            dextraposition of aorta,
            and hypertrophy of
            right ventricle Q21.3
        in tetralogy of Fallot Q21.3
  skull Q75.0
    with
      anencephaly Q00.0
      encephalocele—*see* Encephalocele
      hydrocephalus Q03.9
        with spina bifida—*see* Spina bifida, by site,
            with hydrocephalus
      microcephaly Q02
    spine (with meningocele)—*see* Spina bifida
    vitelline duct Q43.0
  posture R29.3
  rotation, intestine Q43.3
  septum, ventricular Q21.0
Imperfectly descended testis—*see* Cryptorchid
Imperforate (congenital)—*see also* Atresia
  anus Q42.3
    with fistula Q42.2
  esophagus Q39.0
    with tracheoesophageal fistula Q39.1
  hymen Q52.3
  jejunum Q41.1
  rectum Q42.1
    with fistula Q42.0
Impervious (congenital)—*see also* Atresia
  anus Q42.3
    with fistula Q42.2
  bile duct Q44.2
  esophagus Q39.0
    with tracheoesophageal fistula Q39.1
  intestine (small) Q41.9
    large Q42.9
      specified NEC Q42.8
  rectum Q42.1
    with fistula Q42.0
Impetigo (any organism) (any site) (circinate) (contagiosa)
          (simplex) (vulgaris)
          L01.00
  external ear L01.00 *[H62.40]*
Implantation
  cyst
    vagina N89.8
Impression, basilar Q75.8
Improper care (child) (newborn)—*see* Maltreatment
Improperly tied umbilical cord (causing hemorrhage) P51.8
Impulsiveness (impulsive) R45.87
Inability to swallow—*see* Aphagia
Inadequate, inadequacy
  development
    child R62.50
    genitalia
      after puberty NEC E30.0
      congenital
        female Q52.8
          external Q52.79
          internal Q52.8
        male Q55.8
    lungs Q33.6
      associated with short gestation P28.0
    organ or site not listed—*see* Anomaly, by site
  eating habits Z72.4
  environment, household Z59.1
  family support Z63.8
  household care, due to
    family member
      handicapped or ill Z74.2
      temporarily away from home Z74.2
  housing (heating) (space) Z59.1
  intrafamilial communication Z63.8
  mental—*see* Disability, intellectual
  pulmonary
    function R06.89
      newborn P28.5
    ventilation, newborn P28.5
Inanition R64
  fever R50.9

Inappropriate
  diet or eating habits Z72.4
  secretion
    antidiuretic hormone (ADH) (excessive) E22.2
    pituitary (posterior) E22.2
Inattention at or after birth—*see* Neglect
Incarceration, incarcerated
  exomphalos K42.0
    gangrenous K42.1
  hernia—*see also* Hernia, by site, with obstruction
    with gangrene—*see* Hernia, by site, with gangrene
  omphalocele K42.0
  rupture—*see* Hernia, by site
  sarcoepiplomphalocele K42.0
    with gangrene K42.1
Incision, incisional
  hernia K43.2
    with
      gangrene (and obstruction) K43.1
      obstruction K43.0
Inclusion
  blennorrhea (neonatal) (newborn) P39.1
  gallbladder in liver (congenital) Q44.1
Incompatibility
  ABO
    affecting management of pregnancy O36.11-
      anti-A sensitization O36.11-
      anti-B sensitization O36.19-
      specified NEC O36.19-
    infusion or transfusion reaction—*see* Complication(s),
           transfusion,
           incompatibility reaction,
           ABO
    newborn P55.1
  blood (group) (Duffy) (K(ell)) (Kidd) (Lewis) (M) (S)NEC
    affecting management of pregnancy O36.11-
      anti-A sensitization O36.11-
      anti-B sensitization O36.19-
    infusion or transfusion reaction T80.89
    newborn P55.8
  Rh (blood group) (factor) Z31.82
    affecting management of pregnancy NEC O36.09-
      anti-D antibody O36.01-
    infusion or transfusion reaction—*see* Complication(s),
           transfusion,
           incompatibility reaction,
           Rh (factor)
    newborn P55.0
  rhesus—*see* Incompatibility, Rh
Incompetency, incompetent, incompetence
  annular
    aortic (valve)—*see* Insufficiency, aortic
    mitral (valve) I34.0
    pulmonary valve (heart) I37.1
  aortic (valve)—*see* Insufficiency, aortic
  cardiac valve—*see* Endocarditis
  pulmonary valve (heart) I37.1
    congenital Q22.3
Incomplete—*see also* condition
  bladder, emptying R33.9
  defecation R15.0
  expansion lungs (newborn) NEC—*see* Atelectasis
  rotation, intestine Q43.3
Incontinence R32
  anal sphincter R15.9
  feces R15.9
    nonorganic origin F98.1
  psychogenic F45.8
  rectal R15.9
  urethral sphincter R32
  urine (urinary) R32
    nocturnal N39.44
    nonorganic origin F98.0
Increase, increased
  abnormal, in development R63.8
  function
    adrenal
      cortex—*see* Cushing's, syndrome
    pituitary (gland) (anterior) (lobe) E22.9
      posterior E22.2
  intracranial pressure (benign) G93.2
  pressure, intracranial G93.2

Indeterminate sex Q56.4
India rubber skin Q82.8
Indigestion (acid) (bilious) (functional) K30
    due to decomposed food NOS A05.9
    nervous F45.8
    psychogenic F45.8
Induration
    brain G93.89
    breast (fibrous) N64.51
    chancre
        congenital A50.07
        extragenital NEC A51.2
Inertia
    stomach K31.89
        psychogenic F45.8
Infancy, infantile, infantilism—*see also* condition
    celiac K90.0
    genitalia, genitals (after puberty) E30.0
    Herter's (nontropical sprue) K90.0
    intestinal K90.0
    uterus—*see* Infantile, genitalia
Infant (s)—*see also* Infancy
    excessive crying R68.11
    irritable child R68.12
    lack of care—*see* Neglect
    liveborn (singleton) Z38.2
        born in hospital Z38.00
            by cesarean Z38.01
        born outside hospital Z38.1
        multiple NEC Z38.8
            born in hospital Z38.68
                by cesarean Z38.69
            born outside hospital Z38.7
        quadruplet Z38.8
            born in hospital Z38.63
                by cesarean Z38.64
            born outside hospital Z38.7
        quintuplet Z38.8
            born in hospital Z38.65
                by cesarean Z38.66
            born outside hospital Z38.7
        triplet Z38.8
            born in hospital Z38.61
                by cesarean Z38.62
            born outside hospital Z38.7
        twin Z38.5
            born in hospital Z38.30
                by cesarean Z38.31
            born outside hospital Z38.4
    of diabetic mother (syndrome of) P70.1
        gestational diabetes P70.0
Infantile—*see also* condition
    genitalia, genitals E30.0
    os, uterine E30.0
    penis E30.0
    testis E29.1
    uterus E30.0
Infantilism—*see* Infancy
Infarct, infarction
    adrenal (capsule) (gland) E27.49
    intestine, part unspecified
        diffuse acute K55.062
        focal (segmental) K55.061
        unspecified extent K55.069
    large intestine
        diffuse acute K55.042
        focal (segmental) K55.041
        unspecified extent K55.049
    myocardium, myocardial (acute) (with stated duration of
                4 weeks or less) I21.3
        postprocedural
            following cardiac surgery I97.190
            following other surgery I97.191
    small intestine
        diffuse acute K55.022
        focal (segmental) K55.021
        unspecified extent K55.029
    suprarenal (capsule) (gland) E27.49
Infection
    with
        drug resistant organism—*see* Resistance (to), drug—
                see also specific
                organism

Infection, *continued*
    organ dysfunction (acute) R65.20
        with septic shock R65.21
    acromioclavicular M00.9
    adenoid (and tonsil) J03.90
        chronic J35.02
    adenovirus NEC
        as cause of disease classified elsewhere B97.0
        unspecified nature or site B34.0
    alveolus, alveolar (process) K04.7
    antrum (chronic)—*see* Sinusitis, maxillary
    anus, anal (papillae) (sphincter) K62.89
    axillary gland (lymph) L04.2
    bacterial NOS A49.9
        as cause of disease classified elsewhere B96.89
            Enterococcus B95.2
            Escherichia coli [E. coli] (*see also* Escherichia coli)
                B96.20
            Helicobacter pylori [H. pylori] B96.81
            Hemophilus influenzae [H. influenzae] B96.3
            Mycoplasma pneumoniae [M. pneumoniae] B96.0
            Proteus (mirabilis) (morganii) B96.4
            Pseudomonas (aeruginosa) (mallei) (pseudomallei)
                B96.5
            Staphylococcus B95.8
                aureus (methicillin susceptible) (MSSA) B95.61
                methicillin resistant (MRSA) B95.62
                specified NEC B95.7
            Streptococcus B95.5
                group A B95.0
                group B B95.1
                pneumoniae B95.3
                specified NEC B95.4
        specified NEC A48.8
    Borrelia burgdorferi A69.20
    brain (*see also* Encephalitis) G04.90
        membranes—*see* Meningitis
        septic G06.0
            meninges—*see* Meningitis, bacterial
    buttocks (skin) L08.9
    Campylobacter, intestinal A04.5
        as cause of disease classified elsewhere B96.81
    Candida (albicans) (tropicalis)—*see* Candidiasis
    candiru B88.8
    central line-associated T80.219
        bloodstream (CLABSI) T80.211
        specified NEC T80.218
    cervical gland (lymph) L04.0
    Chlamydia, chlamydial A74.9
        anus A56.3
        genitourinary tract A56.2
            lower A56.00
            specified NEC A56.19
        pharynx A56.4
        rectum A56.3
        sexually transmitted NEC A56.8
    Clostridium NEC
        botulinum (food poisoning) A05.1
            infant A48.51
            wound A48.52
        difficile
            sepsis A41.4
        perfringens
            due to food A05.2
            foodborne (disease) A05.2
            necrotizing enterocolitis A05.2
            sepsis A41.4
        welchii
            foodborne (disease) A05.2
            sepsis A41.4
    congenital P39.9
        Candida (albicans) P37.5
        cytomegalovirus P35.1
        herpes simplex P35.2
        infectious or parasitic disease P37.9
            specified NEC P37.8
        listeriosis (disseminated) P37.2
        rubella P35.0
        toxoplasmosis (acute) (subacute) (chronic) P37.1
        urinary (tract) P39.3
    cytomegalovirus, cytomegaloviral B25.9
        congenital P35.1

Infection, *continued*
    maternal, maternal care for (suspected) damage to
                fetus O35.3
        mononucleosis B27.10
            with
                complication NEC B27.19
                meningitis B27.12
                polyneuropathy B27.11
    dental (pulpal origin) K04.7
    due to or resulting from
        central venous catheter T80.219
            bloodstream T80.211
            exit or insertion site T80.212
            localized T80.212
            port or reservoir T80.212
            specified NEC T80.218
            tunnel T80.212
        device, implant or graft (*see also* Complications, by site
                and type, infection or
                inflammation) T85.79
            arterial graft NEC T82.7
            catheter NEC T85.79
                dialysis (renal) T82.7
                    intraperitoneal T85.71
                infusion NEC T82.7
        Hickman catheter T80.219
            bloodstream T80.211
            localized T80.212
            specified NEC T80.218
        immunization or vaccination T88.0
        infusion, injection or transfusion NEC T80.29
            acute T80.22
        peripherally inserted central catheter (PICC) T80.219
            bloodstream T80.211
            localized T80.212
            specified NEC T80.218
        portacath (port-a-cath) T80.219
            bloodstream T80.211
            localized T80.212
            specified NEC T80.218
        triple lumen catheter T80.219
            bloodstream T80.211
            localized T80.212
            specified NEC T80.218
        umbilical venous catheter T80.219
            bloodstream T80.211
            localized T80.212
            specified NEC T80.218
    ear (middle)—*see also* Otitis media
        external—*see* Otitis, externa, infective
        inner—*see* subcategory H83.0
    echovirus
        as cause of disease classified elsewhere B97.12
        unspecified nature or site B34.1
    endocardium I33.0
    Enterobius vermicularis B80
    enterovirus B34.1
        as cause of disease classified elsewhere B97.10
            coxsackievirus B97.11
            echovirus B97.12
            specified NEC B97.19
    erythema infectiosum B08.3
    Escherichia (E.) coli NEC A49.8
        as cause of disease classified elsewhere (*see also*
                Escherichia coli)
                B96.20
        congenital P39.8
            sepsis P36.4
        generalized A41.51
        intestinal—*see* Enteritis, infectious, due to,
                Escherichia coli
    eyelid H01.9
        abscess—*see* Abscess, eyelid
        blepharitis—*see* Blepharitis
        chalazion—*see* Chalazion
        dermatosis (noninfectious)—*see* Dermatosis, eyelid
        hordeolum—*see* Hordeolum
        specified NEC H01.8
    finger (skin) L08.9
        nail L03.01-
            fungus B35.1

Infection, *continued*
  focal
    teeth (pulpal origin) K04.7
    tonsils J35.01
  foot (skin) L08.9
    dermatophytic fungus B35.3
  fungus NOS B49
    beard B35.0
    dermatophytic—*see* Dermatophytosis
    foot B35.3
    groin B35.6
    hand B35.2
    nail B35.1
    perianal (area) B35.6
    scalp B35.0
    skin B36.9
      foot B35.3
      hand B35.2
      toenails B35.1
  Giardia lamblia A07.1
  gingiva (chronic) K05.10
    acute K05.00
      plaque induced K05.00
  gram-negative bacilli NOS A49.9
  gum (chronic) K05.10
    acute K05.00
      plaque induced K05.00
  Helicobacter pylori A04.8
    as the cause of disease classified elsewhere B96.81
  Hemophilus
    influenzae NEC A49.2
      as cause of disease classified elsewhere B96.3
    generalized A41.3
  herpes (simplex)—*see also* Herpes
    congenital P35.2
    disseminated B00.7
    zoster B02.9
  herpesvirus, herpesviral—*see* Herpes
  hip (joint) NEC M00.9
    skin NEC L08.9
  human
    papilloma virus A63.0
  hydrocele N43.0
  inguinal (lymph) glands L04.1
  joint NEC M00.9
  knee (joint) NEC M00.9
    joint M00.9
    skin L08.9
  leg (skin) NOS L08.9
  listeria monocytogenes—*see also* Listeriosis
    congenital P37.2
  local, skin (staphylococcal) (streptococcal) L08.9
    abscess—*code by* site under Abscess
    cellulitis—*code by* site under Cellulitis
    specified NEC L08.89
    ulcer—*see* Ulcer, skin
  lung (*see also* Pneumonia) J18.9
    virus—*see* Pneumonia, viral
  lymph gland—*see also* Lymphadenitis, acute
    mesenteric I88.0
  lymphoid tissue, base of tongue or posterior pharynx, NEC (chronic) J35.03
  Malassezia furfur B36.0
  mammary gland N61.0
  meningococcal (*see also* condition) A39.9
    cerebrospinal A39.0
    meninges A39.0
    meningococcemia A39.4
      acute A39.2
      chronic A39.3
  mesenteric lymph nodes or glands NEC I88.0
  metatarsophalangeal M00.9
  mouth, parasitic B37.0
  Mycoplasma NEC A49.3
    pneumoniae, as cause of disease classified elsewhere B96.0
  myocardium NEC I40.0
  nail (chronic)
    with lymphangitis—*see* Lymphangitis, acute, digit
    finger L03.01-
      fungus B35.1
    ingrowing L60.0

Infection, *continued*
  toe L03.03-
    fungus B35.1
  newborn P39.9
    intra-amniotic NEC P39.2
    skin P39.4
    specified type NEC P39.8
  nipple N61.0
  Oidium albicans B37.9
  Oxyuris vermicularis B80
  pancreas (acute) K85.92
    abscess—*see* Pancreatitis, acute
    specified NEC K85.82
  parameningococcus A39.9
  paraurethral ducts N34.2
  parvovirus NEC B34.3
    as the cause of disease classified elsewhere B97.6
  Pasteurella NEC A28.0
    multocida A28.0
    pseudotuberculosis A28.0
    septica (cat bite) (dog bite) A28.0
  perinatal period P39.9
    specified type NEC P39.8
  perirectal K62.89
  perirenal—*see* Infection, kidney
  peritoneal—*see* Peritonitis
  pharynx—*see also* pharyngitis
    coxsackievirus B08.5
    posterior, lymphoid (chronic) J35.03
  pinworm B80
  pityrosporum furfur B36.0
  pleuro-pneumonia-like organism (PPLO) NEC A49.3
    as cause of disease classified elsewhere B96.0
  pneumococcus, pneumococcal NEC A49.1
    as cause of disease classified elsewhere B95.3
    generalized (purulent) A40.3
      with pneumonia J13
  port or reservoir T80.212
  prepuce NEC N47.7
    with penile inflammation N47.6
  Proteus (mirabilis) (morganii) (vulgaris) NEC A49.8
    as cause of disease classified elsewhere B96.4
  Pseudomonas NEC A49.8
    as cause of disease classified elsewhere B96.5
    pneumonia J15.1
  rectum (sphincter) K62.89
  renal—*see also* Infection, kidney
    pelvis and ureter (cystic) N28.85
  respiratory (tract) NEC J98.8
    acute J22
    rhinovirus J00
    upper (acute)NOS J06.9
      streptococcal J06.9
      viral NOS J06.9
  rhinovirus
    as cause of disease classified elsewhere B97.89
    unspecified nature or site B34.8
  roundworm (large) NEC B82.0
    Ascariasis (*see also* Ascariasis) B77.9
  Salmonella (aertrycke) (arizonae) (callinarum) (choleraesuis) (enteritidis) (suipestifer) (typhimurium)
    with
      (gastro) enteritis A02.0
      specified manifestation NEC A02.8
    due to food (poisoning) A02.9
  scabies B86
  Shigella A03.9
    boydii A03.2
    dysenteriae A03.0
    flexneri A03.1
    group
      A A03.0
      B A03.1
      C A03.2
      D A03.3
  shoulder (joint) NEC M00.9
    skin NEC L08.9
  skin (local) (staphylococcal) (streptococcal) L08.9
    abscess—*code by* site under Abscess
    cellulitis—*code by* site under Cellulitis

Infection, *continued*
  spinal cord NOS (*see also* Myelitis) G04.91
    abscess G06.1
    meninges—*see* Meningitis
    streptococcal G04.89
  staphylococcal, unspecified site
    aureus (methicillin susceptible) (MSSA) A49.01
      methicillin resistant (MRSA) A49.02
    as cause of disease classified elsewhere B95.8
      aureus (methicillin susceptible) (MSSA) B95.61
        methicillin resistant (MRSA) B95.62
      specified NEC B95.7
    food poisoning A05.0
    generalized (purulent) A41.2
    pneumonia—*see* Pneumonia, staphylococcal
  streptococcal NEC A49.1
    as the cause of disease classified elsewhere B95.5
    congenital
      sepsis P36.10
        group B P36.0
        specified NEC P36.19
    generalized (purulent) A40.9
  subcutaneous tissue, local L08.9
  threadworm B80
  toe (skin) L08.9
    cellulitis L03.03-
      fungus B35.1
    nail L03.03-
      fungus B35.1
  tongue NEC K14.0
    parasitic B37.0
  tooth, teeth K04.7
    periapical K04.7
  TORCH—*see* Infection, congenital
    without active infection P00.2
  Trichomonas A59.9
    cervix A59.09
    specified site NEC A59.8
    urethra A59.03
    urogenitalis A59.00
    vagina A59.01
    vulva A59.01
  Trombicula (irritans) B88.0
  tunnel T80.212
  urinary (tract) N39.0
    bladder—*see* Cystitis
    kidney—*see* Infection, kidney
    newborn P39.3
    urethra—*see* Urethritis
  varicella B01.9
  Vibrio
    parahaemolyticus (food poisoning) A05.3
    vulnificus
      as cause of disease classified elsewhere B96.82
      foodborne intoxication A05.5
  virus, viral NOS B34.9
    adenovirus
      as the cause of disease classified elsewhere B97.0
      unspecified nature or site B34.0
    as the cause of disease classified elsewhere B97.89
      adenovirus B97.0
      coxsackievirus B97.11
      echovirus B97.12
      enterovirus B97.10
        coxsackievirus B97.11
        echovirus B97.12
        specified NEC B97.19
      parvovirus B97.6
      specified NEC B97.89
    central nervous system A89
      atypical A81.9
        specified NEC A81.89
      enterovirus NEC A88.8
        meningitis A87.0
    coxsackie (*see also* Infection, coxsackie) B34.1
      as cause of disease classified elsewhere B97.11
    ECHO
      as cause of disease classified elsewhere B97.12
      unspecified nature or site B34.1

INFECTION–INFECTION

Infection, *continued*
  enterovirus, as cause of disease classified elsewhere
          B97.10
    coxsackievirus B97.11
    echovirus B97.12
    specified NEC B97.19
  exanthem NOS B09
  respiratory syncytial
    as cause of disease classified elsewhere B97.4
    bronchopneumonia J12.1
    common cold syndrome J00
    nasopharyngitis (acute) J00
  rhinovirus
    as the cause of disease specified elsewhere
          B97.89
  specified type NEC B33.8
    as the cause of disease specified elsewhere
          B97.89
  yeast (*see also* Candidiasis) B37.9
  Zika virus A92.5
Infertility
  female N97.9
    associated with
      anovulation N97.0
      Stein-Leventhal syndrome E28.2
    due to
      Stein-Leventhal syndrome E28.2
Infestation B88.9
  Acariasis B88.0
    demodex folliculorum B88.0
    sarcoptes scabiei B86
    trombiculae B88.0
  arthropod NEC B88.2
  Ascaris lumbricoides—*see* Ascariasis
  candiru B88.8
  cestodes B71.9
  chigger B88.0
  chigo, chigoe B88.1
  crab-lice B85.3
  Demodex (folliculorum) B88.0
  Dermanyssus gallinae B88.0
  Enterobius vermicularis B80
  eyelid
    in (due to)
      phthiriasis B85.3
  Giardia lamblia A07.1
  helminth B83.9
    intestinal B82.0
      enterobiasis B80
  intestinal NEC B82.9
  Linguatula B88.8
  Lyponyssoides sanguineus B88.0
  mites B88.9
    scabic B86
  Monilia (albicans)—*see* Candidiasis
  mouth B37.0
  nematode NEC (intestinal) B82.0
    Enterobius vermicularis B80
    physaloptera B80
  Oxyuris vermicularis B80
  parasite, parasitic B89
    eyelid B89
    intestinal NOS B82.9
    mouth B37.0
    skin B88.9
    tongue B37.0
  Pediculus B85.2
    body B85.1
    capitis (humanus) (any site) B85.0
    corporis (humanus) (any site) B85.1
    mixed (classifiable to more than one of the titles
          B85.0–B85.3) B85.4
    pubis (any site) B85.3
  Pentastoma B88.8
  Phthirus (pubis) (any site) B85.3
    with any infestation classifiable to B85.0-B85.2 B85.4
  pinworm B80
  pubic louse B85.3
  red bug B88.0
  sand flea B88.1
  Sarcoptes scabiei B86
  scabies B86

Infestation, *continued*
  Schistosoma B65.9
    cercariae B65.3
  skin NOS B88.9
  specified type NEC B88.8
  tapeworm B71.9
  Tetranychus molestissimus B88.0
  threadworm B80
  tongue B37.0
  Trombicula (irritans) B88.0
  Tunga penetrans B88.1
  Vandella cirrhosa B88.8
Infiltrate, infiltration
  leukemic—*see* Leukemia
  lung R91.8
  lymphatic (*see also* Leukemia, lymphatic) C91.9-
    gland I88.9
  on chest x-ray R91.8
  pulmonary R91.8
  vesicant agent
    antineoplastic chemotherapy T80.810
    other agent NEC T80.818
Inflammation, inflamed, inflammatory (with exudation)
  anal canal, anus K62.89
  areola N61.0
  areolar tissue NOS L08.9
  breast N61.0
  bronchi—*see* Bronchitis
  catarrhal J00
  cerebrospinal
    meningococcal A39.0
  due to device, implant or graft—*see also* Complications,
          by site and type,
          infection or
          inflammation
    arterial graft T82.7
    catheter T85.79
      dialysis (renal) T82.7
        intraperitoneal T85.71
      infusion T82.7
      cardiac T82.7
    vascular NEC T82.7
  duodenum K29.80
    with bleeding K29.81
  esophagus K20.9
  follicular, pharynx J31.2
  gland (lymph)—*see* Lymphadenitis
  glottis—*see* Laryngitis
  granular, pharynx J31.2
  leg NOS L08.9
  lip K13.0
  mouth K12.1
  nipple N61.0
  orbit (chronic) H05.10
    acute H05.00
      abscess—*see* Abscess, orbit
      cellulitis—*see* Cellulitis, orbit
      osteomyelitis—*see* Osteomyelitis, orbit
      periostitis—*see* Periostitis, orbital
      tenonitis—*see* Tenonitis, eye
      granuloma—*see* Granuloma, orbit
      myositis—*see* Myositis, orbital
  parotid region L08.9
  perianal K62.89
  pericardium—*see* Pericarditis
  perineum (female) (male) L08.9
  perirectal K62.89
  peritoneum—*see* Peritonitis
  polyp, colon (*see also* Polyp, colon, inflammatory) K51.40
  rectum (*see also* Proctitis) K62.89
  respiratory, upper (*see also* Infection, respiratory, upper)
          J06.9
  skin L08.9
  subcutaneous tissue L08.9
  tongue K14.0
  tonsil—*see* Tonsillitis
  vein—*see also* Phlebitis
    intracranial or intraspinal (septic) G08
    thrombotic I80.9
      leg—*see* Phlebitis, leg
      lower extremity—*see* Phlebitis, leg

Influenza (bronchial) (epidemic) (respiratory (upper))
          (unidentified influenza
          virus) J11.1
  with
    digestive manifestations J11.2
    encephalopathy J11.81
    enteritis J11.2
    gastroenteritis J11.2
    gastrointestinal manifestations J11.2
    laryngitis J11.1
    myocarditis J11.82
    otitis media J11.83
    pharyngitis J11.1
    pneumonia J11.00
      specified type J11.08
    respiratory manifestations NEC J11.1
    specified manifestation NEC J11.89
  A/H5N1 (*see also* Influenza, due to, identified novel
          influenza A virus)
          J09.X2
  avian (*see also* Influenza, due to, identified novel influenza
          A virus) J09.X2
  bird (*see also* Influenza, due to, identified novel influenza A
          virus) J09.X2
  novel (2009) H1N1 influenza (*see also* Influenza, due to,
          identified influenza
          virus NEC) J10.1
  novel influenza A/H1N1 (*see also* Influenza, due to,
          identified influenza
          virus NEC) J10.1
  due to
    avian (*see also* Influenza, due to, identified novel
          influenza A virus)
          J09.X2
    identified influenza virus NEC J10.1
      with
        digestive manifestations J10.2
        encephalopathy J10.81
        enteritis J10.2
        gastroenteritis J10.2
        gastrointestinal manifestations J10.2
        laryngitis J10.1
        myocarditis J10.82
        otitis media J10.83
        pharyngitis J10.1
        pneumonia (unspecified type) J10.00
          with same identified influenza virus J10.01
          specified type NEC J10.08
        respiratory manifestations NEC J10.1
        specified manifestation NEC J10.89
    identified novel influenza A virus J09.X2
      with
        digestive manifestations J09.X3
        encephalopathy J09.X9
        enteritis J09.X3
        gastroenteritis J09.X3
        gastrointestinal manifestations J09.X3
        laryngitis J09.X2
        myocarditis J09.X9
        otitis media J09.X9
        pharyngitis J09.X2
        pneumonia J09.X1
        respiratory manifestations NEC J09.X2
        specified manifestation NEC J09.X9
        upper respiratory symptoms J09.X2
    of other animal origin, not bird or swine (*see also*
          Influenza, due to,
          identified novel
          influenza A virus)
          J09.X2
    swine (viruses that normally cause infections in pigs)
          (*see also* Influenza,
          due to, identified novel
          influenza A virus)
          J09.X2
Influenza-like disease—*see* Influenza
Influenzal—*see* Influenza

Ingestion
chemical—*see* Table of Drugs and Chemicals, by
        substance, poisoning
drug or medicament
    correct substance properly administered—*see*
        Table of Drugs and
        Chemicals, by drug,
        adverse effect
    overdose or wrong substance given or taken—*see*
        Table of Drugs and
        Chemicals, by drug,
        poisoning
foreign body—*see* Foreign body, alimentary tract
tularemia A21.3
Ingrowing
hair (beard) L73.1
nail (finger) (toe) L60.0
Inguinal—*see also* condition
testicle Q53.9
    bilateral Q53.21
    unilateral Q53.11
Inhalation
anthrax A22.1
gases, fumes, or vapors NEC T59.9-
    specified agent—*see* Table of Drugs and Chemicals,
        by substance
liquid or vomitus—*see* Asphyxia
meconium (newborn) P24.00
    with
        pneumonia (pneumonitis) P24.01
        with respiratory symptoms P24.01
mucus—*see* Asphyxia, mucus
oil or gasoline (causing suffocation)—*see* Foreign body,
        by site
smoke J70.5
Injury (*see also* specified type of injury) T14.90
ankle S99.91-
    specified type NEC S99.81-
brachial plexus S14.3
    newborn P14.3
cord
    spermatic (pelvic region) S37.898
        scrotal region S39.848
eye S05.9-
    conjunctiva S05.0-
    cornea
        abrasion S05.0-
foot S99.92-
    specified type NEC S99.82-
genital organ (s)
    external S39.94
        specified NEC S39.848
head S09.90
    with loss of consciousness S06.9-
    specified NEC S09.8
internal T14.8
    pelvis, pelvic (organ) S39.90
    specified NEC S39.83
intra-abdominal S36.90
intracranial (traumatic) S06.9-
    cerebellar hemorrhage, traumatic—*see* Injury,
        intracranial, focal
    intracerebral hemorrhage, traumatic S06.36-
        left side S06.35-
        right side S06.34-
        intracranial (trauma)
            epidural, hemorrhage (traumatic) S06.4X
    subarachnoid hemorrhage, traumatic S06.6X-
    subdural hemorrhage, traumatic S06.5X-
intrathoracic S27.9
    lung S27.309
        aspiration J69.0
        bilateral S27.302
        contusion S27.329
            bilateral S27.322
            unilateral S27.321
        unilateral S27.301
        pneumothorax S27.0-
kidney S37.00-
    acute (nontraumatic) N17.9
    contusion—*see* Contusion, kidney
    laceration—*see* Laceration, kidney
    specified NEC S37.09-

Injury, *continued*
lung—*see also* Injury, intrathoracic, lung
    aspiration J69.0
    transfusion-related (TRALI) J95.84
nerve NEC T14.8
    facial S04.5-
        newborn P11.3
pelvis, pelvic (floor) S39.93
    specified NEC S39.83
postcardiac surgery (syndrome) I97.0
rectovaginal septum NEC S39.83
scalp S09.90
    newborn (birth injury) P12.9
        due to monitoring (electrode) (sampling incision)
            P12.4
    specified NEC P12.89
        caput succedaneum P12.81
spermatic cord (pelvic region) S37.898
    scrotal region S39.848
spinal (cord)
    cervical (neck) S14.109
        C1 level S14.101
        C2 level S14.102
        C3 level S14.103
        C4 level S14.104
        C5 level S14.105
        C6 level S14.106
        C7 level S14.107
        C8 level S14.108
    lumbar S34.109
        complete lesion S34.119
            L1 level S34.111
            L2 level S34.112
            L3 level S34.113
            L4 level S34.114
            L5 level S34.115
        incomplete lesion S34.129
            L1 level S34.121
            L2 level S34.122
            L3 level S34.123
            L4 level S34.124
            L5 level S34.125
        L1 level S34.101
        L2 level S34.102
        L3 level S34.103
        L4 level S34.104
        L5 level S34.105
    sacral S34.139
        complete lesion S34.131
        incomplete lesion S34.132
    thoracic S24.109
        T1 level S24.101
        T2-T6 level S24.102
        T7-T10 level S24.103
        T11-T12 level S24.104
spleen S36.00
    superficial (capsular) (minor) S36.030
toe S99.92-
    specified type NEC S99.82-
transfusion-related acute lung (TRALI) J95.84
vagina S39.93
    abrasion S30.814
    bite S31.45
        insect S30.864
        superficial NEC S30.874
    contusion S30.23
    crush S38.03
    external constriction S30.844
    insect bite S30.864
    laceration S31.41
        with foreign body S31.42
    open wound S31.40
    puncture S31.43
        with foreign body S31.44
    superficial S30.95
        foreign body S30.854
vulva S39.94
    abrasion S30.814
    bite S31.45
        insect S30.864
        superficial NEC S30.874
    contusion S30.23

Injury, *continued*
    crush S38.03
    external constriction S30.844
    insect bite S30.864
    laceration S31.41
        with foreign body S31.42
    open wound S31.40
    puncture S31.43
        with foreign body S31.44
    superficial S30.95
        foreign body S30.854
    whiplash (cervical spine) S13.4
Insensitivity
adrenocorticotropin hormone (ACTH) E27.49
androgen E34.50
    complete E34.51
    partial E34.52
Inspissated bile syndrome (newborn) P59.1
Insolation (sunstroke) T67.0
Insomnia (organic) G47.00
behavioral, of childhood Z73.819
    combined type Z73.812
    limit setting type Z73.811
    sleep-onset association type Z73.810
childhood Z73.819
Instability
vasomotor R55
Insufficiency, insufficient
adrenal (gland) E27.40
    primary E27.1
adrenocortical E27.40
    primary E27.1
anus K62.89
aortic (valve) I35.1
    with
        mitral (valve) disease I08.0
            with tricuspid (valve) disease I08.3
        stenosis I35.2
        tricuspid (valve) disease I08.2
            with mitral (valve) disease I08.3
    congenital Q23.1
    rheumatic I06.1
        with
            mitral (valve) disease I08.0
                with tricuspid (valve) disease I08.3
            stenosis I06.2
                with mitral (valve) disease I08.0
                    with tricuspid (valve) disease I08.3
            tricuspid (valve) disease I08.2
                with mitral (valve) disease I08.3
    specified cause NEC I35.1
cardiac—*see also* Insufficiency, myocardial
    due to presence of (cardiac) prosthesis I97.11-
    postprocedural I97.11-
corticoadrenal E27.40
    primary E27.1
kidney N28.9
    acute N28.9
    chronic N18.9
mitral (valve) I34.0
    with
        aortic valve disease I08.0
            with tricuspid (valve) disease I08.3
        obstruction or stenosis I05.2
            with aortic valve disease I08.0
        tricuspid (valve) disease I08.1
            with aortic (valve) disease I08.3
    congenital Q23.3
    rheumatic I05.1
        with
            aortic valve disease I08.0
                with tricuspid (valve) disease I08.3
            obstruction or stenosis I05.2
                with aortic valve disease I08.0
                    with tricuspid (valve) disease I08.3
            tricuspid (valve) disease I08.1
                with aortic (valve) disease I08.3
    active or acute I01.1
        with chorea, rheumatic (Sydenham's) I02.0
    specified cause, except rheumatic I34.0
muscle—*see also* Disease, muscle
    heart—*see* Insufficiency, myocardial
    ocular NEC H50.9

Insufficiency, insufficient, *continued*
  myocardial, myocardium (with arteriosclerosis) I50.9
    with
      rheumatic fever (conditions in I00) I09.0
        active, acute or subacute I01.2
          with chorea I02.0
        inactive or quiescent (with chorea) I09.0
    congenital Q24.8
    newborn P29.0
    rheumatic I09.0
      active, acute, or subacute I01.2
  placental (mother) O36.51
  pulmonary J98.4
    newborn P28.5
    valve I37.1
      with stenosis I37.2
      congenital Q22.2
      rheumatic I09.89
        with aortic, mitral or tricuspid (valve)disease
                I08.8
  renal (acute) N28.9
    chronic N18.9
  respiratory R06.89
    newborn P28.5
  rotation—*see* Malrotation
  suprarenal E27.40
    primary E27.1
  thyroid (gland) (acquired) E03.9
    congenital E03.1
  tricuspid (valve) (rheumatic) I07.1
    with
      aortic (valve) disease I08.2
        with mitral (valve) disease I08.3
      mitral (valve) disease I08.1
        with aortic (valve) disease I08.3
      obstruction or stenosis I07.2
        with aortic (valve) disease I08.2
          with mitral (valve) disease I08.3
    congenital Q22.8
    nonrheumatic I36.1
      with stenosis I36.2
  urethral sphincter R32
  velopharyngeal
    acquired K13.79
    congenital Q38.8
Intertrigo L30.4
  labialis K13.0
Intolerance
  carbohydrate K90.49
  disaccharide, hereditary E73.0
  fat NEC K90.49
    pancreatic K90.3
  food K90.49
    dietary counseling and surveillance Z71.3
  gluten
    celiac K90.0
    non-celiac K90.41
  lactose E73.9
    specified NEC E73.8
  milk NEC K90.49
    lactose E73.9
  protein K90.49
  starch NEC K90.49
Intoxication
  drug
    acute (without dependence)—*see* Abuse, drug, by type
             with intoxication
      with dependence—*see* Dependence, drug, by type
             with intoxication
    addictive
      via placenta or breast milk—*see* Absorption, drug,
            addictive, through
            placenta
    newborn P93.8
      gray baby syndrome P93.0
    overdose or wrong substance given or taken—*see*
            Table of Drugs and
            Chemicals, by drug,
            poisoning
  foodborne A05.9
    bacterial A05.9
    classical (Clostridium botulinum) A05.1
    due to

Intoxication, *continued*
    Bacillus cereus A05.4
    bacterium A05.9
      specified NEC A05.8
    Clostridium
      botulinum A05.1
      perfringens A05.2
      welchii A05.2
    Salmonella A02.9
      with
        (gastro) enteritis A02.0
        specified manifestation NEC A02.8
    Staphylococcus A05.0
    Vibrio
      parahaemolyticus A05.3
      vulnificus A05.5
    enterotoxin, staphylococcal A05.0
    noxious—*see* Poisoning, food, noxious
  meaning
    inebriation—*see* category F10
    poisoning—*see* Table of Drugs and Chemicals
  serum (*see also* Reaction, serum) T80.69
Intrahepatic gallbladder Q44.1
Intrauterine contraceptive device
  checking Z30.431
  insertion Z30.430
    immediately following removal Z30.433
  in situ Z97.5
  management Z30.431
  reinsertion Z30.433
  removal Z30.432
  replacement Z30.433
Intussusception (bowel) (colon) (enteric) (ileocecal) (ileocolic)
                (intestine) (rectum)
                K56.1
Invagination (bowel, colon, intestine or rectum) K56.1
Inversion
  albumin-globulin (A-G) ratio E88.09
  nipple N64.59
  testis (congenital) Q55.29
Investigation (*see also* Examination) Z04.9
  clinical research subject (control) (normal comparison)
                (participant) Z00.6
I. Q.
  under 20 F73
  20–34 F72
  35–49 F71
  50–69 F70
IRDS (type I) P22.0
  type II P22.1
Iritis—*see also* Iridocyclitis
  diabetic—*see* E08–E13 with .39
Irradiated enamel (tooth, teeth) K03.89
Irradiation effects, adverse T66
Irregular, irregularity
  action, heart I49.9
  bleeding N92.6
  breathing R06.89
  menstruation (cause unknown) N92.6
  periods N92.6
  respiratory R06.89
  septum (nasal) J34.2
Irritable, irritability R45.4
  bladder N32.89
  bowel (syndrome) K58.9
    with constipation K58.1
    with diarrhea K58.0
    mixed K58.2
    other K58.8
    psychogenic F45.8
  colon K58.9
    with constipation K58.1
    with diarrhea K58.0
    mixed K58.2
    other K58.8
    psychogenic F45.8
  heart (psychogenic) F45.8
  infant R68.12
  stomach K31.89
    psychogenic F45.8

Irritation
  anus K62.89
  bladder N32.89
  gastric K31.89
    psychogenic F45.8
  nervous R45.0
  perineum NEC L29.3
  stomach K31.89
    psychogenic F45.8
  vaginal N89.8
Ischemia, ischemic I99.8
  brain—*see* Ischemia, cerebral
  cerebral (chronic) (generalized) I67.82
    intermittent G45.9
    newborn P91.0
    recurrent focal G45.8
    transient G45.9
  intestine, unspecified part
    diffuse acute (reversible) K55.052
    focal(segmental) acute (reversible) K55.051
    unspecified extent K55.059
  large intestine
    diffuse acute (reversible) K55.032
    focal(segmental) acute (reversible) K55.031
    unspecified extent K55.039
  small intestine
    diffuse acute (reversible) K55.012
    focal(segmental) acute (reversible) K55.011
    unspecified extent K55.019
Ischuria R34
Isoimmunization NEC—*see also* Incompatibility
  affecting management of pregnancy (ABO) (with hydrops
                fetalis) O36.11-
    anti-A sensitization O36.11-
    anti-B sensitization O36.19-
    anti-c sensitization O36.09-
    anti-C sensitization O36.09-
    anti-e sensitization O36.09-
    anti-E sensitization O36.09-
    Rh NEC O36.09-
      anti-D antibody O36.01-
    specified NEC O36.19-
  newborn P55.9
    with
      hydrops fetalis P56.0
      kernicterus P57.0
    ABO (blood groups) P55.1
    Rhesus (Rh)factor P55.0
    specified type NEC P55.8
Isolation, isolated
  family Z63.79
Issue of
  medical certificate Z02.79
    for disability determination Z02.71
  repeat prescription (appliance) (glasses) (medicinal
            substance,
            medicament, medicine)
            Z76.0
    contraception—*see* Contraception
Itch, itching—*see also* Pruritus
  baker's L23.6
  barber's B35.0
  cheese B88.0
  clam digger's B65.3
  copra B88.0
  dhobi B35.6
  grain B88.0
  grocer's B88.0
  harvest B88.0
  jock B35.6
  Malabar B35.5
    beard B35.0
    foot B35.3
    scalp B35.0
  meaning scabies B86
  Norwegian B86
  perianal L29.0
  poultrymen's B88.0
  sarcoptic B86
  scabies B86
  scrub B88.0

INSUFFICIENCY, INSUFFICIENT–ITCH, ITCHING

Itch, itching, *continued*
  straw B88.0
  swimmer's B65.3
  winter L29.8
Ixodiasis NEC B88.8

J

Jacquet's dermatitis (diaper dermatitis) L22
Jamaican
  neuropathy G92
  paraplegic tropical ataxic-spastic syndrome G92
Jaundice (yellow) R17
  breast-milk (inhibitor) P59.3
  catarrhal (acute) B15.9
  cholestatic (benign) R17
  due to or associated with
    delayed conjugation P59.8
      associated with (due to)preterm delivery P59.0
    preterm delivery P59.0
  epidemic (catarrhal) B15.9
  familial nonhemolytic (congenital) (Gilbert) E80.4
    Crigler-Najjar E80.5
  febrile (acute) B15.9
  infectious (acute) (subacute) B15.9
  neonatal—*see* Jaundice, newborn
  newborn P59.9
    due to or associated with
      ABO
        antibodies P55.1
        incompatibility, maternal/fetal P55.1
        isoimmunization P55.1
      breast milk inhibitors to conjugation P59.3
        associated with preterm delivery P59.0
      Crigler-Najjar syndrome E80.5
      delayed conjugation P59.8
        associated with preterm delivery P59.0
      Gilbert syndrome E80.4
      hemolytic disease P55.9
        ABO isoimmunization P55.1
      hepatocellular damage P59.20
        specified NEC P59.29
      hypothyroidism, congenital E03.1
      inspissated bile syndrome P59.1
      mucoviscidosis E84.9
      preterm delivery P59.0
      spherocytosis (congenital) D58.0
    nonhemolytic congenital familial (Gilbert) E80.4
    symptomatic R17
      newborn P59.9
Jealousy
  childhood F93.8
  sibling F93.8
Jejunitis—*see* Enteritis
Jejunostomy status Z93.4
Jejunum, jejunal—*see* condition
Jerks, myoclonic G25.3
Jervell-Lange-Nielsen syndrome I45.81
Jigger disease B88.1
Job's syndrome (chronic granulomatous disease) D71
Joseph-Diamond-Blackfan anemia (congenital hypoplastic)
                                    D61.01

K

Kaposi's
  vaccinia T88.1
Kartagener's syndrome or triad (sinusitis, bronchiectasis,
                                    situs inversus) Q89.3
Karyotype
  47,XXX Q97.0
  47,XYY Q98.5
Kawasaki's syndrome M30.3
Kaznelson's syndrome (congenital hypoplastic anemia)
                                    D61.01
Kelis L91.0
Keloid, cheloid L91.0
  Hawkin's L91.0
  scar L91.0
Keloma L91.0
Keratitis (nodular) (nonulcerative) (simple) (zonular) H16.9
  dendritic (a) (herpes simplex) B00.52
  disciform (is) (herpes simplex) B00.52
    varicella D01.01

Keratitis, *continued*
  gonococcal (congenital or prenatal) A54.33
  herpes, herpetic (simplex) B00.52
    zoster B02.33
  in (due to)
    exanthema (*see also* Exanthem) B09
    herpes (simplex) virus B00.52
    measles B05.81
    postmeasles B05.81
Keratoconjunctivitis H16.20-
  herpes, herpetic (simplex) B00.52
    zoster B02.33
  in exanthema (*see also* Exanthem) B09
  postmeasles B05.81
Keratoderma, keratodermia (congenital) (palmaris et
                                    plantaris) (symmetrical)
                                    Q82.8
Keratoglobus H18.79
  congenital Q15.8
    with glaucoma Q15.0
Keratoma L57.0
  palmaris and plantaris hereditarium Q82.8
Keratosis L57.0
  congenital, specified NEC Q80.8
  female genital NEC N94.89
  follicularis Q82.8
    congenita Q82.8
    spinulosa (decalvans) Q82.8
  gonococcal A54.89
  nigricans L83
  palmaris et plantaris (inherited) (symmetrical) Q82.8
    acquired L85.1
  tonsillaris J35.8
  vegetans Q82.8
Kerion (celsi) B35.0
Kink, kinking
  ureter (pelvic junction) N13.5
    with
      hydronephrosis N13.1
Klinefelter's syndrome Q98.4
Klumpke (-Déjerine) palsy, paralysis (birth) (newborn) P14.1
Knee—*see* condition
Knock knee (acquired) M21.06-
  congenital Q74.1
Knot (s)
  intestinal, syndrome (volvulus) K56.2
Knotting (of)
  intestine K56.2
Köebner's syndrome Q81.8
Kozhevnikof's epilepsy G40.109
  intractable G40.119
    with status epilepticus G40.111
    without status epilepticus G40.119
  not intractable G40.109
    with status epilepticus G40.101
    without status epilepticus G40.109
Koplik's spots B05.9
Kraft-Weber-Dimitri disease Q85.8
Kraurosis
  ani K62.89
Kreotoxism A05.9
Kyphoscoliosis, kyphoscoliotic (acquired) (*see also*
                                    Scoliosis) M41.9
  congenital Q67.5
  heart (disease) I27.1
Kyphosis, kyphotic (acquired) M40.209
  Morquio-Brailsford type (spinal) (*see also* subcategory
                                    M49.8) E76.219

L

Labile
  blood pressure R09.89
Labium leporinum—*see* Cleft, lip
Labyrinthitis (circumscribed) (destructive) (diffuse) (inner
                                    ear) (latent) (purulent)
                                    (suppurative) (*see also*
                                    subcategory) H83.0
Laceration
  abdomen, abdominal
    wall S31.119
      with
        foreign body S31.129

Laceration, *continued*
  epigastric region S31.112
    with
      foreign body S31.122
    left
      lower quadrant S31.114
        with
          foreign body S31.124
      upper quadrant S31.111
        with
          foreign body S31.121
    periumbilic region S31.115
      with
        foreign body S31.125
    right
      lower quadrant S31.113
        with
          foreign body S31.123
      upper quadrant S31.110
        with
          foreign body S31.120
  Achilles tendon S86.02-
  ankle S91.01-
    with
      foreign body S91.02-
  antecubital space—*see* Laceration, elbow
  anus (sphincter) S31.831
    with
      foreign body S31.832
    nontraumatic, nonpuerperal—*see* Fissure, anus
  arm (upper) S41.11-
    with foreign body S41.12-
    lower—*see* Laceration, forearm
  auditory canal (external) (meatus)—*see* Laceration, ear
  auricle, ear—*see* Laceration, ear
  axilla—*see* Laceration, arm
  back—*see also* Laceration, thorax, back
    lower S31.010
      with
        foreign body S31.020
  brain (any part) (cortex) (diffuse) (membrane)—*see also*
                                    Injury, intracranial,
                                    diffuse
    during birth P10.8
      with hemorrhage P10.1
  breast S21.01-
    with foreign body S21.02-
  buttock S31.801
    with foreign body S31.802
    left S31.821
      with foreign body S31.822
    right S31.811
      with foreign body S31.812
  calf—*see* Laceration, leg
  canaliculus lacrimalis—*see* Laceration, eyelid
  canthus, eye—*see* Laceration, eyelid
  capsule, joint—*see* Sprain
  cerebral S06.33-
    left side S06.32-
    during birth P10.8
      with hemorrhage P10.1
    right side S06.31-
  cheek (external) S01.41-
    with foreign body S01.42-
    internal—*see* Laceration, oral cavity
  chest wall—*see* Laceration, thorax
  chin—*see* Laceration, head, specified site NEC
  digit (s)
    hand—*see* Laceration, finger
    foot—*see* Laceration, toe
  ear (canal) (external) S01.31-
    with foreign body S01.32-
    drum S09.2-
  epididymis—*see* Laceration, testis
  epigastric region—*see* Laceration, abdomen, wall,
                                    epigastric region
  eyebrow—*see* Laceration, eyelid
  eyelid S01.11-
    with foreign body S01.12-
  face NEC—*see* Laceration, head, specified site NEC
  finger (s) S61.219
    with
      damage to nail S61.319

LACERATION–LACERATION

Laceration, continued
with
foreign body S61.329
foreign body S61.229
index S61.218
with
damage to nail S61.318
with
foreign body S61.328
foreign body S61.228
left S61.211
with
damage to nail S61.311
with
foreign body S61.321
foreign body S61.221
right S61.210
with
damage to nail S61.310
with
foreign body S61.320
foreign body S61.220
little S61.218
with
damage to nail S61.318
with
foreign body S61.328
foreign body S61.228
left S61.217
with
damage to nail S61.317
with
foreign body S61.327
foreign body S61.227
right S61.216
with
damage to nail S61.316
with
foreign body S61.326
foreign body S61.226
middle S61.218
with
damage to nail S61.318
with
foreign body S61.328
foreign body S61.228
left S61.213
with
damage to nail S61.313
with
foreign body S61.323
foreign body S61.223
right S61.212
with
damage to nail S61.312
with
foreign body S61.322
foreign body S61.222
ring S61.218
with
damage to nail S61.318
with
foreign body S61.328
foreign body S61.228
left S61.215
with
damage to nail S61.315
with
foreign body S61.325
foreign body S61.225
right S61.214
with
damage to nail S61.314
with
foreign body S61.324
foreign body S61.224
flank S31.119
with foreign body S31.129
foot (except toe(s) alone) S91.319
with foreign body S91.329
left S91.312
with foreign body S91.322

Laceration, continued
right S91.311
with foreign body S91.321
toe—see Laceration, toe
forearm S51.819
with
foreign body S51.829
elbow only—see Laceration, elbow
left S51.812
with
foreign body S51.822
right S51.811
with
foreign body S51.821
forehead S01.81
with foreign body S01.82
gum—see Laceration, oral cavity
hand S61.419
with
foreign body S61.429
finger—see Laceration, finger
left S61.412
with
foreign body S61.422
right S61.411
with
foreign body S61.421
thumb—see Laceration, thumb
head S01.91
with foreign body S01.92
cheek—see Laceration, cheek
ear—see Laceration, ear
eyelid—see Laceration, eyelid
lip—see Laceration, lip
nose—see Laceration, nose
oral cavity—see Laceration, oral cavity
scalp S01.01
with foreign body S01.02
specified site NEC S01.81
with foreign body S01.82
temporomandibular area—see Laceration, cheek
heel—see Laceration, foot
hip S71.019
with foreign body S71.029
left S71.012
with foreign body S71.022
right S71.011
with foreign body S71.021
hypochondrium—see Laceration, abdomen, wall
hypogastric region—see Laceration, abdomen, wall
inguinal region—see Laceration, abdomen, wall
instep—see Laceration, foot
interscapular region—see Laceration, thorax, back
jaw—see Laceration, head, specified site NEC
joint capsule—see Sprain, by site
knee S81.01-
with foreign body S81.02-
labium (majus) (minus)—see Laceration, vulva
lacrimal duct—see Laceration, eyelid
leg (lower) S81.819
with foreign body S81.829
foot—see Laceration, foot
knee—see Laceration, knee
left S81.812
with foreign body S81.822
right S81.811
with foreign body S81.821
upper—see Laceration, thigh
ligament—see Sprain
lip S01.511
with foreign body S01.521
loin—see Laceration, abdomen, wall
lower back—see Laceration, back, lower
lumbar region—see Laceration, back, lower
malar region—see Laceration, head, specified site NEC
mammary—see Laceration, breast
mastoid region—see Laceration, head, specified site NEC
meninges—see Injury, intracranial, diffuse
meniscus—see Tear, meniscus
mouth—see Laceration, oral cavity
muscle—see Injury, muscle, by site, laceration

Laceration, continued
nail
finger—see Laceration, finger, with damage to nail
toe—see Laceration, toe, with damage to nail
nasal (septum) (sinus)—see Laceration, nose
nasopharynx—see Laceration, head, specified site NEC
neck S11.91
with foreign body S11.92
nerve—see Injury, nerve
nose (septum) (sinus) S01.21
with foreign body S01.22
ocular NOS S05.3-
adnexa NOS S01.11-
oral cavity S01.512
with foreign body S01.522
palate—see Laceration, oral cavity
palm—see Laceration, hand
pelvic S31.010
with
foreign body S31.020
penis S31.21
with foreign body S31.22
perineum
female S31.41
with
foreign body S31.42
male S31.119
with foreign body S31.129
periocular area (with or without lacrimal passages)—see Laceration, eyelid
periumbilic region—see Laceration, abdomen, wall, periumbilic
periurethral tissue—see Laceration, urethra
phalanges
finger—see Laceration, finger
toe—see Laceration, toe
pinna—see Laceration, ear
popliteal space—see Laceration, knee
prepuce—see Laceration, penis
prostate S37.823
pubic region S31.119
with foreign body S31.129
pudendum—see Laceration, genital organs, external
rectovaginal septum—see Laceration, vagina
rectum S36.63
sacral region—see Laceration, back, lower
sacroiliac region—see Laceration, back, lower
salivary gland—see Laceration, oral cavity
scalp S01.01
with foreign body S01.02
scapular region—see Laceration, shoulder
scrotum S31.31
with foreign body S31.32
shin—see Laceration, leg
shoulder S41.019
with foreign body S41.029
left S41.012
with foreign body S41.022
right S41.011
with foreign body S41.021
spleen S36.039
superficial (minor) S36.030
submaxillary region—see Laceration, head, specified site NEC
submental region—see Laceration, head, specified site NEC
subungual
finger (s)—see Laceration, finger, with damage to nail
toe (s)—see Laceration, toe, with damage to nail
temple, temporal region—see Laceration, head, specified site NEC
temporomandibular area—see Laceration, cheek
tendon—see Injury, muscle, by site, laceration
Achilles S86.02-
tentorium cerebelli—see Injury, intracranial, diffuse
testis S31.31
with foreign body S31.32
thigh S71.11-
with foreign body S71.12-
thorax, thoracic (wall) S21.91
with foreign body S21.92
back S21.22-
front S21.12-

Laceration, *continued*
   back S21.21-
      with
         foreign body S21.22-
   breast—*see* Laceration, breast
   front S21.11-
      with
         foreign body S21.12-
   thumb S61.019
      with
         damage to nail S61.119
            with
               foreign body S61.129
         foreign body S61.029
     left S61.012
      with
         damage to nail S61.112
            with
               foreign body S61.122
         foreign body S61.022
     right S61.011
      with
         damage to nail S61.111
            with
               foreign body S61.121
         foreign body S61.021
   toe (s) S91.119
      with
         damage to nail S91.219
            with
               foreign body S91.229
         foreign body S91.129
     great S91.113
      with
         damage to nail S91.213
            with
               foreign body S91.223
         foreign body S91.123
     left S91.112
      with
         damage to nail S91.212
            with
               foreign body S91.222
         foreign body S91.122
     right S91.111
      with
         damage to nail S91.211
            with
               foreign body S91.221
         foreign body S91.121
     lesser S91.116
      with
         damage to nail S91.216
            with
               foreign body S91.226
         foreign body S91.126
     left S91.115
      with
         damage to nail S91.215
            with
               foreign body S91.225
         foreign body S91.125
     right S91.114
      with
         damage to nail S91.214
            with
               foreign body S91.224
         foreign body S91.124
   tongue—*see* Laceration, oral cavity
   tunica vaginalis—*see* Laceration, testis
   tympanum, tympanic membrane—*see* Laceration, ear,
                       drum
   umbilical region S31.115
     with foreign body S31.125
   uvula—*see* Laceration, oral cavity
   vagina S31.41
     with
        foreign body S31.42
     nonpuerperal, nontraumatic N89.8
     old (postpartal) N89.8
   vulva S31.41
     with
        foreign body S31.42

Laceration, *continued*
   wrist S61.519
     with
        foreign body S61.529
     left S61.512
      with
         foreign body S61.522
     right S61.511
      with
         foreign body S61.521
Lack of
   appetite (*see* Anorexia) R63.0
   care
     in home Z74.2
     of infant (at or after birth) T76.02
        confirmed T74.02
   coordination R27.9
     ataxia R27.0
     specified type NEC R27.8
   development (physiological) R62.50
     failure to thrive (child over 28 days old) R62.51
        newborn P92.6
     short stature R62.52
     specified type NEC R62.59
   energy R53.83
   growth R62.52
   heating Z59.1
   housing (permanent) (temporary) Z59.0
     adequate Z59.1
   ovulation N97.0
   person able to render necessary care Z74.2
   physical exercise Z72.3
   shelter Z59.0
Lactation, lactating (breast) (puerperal, postpartum)
   mastitis NEC N61.1
   mother (care and/or examination) Z39.1
   nonpuerperal N64.3
Lacunar skull Q75.8
Lalling F80.0
Lambliasis, lambliosis A07.1
Landouzy-Déjérine dystrophy or facioscapulohumeral
                    atrophy G71.0
Lapsed immunization schedule status Z28.3
Large
   baby (regardless of gestational age) (4000g-4499g) P08.1
Large-for-dates (infant) (4000g to 4499g) P08.1
   affecting management of pregnancy O36.6-
   exceptionally (4500g or more) P08.0
Larsen-Johansson disease or osteochondrosis—*see*
                    Osteochondrosis,
                    juvenile, patella
Laryngismus (stridulus) J38.5
   congenital P28.89
Laryngitis (acute) (edematous) (fibrinous) (infective)
                    (infiltrative) (malignant)
                    (membranous)
                    (phlegmonous)
                    (pneumococcal)
                    (pseudomembranous)
                    (septic) (subglottic)
                    (suppurative)
                    (ulcerative) J04.0
   with
     influenza, flu, or grippe—*see* Influenza, with, laryngitis
     tracheitis (acute)—*see* Laryngotracheitis
   atrophic J37.0
   catarrhal J37.0
   chronic J37.0
     with tracheitis (chronic) J37.1
   Hemophilus influenzae J04.0
   H. influenzae J04.0
   hypertrophic J37.0
   influenzal—*see* Influenza, with, respiratory manifestations
                    NEC
   obstructive J05.0
   sicca J37.0
   spasmodic J05.0
     acute J04.0
   streptococcal J04.0
   stridulous J05.0
Laryngomalacia (congenital) Q31.5
Laryngopharyngitis (acute) J06.0
   chronic J37.0

Laryngoplegia J38.00
   bilateral J38.02
   unilateral J38.01
Laryngotracheitis (acute) (Infectional) (infective) (viral) J04.2
   atrophic J37.1
   catarrhal J37.1
   chronic J37.1
   Hemophilus influenzae J04.2
   hypertrophic J37.1
   influenzal—*see* Influenza, with, respiratory manifestations
                    NEC
   sicca J37.1
   spasmodic J38.5
     acute J05.0
   streptococcal J04.2
Laryngotracheobronchitis—*see* Bronchitis
Late
   talker R62.0
   walker R62.0
Late effects—*see* Sequela
Launois' syndrome (pituitary gigantism) E22.0
Lax, laxity—*see also* Relaxation
   skin (acquired) L57.4
     congenital Q82.8
Lazy leukocyte syndrome D70.8
Leak, leakage
   air NEC J93.82
     postprocedural J95.812
   device, implant or graft—*see also* Complications, by site
                   and type, mechanical
     persistent air J93.82
Leaky heart—*see* Endocarditis
Learning defect (specific) F81.9
Leber's
   congenital amaurosis H35.50
Legg (-Calvé)-**Perthes disease, syndrome or**
                  osteochondrosis
                  M91.1-
Leiner's disease L21.1
Lenegre's disease I44.2
Lengthening, leg—*see* Deformity, limb, unequal length
Lennox-Gastaut syndrome G40.812
   intractable G40.814
     with status epilepticus G40.813
     without status epilepticus G40.814
   not intractable G40.812
     with status epilepticus G40.811
     without status epilepticus G40.812
Lentigo (congenital) L81.4
Leptocytosis, hereditary D56.9
Leptomeningitis (chronic) (circumscribed) (hemorrhagic)
                  (nonsuppurative)—*see*
                  Meningitis
Leptus dermatitis B88.0
Lesion(s) (nontraumatic)
   angiocentric immunoproliferative D47.Z9
   anorectal K62.9
   aortic (valve) I35.9
   brain G93.9
       hypertensive I67.4
   buccal cavity K13.79
   cardiac (*see also* Disease, heart) I51.9
     congenital Q24.9
   cerebrovascular I67.9
     degenerative I67.9
     hypertensive I67.4
   chorda tympani G51.8
   joint—*see* Disorder, joint
     sacroiliac (old) M53.3
   lip K13.0
   maxillary sinus J32.0
   mitral I05.9
   motor cortex NEC G93.89
   mouth K13.79
   nervous system, congenital Q07.9
   nose (internal) J34.89
   oral mucosa K13.70
   peptic K27.9
   primary (*see also* Syphilis, primary) A51.0
     carate A67.0
     pinta A67.0
     yaws A66.0

LESION(S)-LOSS

Lesion(s), *continued*
  pulmonary J98.4
    valve I37.9
  sacroiliac (joint) (old) M53.3
  sinus (accessory) (nasal) J34.89
  skin L98.9
    suppurative L08.0
  tonsillar fossa J35.9
  tricuspid (valve) I07.9
    nonrheumatic I36.9
  vascular I99.9
Lethargy R53.83
Leukemia, leukemic C95.9-
  acute lymphoblastic C91.0-
  acute myeloblastic (minimal differentiation) (with
                            maturation) C92.0-
  AML (1/ETO) (M0) (M1) (M2) (without a FAB classification)
                            C92.0-
  chronic myelomonocytic C93.1-
  CMML (-1) (-2) (with eosinophilia) C93.1-
  juvenile myelomonocytic C93.3-
  lymphoid C91.9-
  monocytic (subacute) C93.9-
  myelogenous (*see also* Category C92) C92.9-
  myeloid C92.9-
  subacute lymphocytic C91.9-
Leukemoid reaction (*see also* Reaction, leukemoid)
                            D72.823-
Leukocytopenia D72.819
Leukocytosis D72.829
  eosinophilic D72.1
Leukoencephalitis G04.81
  acute (subacute) hemorrhagic G36.1
    postimmunization or postvaccinal G04.02
  postinfectious G04.01
Leukoencephalopathy (*see also* Encephalopathy) G93.49
  postimmunization and postvaccinal G04.02
  reversible, posterior G93.6
Leukomalacia, cerebral, newborn P91.2
  periventricular P91.2
Leukonychia (punctata) (striata) L60.8
  congenital Q84.4
Leukopathia unguium L60.8
  congenital Q84.4
Leukopenia D72.819
  basophilic D72.818
  chemotherapy (cancer) induced D70.1
  congenital D70.0
  cyclic D70.0
  drug induced NEC D70.2
    due to cytoreductive cancer chemotherapy D70.1
  eosinophilic D72.818
  familial D70.0
  infantile genetic D70.0
  malignant D70.9
  periodic D70.0
  transitory neonatal P61.5
Leukoplakia
  anus K62.89
  rectum K62.89
Leukorrhea N89.8
  due to Trichomonas (vaginalis) A59.00
  trichomonal A59.00
Leukosarcoma C85.9-
Levocardia (isolated) Q24.1
  with situs inversus Q89.3
Lev's disease or syndrome (acquired complete heart block)
                            I44.2
Leyden-Moebius dystrophy G71.0
Libman-Sacks disease M32.11
Lice (infestation) B85.2
  body (Pediculus corporis) B85.1
  crab B85.3
  head (Pediculus corporis) B85.0
  mixed (classifiable to more than one of the titles B85.0–
                            B85.3) B85.4
  pubic (Phthirus pubis) B85.3
Lichen L28.0
  congenital Q82.8
  pilaris Q82.8
    acquired L85.8

Light
  for gestational age—*see* Light for dates
  headedness R42
Light-for-dates (infant) P05.00
  with weight of
    499 grams or less P05.01
    500–749 grams P05.02
    750–999 grams P05.03
    1000–1249 grams P05.04
    1250–1499 grams P05.05
    1500–1749 grams P05.06
    1750–1999 grams P05.07
    2000–2499 grams P05.08
    2,500 g and over P05.09
  and small-for-dates—*see* Small for dates
  affecting management of pregnancy O36.59-
Lindau (-von Hippel) **disease** Q85.8
Line (s)
  Beau's L60.4
  Harris'—*see* Arrest, epiphyseal
Lingua
  geographica K14.1
Linguatulosis B88.8
Lipochondrodystrophy E76.01
Lipochrome histiocytosis (familial) D71
Lipodystrophy (progressive) E88.1
  intestinal K90.81
Lipoid—*see also* condition
  histiocytosis D76.3
  nephrosis N04.9
Lipoma D17.9
  infiltrating D17.9
  intramuscular D17.9
  pleomorphic D17.9
  site classification
    arms (skin) (subcutaneous) D17.2-
    connective tissue D17.30
      intra-abdominal D17.5
      intrathoracic D17.4
      peritoneum D17.79
      retroperitoneum D17.79
      specified site NEC D17.39
      spermatic cord D17.6
    face (skin) (subcutaneous) D17.0
    genitourinary organ NEC D17.72
    head (skin) (subcutaneous) D17.0
    intra-abdominal D17.5
    intrathoracic D17.4
    kidney D17.71
    legs (skin) (subcutaneous) D17.2-
    neck (skin) (subcutaneous) D17.0
    peritoneum D17.79
    retroperitoneum D17.79
    skin D17.30
      specified site NEC D17.39
    specified site NEC D17.79
    spermatic cord D17.6
    subcutaneous D17.30
      specified site NEC D17.39
    trunk (skin) (subcutaneous) D17.1
    unspecified D17.9
  spindle cell D17.9
Lipoproteinemia E78.5
  broad-beta E78.2
  floating-beta E78.2
Lisping F80.0
Listeriosis, Listerellosis A32.9
  congenital (disseminated) P37.2
  cutaneous A32.0
  neonatal, newborn (disseminated) P37.2
  oculoglandular A32.81
  specified NEC A32.89
Little leaguer's elbow—*see* Epicondylitis, medial
Little's disease G80.9
Livedo (annularis) (racemosa) (reticularis) R23.1
Living alone (problems with) Z60.2
  with handicapped person Z74.2
Lobstein (-Ekman) disease or syndrome Q78.0
Lone Star fever A77.0
Long
  QT syndrome I45.81

Long-term (current) (prophylactic) **drug therapy** (use of)
  antibiotics Z79.2
    short-term use—omit code
  anti-inflammatory, non-steroidal (NSAID) Z79.1
  aspirin Z79.82
  drug, specified NEC Z79.899
  hypoglycemic, oral, drugs Z79.84
  insulin Z79.4
  non-steroidal anti-inflammatories (NSAID) Z79.1
  steroids
    inhaled Z79.51
    systemic Z79.52
Longitudinal stripes or grooves, nails L60.8
  congenital Q84.6
Lordosis M40.50
  acquired—*see* Lordosis, specified type NEC
  congenital Q76.429
    lumbar region Q76.426
    lumbosacral region Q76.427
    sacral region Q76.428
    sacrococcygeal region Q76.428
    thoracolumbar region Q76.425
  lumbar region M40.56
  lumbosacral region M40.57
  postural—*see* Lordosis, specified type NEC
  specified type NEC M40.40
    lumbar region M40.46
    lumbosacral region M40.47
    thoracolumbar region M40.45
  thoracolumbar region M40.55
Loss (of)
  appetite (*see* Anorexia) R63.0
    hysterical F50.89
    nonorganic origin F50.89
    psychogenic F50.89
  blood—*see* hemorrhage
  consciousness, transient R55
    traumatic—*see* Injury, intracranial
  control, sphincter, rectum R15.9
    nonorganic origin F98.1
  fluid (acute) E86.9
    with
      hypernatremia E87.0
      hyponatremia E87.1
  hearing—*see also* Deafness
    central NOS H90.5
    conductive H90.2
      bilateral H90.0
      unilateral
        with
          restricted hearing on the contralateral side
                            H90.A1-
          unrestricted hearing on the contralateral
                            side H90.1-
    mixed conductive and sensorineural hearing loss H90.8
      bilateral H90.6
      unilateral
        with
          restricted hearing on the contralateral side
                            H90.A3-
          unrestricted hearing on the contralateral
                            side H90.7-
    neural NOS H90.5
    perceptive NOS H90.5
    sensorineural NOS H90.5
      bilateral H90.3
      unilateral
        with
          restricted hearing on the contralateral side
                            H90.A2-
          unrestricted hearing on the contralateral
                            side H90.4-
    sensory NOS H90.5
  parent in childhood Z63.4
  self-esteem, in childhood Z62.898
  sense of
    smell—*see* Disturbance, sensation, smell
    taste—*see* Disturbance, sensation, taste
    touch R20.8
  sensory R44.9
    dissociative F44.6
  vision, visual H54.7
  weight (abnormal) (cause unknown) R63.4

Louis-Bar syndrome (ataxia-telangiectasia) G11.3
Louping ill (encephalitis) A84.8
Louse, lousiness—*see* Lice
Low
achiever, school Z55.3
birthweight (2499 grams or less) P07.10
with weight of
1000–1249 grams P07.14
1250–1499 grams P07.15
1500–1749 grams P07.16
1750–1999 grams P07.17
2000–2499 grams P07.18
extreme (999 grams or less) P07.00
with weight of
499 grams or less P07.01
500–749 grams P07.02
750–999 grams P07.03
for gestational age—*see* Light for dates
blood pressure—*see also* Hypotension
reading (incidental) (isolated) (nonspecific) R03.1
cardiac reserve—*see* Disease, heart
hematocrit D64.9
hemoglobin D64.9
salt syndrome E87.1
self-esteem R45.81
Low-density-lipoprotein-type (LDL) hyperlipoproteinemia E78.00
Lowe's syndrome E72.03
Lown-Ganong-Levine syndrome I45.6
Ludwig's angina or disease K12.2
Luetscher's syndrome E86.0
Lumbago, lumbalgia M54.5
with sciatica M54.4-
Lumbermen's itch B88.0
Lupoid (miliary) **of Boeck** D86.3
Lupus
anticoagulant D68.62
with
hemorrhagic disorder D68.312
erythematosus (discoid) (local) L93.0
disseminated M32.9
systemic M32.9
with organ or system involvement M32.10
endocarditis M32.11
lung M32.13
pericarditis M32.12
renal (glomerular) M32.14
tubulo-interstitial M32.15
specified organ or system NEC M32.19
drug-induced M32.0
inhibitor (presence of) D68.62
with
hemorrhagic disorder D68.312
nephritis (chronic) M32.14
Lutembacher's disease or syndrome (atrial septal defect with mitral stenosis) Q21.1
Luxation—*see also* Dislocation
eyeball (nontraumatic) H44.82-
birth injury P15.3
Lyell's syndrome L51.2
due to drug L51.2
correct substance properly administered—*see* Table of Drugs and Chemicals, by drug, adverse effect
overdose or wrong substance given or taken—*see* Table of Drugs and Chemicals, by drug, poisoning
Lyme disease A69.20
Lymphadenitis I88.9
acute L04.9
axilla L04.2
face L04.0
head L04.0
hip L04.3
limb
lower L04.3
upper L04.2
neck L04.0
shoulder L04.2
specified site NEC L04.8
trunk L04.1

Lymphadenitis, *continued*
any site, except mesenteric I88.9
chronic I88.1
subacute I88.1
chronic I88.1
mesenteric I88.0
due to
chlamydial lymphogranuloma A55
gonorrheal A54.89
infective—*see* Lymphadenitis, acute
mesenteric (acute) (chronic) (nonspecific) (subacute) I88.0
due to Salmonella typhi A01.09
tuberculous A18.39
mycobacterial A31.8
purulent—*see* Lymphadenitis, acute
pyogenic—*see* Lymphadenitis, acute
regional, nonbacterial I88.8
septic—*see* Lymphadenitis, acute
subacute, unspecified site I88.1
suppurative—*see* Lymphadenitis, acute
syphilitic (early) (secondary) A51.49
late A52.79
venereal (chlamydial) A55
Lymphadenopathy (generalized) R59.1
due to toxoplasmosis (acquired) B58.89
congenital (acute) (subacute) (chronic) P37.1
Lymphadenosis R59.1
Lymphangitis I89.1
with
abscess—*code by* site under Abscess
cellulitis—*code by* site under Cellulitis
acute L03.91
abdominal wall L03.321
auricle (ear)—*see* Lymphangitis, acute, ear
axilla L03.12-
back (any part) L03.322
buttock L03.327
cervical (meaning neck) L03.222
cheek (external) L03.212
chest wall L03.323
digit
finger—*see* Cellulitis, finger
toe—*see* Cellulitis, toe
ear (external) H60.1-
eyelid—*see* Abscess, eyelid
face NEC L03.212
finger (intrathecal) (periosteal) (subcutaneous) (subcuticular) L03.02-
gluteal (region) L03.327
groin L03.324
head NEC L03.891
face (any part, except ear, eye and nose) L03.212
jaw (region) L03.212
lower limb L03.12-
navel L03.326
neck (region) L03.222
orbit, orbital—*see* Cellulitis, orbit
pectoral (region) L03.323
perineal, perineum L03.325
scalp (any part) L03.891
specified site NEC L03.898
toe (intrathecal) (periosteal) (subcutaneous) (subcuticular) L03.04-
trunk L03.329
abdominal wall L03.321
back (any part) L03.322
buttock L03.327
chest wall L03.323
groin L03.324
perineal, perineum L03.325
umbilicus L03.326
umbilicus L03.326
upper limb L03.12-
strumous tuberculous A18.2
subacute (any site) I89.1
Lymphocytoma, benign cutis L98.8
Lymphocytopenia D72.810
Lymphocytosis (symptomatic) D72.820
infectious (acute) B33.8

Lymphogranuloma (malignant)—*see also* Lymphoma, Hodgkin
chlamydial A55
inguinal A55
venereum (any site) (chlamydial) (with stricture of rectum) A55
Lymphogranulomatosis (malignant)—*see also* Lymphoma, Hodgkin
benign (Boeck's sarcoid) (Schaumann's) D86.1
Lymphohistiocytosis, hemophagocytic (familial) D76.1
Lymphoma (of) (malignant) C85.90
diffuse large cell C83.3-
anaplastic C83.3-
B-cell C83.3-
CD30-positive C83.3-
centroblastic C83.3-
immunoblastic C83.3-
plasmablastic C83.3-
subtype not specified C83.3-
T-cell rich C83.3-
histiocytic C85.9-
true C96.A
Hodgkin C81.9
classical C81.7-
lymphocyte-rich C81.4-
lymphocyte depleted C81.3-
mixed cellularity C81.2-
nodular sclerosis C81.1-
specified NEC C81.7-
lymphocyte-rich classical C81.4-
lymphocyte depleted classical C81.3-
mixed cellularity classical C81.2-
nodular
lymphocyte predominant C81.0-
sclerosis classical C81.1-
Lennert's C84.4-
lymphoepithelioid C84.4-
mature T-cell NEC C84.4-
non-Hodgkin (*see also* Lymphoma, by type) C85.9-
specified NEC C85.8-
peripheral T-cell, not classified C84.4-
Lymphopenia D72.810
Lymphoplasmacytic leukemia—*see* Leukemia, chronic lymphocytic, B-cell type
Lymphosarcoma (diffuse) (*see also* Lymphoma) C85.9-

M

Macrocolon (*see also* Megacolon) Q43.1
Macrocornea Q15.8
with glaucoma Q15.0
Macrodactylia, macrodactylism (fingers) (thumbs) Q74.0
toes Q74.2
Macrogenitosomia (adrenal) (male) (praecox) E25.9
congenital E25.0
Macrophthalmos Q11.3
in congenital glaucoma Q15.0
Macrosigmoid K59.39
congenital Q43.2
toxic K59.31
Macrospondylitis, acromegalic E22.0
Maculae ceruleae B85.1
Madelung's
deformity (radius) Q74.0
disease
radial deformity Q74.0
Main en griffe (acquired)—*see also* Deformity, limb, clawhand
congenital Q74.0
Maintenance (encounter for)
antineoplastic chemotherapy Z51.11
antineoplastic radiation therapy Z51.0
Malabsorption K90.9
calcium K90.89
carbohydrate K90.49
disaccharide E73.9
fat K90.49
intestinal K90.9
specified NEC K90.89
lactose E73.9
postgastrectomy K91.2
postsurgical K91.2
protein K90.49

Malabsorption, *continued*
starch K90.49
syndrome K90.9
postsurgical K91.2
Maladaptation—*see* Maladjustment
Maladie de Roger Q21.0
Maladjustment
educational Z55.4
family Z63.9
social Z60.9
due to
acculturation difficulty Z60.3
Malaise R53.81
Malaria, malarial (fever) B54
with
blackwater fever B50.8
hemoglobinuric (bilious) B50.8
hemoglobinuria B50.8
accidentally induced (therapeutically)—*code by* type
under Malaria
algid B50.9
cerebral B50.0 [G94]
clinically diagnosed (without parasitological confirmation)
B54
congenital NEC P37.4
falciparum P37.3
congestion, congestive B54
continued (fever) B50.9
estivo-autumnal B50.9
falciparum B50.9
with complications NEC B50.8
cerebral B50.0 [G94]
severe B50.8
hemorrhagic B54
malariae B52.9
with
complications NEC B52.8
glomerular disorder B52.0
malignant (tertian)—*see* Malaria, falciparum
mixed infections—*code to* first listed type in B50-B53
ovale B53.0
parasitologically confirmed NEC B53.8
pernicious, acute—*see* Malaria, falciparum
Plasmodium (P.)
falciparum NEC—*see* Malaria, falciparum
malariae NEC B52.9
with Plasmodium
falciparum (and or vivax)—*see* Malaria,
falciparum
vivax—*see also* Malaria, vivax
and falciparum—*see* Malaria, falciparum
ovale B53.0
with Plasmodium malariae—*see also* Malaria,
malariae
and vivax—*see also* Malaria, vivax
and falciparum—*see* Malaria, falciparum
simian B53.1
with Plasmodium malariae—*see also* Malaria,
malariae
and vivax—*see also* Malaria, vivax
and falciparum—*see* Malaria, falciparum
vivax NEC B51.9
with Plasmodium falciparum—*see* Malaria,
falciparum
quartan—*see* Malaria, malariae
quotidian—*see* Malaria, falciparum
recurrent B54
remittent B54
specified type NEC (parasitologically confirmed) B53.8
spleen B54
subtertian (fever)—*see* Malaria, falciparum
tertian (benign)—*see also* Malaria, vivax
malignant B50.9
tropical B50.9
typhoid B54
vivax B51.9
with
complications NEC B51.8
ruptured spleen B51.0
Malassimilation K90.9
Mal de mer T75.3

Maldescent, testis Q53.9
bilateral Q53.20
abdominal Q53.21
perineal Q53.22
unilateral Q53.10
abdominal Q53.11
perineal Q53.12
Maldevelopment—*see also* Anomaly
brain Q07.9
hip Q74.2
congenital dislocation Q65.2
bilateral Q65.1
unilateral Q65.0-
mastoid process Q75.8
toe Q74.2
Male type pelvis Q74.2
Malformation (congenital)—*see also* Anomaly
alimentary tract Q45.9
specified type NEC Q45.8
upper Q40.9
specified type NEC Q40.8
aorta Q25.40
absence Q25.41
aneurysm, congenital Q25.43
aplasia Q25.41
atresia Q25.29
aortic arch Q25.21
coarctation (preductal) (postductal) Q25.1
dilatation, congenital Q25.44
hypoplasia Q25.42
patent ductus arteriosus Q25.0
specified type NEC Q25.49
stenosis Q25.1
supravalvular Q25.3
bile duct Q44.5
bone Q79.9
face Q75.9
specified type NEC Q75.8
skull Q75.9
specified type NEC Q75.8
bursa Q79.9
corpus callosum (congenital) Q04.0
digestive system NEC, specified type NEC Q45.8
dura Q07.9
brain Q04.9
spinal Q06.9
ear Q17.9
external Q17.9
eye Q15.9
lid Q10.3
specified NEC Q15.8
great
vein Q26.9
anomalous
pulmonary venous connection Q26.4
partial Q26.3
total Q26.2
heart Q24.9
specified type NEC Q24.8
integument Q84.9
joint Q74.9
ankle Q74.2
sacroiliac Q74.2
kidney Q63.9
accessory Q63.0
giant Q63.3
horseshoe Q63.1
hydronephrosis (congenital) Q62.0
malposition Q63.2
specified type NEC Q63.8
meninges or membrane (congenital) Q07.9
cerebral Q04.8
spinal (cord) Q06.9
multiple types NEC Q89.7
musculoskeletal system Q79.9
nervous system (central) Q07.9
parathyroid gland Q89.2
penis Q55.69
aplasia Q55.5
curvature (lateral) Q55.61
hypoplasia Q55.62

Malformation, *continued*
pulmonary
arteriovenous Q25.72
artery Q25.9
atresia Q25.5
specified type NEC Q25.79
respiratory system Q34.9
scrotum—*see* Malformation, testis and scrotum
sense organs NEC Q07.9
specified NEC Q89.8
tendon Q79.9
testis and scrotum Q55.20
aplasia Q55.0
hypoplasia Q55.1
polyorchism Q55.21
retractile testis Q55.22
scrotal transposition Q55.23
specified NEC Q55.29
thyroid gland Q89.2
tongue (congenital) Q38.3
hypertrophy Q38.2
tie Q38.1
urinary system Q64.9
Malibu disease L98.8
Malignancy—*see also* Neoplasm, malignant, by site
unspecified site (primary) C80.1
Malignant—*see* condition
Malingerer, malingering Z76.5
Mallet finger (acquired) M20.01-
congenital Q74.0
Malnutrition E46
following gastrointestinal surgery K91.2
lack of care, or neglect (child) (infant) T76.02
confirmed T74.02
protein E46
calorie E46
energy E46
Malocclusion (teeth) M26.4
temporomandibular (joint) M26.69
Malposition
alimentary tract Q45.8
lower Q43.8
upper Q40.8
arterial trunk Q20.0
cervix—*see* Malposition, uterus
congenital
aorta Q25.4
artery (peripheral) Q27.8
pulmonary Q25.79
biliary duct or passage Q44.5
clavicle Q74.0
digestive organ or tract NEC Q45.8
lower Q43.8
upper Q40.8
endocrine (gland) NEC Q89.2
finger (s) Q68.1
supernumerary Q69.0
gallbladder Q44.1
gastrointestinal tract Q45.8
genitalia, genital organ (s)or tract
female Q52.8
external Q52.79
internal NEC Q52.8
male Q55.8
heart Q24.8
dextrocardia Q24.0
with complete transposition of viscera Q89.3
hepatic duct Q44.5
hip (joint) Q65.89
parathyroid (gland) Q89.2
pituitary (gland) Q89.2
scapula Q74.0
shoulder Q74.0
symphysis pubis Q74.2
thymus (gland) Q89.2
thyroid (gland) (tissue) Q89.2
cartilage Q31.8
toe (s) Q66.9
supernumerary Q69.2
gastrointestinal tract, congenital Q45.8
Malposture R29.3

Maltreatment
  child
    abandonment
      confirmed T74.02
      suspected T76.02
    confirmed T74.92
    history of—*see* History, personal (of), abuse
    neglect
      confirmed T74.02
      history of—*see* History, personal (of), abuse
      suspected T76.02
    physical abuse
      confirmed T74.12
      history of—*see* History, personal (of), abuse
      suspected T76.12
    psychological abuse
      confirmed T74.32
      history of—*see* History, personal (of), abuse
      suspected T76.32
    sexual abuse
      confirmed T74.22
      history of—*see* History, personal (of), abuse
      suspected T76.22
    suspected T76.92
    personal history of Z91.89
Mammillitis N61.0
Mammitis—*see* Mastitis
Mammogram (examination) Z12.39
  routine Z12.31
Mammoplasia N62
Maple-syrup-urine disease E71.0
Marchesani (-Weill) syndrome Q87.0
Marie's
  cerebellar ataxia (late-onset) G11.2
  disease or syndrome (acromegaly) E22.0
Marion's disease (bladder neck obstruction) N32.0
Mark
  port wine Q82.5
  raspberry Q82.5
  strawberry Q82.5
  tattoo L81.8
Maroteaux-Lamy syndrome (mild) (severe) E76.29
Marrow (bone)
  arrest D61.9
Masculinization (female) with adrenal hyperplasia E25.9
  congenital E25.0
Mass
  abdominal R19.00
    epigastric R19.06
    generalized R19.07
    left lower quadrant R19.04
    left upper quadrant R19.02
    periumbilic R19.05
    right lower quadrant R19.03
    right upper quadrant R19.01
    specified site NEC R19.09
  breast N63
  chest R22.2
  cystic—*see* Cyst
  ear H93.8-
  head R22.0
  intra-abdominal (diffuse) (generalized)—*see* Mass, abdominal
  kidney N28.89
  liver R16.0
  localized (skin) R22.9
    chest R22.2
    head R22.0
    limb
      lower R22.4-
      upper R22.3-
    neck R22.1
    trunk R22.2
  lung R91.8
  malignant—*see* Neoplasm, malignant, by site
  neck R22.1
  pelvic (diffuse) (generalized)—*see* Mass, abdominal
  specified organ NEC—*see* Disease, by site
  splenic R16.1
  substernal thyroid—*see* Goiter
  superficial (localized) R22.9
  umbilical (diffuse) (generalized) R19.09
Mastalgia N64.4

Mastitis (acute) (diffuse) (nonpuerperal) (subacute) N61.0
  infective N61.0
  newborn P39.0
  neonatal (noninfective) P83.4
    infective P39.0
Mastodynia N64.4
Mastoidalgia—*see* subcategory H92.0
Mastoplasia, mastoplastia N62
Masturbation (excessive) F98.8
McQuarrie's syndrome (idiopathic familial hypoglycemia) E16.2
Measles (black) (hemorrhagic) (suppressed) B05.9
  with
    complications NEC B05.89
    encephalitis B05.0
    intestinal complications B05.4
    keratitis (keratoconjunctivitis) B05.81
    meningitis B05.1
    otitis media B05.3
    pneumonia B05.2
  French—*see* Rubella
  German—*see* Rubella
  Liberty—*see* Rubella
Meckel-Gruber syndrome Q61.9
Meckel's diverticulitis, diverticulum (displaced) (hypertrophic) Q43.0
Meconium
  ileus, newborn P76.0
    in cystic fibrosis E84.11
    meaning meconium plug (without cystic fibrosis) P76.0
  obstruction, newborn P76.0
    due to fecaliths P76.0
    in mucoviscidosis E84.11
  plug syndrome (newborn)NEC P76.0
Mediastinopericarditis—*see also* Pericarditis
  acute I30.9
  adhesive I31.0
  chronic I31.8
    rheumatic I09.2
Medulloblastoma
  desmoplastic C71.6
  specified site—*see* Neoplasm, malignant, by site
  unspecified site C71.6
Medullomyoblastoma
  specified site—*see* Neoplasm, malignant, by site
  unspecified site C71.6
Meekeren-Ehlers-Danlos syndrome Q79.6
Megacolon (acquired) (functional) (not Hirschsprung's disease) (in) K59.39
  congenital, congenitum (aganglionic) Q43.1
  Hirschsprung's (disease) Q43.1
  toxic K59.31
Megalerythema (epidemic) B08.3
Megalocornea Q15.8
  with glaucoma Q15.0
Megalodactylia (fingers) (thumbs) (congenital) Q74.0
  toes Q74.2
Megarectum K62.89
Megasigmoid K59.39
  congenital Q43.2
  toxic K59.31
Melancholia F32.9
  hypochondriac F45.29
  intermittent (single episode) F32.89
    recurrent episode F33.9
Melanocytosis, neurocutaneous Q82.8
Melanoderma, melanodermia L81.4
Melanodontia, infantile K03.89
Melanodontoclasia K03.89
Melanosis L81.4
  Riehl's L81.4
  tar L81.4
  toxic L81.4
MELAS syndrome E88.41
Melena K92.1
  with ulcer—*code by* site under Ulcer, with hemorrhage K27.4
  due to swallowed maternal blood P78.2
  newborn, neonatal P54.1
    due to swallowed maternal blood P78.2
Membrane (s), membranous—*see also* condition
  over face of newborn P28.9

Menarche
  delayed E30.0
  precocious E30.1
Meningism—*see* Meningismus
Meningismus (infectional) (pneumococcal) R29.1
  due to serum or vaccine R29.1
  influenzal—*see* Influenza, with, manifestations NEC
Meningitis (basal) (basic) (brain) (cerebral) (cervical) (congestive) (diffuse) (hemorrhagic) (infantile) (membranous) (metastatic) (nonspecific) (pontine) (progressive) (simple) (spinal) (subacute) (sympathetic) (toxic) G03.9
  abacterial G03.0
  arbovirus A87.8
  aseptic G03.0
  bacterial G00.9
    Escherichia Coli (E. coli) G00.8
    gram-negative G00.9
    H. influenzae G00.0
    pneumococcal G00.1
    specified organism NEC G00.8
    streptococcal (acute) G00.2
  candidal B37.5
  caseous (tuberculous) A17.0
  cerebrospinal A39.0
  clear cerebrospinal fluid NEC G03.0
  coxsackievirus A87.0
  diplococcal (gram positive) A39.0
  echovirus A87.0
  enteroviral A87.0
  epidemic NEC A39.0
  Escherichia Coli (E. coli) G00.8
  fibrinopurulent G00.9
    specified organism NEC G00.8
  gram-negative cocci G00.9
  gram-positive cocci G00.9
  Haemophilus (influenzae) G00.0
  H. influenzae G00.0
  in (due to)
    bacterial disease NEC A48.8 *[G01]*
    chickenpox B01.0
    Diplococcus pneumoniae G00.1
    enterovirus A87.0
    herpes (simplex) virus B00.3
      zoster B02.1
    infectious mononucleosis B27.92
    Lyme disease A69.21
    measles B05.1
    Streptococcal pneumoniae G00.1
    varicella B01.0
    viral disease NEC A87.8
    whooping cough A37.90
    zoster B02.1
  infectious G00.9
  influenzal (H. influenzae) G00.0
  meningococcal A39.0
  monilial B37.5
  Neisseria A39.0
  nonbacterial G03.0
  nonpyogenic G03.0
  pneumococcal streptococcus pneumoniae G00.1
  postmeasles B05.1
  purulent G00.9
    specified organism NEC G00.8
  pyogenic G00.9
    specified organism NEC G00.8
  septic G00.9
    specified organism NEC G00.8
  serosa circumscripta NEC G03.0
  serous NEC G93.2
  specified organism NEC G00.8
  sterile G03.0
  streptococcal (acute) G00.2
  suppurative G00.9
    specified organism NEC G00.8
  traumatic (complication of injury) T79.8
  tuberculous A17.0
  viral NEC A87.9

MENINGOCOCCEMIA–MONOSOMY

Meningococcemia A39.4
  acute A39.2
  chronic A39.3
Meningococcus, meningococcal (*see also* condition) A39.9
  carrier (suspected) of Z22.31
  meningitis (cerebrospinal) A39.0
Meningoencephalitis (*see also* Encephalitis) G04.90
  acute NEC (*see also* Encephalitis, viral) A86
    disseminated G04.00
      postimmunization or postvaccination G04.02
  California A83.5
  herpesviral, herpetic B00.4
    due to herpesvirus 7 B10.09
    specified NEC B10.09
  in (due to)
    diseases classified elsewhere G05.3
    Hemophilus influenzae (H. Influenzae) G00.0
    herpes B00.4
      due to herpesvirus 7 B10.09
      specified NEC B10.09
    H. influenzae G00.0
    Lyme disease A69.22
    toxoplasmosis (acquired) B58.2
      congenital P37.1
  infectious (acute) (viral) A86
  parasitic NEC B89 *[G05.3]*
  pneumococcal G04.2
  toxic NEC G92
  virus NEC A86
Meningoencephalomyelitis—*see also* Encephalitis
  acute NEC (viral) A86
    disseminated G04.00
      postimmunization or postvaccination G04.02
      postinfectious G04.01
  due to
    Toxoplasma or toxoplasmosis (acquired) B58.2
      congenital P37.1
  postimmunization or postvaccination G04.02
Meningomyelitis—*see also* Meningoencephalitis
  in diseases classified elsewhere G05.4
Menkes' disease or syndrome E83.09
  meaning maple-syrup-urine disease E71.0
Menometrorrhagia N92.1
Menorrhagia (primary) N92.0
  pubertal (menses retained) N92.2
Menostaxis N92.0
Menses, retention N94.89
Menstrual—*see* Menstruation
Menstruation
  absent—*see* Amenorrhea
  anovulatory N97.0
  cycle, irregular N92.6
  during pregnancy O20.8
  excessive (with regular cycle) N92.0
    with irregular cycle N92.1
      at puberty N92.2
  frequent N92.0
  infrequent—*see* Oligomenorrhea
  irregular N92.6
    specified NEC N92.5
  latent N92.5
  membranous N92.5
  painful (*see also* Dysmenorrhea) N94.6
    primary N94.4
    psychogenic F45.8
    secondary N94.5
  passage of clots N92.0
  precocious E30.1
  protracted N92.5
  rare—*see* Oligomenorrhea
  retained N94.89
  retrograde N92.5
  scanty—*see* Oligomenorrhea
  suppression N94.89
  vicarious (nasal) N94.89
Mental—*see also* condition
  observation without need for further medical care Z03.89
MERRF syndrome (myoclonic epilepsy associated with
                    ragged-red fiber)
                    E88.42

Metabolic syndrome E88.81
Metal
  pigmentation L81.8
Metatarsus, metatarsal—*see also* condition
  valgus (abductus), congenital Q66.6
  varus (adductus) (congenital) Q66.22
    primus Q66.21
Methemoglobinemia D74.9
  congenital D74.0
  enzymatic (congenital) D74.0
  Hb M disease D74.0
  hereditary D74.0
  toxic D74.8
Metropathia hemorrhagica N93.8
Metrorrhagia N92.1
  psychogenic F45.8
Metrostaxis N93.8
Meyer-Schwickerath and Weyers syndrome Q87.0
Mibelli's disease (porokeratosis) Q82.8
Micrencephalon, micrencephaly Q02
Microalbuminuria R80.9
Microcephalus, microcephalic, microcephaly Q02
  due to toxoplasmosis (congenital) P37.1
Microdeletions NEC Q93.88
Microdrepanocytosis D57.40
  with crisis (vaso-occlusive pain) D57.419
    with
      acute chest syndrome D57.411
      splenic sequestration D57.412
Microencephalon Q02
Microgenitalia, congenital
  female Q52.8
  male Q55.8
Microophthalmos, microphthalmia (congenital) Q11.2
  due to toxoplasmosis P37.1
Micropenis Q55.62
Microsporon furfur infestation B36.0
Micturition
  disorder NEC R39.198
    psychogenic F45.8
  frequency R35.0
    psychogenic F45.8
  hesitancy R39.11
  need to immediately re-void R39.191
  painful R30.9
    dysuria R30.0
    psychogenic F45.8
    tenesmus R30.1
  poor stream R39.12
  position dependent R39.192
  urgency R39.15
Migraine (idiopathic) G43.909
  with aura (acute-onset) (prolonged) (typical) (without
                            headache) G43.109
    with refractory migraine G43.119
      with status migrainosus G43.111
      without status migrainosus G43.119
    not intractable G43.109
      with status migrainosus G43.101
      without status migrainosus G43.109
    without mention of refractory migraine G43.109
      with status migrainosus G43.101
      without status migrainosus G43.109
  basilar—*see* Migraine, with aura
  classical—*see* Migraine, with aura
  common—*see* Migraine, without aura
  complicated G43.109
  equivalents—*see* Migraine, with aura
  transformed—*see* Migraine, without aura, chronic
  triggered seizures—*see* Migraine, with aura
  without aura G43.009
    with refractory migraine G43.019
      with status migrainosus G43.011
      without status migrainosus G43.019
    not intractable
      with status migrainosus G43.001
      without status migrainosus G43.009
    without mention of refractory migraine G43.009
      with status migrainosus G43.001
      without status migrainosus G43.009
Migrant, social Z59.0
Migration, anxiety concerning Z60.3

Migratory, migrating—*see also* condition
  person Z59.0
  testis Q55.29
Miliaria L74.3
  alba L74.1
  crystallina L74.1
  rubra L74.0
Milk
  crust L21.0
  poisoning—*see* Poisoning, food, noxious
  sickness—*see* Poisoning, food, noxious
  spots I31.0
Milk-alkali disease or syndrome E83.52
Minot's disease (hemorrhagic disease), **newborn** P53
Mirror writing F81.0
Miscarriage O03.9
Missed
  delivery O36.4
Missing—*see* Absence
Mite(s) (infestation) B88.9
  diarrhea B88.0
  grain (itch) B88.0
  hair follicle (itch) B88.0
  in sputum B88.0
Mittelschmerz N94.0
Mixed—*see* condition
MNGIE (Mitochondrial Neurogastrointestinal Encephalopathy)
                      syndrome E88.49
Mobile, mobility
  gallbladder, congenital Q44.1
Mobitz heart block (atrioventricular) I44.1
Moebius, Möbius
  syndrome Q87.0
    congenital oculofacial paralysis (with other anomalies)
                      Q87.0
Moeller's glossitis K14.0
Mohr's syndrome (Types I and II) Q87.0
Molding, head (during birth)—omit code
Mole (pigmented)—*see also* Nevus
  tubal O00.10
    with intrauterine pregnancy O00.11
Molimen, molimina (menstrual) N94.3
Molluscum contagiosum (epitheliale) B08.1
Moniliasis (*see also* Candidiasis) B37.9
  neonatal P37.5
Monitoring (encounter for)
  therapeutic drug level Z51.81
Monocytopenia D72.818
Monocytosis (symptomatic) D72.821
Mononucleosis, infectious B27.90
  with
    complication NEC B27.99
      meningitis B27.92
      polyneuropathy B27.91
  cytomegaloviral B27.10
    with
      complication NEC B27.19
        meningitis B27.12
        polyneuropathy B27.11
  Epstein-Barr (virus) B27.00
    with
      complication NEC B27.09
        meningitis B27.02
        polyneuropathy B27.01
  gammaherpesviral B27.00
    with
      complication NEC B27.09
        meningitis B27.02
        polyneuropathy B27.01
  specified NEC B27.80
    with
      complication NEC B27.89
        meningitis B27.82
        polyneuropathy B27.81
Mononeuropathy G58.9
Monoplegia G83.3-
  hysterical (transient) F44.4
  psychogenic (conversion reaction) F44.4
Monorchism, monorchidism Q55.0
Monosomy (*see also* Deletion, chromosome) Q93.9
  specified NEC Q93.89
  X Q96.9

Monster, monstrosity (single) Q89.7
Monteggia's fracture (-dislocation) S52.27-
Morbidity not stated or unknown R69
Morbilli—*see* Measles
Morbus—*see also* Disease
    angelicus, anglorum E55.0
    celiacus K90.0
    hemorrhagicus neonatorum P53
    maculosus neonatorum P54.5
Morgagni's
    cyst, organ, hydatid, or appendage
        male (epididymal) Q55.4
            testicular Q55.29
Morgagni-Stokes-Adams syndrome I45.9
Morgagni-Turner (-Albright) **syndrome** Q96.9
Moron (I.Q.50-69) F70
Morvan's disease or syndrome G60.8
Mosaicism, mosaic (autosomal) (chromosomal)
    45,X/other cell lines NEC with abnormal sex chromosome
                Q96.4
    45,X/46,XX Q96.3
    sex chromosome
        female Q97.8
        lines with various numbers of X chromosomes Q97.2
        male Q98.7
        XY Q96.3
Motion sickness (from travel, any vehicle) (from roundabouts
              or swings) T75.3
Mountain
    sickness T70.29
        with polycythemia, acquired (acute) D75.1
MRSA (Methicillin resistant Staphylococcus aureus)
    infection A49.02
    as the cause of disease classified elsewhere B95.62
    sepsis A41.02
MSSA (Methicillin susceptible Staphylococcus aureus)
    infection A49.02
    as the cause of disease classified elsewhere B95.61
    sepsis A41.01
Mucinosis (cutaneous) (focal) (papular) (reticular
              erythematosus) (skin)
              L98.5
    oral K13.79
Mucocele
    buccal cavity K13.79
    nasal sinus J34.1
    nose J34.1
    sinus (accessory) (nasal) J34.1
    turbinate (bone) (middle) (nasal) J34.1
Mucositis (ulcerative) K12.30
    nasal J34.81
Mucopolysaccharidosis E76.3
    beta-gluduronidase deficiency E76.29
    cardiopathy E76.3 *[152]*
    Hunter's syndrome E76.1
    Hurler's syndrome E76.01
    Maroteaux-Lamy syndrome E76.29
    Morquio syndrome E76.219
        A E76.210
        B E76.211
        classic E76.210
    Sanfilippo syndrome E76.22
    specified NEC E76.29
    type
        I
            Hurler's syndrome E76.01
            Hurler-Scheie syndrome E76.02
            Scheie's syndrome E76.03
        II E76.1
        III E76.22
        IV E76.219
        IVA E76.210
        IVB E76.211
        VI E76.29
        VII E76.29
Mucoviscidosis E84.9
    with meconium obstruction E84.11
Mucus
    asphyxiation or suffocation—*see* Asphyxia, mucus
    in stool R19.5
    plug—*see* Asphyxia, mucus
Muguet B37.0

Multicystic kidney (development) Q61.4
Mumps B26.9
Murmur (cardiac) (heart) (organic) R01.1
    aortic (valve)—*see* Endocarditis, aortic
    benign R01.0
    diastolic—*see* Endocarditis
    Flint I35.1
    functional R01.0
    Graham Steell I37.1
    innocent R01.0
    mitral (valve)—*see* Insufficiency, mitral
    nonorganic R01.0
    presystolic, mitral—*see* Insufficiency, mitral
    pulmonic (valve) I37.8
    systolic R01.1
    tricuspid (valve) I07.9
    valvular—*see* Endocarditis
Muscle, muscular—*see also* condition
    carnitine (palmityltransferase) deficiency E71.314
Mutation (s)
    surfactant, of lung J84.83
Mutism—*see also* Aphasia
    deaf (acquired) (congenital) NEC H91.3
    elective (adjustment reaction) (childhood) F94.0
    hysterical F44.4
    selective (childhood) F94.0
Myalgia M79.1
    traumatic NEC T14.8
Myasthenia G70.9
    congenital G70.2
    cordis—*see* Failure, heart
    developmental G70.2
    gravis G70.00
        with exacerbation (acute) G70.01
        in crisis G70.01
        neonatal, transient P94.0
        pseudoparalytica G70.00
            with exacerbation (acute) G70.01
            in crisis G70.01
    stomach, psychogenic F45.8
    syndrome
        in
            diabetes mellitus—*see* E08-E13 with .44
            neoplastic disease (*see also* Neoplasm) D49.9
                [G73.3]
            thyrotoxicosis E05.90 *[G73.3]*
            with thyroid storm E05.91 *[G73.3]*
Myasthenic M62.81
Mycoplasma (M.) pneumoniae, as cause of disease
              classified elsewhere
              B96.0
Mycosis, mycotic B49
    mouth B37.0
    nails B35.1
    stomatitis B37.0
    vagina, vaginitis (candidal) B37.3
Myelitis (acute) (ascending) (childhood) (chronic)
              (descending) (diffuse)
              (disseminated)
              (idiopathic) (pressure)
              (progressive) (spinal
              cord) (subacute) (*see
              also Encephalitis)
              G04.91
    in diseases classified elsewhere G05.4
    postchickenpox B01.12
    postimmunization G04.02
    postinfectious G04.89
    postvaccinal G04.02
    specified NEC G04.89
    toxic G92
    varicella B01.12
Myelogenous—*see* condition
Myeloid—*see* condition
Myelokathexis D70.9
Myelopathy (spinal cord) G95.9
    in (due to)
        infection—*see* Encephalitis
        mercury—*see* subcategory T56.1
        neoplastic disease (*see also* Neoplasm) D49.9 *[G99.2]*
Myelophthisis D61.82

Myelosis
    acute C92.0-
    aleukemic C92.9-
    nonleukemic D72.828
    subacute C92.9-
Myocardiopathy (congestive) (constrictive) (familial)
              (hypertrophic
              nonobstructive)
              (idiopathic) (infiltrative)
              (obstructive)
              (primary) (restrictive)
              (sporadic) (*see also*
              Cardiomyopathy) I42.9
    hypertrophic obstructive I42.1
    in (due to)
        Friedreich's ataxia G11.1 *[I43]*
        progressive muscular dystrophy G71.0 *[I43]*
    secondary I42.9
    thyrotoxic E05.90 *[I43]*
        with storm E05.91 *[I43]*
Myocarditis (with arteriosclerosis) (chronic) (fibroid)
              (interstitial) (old)
              (progressive) (senile)
              I51.4
    with
        rheumatic fever (conditions in I00) I09.0
            active—*see* Myocarditis, acute, rheumatic
            inactive or quiescent (with chorea) I09.0
    active I40.9
        rheumatic I01.2
            with chorea (acute) (rheumatic) (Sydenham's) I02.0
    acute or subacute (interstitial) I40.9
        due to
            streptococcus (beta-hemolytic) I01.2
        idiopathic I40.1
        rheumatic I01.2
            with chorea (acute) (rheumatic) (Sydenham's) I02.0
        specified NEC I40.8
    bacterial (acute) I40.0
    eosinophilic I40.1
    epidemic of newborn (Coxsackie) B33.22
    Fiedler's (acute) (isolated) I40.1
    giant cell (acute) (subacute) I40.1
    granulomatous (idiopathic) (isolated) (nonspecific) I40.1
    idiopathic (granulomatous) I40.1
    in (due to)
        Lyme disease A69.29
        sarcoidosis D86.85
    infective I40.0
    influenzal—*see* Influenza, with, myocarditis
    isolated (acute) I40.1
    nonrheumatic, active I40.9
    parenchymatous I40.9
    pneumococcal I40.0
    rheumatic (chronic) (inactive) (with chorea) I09.0
        active or acute I01.2
            with chorea (acute) (rheumatic) (Sydenham's) I02.0
    septic I40.0
    staphylococcal I40.0
    suppurative I40.0
    toxic I40.8
    virus, viral I40.0
        of newborn (Coxsackie) B33.22
Myoclonus, myoclonic, myoclonia (familial) (essential)
              (multifocal) (simplex)
              G25.3
    drug-induced G25.3
    epilepsy (*see also* Epilepsy, generalized, specified NEC)
              G40.4-
        familial (progressive) G25.3
    familial progressive G25.3
    Friedreich's G25.3
    jerks G25.3
    massive G25.3
    palatal G25.3
    pharyngeal G25.3
Myofibromatosis D48.1
    infantile Q89.8
Myopathy G72.9
    distal G71.0
    facioscapulohumeral G71.0
    in (due to)

Myopathy, *continued*
Cushing's syndrome E24.9 *[G73.7]*
hyperadrenocorticism E24.9 *[G73.7]*
hypothyroidism E03.9 *[G73.7]*
myxedema E03.9 *[G73.7]*
sarcoidosis D86.87
scarlet fever A38.1
systemic lupus erythematosus M32.19
thyrotoxicosis (hyperthyroidism) E05.90 *[G73.7]*
with thyroid storm E05.91 *[G73.7]*
limb-girdle G71.0
ocular G71.0
oculopharyngeal G71.0
scapulohumeral G71.0
Myositis M60.9
in (due to)
sarcoidosis D86.87
infective M60.009
arm M60.002
left M60.001
right M60.000
leg M60.005
left M60.004
right M60.003
lower limb M60.005
ankle M60.07-
foot M60.07-
lower leg M60.06-
thigh M60.05-
toe M60.07-
multiple sites M60.09
specified site NEC M60.08
upper limb M60.002
finger M60.04-
forearm M60.03-
hand M60.04-
shoulder region M60.01-
upper arm M60.02-
Myospasia impulsiva F95.2
Myotonia (acquisita) (intermittens) M62.89
congenita (acetazolamide responsive) (dominant)
(recessive) G71.12
levior G71.12
Myriapodiasis B88.2
Myringitis H73.2-
with otitis media—*see* Otitis, media
acute H73.00-
bullous H73.01-
specified NEC H73.09-
bullous—*see* Myringitis, acute, bullous
chronic H73.1-
Myxadenitis labialis K13.0
Myxedema (adult) (idiocy) (infantile) (juvenile) (*see also*
Hypothyroidism) E03.9
circumscribed E05.90
with storm E05.91
coma E03.5
congenital E00.1
cutis L98.5
localized (pretibial) E05.90
with storm E05.91
Myxolipoma D17.9

N

Naegeli's
disease Q82.8
Nail—*see also* condition
biting F98.8
Nanism, nanosomia—*see* Dwarfism
Napkin rash L22
Narcosis R06.89
Narcotism—*see* Dependence
NARP (Neuropathy, Ataxia and Retinitis pigmentosa)
syndrome E88.49
Nasopharyngeal—*see also* condition
pituitary gland Q89.2
torticollis M43.6
Nasopharyngitis (acute) (infective) (streptococcal) (subacute)
J00
chronic (suppurative) (ulcerative) J31.1

Nasopharynx, nasopharyngeal—*see* condition
Natal tooth, teeth K00.6
Nausea (without vomiting) R11.0
with vomiting R11.2
marina T75.3
navalis T75.3
Near drowning T75.1
Nearsightedness—*see* Myopia
Near-syncope R55
Necrolysis, toxic epidermal L51.2
due to drug
correct substance properly administered—*see* Table of
Drugs and Chemicals,
by drug, adverse effect
overdose or wrong substance given or taken—*see*
Table of Drugs and
Chemicals, by drug,
poisoning
Necrosis, necrotic (ischemic)—*see also* Gangrene
adrenal (capsule) (gland) E27.49
antrum J32.0
bone (*see also* Osteonecrosis) M87.9
ethmoid J32.2
cortical (acute) (renal) N17.1
ethmoid (bone) J32.2
fat, fatty (generalized)—*see also* Disorder, soft tissue,
specified type NEC
skin (subcutaneous), newborn P83.0
subcutaneous due to birth injury P15.6
kidney (bilateral) N28.0
acute N17.9
cortical (acute) (bilateral) N17.1
medullary (bilateral) (in acute renal failure) (papillary)
N17.2
papillary (bilateral) (in acute renal failure) N17.2
tubular N17.0
traumatic T79.5
medullary (acute) (renal) N17.2
papillary (acute) (renal) N17.2
pharynx J02.9
in granulocytopenia—*see* Neutropenia
subcutaneous fat, newborn P83.8
suprarenal (capsule) (gland) E27.49
tonsil J35.8
tubular (acute) (anoxic) (renal) (toxic) N17.0
postprocedural N99.0
Need (for)
Need (for)
care provider because (of)
assistance with personal care Z74.1
continuous supervision required Z74.3
impaired mobility Z74.09
no other household member able to render care Z74.2
specified reason NEC Z74.8
immunization—*see* Vaccination
vaccination—*see* Vaccination
Neglect
child (childhood)
confirmed T74.02
history of Z62.812
suspected T76.02
emotional, in childhood Z62.898
Nelaton's syndrome G60.8
Neonatal—*see also* Newborn
acne L70.4
bradycardia P29.12
screening, abnormal findings on P09
tachycardia P29.11
tooth, teeth K00.6
Neonatorum—*see* condition
Neoplasia
intraepithelial (histologically confirmed)
anal (AIN) (histologically confirmed) K62.82
grade I K62.82
grade II K62.82
severe D01.3
Neoplasm, neoplastic—*see also* Table of Neoplasms
lipomatous, benign—*see* Lipoma
Nephralgia N23

Nephritis, nephritic (albuminuric) (azotemic) (congenital)
(disseminated)
(epithelial) (familial)
(focal) (granulomatous)
(hemorrhagic) (infantile)
(nonsuppurative,
excretory) (uremic)
N05.9
acute N00.9
with
dense deposit disease N00.6
diffuse
crescentic glomerulonephritis N00.7
endocapillary proliferative glomerulonephritis
N00.4
membranous glomerulonephritis N00.2
mesangial proliferative glomerulonephritis
N00.3
mesangiocapillary glomerulonephritis N00.5
focal and segmental glomerular lesions N00.1
minor glomerular abnormality N00.0
specified morphological changes NEC N00.8
croupous N00.9
due to
diabetes mellitus—*see* E08-E13 with .21
subacute bacterial endocarditis I33.0
systemic lupus erythematosus (chronic) M32.14
in
diabetes mellitus—*see* E08–E13 with .21
polycystic Q61.3
autosomal
dominant Q61.2
recessive NEC Q61.19
childhood type NEC Q61.19
infantile type NEC Q61.19
poststreptococcal N05.9
acute N00.9
chronic N03.9
tubulo-interstitial (in) N12
acute (infectious) N10
war N00.9
Nephroblastoma (epithelial) (mesenchymal) C64.-
Nephrocystitis, pustular—*see* Nephritis, tubulo-interstitial
Nephroma C64-
mesoblastic D41.0-
Nephronephritis—*see* Nephrosis
Nephronophthisis Q61.5
Nephropathy (*see also* Nephritis) N28.9
analgesic N14.0
with medullary necrosis, acute N17.2
diabetic—*see* E08–E13 with .21
obstructive N13.8
phenacetin N17.2
vasomotor N17.0
Nephrosis, nephrotic (Epstein's) (syndrome) (congenital)
N04.9
with
glomerular lesion N04.1
hypocomplementemic N04.5
acute N04.9
anoxic—*see* Nephrosis, tubular
chemical—*see* Nephrosis, tubular
Finnish type (congenital) Q89.8
hemoglobin N10
hemoglobinuric—*see* Nephrosis, tubular
in
diabetes mellitus—*see* E08–E13 with .21
lipoid N04.9
minimal change N04.0
myoglobin N10
radiation N04.9
toxic—*see* Nephrosis, tubular
tubular (acute) N17.0
postprocedural N99.0
radiation N04.9
Nerves R45.0
Nervous (*see also* condition) R45.0
heart F45.8
stomach F45.8
tension R45.0
Nervousness R45.0

Neuralgia, neuralgic (acute) M79.2
  ciliary G44.009
    intractable G44.001
    not intractable G44.009
  ear—see subcategory H92.0
  migrainous G44.009
    intractable G44.001
    not intractable G44.009
  perineum R10.2
  pubic region R10.2
  scrotum R10.2
  spermatic cord R10.2
Neurasthenia F48.8
  cardiac F45.8
  gastric F45.8
  heart F45.8
Neuritis (rheumatoid) M79.2
  cranial nerve
    due to Lyme disease A69.22
    seventh or facial G51.8
      newborn (birth injury) P11.3
    fifth or trigeminal G51.0
    sixth or abducent—see Strabismus, paralytic, sixth
                  nerve
  facial G51.8
    newborn (birth injury) P11.3
  serum (see also Reaction, serum) T80.69
Neuroblastoma
  specified site—see Neoplasm, malignant, by site
  unspecified site C74.90
Neurodermatitis (circumscribed) (circumscripta) (local) L28.0
  atopic L20.81
  diffuse (Brocq) L20.81
  disseminated L20.81
Neurofibromatosis (multiple) (nonmalignant) Q85.00
  acoustic Q85.02
  malignant—see Neoplasm, nerve, malignant
  specified NEC Q85.09
  type 1 (von Recklinghausen) Q85.01
  type 2 Q85.02
Neurocirculatory asthenia F45.8
Neurogenic—see also condition
  bladder (see also Dysfunction, bladder, neuromuscular)
                  N31.9
    cauda equina syndrome G83.4
  bowel NEC K59.2
  heart F45.8
Neuromyopathy G70.9
  paraneoplastic D49.9 [G13.0]
Neuropathy, neuropathic G62.9
  hereditary G60.9
    motor and sensory (types I-IV) G60.0
    sensory G60.8
    specified NEC G60.8
  idiopathic G60.9
    progressive G60.3
    specified NEC G60.8
  peripheral (nerve) (see also Polyneuropathy) G62.9
    autonomic G90.9
    in (due to)
      hyperthyroidism E05.90 [G99.0]
        with thyroid storm E05.91 [G99.0]
Neurosis, neurotic F48.9
  anankastic F42.8
  anxiety (state) F41.1
    panic type F41.0
  bladder F45.8
  cardiac (reflex) F45.8
  cardiovascular F45.8
  character F60.9
  colon F45.8
  compulsive, compulsion F42.9
  conversion F44.9
  cutaneous F45.8
  excoriation F42.4
  gastric F45.8
  gastrointestinal F45.8
  heart F45.8
  hysterical F44.9
  incoordination F45.8
    larynx F45.8
    vocal cord F45.8

Neurosis, neurotic, *continued*
  intestine F45.8
  larynx (sensory) F45.8
    hysterical F44.4
  mixed NEC F48.8
  musculoskeletal F45.8
  obsessional F42.9
  obsessive-compulsive F42.9
  ocular NEC F45.8
  pharynx F45.8
  phobic F40.9
  posttraumatic (situational) F43.10
    acute F43.11
    chronic F43.12
  rectum F45.8
  respiratory F45.8
  rumination F45.8
  sexual F65.9
  state F48.9
  stomach F45.8
  traumatic F43.10
    acute F43.11
    chronic F43.12
  vasomotor F45.8
  visceral F45.8
Neurospongioblastosis diffusa Q85.1
Neutropenia, neutropenic (chronic) (genetic) (idiopathic)
                    (immune) (infantile)
                    (malignant) (pernicious)
                    (splenic) D70.9
  congenital (primary) D70.0
  cyclic D70.4
  cytoreductive cancer chemotherapy sequela D70.1
  drug-induced D70.2
    due to cytoreductive cancer chemotherapy D70.1
  due to infection D70.3
  fever D70.9
  neonatal, transitory (isoimmune) (maternal transfer) P61.5
  periodic D70.4
  secondary (cyclic) (periodic) (splenic) D70.4
    drug-induced D70.2
      due to cytoreductive cancer chemotherapy D70.1
  toxic D70.8
Nevus D22.9
  achromic—see Neoplasm, skin, benign
  amelanotic—see Neoplasm, skin, benign
  angiomatous D18.00
    skin D18.01
    specified site NEC D18.09
  araneus I78.1
  bathing trunk D48.5
  blue—(see Neoplasm, skin, benign for blue, cellular, giant,
                  or Jadassohn's or other
                  than malignant)
    malignant—see Melanoma
  capillary D18.00
    skin D18.01
    specified site NEC D18.09
  cavernous D18.00
    skin D18.01
    specified site NEC D18.09
  cellular—see Neoplasm, skin, benign
    blue—see Neoplasm, skin, benign
  comedonicus Q82.5
  dermal—see Neoplasm, skin, benign
    with epidermal nevus—see Neoplasm, skin, benign
  dysplastic—see Neoplasm, skin, benign
  flammeus Q82.5
  hemangiomatous D18.00
    skin D18.01
    specified site NEC D18.09
  lymphatic D18.1
  meaning hemangioma D18.00
    skin D18.01
    specified site NEC D18.09
  multiplex Q85.1
  non-neoplastic I78.1
  portwine Q82.5
  sanguineous Q82.5
  spider I78.1
  stellar I78.1
  strawberry Q82.5

Nevus, *continued*
  unius lateris Q82.5
  Unna's Q82.5
  vascular Q82.5
  verrucous Q82.5
Newborn (infant) (liveborn) (singleton) Z38.2
  abstinence syndrome P96.1
  acne L70.4
  affected by
    abruptio placenta P02.1
    amniocentesis (while in utero) P00.6
    amnionitis P02.7
    apparent life threatening event (ALTE) R68.13
    bleeding (into)
      cerebral cortex P52.22
      germinal matrix P52.0
      ventricles P52.1
    breech delivery P03.0
    cardiac arrest P29.81
    cerebral ischemia P91.0
    Cesarean delivery P03.4
    chemotherapy agents P04.1
    chorioamnionitis P02.7
    cocaine (crack) P04.41
    complications of labor and delivery P03.9
      specified NEC P03.89
    compression of umbilical cord NEC P02.5
    contracted pelvis P03.1
    delivery P03.9
      Cesarean P03.4
      forceps P03.2
      vacuum extractor P03.3
    entanglement (knot)in umbilical cord P02.5
    fetal (intrauterine)
      growth retardation P05.9
    forceps delivery P03.2
    heart rate abnormalities
      bradycardia P29.12
      intrauterine P03.819
        before onset of labor P03.810
        during labor P03.811
      tachycardia P29.11
    hemorrhage (antepartum) P02.1
      intraventricular (nontraumatic) P52.3
        grade 1 P52.0
        grade 2 P52.1
        grade 3 P52.21
        grade 4 P52.22
        subependymal P52.0
          with intracerebral extension P52.22
          with intraventricular extension P52.1
            with enlargement of ventricles P52.21
          without intraventricular extension P52.0
    hypoxic ischemic encephalopathy [HIE] P91.60
      mild P91.61
      moderate P91.62
      severe P91.63
    induction of labor P03.89
    intrauterine (fetal)blood loss P50.9
    intrauterine (fetal) hemorrhage P50.9
    malpresentation (malposition)NEC P03.1
    maternal (complication of) (use of)
      alcohol P04.3
      analgesia (maternal) P04.0
      anesthesia (maternal) P04.0
      blood loss P02.1
      circulatory disease P00.3
      condition P00.9
        specified NEC P00.89
      delivery P03.9
        Cesarean P03.4
        forceps P03.2
        vacuum extractor P03.3
      diabetes mellitus (pre-existing) P70.1
      disorder P00.9
        specified NEC P00.89
      drugs (addictive) (illegal)NEC P04.49
      hemorrhage P02.1
      incompetent cervix P01.0
      infectious disease P00.2
      malpresentation before labor P01.7
      medical procedure P00.7

Newborn, *continued*

medication P04.1
parasitic disease P00.2
placenta previa P02.0
premature rupture of membranes P01.1
respiratory disease P00.3
surgical procedure P00.6
medication (legal) (maternal use) (prescribed) P04.1
membranitis P02.7
methamphetamine (s) P04.49
mixed metabolic and respiratory acidosis P84
neonatal abstinence syndrome P96.1
noxious substances transmitted via placenta or breast milk P04.9
specified NEC P04.8
placenta previa P02.0
placental
abnormality (functional) (morphological) P02.20
specified NEC P02.29
dysfunction P02.29
infarction P02.29
insufficiency P02.29
separation NEC P02.1
transfusion syndromes P02.3
placentitis P02.7
prolapsed cord P02.4
respiratory arrest P28.81
slow intrauterine growth P05.9
tobacco P04.2
twin to twin transplacental transfusion P02.3
umbilical cord (tightly)around neck P02.5
umbilical cord condition P02.60
short cord P02.69
specified NEC P02.69
uterine contractions (abnormal) P03.6
vasa previa P02.69
from intrauterine blood loss P50.0
apnea P28.4
primary P28.3
obstructive P28.4
sleep (central) (obstructive) (primary) P28.3
born in hospital Z38.00
by cesarean Z38.01
born outside hospital Z38.1
breast buds P96.89
breast engorgement P83.4
check-up—*see* Newborn, examination
convulsion P90
dehydration P74.1
examination
8 to 28 days old Z00.111
under 8 days old Z00.110
fever P81.9
environmentally-induced P81.0
hyperbilirubinemia P59.9
of prematurity P59.0
infection P39.9
candidal P37.5
specified NEC P39.8
urinary tract P39.3
jaundice P59.9
due to
breast milk inhibitor P59.3
hepatocellular damage P59.20
specified NEC P59.29
preterm delivery P59.0
of prematurity P59.0
specified NEC P59.8
mastitis P39.0
infective P39.0
noninfective P83.4
multiple born NEC Z38.8
born in hospital Z38.68
by cesarean Z38.69
born outside hospital Z38.7
omphalitis P38.9
with mild hemorrhage P38.1
without hemorrhage P38.9
post-term P08.21
prolonged gestation (over 42 completed weeks) P08.22

Newborn, *continued*

quadruplet Z38.8
born in hospital Z38.63
by cesarean Z38.64
born outside hospital Z38.7
quintuplet Z38.8
born in hospital Z38.65
by cesarean Z38.66
born outside hospital Z38.7
seizure P90
sepsis (congenital) P36.9
due to
anaerobes NEC P36.5
Escherichia coli P36.4
Staphylococcus P36.30
aureus P36.2
specified NEC P36.39
Streptococcus P36.10
group B P36.0
specified NEC P36.19
specified NEC P36.8
triplet Z38.8
born in hospital Z38.61
by cesarean Z38.62
born outside hospital Z38.7
twin Z38.5
born in hospital Z38.30
by cesarean Z38.31
born outside hospital Z38.4
vomiting P92.09
bilious P92.01
weight check Z00.111

Night

blindness—*see* Blindness, night
sweats R61
terrors (child) F51.4
Nightmares (REM sleep type) F51.5
Nipple—*see* condition
Nitrosohemoglobinemia D74.8
Nocturia R35.1
psychogenic F45.8
Nocturnal—*see* condition
Node (s)—*see also* Nodule
Osler's I33.0
Nodule (s), nodular
breast NEC N63
cutaneous—*see* Swelling, localized
inflammatory—*see* Inflammation
lung, solitary (subsegmental branch of the bronchial tree) R91.1
multiple R91.8
retrocardiac R09.89
solitary, lung (subsegmental branch of the bronchial tree) R91.1
multiple R91.8
subcutaneous—*see* Swelling, localized
Nonclosure—*see also* Imperfect, closure
ductus arteriosus (Botallo's) Q25.0
foramen
botalli Q21.1
ovale Q21.1
Noncompliance Z91.19
with
dietary regimen Z91.11
medical treatment Z91.19
medication regimen NEC Z91.14
underdosing (*see also* Table of Drugs and Chemicals, categories T36–T50, with final character 6) Z91.14
intentional NEC Z91.128
due to financial hardship of patient Z91.120
unintentional NEC Z91.138
Nondescent (congenital)—*see also* Malposition, congenital
testicle Q53.9
bilateral Q53.20
abdominal Q53.21
perineal Q53.22
unilateral Q53.10
abdominal Q53.11
perineal Q53.12

Nondevelopment

brain Q02
part of Q04.3
heart Q24.8
organ or site, congenital NEC—*see* Hypoplasia
Nonexpansion, lung (newborn) P28.0
Nonovulation N97.0
Nonpneumatization, lung NEC P28.0
Nonunion
fracture—*see* Fracture, by site
organ or site, congenital NEC—*see* Imperfect, closure
symphysis pubis, congenital Q74.2
Noonan's syndrome Q87.1
Normocytic anemia (infectional) due to blood loss (chronic) D50.0
acute D62
Norwegian itch B86
Nose, nasal—*see* condition
Nosebleed R04.0
Nose-picking F98.8
Nosophobia F45.22
Nostalgia F43.20
Nothnagel's
syndrome—*see* Strabismus, paralytic, third nerve
vasomotor acroparesthesia I73.89
Noxious
foodstuffs, poisoning by—*see* Poisoning, food, noxious, plant
substances transmitted through placenta or breast milk P04.9
Nursemaid's elbow S53.03-
Nutrition deficient or insufficient (*see also* Malnutrition) E46
due to
insufficient food T73.0
lack of
care (child) T76.02
food T73.0
Nycturia R35.1
psychogenic F45.8
Nystagmus H55.00
benign paroxysmal—*see* Vertigo, benign paroxysmal
congenital H55.01
dissociated H55.04
latent H55.02
miners' H55.09
specified form NEC H55.09
visual deprivation H55.03

O

Obesity E66.9
with alveolar hypoventilation E66.2
constitutional E66.8
dietary counseling and surveillance Z71.3
drug-induced E66.1
due to
drug E66.1
excess calories E66.09
morbid E66.01
severe E66.01
endocrine E66.8
endogenous E66.8
familial E66.8
glandular E66.8
hypothyroid—*see* Hypothyroidism
morbid E66.01
with alveolar hypoventilation E66.2
due to excess calories E66.01
with obesity hypoventilation syndrome (OHS) E66.2
nutritional E66.09
pituitary E23.6
severe E66.01
specified type NEC E66.8
Observation (following) (for) (without need for further medical care) Z04.9
accident NEC Z04.3
at work Z04.2
transport Z04.1
adverse effect of drug Z03.6
alleged rape or sexual assault (victim), ruled out
child Z04.42
criminal assault Z04.8

Observation, *continued*
    development state
        adolescent Z00.3
        period of rapid growth in childhood Z00.2
        puberty Z00.3
    disease, specified NEC Z03.89
    following work accident Z04.2
    newborn (for suspected condition, ruled out)—*see*
                            Newborn, affected
                            by (suspected to be),
                            maternal (complication
                            of) (use of)
    suicide attempt, alleged NEC Z03.89
        self-poisoning Z03.6
    suspected, ruled out—*see also* Suspected condition,
                            ruled out
      abuse, physical
        child Z04.72
      accident at work Z04.2
      child battering victim Z04.72
      condition NEC Z03.89
      drug poisoning or adverse effect Z03.6
      exposure (to)
        anthrax Z03.810
        biological agent NEC Z03.818
      inflicted injury NEC Z04.8
      newborn, ruled-out
        cardiac condition Z05.0
        connective tissue condition Z05.73
        gastrointestinal condition Z05.5
        genetic condition Z05.41
        genitourinary condition Z05.6
        immunologic condition Z05.43
        infectious condition Z05.1
        metabolic condition Z05.42
        musculoskeletal condition Z05.72
        neurological condition Z05.2
        other condition Z05.8
        respiratory condition Z05.3
        skin and subcutaneous tissue condition Z05.71
        unspecified suspected condition Z05.9
      suicide attempt, alleged Z03.89
        self-poisoning Z03.6
      toxic effects from ingested substance (drug) (poison)
                        Z03.6
    toxic effects from ingested substance (drug) (poison)
                    Z03.6

Obsession, obsessional state F42
Obsessive-compulsive neurosis or reaction F42.8
    mixed thoughts and acts F42.2
Obstruction, obstructed, obstructive
    airway J98.8
      with
        allergic alveolitis J67.9
        asthma J45.909
          with
            exacerbation (acute) J45.901
            status asthmaticus J45.902
    aqueduct of Sylvius G91.1
      congenital Q03.0
        with spina bifida—*see* Spina bifida, by site, with
                          hydrocephalus
    artery (*see also* Embolism, artery) I74.9
    bile duct or passage (common) (hepatic) (noncalculous)
                      K83.1
      with calculus K80.51
      congenital (causing jaundice) Q44.3
    bladder-neck (acquired) N32.0
      congenital Q64.31
    cystic duct—*see also* Obstruction, gallbladder
      with calculus K80.21
    device, implant or graft (*see also* Complications, by site
                  and type, mechanical)
                  T85.698
      ventricular intracranial shunt T85.09
    fecal K56.41
      with hernia—*see* Hernia, by site, with obstruction
    foramen of Monro (congenital) Q03.8
      with spina bifida—*see* Spina bifida, by site, with
                      hydrocephalus
    foreign body—*see* Foreign body

Obstruction, obstructed, obstructive, *continued*
    gallbladder K82.0
      with calculus, stones K80.21
      congenital Q44.1
    intestine K56.60
      adynamic K56.0
      congenital (small) Q41.9
        large Q42.9
          specified part NEC Q42.8
      neurogenic K56.0
        Hirschsprung's disease or megacolon Q43.1
      newborn P76.9
        due to
          fecaliths P76.8
          inspissated milk P76.2
          meconium (plug) P76.0
            in mucoviscidosis E84.11
        specified NEC P76.8
      reflex K56.0
      specified NEC K56.69
      volvulus K56.2
    lacrimal (passages) (duct)
      by
        dacryolith—*see* Dacryolith
        stenosis—*see* Stenosis, lacrimal
      congenital Q10.5
      neonatal H04.53-
    lacrimonasal duct—*see* Obstruction, lacrimal
    meconium (plug)
      newborn P76.0
        due to fecaliths P76.0
        in mucoviscidosis E84.11
    nasal J34.89
    nose J34.89
    portal (circulation) (vein) I81
    pulmonary valve (heart) I37.0
    pylorus
      congenital or infantile Q40.0
    rectum K62.4
    renal N28.89
      outflow N13.8
      pelvis, congenital Q62.39
    sinus (accessory) (nasal) J34.89
    stomach NEC K31.89
      congenital Q40.2
      due to pylorospasm K31.3
    ureter (functional) (pelvic junction) NEC N13.5
      with
        hydronephrosis N13.0
    urinary (moderate) N13.9
      organ or tract (lower) N13.9
      specified NEC N13.8
    uropathy N13.9
    vagina N89.5
    vesical NEC N32.0
    vesicourethral orifice N32.0
      congenital Q64.31
Occlusion, occluded
    anus K62.4
      congenital Q42.3
        with fistula Q42.2
    aqueduct of Sylvius G91.1
      congenital Q03.0
        with spina bifida—*see* Spina bifida, by site, with
                        hydrocephalus
    artery (*see also* Embolism, artery) I74.9
    choanal Q30.0
    gallbladder—*see also* Obstruction, gallbladder
      congenital (causing jaundice) Q44.1
    hymen N89.6
      congenital Q52.3
    nose J34.89
      congenital Q30.0
    posterior lingual, of mandibular teeth M26.29
    teeth (mandibular) (posterior lingual) M26.29
    ureter (complete) (partial) N13.5
      congenital Q62.10
    ureteropelvic junction N13.5
      congenital Q62.11
    ureterovesical orifice N13.5
      congenital Q62.12
    vagina N89.5
    ventricle (brain) NEC G91.1

Occult
    blood in feces (stools) R19.5
Oculogyric crisis or disturbance H51.8
    psychogenic F45.8
Odontoclasia K03.89
Oligoastrocytoma
    specified site—*see* Neoplasm, malignant, by site
    unspecified site C71.9
Oligocythemia D64.9
Oligodendroblastoma
    specified site—*see* Neoplasm, malignant
    unspecified site C71.9
Oligodendroglioma
    anaplastic type
      specified site—*see* Neoplasm, malignant, by site
      unspecified site C71.9
    specified site—*see* Neoplasm, malignant, by site
    unspecified site C71.9
Oligodontia—*see* Anodontia
Oligoencephalon Q02
Oligohydramnios O41.0-
Oligophrenia—*see also* Disability, intellectual
    phenylpyruvic E70.0
Oliguria R34
    postprocedural N99.0
Omphalitis (congenital) (newborn) P38.9
    with mild hemorrhage P38.1
    without hemorrhage P38.9
Omphalocele Q79.2
Omphalomesenteric duct, persistent Q43.0
Omphalorrhagia, newborn P51.9
Onanism (excessive) F98.8
Onychia—*see also* Cellulitis, digit
    with lymphangitis—*see* Lymphangitis, acute, digit
    candidal B37.2
    dermatophytic B35.1
Onychocryptosis L60.0
Onycholysis L60.1
Onychomadesis L60.8
Onychomycosis (finger) (toe) B35.1
Onychophagia F98.8
Onychophosis L60.8
Onychoptosis L60.8
Onyxis (finger) (toe) L60.0
Oophoritis (cystic) (infectional) (interstitial) N70.92
    with salpingitis N70.93
Ophthalmia (*see also* Conjunctivitis) H10.9
    blennorrhagic (gonococcal) (neonatorum) A54.31
    gonococcal (neonatorum) A54.31
    neonatorum, newborn P39.1
      gonococcal A54.31
Orchitis (gangrenous) (nonspecific) (septic) (suppurative)
                      N45.2
    blennorrhagic (gonococcal) (acute) (chronic) A54.23
    chlamydial A56.19
    gonococcal (acute) (chronic) A54.23
    mumps B26.0
    syphilitic A52.76
Orthopnea R06.01
Osgood-Schlatter disease or osteochondrosis M92.5-
Osler (-Weber)-Rendu disease I78.0
Osler's nodes I33.0
Ossification
    diaphragm J98.6
Osteitis—*see also* Osteomyelitis
    deformans M88.9
    fragilitans Q78.0
    in (due to)
      malignant neoplasm of bone C41.9 *[M90.60]*
      neoplastic disease (*see also* Neoplasm) D49.9
                     [M90.60]
        carpus D49.9 *[M90.64-]*
        clavicle D49.9 *[M90.61-]*
        femur D49.9 *[M90.65-]*
        fibula D49.9 *[M90.66-]*
        finger D49.9 *[M90.64-]*
        humerus D49.9 *[M90.62-]*
        ilium D49.9 *[M90.65-]*
        ischium D49.9 *[M90.65-]*
        metacarpus D49.9 *[M90.64-]*
        metatarsus D49.9 *[M90.67-]*
        multiple sites D49.9 *[M90.69]*
        neck D49.9 *[M90.68]*

Osteitis, *continued*
   radius D49.9 *[M90.63-]*
   rib D49.9 *[M90.68]*
   scapula D49.9 *[M90.61-]*
   skull D49.9 *[M90.68]*
   tarsus D49.9 *[M90.67-]*
   tibia D49.9 *[M90.66-]*
   toe D49.9 *[M90.67-]*
   ulna D49.9 *[M90.63-]*
   vertebra D49.9 *[M90.68]*
  skull M88.0
  specified NEC—*see* Paget's disease, bone, by site
  vertebra M88.1
 tuberculosa A18.09
  cystica D86.89
  multiplex cystoides D86.89
Osteochondritis—*see also* Osteochondropathy, by site
 juvenile M92.9
  patellar M92.4-
Osteochondropathy M93.90
 slipped upper femoral epiphysis—*see* Slipped, epiphysis, upper femoral
Osteochondrosis—*see also* Osteochondropathy, by site
 acetabulum (juvenile) M91.0
 astragalus (juvenile) M92.6-
 Blount's M92.5-
 Buchanan's M91.0
 Burns' M92.1-
 calcaneus (juvenile) M92.6-
 capitular epiphysis (femur) (juvenile) M91.1-
 carpal (juvenile) (lunate) (scaphoid) M92.21-
 coxae juvenilis M91.1-
 deformans juvenilis, coxae M91.1-
 Diaz's M92.6-
 dissecans (knee) (shoulder)—*see* Osteochondritis, dissecans
 femoral capital epiphysis (juvenile) M91.1-
 femur (head), juvenile M91.1-
 fibula (juvenile) M92.5-
 foot NEC (juvenile) M92.8
 Freiberg's M92.7-
 Haas' (juvenile) M92.0-
 Haglund's M92.6-
 hip (juvenile) M91.1-
 humerus (capitulum) (head) (juvenile) M92.0-
 ilium, iliac crest (juvenile) M91.0
 ischiopubic synchondrosis M91.0
 Iselin's M92.7-
 juvenile, juvenilis M92.9
  after congenital dislocation of hip reduction M91.8-
  arm M92.3-
  capitular epiphysis (femur) M91.1-
  clavicle, sternal epiphysis M92.3-
  coxae M91.1-
  deformans M92.9
  fibula M92.5-
  foot NEC M92.8
  hand M92.20-
   carpal lunate M92.21-
   metacarpal head M92.22-
   specified site NEC M92.29-
  head of femur M91.1-
  hip and pelvis M91.9-
   coxa plana—*see* Coxa, plana
   femoral head M91.1-
   pelvis M91.0
   pseudocoxalgia—*see* Pseudocoxalgia
   specified NEC M91.8-
  humerus M92.0-
  limb
   lower NEC M92.8
   upper NEC M92.3-
  medial cuneiform bone M92.6-
  metatarsus M92.7-
  patella M92.4-
  radius M92.1-
  specified site NEC M92.8
  tarsus M92.6-
  tibia M92.5-
  ulna M92.1-
  upper limb NEC M92.3-
 Kienböck's M92.21-

Osteochondrosis, *continued*
 Köhler's
  patellar M92.4-
  tarsal navicular M92.6-
 Legg-Perthes (-Calvé) (-Waldenström) M91.1-
 limb
  lower NEC (juvenile) M92.8
  upper NEC (juvenile) M92.3-
 lunate bone (carpal) (juvenile) M92.21-
 Mauclaire's M92.22-
 metacarpal (head) (juvenile) M92.22-
 metatarsus (fifth) (head) (juvenile) (second) M92.7-
 navicular (juvenile) M92.6-
 os
  calcis (juvenile) M92.6-
  tibiale externum (juvenile) M92.6-
 Osgood-Schlatter M92.5-
 Panner's M92.0-
 patellar center (juvenile) (primary) (secondary) M92.4-
 pelvis (juvenile) M91.0
 Pierson's M91.0
 radius (head) (juvenile) M92.1-
 Sever's M92.6-
 Sinding-Larsen M92.4-
 symphysis pubis (juvenile) M91.0
 talus (juvenile) M92.6-
 tarsus (navicular) (juvenile) M92.6-
 tibia (proximal) (tubercle) (juvenile) M92.5-
 ulna (lower) (juvenile) M92.1-
 van Neck's M91.0
Osteogenesis imperfecta Q78.0
Osteomyelitis (general) (infective) (localized) (neonatal) (purulent) (septic) (staphylococcal) (streptococcal) (suppurative) (with periostitis) M86.9
 acute M86.10
  carpus M86.14-
  clavicle M86.11-
  femur M86.15-
  fibula M86.16-
  finger M86.14-
  humerus M86.12-
  ilium M86.159
  ischium M86.159
  metacarpus M86.14-
  metatarsus M86.17-
  multiple sites M86.19
  neck M86.18
  radius M86.13-
  rib M86.18
  scapula M86.11-
  skull M86.18
  tarsus M86.17-
  tibia M86.16-
  toe M86.17-
  ulna M86.13-
Osteonecrosis M87.9
 secondary
  due to
   hemoglobinopathy NEC D58.2 [M90.50]
    carpus D58.2 *[M90.54-]*
    clavicle D58.2 *[M90.51-]*
    femur D58.2 *[M90.55-]*
    fibula D58.2 *[M90.56-]*
    finger D58.2 *[M90.54-]*
    humerus D58.2 *[M90.52-]*
    ilium D58.2 *[M90.55-]*
    ischium D58.2 *[M90.55-]*
    metacarpus D58.2 *[M90.54-]*
    metatarsus D58.2 *[M90.57-]*
    multiple sites D58.2 *[M90.58]*
    neck D58.2 *[M90.58]*
    radius D58.2 *[M90.53-]*
    rib D58.2 *[M90.58]*
    scapula D58.2 *[M90.51-]*
    skull D58.2 *[M90.58]*
    tarsus D58.2 *[M90.57-]*
    tibia D58.2 *[M90.56-]*
    toe D58.2 *[M90.57-]*
    ulna D58.2 *[M90.53-]*
    vertebra D58.2 *[M90.58]*

Osteophyte M25.70
 ankle M25.77-
 elbow M25.72-
 foot joint M25.77-
 hand joint M25.74-
 hip M25.75-
 knee M25.76-
 shoulder M25.71-
 spine M25.78
 vertebrae M25.78
 wrist M25.73-
Osteopsathyrosis (idiopathica) Q78.0
Osteosis
 cutis L94.2
Ostium
 atrioventriculare commune Q21.2
 primum (arteriosum) (defect) (persistent) Q21.2
 secundum (arteriosum) (defect) (patent) (persistent) Q21.1
Ostrum-Furst syndrome Q75.8
Otalgia—*see* subcategory H92.0
Otitis (acute) H66.90
 with effusion—*see also* Otitis, media, nonsuppurative
  purulent—*see* Otitis, media, suppurative
 chronic—*see also* Otitis, media, chronic
  with effusion—*see also* Otitis, media, nonsuppurative, chronic
 externa H60.9-
  abscess—*see also* Abscess, ear, external
  acute (noninfective) H60.50-
   infective—*see* Otitis, externa, infective
  cellulitis—*see* Cellulitis, ear
  in (due to)
   aspergillosis B44.89
   candidiasis B37.84
   erysipelas A46 *[H62.40]*
   herpes (simplex) virus infection B00.1
    zoster B02.8
   impetigo L01.00 *[H62.40]*
   infectious disease NEC B99 *[H62.4-]*
   mycosis NEC B36.9 *[H62.40]*
   parasitic disease NEC B89 *[H62.40]*
   viral disease NEC B34.9 *[H62.40]*
   zoster B02.8
  infective NEC H60.39-
   abscess—*see* Abscess, ear, external
   cellulitis—*see* Cellulitis, ear
   swimmer's ear H60.33-
  malignant H60.2-
  mycotic NEC B36.9 *[H62.40]*
   in
    aspergillosis B44.89
    candidiasis B37.84
    moniliasis B37.84
  specified NEC—*see* subcategory H60.8
  tropical NEC B36.8
   in
    aspergillosis B44.89
    candidiasis B37.84
    moniliasis B37.84
 insidiosa—*see* Otosclerosis
 interna—*see* subcategory H83.0
 media (hemorrhagic) (staphylococcal) (streptococcal) H66.9-
  with effusion (nonpurulent)—*see* Otitis, media, nonsuppurative
  acute, subacute H66.90
   allergic—*see* Otitis, media, nonsuppurative, acute, allergic
   exudative—*see* Otitis, media, nonsuppurative, acute
   mucoid—*see* Otitis, media, nonsuppurative, acute
   necrotizing—*see also* Otitis, media, suppurative, acute
    in
     measles B05.3
     scarlet fever A38.0
   nonsuppurative NEC—*see* Otitis, media, nonsuppurative, acute
   purulent—*see* Otitis, media, suppurative, acute
   sanguinous—*see* Otitis, media, nonsuppurative, acute
   secretory—*see* Otitis, media, nonsuppurative, acute, serous

Otitis, *continued*

seromucinous—*see* Otitis, media, nonsuppurative,
acute
serous—*see* Otitis, media, nonsuppurative, acute,
serous
suppurative—*see* Otitis, media, suppurative, acute
allergic—*see* Otitis, media, nonsuppurative
catarrhal—*see* Otitis, media, nonsuppurative
chronic H66.90
with effusion (nonpurulent)—*see* Otitis, media,
nonsuppurative,
chronic
allergic—*see* Otitis, media, nonsuppurative,
chronic, allergic
benign suppurative—*see* Otitis, media,
suppurative, chronic,
tubotympanic
catarrhal—*see* Otitis, media, nonsuppurative,
chronic, serous
exudative—*see* Otitis, media, suppurative, chronic
mucinous—*see* Otitis, media, nonsuppurative,
chronic, mucoid
mucoid—*see* Otitis, media, nonsuppurative,
chronic, mucoid
nonsuppurative NEC—*see* Otitis, media,
nonsuppurative,
chronic
purulent—*see* Otitis, media, suppurative, chronic
secretory—*see* Otitis, media, nonsuppurative,
chronic, mucoid
seromucinous—*see* Otitis, media, nonsuppurative,
chronic
serous—*see* Otitis, media, nonsuppurative,
chronic, serous
suppurative—*see* Otitis, media, suppurative,
chronic
transudative—*see* Otitis, media, nonsuppurative,
chronic, mucoid
exudative—*see* Otitis, media, suppurative
in (due to) (with)
influenza—*see* Influenza, with, otitis media
measles B05.3
scarlet fever A38.0
tuberculosis A18.6
viral disease NEC B34.- *[H67.-]*
mucoid—*see* Otitis, media, nonsuppurative
nonsuppurative H65.9-
acute or subacute NEC H65.19- (6th characters
1—3, 9)
allergic H65.11- (6th characters 1—3, 9)
recurrent H65.11- (6th characters 4—7)
recurrent H65.19- (6th characters 4—7)
secretory—*see* Otitis, media, nonsuppurative,
serous
serous H65.0- (6th characters 0—3)
recurrent H65.0- (6th characters 4—7)
chronic H65.49-
allergic H65.41-
mucoid H65.3-
serous H65.2-
postmeasles B05.3
purulent—*see* Otitis, media, suppurative
secretory—*see* Otitis, media, nonsuppurative
seromucinous—*see* Otitis, media, nonsuppurative
serous—*see* Otitis, media, nonsuppurative
suppurative H66.4-
acute H66.00- (6th characters 1–3, 9)
with rupture of ear drum H66.01- (6th
characters 1–3, 9)
recurrent H66.00- (6th characters 4–7)
with rupture of ear drum H66.01- (6th
characters 4–7)
chronic (*see also* subcategory) H66.3
atticoantral H66.2-
benign—*see* Otitis, media, suppurative,
chronic, tubotympanic
tubotympanic H66.1-
transudative—*see* Otitis, media, nonsuppurative
tuberculous A18.6

Otomycosis (diffuse) NEC B36.9 [H62.40]
in
aspergillosis B44.89
candidiasis B37.84
moniliasis B37.84
Otorrhea H92.1-
Ovary, ovarian—*see also* condition
vein syndrome N13.8
Overactive—*see also* Hyperfunction
bladder N32.81
Overactivity R46.3
child—*see* Disorder, attention-deficit hyperactivity
Overbite (deep) (excessive) (horizontal) (vertical) M26.29
Overeating R63.2
nonorganic origin F50.89
psychogenic F50.89
Overlapping toe (acquired)—*see also* Deformity, toe,
specified NEC
congenital (fifth toe) Q66.89
Overload
circulatory, due to transfusion (blood) (blood components)
(TACO) E87.71
fluid E87.70
due to transfusion (blood) (blood components) E87.71
specified NEC E87.79
iron, due to repeated red blood cell transfusions E83.111
potassium (K) E87.5
sodium (Na) E87.0
Overnutrition—*see* Hyperalimentation
Overproduction—*see also* Hypersecretion
growth hormone E22.0
Overriding
toe (acquired)—*see also* Deformity, toe, specified NEC
congenital Q66.89
Overstrained R53.83
Overweight E66.3
Overworked R53.83
Ovulation (cycle)
failure or lack of N97.0
pain N94.0
Oxyuriasis B80
Oxyuris vermicularis (infestation) B80
Ozena J31.0

P

Pachydermatocele (congenital) Q82.8
Paget's disease
bone M88.9
carpus M88.84-
clavicle M88.81-
femur M88.85-
fibula M88.86-
finger M88.84-
humerus M88.82-
ilium M88.85-
in neoplastic disease—*see* Osteitis, deformans, in
neoplastic disease
ischium M88.85-
metacarpus M88.84-
metatarsus M88.87-
multiple sites M88.89
neck M88.88
radius M88.83-
rib M88.88
scapula M88.81-
skull M88.0
tarsus M88.87-
tibia M88.86-
toe M88.87-
ulna M88.83-
vertebra M88.88
osteitis deformans—*see* Paget's disease, bone
Pain(s) (*see also* Painful) R52
abdominal R10.9
colic R10.83
generalized R10.84
with acute abdomen R10.0
lower R10.30
left quadrant R10.32
pelvic or perineal R10.2
periumbilical R10.33
right quadrant R10.31

Pain(s), *continued*

rebound—*see* Tenderness, abdominal, rebound
severe with abdominal rigidity R10.0
tenderness—*see* Tenderness, abdominal
upper R10.10
epigastric R10.13
left quadrant R10.12
right quadrant R10.11
acute R52
due to trauma G89.11
neoplasm related G89.3
postprocedural NEC G89.18
adnexa (uteri) R10.2
anus K62.89
axillary (axilla) M79.62-
back (postural) M54.9
bladder R39.89
associated with micturition—*see* Micturition, painful
chronic R39.82
breast N64.4
broad ligament R10.2
cancer associated (acute) (chronic) G89.3
chest (central) R07.9
chronic G89.29
neoplasm related G89.3
coccyx M53.3
due to cancer G89.3
due to malignancy (primary) (secondary) G89.3
ear—*see* subcategory H92.0
epigastric, epigastrium R10.13
face, facial R51
atypical G50.1
female genital organs NEC N94.89
gastric—*see* Pain, abdominal
generalized NOS R52
genital organ
female N94.89
male
scrotal N50.82
testicular N50.81-
groin—*see* Pain, abdominal, lower
hand M79.64-
joints M25.54-
head—*see* Headache
heart—*see* Pain, precordial
infra-orbital—*see* Neuralgia, trigeminal
intermenstrual N94.0
jaw R68.84
joint M25.50
ankle M25.57-
elbow M25.52-
finger M25.54-
foot M25.57-
hand M79.64-
hip M25.55-
knee M25.56-
shoulder M25.51-
toe M25.57-
wrist M25.53-
kidney N23
laryngeal R07.0
limb M79.609
lower M79.60-
foot M79.67-
lower leg M79.66-
thigh M79.65-
toe M79.67-
upper M79.60-
axilla M79.62-
finger M79.64-
forearm M79.63-
hand M79.64-
upper arm M79.62-
mandibular R68.84
mastoid—*see* subcategory H92.0
maxilla R68.84
menstrual (*see also* Dysmenorrhea) N94.6
mouth K13.79
muscle—*see* Myalgia
musculoskeletal (*see also* Pain, by site) M79.1
myofascial M79.1
nasal J34.89

Pain(s), *continued*
  nasopharynx J39.2
  neck NEC M54.2
  nose J34.89
  ocular H57.1-
  ophthalmic H57.1-
  orbital region H57.1-
  ovary N94.89
  over heart—*see* Pain, precordial
  ovulation N94.0
  pelvic (female) R10.2
  perineal, perineum R10.2
  postoperative NOS G89.18
  postprocedural NOS G89.18
  premenstrual F32.81
  rectum K62.89
  round ligament (stretch) R10.2
  sacroiliac M53.3
  scrotal N50.82
  shoulder M25.51-
  spine M54.9
    cervical M54.2
    low back M54.5
      with sciatica M54.4-
  temporomandibular (joint) M26.62-
  testicular N50.81-
  throat R07.0
  tibia M79.66-
  toe M79.67-
  tumor associated G89.3
  ureter N23
  urinary (organ) (system) N23
  uterus NEC N94.89
  vagina R10.2
  vesical R39.89
    associated with micturition—*see* Micturition, painful
  vulva R10.2
Painful—*see also* Pain
  menstruation—*see* Dysmenorrhea
    psychogenic F45.8
  micturition—*see* Micturition, painful
  scar NEC L90.5
  wire sutures T81.89
Painter's colic—*see* subcategory T56.0
Palate—*see* condition
Palatoplegia K13.79
Palatoschisis—*see* Cleft, palate
Palliative care Z51.5
Pallor R23.1
Palpitations (heart) R00.2
  psychogenic F45.8
Palsy (*see also* Paralysis) G83.9
  Bell's—*see also* Palsy, facial
    newborn P11.3
  brachial plexus NEC G54.0
    newborn (birth injury) P14.3
  cerebral (congenital) G80.9
  cranial nerve—*see also* Disorder, nerve, cranial
    multiple G52.7
    in
      neoplastic disease (*see also* Neoplasm) D49.9
          [G53]
      sarcoidosis D86.82
  Erb's P14.0
  facial G51.0
    newborn (birth injury) P11.3
  Klumpke (-Déjérine) P14.1
  lead—*see* subcategory T56.0
  seventh nerve—*see also* Palsy, facial
    newborn P11.3
Pancake heart R93.1
  with cor pulmonale (chronic) I27.81
Pancarditis (acute) (chronic) I51.89
  rheumatic I09.89
    active or acute I01.8
Pancolitis, ulcerative (chronic) K51.00
  with
    complication K51.019
    abscess K51.014
    fistula K51.013
    obstruction K51.012
    rectal bleeding K51.011
    specified complication NEC K51.018

Pancreatitis (annular) (apoplectic) (calcareous) (edematous)
        (hemorrhagic)
        (malignant) (recurrent)
        (subacute)(suppurative)
        K85.90
  acute K85.90
  idiopathic K85.00
    with infected necrosis K85.02
    with uninfected necrosis K85.01
    with infected necrosis K85.92
    with uninfected necrosis K85.91
Pancytopenia (acquired) D61.818
  with
    malformations D61.09
    myelodysplastic syndrome—*see* Syndrome,
        myelodysplastic
  antineoplastic chemotherapy induced D61.810
  congenital D61.09
  drug-induced NEC D61.811
Panhematopenia D61.9
  congenital D61.09
  constitutional D61.09
Panhemocytopenia D61.9
  congenital D61.09
  constitutional D61.09
Panic (attack) (state) F41.0
  reaction to exceptional stress (transient) F43.0
Panmyelopathy, familial, constitutional D61.09
Panmyelophthisis D61.82
  congenital D61.09
Pansinusitis (chronic) (hyperplastic) (nonpurulent) (purulent)
        J32.4
  acute J01.40
    recurrent J01.41
Papanicolaou smear, cervix Z12.4
  as part of routine gynecological examination Z01.419
    with abnormal findings Z01.411
  for suspected neoplasm Z12.4
  nonspecific abnormal finding R87.619
  routine Z01.419
    with abnormal findings Z01.411
Papilledema (choked disc) H47.10
  associated with
    decreased ocular pressure H47.12
    increased intracranial pressure H47.11
    retinal disorder H47.13
  Foster-Kennedy syndrome H47.14-
Papillitis H46.00
  anus K62.89
  necrotizing, kidney N17.2
  renal, necrotizing N17.2
  tongue K14.0
Papilloma—*see also* Neoplasm, benign, by site
  acuminatum (female) (male) (anogenital) A63.0
  choroid plexus (lateral ventricle) (third ventricle) D33.0
    anaplastic C71.5
    fourth ventricle D33.1
    malignant C71.5
  rectum K62.89
Papillomatosis—*see also* Neoplasm, benign, by site
  confluent and reticulated L83
Papillon-Léage and Psaume syndrome Q87.0
Para-albuminemia E88.09
Paracephalus Q89.7
Parageusia R43.2
  psychogenic F45.8
Paralysis, paralytic (complete) (incomplete) G83.9
  anus (sphincter) K62.89
  asthenic bulbar G70.00
    with exacerbation (acute) G70.01
    in crisis G70.01
  Bell's G51.0
    newborn P11.3
  bowel, colon or intestine K56.0
  brachial plexus G54.0
    birth injury P14.3
    newborn (birth injury) P14.3
  brain G83.9
  bulbospinal G70.00
    with exacerbation (acute) G70.01
    in crisis G70.01
  cardiac (*see also* Failure, heart) I50.9
  Clark's G80.9

Paralysis, paralytic, *continued*
  colon K56.0
  deglutition R13.0
    hysterical F44.4
  diaphragm (flaccid) J98.6
    due to accidental dissection of phrenic nerve during
        procedure—*see*
        Puncture, accidental
        complicating surgery
  Duchenne's
    birth injury P14.0
    due to or associated with
      muscular dystrophy G71.0
  due to intracranial or spinal birth injury—*see* Palsy,
      cerebral
  Erb (-Duchenne) (birth) (newborn) P14.0
  facial (nerve) G51.0
    birth injury P11.3
    congenital P11.3
    following operation NEC—*see* Puncture, accidental
      complicating surgery
    newborn (birth injury) P11.3
  gait R26.1
  glottis J38.00
    bilateral J38.02
    unilateral J38.01
  Hoppe-Goldflam G70.00
    with exacerbation (acute) G70.01
    in crisis G70.01
  hysterical F44.4
  ileus K56.0
  inferior nuclear G83.9
  intestine K56.0
  Klumpke (-Déjérine) (birth) (newborn) P14.1
  laryngeal nerve (recurrent) (superior) (unilateral) J38.00
    bilateral J38.02
    unilateral J38.01
  larynx J38.00
    bilateral J38.02
    unilateral J38.01
  lead—*see* subcategory T56.0
  left side—*see* Hemiplegia
  leg G83.1-
    both—*see* Paraplegia
    hysterical F44.4
    psychogenic F44.4
  lip K13.0
  monoplegic—*see* Monoplegia
  motor G83.9
  muscle, muscular NEC G72.89
    pseudohypertrophic G71.0
  nerve—*see also* Disorder, nerve
    facial G51.0
      birth injury P11.3
      congenital P11.3
      newborn (birth injury) P11.3
    seventh or facial G51.0
      newborn (birth injury) P11.3
  oculofacial, congenital (Moebius) Q87.0
  palate (soft) K13.79
  pseudohypertrophic (muscle) G71.0
  psychogenic F44.4
  radicular NEC—*see* Radiculopathy
    upper limbs, newborn (birth injury) P14.3
  respiratory (muscle) (system) (tract) R06.81
    center NEC G93.89
    congenital P28.89
    newborn P28.89
  right side—*see* Hemiplegia
  saturnine—*see* subcategory T56.0
  spastic G83.9
    cerebral—*see* Palsy, cerebral, spastic
    congenital (cerebral)—*see* Palsy, cerebral, spastic
  spinal (cord) G83.9
  syndrome G83.9
    specified NEC G83.89
  uveoparotitic D86.89
  uvula K13.79
  velum palate K13.79
  vocal cords J38.00
    bilateral J38.02
    unilateral J38.01

Paramenia N92.6
Paramyoclonus multiplex G25.3
Paraphilia F65.9
Paraphimosis (congenital) N47.2
Paraplegia (lower) G82.20
  ataxic—see Degeneration, combined, spinal cord
  complete G82.21
  functional (hysterical) F44.4
  hysterical F44.4
  incomplete G82.22
  psychogenic F44.4
Parasitic—see also condition
  disease NEC B89
  sycosis (beard) (scalp) B35.0
  stomatitis B37.0
Parasitism B89
  intestinal B82.9
  skin B88.9
  specified—see Infestation
Paraspadias Q54.9
Paraspasmus facialis G51.8
Parasuicide (attempt)
  history of (personal) Z91.5
    in family Z81.8
Paratrachoma A74.0
Parencephalitis—see also Encephalitis
  sequelae G09
Parent-child conflict—see Conflict, parent-child
  estrangement NEC Z62.890
Paresis—see also Paralysis
  bowel, colon or intestine K56.0
  pseudohypertrophic G71.0
Paronychia—see also Cellulitis, digit
  with lymphangitis—see Lymphangitis, acute, digit
  candidal (chronic) B37.2
Parorexia (psychogenic) F50.89
Parosmia R43.1
  psychogenic F45.8
Parry-Romberg syndrome G51.8
Particolored infant Q82.8
Parulis K04.7
Parvovirus, as the cause of disease classified elsewhere
        B97.6
Passage
  meconium (newborn) during delivery P03.82
  of sounds or bougies—see Attention to, artificial, opening
Passive—see condition
  smoking Z77.22
Pasteurella septica A28.0
PAT (paroxysmal atrial tachycardia) I47.1
Patent—see also Imperfect, closure
  ductus arteriosus or Botallo's Q25.0
  foramen
    botalli Q21.1
    ovale Q21.1
  interauricular septum Q21.1
  interventricular septum Q21.0
  omphalomesenteric duct Q43.0
  ostium secundum Q21.1
  vitelline duct Q43.0
Pathologic, pathological—see also condition
  asphyxia R09.01
Patulous—see also Imperfect, closure (congenital)
  alimentary tract Q45.8
    lower Q43.8
    upper Q40.8
Pause, sinoatrial I49.5
Pectenosis K62.4
Pectus
  carinatum (congenital) Q67.7
  excavatum (congenital) Q67.6
  recurvatum (congenital) Q67.6
Pediculosis (infestation) B85.2
  capitis (head-louse) (any site) B85.0
  corporis (body-louse) (any site) B85.1
  eyelid B85.0
  mixed (classifiable to more than one of the titles
        B85.0–B85.3) B85.4
  pubis (pubic louse) (any site) B85.3
  vestimenti B85.1
  vulvae B85.3
Pediculus (infestation)—see Pediculosis

Pelvic—see also condition
  examination (periodic) (routine) Z01.419
    with abnormal findings Z01.411
  kidney, congenital Q63.2
Pelviperitonitis—see also Peritonitis, pelvic
  gonococcal A54.24
Pemphigus L10.9
  benign familial (chronic) Q82.8
Perforation, perforated (nontraumatic) (of)
  accidental during procedure (blood vessel) (nerve)
        (organ)—see
        Complication,
        accidental puncture or
        laceration
  antrum—see Sinusitis, maxillary
  appendix K35.2
  atrial septum, multiple Q21.1
  by
    device, implant or graft (see also Complications, by site
        and type, mechanical)
        T85.628
    ventricular intracranial shunt T85.09
    instrument (any) during a procedure, accidental—see
        Puncture, accidental
        complicating surgery
  cecum K35.2
  ear drum—see Perforation, tympanum
  nasal
    septum J34.89
      congenital Q30.3
    sinus J34.89
      congenital Q30.8
      due to sinusitis—see Sinusitis
  palate (see also Cleft, palate) Q35.9
  palatine vault (see also Cleft, palate, hard) Q35.1
  sinus (accessory) (chronic) (nasal) J34.89
  sphenoidal sinus—see Sinusitis, sphenoidal
  tympanum, tympanic (membrane) (persistent
        post- traumatic)
        (postinflammatory)
        H72.9-
    attic H72.1-
      multiple H72.81-
      total H72.82-
    central H72.0-
      multiple H72.81-
      total H72.82-
    marginal NEC—see subcategory H72.2
    multiple H72.81-
    pars flaccida—see Perforation, tympanum, attic
    total H72.82-
    traumatic, current episode S09.2-
  uvula K13.79
Periadenitis mucosa necrotica recurrens K12.0
Pericarditis (with decompensation) (with effusion) I31.9
  with rheumatic fever (conditions in I00)
    active—see Pericarditis, rheumatic
    inactive or quiescent I09.2
  acute (hemorrhagic) (nonrheumatic) (Sicca) I30.9
    with chorea (acute) (rheumatic) (Sydenham's) I02.0
    benign I30.8
    nonspecific I30.0
    rheumatic I01.0
      with chorea (acute) (Sydenham's) I02.0
    adhesive or adherent (chronic) (external) (internal) I31.0
    acute—see Pericarditis, acute
    rheumatic I09.2
  bacterial (acute) (subacute) (with serous or seropurulent
        effusion) I30.1
  calcareous I31.1
  cholesterol (chronic) I31.8
    acute I30.9
  chronic (nonrheumatic) I31.9
    rheumatic I09.2
  constrictive (chronic) I31.1
  coxsackie B33.23
  fibrinopurulent I30.1
  fibrinous I30.8
  fibrous I31.0
  idiopathic I30.0
  in systemic lupus erythematosus M32.12
  infective I30.1

Pericarditis, continued
  meningococcal A39.53
  neoplastic (chronic) I31.8
    acute I30.9
  obliterans, obliterating I31.0
  plastic I31.0
  pneumococcal I30.1
  purulent I30.1
  rheumatic (active) (acute) (with effusion) (with pneumonia)
        I01.0
    with chorea (acute) (rheumatic) (Sydenham's) I02.0
    chronic or inactive (with chorea) I09.2
  septic I30.1
  serofibrinous I30.8
  staphylococcal I30.1
  streptococcal I30.1
  suppurative I30.1
  syphilitic A52.06
  tuberculous A18.84
  viral I30.1
Perichondritis
  nose J34.89
Periepididymitis N45.1
Perilabyrinthitis (acute)—see subcategory H83.0
Periods—see also Menstruation
  heavy N92.0
  irregular N92.6
  shortened intervals (irregular) N92.1
Periorchitis N45.2
Periproctitis K62.89
Peritonitis (adhesive) (bacterial) (fibrinous) (hemorrhagic)
        (idiopathic) (localized)
        (perforative) (primary)
        (with adhesions)(with
        effusion) K65.9
  with or following
    abscess K65.1
    appendicitis K35.2
      with perforation or rupture K35.2
      generalized K35.2
      localized K35.3
  acute (generalized) K65.0
  chlamydial A74.81
  diaphragmatic K65.0
  diffuse K65.0
  disseminated K65.0
  eosinophilic K65.8
    acute K65.0
  fibropurulent K65.0
  general (ized) K65.0
  meconium (newborn) P78.0
  neonatal P78.1
    meconium P78.0
  pancreatic K65.0
  pelvic
    female N73.5
      acute N73.3
      chronic N73.4
        with adhesions N73.6
    male K65.0
  purulent K65.0
  septic K65.0
  specified NEC K65.8
  spontaneous bacterial K65.2
  subdiaphragmatic K65.0
  subphrenic K65.0
  suppurative K65.0
Peritonsillitis J36
Perlèche NEC K13.0
  due to
    candidiasis B37.83
    moniliasis B37.83
Persistence, persistent (congenital)
  anal membrane Q42.3
    with fistula Q42.2
  atrioventricular canal Q21.2
  fetal
    circulation P29.3
    hemoglobin, hereditary (HPFH) D56.4
  foramen
    Botalli Q21.1
    ovale Q21.1

Persistence, persistent, *continued*
  hemoglobin, fetal (hereditary) (HPFH) D56.4
  Meckel's diverticulum Q43.0
  omphalomesenteric duct Q43.0
  ostium
    atrioventriculare commune Q21.2
    primum Q21.2
    secundum Q21.1
  primary (deciduous)
    teeth K00.6
  sinus
    urogenitalis
      female Q52.8
      male Q55.8
  thyroglossal duct Q89.2
  thyrolingual duct Q89.2
  truncus arteriosus or communis Q20.0
  vitelline duct Q43.0
Person (with)
  concern (normal) about sick person in family Z63.6
  consulting on behalf of another Z71.0
  feigning illness Z76.5
  living (in)
    without
      adequate housing (heating) (space) Z59.1
      housing (permanent) (temporary) Z59.0
      person able to render necessary care Z74.2
      shelter Z59.0
Personality (disorder) F60.9
  pathologic F60.9
  pattern defect or disturbance F60.9
Perthes' disease M91.1-
Pertussis (*see also* Whooping cough) A37.90
Perversion, perverted
  appetite F50.89
    psychogenic F50.89
  function
    pituitary gland E23.2
      posterior lobe E22.2
  sense of smell and taste R43.8
    psychogenic F45.8
  sexual—*see* Deviation, sexual
Pervious, congenital—*see also* Imperfect, closure
  ductus arteriosus Q25.0
Pes (congenital)—*see also* Talipes
  adductus Q66.89
  cavus Q66.7
  valgus Q66.6
Petechia, petechiae R23.3
  newborn P54.5
Petit mal seizure—*see* Epilepsy, generalized, specified NEC
Petit's hernia—*see* Hernia, abdomen, specified site NEC
  Peutz-Jeghers disease or syndrome Q85.8
Phakomatosis (*see also* specific eponymous syndromes)
              Q85.9
  Bourneville's Q85.1
  specified NEC Q85.8
Pfeiffer's disease—*see* Mononucleosis, infectious
Phagedena (dry) (moist) (sloughing)—*see also* Gangrene
  geometric L88
Pharyngeal pouch syndrome D82.1
Pharyngitis (acute) (catarrhal) (gangrenous) (infective)
              (malignant)
              (membranous)
              (phlegmonous)
              (pseudomembranous)
              (simple) (subacute)
              (suppurative)
              (ulcerative) (viral) J02.9
  aphthous B08.5
  atrophic J31.2
  chlamydial A56.4
  chronic (atrophic) (granular) (hypertrophic) J31.2
  coxsackievirus B08.5
  enteroviral vesicular B08.5
  follicular (chronic) J31.2
  granular (chronic) J31.2
  herpesviral B00.2
  hypertrophic J31.2
  infectional, chronic J31.2
  influenzal—*see* Influenza, with, respiratory manifestations
              NEC
  pneumococcal J02.8

Pharyngitis, *continued*
  purulent J02.9
  putrid J02.9
  septic J02.0
  sicca J31.2
  specified organism NEC J02.8
  staphylococcal J02.8
  streptococcal J02.0
  vesicular, enteroviral B08.5
  viral NEC J02.8
Pharyngolaryngitis (acute) J06.0
  chronic J37.0
Pharyngotonsillitis, herpesviral B00.2
Phenomenon
  vasomotor R55
  vasovagal R55
  Wenckebach's I44.1
Phenylketonuria E70.1
  classical E70.0
Phimosis (congenital) (due to infection) N47.1
Phlebitis (infective) (pyemic) (septic) (suppurative) I80.9
  femoral vein (superficial) I80.1-
  femoropopliteal vein I80.0-
  hepatic veins I80.8
  iliofemoral—*see* Phlebitis, femoral vein
  leg I80.3
    deep (vessels)NEC I80.20-
      iliac I80.21-
      popliteal vein I80.22-
      specified vessel NEC I80.29-
      tibial vein I80.23-
    femoral vein (superficial) I80.1-
    superficial (vessels) I80.0-
  lower limb—*see* Phlebitis, leg
  popliteal vein—*see* Phlebitis, leg, deep, popliteal
  saphenous (accessory) (great) (long) (small)—*see*
              Phlebitis, leg,
              superficial
  specified site NEC I80.8
  tibial vein—*see* Phlebitis, leg, deep, tibial
  ulcerative I80.9
    leg—*see* Phlebitis, leg
  umbilicus I80.8
Phobia, phobic F40.9
  reaction F40.9
  state F40.9
Photodermatitis (sun) L56.8
  chronic L57.8
  due to drug L56.8
  light other than sun L59.8
Photosensitivity, photosensitization (sun) skin L56.8
  light other than sun L59.8
Phthiriasis (pubis) B85.3
  with any infestation classifiable to B85.0–B85.2 B85.4
Physical restraint status Z78.1
Pica F50.89
  in adults F50.89
  infant or child F98.3
Picking, nose F98.8
Pickwickian syndrome E66.2
Pierre Robin deformity or syndrome Q87.0
Pig-bel A05.2
Pigeon
  breast or chest (acquired) M95.4
    congenital Q67.7
Pigmentation (abnormal) (anomaly) L81.9
  iron L81.8
  lids, congenital Q82.8
  metals L81.8
  optic papilla, congenital Q14.2
  retina, congenital (grouped) (nevoid) Q14.1
  scrotum, congenital Q82.8
  tattoo L81.8
Piles (*see also* Hemorrhoids) K64.9
Pinhole meatus (*see also* Stricture, urethra) N35.9
Pink
  eye—*see* Conjunctivitis, acute, mucopurulent
Pinworm (disease) (infection) (infestation) B80
Pithecoid pelvis Q74.2
Pitting (*see also* Edema) R60.9
  lip R60.0
  nail L60.8

Pityriasis (capitis) L21.0
  circinata (et maculata) L42
  furfuracea L21.0
  rosea L42
  versicolor (scrotal) B36.0
Plagiocephaly
  aquired M95.2
  congenital Q67.3
Plaque (s)
  epicardial I31.8
Planning, family
  contraception Z30.9
  procreation Z31.69
Plasmacytopenia D72.818
Plasmacytosis D72.822
Platybasia Q75.8
Platyonychia (congenital) Q84.6
  acquired L60.8
Platypelloid pelvis M95.5
  congenital Q74.2
Plethora R23.2
  newborn P61.1
Pleurisy (acute) (adhesive) (chronic) (costal) (diaphragmatic)
              (double) (dry) (fibrinous)
              (fibrous) (interlobar)
              (latent) (plastic)
              (primary) (residual)
              (sicca) (sterile)
              (subacute) (unresolved)
              R09.1
  with
    adherent pleura J86.0
    effusion J90
    pneumococcal J90
    purulent—*see* Pyothorax
    septic—*see* Pyothorax
    serofibrinous—*see* Pleurisy, with effusion
    seropurulent—*see* Pyothorax
    serous—*see* Pleurisy, with effusion
    staphylococcal J86.9
    streptococcal J90
    suppurative—*see* Pyothorax
    traumatic (post) (current)—*see* Injury, intrathoracic, pleura
Pleuropericarditis—*see also* Pericarditis
  acute I30.9
Pleuro-pneumonia-like organism (PPLO), as the cause
              of disease classified
              elsewhere B96.0
Plica
  polonica B85.0
  tonsil J35.8
Plug
  meconium (newborn) NEC syndrome P76.0
  mucus—*see* Asphyxia, mucus
Plumbism—*see* subcategory T56.0
Pneumatocele (lung) J98.4
  intracranial G93.89
Pneumaturia R39.89
Pneumocephalus G93.89
Pneumococcemia A40.3
Pneumococcus, pneumococcal—*see* condition
Pneumohemopericardium I31.2
Pneumomediastinum J98.2
  congenital or perinatal P25.2
Pneumonia (acute) (double) (migratory) (purulent) (septic)
              (unresolved) J18.9
  with
    due to specified organism—*see* Pneumonia, in
              (due to)
    influenza—*see* Influenza, with, pneumonia
  anaerobes J15.8
  anthrax A22.1
  Ascaris B77.81
  aspiration J69.0
    due to
      aspiration of microorganisms
        bacterial J15.9
        viral J12.9
      food (regurgitated) J69.0
      gastric secretions J69.0
      milk (regurgitated) J69.0
      oils, essences J69.1

Pneumothorax NOS, *continued*
    newborn P25.1
    primary J93.11
    secondary J93.12
    tension J93.0
  tense valvular, infectional J93.0
  tension (spontaneous) J93.0
  traumatic S27.0
Poikiloderma L81.6
  congenital Q82.8
Pointed ear (congenital) Q17.3
Poison ivy, oak, sumac or other plant dermatitis (allergic)
           (contact) L23.7
Poisoning (acute)—*see also* Table of Drugs and Chemicals
  algae and toxins T65.82-
  Bacillus B (aertrycke) (cholerae (suis)) (paratyphosus)
         (suipestifer) A02.9
    botulinus A05.1
  bacterial toxins A05.9
  berries, noxious—*see* Poisoning, food, noxious, berries
  botulism A05.1
  ciguatera fish T61.0-
  Clostridium botulinum A05.1
  drug—*see* Table of Drugs and Chemicals, by drug,
         poisoning
  epidemic, fish (noxious)—*see* Poisoning, seafood
    bacterial A05.9
  fava bean D55.0
  food (acute) (diseased) (infected) (noxious)NEC T62.9-
    bacterial—*see* Intoxication, foodborne, by agent
    due to
      Bacillus (aertrycke) (choleraesuis) (paratyphosus)
          (suipestifer) A02.9
        botulinus A05.1
      Clostridium (perfringens) (Welchii) A05.2
      salmonella (aertrycke) (callinarum) (choleraesuis)
         (enteritidis) (paratyphi)
         (suipestifer) A02.9
      with
        gastroenteritis A02.0
        sepsis A02.1
      staphylococcus A05.0
      Vibrio
        parahaemolyticus A05.3
        vulnificus A05.5
    noxious or naturally toxic T62.9-
      berries—*see* subcategory T62.1-
      fish—*see* Poisoning, seafood
      mushrooms—*see* subcategory T62.0X-
      plants NEC—*see* subcategory T62.2X-
      seafood—*see* Poisoning, seafood
      specified NEC—*see* subcategory T62.8X-
    kreotoxism, food A05.9
    lead T56.0-
    mushroom—*see* Poisoning, food, noxious, mushroom
    mussels—*see also* Poisoning, shellfish
      bacterial—*see* Intoxication, foodborne, by agent
    Staphylococcus, food A05.0
Pollakiuria R35.0
  psychogenic F45.8
Pollinosis J30.1
Pollitzer's disease L73.2
Polycystic (disease)
  degeneration, kidney Q61.3
    autosomal recessive (infantile type) NEC Q61.19
  kidney Q61.3
    autosomal
      recessive NEC Q61.19
    autosomal recessive (childhood type) NEC Q61.19
    infantile type NEC Q61.19
  ovary, ovaries E28.2
Polycythemia (secondary) D75.1
  acquired D75.1
  due to
    donor twin P61.1
    erythropoietin D75.1
    fall in plasma volume D75.1
    high altitude D75.1
    maternal-fetal transfusion P61.1
    stress D75.1
  emotional D75.1
  erythropoietin D75.1

Polycythemia, *continued*
  Gaisböck's (hypertonica) D75.1
  high altitude D75.1
  hypertonica D75.1
  hypoxemic D75.1
  neonatorum P61.1
  nephrogenous D75.1
  relative D75.1
  secondary D75.1
  spurious D75.1
  stress D75.1
Polycytosis cryptogenica D75.1
Polydactylism, polydactyly Q69.9
  toes Q69.2
Polydipsia R63.1
Polyhydramnios O40.-
Polymenorrhea N92.0
Polyneuritis, polyneuritic—*see also* Polyneuropathy
  cranialis G52.7
Polyneuropathy (peripheral) G62.9
  hereditary G60.9
    specified NEC G60.8
  in (due to)
    hypoglycemia E16.2 *[G63]*
    infectious
      disease NEC B99 *[G63]*
      mononucleosis B27.91
    Lyme disease A69.22
    neoplastic disease (*see also* Neoplasm) D49.9 *[G63]*
    sarcoidosis D86.89
    systemic
      lupus erythematosus M32.19
  sensory (hereditary) (idiopathic) G60.8
Polyopia H53.8
Polyorchism, polyorchidism Q55.21
Polyp, polypus
  accessory sinus J33.8
  adenoid tissue J33.0
  antrum J33.8
  anus, anal (canal) K62.0
  choanal J33.0
  colon K63.5
    adenomatous D12.6
    ascending D12.2
    cecum D12.0
    descending D12.4
    inflammatory K51.40
      with
        abscess K51.414
        complication K51.419
          specified NEC K51.418
        fistula K51.413
        intestinal obstruction K51.412
        rectal bleeding K51.411
    sigmoid D12.5
    transverse D12.3
  ethmoidal (sinus) J33.8
  frontal (sinus) J33.8
  maxillary (sinus) J33.8
  nares
    anterior J33.9
    posterior J33.0
  nasal (mucous) J33.9
    cavity J33.0
    septum J33.0
  nasopharyngeal J33.0
  nose (mucous) J33.9
  rectum (nonadenomatous) K62.1
    adenomatous—*see* Polyp, adenomatous
  septum (nasal) J33.0
  sinus (accessory) (ethmoidal) (frontal) (maxillary)
         (sphenoidal) J33.8
  sphenoidal (sinus) J33.8
  turbinate, mucous membrane J33.8
Polyposis—*see also* Polyp
  coli (adenomatous) D12.6
  colon (adenomatous) D12.6
  familial D12.6
  intestinal (adenomatous) D12.6
  multiple, adenomatous (*see also* Neoplasm, benign) D36.9
Polyserositis
  due to pericarditis I31.1
  pericardial I31.1

Polysyndactyly (*see also* Syndactylism, syndactyly) Q70.4
Polyuria R35.8
  nocturnal R35.1
  psychogenic F45.8
Pomphylox L30.1
Poor
  urinary stream R39.12
  vision NEC H54.7
Porencephaly (congenital) (developmental) (true) Q04.6
  acquired G93.0
  nondevelopmental G93.0
  traumatic (post) F07.89
Porocephaliasis B88.8
Porokeratosis Q82.8
Port wine nevus, mark, or stain Q82.5
Positive
  culture (nonspecific)
    blood R78.81
    bronchial washings R84.5
    cerebrospinal fluid R83.5
    nose R84.5
      staphylococcus (Methicillin susceptible) Z22.321
        Methicillin resistant Z22.322
    urine R82.79
  PPD (skin test) R76.11
  serology for syphilis A53.0
    false R76.8
    with signs or symptoms—*code as* Syphilis, by site
        and stage
  skin test, tuberculin (without active tuberculosis) R76.11
  test, human immunodeficiency virus (HIV) R75
  VDRL A53.0
    with signs and symptoms—*code by* site and stage
        under Syphilis A53.9
  Wassermann reaction A53.0
Postcardiotomy syndrome I97.0
Postcommissurotomy syndrome I97.0
Postconcussional syndrome F07.81
Postcontusional syndrome F07.81
Posthemorrhagic anemia (chronic) D50.0
  acute D62
  newborn P61.3
Postmaturity, postmature (over 42 weeks)
  newborn P08.22
Postmeasles complication NEC (*see also* condition) B05.89
Postnasal drip R09.82
  due to
    allergic rhinitis—*see* Rhinitis, allergic
    common cold J00
    gastroesophageal reflux—*see* Reflux,
        gastroesophageal
    nasopharyngitis—*see* Nasopharyngitis
    other know condition—*code to* condition
    sinusitis—*see* Sinusitis
Postoperative (postprocedural)—*see* Complication,
        postoperative
  state NEC Z98.890
Post-term (40-42 weeks) (pregnancy) (mother) O48.0
  infant P08.21
Post-traumatic brain syndrome, nonpsychotic F07.81
Postvaccinal reaction or complication—*see* Complications,
        vaccination
Postvalvulotomy syndrome I97.0
Poultrymen's itch B88.0
Poverty NEC Z59.6
  extreme Z59.5
Prader-Willi syndrome Q87.1
Precocious
  adrenarche E30.1
  menarche E30.1
  menstruation E30.1
  pubarche E30.1
  puberty E30.1
    central E22.8
  sexual development NEC E30.1
Precocity, sexual (constitutional) (female) (idiopathic) (male)
        E30.1
  with adrenal hyperplasia E25.9
    congenital E25.0
Prediabetes, prediabetic R73.03

Pre-eclampsia O14.9
  with pre-existing hypertension—*see* Hypertension, complicating pregnancy, pre-existing, with, pre-eclampsia
  mild O14.0-
  moderate O14.0-
  severe O14.1-
    with hemolysis, elevated liver enzymes and low platelet count (HELLP) O14.2-
Pre-excitation atrioventricular conduction I45.6
Pregnancy (single) (uterine)—*see also* Delivery and Puerperal
Note: The Tabular must be reviewed for assignment of the appropriate character indicating the trimester of the pregnancy
Note: The Tabular must be reviewed for assignment of appropriate seventh character for multiple gestation codes in Chapter 15

  abdominal (ectopic) O00.00
    with uterine pregnancy O00.01
    with viable fetus O36.7-
  ampullar O00.10
  broad ligament O00.80
  cervical O00.80
  complicated by (care of) (management affected by)
    abnormal, abnormality
      findings on antenatal screening of mother O28.9
        biochemical O28.1
        cytological O28.2
        chromosomal O28.5
        genetic O28.5
        hematological O28.0
        radiological O28.4
        specified NEC O28.8
        ultrasonic O28.3
    conjoined twins O30.02-
    death of fetus (near term) O36.4
      early pregnancy O02.1
      of one fetus or more in multiple gestation O31.2-
    decreased fetal movement O36.81-
    diabetes (mellitus) O24.91-
      gestational (pregnancy induced—*see* Diabetes, gestational
      pre-existing O24.31-
        specified NEC O24.81-
        type 1 O24.01-
        type 2 O24.11-
    edema O12.0-
      with
        gestational hypertension, mild (*see also* Pre-eclampsia) O14.0-
    fetal (maternal care for)
      abnormality or damage O35.9
        specified type NEC O35.8
      anemia and thrombocytopenia O36.82-
      anencephaly O35.0
      chromosomal abnormality (conditions in Q90–Q99) O35.1
      conjoined twins O30.02-
      damage from
        amniocentesis O35.7
        biopsy procedures O35.7
        drug addiction O35.5
        hematological investigation O35.7
        intrauterine contraceptive device O35.7
        maternal
          alcohol addiction O35.4
          cytomegalovirus infection O35.3
          disease NEC O35.8
          drug addiction O35.5
          listeriosis O35.8
          rubella O35.3
          toxoplasmosis O35.8
          viral infection O35.3
        medical procedure NEC O35.7
        radiation O35.6
      death (near term) O36.4
        early pregnancy O02.1

Pregnancy, *continued*
  decreased movement O36.81-
  disproportion due to deformity (fetal) O33.7
  excessive growth (large for dates) O36.6-
  growth retardation O36.59-
    light for dates O36.59-
    small for dates O36.59-
  hereditary disease O35.2
  hydrocephalus O35.0
  intrauterine death O36.4
  poor growth O36.59-
    light for dates O36.59-
    small for dates O36.59-
  problem O36.9-
    specified NEC O36.89-
  spina bifida O35.0
  thrombocytopenia O36.82-
  HELLP syndrome (hemolysis, elevated liver enzymes and low platelet count) O14.2-
  hemorrhage
    before 20 completed weeks gestation O20.9
      specified NEC O20.8
    early O20.9
      specified NEC O20.8
    threatened abortion O20.0
  hydramnios O40.-
  hydrops
    amnii O40.-
    fetalis O36.2-
      associated with isoimmunization (*see also* Pregnancy, complicated by, isoimmunization) O36.11-
  hydrorrhea O42.90
  inconclusive fetal viability O36.80
  insulin resistance O26.89
  intrauterine fetal death (near term) O36.4
    early pregnancy O02.1
  isoimmunization O36.11-
    anti-A sensitization O36.11-
    anti-B sensitization O36.19-
    Rh O36.09-
      anti-D antibody O36.01-
    specified NEC O36.19-
  missed
    abortion O02.1
    delivery O36.4
  multiple gestations O30.9-
    conjoined twins O30.02-
    specified number of multiples NEC—*see* Pregnancy, multiple (gestation), specified NEC
    quadruplet—*see* Pregnancy, quadruplet
    specified complication NEC O31.8X-
    triplet—*see* Pregnancy, triplet
    twin—*see* Pregnancy, twin
  oligohydramnios O41.0-
    with premature rupture of membranes (*see also* Pregnancy, complicated by, premature rupture of membranes) O42.-
  placental insufficiency O36.51-
  polyhydramnios O40.-
  pre-eclampsia O14.9-
    mild O14.0-
    moderate O14.0-
    severe O14.1-
      with hemolysis, elevated liver enzymes and low platelet count (HELLP) O14.2-
  premature rupture of membranes O42.90
    full-term, unspec as to length of time between rupture and onset of labor O42.92
    with onset of labor
      within 24 hours O42.00
        at or after 37 weeks gestation O42.02
        pre-term (before 37 completed weeks of gestation) O42.01-

Pregnancy, *continued*
      after 24 hours O42.10
        at or after 37 weeks gestation O42.12
        pre-term (before 37 completed weeks of gestation) O42.11-
    after 37 weeks gestation O42.92
    pre-term (before 37 completed weeks of gestation) O42.91-
  preterm labor
    second trimester
      without delivery O60.02
    third trimester
      without delivery O60.03
    without delivery O60.00
      second trimester O60.02
      third trimester O60.03
  Rh immunization, incompatibility or sensitization NEC O36.09-
    anti-D antibody O36.01-
  threatened
    abortion O20.0
  young mother
    multigravida O09.62-
    primigravida O09.61-
  cornual O00.8-
  ectopic (ruptured) O00.9-
    abdominal O00.00
      with uterine pregnancy O00.01
      with viable fetus O36.7-
    cervical O00.8-
    cornual O00.8-
    intraligamentous O00.8-
    mural O00.8-
    ovarian O00.2-
    specified site NEC O00.8-
    tubal (ruptured) O00.10
      with intrauterine pregnancy O00.11
  fallopian O00.10
    with intrauterine pregnancy O00.11
  incidental finding Z33.1
  interstitial O00.8-
  intraligamentous O00.8-
  intramural O00.8-
  intraperitoneal O00.00
    with intrauterine pregnancy O00.01
  isthmian O00.10
  mesometric (mural) O00.8-
  mural O00.8-
  ovarian O00.2-
  quadruplet O30.20-
    with
      two or more monoamniotic fetuses O30.22-
      two or more monochorionic fetuses O30.21-
      two or more monoamniotic fetuses O30.22-
      two or more monochorionic fetuses O30.21-
      unable to determine number of placenta and number of amniotic sacs O30.29-
      unspecified number of placenta and unspecified number of amniotic sacs O30.20-
  quintuplet—*see* Pregnancy, multiple (gestation), specified NEC
  sextuplet—*see* Pregnancy, multiple (gestation), specified NEC
  supervision of
    young mother
      multigravida O09.62-
      primigravida O09.61-
  triplet O30.10-
    with
      two or more monoamniotic fetuses O30.12-
      two or more monochrorionic fetuses O30.11-
      two or more monoamniotic fetuses O30.12-
      two or more monochrorionic fetuses O30.11-
      unable to determine number of placenta and number of amniotic sacs O30.19-
      unspecified number of placenta and unspecified number of amniotic sacs O30.10-
  tubal (with abortion) (with rupture) O00.10
    with intrauterine pregnancy O00.11

PREGNANCY–PROBLEM (WITH) (RELATED TO)

Pregnancy, *continued*
  twin O30.00-
    conjoined O30.02-
    dichorionic/diamniotic (two placentae, two amniotic sacs) O30.04-
    monochorionic/diamniotic (one placenta, two amniotic sacs) O30.03-
    monochorionic/monoamniotic (one placenta, one amniotic sac) O30.01-
    unable to determine number of placenta and number of amniotic sacs O30.09-
    unspecified number of placenta and unspecified number of amniotic sacs O30.00-
  unwanted Z64.0
  weeks of gestation
    8 weeks Z3A.08
    9 weeks Z3A.09
    10 weeks Z3A.10
    11 weeks Z3A.11
    12 weeks Z3A.12
    13 weeks Z3A.13
    14 weeks Z3A.14
    15 weeks Z3A.15
    16 weeks Z3A.16
    17 weeks Z3A.17
    18 weeks Z3A.18
    19 weeks Z3A.19
    20 weeks Z3A.20
    21 weeks Z3A.21
    22 weeks Z3A.22
    23 weeks Z3A.23
    24 weeks Z3A.24
    25 weeks Z3A.25
    26 weeks Z3A.26
    27 weeks Z3A.27
    28 weeks Z3A.28
    29 weeks Z3A.29
    30 weeks Z3A.30
    31 weeks Z3A.31
    32 weeks Z3A.32
    33 weeks Z3A.33
    34 weeks Z3A.34
    35 weeks Z3A.35
    36 weeks Z3A.36
    37 weeks Z3A.37
    38 weeks Z3A.38
    39 weeks Z3A.39
    40 weeks Z3A.40
    41 weeks Z3A.41
    42 weeks Z3A.42
    greater than 42 weeks Z3A.49
    less than 8 weeks Z3A.01
    not specified Z3A.00
Premature—*see also* condition
  beats I49.40
    atrial I49.1
    auricular I49.1
    supraventricular I49.1
  birth NEC—*see* Preterm, newborn
  closure, foramen ovale Q21.8
  contraction
    atrial I49.1
    auricular I49.1
    auriculoventricular I49.49
    heart (extrasystole) I49.49
  lungs P28.0
  newborn
    extreme (less than 28 completed weeks)—*see* Immaturity, extreme
    less than 37 completed weeks—*see* Preterm, newborn
  puberty E30.1
Premenstrual
  dysphoric disorder (PMDD) F32.81
  tension N94.3
Prenatal
  teeth K00.6
Preponderance, left or right ventricular I51.7
Prescription of contraceptives (initial) Z30.019
  barrier Z30.018
  diaphragm Z30.018

Prescription of contraceptives, *continued*
  emergency (postcoital) Z30.012
  implantable subdermal Z30.017
  injectable Z30.013
  intrauterine contraceptive device Z30.014
  pills Z30.011
  postcoital (emergency) Z30.012
  repeat Z30.40
    barrier Z30.49
    diaphragm Z30.49
    implantable subdermal Z30.46
    injectable Z30.42
    pills Z30.41
    specified type NEC Z30.49
    transdermal patch Z30.45
    vaginal ring Z30.44
  specified type NEC Z30.018
  transdermal patch Z30.016
  vaginal ring Z30.015
Presence (of)
  arterial-venous shunt (dialysis) Z99.2
  artificial
    heart (fully implantable) (mechanical) Z95.812
      valve Z95.2
    cardiac
      pacemaker Z95.0
  cerebrospinal fluid drainage device Z98.2
  CSF shunt Z98.2
  heart valve implant (functional) Z95.2
    prosthetic Z95.2
    specified type NEC Z95.4
    xenogenic Z95.3
  implanted device (artificial) (functional) (prosthetic) Z96.9
    cardiac pacemaker Z95.0
    heart valve Z95.2
      prosthetic Z95.2
      specified NEC Z95.4
      xenogenic Z95.3
Prespondylolisthesis (congenital) Q76.2
Pressure
  area, skin—*see* Ulcer, pressure, by site
  increased
    intracranial (benign) G93.2
      injury at birth P11.0
Pre-syncope R55
Preterm
  newborn (infant) P07.30
    gestational age
      28 completed weeks (28 weeks, 0 days through 28 weeks, 6 days) P07.31
      29 completed weeks (29 weeks, 0 days through 29 weeks, 6 days) P07.32
      30 completed weeks (30 weeks, 0 days through 30 weeks, 6 days) P07.33
      31 completed weeks (31 weeks, 0 days through 31 weeks, 6 days) P07.34
      32 completed weeks (32 weeks, 0 days through 32 weeks, 6 days) P07.35
      33 completed weeks (33 weeks, 0 days through 33 weeks, 6 days) P07.36
      34 completed weeks (34 weeks, 0 days through 34 weeks, 6 days) P07.37
      35 completed weeks (35 weeks, 0 days through 35 weeks, 6 days) P07.38
      36 completed weeks (36 weeks, 0 days through 36 weeks, 6 days) P07.39
Priapism N48.30
  due to
    disease classified elsewhere N48.32
    drug N48.33
    specified cause NEC N48.39
    trauma N48.31
Prickly heat L74.0
Primus varus (bilateral) Q66.21
Pringle's disease (tuberous sclerosis) Q85.1
Problem (with) (related to)
  academic Z55.8
  acculturation Z60.3
  adopted child Z62.821
  alcoholism in family Z63.72
  atypical parenting situation Z62.9
  behavioral (adult) F69
    drug seeking Z76.5

Problem (with) (related to), *continued*
  birth of sibling affecting child Z62.898
  care (of)
    child
      abuse (affecting the child)—*see* Maltreatment, child
      custody or support proceedings Z65.3
      in welfare custody Z62.21
      in care of non-parental family member Z62.21
      in foster care Z62.21
      living in orphanage or group home Z62.22
  conflict or discord (with)
    classmates Z55.4
    counselor Z64.4
    family Z63.9
      specified NEC Z63.8
    probation officer Z64.4
    social worker Z64.4
    teachers Z55.4
  drug addict in family Z63.72
  education Z55.9
    specified NEC Z55.8
  enuresis, child F98.0
  failed examinations (school) Z55.2
  falling Z91.81
  family (*see also* Disruption, family) Z63.9-
    specified NEC Z63.8
  feeding (elderly) (infant) R63.3
    newborn P92.9
      breast P92.5
      overfeeding P92.4
      slow P92.2
      specified NEC P92.8
      underfeeding P92.3
    nonorganic F50.89
  foster child Z62.822
  genital NEC
    female N94.9
    male N50.9
  homelessness Z59.0
  housing Z59.9
    inadequate Z59.1
  identity (of childhood) F93.8
  intrafamilial communication Z63.8
  jealousy, child F93.8
  language (developmental) F80.9
  learning (developmental) F81.9
  lifestyle Z72.9
    gambling Z72.6
    high-risk sexual behavior (heterosexual) Z72.51
      bisexual Z72.53
      homosexual Z72.5
    inappropriate eating habits Z72.4
    self-damaging behavior NEC Z72.89
    specified NEC Z72.89
    tobacco use Z72.0
  literacy Z55.9
    low level Z55.0
    specified NEC Z55.8
  mental F48.9
  presence of sick or disabled person in family or household Z63.79
    needing care Z63.6
  primary support group (family) Z63.9
    specified NEC Z63.8
  psychosocial Z65.9
    specified NEC Z65.8
  relationship Z63.9
    childhood F93.8
  seeking and accepting known hazardous and harmful
    behavioral or psychological interventions Z65.8
    chemical, nutritional or physical interventions Z65.8
  sight H54.7
  speech R47.9
    developmental F80.9
    specified NEC R47.89
  swallowing—*see* Dysphagia
  taste—*see* Disturbance, sensation, taste
  tic, child F95.0
  underachievement in school Z55.3
  voice production R47.89

Procedure (surgical)
for purpose other than remedying health state Z41.9
specified NEC Z41.8
not done Z53.9
because of
administrative reasons Z53.8
contraindication Z53.09
smoking Z53.01
patient's decision Z53.20
for reasons of belief or group pressure Z53.1
left against medical advice (AMA) Z53.21
specified reason NEC Z53.29
specified reason NEC Z53.8
Proctalgia K62.89
Proctitis K62.89
amebic (acute) A06.0
chlamydial A56.3
gonococcal A54.6
granulomatous—see Enteritis, regional, large intestine
herpetic A60
ulcerative (chronic) K51.20
with
complication K51.219
abscess K51.214
fistula K51.213
obstruction K51.212
rectal bleeding K51.211
specified NEC K51.218
Proctocele
male K62.3
Proctoptosis K62.3
Proctorrhagia K62.5
Proctospasm K59.4
psychogenic F45.8
Prolapse, prolapsed
anus, anal (canal) (sphincter) K62.2
bladder (mucosa) (sphincter) (acquired)
congenital Q79.4
rectum (mucosa) (sphincter) K62.3
Prolonged, prolongation (of)
bleeding (time) (idiopathic) R79.1
coagulation (time) R79.1
gestation (over 42 completed weeks)
newborn P08.22
interval I44.0
partial thromboplastin time (PTT) R79.1
prothrombin time R79.1
QT interval I45.81
Pronation
ankle—see Deformity, limb, foot, specified NEC
foot—see also Deformity, limb, foot, specified NEC
congenital Q74.2
Prophylactic
administration of
antibiotics, long-term Z79.2
antivenin Z29.12
short-term use—omit code
drug (see also Long-term (current) drug therapy (use
of)) Z79.899-
fluoride varnish application Z29.3
other specified Z29.8
rabies immune therapy Z29.14
respiratory syncytial virus immune globulin Z29.11
Rho (D) immune globulin Z29.13
unspecified Z29.9
medication Z79.899
vaccination Z23
Prostatitis (congestive) (suppurative) (with cystitis) N41.9
acute N41.0
Prostration R53.83
heat—see also Heat, exhaustion
anhydrotic T67.3
due to
salt (and water)depletion T67.4
water depletion T67.3
Protein
sickness (see also Reaction, serum) T80.69
Proteinuria R80.9
isolated R80.0
with glomerular lesion N06.9
orthostatic R80.2
with glomerular lesion—see Proteinuria, isolated, with
glomerular lesion

Proteinuria, continued
postural R80.2
with glomerular lesion—see Proteinuria, isolated, with
glomerular lesion
Proteolysis, pathologic D65
Proteus (mirabilis) (morganii), **as the cause of disease
classified elsewhere**
B96.4
Protrusion, protrusio
device, implant or graft (see also Complications, by site
and type, mechanical)
T85.698
ventricular intracranial shunt T85.09
Prune belly (syndrome) Q79.4
Prurigo (ferox) (gravis) (Hebrae) (Hebra's) (mitis) (simplex)
L28.2
Besnier's L20.0
psychogenic F45.8
Pruritus, pruritic (essential) L29.9
ani, anus L29.0
psychogenic F45.8
anogenital L29.3
psychogenic F45.8
hiemalis L29.8
neurogenic (any site) F45.8
perianal L29.0
psychogenic (any site) F45.8
scroti, scrotum L29.1
psychogenic F45.8
specified NEC L29.8
psychogenic F45.8
Trichomonas A59.9
vulva, vulvae L29.2
psychogenic F45.8
Pseudoangioma I81
Pseudarthrosis, pseudoarthrosis (bone)—see Nonunion,
fracture
clavicle, congenital Q74.0
Pseudocirrhosis, liver, pericardial I31.1
Pseudocyesis F45.8
Pseudohermaphroditism Q56.3
adrenal E25.8
female Q56.2
with adrenocortical disorder E25.8
without adrenocortical disorder Q56.2
adrenal, congenital E25.0
male Q56.1
with
androgen resistance E34.51
feminizing testis E34.51
Pseudohydrocephalus G93.2
Pseudohypertrophic muscular dystrophy (Erb's) G71.0
Pseudohypertrophy, muscle G71.0
Pseudomonas
aeruginosa, as cause of disease classified elsewhere
B96.5
mallei infection A24.0
as cause of disease classified elsewhere B96.5
pseudomallei, as cause of disease classified elsewhere
B96.5
Pseudoparalysis
atonic, congenital P94.2
Pseudopolycythemia D75.1
Pseudopuberty, precocious
female heterosexual E25.8
male isosexual E25.8
Pseudorubella B08.20
Pseudosclerema, newborn P83.8
Pseudotuberculosis A28.2
enterocolitis A04.8
pasteurella (infection) A28.0
Pseudotumor
cerebri G93.2
Pseudoxanthoma elasticum Q82.8
Psilosis (sprue) (tropical) K90.1
nontropical K90.0
Psoriasis L40.9
flexural L40.8
specified NEC L40.8
Psychoneurosis, psychoneurotic—see also Neurosis
hysteria F44.9

Psychopathy, psychopathic
autistic F84.5
constitution, post-traumatic F07.81
personality—see Disorder, personality
Psychosexual identity disorder of childhood F64.2
Psychosis, psychotic F29
acute (transient) F23
hysterical F44.9
affective—see Disorder, mood
childhood F84.0
atypical F84.8
exhaustive F43.0
hysterical (acute) F44.9
infantile F84.0
atypical F84.8
Ptosis—see also Blepharoptosis
eyelid—see Blepharoptosis
congenital Q10.0
PTP D69.51
Ptyalism (periodic) K11.7
hysterical F45.8
Pubarche, precocious E30.1
Pubertas praecox E30.1
Puberty (development state) Z00.3
bleeding (excessive) N92.2
delayed E30.0
precocious (constitutional) (cryptogenic) (idiopathic) E30.1
central E22.8
due to
ovarian hyperfunction E28.1
estrogen E28.0
testicular hyperfunction E29.0
premature E30.1
due to
adrenal cortical hyperfunction E25.8
pineal tumor E34.8
pituitary (anterior) hyperfunction E22.8
Puente's disease (simple glandular cheilitis) K13.0
Pulse
alternating R00.8
bigeminal R00.8
fast R00.0
feeble, rapid due to shock following injury T79.4
rapid R00.0
weak R09.89
Punch drunk F07.81
Punctum lacrimale occlusion—see Obstruction, lacrimal
Puncture
abdomen, abdominal
wall S31.139
with
foreign body S31.149
penetration into peritoneal cavity S31.639
with foreign body S31.649
epigastric region S31.132
with
foreign body S31.142
penetration into peritoneal cavity S31.632
with foreign body S31.642
left
lower quadrant S31.134
with
foreign body S31.144
penetration into peritoneal cavity
S31.634
with foreign body S31.644
upper quadrant S31.131
with
foreign body S31.141
penetration into peritoneal cavity
S31.631
with foreign body S31.641
periumbilic region S31.135
with
foreign body S31.145
penetration into peritoneal cavity S31.635
with foreign body S31.645
right
lower quadrant S31.133
with
foreign body S31.143

Puncture, *continued*

penetration into peritoneal cavity
S31.633
with foreign body S31.643
upper quadrant S31.130
with
foreign body S31.140
penetration into peritoneal cavity
S31.630
with foreign body S31.640
accidental, complicating surgery—*see* Complication,
accidental puncture or
laceration
alveolar (process)—*see* Puncture, oral cavity
ankle S91.039
with
foreign body S91.049
left S91.032
with
foreign body S91.042
right S91.031
with
foreign body S91.041
anus S31.833
with foreign body S31.834
arm (upper) S41.139
with foreign body S41.149
left S41.132
with foreign body S41.142
lower—*see* Puncture, forearm
right S41.131
with foreign body S41.141
auditory canal (external) (meatus)—*see* Puncture, ear
auricle, ear—*see* Puncture, ear
axilla—*see* Puncture, arm
back—*see also* Puncture, thorax, back
lower S31.030
with
foreign body S31.040
with penetration into retroperitoneal space
S31.041
penetration into retroperitoneal space S31.031
bladder (traumatic) S37.29
nontraumatic N32.89
breast S21.039
with foreign body S21.049
left S21.032
with foreign body S21.042
right S21.031
with foreign body S21.041
buttock S31.803
with foreign body S31.804
left S31.823
with foreign body S31.824
right S31.813
with foreign body S31.814
by
device, implant or graft—*see* Complications, by site
and type, mechanical
foreign body left accidentally in operative wound
T81.539
instrument (any) during a procedure, accidental—*see*
Puncture, accidental
complicating surgery
calf—*see* Puncture, leg
canaliculus lacrimalis—*see* Puncture, eyelid
canthus, eye—*see* Puncture, eyelid
cervical esophagus S11.23
with foreign body S11.24
cheek (external) S01.439
with foreign body S01.449
left S01.432
with foreign body S01.442
right S01.431
with foreign body S01.441
internal—*see* Puncture, oral cavity
chest wall—*see* Puncture, thorax
chin—*see* Puncture, head, specified site NEC
clitoris—*see* Puncture, vulva
costal region—*see* Puncture, thorax
digit (s)
hand—*see* Puncture, finger
foot—*see* Puncture, toe

Puncture, *continued*

ear (canal) (external) S01.339
with foreign body S01.349
left S01.332
with foreign body S01.342
right S01.331
with foreign body S01.341
drum S09.2-
elbow S51.039
with
foreign body S51.049
left S51.032
with
foreign body S51.042
right S51.031
with
foreign body S51.041
epididymis—*see* Puncture, testis
epigastric region—*see* Puncture, abdomen, wall, epigastric
epiglottis S11.83
with foreign body S11.84
esophagus
cervical S11.23
with foreign body S11.24
thoracic S27.818
eyeball S05.6-
with foreign body S05.5-
eyebrow—*see* Puncture, eyelid
eyelid S01.13-
with foreign body S01.14-
left S01.132
with foreign body S01.142
right S01.131
with foreign body S01.141
face NEC—*see* Puncture, head, specified site NEC
finger (s) S61.239
with
damage to nail S61.339
with
foreign body S61.349
foreign body S61.249
index S61.238
with
damage to nail S61.338
with
foreign body S61.348
foreign body S61.248
left S61.231
with
damage to nail S61.331
with
foreign body S61.341
foreign body S61.241
right S61.230
with
damage to nail S61.330
with
foreign body S61.340
foreign body S61.240
little S61.238
with
damage to nail S61.338
with
foreign body S61.348
foreign body S61.248
left S61.237
with
damage to nail S61.337
with
foreign body S61.347
foreign body S61.247
right S61.236
with
damage to nail S61.336
with
foreign body S61.346
foreign body S61.246
middle S61.238
with
damage to nail S61.338
with
foreign body S61.348
foreign body S61.248

Puncture, *continued*

left S61.233
with
damage to nail S61.333
with
foreign body S61.343
foreign body S61.243
right S61.232
with
damage to nail S61.332
with
foreign body S61.342
foreign body S61.242
ring S61.238
with
damage to nail S61.338
with
foreign body S61.348
foreign body S61.248
left S61.235
with
damage to nail S61.335
with
foreign body S61.345
foreign body S61.245
right S61.234
with
damage to nail S61.334
with
foreign body S61.344
foreign body S61.244
flank S31.139
with foreign body S31.149
foot (except toe(s) alone) S91.339
with foreign body S91.349
left S91.332
with foreign body S91.342
right S91.331
with foreign body S91.341
toe—*see* Puncture, toe
forearm S51.839
with
foreign body S51.849
elbow only—*see* Puncture, elbow
left S51.832
with
foreign body S51.842
right S51.831
with
foreign body S51.841
forehead—*see* Puncture, head, specified site NEC
genital organs, external
female (*code to* Puncture by specific site for vagina or
vulva) S31.532
with foreign body S31.542
male (*code to* Puncture by specific site for penis,
scrotum, or testis)
S31.531
with foreign body S31.541
groin—*see* Puncture, abdomen, wall
gum—*see* Puncture, oral cavity
hand (*code to* Puncture by specific site for finger or
thumb) S61.439
with
foreign body S61.449
left S61.432
with
foreign body S61.442
right S61.431
with
foreign body S61.441
head (*code to* Puncture by specific site for cheek/
temporomandibular
area, ear, eyelid, nose,
or oral cavity) S01.93
with foreign body S01.94
scalp S01.03
with foreign body S01.04
specified site NEC S01.83
with foreign body S01.84
heel—*see* Puncture, foot
hip S71.039

Puncture, *continued*
> with foreign body S71.049
>> left S71.032
>>> with foreign body S71.042
>> right S71.031
>>> with foreign body S71.041
> hypochondrium—*see* Puncture, abdomen, wall
> hypogastric region—*see* Puncture, abdomen, wall
> inguinal region—*see* Puncture, abdomen, wall
> instep—*see* Puncture, foot
> interscapular region—*see* Puncture, thorax, back
> jaw—*see* Puncture, head, specified site NEC
> knee S81.039
>> with foreign body S81.049
>> left S81.032
>>> with foreign body S81.042
>> right S81.031
>>> with foreign body S81.041
> leg (lower) (*code to* Puncture by specified site for foot, knee, or upper leg/thigh) S81.839
>> with foreign body S81.849
>> left S81.832
>>> with foreign body S81.842
>> right S81.831
>>> with foreign body S81.841
> lip S01.531
>> with foreign body S01.541
> loin—*see* Puncture, abdomen, wall
> lower back—*see* Puncture, back, lower
> lumbar region—*see* Puncture, back, lower
> malar region—*see* Puncture, head, specified site NEC
> mammary—*see* Puncture, breast
> mastoid region—*see* Puncture, head, specified site NEC
> mouth—*see* Puncture, oral cavity
> nail
>> finger—*see* Puncture, finger, with damage to nail
>> toe—*see* Puncture, toe, with damage to nail
> nasal (septum) (sinus)—*see* Puncture, nose
> nasopharynx—*see* Puncture, head, specified site NEC
> neck S11.93
>> with foreign body S11.94
> nose (septum) (sinus) S01.23
>> with foreign body S01.24
> oral cavity S01.532
>> with foreign body S01.542
> palate—*see* Puncture, oral cavity
> palm—*see* Puncture, hand
> penis S31.23
>> with foreign body S31.24
> perineum
>> female S31.43
>>> with foreign body S31.44
>> male S31.139
>>> with foreign body S31.149
> phalanges
>> finger—*see* Puncture, finger
>> toe—*see* Puncture, toe
> pinna—*see* Puncture, ear
> popliteal space—*see* Puncture, knee
> scalp S01.03
>> with foreign body S01.04
> scapular region—*see* Puncture, shoulder
> scrotum S31.33
>> with foreign body S31.34
> shin—*see* Puncture, leg
> shoulder S41.039
>> with foreign body S41.049
>> left S41.032
>>> with foreign body S41.042
>> right S41.031
>>> with foreign body S41.041
> subungual
>> finger (s)—*see* Puncture, finger, with damage to nail
>> toe—*see* Puncture, toe, with damage to nail
> thigh S71.139
>> with foreign body S71.149
>> left S71.132
>>> with foreign body S71.142
>> right S71.131
>>> with foreign body S71.141

Puncture, *continued*
> thorax, thoracic (wall) S21.93
>> with foreign body S21.94
>> back S21.23-
>>> with
>>>> foreign body S21.24-
>>>>> with penetration S21.44
>>>> penetration S21.43
>> breast—*see* Puncture, breast
>> front S21.13-
>>> with
>>>> foreign body S21.14-
>>>>> with penetration S21.34
>>>> penetration S21.33
> throat—*see* Puncture, neck
> thumb S61.039
>> with
>>> damage to nail S61.139
>>>> with
>>>>> foreign body S61.149
>>> foreign body S61.049
>> left S61.032
>>> with
>>>> damage to nail S61.132
>>>>> with
>>>>>> foreign body S61.142
>>>> foreign body S61.042
>> right S61.031
>>> with
>>>> damage to nail S61.131
>>>>> with
>>>>>> foreign body S61.141
>>>> foreign body S61.041
> toe (s) S91.139
>> with
>>> damage to nail S91.239
>>>> with
>>>>> foreign body S91.249
>>> foreign body S91.149
>> great S91.133
>>> with
>>>> damage to nail S91.233
>>>>> with
>>>>>> foreign body S91.243
>>>> foreign body S91.143
>>> left S91.132
>>>> with
>>>>> damage to nail S91.232
>>>>>> with
>>>>>>> foreign body S91.242
>>>>> foreign body S91.142
>>> right S91.131
>>>> with
>>>>> damage to nail S91.231
>>>>>> with
>>>>>>> foreign body S91.241
>>>>> foreign body S91.141
>> lesser S91.136
>>> with
>>>> damage to nail S91.236
>>>>> with
>>>>>> foreign body S91.246
>>>> foreign body S91.146
>>> left S91.135
>>>> with
>>>>> damage to nail S91.235
>>>>>> with
>>>>>>> foreign body S91.245
>>>>> foreign body S91.145
>>> right S91.134
>>>> with
>>>>> damage to nail S91.234
>>>>>> with
>>>>>>> foreign body S91.244
>>>>> foreign body S91.144
> tympanum, tympanic membrane S09.2-
> umbilical region S31.135
>> with foreign body S31.145
> vagina S31.43
>> with foreign body S31.44
> vulva S31.43
>> with foreign body S31.44

Puncture, *continued*
> wrist S61.539
>> with
>>> foreign body S61.549
>> left S61.532
>>> with
>>>> foreign body S61.542
>> right S61.531
>>> with
>>>> foreign body S61.541
PUO (pyrexia of unknown origin) R50.9
Purpura D69.2
> abdominal D69.0
> allergic D69.0
> anaphylactoid D69.0
> arthritic D69.0
> autoerythrocyte sensitization D69.2
> autoimmune D69.0
> bacterial D69.0
> Bateman's (senile) D69.2
> capillary fragility (hereditary) (idiopathic) D69.8
> Devil's pinches D69.2
> fibrinolytic—*see* Fibrinolysis
> fulminans, fulminous D65
> gangrenous D65
> hemorrhagic, hemorrhagica D69.3
>> not due to thrombocytopenia D69.0
> Henoch (-Schönlein) (allergic) D69.0
> idiopathic (thrombocytopenic) D69.3
>> nonthrombocytopenic D69.0
> immune thrombocytopenic D69.3
> infectious D69.0
> malignant D69.0
> neonatorum P54.5
> nervosa D69.0
> newborn P54.5
> nonthrombocytopenic D69.2
>> hemorrhagic D69.0
>> idiopathic D69.0
> nonthrombopenic D69.2
> peliosis rheumatica D69.0
> posttransfusion (post-transfusion) (from (fresh) whole blood or blood products) D69.51
> primary D69.49
> red cell membrane sensitivity D69.2
> rheumatica D69.0
> Schönlein (-Henoch) (allergic) D69.0
> *scorbutic* E54 [D77]
> senile D69.2
> simplex D69.2
> symptomatica D69.0
> telangiectasia annularis L81.7
> thrombocytopenic D69.49
>> congenital D69.42
>> hemorrhagic D69.3
>> hereditary D69.42
>> idiopathic D69.3
>> immune D69.3
>> neonatal, transitory P61.0
>> thrombotic M31.1
> thrombohemolytic—*see* Fibrinolysis
> thrombolytic—*see* Fibrinolysis
> thrombopenic D69.49
> thrombotic, thrombocytopenic M31.1
> toxic D69.0
> vascular D69.0
> visceral symptoms D69.0
Purpuric spots R23.3
Purulent—*see* condition
Pus
> in
>> stool R19.5
>> urine N39.0
> tube (rupture)—*see* Salpingo-oophoritis
Pustular rash L08.0
Pustule (nonmalignant) L08.9
> malignant A22.0
Pyelectasis—*see* Hydronephrosis
Pyelitis (congenital) (uremic)—*see also* Pyelonephritis
> with
>> calculus—*see* category N20
>>> with hydronephrosis N13.2

Pyelitis, *continued*
  acute N10
  chronic N11.9
    with calculus—*see* category N20
      with hydronephrosis N13.2
Pyelonephritis—*see also* Nephritis, tubulo-interstitial
  with
    calculus—*see* category N20
      with hydronephrosis N13.2
  acute N10
  calculous—*see* category N20
    with hydronephrosis N13.2
  chronic N11.9
    with calculus—*see* category N20
      with hydronephrosis N13.2
  in (due to)
    lymphoma NEC C85.90 *[N16]*
    sarcoidosis D86.84
    sepsis A41.9 *[N16]*
    transplant rejection T86.91 *[N16]*
Pyelophlebitis I80.8
Pyemia, pyemic (fever) (infection) (purulent)—*see also*
                                    Sepsis
  pneumococcal
  specified organism NEC A41.89
Pyknolepsy G40.A09
  intractable G40.A19
    with status epilepticus G40.A11
    without status epilepticus G40.A19
  not intractable G40.A09
    with status epilepticus G40.A01
    without status epilepticus G40.A09
Pyloritis K29.90
  with bleeding K29.91
Pylorospasm (reflex) NEC K31.3
  congenital or infantile Q40.0
  newborn Q40.0
  neurotic F45.8
  psychogenic F45.8
Pylorus, pyloric—*see* condition
Pyoarthrosis—*see* Arthritis, pyogenic or pyemic
Pyocele
  mastoid—*see* Mastoiditis, acute
  sinus (accessory)—*see* Sinusitis
  turbinate (bone) J32.9
Pyoderma, pyodermia L08.0
  gangrenosum L88
  newborn P39.4
  phagedenic L88
  vegetans L08.81
Pyodermatitis L08.0
  vegetans L08.81
Pyopericarditis, pyopericardium I30.1
Pyopneumopericardium I30.1
Pyopneumothorax (infective) J86.9
  with fistula J86.0
Pyothorax J86.9
  with fistula J86.0
Pyrexia (of unknown origin) R50.9
  atmospheric T67.0
  heat T67.0
  newborn P81.9
    environmentally-induced P81.0
  persistent R50.9
Pyroglobulinemia NEC E88.09
Pyrosis R12
Pyuria (bacterial) N39.0
Pityriasis (capitis) L21.0
  furfuracea L21.0

Q

Quadriparesis—*see* Quadriplegia
  meaning muscle weakness M62.81
Quadriplegia G82.50
  complete
    C1–C4 level G82.51
    C5–C7 level G82.53
  incomplete
    C1–C4 level G82.52
    C5–C7 level G82.54
  traumatic *code to* injury with seventh character S
    current episode—*see* Injury, spinal (cord), cervical

Quincke's disease or edema T78.3
Quinsy (gangrenous) J36

R

Rabies A82.9
  contact Z20.3
  exposure to Z20.3
  inoculation reaction—*see* Complications, vaccination
Radiation
  therapy, encounter for Z51.0
Radiotherapy session Z51.0
Rag picker's disease A22.1
Rag sorter's disease A22.1
Rales R09.89
Ramsay-Hunt disease or syndrome (*see also* Hunt's
                                    disease) B02.21
  meaning dyssynergia cerebellaris myoclonica G11.1
Rape
  alleged, observation or examination, ruled out
    child Z04.42
  child
    confirmed T74.22
    suspected T76.22
Rapid
  feeble pulse, due to shock, following injury T79.4
  heart (beat) R00.0
    psychogenic F45.8
Rash (toxic) R21
  canker A38.9
  diaper L22
  drug (internal use) L27.0
    contact (*see also* Dermatitis, due to, drugs, external)
                                    L25.1
  following immunization T88.1-
  food—*see* Dermatitis, due to, food
  heat L74.0
  napkin (psoriasiform) L22
  nettle—*see* Urticaria
  pustular L08.0
  rose R21
    epidemic B06.9
  scarlet A38.9
  serum (*see also* Reaction, serum) T80.69
  wandering tongue K14.1
RDS (newborn) (type I) P22.0
  type II P22.1
Reaction—*see also* Disorder
  adverse
    food (any) (ingested)NEC T78.1
      anaphylactic—*see* Shock, anaphylactic, due to
                                    food
  allergic—*see* Allergy
  anaphylactic—*see* Shock, anaphylactic
  anaphylactoid—*see* Shock, anaphylactic
  anesthesia—*see* Anesthesia, complication
  antitoxin (prophylactic) (therapeutic)—*see* Complications,
                                    vaccination
  combat and operational stress F43.0
  compulsive F42.8
  conversion F44.9
  crisis, acute F43.0
  deoxyribonuclease (DNA) (DNase)hypersensitivity D69.2
  depressive (single episode) F32.9
    psychotic F32.3
    recurrent—*see* Disorder, depressive, recurrent
  dissociative F44.9
  drug NEC T88.7
    allergic—*see* Allergy, drug
    newborn P93.8
      gray baby syndrome P93.0
    overdose or poisoning (by accident)—*see* Table of
                                    Drugs and Chemicals,
                                    by drug, poisoning
    photoallergic L56.1
    phototoxic L56.0
    withdrawal—*see* Dependence, by drug, with,
                                    withdrawal
      infant of dependent mother P96.1
      newborn P96.1

Reaction, *continued*
    wrong substance given or taken (by accident)—*see*
                                    Table of Drugs and
                                    Chemicals, by drug,
                                    poisoning
  fear F40.9
    child (abnormal) F93.8
  febrile nonhemolytic transfusion (FNHTR) R50.84
  hysterical F44.9
  immunization—*see* Complications, vaccination
  leukemoid D72.823
    basophilic D72.823
    lymphocytic D72.823
    monocytic D72.823
    myelocytic D72.823
    neutrophilic D72.823
  neurogenic—*see* Neurosis
  neurotic F48.9
  nonspecific
    to
      cell mediated immunity measurement of gamma
                                    interferon antigen
                                    response without active
                                    tuberculosis R76.12
      QuantiFERON-TB test (QFT) without active
                                    tuberculosis R76.12
      tuberculin test (*see also* Reaction, tuberculin skin
                                    test) R76.11
  obsessive-compulsive F42.8
  phobic F40.9
  psychoneurotic—*see also* Neurosis
    compulsive F42
    obsessive F42
  psychophysiologic—*see* Disorder, somatoform
  psychosomatic—*see* Disorder, somatoform
  psychotic—*see* Psychosis
  scarlet fever toxin—*see* Complications, vaccination
  serum T80.69-
    anaphylactic (immediate) (*see also* Shock,
                                    anaphylactic) T80.59-
    specified reaction NEC
      due to
        administration of blood and blood products
                                    T80.61-
        immunization T80.62-
    serum specified NEC T80.69-
    vaccination T80.62-
  stress (severe) F43.9
    acute (agitation) ("daze") (disorientation) (disturbance
                                    of consciousness)
                                    (flight reaction) (fugue)
                                    F43.0
    specified NEC F43.8
  surgical procedure—*see* Complications, surgical
                                    procedure
  tetanus antitoxin—*see* Complications, vaccination
  toxic, to local anesthesia T81.89
  toxin-antitoxin—*see* Complications, vaccination
  tuberculin skin test, abnormal R76.11
  withdrawing, child or adolescent F93.8
Reactive airway disease—*see* Asthma
Reactive depression—*see* Reaction, depressive
Recklinghausen disease Q85.01
  bones E21.0
Rectalgia K62.89
Rectitis K62.89
Rectocele
  male K62.3
Rectosigmoiditis K63.89
  ulcerative (chronic) K51.30
    with
      complication K51.319
        abscess K51.314
        fistula K51.313
        obstruction K51.312
        rectal bleeding K51.311
        specified NEC K51.318
Red bugs B88.0
Redundant, redundancy
  foreskin (congenital) N47.8
  prepuce (congenital) N47.8
Reflex R29.2
  vasovagal R55

Reflux K21.9
  acid K21.9
  esophageal K21.9
    with esophagitis K21.0
    newborn P78.83
  gastroesophageal K21.9
    with esophagitis K21.0
  vesicoureteral (with scarring) N13.70
    without nephropathy N13.71
Refusal of
  food, psychogenic F50.89
Regurgitation R11.10
  aortic (valve)—*see* Insufficiency, aortic
  food—*see also* Vomiting
    with reswallowing—*see* Rumination
    newborn P92.1
  gastric contents—*see* Vomiting
  heart—*see* Endocarditis
  mitral (valve)—*see* Insufficiency, mitral
    congenital Q23.3
  myocardial—*see* Endocarditis
  pulmonary (valve) (heart) I37.1
    congenital Q22.2
    syphilitic A52.03
  tricuspid—*see* Insufficiency, tricuspid
  valve, valvular—*see* Endocarditis
    congenital Q24.8
Reifenstein syndrome E34.52
Reinsertion
  implantable subdermal contraceptive Z30.46
  intrauterine contraceptive device Z30.433
Rejection
  food, psychogenic F50.89
  transplant T86.91
    bone T86.830
      marrow T86.01
    heart T86.21
      with lung (s) T86.31
    kidney T86.11
    liver T86.41
    lung (s) T86.810
      with heart T86.31
    organ (immune or nonimmune cause) T86.91
    stem cell (peripheral blood) (umbilical cord) T86.5
Relaxation
  anus (sphincter) K62.89
    psychogenic F45.8
  cardioesophageal K21.9
  diaphragm J98.6
  posture R29.3
  rectum (sphincter) K62.89
Remittent fever (malarial) B54
Remnant
  fingernail L60.8
    congenital Q84.6
  thyroglossal duct Q89.2
  tonsil J35.8
    infected (chronic) J35.01
Removal (from) (of)
  device
    contraceptive Z30.432
      implantable subdermal Z30.46
  dressing (nonsurgical) Z48.00
    surgical Z48.01
  home in childhood (to foster home or institution) Z62.29
  staples Z48.02
  suture Z48.02
Rendu-Osler-Weber disease or syndrome I78.0
Replacement by artificial or mechanical device or
                prosthesis of
  heart Z95.812
    valve Z95.2
      prosthetic Z95.2
      specified NEC Z95.4
      xenogenic Z95.3
  organ replacement
    by artificial or mechanical device or prosthesis of
      heart Z95.812
        valve Z95.2
Request for expert evidence Z04.8
Residual—*see also* condition
  urine R39.198

Resistance, resistant (to)
  insulin E88.81
  organism (s)
    to
      drug Z16.30
        aminoglycosides Z16.29
        amoxicillin Z16.11
        ampicillin Z16.11
        antibiotic (s) Z16.20
          multiple Z16.24
          specified NEC Z16.29
        antimicrobial (single) Z16.30
          multiple Z16.35
          specified NEC Z16.39
        beta lactam antibiotics Z16.10
          specified NEC Z16.19
        cephalosporins Z16.19
        extended beta lactamase (ESBL) Z16.12
        macrolides Z16.29
        methicillin—*see* MRSA
        multiple drugs (MDRO)
          antibiotics Z16.24
          antimycobacterial (single) Z16.341
        penicillins Z16.11
        sulfonamides Z16.29
        tetracyclines Z16.29
        vancomycin Z16.21
          related antibiotics Z16.22
Respiration
  Cheyne-Stokes R06.3
  decreased due to shock, following injury T79.4
  disorder of, psychogenic F45.8
  insufficient, or poor R06.89
    newborn P28.5
  painful R07.1
  sighing, psychogenic F45.8
Respiratory—*see also* condition
  distress syndrome (newborn) (type I) P22.0
    type II P22.1
  syncytial virus, as cause of disease classified elsewhere
                       B97
Retained—*see also* Retention
  foreign body fragments (type of) Z18.9
    acrylics Z18.2
    animal quill (s) or spines Z18.31
    cement Z18.83
    concrete Z18.83
    crystalline Z18.83
    diethylhexylphthalates Z18.2
    glass Z18.81
    isocyanate Z18.2
    magnetic metal Z18.11
    metal Z18.10
    nonmagnetic metal Z18.12
    organic NEC Z18.39
    plastic Z18.2
    quill (s) (animal) Z18.31
    specified NEC Z18.89
    spine (s) (animal) Z18.31
    stone Z18.83
    tooth (teeth) Z18.32
    wood Z18.33
  fragments (type of) Z18.9
    acrylics Z18.2
    animal quill (s) or spines Z18.31
    cement Z18.83
    concrete Z18.83
    crystalline Z18.83
    diethylhexylphthalates Z18.2
    glass Z18.81
    isocyanate Z18.2
    magnetic metal Z18.11
    metal Z18.10
    nonmagnetic metal Z18.12
    organic NEC Z18.39
    plastic Z18.2
    quill (s) (animal) Z18.31
    specified NEC Z18.89
    spine (s) (animal) Z18.31
    stone Z18.83
    tooth (teeth) Z18.32
    wood Z18.33

Retardation
  development, developmental, specific—*see* Disorder,
                developmental
  endochondral bone growth—*see* Disorder, bone,
                development or growth
  growth R62.50
    due to malnutrition E45
  mental—*see* Disability, intellectual
  motor function, specific F82
  physical (child) R62.52
    due to malnutrition E45
  reading (specific) F81.0
  spelling (specific) (without reading disorder) F81.81
Retching—*see* Vomiting
Retention—*see also* Retained
  cyst—*see* Cyst
  dead
    fetus (at or near term) (mother) O36.4
  deciduous tooth K00.6
  fetus
    dead O36.4
  fluid R60.9
  foreign body—*see also* Foreign body, retained
    current trauma—*code as* Foreign body, by site or type
  menses N94.89
  urine R33.9
    psychogenic F45.8
Reticulohistiocytoma (giant-cell) D76.3
Reticulosis (skin)
  hemophagocytic, familial D76.1
Retina, retinal—*see also* condition
  dark area D49.81
Retinoblastoma C69.2-
  differentiated C69.2-
  undifferentiated C69.2-
Retinopathy (background) H35.00
  of prematurity H35.10-
    stage 0 H35.11-
    stage 1 H35.12-
    stage 2 H35.13-
    stage 3 H35.14-
    stage 4 H35.15-
    stage 5 H35.16-
Retractile testis Q55.22
Retraction
  nipple N64.53
    associated with
      lactation O92.03
    congenital Q83.8
Retrograde menstruation N92.5
Retrosternal thyroid (congenital) Q89.2
Retroversion, retroverted
  testis (congenital) Q55.29
Rett's disease or syndrome F84.2
Rh (factor)
  hemolytic disease (newborn) P55.0
  incompatibility, immunization or sensitization
    affecting management of pregnancy NEC O36.09-
      anti-D antibody O36.01-
    newborn P55.0
    transfusion reaction—*see* Complication(s), transfusion,
                incompatibility reaction,
                Rh (factor)
  negative mother affecting newborn P55.0
  titer elevated—*see* Complication(s), transfusion,
                incompatibility reaction,
                Rh (factor)
  transfusion reaction—*see* Complication(s), transfusion,
                incompatibility reaction,
                Rh (factor)
Rhabdomyolysis (idiopathic) **NEC** M62.82
  traumatic T79.6
Rheumatic (acute) (subacute) (chronic)
  coronary arteritis I01.9
  fever (acute)—*see* Fever, rheumatic
  heart—*see* Disease, heart, rheumatic
  myocardial degeneration—*see* Degeneration,
                myocardium
  myocarditis (chronic) (inactive) (with chorea) I09.0
    active or acute I01.2
      with chorea (acute) (rheumatic) (Sydenham's) I02.0
  pancarditis, acute I01.8
    with chorea (acute (rheumatic) Sydenham's) I02.0

Rheumatic, *continued*
    pericarditis (active) (acute) (with effusion) (with pneumonia) I01.0
        with chorea (acute) (rheumatic) (Sydenham's) I02.0
        chronic or inactive I09.2
    pneumonia I00 *[J17]*
    torticollis M43.6
Rheumatism (articular) (neuralgic) (nonarticular) M79.0
    intercostal, meaning Tietze's disease M94.0
    sciatic M54.4-
Rhinitis (atrophic) (catarrhal) (chronic) (croupous) (fibrinous) (granulomatous) (hyperplastic) (hypertrophic) (membranous) (obstructive) (purulent) (suppurative) (ulcerative) J31.0
    with
        sore throat—*see* Nasopharyngitis
    acute J00
    allergic J30.9
        with asthma J45.909
            with
                exacerbation (acute) J45.901
                status asthmaticus J45.902
        due to
            food J30.5
            pollen J30.1
        nonseasonal J30.89
        perennial J30.89
        seasonal NEC J30.2
        specified NEC J30.89
    infective J00
    pneumococcal J00
    vasomotor J30.0
Rhinoantritis (chronic)—*see* Sinusitis, maxillary
Rhinodacryolith—*see* Dacryolith
Rhinolith (nasal sinus) J34.89
Rhinomegaly J34.89
Rhinopharyngitis (acute) (subacute)—*see also* Nasopharyngitis
Rhinorrhea J34.89
    paroxysmal—*see* Rhinitis, allergic
    spasmodic—*see* Rhinitis, allergic
Rhinovirus infection NEC B34.8
Rhizomelic chondrodysplasia punctata E71.540
Rhythm
    disorder I49.9
    escape I49.9
    heart, abnormal I49.9
    idioventricular I44.2
Rhytidosis facialis L98.8
Rickets (active) (acute) (adolescent) (chest wall) (congenital) (current) (infantile) (intestinal) E55.0
    celiac K90.0
    hypophosphatemic with nephrotic-glycosuric dwarfism E72.09
    inactive E64.3
    sequelae, any E64.3
Riehl's melanosis L81.4
Rietti-Greppi-Micheli anemia D56.9
Rieux's hernia—*see* Hernia, abdomen, specified site NEC
Riga (-Fede) **disease** K14.0
Right middle lobe syndrome J98.11
Rigid, rigidity—*see also* condition
    abdominal R19.30
        with severe abdominal pain R10.0
    nuchal R29.1
Rigors R68.89
    with fever R50.9
Ringworm B35.9
    beard B35.0
    black dot B35.0
    body B35.4
    corporeal B35.4
    foot B35.3
    groin B35.6
    hand B35.2
    honeycomb B35.0
    nails B35.1
    perianal (area) B35.6

Ringworm, *continued*
    scalp B35.0
    specified NEC B35.8
Risk, suicidal
    meaning personal history of attempted suicide Z91.5
    meaning suicidal ideation—*see* Ideation, suicidal
Ritter's disease L00
Robert's pelvis Q74.2
Robin (-Pierre) syndrome Q87.0
Robinow-Silvermann-Smith syndrome Q87.1
Rocky Mountain (spotted) **fever** A77.0
Roger's disease Q21.0
Rolando's fracture (displaced) S62.22-
    nondisplaced S62.22-
Romano-Ward (prolonged QT interval) **syndrome** I45.81
Romberg's disease or syndrome G51.8
Roof, mouth—*see* condition
Rosary, rachitic E55.0
Roseola B09
    infantum B08.20
        due to human herpesvirus 6 B08.21
        due to human herpesvirus 7 B08.22
Rossbach's disease K31.89
    psychogenic F45.8
Rothmund (-Thomson) **syndrome** Q82.8
Round
    worms (large) (infestation) NEC B82.0
        Ascariasis (*see also* Ascariasis) B77.9
Rose
    cold J30.1
    fever J30.1
    rash R21
        epidemic B06.9
Rotor's disease or syndrome E80.6
Rubella (German measles) B06.9
    complication NEC B06.09
        neurological B06.00
    congenital P35.0
    contact Z20.4
    exposure to Z20.4
    maternal
        manifest rubella in infant P35.0
        care for (suspected) damage to fetus O35.3
        suspected damage to fetus affecting management of pregnancy O35.3
    specified complications NEC B06.09
Rubeola (meaning measles)—*see* Measles
    meaning rubella—*see* Rubella
Rudimentary (congenital)—*see also* Agenesis
    bone Q79.9
Ruled out condition—*see* Observation, suspected
Rumination R11.10
    with nausea R11.2
    disorder of infancy F98.21
    neurotic F42.8
    newborn P92.1
    obsessional F42.8
    psychogenic F42.8
Runny nose R09.89
Rupture, ruptured
    abscess (spontaneous)—*code by* site under Abscess
    aorta, aortic I71.8
        valve or cusp (*see also* Endocarditis, aortic) I35.8
    appendix (with peritonitis) K35.2
        with localized peritonitis K35.3
    arteriovenous fistula, brain I60.8
    cardiac (auricle) (ventricle) (wall) I23.3
        with hemopericardium I23.0
        infectional I40.9
        traumatic—*see* Injury, heart
    cecum (with peritonitis) K65.0
        with peritoneal abscess K35.3
    cerebral aneurysm (congenital) (*see* Hemorrhage, intracranial, subarachnoid)
    circle of Willis I60.6
    corpus luteum (infected) (ovary) N83.1-
    cyst—*see* Cyst
    ear drum (nontraumatic)—*see also* Perforation, tympanum
        traumatic S09.2-
            due to blast injury—*see* Injury, blast, ear

Rupture, ruptured, *continued*
    fallopian tube NEC (nonobstetric) (nontraumatic) N83.8
        due to pregnancy O00.10
    gastric—*see also* Rupture, stomach
        vessel K92.2
    graafian follicle (hematoma) N83.0-
    hymen (nontraumatic) (nonintentional) N89.8
    kidney (traumatic) S37.06-
        birth injury P15.8
    meningeal artery I60.8
    ovary, ovarian N83.8
        corpus luteum cyst N83.1-
        follicle (graafian) N83.0-
    oviduct (nonobstetric) (nontraumatic) N83.8
        due to pregnancy O00.10
    pulmonary
        valve (heart) I37.8
    rotator cuff (nontraumatic) M75.10-
        complete M75.12-
        incomplete M75.11-
    spleen (traumatic) S36.09
        birth injury P15.1
    tonsil J35.8
    traumatic
        kidney S37.06-
        spleen S36.09
    tricuspid (heart) (valve) I07.8
    tube, tubal (nonobstetric) (nontraumatic) N83.8
        abscess—*see* Salpingitis
        due to pregnancy O00.10
    tympanum, tympanic (membrane) (nontraumatic) (*see also* Perforation, tympanic membrane) H72.9-
        traumatic—*see* Rupture, ear drum, traumatic
    viscus R19.8
Russell-Silver syndrome Q87.1
Ruvalcaba-Myhre-Smith syndrome E71.440
Rytand-Lipsitch syndrome I44.2

S

Saccharomyces infection B37.9
Sachs' amaurotic familial idiocy or disease E75.02
Sachs-Tay disease E75.02
Sacks-Libman disease M32.11
Sacralgia M53.3
Sacrodynia M53.3
Saint
    Anthony's fire—*see* Erysipelas
Salmonella—*see* Infection, Salmonella
Salmonellosis A02.0
Salpingitis (catarrhal) (fallopian tube) (nodular) (pseudofollicular) (purulent) (septic) N70.91
    with oophoritis N70.93
    acute N70.01
        with oophoritis N70.03
    chlamydial A56.11
    chronic N70.11
        with oophoritis N70.13
    ear—*see* Salpingitis, eustachian
    eustachian (tube) H68.00-
        acute H68.01-
        chronic H68.02-
    gonococcal (acute) (chronic) A54.24
    specific (gonococcal) (acute) (chronic) A54.24
    venereal (gonococcal) (acute) (chronic) A54.24
Salpingo-oophoritis (catarrhal) (purulent) (ruptured) (septic) (suppurative) N70.93
    acute N70.03
        gonococcal A54.24
    chronic N70.13
    gonococcal (acute) (chronic) A54.24
    specific (gonococcal) (acute) (chronic) A54.24
    venereal (gonococcal) (acute) (chronic) A54.24
Sanfilippo (Type B) (Type C) (Type D) syndrome E76.22
Sanger-Brown ataxia G11.2
Sao Paulo fever or typhus A77.0
Sarcoepiplocele—*see* Hernia
Sarcoepiplomphalocele Q79.2

Sarcoid—*see also* Sarcoidosis
  arthropathy D86.86
  Boeck's D86.9
  Darier-Roussy D86.3
  iridocyclitis D86.83
  meningitis D86.81
  myocarditis D86.85
  myositis D86.87
  pyelonephritis D86.84
  Spiegler-Fendt L08.89
Sarcoidosis D86.9
  with
      cranial nerve palsies D86.82
      hepatic granuloma D86.89
      polyarthritis D86.86
      tubulo-interstitial nephropathy D86.84
  combined sites NEC D86.89
  lung D86.0
      and lymph nodes D86.2
  lymph nodes D86.1
      and lung D86.2
  meninges D86.81
  skin D86.3
  specified type NEC D86.89
Sarcoma (of)—*see also* Neoplasm, connective tissue,
                                        malignant
  cerebellar C71.6
      circumscribed (arachnoidal) C71.6
  circumscribed (arachnoidal) cerebellar C71.6
  clear cell—*see also* Neoplasm, connective tissue,
                                        malignant
      kidney C64.-
  monstrocellular
      specified site—*see* Neoplasm, malignant, by site
      unspecified site C71.9
SBE (subacute bacterial endocarditis) I33.0
Scabies (any site) B86
Scaglietti-Dagnini syndrome E22.0
Scald—*see* Burn
Scapulohumeral myopathy G71.0
Scar, scarring (*see also* Cicatrix) L90.5
  adherent L90.5
  atrophic L90.5
  cheloid L91.0
  hypertrophic L91.0
  keloid L91.0
  painful L90.5
  vagina N89.8
      postoperative N99.2
  vulva N90.89
Scarabiasis B88.2
Scarlatina (anginosa) (maligna) (ulcerosa) A38.9
  myocarditis (acute) A38.1
      old—*see* Myocarditis
  otitis media A38.0
Scarlet fever (albuminuria) (angina) A38.9
Schaumann's
  benign lymphogranulomatosis D86.1
  disease or syndrome—*see* Sarcoidosis
Schistosomiasis B65.9
  cutaneous B65.3
Schizencephaly Q04.6
Schizophrenia, schizophrenic F20.9
  childhood type F84.5
  syndrome of childhood F84.5
Schlatter-Osgood disease or osteochondrosis M92.5-
Schlatter's tibia M92.5-
Schmorl's disease or nodes
  sacrococcygeal region M53.3
Schönlein (-Henoch) disease or purpura (primary)
                                        (rheumatic) D69.0
Schultze's type acroparesthesia, simple I73.89
Schwannomatosis Q85.03
Schwartz-Bartter syndrome E22.2
Sciatica (infective)
  with lumbago M54.4-
Scleredema
  newborn P83.0
Sclerema (adiposum) (edematosum) (neonatorum) (newborn)
                                        P83.0
Sclerocystic ovary syndrome E28.2

Scleroderma, sclerodermia (acrosclerotic) (diffuse)
                                        (generalized)
                                        (progressive)
                                        (pulmonary) (*see also*
                                        Sclerosis, systemic)
                                        M34.9-
  newborn P83.8
Sclerosis, sclerotic
  brain (generalized) (lobular) G37.9
      tuberous Q85.1
  Friedreich's (spinal cord) G11.1
  hereditary
      spinal (Friedreich's ataxia) G11.1
  hippocampal G93.81
  mesial temporal G93.81
  mitral I05.8
  pulmonary—*see* Fibrosis, lung
      artery I27.0
  spinal (cord) (progressive) G95.89
      hereditary (Friedreich's) (mixed form) G11.1
  temporal (mesial) G93.81
  tricuspid (heart) (valve) I07.8
  tuberous (brain) Q85.1
Scoliosis (acquired) (postural) M41.9
  adolescent (idiopathic)—*see* Scoliosis, idiopathic, juvenile
  congenital Q67.5
      due to bony malformation Q76.3
  idiopathic M41.20
      adolescent M41.129
          cervical region M41.122
          cervicothoracic region M41.123
          lumbar region M41.126
          lumbosacral region M41.127
          thoracic region M41.124
          thoracolumbar region M41.125
      cervical region M41.22
      cervicothoracic region M41.23
      infantile M41.00
          cervical region M41.02
          cervicothoracic region M41.03
          lumbar region M41.06
          lumbosacral region M41.07
          sacrococcygeal region M41.08
          thoracic region M41.04
          thoracolumbar region M41.05
      juvenile M41.119
          cervical region M41.112
          cervicothoracic region M41.113
          lumbar region M41.116
          lumbosacral region M41.117
          thoracic region M41.114
          thoracolumbar region M41.115
  sciatic M54.4-
Scratch—*see* Abrasion
Scratchy throat R09.89
Screening (for) Z13.9
  anemia Z13.0
  cardiovascular disorder Z13.6
  chlamydial diseases Z11.8
  chromosomal abnormalities (nonprocreative) NEC Z13.79
  congenital
      dislocation of hip Z13.89
      eye disorder Z13.5
      malformation or deformation Z13.89
  cystic fibrosis Z13.228
  depression Z13.89
  developmental handicap Z13.4
      in early childhood Z13.4
  diabetes mellitus Z13.1
  disability, intellectual Z13.4
  disease or disorder Z13.9
      bacterial NEC Z11.2
          intestinal infectious Z11.0
          respiratory tuberculosis Z11.1
      blood or blood-forming organ Z13.0
      cardiovascular Z13.6
      chlamydial Z11.8
      dental Z13.89
      developmental Z13.4
      endocrine Z13.29
      heart Z13.6
      human immunodeficiency virus (HIV) infection Z11.4
      immunity Z13.0

Screening, *continued*
  infectious Z11.9
  mental Z13.89
  metabolic Z13.228
  neurological Z13.89
  nutritional Z13.21
      metabolic Z13.228
          lipoid disorders Z13.220
  respiratory Z13.83
  rheumatic Z13.828
  rickettsial Z11.8
  sexually-transmitted NEC Z11.3
      human immunodeficiency virus (HIV) Z11.4
  sickle cell trait Z13.0
  spirochetal Z11.8
  thyroid Z13.29
  venereal Z11.3
  viral NEC Z11.59
      human immunodeficiency virus (HIV) Z11.4
  elevated titer Z13.89
  galactosemia Z13.228
  gonorrhea Z11.3
  hematopoietic malignancy Z12.89
  hemoglobinopathies Z13.0
  Hodgkin disease Z12.89
  human immunodeficiency virus (HIV) Z11.4
  human papillomavirus Z11.51
  hypertension Z13.6
  immunity disorders Z13.0
  infection
      mycotic Z11.8
      parasitic Z11.8
  intellectual disability Z13.4
  leukemia Z12.89
  lymphoma Z12.89
  malaria Z11.6
  measles Z11.59
  mental disorder Z13.89
  metabolic errors, inborn Z13.228
  musculoskeletal disorder Z13.828
  mycoses Z11.8
  neoplasm (malignant) (of) Z12.9
      blood Z12.89
      breast Z12.39
          routine mammogram Z12.31
      cervix Z12.4
      hematopoietic system Z12.89
      lymph (glands) Z12.89
      nervous system Z12.82
  nephropathy Z13.89
  nervous system disorders NEC Z13.858
  neurological condition Z13.89
  parasitic infestation Z11.9
      specified NEC Z11.8
  phenylketonuria Z13.228
  poisoning (chemical) (heavy metal) Z13.88
  postnatal, chromosomal abnormalities Z13.89
  rheumatoid arthritis Z13.828
  sexually-transmitted disease NEC Z11.3
      human immunodeficiency virus (HIV) Z11.4
  sickle-cell disease or trait Z13.0
  special Z13.9
      specified NEC Z13.89
  syphilis Z11.3
  traumatic brain injury Z13.850
  venereal disease Z11.3
  viral encephalitis (mosquito- or tick-borne) Z11.59
  whooping cough Z11.2
Scrofula, scrofulosis (tuberculosis of cervical lymph glands)
                                        A18.2
Scurvy, scorbutic E54
  anemia D53.2
  gum E54
  infantile E54
  rickets E55.0 *[M90.80]*
Seasickness T75.3
Seatworm (infection) (infestation) B80
Seborrhea, seborrheic L21.9
  capillitii R23.8
  capitis L21.0
  dermatitis L21.9
      infantile L21.1

Seborrhea, seborrheic, *continued*
   eczema L21.9
      infantile L21.1
   sicca L21.0
Seckel's syndrome Q87.1
Second hand tobacco smoke exposure (acute) (chronic) Z77.22
   in the perinatal period P96.81
Secretion
   antidiuretic hormone, inappropriate E22.2
   hormone
      antidiuretic, inappropriate (syndrome) E22.2
   urinary
      excessive R35.8
      suppression R34
Seitelberger's syndrome (infantile neuraxonal dystrophy) G31.89
Seizure(s) (*see also* Convulsions) R56.9
   akinetic—*see* Epilepsy, generalized, specified NEC
   atonic—*see* Epilepsy, generalized, specified NEC
   convulsive—*see* Convulsions
   disorder (*see also* Epilepsy) G40.909
   epileptic—*see* Epilepsy
   febrile (simple) R56.00
      with status epilepticus G40.901
      complex (atypical) (complicated) R56.01
         with status epilepticus G40.901
   intractable G40.919
      with status epilepticus G40.911
   newborn P90
   nonspecific epileptic
      atonic—*see* Epilepsy, generalized, specified NEC
      clonic—*see* Epilepsy, generalized, specified NEC
      myoclonic—*see* Epilepsy, generalized, specified NEC
      tonic—*see* Epilepsy, generalized, specified NEC
      tonic-clonic—*see* Epilepsy, generalized, specified NEC
   partial, developing into secondarily generalized seizures
      complex—*see* Epilepsy, localization-related, symptomatic, with complex partial seizures
      simple—*see* Epilepsy, localization-related, symptomatic, with simple partial seizures
   post traumatic R56.1
   recurrent G40.909
   specified NEC G40.89
Self-damaging behavior (life-style) Z72.89
Self-harm (attempted)
   history (personal) Z91.5
      in family Z81.8
Self-mutilation (attempted)
   history (personal) Z91.5
      in family Z81.8
Self-poisoning
   history (personal) Z91.5
      in family Z81.8
   observation following (alleged) attempt Z03.6
Semicoma R40.1
Sensitive, sensitivity—*see also* Allergy
   child (excessive) F93.8
   gluten (non-celiac) K90.41
   dentin K03.89
   methemoglobin D74.8
   tuberculin, without clinical or radiological symptoms R76.11
Sensitization, auto-erythrocytic D69.2
Separation
   anxiety, abnormal (of childhood) F93.0
   apophysis, traumatic—*code as* Fracture, by site
   epiphysis, epiphyseal
      nontraumatic—*see also* Osteochondropathy, specified type NEC
      upper femoral—*see* Slipped, epiphysis, upper femoral
      traumatic—*code as* Fracture, by site
Sepsis (generalize) (unspecified organism) A41.9
   with
      organ dysfunction (acute) (multiple) R65.20
         with septic shock R65.21
   anaerobic A41.4
   candidal B37.7
   cryptogenic A41.9

Sepsis, *continued*
   due to device, implant or graft T85.79
      catheter NEC T85.79
         dialysis (renal) T82.7
            intraperitoneal T85.71
         infusion NEC T82.7
         vascular T82.7
   Enterococcus A41.81
   Escherichia coli (E. coli) A41.51
   following
      immunization T88.0
      infusion, therapeutic injection or transfusion NEC T80.29
   gangrenous A41.9
   Gram-negative (organism) A41.5-
      anaerobic A41.4
   Haemophilus influenzae A41.3
   meningeal—*see* meningitis
   meningococcal A39.4
      acute A39.2
      chronic A39.3
   MSSA (Methicillin susceptible Staphylococcus aureus) A41.01
   newborn P36.9
      due to
         anaerobes NEC P36.5
         Escherichia coli P36.4
         Staphylococcus P36.30
            aureus P36.2
            specified NEC P36.39
         Streptococcus P36.10
            group B P36.0
            specified NEC P36.19
         specified NEC P36.8
   Pasteurella multocida A28.0
   pneumococcal A40.3
   severe R65.20
      with septic shock R65.21
   Shigella (*see also* Dysentery, bacillary) A03.9
   skin, localized—*see* Abscess
   specified organism NEC A41.89
   Staphylococcus, staphylococcal A41.2
      aureus (methicillin susceptible) (MSSA) A41.01
         methicillin resistant (MRSA) A41.02
      coagulase-negative A41.1
      specified NEC A41.1
   Streptococcus, streptococcal A40.9
      group
         D A41.81
      neonatal P36.10
         group B P36.0
         specified NEC P36.19
      pneumoniae A40.3
Septic—*see* condition
   gallbladder (acute) K81.0
   sore—*see also* Abscess
      throat J02.0
         streptococcal J02.0
   tonsils, chronic J35.01
      with adenoiditis J35.03
Septicemia A41.9
   meaning sepsis—*see* Sepsis
Septum, septate (congenital)—*see also* Anomaly, by site
   anal Q42.3
      with fistula Q42.2
   aqueduct of Sylvius Q03.0
      with spina bifida—*see* Spina bifida, by site, with hydrocephalus
   vaginal, longitudinal Q52.129
      microperforate
         left side Q52.124
         right side Q52.123
      nonobstructing Q52.120
      obstructing
         left side Q52.122
         right side Q52.121
Serology for syphilis
   doubtful
      with signs or symptoms—*code by* site and stage under Syphilis
   reactivated A53.0
Serositis, multiple K65.8
   pericardial I31.1

Serum
   allergy, allergic reaction (*see also* Reaction, serum) T80.69
      shock (*see also* Shock, anaphylactic) T80.59
   arthritis (*see also* Reaction, serum) T80.69
   complication or reaction NEC (*see also* Reaction, serum) T80.69
   disease NEC (*see also* Reaction, serum) T80.69
   hepatitis—*see also* Hepatitis, viral, type B
      carrier (suspected) of B18.1
   intoxication (*see also* Reaction, serum) T80.69
   neuritis (*see also* Reaction, serum) T80.69
   poisoning NEC (*see also* Reaction, serum) T80.69
   rash NEC (*see also* Reaction, serum) T80.69
   reaction NEC (*see also* Reaction, serum) T80.69
   sickness NEC (*see also* Reaction, serum) T80.69
   urticaria (*see also* Reaction, serum) T80.69
Severe sepsis R65.20
   with septic shock R65.21
Sexual
   immaturity (female) (male) E30.0
   precocity (constitutional) (cryptogenic) (female) (idiopathic) (male) E30.1
Shadow lung R91.8
Shedding
   nail L60.8
   premature, primary (deciduous) teeth K00.6
Shelf, rectal K62.89
Shellshock (current) F43.0
   lasting state—*see* Disorder, post-traumatic stress
Shigellosis A03.9
   Group A A03.0
   Group B A03.1
   Group C A03.2
   Group D A03.3
Shingles—*see* Herpes, zoster
Shock R57.9
   adverse food reaction (anaphylactic)—*see* Shock, anaphylactic, due to food
   allergic—*see* Shock, anaphylactic
   anaphylactic T78.2
      chemical—*see* Table of Drugs and Chemicals
      due to drug or medicinal substance
         correct substance properly administered T88.6-
         overdose or wrong substance given or taken (by accident)—*see* Table of Drugs and Chemicals, by drug, poisoning
      due to food (nonpoisonous) T78.00
         additives T78.06
         dairy products T78.07
         eggs T78.08
         fish T78.03
            shellfish T78.02
         fruit T78.04
         milk T78.07
         nuts T78.05
            peanuts T78.01
         peanuts T78.01
         seeds T78.05
         specified type NEC T78.09
         vegetable T78.04
      following sting (s)—*see* Table of Drugs and Chemicals, by animal or substance, poisoning
      immunization T80.52-
      serum T80.59-
         blood and blood products T80.51-
         immunization T80.52-
         specified NEC T80.59-
         vaccination T80.52-
   anaphylactoid—*see* Shock, anaphylactic
   cardiogenic R57.0
   chemical substance—*see* Table of Drugs and Chemicals
   culture—*see* Disorder, adjustment
   drug
      due to correct substance properly administered T88.6
      overdose or wrong substance given or taken (by accident)—*see* Table of Drugs and Chemicals, by drug, poisoning
   electric T75.4
      (taser) T75.4

Shock, *continued*
  endotoxic R65.21
    postprocedural (during or resulting from a procedure,
                not elsewhere
                classified) T81.12-
  following
    injury (immediate) (delayed) T79.4
  food (anaphylactic)—*see* Shock, anaphylactic, due to food
  from electroshock gun (taser) T75.4
  gram-negative R65.21
    postprocedural (during or resulting from a procedure,
                NEC) T81.12
  hematologic R57.8
  hemorrhagic
    surgery (intraoperative) (postoperative) T81.19
    trauma T79.4
  hypovolemic R57.1
    surgical T81.19
    traumatic T79.4
  kidney N17.0
    traumatic (following crushing) T79.5
  lung J80
  pleural (surgical) T81.19
    due to trauma T79.4
  postprocedural (postoperative) T81.10
    cardiogenic T81.11
    endotoxic T81.12-
    gram-negative T81.12-
    hypovolemic T81.19
    septic T81.12-
    specified type NEC T81.19
  psychic F43.0
  septic (due to severe sepsis) R65.21
  specified NEC R57.8
  surgical T81.10
  taser gun (taser) T75.4
  therapeutic misadventure NEC T81.10
  toxic, syndrome A48.3
  transfusion—*see* Complications, transfusion
  traumatic (immediate) (delayed) T79.4
Short, shortening, shortness
  arm (acquired)—*see also* Deformity, limb, unequal length
    congenital Q71.81-
  breath R06.02
  bowel syndrome K91.2
  common bile duct, congenital Q44.5
  cystic duct, congenital Q44.5
  frenum, frenulum, linguae (congenital) Q38.1
  hip (acquired)—*see also* Deformity, limb, unequal length
    congenital Q65.89
  leg (acquired)—*see also* Deformity, limb, unequal length
    congenital Q72.81-
  lower limb (acquired)—*see also* Deformity, limb, unequal
                length
    congenital Q72.81-
  stature (child) (hereditary) (idiopathic) NEC R62.52
    constitutional E34.3
    due to endocrine disorder E34.3
    Laron-type E34.3
  tendon—*see also* Contraction, tendon
    with contracture of joint—*see* Contraction, joint
    Achilles (acquired) M67.0-
      congenital Q66.89
    congenital Q79.8
Shunt
  arterial-venous (dialysis) Z99.2
  arteriovenous, pulmonary (acquired) I28.0
    congenital Q25.72
  cerebral ventricle (communicating)in situ Z98.2
Sialitis, silitis (any gland) (chronic) (suppurative)—*see*
                Sialoadenitis
Sialoadenitis (any gland) (periodic) (suppurative) K11.20
  acute K11.21
    recurrent K11.22
  chronic K11.23
Sibling rivalry Z62.891
Sicard's syndrome G52.7
Sick R69
  or handicapped person in family Z63.79
    needing care at home Z63.6
  sinus (syndrome) I49.5

Sickle-cell
  anemia—*see* Disease, sickle-cell
  trait D57.3
Sicklemia—*see also* Disease, sickle-cell
  trait D57.3
Sickness
  air (travel) T75.3
  airplane T75.3
  car T75.3
  green D50.8
  milk—*see* Poisoning, food, noxious
  motion T75.3
  mountain T70.29
    acute D75.1
  protein (*see also* Reaction, serum) T80.69
  roundabout (motion) T75.3
  sea T75.3
  serum NEC (*see also* Reaction, serum) T80.69
  swing (motion) T75.3
  train (railway) (travel) T75.3
  travel (any vehicle) T75.3
Siemens' syndrome (ectodermal dysplasia) Q82.8
Sighing R06.89
  psychogenic F45.8
Sigmoiditis (*see also* Enteritis) K52.9
  infectious A09
  noninfectious K52.9
Silver's syndrome Q87.1
Simple, simplex—*see* condition
Simulation, conscious (of illness) Z76.5
Single
  atrium Q21.2
  umbilical artery Q27.0
Sinus—*see also* Fistula
  bradycardia R00.1
  tachycardia R00.0
    paroxysmal I47.1
  tarsi syndrome—M25.57-
Sinusitis (accessory) (chronic) (hyperplastic) (nasal)
                (nonpurulent) (purulent)
                J32.9
  acute J01.90
    ethmoidal J01.20
      recurrent J01.21
    frontal J01.10
      recurrent J01.11
    involving more than one sinus, other than pansinusitis
                J01.80
      recurrent J01.81
    maxillary J01.00
      recurrent J01.01
    pansinusitis J01.40
      recurrent J01.41
    recurrent J01.91
    specified NEC J01.80
      recurrent J01.81
    sphenoidal J01.30
      recurrent J01.31
  allergic—*see* Rhinitis, allergic
  ethmoidal J32.2
    acute J01.20
      recurrent J01.21
  frontal J32.1
    acute J01.10
      recurrent J01.11
  influenzal—*see* Influenza, with, respiratory manifestations
                NEC
  involving more than one sinus but not pansinusitis J32.8
    acute J01.80
      recurrent J01.81
  maxillary J32.0
    acute J01.00
      recurrent J01.01
  sphenoidal J32.3
    acute J01.30
      recurrent J01.31
Sinusitis-bronchiectasis-situs inversus (syndrome) (triad)
                Q89.3
Siriasis T67.0
Situation, psychiatric F99
Situational
  disturbance (transient)—*see* Disorder, adjustment
    acute F43.0

Situational, *continued*
  maladjustment—*see* Disorder, adjustment
  reaction—*see* Disorder, adjustment
    acute F43.0
Situs inversus or transversus (abdominalis) (thoracis) Q89.3
Sixth disease B08.20
  due to human herpesvirus 6 B08.21
  due to human herpesvirus 7 B08.22
Sjögren-Larsson syndrome Q87.1
Skin—*see also* condition
  clammy R23.1
Sleep
  disorder or disturbance G47.9
    child F51.9
      nonorganic origin F51.9
      specified NEC G47.8
  disturbance G47.9
    nonorganic origin F51.9
  drunkenness F51.9
  rhythm inversion G47.2-
  terrors F51.4
  walking F51.3
    hysterical F44.89
Slim disease (in HIV infection) B20
Slipped, slipping
  epiphysis (traumatic)—*see also* Osteochondropathy,
                specified type NEC
    capital femoral (traumatic)
      acute (on chronic) S79.01-
    current traumatic—*code as* Fracture, by site
    upper femoral (nontraumatic) M93.00-
      acute M93.01-
        on chronic M93.03-
      chronic M93.02-
  ligature, umbilical P51.8
Slow
  feeding, newborn P92.2
  heart (beat) R00.1
Slowing, urinary stream R39.198
Small-and-light-for-dates—*see* Small for dates
Small-for-dates (infant) P05.10
  with weight of
    499 grams or less P05.11
    500–749 grams P05.12
    750–999 grams P05.13
    1000–1249 grams P05.14
    1250–1499 grams P05.15
    1500–1749 grams P05.16
    1750–1999 grams P05.17
    2000–2499 grams P05.18
    2500 grams and over P05.19
Smearing, fecal R15.1
Smith's fracture S52.54-
Smoker—*see* Dependence, drug, nicotine
Smoking
  passive Z77.22
Smothering spells R06.81
Sneezing (intractable) R06.7
Sniffing
  cocaine
    abuse—*see* Abuse, drug, cocaine
    dependence—*see* Dependence, drug, cocaine
  gasoline
    abuse—*see* Abuse, drug, inhalant
    dependence—*see* Dependence, drug, inhalant
  glue (airplane)
    abuse—*see* Abuse, drug, inhalant
    drug dependence—*see* Dependence, drug, inhalant
Sniffles
  newborn P28.89
Snoring R06.83
Snow blindness—*see* Photokeratitis
Snuffles (non-syphilitic) R06.5
  newborn P28.89
Social
  exclusion Z60.4
  migrant Z59.0
    acculturation difficulty Z60.3
  skills inadequacy NEC Z73.4
  transplantation Z60.3
Softening
  brain (necrotic) (progressive) G93.89
    congenital Q04.8

Softening, *continued*
  cartilage M94.2-
    patella M22.4-
Soldier's
  heart F45.8
  patches I31.0
Solitary
  cyst, kidney N28.1
  kidney, congenital Q60.0
Soor B37.0
Sore
  mouth K13.79
    canker K12.0
  muscle M79.1
  skin L98.9
  throat (acute)—*see also* Pharyngitis
    with influenza, flu, or grippe—*see* Influenza,
                with, respiratory
                manifestations NEC
    chronic J31.2
    coxsackie (virus) B08.5
    herpesviral B00.2
    influenzal—*see* Influenza, with, respiratory
                manifestations NEC
    septic J02.0
    streptococcal (ulcerative) J02.0
    viral NEC J02.8
      coxsackie B08.5
Soto's syndrome (cerebral gigantism) Q87.3
Spading nail L60.8
  congenital Q84.6
Spanish collar N47.1
Spasm(s), spastic, spasticity (*see also* condition) R25.2
  artery I73.9
    cerebral G45.9
  anus, ani (sphincter) (reflex) K59.4
    psychogenic F45.8
  bladder (sphincter, external or internal) N32.89
    psychogenic F45.8
  bronchus, bronchiole J98.01
  cerebral (arteries) (vascular) G45.9
  colon K58.9
    with constipation K58.1
    with diarrhea K58.0
    mixed K58.2
    other K58.8
    psychogenic F45.8
  diaphragm (reflex) R06.6
    psychogenic F45.8
  esophagus (diffuse) K22.4
    psychogenic F45.8
  gastrointestinal (tract) K31.89
    psychogenic F45.8
  glottis J38.5
    hysterical F44.4
    psychogenic F45.8
      conversion reaction F44.4
    reflex through recurrent laryngeal nerve J38.5
  habit—*see* Tic
  hysterical F44.4
  intestinal (*see also* Syndrome, irritable bowel) K58.9
    psychogenic F45.8
  larynx, laryngeal J38.5
    hysterical F44.4
    psychogenic F45.8
      conversion reaction F44.4
  muscle NEC M62.838
    back M62.830
  nerve, trigeminal G51.0
  nervous F45.8
  nodding F98.4
  oculogyric H51.8
    psychogenic F45.8
  perineal, female N94.89
  pharynx (reflex) J39.2
    hysterical F45.8
    psychogenic F45.8
  psychogenic F45.8
  pylorus NEC K31.3
    congenital or infantile Q40.0
    psychogenic F45.8
  rectum (sphincter) K59.4
    psychogenic F45.8

Spasm(s), spastic, spasticity, *continued*
  sigmoid (*see also* Syndrome, irritable bowel) K58.9
    psychogenic F45.8
  stomach K31.89
    neurotic F45.8
  throat J39.2
    hysterical F45.8
    psychogenic F45.8
  tic F95.9
    chronic F95.1
    transient of childhood F95.0
  urethra (sphincter) N35.9
Spasmodic—*see* condition
Spasmus nutans F98.4
Spastic, spasticity—*see also* Spasm
  child (cerebral) (congenital) (paralysis) G80.1
Specific, specified—*see* condition
Speech
  defect, disorder, disturbance, impediment R47.9
    psychogenic, in childhood and adolescence F98.8
    slurring R47.81
    specified NEC R47.89
Spens' syndrome (syncope with heart block) I45.9
Spermatocele N43.40
  congenital Q55.4
  multiple N43.42
  single N43.41
Spherocytosis (congenital) (familial) (hereditary) D58.0
  hemoglobin disease D58.0
  sickle-cell (disease) D57.8-
Spider
  bite—*see* Table of Drugs and Chemicals, by animal or
                substance, poisoning
  fingers—*see* Syndrome, Marfan's
  nevus I78.1
  toes—*see* Syndrome, Marfan's
  vascular I78.1
Spiegler-Fendt
  benign lymphocytoma L98.8
Spina bifida (aperta) Q05.9
  with hydrocephalus NEC Q05.4
  cervical Q05.5
    with hydrocephalus Q05.0
  dorsal Q05.6
    with hydrocephalus Q05.1
  lumbar Q05.7
    with hydrocephalus Q05.2
  lumbosacral Q05.7
    with hydrocephalus Q05.2
  occulta Q76.0
  sacral Q05.8
    with hydrocephalus Q05.3
  thoracic Q05.6
    with hydrocephalus Q05.1
  thoracolumbar Q05.6
    with hydrocephalus Q05.1
Splenitis (interstitial) (malignant) (nonspecific) D73.89
  malarial (*see also* Malaria) B54 *[D77]*
  tuberculous A18.85
Splenomegaly, splenomegalia (Bengal) (cryptogenic)
                (idiopathic) (tropical)
                R16.1
  with hepatomegaly R16.2
  malarial (*see also* Malaria) B54 *[D77]*
  neutropenic D73.81
Spondylolisthesis (acquired) (degenerative) M43.10
  congenital Q76.2
Spondylolysis (acquired) M43.00
  congenital Q76.2
Spongioblastoma (any type)—*see* Neoplasm, malignant,
                by site
  specified site—*see* Neoplasm, malignant, by site
  unspecified site C71.9
Spongioneuroblastoma—*see* Neoplasm, malignant, by site
Spontaneous—*see also* condition
  fracture (cause unknown)—*see* Fracture, pathological
Sporadic—*see* condition
Spots, spotting (in) (of)
  café au lait L81.3
  Cayenne pepper I78.1
  de Morgan's (senile angiomas) I78.1
  intermenstrual (regular) N92.0
    irregular N92.1

Spots, spotting, *continued*
  liver L81.4
  purpuric R23.3
  ruby I78.1
Sprain (joint) (ligament)
  ankle S93.40-
    calcaneofibular ligament S93.41-
    deltoid ligament S93.42-
    internal collateral ligament S93.49-
    specified ligament NEC S93.49-
    talofibular ligament S93.49-
    tibiofibular ligament S93.43-
  anterior longitudinal, cervical S13.4
  atlas, atlanto-axial, atlanto-occipital S13.4
  cervical, cervicodorsal, cervicothoracic S13.4
  elbow S53.40-
    radial collateral ligament S53.43-
    radiohumeral S53.41-
    specified type NEC S53.49-
    ulnar collateral ligament S53.44-
    ulnohumeral S53.42-
  finger (s) S63.61-
    index S63.61-
    interphalangeal (joint) S63.63-
      index S63.63-
      little S63.63-
      middle S63.63-
      ring S63.63-
    little S63.61-
    middle S63.61-
    ring S63.61-
    metacarpophalangeal (joint) S63.65-
    specified site NEC S63.69-
      index S63.69-
      little S63.69-
      middle S63.69-
      ring S63.69-
  foot S93.60-
    specified ligament NEC S93.69-
    tarsal ligament S93.61-
    tarsometatarsal ligament S93.62-
  hand S63.9-
    specified site NEC—*see* subcategory S63.8
  innominate
    sacral junction S33.6
  jaw (articular disc) (cartilage) (meniscus) S03.4-
    old M26.69
  knee S83.9-
    collateral ligament S83.40-
      lateral (fibular) S83.42-
      medial (tibial) S83.41-
    cruciate ligament S83.50-
      anterior S83.51-
      posterior S83.52-
  lumbar (spine) S33.5
  lumbosacral S33.9
  mandible (articular disc) S03.4-
    old M26.69
  meniscus
    jaw S03.4-
      old M26.69
    mandible S03.4
      old M26.69
  neck S13.9
    anterior longitudinal cervical ligament S13.4
    atlanto-axial joint S13.4
    atlanto-occipital joint S13.4
    cervical spine S13.4
  pelvis NEC S33.8
  rotator cuff (capsule) S43.42-
  sacroiliac (region)
    joint S33.6
  spine
    cervical S13.4
    lumbar S33.5
  symphysis
    jaw S03.4-
      old M26.69
    mandibular S03.4-
      old M26.69
  talofibular S93.49-
  tarsal—*see* Sprain, foot, specified site NEC
  tarsometatarsal—*see* Sprain, foot, specified site NEC

Sprain (joint) (ligament), *continued*
temporomandibular S03.4-
old M26.69
thumb S63.60-
interphalangeal (joint) S63.62-
metacarpophalangeal (joint) S63.64-
specified site NEC S63.68-
toe (s) S93.50-
great S93.50-
interphalangeal joint S93.51-
great S93.51-
lesser S93.51-
lesser S93.50-
metatarsophalangeal joint S93.52-
great S93.52-
lesser S93.52-
wrist S63.50-
carpal S63.51-
radiocarpal S63.52-
specified site NEC S63.59-
Sprengel's deformity (congenital) Q74.0
Sprue (tropical) K90.1
celiac K90.0
idiopathic K90.49
meaning thrush B37.0
nontropical K90.0
Spur, bone—*see also* Enthesopathy
nose (septum) J34.89
Spurway's syndrome Q78.0
Sputum
abnormal (amount) (color) (odor) (purulent) R09.3
blood-stained R04.2
excessive (cause unknown) R09.3
Squashed nose M95.0
congenital Q67.4
St. Hubert's disease A82.9
Staggering gait R26.0
hysterical F44.4
Stain, staining
meconium (newborn) P96.83
port wine Q82.5
Stammering (*see also* Disorder, fluency) F80.81
Staphylitis (acute) (catarrhal) (chronic) (gangrenous)
(membranous)
(suppurative)
(ulcerative) K12.2
Staphylococcal scalded skin syndrome L00
Staphylococcemia A41.2
Staphylococcus, staphylococcal—*see also* condition
as cause of disease classified elsewhere B95.8
aureus (methicillin susceptible) (MSSA) B95.61
methicillin resistant (MRSA) B95.62
specified NEC, as the cause of disease classified
elsewhere B95.7

Stasis
renal N19
tubular N17.0
State (of)
agitated R45.1
acute reaction to stress F43.0
compulsive F42.8
mixed with obsessional thoughts F42.2
crisis F43.0
depressive F32.9
dissociative F44.9
neurotic F48.9
obsessional F42.8
panic F41.0
persistent vegetative R40.3
pregnant, incidental Z33.1
phobic F40.9
tension (mental) F48.9
specified NEC F48.8
vegetative, persistent R40.3
withdrawal—*see* Withdrawal, state
Status (post)—*see also* Presence (of)
absence, epileptic—*see* Epilepsy, by type, with status
epilepticus
asthmaticus—*see* Asthma, by type, with status
asthmaticus
awaiting organ transplant Z76.82
colectomy (complete) (partial) Z90.49
colonization *see* Carrier (suspected) of

Status (post), *continued*
delinquent immunization Z28.3
dialysis (hemodialysis) (peritoneal) Z99.2
do not resuscitate (DNR) Z66
donor—*see* Donor
epileptic, epilepticus (*see also* Epilepsy, by type, with
status epilepticus)
G40.901
gastrostomy Z93.1
human immunodeficiency virus (HIV) infection,
asymptomatic Z21
lapsed immunization schedule Z28.3
nephrectomy (unilateral) (bilateral) Z90.5
pacemaker
cardiac Z95.0
physical restraint Z78.1
postcommotio cerebri F07.81
postoperative (postprocedural) NEC Z98.890
postsurgical (postprocedural) NEC Z98.890
pregnant, incidental Z33.1
retained foreign body—*see* Retained, foreign body
fragments (type of)
renal dialysis (hemodialysis) (peritoneal) Z99.2
shunt
arteriovenous (for dialysis) Z99.2
cerebrospinal fluid Z98.2
transplant—*see* Transplant
organ removed Z98.85
underimmunization Z28.3
ventricular (communicating) (for drainage) Z98.2
Stealing
child problem F91.8
in company with others Z72.810
Steam burn—*see* Burn
Steatoma L72.3
eyelid (cystic)—*see* Dermatosis, eyelid
infected—*see* Hordeolum
Steatorrhea (chronic) K90.49
idiopathic (adult) (infantile) K90.9
primary K90.0
Stein-Leventhal syndrome E28.2
Stein's syndrome E28.2
Stenocephaly Q75.8
Stenosis, stenotic (cicatricial)—*see also* Stricture
anus, anal (canal) (sphincter) K62.4
and rectum K62.4
congenital Q42.3
with fistula Q42.2
aorta (ascending) (supraventricular) (congenital) Q25.1
aortic (valve) I35.0
with insufficiency I35.2
congenital Q23.0
rheumatic I06.0
with
incompetency, insufficiency or regurgitation I06.2
with mitral (valve) disease I08.0
with tricuspid (valve) disease I08.3
mitral (valve) disease I08.0
with tricuspid (valve) disease I08.3
tricuspid (valve) disease I08.2
with mitral (valve) disease I08.3
specified cause NEC I35.0
aqueduct of Sylvius (congenital) Q03.0
with spina bifida—*see* Spina bifida, by site, with
hydrocephalus
acquired G91.1
bile duct (common) (hepatic) K83.1
congenital Q44.3
brain G93.89
colon—*see also* Obstruction, intestine
congenital Q42.9
specified NEC Q42.8
common (bile) duct K83.1
congenital Q44.3
heart valve (congenital) Q24.8
aortic Q23.0
pulmonary Q22.1
hypertrophic subaortic (idiopathic) I42.1
intestine—*see also* Obstruction, intestine
congenital (small) Q41.9
large Q42.9
specified NEC Q42.8
specified NEC Q41.8

Stenosis, stenotic, *continued*
mitral (chronic) (inactive) (valve) I05.0
with
aortic valve disease I08.0
incompetency, insufficiency or regurgitation I05.2
active or acute I01.1
with rheumatic or Sydenham's chorea I02.0
congenital Q23.2
specified cause, except rheumatic I34.2
myocardium, myocardial—*see also* Degeneration,
myocardial
hypertrophic subaortic (idiopathic) I42.1
nares (anterior) (posterior) J34.89
congenital Q30.0
pulmonary (artery) (congenital) Q25.6
with ventricular septal defect, transposition of aorta,
and hypertrophy of
right ventricle Q21.3
in tetralogy of Fallot Q21.3
infundibular Q24.3
subvalvular Q24.3
supravalvular Q25.6
valve I37.0
with insufficiency I37.2
congenital Q22.1
rheumatic I09.89
with aortic, mitral or tricuspid (valve) disease
I08.8
pulmonic (congenital) Q22.1
pylorus (hypertrophic) (acquired) K31.1
congenital Q40.0
infantile Q40.0
subaortic (congenital) Q24.4
hypertrophic (idiopathic) I42.1
tricuspid (valve) I07.0
with
aortic (valve) disease I08.2
incompetency, insufficiency or regurgitation I07.2
with aortic (valve) disease I08.2
with mitral (valve) disease I08.3
mitral (valve) disease I08.1
with aortic (valve) disease I08.3
congenital Q22.4
nonrheumatic I36.0
with insufficiency I36.2
ureteropelvic junction, congenital Q62.11
ureterovesical orifice, congenital Q62.12
vagina N89.5
congenital Q52.4
valve (cardiac) (heart) (*see also* Endocarditis) I38
congenital Q24.8
aortic Q23.0
pulmonary Q22.1
Stercolith (impaction) K56.41
Stercoraceous, stercoral ulcer K63.3
anus or rectum K62.6
Stereotypies NEC F98.4
Steroid
effects (adverse) (adrenocortical) (iatrogenic)
cushingoid E24.2
correct substance properly administered—*see*
Table of Drugs and
Chemicals, by drug,
adverse effect
overdose or wrong substance given or taken—*see*
Table of Drugs and
Chemicals, by drug,
poisoning
Stevens-Johnson disease or syndrome L51.1
toxic epidermal necrolysis overlap L51.3
Sticker's disease B08.3
Stiffness, joint NEC M25.60-
ankle M25.67-
ankylosis—*see* Ankylosis, joint
contracture—*see* Contraction, joint
elbow M25.62-
foot M25.67-
hand M25.64-
hip M25.65-
knee M25.66-
shoulder M25.61-
wrist M25.63-

Stokes-Adams disease or syndrome I45.9
Stomatitis (denture) (ulcerative) K12.1
  angular K13.0
    due to dietary or vitamin deficiency E53.0
  aphthous K12.0
  bovine B08.61
  candidal B37.0
  catarrhal K12.1
  due to
    dietary deficiency E53.0
    thrush B37.0
  follicular K12.1
  herpesviral, herpetic B00.2
  herpetiformis K12.0
  malignant K12.1
  membranous acute K12.1
  monilial B37.0
  mycotic B37.0
  parasitic B37.0
  septic K12.1
  suppurative (acute) K12.2
  vesicular K12.1
    with exanthem (enteroviral) B08.4
Stomatomycosis B37.0
Stomatorrhagia K13.79
Stovkis (-Talma) **disease** D74.8
Strabismus (congenital) (nonparalytic) H50.9
  concomitant H50.40
    convergent—*see* Strabismus, convergent concomitant
    divergent—*see* Strabismus, divergent concomitant
  convergent concomitant H50.00
    accommodative component H50.43
    alternating H50.05
      with
        A pattern H50.06
        specified nonconcomitances NEC H50.08
        V pattern H50.07
      monocular H50.01-
        with
          A pattern H50.02-
          specified nonconcomitances NEC H50.04-
          V pattern H50.03-
        intermittent H50.31-
          alternating H50.32
  cyclotropia H50.41
  divergent concomitant H50.10
    alternating H50.15
      with
        A pattern H50.16
        specified noncomitances NEC H50.18
        V pattern H50.17
      monocular H50.11-
        with
          A pattern H50.12-
          specified noncomitances NEC H50.14-
          V pattern H50.13-
        intermittent H50.33
          alternating H50.34
  Duane's syndrome H50.81-
  due to adhesions, scars H50.69
  heterophoria H50.50
    alternating H50.55
    cyclophoria H50.54
    esophoria H50.51
    exophoria H50.52
    vertical H50.53
  heterotropia H50.40
    intermittent H50.30
  hypertropia H50.2-
  hypotropia—*see* Hypertropia
  latent H50.50
  mechanical H50.60
    Brown's sheath syndrome H50.61-
    specified type NEC H50.69
  monofixation syndrome H50.42
  paralytic H49.9
    abducens nerve H49.2-
    fourth nerve H49.1-
    Kearns-Sayre syndrome H49.81-
    ophthalmoplegia (external)
      progressive H49.4-
        with pigmentary retinopathy H49.81-
      total H49.3-

Strabismus, *continued*
    sixth nerve H49.2-
    specified type NEC H49.88-
    third nerve H49.0-
    trochlear nerve H49.1-
  specified type NEC H50.89
  vertical H50.2-
Strangulation, strangulated—*see also* Asphyxia, traumatic
  bladder-neck N32.0
  bowel or colon K56.2
  intestine (large) (small) K56.2
    with hernia—*see also* Hernia, by site, with obstruction
      with gangrene—*see* Hernia, by site, with gangrene
  mesentery K56.2
  omentum K56.2
  organ or site, congenital NEC—*see* Atresia, by site
  vesicourethral orifice N32.0
Strangury R30.0
Strawberry
  mark Q82.5
Straw itch B88.0
Strephosymbolia F81.0
  secondary to organic lesion R48.8
Streptococcus, streptococcal—*see also* condition
  as cause of disease classified elsewhere B95.5
  group
    A, as cause of disease classified elsewhere B95.0
    B, as cause of disease classified elsewhere B95.1
    D, as cause of disease classified elsewhere B95.2
    pneumoniae, as cause of disease classified elsewhere B95.3
    specified NEC, as cause of disease classified elsewhere B95.4
Stress F43.9
  family—*see* Disruption, family
  fetal P84
  polycythemia D75.1
  reaction (*see also* Reaction, stress) F43.9
Stricture—*see also* Stenosis
  anus (sphincter) K62.4
    congenital Q42.3
      with fistula Q42.2
    infantile Q42.3
      with fistula Q42.3
  aorta (ascending) (congenital) Q25.1
  aortic (valve)—*see* Stenosis, aortic
  aqueduct of Sylvius (congenital) Q03.0
    with spina bifida—*see* Spina bifida, by site, with hydrocephalus
    acquired G91.1
  artery I77.1
    congenital (peripheral) Q27.8
      umbilical Q27.0
  bile duct (common) (hepatic) K83.1
    congenital Q44.3
  bladder N32.89
    neck N32.0
  brain G93.89
  colon—*see also* Obstruction, intestine
    congenital Q42.9
      specified NEC Q42.8
  digestive organs NEC, congenital Q45.8
  fallopian tube N97.1
    gonococcal A54.24
  heart—*see also* Disease, heart
    valve (*see also* Endocarditis) I38
      aortic Q23.0
      mitral Q23.4
      pulmonary Q22.1
  intestine—*see also* Obstruction, intestine
    congenital (small) Q41.9
      large Q42.9
        specified NEC Q42.8
      specified NEC Q41.8
    ischemic K55.1
  myocardium, myocardial I51.5
    hypertrophic subaortic (idiopathic) I42.1
  nares (anterior) (posterior) J34.89
    congenital Q30.0
  nose J34.89
    congenital Q30.0
  nostril (anterior) (posterior) J34.89
    congenital Q30.0

Stricture, *continued*
  pelviureteric junction (congenital) Q62.11
  pulmonary, pulmonic
    artery (congenital) Q25.6
      infundibulum (congenital) Q24.3
    valve I37.0
      congenital Q22.1
  punctum lacrimale—*see also* Stenosis, lacrimal, punctum
    congenital Q10.5
  pylorus (hypertrophic) K31.1
    congenital Q40.0
    infantile Q40.0
  rectum (sphincter) K62.4
    congenital Q42.1
      with fistula Q42.0
    due to
      chlamydial lymphogranuloma A55
      lymphogranuloma venereum A55
    gonococcal A54.6
    inflammatory (chlamydial) A55
    syphilitic A52.74
  subaortic Q24.4
    hypertrophic (acquired) (idiopathic) I42.1
  ureter (postoperative) N13.5
    with
      hydronephrosis N13.1
  ureteropelvic junction N13.0
    congenital Q62.11
  urethra (organic) (spasmodic) N35.9
    congenital Q64.39
      valvular (posterior) Q64.2
    gonococcal, gonorrheal A54.01
    postinfective NEC
      female N35.12
      male N35.119
        anterior urethra N35.114
        bulbous urethra N35.112
        meatal N35.111
        membranous urethra N35.113
    post-traumatic
      female N35.028
      male N35.014
        anterior urethra N35.013
        bulbous urethra N35.011
        meatal N35.010
        membranous urethra N35.012
    specified cause NEC N35.8
  valve (cardiac) (heart)—*see also* Endocarditis
    congenital
      aortic Q23.0
      pulmonary Q22.1
  vesicourethral orifice N32.0
    congenital Q64.31
Stridor R06.1
  congenital (larynx) P28.89
Stroke (apoplectic) (brain) (embolic) (ischemic) (paralytic) (thrombotic) I63.9
  epileptic—*see* Epilepsy
  heat T67.0
Struma—*see also* Goiter
  nodosa (simplex) E04.9
    endemic E01.2
    multinodular E01.1
Stupor (catatonic) R40.1
  reaction to exceptional stress (transient) F43.0
Sturge (-Weber) (-Dimitri) (-Kalischer) **disease or syndrome** Q85.8
Stuttering F80.81
  childhood onset F80.81
  in conditions classified elsewhere R47.82
Sty, stye (external) (internal) (meibomian) (zeisian)—*see* Hordeolum
Subacidity, gastric K31.89
  psychogenic F45.8
Subacute—*see* condition
Subarachnoid—*see* condition
Subcortical—*see* condition
Subglossitis—*see* Glossitis
Subhemophilia D66
Subluxation—*see also* Dislocation
  finger S63.20-
    index S63.20-
      interphalangeal S63.22-

Subluxation, *continued*
distal S63.24-
index S63.24-
little S63.24-
middle S63.24-
ring S63.24-
index S63.22-
little S63.22-
middle S63.22-
proximal S63.23-
index S63.23-
little S63.23-
middle S63.23-
ring S63.23-
ring S63.22-
little S63.20-
metacarpophalangeal (joint) S63.21-
index S63.26-
little S63.26-
middle S63.26-
ring S63.26-
middle S63.20-
ring S63.20
hip S73.00-
anterior S73.03-
obturator S73.02-
central S73.04-
posterior S73.01-
interphalangeal (joint)
finger S63.22-
distal joint S63.24-
index S63.24-
little S63.24-
middle S63.24-
ring S63.24-
index S63.22-
little S63.22-
middle S63.22-
proximal joint S63.23-
index S63.23-
little S63.23-
middle S63.23-
ring S63.23-
ring S63.22-
thumb S63.12-
distal joint S63.14-
proximal joint S63.13-
knee S83.10-
cap—*see* Subluxation, patella
patella—*see* Subluxation, patella
proximal tibia
anteriorly S83.11-
laterally S83.14-
medially S83.13-
posteriorly S83.12-
specified type NEC S83.19-
metacarpal (bone)
proximal end S63.06-
metacarpophalangeal (joint)
finger S63.21-
index S63.21-
little S63.21-
middle S63.21-
ring S63.21-
thumb S63.11-
patella S83.00-
lateral S83.01-
recurrent (nontraumatic) M22.1-
specified type NEC S83.09-
radial head S53.00-
nursemaid's elbow S53.03-
specified type NEC S53.09-
thumb S63.103
interphalangeal joint—*see* Subluxation,
interphalangeal (joint),
thumb
metacarpophalangeal joint S63.11-
Submersion (fatal) (nonfatal) T75.1
Substernal thyroid E04.9
congenital Q89.2
Substitution disorder F44.9
Subthyroidism (acquired)—*see also* Hypothyroidism
congenital E03.1

Sucking thumb, child (excessive) F98.8
Sudamen, sudamina L74.1
Sugar
blood
high (transient) R73.9
low (transient) E16.2
in urine R81
Suicide, suicidal (attempted) T14.91
by poisoning—*see* Table of Drugs and Chemicals
history of (personal) Z91.5
in family Z81.8
ideation—*see* Ideation, suicidal
risk
meaning personal history of attempted suicide Z91.5
meaning suicidal ideation—*see* Ideation, suicidal
tendencies
meaning personal history of attempted suicide Z91.5
meaning suicidal ideation—*see* Ideation, suicidal
trauma—*see* nature of injury by site
Sulfhemoglobinemia, sulphemoglobinemia (acquired) (with
methemoglobinemia)
D74.8
Sunburn L55.9
due to
tanning bed (acute) L56.8
first degree L55.0
second degree L55.1
third degree L55.2
Sunstroke T67.0
Supernumerary (congenital)
carpal bones Q74.0
finger Q69.0
nipple (s) Q83.3
tarsal bones Q74.2
testis Q55.29
thumb Q69.1
toe Q69.2
Supervision (of)
contraceptive—*see* Prescription, contraceptives
dietary (for) Z71.3
allergy (food) Z71.3
colitis Z71.3
diabetes mellitus Z71.3
food allergy or intolerance Z71.3
gastritis Z71.3
hypercholesterolemia Z71.3
hypoglycemia Z71.3
intolerance (food) Z71.3
obesity Z71.3
specified NEC Z71.3
healthy infant or child Z76.2
foundling Z76.1
lactation Z39.1
Suppression
menstruation N94.89
urine, urinary secretion R34
Suppuration, suppurative—*see also* condition
accessory sinus (chronic)—*see* Sinusitis
antrum (chronic)—*see* Sinusitis, maxillary
bladder—*see* Cystitis
brain G06.0
sequelae G09
breast N61.1
ear (middle)—*see also* Otitis, media
external NEC—*see* Otitis, externa, infective
internal—*see* subcategory H83.0
ethmoidal (chronic) (sinus)—*see* Sinusitis, ethmoidal
frontal (chronic) (sinus)—*see* Sinusitis, frontal
gallbladder (acute) K81.0
intracranial G06.0
joint—*see* Arthritis, pyogenic or pyemic
labyrinthine—*see* subcategory H83.0
mammary gland N61.1
maxilla, maxillary M27.2
sinus (chronic)—*see* Sinusitis, maxillary
muscle—*see* Myositis, infective
nasal sinus (chronic)—*see* Sinusitis
pelvis, pelvic
female—*see* Disease, pelvis, inflammatory
male K65.0
sinus (accessory) (chronic) (nasal)—*see* Sinusitis
sphenoidal sinus (chronic)—*see* Sinusitis, sphenoidal
thyroid (gland) E06.0

Suppuration, suppurative, *continued*
tonsil—*see* Tonsillitis
uterus—*see* Endometritis
Supraglottitis J04.30
with obstruction J04.31
Surgical
shock T81.10
Surveillance (of) (for)—*see also* Observation
alcohol abuse Z71.41
contraceptive—*see* Prescription, contraceptives
dietary Z71.3
drug abuse Z71.51
Suspected condition, ruled out—*see also* Observation,
suspected
fetal anomaly Z03.73
fetal growth Z03.74
newborn—*see* Observation, newborn, suspected
condition ruled out
Z09.5
Suture
burst (in operation wound) T81.31
external operation wound T81.31
removal Z48.02
Swearing, compulsive F42.8
in Gilles de la Tourette's syndrome F95.2
Sweat, sweats
night R61
Sweating, excessive R61
Swelling (of) R60.9
abdomen, abdominal (not referable to any particular
organ)—*see* Mass,
abdominal
ankle—*see* Effusion, joint, ankle
arm M79.89
forearm M79.89
breast N63
chest, localized R22.2
extremity (lower) (upper)—*see* Disorder, soft tissue,
specified type NEC
finger M79.89
foot M79.89
glands R59.9
generalized R59.1
localized R59.0
hand M79.89
head (localized) R22.0
inflammatory—*see* Inflammation
intra-abdominal—*see* Mass, abdominal
joint—*see* Effusion, joint
leg M79.89
lower M79.89
limb—*see* Disorder, soft tissue, specified type NEC
localized (skin) R22.9
chest R22.2
head R22.0
limb
lower—*see* Mass, localized, limb, lower
upper—*see* Mass, localized, limb, upper
neck R22.1
trunk R22.2
neck (localized) R22.1
pelvic—*see* Mass, abdominal
scrotum N50.89
splenic—*see* Splenomegaly
testis N50.89
toe M79.89
umbilical R19.09
Swimmer's
cramp T75.1
ear H60.33-
itch B65.3
Swimming in the head R42
Swollen—*see* Swelling
Sycocis L73.8
barbae (not parasitic) L73.8
contagiosa (mycotic) B35.0
lupoides L73.8
mycotic B35.0
parasitic B35.0
vulgaris L73.8
Symond's syndrome G93.2
Sympathetic—*see* condition

Sympathicoblastoma
  specified site—*see* Neoplasm, malignant, by site
  unspecified site C74.90
Sympathogonioma—*see* Sympathicoblastoma
Symphalangy (fingers) (toes) Q70.9
Symptoms NEC R68.89
  breast NEC N64.59
  development NEC R63.8
  genital organs, female R10.2
  involving
    abdomen NEC R19.8
    awareness R41.9
      altered mental status R41.82
    cardiovascular system NEC R09.89
    chest NEC R09.89
    circulatory system NEC R09.89
    cognitive functions R41.9
      altered mental status R41.82
    development NEC R62.50
    digestive system R19.8
    food and fluid intake R63.8
    general perceptions and sensations R44.9
      specified NEC R44.8
    musculoskeletal system R29.91
      specified NEC R29.898
    nervous system R29.90
      specified NEC R29.818
    pelvis R19.8
    respiratory system NEC R09.89
  metabolism NEC R63.8
  of infancy R68.19
  pelvis NEC, female R10.2
Sympus Q74.2
Syncope (near) (pre-) R55
  bradycardia R00.1
  cardiac R55
  heart R55
  heat T67.1
  laryngeal R05
  psychogenic F48.8
  tussive R05
  vasoconstriction R55
  vasodepressor R55
  vasomotor R55
  vasovagal R55
Syndactylism, syndactyly Q70.9
  complex (with synostosis)
    fingers Q70.0-
    toes Q70.2-
  simple (without synostosis)
    fingers Q70.1-
    toes Q70.3-
Syndrome—*see also* Disease
  abdominal
    acute R10.0
    muscle deficiency Q79.4
  abstinence, neonatal P96.1
  acquired immunodeficiency—*see* Human,
                    immunodeficiency virus
                    (HIV) disease
  acute abdominal R10.0
  acute respiratory distress (adult) (child) J80
    idiopathic J84.114
  Adair-Dighton Q78.0
  Adams-Stokes (-Morgagni) I45.9
  adrenocortical—*see* Cushing's, syndrome
  adrenogenital E25.9
    congenital, associated with enzyme deficiency E25.0
  Aldrich (-Wiskott) D82.0
  Alport Q87.81
  alveolar hypoventilation E66.2
  androgen insensitivity E34.50
    complete E34.51
    partial E34.52
  androgen resistance (*see also* Syndrome, androgen
                    insensitivity) E34.50
  ankyloglossia superior Q38.1
  antibody deficiency D80.9
    agammaglobulinemic D80.1
      hereditary D80.0
    congenital D80.0
    hypogammaglobulinemic D80.1
      hereditary D80.0

Syndrome, *continued*
  Arnold-Chiari—*see* Arnold-Chiari disease
  Arrillaga-Ayerza I27.0
  arterial tortuosity Q87.82
  aspiration, of newborn—*see* Aspiration, by substance,
                    with pneumonia
    meconium P24.01
  ataxia-telangiectasia G11.3
  autoerythrocyte sensitization (Gardner-Diamond) D69.2
  autoimmune lymphoproliferative *[ALPS]* D89.82
  Ayerza (-Arrillaga) I27.0
  Beals Q87.40
  Bernheim's I50.9
  bilateral polycystic ovarian E28.2
  black
    widow spider bite—*see* Table of Drugs and Chemicals,
                    by animal or substance,
                    poisoning
  Blackfan-Diamond D61.01
  blind loop K90.2
    congenital Q43.8
    postsurgical K91.2
  blue sclera Q78.0
  Boder-Sedgewick G11.3
  Borjeson Forssman Lehmann Q89.8
  Bouillaud's I01.9
  Bourneville (-Pringle) Q85.1
  bradycardia-tachycardia I49.5
  brain (nonpsychotic) F09
    with psychosis, psychotic reaction F09
    acute or subacute—*see* Delirium
    congenital—*see* Disability, intellectual
    organic F09
      post-traumatic (nonpsychotic) F07.81
    postcontusional F07.81
    post-traumatic, nonpsychotic F07.81
  Brock's J98.11
  bronze baby P83.8
  Burnett's (milk-alkali) E83.52
  cardiacos negros I27.0
  cardiopulmonary-obesity E66.2
  cardiorespiratory distress (idiopathic), newborn P22.0
  cat cry Q93.4
  celiac K90.0
  cerebral
    gigantism E22.0
  CHARGE Q89.8
  child maltreatment—*see* Maltreatment, child
  chondrocostal junction M94.0
  chromosome 5 short arm deletion Q93.4
  Clerambault's automatism G93.89
  clumsiness, clumsy child F82
  cluster headache G44.009
    intractable G44.001
    not intractable G44.009
  Coffin-Lowry Q89.8
  combined immunity deficiency D81.9
  concussion F07.81
  congenital
    facial diplegia Q87.0
    oculo-auriculovertebral Q87.0
    oculofacial diplegia (Moebius) Q87.0
    rubella (manifest) P35.0
  congestive dysmenorrhea N94.6
  Costen's (complex) M26.69
  costochondral junction M94.0
  costovertebral E22.0
  Cowden Q85.8
  cri-du-chat Q93.4
  crib death R99
  croup J05.0
  Cushing's E24.9
    due to
      drugs E24.2
      overproduction of pituitary ACTH E24.0
    drug-induced E24.2
    overdose or wrong substance given or taken—*see*
                    Table of Drugs and
                    Chemicals, by drug,
                    poisoning
    pituitary-dependent E24.0
    specified type NEC E24.8
  cryptophthalmos Q87.0

Syndrome, *continued*
  Dandy-Walker Q03.1
    with spina bifida Q07.01
  defibrination—*see also* Fibrinolysis
    newborn P60
  dependence—*see* F10-F19 with fourth character .2
  De Quervain E34.51
  diabetes mellitus in newborn infant P70.2
  Diamond-Blackfan D61.01
  Diamond-Gardener D69.2
  DIC (diffuse or disseminated intravascular coagulopathy)
                    D65
  di George's D82.1
  Dighton's Q78.0
  disequilibrium E87.8
  Down (*see also* Down syndrome) Q90.9
  Dressler's (postmyocardial infarction) I24.1
    postcardiotomy I97.0
  drug withdrawal, infant of dependent mother P96.1
  due to abnormality
    chromosomal Q99.9
      sex
        female phenotype Q97.9
        male phenotype Q98.9
        specified NEC Q99.8
  Dupré's (meningism) R29.1
  dysmetabolic X E88.81
  dyspraxia, developmental F82
  Eagle-Barrett Q79.4
  eczema-thrombocytopenia D82.0
  Eddowes' Q78.0
  effort (psychogenic) F45.8
  Ehlers-Danlos Q79.6
  Eisenmenger's I27.89
  Ekman's Q78.0
  eosinophilia-myalgia M35.8
  epileptic—*see also* Epilepsy, by type
    absence G40.A09
      intractable G40.A19
        with status epilepticus G40.A11
        without status epilepticus G40.A19
      not intractable G40.A09
        with status epilepticus G40.A01
        without status epilepticus G40.A09
  Erdheim's E22.0
  Evans D69.41
  eye retraction—*see* Strabismus
  eyelid-malar-mandible Q87.0
  Fallot's Q21.3
  familial eczema-thrombocytopenia (Wiskott-Aldrich) D82.0
  Fanconi's (anemia) (congenital pancytopenia) D61.09
  fatigue
    chronic R53.82
  faulty bowel habit K59.39
  fetal
    alcohol (dysmorphic) Q86.0
  Fiedler's I40.1
  first arch Q87.0
  fish odor E72.8
  floppy
    baby P94.2
  food protein-induced enterocolitis K52.21
  fragile X Q99.2
  Fukuhara E88.49
  functional
    bowel K59.9
  Gaisböck's D75.1
  Gardner-Diamond D69.2
  Gee-Herter-Heubner K90.0
  Gianotti-Crosti L44.4
  Gilles de la Tourette's F95.2
  Goldberg Q89.8
  Goldberg-Maxwell E34.51
  Gouley's I31.1
  Gower's R55
  hand-foot L27.1
  hemophagocytic, infection-associated D76.2
  Henoch-Schönlein D69.0
  hepatopulmonary K76.81
  Herter (-Gee) (nontropical sprue) K90.0
  Heubner-Herter K90.0
  histamine-like (fish poisoning)—*see* Poisoning, fish
  histiocytic D76.3

SYMPATHICOBLASTOMA-SYNDROME

Syndrome, *continued*
- histiocytosis NEC D76.3
- HIV infection, acute B20
- Hoffmann-Werdnig G12.0
- hypereosinophilic (idiopathic) D72.1
- hyperkinetic—*see* Hyperkinesia
- hypernatremia E87.0
- hyperosmolarity E87.0
- hypertransfusion, newborn P61.1
- hyperventilation F45.8
- hyperviscosity (of serum)
    - polycythemic D75.1
- hypoglycemic (familial) (neonatal) E16.2
- hyponatremic E87.1
- hypoplastic left-heart Q23.4
- hyposmolality E87.1
- hypothenar hammer I73.89
- ICF (intravascular coagulation-fibrinolysis) D65
- idiopathic
    - cardiorespiratory distress, newborn P22.0
    - nephrotic (infantile) N04.9
- immunity deficiency, combined D81.9
- immunodeficiency
    - acquired—*see* Human, immunodeficiency virus (HIV) disease
    - combined D81.9
- inappropriate secretion of antidiuretic hormone E22.2
- inspissated bile (newborn) P59.1
- intestinal
    - knot K56.2
- intravascular coagulation-fibrinolysis (ICF) D65
- IRDS (idiopathic respiratory distress, newborn) P22.0
- irritable
    - bowel K58.9
        - with constipation K58.1
        - with diarrhea K58.0
        - mixed K58.2
        - other K58.8
        - psychogenic F45.8
    - heart (psychogenic) F45.8
- IVC (intravascular coagulopathy) D65
- Jervell-Lange-Nielsen I45.81
- Job's D71
- Joseph-Diamond-Blackfan D61.01
- jugular foramen G52.7
- Kabuki Q89.8
- Kanner's (autism) F84.0
- Kartagener's Q89.3
- Kostmann's D70.0
- Launois' E22.0
- lazy
    - leukocyte D70.8
- Lemiere I80.8
- Lennox-Gastaut G40.812
    - intractable G40.814
        - with status epilepticus G40.813
        - without status epilepticus G40.814
    - not intractable G40.812
        - with status epilepticus G40.811
        - without status epilepticus G40.812
- Leopold-Levi's E05.90
- Lev's I44.2
- long arm 18 or 21 deletion Q93.89
- long QT I45.81
- Louis-Barré G11.3
- low
    - output (cardiac) I50.9
- Luetscher's (dehydration) E86.0
- Lutembacher's Q21.1
- macrophage activation D76.1
    - due to infection D76.2
- Mal de Debarquement R42
- malabsorption K90.9
    - postsurgical K91.2
- malformation, congenital, due to
    - alcohol Q86.0
- maple-syrup-urine E71.0
- Marfan's Q87.40
    - with
        - cardiovascular manifestations Q87.418
            - aortic dilation Q87.410
        - ocular manifestations Q87.42
        - skeletal manifestations Q87.43

Syndrome, *continued*
- Marie's E22.0
- mast cell activation D89.40
    - idiopathic D89.42
    - monoclonal D89.41
    - other D89.49
    - secondary D89.43
- McQuarrie's E16.2
- meconium plug (newborn) P76.0
- Meekeren-Ehlers-Danlos Q79.6
- MELAS E88.41
- MERRF (myoclonic epilepsy associated with ragged-red fibers) E88.42
- metabolic E88.81
- micrognathia-glossoptosis Q87.0
- midbrain NEC G93.89
- milk-alkali E83.52
- Miller-Dieker Q93.88
- Minkowski-Chauffard D58.0
- MNGIE (Mitochondrial Neurogastrointestinal Encephalopathy) E88.49
- Morgagni-Adams-Stokes I45.9
- mucocutaneous lymph node (acute febrile) (MCLS) M30.3
- myasthenic G70.9
    - in
        - diabetes mellitus—*see* Diabetes, amyotrophy
        - endocrine disease NEC E34.9 [G73.3]
        - neoplastic disease (*see also* Neoplasm) D49.9 [G73.3]
        - thyrotoxicosis (hyperthyroidism) E05.90 [G73.3]
            - with thyroid storm E05.91 [G73.3]
- myofascial pain M79.1
- NARP (Neuropathy, Ataxia and Retinitis pigmentosa) E88.49
- neonatal abstinence P96.1
- nephritic—*see also* Nephritis
    - with edema—*see* Nephrosis
    - acute N00.9
    - chronic N03.9
- nephrotic (congenital) (*see also* Nephrosis) N04.9
    - with
        - dense deposit disease N04.6
        - diffuse
            - crescentic glomerulonephritis N04.7
            - endocapillary proliferative glomerulonephritis N04.4
            - membranous glomerulonephritis N04.2
            - mesangial proliferative glomerulonephritis N04.3
            - mesangiocapillary glomerulonephritis N04.5
        - focal and segmental glomerular lesions N04.1
        - minor glomerular abnormality N04.0
        - specified morphological changes NEC N04.8
    - diabetic—*see* Diabetes, nephrosis
- Nothnagel's vasomotor acroparesthesia I73.89
- ophthalmoplegia-cerebellar ataxia—*see* Strabismus, paralytic, third nerve
- oral-facial-digital Q87.0
- oro-facial-digital Q87.0
- Osler-Weber-Rendu I78.0
- oto-palatal-digital Q87.0
- ovary
    - polycystic E28.2
    - sclerocystic E28.2
- pain—*see also* Pain
    - complex regional I G90.50
        - lower limb G90.52-
            - specified site NEC G90.59
        - upper limb G90.51-
- painful
    - bruising D69.2
- paralytic G83.9
    - specified NEC G83.89
- pharyngeal pouch D82.1
- Pick's (heart) (liver) I31.1
- Pickwickian E66.2
- pituitary E22.0
- pontine NEC G93.89
- postcardiac injury
    - postcardiotomy I97.0
- postcommissurotomy I97.0
- postconcussional F07.81

Syndrome, *continued*
- postcontusional F07.81
- postvalvulotomy I97.0
- prune belly Q79.4
- pseudoparalytica G70.00
    - with exacerbation (acute) G70.01
    - in crisis G70.01
- pseudo -Turner's Q87.1
- pulmonary
    - arteriosclerosis I27.0
    - dysmaturity (Wilson-Mikity) P27.0
    - hypoperfusion (idiopathic) P22.0
- QT interval prolongation I45.81
- RDS (respiratory distress syndrome, newborn) P22.0
- Reifenstein E34.52
- Rendu-Osler-Weber I78.0
- respiratory
    - distress
        - acute J80
            - child J80
            - idiopathic J84.114
        - newborn (idiopathic) (type I) P22.0
            - type II P22.1
- retinoblastoma (familial) C69.2
- retroviral seroconversion (acute) Z21
- Romano-Ward (prolonged QT interval) I45.81
- rubella (congenital) P35.0
- Ruvalcaba-Myhre-Smith E71.440
- Rytand-Lipsitch I44.2
- salt
    - depletion E87.1
        - due to heat NEC T67.8
            - causing heat exhaustion or prostration T67.4
    - low E87.1
- Scaglietti-Dagnini E22.0
- scapuloperoneal G71.0
- schizophrenic, of childhood NEC F84.5
- Schwartz-Bartter E22.2
- sclerocystic ovary E28.2
- Seitelberger's G31.89
- seroconversion, retroviral (acute) Z21
- serous meningitis G93.2
- severe acute respiratory (SARS) J12.81
- shaken infant T74.4
- shock (traumatic) T79.4
    - kidney N17.0
        - following crush injury T79.5
    - toxic A48.3
- shock-lung J80
- short
    - bowel K91.2
- Shwachman's D70.4
- sick
    - cell E87.1
    - sinus I49.5
- sinus tarsi M25.57-
- sinusitis-bronchiectasis-situs inversus Q89.3
- Smith-Magenis Q93.88
- Soto's Q87.3
- Spen's I45.9
- splenic
    - neutropenia D73.81
- Spurway's Q78.0
- staphylococcal scalded skin L00
- Stein-Leventhal E28.2
- Stein's E28.2
- Stevens-Johnson syndrome L51.1
    - toxic epidermal necrolysis overlap L51.3
- Stickler Q89.8
- stiff baby Q89.8
- Stokes (-Adams) I45.9
- swallowed blood P78.2
- sweat retention L74.0
- Symond's G93.2
- systemic inflammatory response (SIRS), of non-infectious origin (without organ dysfunction) R65.10
    - with acute organ dysfunction R65.11
- tachycardia-bradycardia I49.5
- teething K00.7
- tegmental G93.89
- telangiectasia-pigmentation-cataract Q82.8

SYNDROME-TENSION

Syndrome, *continued*
  temporal pyramidal apex—*see* Otitis, media, suppurative, acute
  temporomandibular joint-pain-dysfunction M26.62-
  testicular feminization (*see also* Syndrome, androgen insensitivity) E34.51
  Tietze's M94.0
  toxic shock A48.3
  triple X, female Q97.0
  trisomy Q92.9
    13 Q91.7
      meiotic nondisjunction Q91.4
    18 Q91.3
      meiotic nondisjunction Q91.0
    21 Q90.9
  tumor lysis (following antineoplastic chemotherapy) (spontaneous) NEC E88.3
  uremia, chronic (*see also* Disease, kidney, chronic) N18.9
  vago-hypoglossal G52.7
  van der Hoeve's Q78.0
  vasovagal R55
  velo-cardio-facial Q93.81
  visual disorientation H53.8
  Werdnig-Hoffman G12.0
  wet
    lung, newborn P22.1
  whiplash S13.4
  whistling face Q87.0
  Wiskott-Aldrich D82.0
  withdrawal—*see* Withdrawal, state
    drug
      infant of dependent mother P96.1
      therapeutic use, newborn P96.2
  Zahorsky's B08.5
  Zellweger syndrome E71.510
  Zellweger-like syndrome E71.541
Synostosis (congenital) Q78.8
  astragalo-scaphoid Q74.2
  radioulnar Q74.0
Syphilis, syphilitic (acquired) A52.79
  age under 2 years NOS—*see also* Syphilis, congenital, early
    acquired A51.9
  anemia (late) A52.79 *[D63.8]*
  asymptomatic—*see* Syphilis, latent
  bubo (primary) A51.0
  chancre (multiple) A51.0
    extragenital A51.2
    Rollet's A51.0
  congenital A50.9
    early, or less than 2 years after birth NEC A50.2
      with manifestations—*see* Syphilis, congenital, early, symptomatic
  contact Z20.2
  cutaneous—*see* Syphilis, skin
  early A51.9
    symptomatic A51.9
      extragenital chancre A51.2
      primary, except extragenital chancre A51.0
  exposure to Z20.2
  genital (primary) A51.0
  inactive—*see* Syphilis, latent
  infantum—*see* Syphilis, congenital
  inherited—*see* Syphilis, congenital
  latent A53.0
    with signs or symptoms—*code by* site and stage under Syphilis
    date of infection unspecified A53.0
    early, or less than 2 years after infection A51.5
    follow-up of latent syphilis A53.0
      date of infection unspecified A53.0
      late, or 2 years or more after infection A52.8
    late, or 2 years or more after infection A52.8
    positive serology (only finding) A53.0
      date of infection unspecified A53.0
      early, or less than 2 years after infection A51.5
      late, or 2 years or more after infection A52.8
  lip A51.39
    chancre (primary) A51.2
    late A52.79
  penis (chancre) A51.0
  primary A51.0

Syphilis, syphilitic, *continued*
  extragenital chancre NEC A51.2
  fingers A51.2
  genital A51.0
  lip A51.2
  specified site NEC A51.2
  tonsils A51.2
  tonsil (lingual) (late) A52.76
    primary A51.2
  vagina A51.0
    late A52.76
  vulva A51.0
    late A52.76
  secondary A51.39
System, systemic—*see also* condition
  inflammatory response syndrome (SIRS) of non-infectious origin (without organ dysfunction) R65.10
    with acute organ dysfunction R65.11
  lupus erythematosus M32.9

T

Tachyalimentation K91.2
Tachyarrhythmia, tachyrhythmia—*see* Tachycardia
Tachycardia R00.0
  atrial (paroxysmal) I47.1
  auricular I47.1
  AV nodal re-entry (re-entrant) I47.1
  junctional (paroxysmal) I47.1
  newborn P29.11
  nodal (paroxysmal) I47.1
  paroxysmal (sustained) (nonsustained) I47.9
    with sinus bradycardia I49.5
    atrial (PAT) I47.1
    atrioventricular (AV) (re-entrant) I47.1
      psychogenic F54
    junctional I47.1
      ectopic I47.1
    nodal I47.1
    supraventricular (sustained) I47.1
  psychogenic F45.8
  sick sinus I49.5
  sinoauricular NOS R00.0
    paroxysmal I47.1
  sinus [sinusal] NOS R00.0
    paroxysmal I47.1
  supraventricular I47.1
  ventricular (paroxysmal) (sustained) I47.2
Tachypnea R06.82
  hysterical F45.8
  newborn (idiopathic) (transitory) P22.1
  psychogenic F45.8
  transitory, of newborn P22.1
TACO (transfusion associated circulatory overload) E87.71
Tag (hypertrophied skin) (infected) L91.8
  adenoid J35.8
  anus K64.4
  hemorrhoidal K64.4
  sentinel K64.4
  skin L91.8
    accessory (congenital) Q82.8
    anus K64.4
    congenital Q82.8
    preauricular Q17.0
  tonsil J35.8
Talipes (congenital) Q66.89
  acquired, planus—*see* Deformity, limb, flat foot
  asymmetric Q66.89
  calcaneovalgus Q66.4
  calcaneovarus Q66.1
  calcaneus Q66.89
  cavus Q66.7
  equinovalgus Q66.6
  equinovarus Q66.0
  equinus Q66.89
  percavus Q66.7
  planovalgus Q66.6
  planus (acquired) (any degree)—*see also* Deformity, limb, flat foot
    congenital Q66.5-
  valgus Q66.6
  varus Q66.3

Tamponade, heart I31.4
Tantrum, child problem F91.8
Tapeworm (infection) (infestation)—*see* Infestation, tapeworm
Tapia's syndrome G52.7
Tattoo (mark) L81.8
Tay-Sachs amaurotic familial idiocy or disease E75.02
TBI (traumatic brain injury) S06.9
Tear, torn (traumatic)—*see also* Laceration
  anus, anal (sphincter) S31.831
    nontraumatic (healed) (old) K62.81
  rotator cuff (nontraumatic) M75.10-
    complete M75.12-
    incomplete M75.11-
    traumatic S46.01-
      capsule S43.42-
  vagina—*see* Laceration, vagina
Teeth—*see also* condition
  grinding
    psychogenic F45.8
    sleep related G47.63
Teething (syndrome) K00.7
Telangiectasia, telangiectasis (verrucous) I78.1
  ataxic (cerebellar) (Louis-Bar) G11.3
  familial I78.0
  hemorrhagic, hereditary (congenital) (senile) I78.0
  hereditary, hemorrhagic (congenital) (senile) I78.0
  spider I78.1
Telescoped bowel or intestine K56.1
  congenital Q43.8
Temperature
  body, high (of unknown origin) R50.9
  cold, trauma from T69.9
    newborn P80.0
    specified effect NEC T69.8
Temporomandibular joint pain-dysfunction syndrome M26.62-
Tendency
  bleeding—*see* Defect, coagulation
  suicide
    meaning personal history of attempted suicide Z91.5
    meaning suicidal ideation—*see* Ideation, suicidal
Tenderness, abdominal R10.819
  epigastric R10.816
  generalized R10.817
  left lower quadrant R10.814
  left upper quadrant R10.812
  periumbilic R10.815
  right lower quadrant R10.813
  right upper quadrant R10.811
  rebound R10.829
    epigastric R10.826
    generalized R10.827
    left lower quadrant R10.824
    left upper quadrant R10.822
    periumbilic R10.825
    right lower quadrant R10.823
    right upper quadrant R10.821
Tendinitis, tendonitis—*see also* Enthesopathy
  Achilles M76.6-
Tenesmus (rectal) R19.8
  vesical R30.1
Tennis elbow—*see* Epicondylitis, lateral
Tenosynovitis (*see also* Synovitis) M65.9
  adhesive—*see* Tenosynovitis, specified type NEC
    shoulder—*see* Capsulitis, adhesive
  shoulder region M65.81-
    adhesive—*see* Capsulitis, adhesive
  specified type NEC M65.88
    ankle M65.87-
    foot M65.87-
    forearm M65.83-
    hand M65.84-
    lower leg M65.86-
    multiple sites M65.89
    pelvic region M65.85-
    shoulder region M65.81-
    specified site NEC M65.88
    thigh M65.85-
    upper arm M65.82-
Tension
  arterial, high—*see also* Hypertension
    without diagnosis of hypertension R03.0

Tension, *continued*
  headache G44.209
    intractable G44.201
    not intractable G44.209
  nervous R45.0
  pneumothorax J93.0
  state (mental) F48.9
Tentorium—*see* condition
Teratencephalus Q89.8
Teratism Q89.7
Terror (s) night (child) F51.4
Test, tests, testing (for)
  blood-alcohol Z04.8
    positive—*see* Findings, abnormal, in blood
  blood-drug Z04.8
    positive—*see* Findings, abnormal, in blood
  hearing Z01.10
    with abnormal findings NEC Z01.118
  HIV (human immunodeficiency virus)
    nonconclusive (in infants) R75
    positive Z21
    seropositive Z21
  immunity status Z01.84
  laboratory (as part of a general medical examination)
        Z00.00
    with abnormal finding Z00.01
    for medicolegal reason NEC Z04.8
  Mantoux (for tuberculosis) Z11.1
    abnormal result R76.11
  skin, diagnostic
    allergy Z01.82
      special screening examination—*see* Screening, by
          name of disease
    Mantoux Z11.1
    tuberculin Z11.1
  specified NEC Z01.89
  tuberculin Z11.1
    abnormal result R76.11
  vision Z01.00
    with abnormal findings Z01.01
  Wassermann Z11.3
    positive—*see* Serology for syphilis, positive
Testicle, testicular, testes—*see also* condition
  feminization syndrome (*see also* Syndrome, androgen
          insensitivity) E34.51
  migrans Q55.29
Tetany (due to) R29.0
  associated with rickets E55.0
  hyperpnea R06.4
    hysterical F44.5
    psychogenic F45.8
  hyperventilation (*see also* Hyperventilation) R06.4
    hysterical F44.5
  neonatal (without calcium or magnesium deficiency) P71.3
  psychogenic (conversion reaction) F44.5
Tetralogy of Fallot Q21.3
Tetraplegia (chronic) (*see also* Quadriplegia) G82.50
Thalassemia (anemia) (disease) D56.9
  with other hemoglobinopathy D56.8
  alpha (major) (severe) (triple gene defect) D56.0
    minor D56.3
    silent carrier D56.3
    trait D56.3
  beta (severe) D56.1
    homozygous D56.1
    major D56.1
    minor D56.3
    trait D56.3
  delta-beta (homozygous) D56.2
    minor D56.3
    trait D56.3
  dominant D56.8
  hemoglobin
    C D56.8
    E-beta D56.5
  intermedia D56.1
  major D56.1
  minor D56.3
  mixed D56.8
  sickle-cell—*see* Disease, sickle-cell, thalassemia
  specified type NEC D56.8
  trait D56.3
  variants D56.8

Thaysen-Gee disease (nontropical sprue) K90.0
Thaysen's disease K90.0
Thelitis N61.0
Therapy
  drug, long-term (current) (prophylactic)
    antibiotics Z79.2
    anti-inflammatory Z79.1
    aspirin Z79.82
    drug, specified NEC Z79.899
    hypoglycemic drugs, oral Z79.84
    insulin Z79.4
    steroids
      inhaled Z79.51
      systemic Z79.52
Thermoplegia T67.0
Thickening
  breast N64.59
Thirst, excessive R63.1
  due to deprivation of water T73.1
Thomsen disease G71.12
Threadworm (infection) (infestation) B80
Threatened
  abortion O20.0
    with subsequent abortion O03.9
  miscarriage O20.0
Thrombocythemia (essential) (hemorrhagic) (idiopathic)
          (primary) D47.3
Thrombocytopenia, thrombocytopenic D69.6
  with absent radius (TAR) Q87.2
  congenital D69.42
  dilutional D69.59
  due to
    drugs D69.59
    extracorporeal circulation of blood D69.59
    (massive) blood transfusion D69.59
    platelet alloimmunization D69.59
  essential D69.3
  hereditary D69.42
  idiopathic D69.3
  neonatal, transitory P61.0
    due to
      exchange transfusion P61.0
      idiopathic maternal thrombocytopenia P61.0
      isoimmunization P61.0
  primary NEC D69.49
    idiopathic D69.3
  secondary D69.59
  transient neonatal P61.0
Thrombocytosis, essential D47.3
  primary D47.3
Thromboembolism—*see* Embolism
Thrombophlebitis I80.9
  femoral vein (superficial) I80.1-
  femoropopliteal vein I80.0-
  hepatic (vein) I80.8
  iliofemoral I80.1-
  leg I80.299
    superficial I80.0-
  lower extremity I80.299
  popliteal vein—*see* Phlebitis, leg, deep, popliteal
  saphenous (greater) (lesser) I80.0-
  specified site NEC I80.8
  tibial vein I80.23-
Thrombosis, thrombotic (bland) (multiple) (progressive)
          (silent) (vessel) I82.90
  anus K64.5
  artery, arteries (postinfectional) I74.9
  genital organ
    female NEC N94.89
  liver (venous) I82.0
    artery I74.8
    portal vein I81
  mesenteric (artery) (with gangrene) K55.0
    vein (inferior) (superior) I81
  perianal venous K64.5
  portal I81
  renal (artery) N28.0
    vein I82.3
  tricuspid I07.8
  vein (acute) I82.90
    perianal K64.5
    renal I82.3
  venous, perianal K64.5

Thrombus—*see* Thrombosis
Thrush—*see also* candidiasis
  oral B37.0
  newborn P37.5
  vagina B37.3
Thumb—*see also* condition
  sucking (child problem) F98.8
Thyroglossal—*see also* condition
  cyst Q89.2
  duct, persistent Q89.2
Thyroid (gland) (body)—*see also* condition
  lingual Q89.2
Thyroiditis E06.9
  acute (nonsuppurative) (pyogenic) (suppurative) E06.0
  pyogenic E06.0
  suppurative E06.0
Thyrolyngual duct, persistent Q89.2
Thyrotoxic
  crisis—*see* Thyrotoxicosis
  heart disease or failure (*see also* Thyrotoxicosis) E05.90
        [143]
    with thyroid storm E05.91 *[143]*
  storm—*see* Thyrotoxicosis
Thyrotoxicosis (recurrent) E05.90
  with
    goiter (diffuse) E05.00
      with thyroid storm E05.01
      adenomatous uninodular E05.10
        with thyroid storm E05.11
      multinodular E05.20
        with thyroid storm E05.21
      nodular E05.20
        with thyroid storm E05.21
      uninodular E05.10
        with thyroid storm E05.11
    heart E05.90 *[143]*
      with thyroid storm E05.91 *[143]*
      failure E05.90 *[143]*
    neonatal (transient) P72.1
Tic (disorder) F95.9
  child problem F95.0
  compulsive F95.1
  de la Tourette F95.2
  disorder
    chronic
      motor F95.1
      vocal F95.1
    combined vocal and multiple motor F95.2
    transient F95.0
  habit F95.9
    transient of childhood F95.0
  lid, transient of childhood F95.0
  motor-verbal F95.2
  orbicularis F95.8
    transient of childhood F95.0
  provisional F95.0
  spasm (motor or vocal) F95.9
    chronic F95.1
    transient of childhood F95.0
Tick-borne—*see* condition
Tietze's disease or syndrome M94.0
Tight, tightness
  anus K62.89
  foreskin (congenital) N47.1
  rectal sphincter K62.89
  urethral sphincter N35.9
Timidity, child F93.8
Tinea (intersecta) (tarsi) B35.9
  asbestina B35.0
  barbae B35.0
  beard B35.0
  black dot B35.0
  capitis B35.0
  corporis B35.4
  cruris B35.6
  flava B36.0
  foot B35.3
  furfuracea B36.0
  imbricata (Tokelau) B35.5
  kerion B35.0
  microsporic—*see* Dermatophytosis
  nodosa—*see* Piedra
  pedis B35.3

Tinea, *continued*
scalp B35.0
specified site NEC B35.8
sycosis B35.0
tonsurans B35.0
trichophytic—*see* Dermatophytosis
unguium B35.1
versicolor B36.0
Tinnitus NOS H93.1-
audible H93.1-
aurium H93.1-
pulsatile H93.A-
subjective H93.1-
Tiredness R53.83
Tobacco (nicotine)
abuse—*see* Tobacco, use
dependence—*see* Dependence, drug, nicotine
harmful use Z72.0
heart—*see* Tobacco, toxic effect
maternal use, affecting newborn P04.2
toxic effect—*see* Table of Drugs and Chemicals, by
substance, poisoning
chewing tobacco—*see* Table of Drugs and Chemicals,
by substance,
poisoning
cigarettes—*see* Table of Drugs and Chemicals, by
substance, poisoning
use Z72.0
counseling and surveillance Z71.6
history Z87.891
withdrawal state—*see* Dependence, drug, nicotine
F17.203
Tongue—*see also* condition
tie Q38.1
Tonsillitis (acute) (catarrhal) (croupous) (follicular)
(gangrenous)
(infective) (lacunar)
(lingual) (malignant)
(membranous)
(parenchymatous)
(phlegmonous)
(pseudomembranous)
(purulent) (septic)
(subacute)
(suppurative) (toxic)
(ulcerative)(vesicular)
(viral) J03.90
chronic J35.01
with adenoiditis J35.03
hypertrophic J35.01
with adenoiditis J35.03
recurrent J03.91
specified organism NEC J03.80
recurrent J03.81
staphylococcal J03.80
recurrent J03.81
streptococcal J03.00
recurrent J03.01
Tooth, teeth—*see* condition
TORCH infection—*see* Infection, congenital
without active infection P00.2
Torsion
appendix epididymis N44.04
appendix testis N44.03
bile duct (common) (hepatic) K83.8
congenital Q44.5
bowel, colon or intestine K56.2
epididymis (appendix) N44.04
gallbladder K82.8
congenital Q44.1
hydatid of Morgagni
male N44.03
Meckel's diverticulum (congenital) Q43.0
mesentery K56.2
omentum K56.2
organ or site, congenital NEC—*see* Anomaly, by site
penis (acquired) N48.82
congenital Q55.63
spermatic cord N44.02
extravaginal N44.01
intravaginal N44.02

Torsion, *continued*
testis, testicle N44.00
appendix N44.03
tibia—*see* Deformity, limb, specified type NEC, lower leg
Torticollis (intermittent) (spastic) M43.6
congenital (sternomastoid) Q68.0
due to birth injury P15.8
hysterical F44.4
ocular R29.891
psychogenic F45.8
conversion reaction F44.4
rheumatic M43.6
traumatic, current S13.4
Tortuous
ureter N13.8
Tourette's syndrome F95.2
Tourniquet syndrome—*see* Constriction, external, by site
Tower skull Q75.0
with exophthalmos Q87.0
Toxemia
erysipelatous—*see* Erysipelas
food—*see* Poisoning, food
staphylococcal, due to food A05.0
Toxic (poisoning) (*see also* condition) T65.91
effect—*see* Table of Drugs and Chemicals, by substance,
poisoning
shock syndrome A48.3
Toxicity—*see* Table of Drugs and Chemicals, by substance,
poisoning
fava bean D55.0
food, noxious—*see* Poisoning, food
from drug or nonmedicinal substance—*see* Table of
Drugs and Chemicals,
by drug
Toxicosis—*see also* Toxemia
capillary, hemorrhagic D69.0
Toxoplasma, toxoplasmosis (acquired) B58.9
with
hepatitis B58.1
meningoencephalitis B58.2
ocular involvement B58.00
other organ involvement B58.89
pneumonia, pneumonitis B58.3
congenital (acute) (subacute) (chronic) P37.1
maternal, manifest toxoplasmosis in infant (acute)
(subacute) (chronic)
P37.1
Tracheitis (catarrhal) (infantile) (membranous) (plastic)
(septal) (suppurative)
(viral) J04.10
with
bronchitis (15 years of age and above) J40
acute or subacute—*see* Bronchitis, acute
under 15 years of age J20.9
laryngitis (acute) J04.2
chronic J37.1
acute J04.10
with obstruction J04.11
chronic J42
with
laryngitis (chronic) J37.1
Tracheomalacia J39.8
congenital Q32.0
Tracheopharyngitis (acute) J06.9
chronic J42
Trachoma, trachomatous A71.9
Türck's J37.0
Train sickness T75.3
Trait
Hb-S D57.3
hemoglobin
abnormal NEC D58.2
with thalassemia D56.3
C—*see* Disease, hemoglobin C
S (Hb-S) D57.3
Lepore D56.3
sickle-cell D57.3
with elliptocytosis or spherocytosis D57.3
Transfusion
associated (red blood cell) hemochromatosis E83.111
reaction (adverse)—*see* Complications, transfusion
related acute lung injury (TRALI) J95.84

Transient (meaning homeless) (*see also* condition) Z59.0
Translocation
balanced autosomal Q95.9
in normal individual Q95.0
chromosomes NEC Q99.8
balanced and insertion in normal individual Q95.0
Down syndrome Q90.2
trisomy
13 Q91.6
18 Q91.2
21 Q90.2
Transplant (ed) (status) Z94.9
awaiting organ Z76.82
candidate Z76.82
heart Z94.1
valve Z95.2
prosthetic Z95.2
specified NEC Z95.4
xenogenic Z95.3
kidney Z94.0
organ (failure) (infection) (rejection) Z94.9
removal status Z98.85
social Z60.3
Transposition (congenital)—*see also* Malposition, congenital
abdominal viscera Q89.3
aorta (dextra) Q20.3
great vessels (complete) (partial) Q20.3
heart Q24.0
with complete transposition of viscera Q89.3
scrotum Q55.23
stomach Q40.2
with general transposition of viscera Q89.3
vessels, great (complete) (partial) Q20.3
viscera (abdominal) (thoracic) Q89.3
Transsexualism F64.0
Transvestism, transvestitism (dual-role) F64.1
fetishistic F65.1
Tremor (s) R25.1
hysterical F44.4
psychogenic (conversion reaction) F44.4
Triad
Kartagener's Q89.3
Trichomoniasis A59.9
bladder A59.03
cervix A59.09
seminal vesicles A59.09
specified site NEC A59.8
urethra A59.03
urogenitalis A59.00
vagina A59.01
vulva A59.01
Trigger finger (acquired) M65.30
congenital Q74.0
Triphalangeal thumb Q74.0
Triple—*see also* Anomaly
X, female Q97.0
Trismus R25.2
Trisomy (syndrome) Q92.9
13 (partial) Q91.7
meiotic nondisjunction Q91.4
18 (partial) Q91.3
meiotic nondisjunction Q91.0
21 (partial) Q90.9
Trombiculosis, trombiculiasis, trombidiosis B88.0
Trouble—*see also* Disease
nervous R45.0
Truancy, childhood
from school Z72.810
Truncus
arteriosus (persistent) Q20.0
communis Q20.0
Trunk—*see* condition
Tuberculoma—*see also* Tuberculosis
brain A17.81
meninges (cerebral) (spinal) A17.1
spinal cord A17.81

Tuberculosis, tubercular, tuberculous (calcification) (calcified) (caseous) (chromogenic acid-fast bacilli) (degeneration) (fibrocaseous) (fistula) (interstitial) (isolated circumscribed lesions) (necrosis) (parenchymatous) (ulcerative) A15.9
- abscess (respiratory) A15.9
  - latent R76.11
  - meninges (cerebral) (spinal) A17.0
  - scrofulous A18.2
- arachnoid A17.0
- axilla, axillary (gland) A18.2
- cachexia A15.9
- cerebrospinal A17.81
  - meninges A17.0
- cervical (lymph gland or node) A18.2
- contact Z20.1
- dura (mater) (cerebral) (spinal) A17.0
  - abscess (cerebral) (spinal) A17.81
- exposure (to) Z20.1
- exudative (*see* Tuberculosis, pulmonary)
- glandular, general A18.2
- immunological findings only A15.7
- infection A15.9
  - without clinical manifestation A15.7
- infraclavicular gland A18.2
- inguinal gland A18.2
- inguinalis A18.2
- latent R76.11
- leptomeninges, leptomeningitis (cerebral) (spinal) A17.0
- lymph gland or node (peripheral) A18.2
  - cervical A18.2
- marasmus A15.9
- neck gland A18.2
- meninges, meningitis (basilar) (cerebral) (cerebrospinal) (spinal) A17.0
- pachymeningitis A17.0
- respiratory A15.9
  - primary A15.7
  - specified site NEC A15.8
- scrofulous A18.2
- senile A15.9
- spine, spinal (column) A18.01
  - cord A17.81
  - medulla A17.81
  - membrane A17.0
  - meninges A17.0
- supraclavicular gland A18.2
- unspecified site A15.9
Tuberous sclerosis (brain) Q85.1
Tumefaction—*see also* Swelling
- liver—*see* Hypertrophy, liver
Tumor—*see also* Neoplasm, unspecified behavior, by site
- Cock's peculiar L72.3
- glomus D18.00
  - skin D18.01
  - specified site NEC D18.09
- Grawitz's C64.-
- neuroectodermal (peripheral)—*see* Neoplasm, malignant, by site
  - primitive
    - specified site—*see* Neoplasm, malignant, by site
    - unspecified site C71.9
- phantom F45.8
- sternomastoid (congenital) Q68.0
- turban D23.4
- Wilms' C64.-
Tumor lysis syndrome (following antineoplastic chemotherapy) (spontaneous) NEC E88.3

Tungiasis B88.1
Typhus (fever) A75.9
- Sao Paulo A77.0
Turban tumor D23.4
Türck's trachoma J37.0
Turner-like syndrome Q87.1
Turner's syndrome Q96.9
Turner-Ullrich syndrome Q96.9

Twist, twisted
- bowel, colon or intestine K56.2
- mesentery K56.2
- omentum K56.2
- organ or site, congenital NEC—*see* Anomaly, by site
Tylosis (acquired) L84
- palmaris et plantaris (congenital) (inherited) Q82.8
  - acquired L85.1
Tympanism R14.0
Tympanites (abdominal) (intestinal) R14.0
Tympanitis—*see* Myringitis
Tympany
- abdomen R14.0
- chest R09.89

U

Ulcer, ulcerated, ulcerating, ulceration, ulcerative
- anorectal K62.6
- anus (sphincter) (solitary) K62.6
- aphthous (oral) (recurrent) K12.0
- bleeding K27.4
- breast N61.1
- buccal (cavity) (traumatic) K12.1
- cervix (uteri) (decubitus) (trophic) N86
  - with cervicitis N72
- Dieulafoy's K25.0
- duodenum, duodenal (eroded) (peptic) K26.9
  - with
    - hemorrhage K26.4
      - and perforation K26.6
    - perforation K26.5
  - acute K26.3
    - with
      - hemorrhage K26.0
        - and perforation K26.2
      - perforation K26.1
  - chronic K26.7
    - with
      - hemorrhage K26.4
        - and perforation K26.6
      - perforation K26.5
- dysenteric A09
- esophagus (peptic) K22.10
  - due to
    - gastrointestinal reflux disease K21.0
- frenum (tongue) K14.0
- hemorrhoid (*see also* Hemorrhoids, by degree) K64.8
- intestine, intestinal K63.3
  - rectum K62.6
- lip K13.0
- meatus (urinarius) N34.2
- Meckel's diverticulum Q43.0
- oral mucosa (traumatic) K12.1
- palate (soft) K12.1
- peptic (site unspecified) K27.9
  - with
    - hemorrhage K27.4
      - and perforation K27.6
    - perforation K27.5
  - acute K27.3
    - with
      - hemorrhage K27.0
        - and perforation K27.2
      - perforation K27.1
  - chronic K27.7
    - with
      - hemorrhage K27.4
        - and perforation K27.6
      - perforation K27.5
  - esophagus K22.10
    - with bleeding K22.11
  - newborn P78.82
- perforating K27.5
  - skin—*see* Ulcer, skin
- peritonsillar J35.8
- pressure (pressure area) L89.9-
  - ankle L89.5-
  - back L89.1-
  - buttock L89.3-
  - coccyx L89.15-
  - contiguous site of back, buttock, hip L89.4-
  - elbow L89.0-

Ulcer, ulcerated, ulcerating, ulceration, ulcerative, *continued*
- face L89.81-
- head L89.81-
- heel L89.6-
- hip L89.2-
- sacral region (tailbone) L89.15-
- specified site NEC L89.89-
- stage 1 (healing) (pre-ulcer skin changes limited to persistent focal edema)
  - ankle L89.5-
  - back L89.1-
  - buttock L89.3-
  - coccyx L89.15-
  - contiguous site of back, buttock, hip L89.4-
  - elbow L89.0-
  - face L89.81-
  - head L89.81-
  - heel L89.6-
  - hip L89.2-
  - sacral region (tailbone) L89.15-
  - specified site NEC L89.89-
- stage 2 (healing) (abrasion, blister, partial thickness skin loss involving epidermis and/or dermis)
  - ankle L89.5-
  - back L89.1-
  - buttock L89.3-
  - coccyx L89.15-
  - contiguous site of back, buttock, hip L89.4-
  - elbow L89.0-
  - face L89.81-
  - head L89.81-
  - heel L89.6-
  - hip L89.2-
  - sacral region (tailbone) L89.15-
  - specified site NEC L89.89-
- stage 3 (healing) (full thickness skin loss involving damage or necrosis of subcutaneous tissue)
  - ankle L89.5-
  - back L89.1-
  - buttock L89.3-
  - coccyx L89.15-
  - contiguous site of back, buttock, hip L89.4-
  - elbow L89.0-
  - face L89.81-
  - head L89.81-
  - heel L89.6-
  - hip L89.2-
  - sacral region (tailbone) L89.15-
  - specified site NEC L89.89-
- stage 4 (healing) (necrosis of soft tissues through to underlying muscle, tendon, or bone)
  - ankle L89.5-
  - back L89.1-
  - buttock L89.3-
  - coccyx L89.15-
  - contiguous site of back, buttock, hip L89.4-
  - elbow L89.0-
  - face L89.81-
  - head L89.81-
  - heel L89.6-
  - hip L89.2-
  - sacral region (tailbone) L89.15-
  - specified site NEC L89.89-
- rectum (sphincter) (solitary) K62.6
  - stercoraceous, stercoral K62.6
- scrofulous (tuberculous) A18.2
- scrotum N50.89
  - varicose I86.1
- solitary, anus or rectum (sphincter) K62.6
- sore throat J02.9
  - streptococcal J02.0
- stercoraceous, stercoral K63.3
  - anus or rectum K62.6
- stomach (eroded) (peptic) (round) K25.9
  - with
    - hemorrhage K25.4
      - and perforation K25.6
    - perforation K25.5

TUBERCULOSIS, TUBERCULAR, TUBERCULOUS-ULCER, ULCERATED, ULCERATING, ULCERATION, ULCERATIVE

Ulcer, ulcerated, ulcerating, ulceration, ulcerative, *continued*
- acute K25.3
  - with
    - hemorrhage K25.0
      - and perforation K25.2
    - perforation K25.1
  - chronic K25.7
    - with
      - hemorrhage K25.4
        - and perforation K25.6
      - perforation K25.5
- stomatitis K12.1
- strumous (tuberculous) A18.2
- tongue (traumatic) K14.0
- tonsil J35.8
- turbinate J34.89
- uterus N85.8
  - cervix N86
    - with cervicitis N72
  - neck N86
    - with cervicitis N72
- valve, heart I33.0
- varicose (lower limb, any part)—*see also* Varix, leg, with, ulcer
  - scrotum I86.1

Ulcerosa scarlatina A38.8
Ulcus—*see also* Ulcer
- durum (syphilitic) A51.0
  - extragenital A51.2

Ulerythema
- ophryogenes, congenital Q84.2
- sycosiforme L73.8

Ullrich (-Bonnevie) (-Turner) syndrome Q87.1
Ullrich-Feichtiger syndrome Q87.0
Unavailability (of)
- medical facilities (at) Z75.3
  - due to
    - lack of services at home Z75.0
    - home Z75.0

Underdevelopment—*see also* Undeveloped
- sexual E30.0

Underdosing (*see also* Table of Drugs and Chemicals, categories T36–T50, with final character 6) Z91.14
- intentional NEC Z91.128
  - due to financial hardship of patient Z91.120
- unintentional NEC Z91.138

Underimmunization status Z28.3
Underweight R63.6
- for gestational age—*see* Light for dates

Underwood's disease P83.0
Undeveloped, undevelopment—*see also* Hypoplasia
- brain (congenital) Q02
- cerebral (congenital) Q02
- heart Q24.8
- lung Q33.6
- testis E29.1
- uterus E30.0

Undiagnosed (disease) R69
Unguis incarnatus L60.0
Unstable
- hip (congenital) Q65.6

Unsteadiness on feet R26.81
Untruthfulness, child problem F91.8
Upbringing, institutional Z62.22
- away from parents NEC Z62.29
- in care of non-parental family member Z62.21
- in foster care Z62.21
- in orphanage or group home Z62.22
- in welfare custody Z62.21

Upper respiratory—*see* condition
Upset
- gastric K30
- gastrointestinal K30
  - psychogenic F45.8
- intestinal (large) (small) K59.9
  - psychogenic F45.8
- mental F48.9
- stomach K30
  - psychogenic F45.8

Uremia, uremic N19
- chronic (*see also* Disease, kidney, chronic) N18.9
- congenital P96.0

Ureteralgia N23
Ureteritis N28.89
- due to calculus N20.1
  - with calculus, kidney N20.2
    - with hydronephrosis N13.2
- nonspecific N28.89

Ureterocele N28.89
- congenital (orthotopic) Q62.31

Urethralgia R39.89
Urethritis (anterior) (posterior) N34.2
- candidal B37.41
- chlamydial A56.01
- diplococcal (gonococcal) A54.01
  - with abscess (accessory gland) (periurethral) A54.1
- gonococcal A54.01
  - with abscess (accessory gland) (periurethral) A54.1
- nongonococcal N34.1
- nonspecific N34.1
- nonvenereal N34.1
- specified NEC N34.2
- trichomonal or due to Trichomonas (vaginalis) A59.03

Urethrorrhea R36.9
Urgency
- fecal R15.2
- urinary R39.15

Urination
- frequent R35.0
- painful R30.9

Urine
- blood in—*see* Hematuria
- discharge, excessive R35.8
- enuresis, nonorganic origin F98.0
- frequency R35.0
- incontinence R32
  - nonorganic origin F98.0
- intermittent stream R39.198
- pus in N39.0
- retention or stasis R33.9
  - psychogenic F45.8
- secretion
  - deficient R34
  - excessive R35.8
  - frequency R35.0
- stream
  - intermittent R39.198
  - slowing R39.198
  - weak R39.12

Urodialysis R34
Uropathy N39.9
- obstructive N13.9
  - specified NEC N13.8
- reflux N13.9
  - specified NEC N13.8

Urticaria L50.9
- with angioneurotic edema T78.3
- allergic L50.0
- chronic L50.8
- due to
  - drugs L50.0
  - food L50.0
  - inhalants L50.0
  - serum (*see also* Reaction, serum) T80.69
- giant T78.3
- gigantea T78.3
- larynx T78.3
- neonatorum P83.8
- recurrent periodic L50.8
- serum (*see also* Reaction, serum) T80.69
- specified type NEC L50.8

Use (of)
- alcohol Z72.89
  - harmful—*see* Abuse, alcohol
- caffeine—*see* Use, stimulant NEC
- cannabis F12.90
- stimulant NEC F15.90
  - with
    - intoxication F15.929
      - uncomplicated F15.920
    - withdrawal F15.93

Use (of), *continued*
- harmful—*see* Abuse, drug, stimulant NEC
- tobacco Z72.0
  - with dependence—*see* Dependence, drug, nicotine
- volatile solvents (*see also* Use, inhalant) F18.90
  - harmful—*see* Abuse, drug, inhalant

Uveitis (anterior)—*see also* Iridocyclitis
- due to toxoplasmosis (acquired) B58.09
  - congenital P37.1

Uveoparotitis D86.89
Uvulitis (acute) (catarrhal) (chronic) (membranous) (suppurative) (ulcerative) K12.2

V

Vaccination (prophylactic)
- complication or reaction—*see* Complications, vaccination
- delayed Z28.9
- encounter for Z23
- not done—*see* Immunization, not done, because (of)

Vaccinia (generalized) (localized) T88.1
- congenital P35.8
- without vaccination B08.011

Vacuum, in sinus (accessory) (nasal) J34.89
Vagabond's disease B85.1
Vaginitis (acute) (circumscribed) (diffuse) (emphysematous) (nonvenereal) (ulcerative) N76.0
- bacterial N76.0
- blennorrhagic (gonococcal) A54.02
- candidal B37.3
- chlamydial A56.02
- chronic N76.1
- due to Trichomonas (vaginalis) A59.01
- gonococcal A54.02
  - with abscess (accessory gland) (periurethral) A54.1
- in (due to)
  - candidiasis B37.3
  - herpesviral (herpes simplex) infection A60.04
  - pinworm infection B80 [N77.1]
- monilial B37.3
- mycotic (candidal) B37.3
- syphilitic (early) A51.0
  - late A52.76
- trichomonal A59.01

Vaginosis—*see* Vaginitis
Valve, valvular (formation)—*see also* condition
- cerebral ventricle (communicating) in situ Z98.2

Van der Hoeve (-de Kleyn) **syndrome** Q78.0
Vapor asphyxia or suffocation T59.9
- specified agent—*see* Table of Drugs and Chemicals

Variants, thalassemic D56.8
Varicella B01.9
- with
  - complications NEC B01.89
  - encephalitis B01.11
  - encephalomyelitis B01.11
  - meningitis B01.0
  - myelitis B01.12
  - pneumonia B01.2
- congenital P35.8

Varices—*see* Varix
Varicocele (scrotum) (thrombosed) I86.1
- spermatic cord (ulcerated) I86.1

Varicose
- ulcer (lower limb, any part)—*see also* Varix, leg, with, ulcer
- anus (*see also* Hemorrhoids) K64.8
- scrotum I86.1

Varix (lower limb) (ruptured) I83.90
- esophagus (idiopathic) (primary) (ulcerated) I85.00
  - bleeding I85.01
  - congenital Q27.8
- scrotum (ulcerated) I86.1

Vascular—*see also* condition
- spider I78.1

Vasculitis I77.6
- allergic D69.0

Vasovagal attack (paroxysmal) R55
- psychogenic F45.8

Vegetation, vegetative
 adenoid (nasal fossa) J35.8
 endocarditis (acute) (any valve) (subacute) I33.0
 heart (mycotic) (valve) I33.0
Venereal
 disease A64
Venom, venomous—*see* Table of Drugs and Chemicals, by
                           animal or substance,
                           poisoning
Ventriculitis (cerebral) (*see also* Encephalitis) G04.90
Ventriculostomy status Z98.2
Vernet's syndrome G52.7
Verruca (due to HPV) (filiformis) (simplex) (viral) (vulgaris)
                           B07.9
 acuminata A63.0
 plana B07.8
 plantaris B07.0
 venereal A63.0
Vertigo R42
 laryngeal R05
Vesiculitis (seminal) N49.0
 trichomonal A59.09
Vestibulitis (ear) (*see also* subcategory) H83.0
 nose (external) J34.89
 vulvar N94.810
Villaret's syndrome G52.7
Virilism (adrenal) E25.9
 congenital E25.0
Virilization (female) (suprarenal) E25.9
 congenital E25.0
 isosexual E28.2
Virus, viral—*see also* condition
 as cause of disease classified elsewhere B97.89
 cytomegalovirus B25.9
 human immunodeficiency (HIV)—*see* Human,
                           immunodeficiency virus
                           (HIV) disease
 infection—*see* Infection, virus
 specified NEC B34.8
 swine influenza (viruses that normally cause infections
                           in pigs) (*see also*
                           Influenza, due to,
                           identified novel
                           influenza A virus)
                           J09.X2
 West Nile (fever) A92.30
  with
    complications NEC A92.39
    cranial nerve disorders A92.32
    encephalitis A92.31
    encephalomyelitis A92.31
    neurologic manifestation NEC A92.32
    optic neuritis A92.32
    polyradiculitis A92.32
 Zika virus disease A92.5
Vision, visual
 blurred, blurring H53.8
  hysterical F44.6
 defect, defective NEC H54.7
 disorientation (syndrome) H53.8
 disturbance H53.9
  hysterical F44.6
 examination Z01.00
  with abnormal findings Z01.01
 field, limitation (defect)—*see* Defect, visual field
 hallucinations R44.1
Vitality, lack or want of R53.83
 newborn P96.89
Vitamin deficiency—*see* Deficiency, vitamin
Vitelline duct, persistent Q43.0
Vitiligo L80
 eyelid H02.739
  left H02.736
   lower H02.735
   upper H02.734
  right H02.733
   lower H02.732
   upper H02.731
Volvulus (bowel) (colon) (intestine) K56.2
 with perforation K56.2
 congenital Q43.8
 duodenum K31.5

Vomiting R11.10
 with nausea R11.2
 bilious (cause unknown) R11.14
  in newborn P92.01
 cyclical G43.A0
  with refractory migraine G43.A1
  intractable G43.A1
  not intractable G43.A0
  psychogenic F50.89
  without refractory migraine G43.A0
 fecal matter R11.13
 following gastrointestinal surgery K91.0
  psychogenic F50.89
 functional K31.89
 hysterical F50.89
 nervous F50.89
 neurotic F50.89
 newborn NEC P92.09
  bilious P92.01
 periodic R11.10
  psychogenic F50.89
 projectile R11.12
 psychogenic F50.89
 without nausea R11.11
Von Hippel (-Lindau) **disease or syndrome** Q85.8
Von Recklinghausen
 disease (neurofibromatosis) Q85.01
  bones E21.0
Vrolik's disease Q78.0
Vulvitis (acute) (allergic) (atrophic) (hypertrophic)
                           (intertriginous) (senile)
                           N76.2
 adhesive, congenital Q52.79
 blennorrhagic (gonococcal) A54.02
 candidal B37.3
 chlamydial A56.02
 gonococcal A54.02
  with abscess (accessory gland) (periurethral) A54.1
 monilial B37.3
 syphilitic (early) A51.0
  late A52.76
 trichomonal A59.01
Vulvodynia N94.819
 specified NEC N94.818
Vulvorectal—*see* condition
Vulvovaginitis (acute)—*see* Vaginitis

W

Waiting list
 for organ transplant Z76.82
Walking
 difficulty R26.2
  psychogenic F44.4
 sleep F51.3
  hysterical F44.89
Wall, abdominal—*see* condition
Wandering
 gallbladder, congenital Q44.1
 in diseases classified elsewhere Z91.83
Wart (due to HPV) (filiform) (infectious) (viral) B07.9
 anogenital region (venereal) A63.0
 common B07.8
 external genital organs (venereal) A63.0
 flat B07.8
 plantar B07.0
 venereal A63.0
Waterbrash R12
Weak, weakening, weakness (generalized) R53.1
 bladder (sphincter) R32
 mind F70
 muscle M62.81
 newborn P96.89
 urinary stream R39.12
Weaver's syndrome Q87.3
Web, webbed (congenital)
 fingers Q70.1-
 toes Q70.3-
Weber-Cockayne syndrome (epidermolysis bullosa) Q81.8
Weber-Osler syndrome I78.0

Weight
 1000–2499 grams at birth (low)—*see* Low, birthweight
 999 grams or less at birth (extremely low)—*see* Low,
                           birthweight, extreme
 and length below 10th percentile for gestational age
                           P05.1-
 below 10th percentile but length above 10th percentile
                           P05.0-
 gain (abnormal) (excessive) R63.5
  in pregnancy—*see* Pregnancy, complicated by,
                           excessive weight gain
  low—*see* Pregnancy, complicated by, insufficient,
                           weight gain
 loss (abnormal) (cause unknown) R63.4
Weil (I)-Marchesani syndrome Q87.1
Wen—*see* Cyst, sebaceous
Wenckebach's block or phenomenon I44.1
Werdnig-Hoffmann syndrome (muscular atrophy) G12.0
Werlhof's disease D69.3
Wernicke's
 developmental aphasia F80.2
West's syndrome—*see* Epilepsy, spasms
Wet
 lung (syndrome), newborn P22.1
Wheal—*see* Urticaria
Wheezing R06.2
Whiplash injury S13.4
Whipple's disease (*see also* subcategory M14.8-) K90.81
Whistling face Q87.0
White—*see also* condition
 kidney, small N03.9
 mouth B37.0
Whitehead L70.0
Whitlow—*see also* Cellulitis, digit
 with lymphangitis—*see* Lymphangitis, acute, digit
 herpesviral B00.89
Whooping cough A37.90
 with pneumonia A37.91
Wilms' tumor C64.-
Wiskott-Aldrich syndrome D82.0
Withdrawal state—*see also* Dependence, drug by type, with
                           withdrawal
 newborn
  correct therapeutic substance properly administered
                           P96.2
  infant of dependent mother P96.1
  therapeutic substance, neonatal P96.2
Witts' anemia D50.8
Wolff-Parkinson-White syndrome I45.6
Wool sorter's disease A22.1
Word
 blindness (congenital) (developmental) F81.0
 deafness (congenital) (developmental) H93.25
Worried well Z71.1
Worries R45.82
Wound, open
*Please see Bite, Laceration, or Puncture by site for these
                           types of wounds not
                           referenced here.*
 abdomen, abdominal
  wall S31.109
   with penetration into peritoneal cavity S31.609
   epigastric region S31.102
    with penetration into peritoneal cavity S31.602
   left
    lower quadrant S31.104
     with penetration into peritoneal cavity
                           S31.604
    upper quadrant S31.101
     with penetration into peritoneal cavity
                           S31.601
   periumbilic region S31.105
    with penetration into peritoneal cavity S31.605
   right
    lower quadrant S31.103
     with penetration into peritoneal cavity
                           S31.603
    upper quadrant S31.100
     with penetration into peritoneal cavity
                           S31.600
 ankle S91.00-
 antecubital space S51.00-

Wound, open, *continued*
    submaxillary region S01.80
    submental region S01.80
    subungual
        finger (s)—*see* Wound, open, finger
        toe (s)—*see* Wound, open, toe
    supraclavicular region—*see* Wound, open, neck, specified
                    site NEC
    temple, temporal region S01.80
    temporomandibular area—*see* Wound, open, cheek
    testis S31.30
        with amputation—*see* Amputation, traumatic, testes
        bite S31.35
    thigh S71.10-
        with amputation—*see* Amputation, traumatic, hip
    thorax, thoracic (wall) S21.90
        back S21.20-
            with penetration S21.40
        breast S21.00-
        front S21.10-
            with penetration S21.30
    throat—*see* Wound, open, neck
    thumb S61.009
        with
            amputation—*see* Amputation, traumatic, thumb
            damage to nail S61.109
        left S61.002
            with
                damage to nail S61.102
        right S61.001
            with
                damage to nail S61.101
    thyroid (gland) S11.10
    toe (s) S91.109
        with
            amputation—*see* Amputation, traumatic, toe
            damage to nail S91.209
        bite—*see* Bite, toe
        great S91.103
            with
                damage to nail S91.203

Wound, open, *continued*
        left S91.102
            with
                damage to nail S91.202
        right S91.101
            with
                damage to nail S91.201
        lesser S91.106
            with
                damage to nail S91.206
        left S91.105
            with
                damage to nail S91.205
        right S91.104
            with
                damage to nail S91.204
    tongue—*see* Wound, open, oral cavity
    trachea (cervical region)—*see* Wound, open, neck,
                    trachea
    tunica vaginalis—*see* Wound, open, testis
    tympanum, tympanic membrane S09.2-
    umbilical region—*see* Wound, open, abdomen, wall,
                    periumbilic region
    uvula—*see* Wound, open, oral cavity
    vagina S31.40
        bite S31.45
    vocal cord S11.039
        laceration S11.031
            with foreign body S11.032
        puncture S11.033
            with foreign body S11.034
    vitreous (humor)—*see* Wound, open, ocular
    vulva S31.40
        with amputation—*see* Amputation, traumatic, vulva
        bite S31.45
    wrist S61.50-
Wound, superficial—*see* Injury—*see also* specified injury
                    type

X

Xanthelasmatosis (essential) E78.2
Xanthoastrocytoma
    specified site—*see* Neoplasm, malignant, by site
    unspecified site C71.9
Xanthogranuloma D76.3
Xanthoma (s), **xanthomatosis** (primary) (familial) (hereditary)
                        E75.5
    with
        hyperlipoproteinemia
            Type III E78.2
    disseminatum (skin) E78.2
    eruptive E78.2
    hypercholesterinemic E78.00
    hypercholesterolemic E78.00
    hyperlipidemic E78.5
    multiple (skin) E78.2
    tubo-eruptive E78.2
    tuberosum E78.2
    tuberous E78.2
X0 syndrome Q96.9
X-ray (of)
    abnormal findings—Abnormal, diagnostic imaging
    breast (mammogram) (routine) Z12.31
    chest
        routine (as part of a general medical examination)
                Z00.00
            with abnormal findings Z00.01
    routine (as part of a general medical examination) Z00.00
        with abnormal findings Z00.01

Y

Yawning R06.89
    psychogenic F45.8
Yeast infection (*see also* Candidiasis) B37.9

Z

Zahorsky's syndrome (herpangina) B08.5
Zika virus NOS A92.5
Zona—*see* Herpes, zoster

Chapter 1. Certain infectious and parasitic diseases (A00–B99)

GUIDELINES

HIV Infections
See category B20.

Coding of Sepsis and Severe Sepsis

SEPSIS
For a diagnosis of sepsis, assign the appropriate code for the underlying systemic infection. If the type of infection or causal organism is not further specified, assign code A41.9, Sepsis, unspecified organism. A code from subcategory R65.2, Severe sepsis, should not be assigned unless severe sepsis or an associated acute organ dysfunction is documented.

Negative or inconclusive blood cultures and sepsis
Negative or inconclusive blood cultures do not preclude a diagnosis of sepsis in patients with clinical evidence of the condition, however, the provider should be queried.

Urosepsis
The term urosepsis is a nonspecific term. It is not to be considered synonymous with sepsis. It has no default code in the Alphabetic Index. Should a provider use this term they should be queried.

Sepsis with organ dysfunction
If a patient has sepsis and associated acute organ dysfunction or multiple organ dysfunction (MOD), follow the instructions for coding severe sepsis.

Acute organ dysfunction that is not clearly associated with the sepsis
If a patient has sepsis and an acute organ dysfunction, but the medical record documentation indicates that the acute organ dysfunction is related to a medical condition other than the sepsis, do not assign a code from subcategory R65.2, Severe sepsis. An acute organ dysfunction must be associated with the sepsis in order to assign the severe sepsis code. If the documentation is not clear as to whether an acute organ dysfunction is related to the sepsis or another medical condition, query the provider.

SEVERE SEPSIS
The coding of severe sepsis requires a minimum of 2 codes: first a code for the underlying systemic infection, followed by a code from subcategory R65.2, Severe sepsis. If the causal organism is not documented, assign code A41.9, Sepsis, unspecified organism, for the infection. Additional code(s) for the associated acute organ dysfunction are also required.

Due to the complex nature of severe sepsis, some cases may require querying the provider prior to assignment of the codes.

Septic shock
Septic shock generally refers to circulatory failure associated with severe sepsis, and therefore, it represents a type of acute organ dysfunction. For cases of septic shock, the code for the systemic infection should be sequenced first, followed by code R65.21, Severe sepsis with septic shock or code T81.12, Postprocedural septic shock. Any additional codes for the other acute organ dysfunctions should also be assigned. As noted in the sequencing instructions in the Tabular List, the code for septic shock cannot be assigned as a principal diagnosis.

Sequencing of severe sepsis
If severe sepsis is present on admission, and meets the definition of principal diagnosis, the underlying systemic infection should be assigned as principal diagnosis followed by the appropriate code from subcategory R65.2 as required by the sequencing rules in the Tabular List. A code from subcategory R65.2 can never be assigned as a principal diagnosis. When severe sepsis develops during an encounter (it was not present on admission) the underlying systemic infection and the appropriate code from subcategory R65.2 should be assigned as secondary diagnoses. Severe sepsis may be present on admission but the diagnosis may not be confirmed until sometime after admission. If the documentation is not clear whether severe sepsis was present on admission, the provider should be queried.

Sepsis and severe sepsis with a localized infection
If the reason for admission is both sepsis or severe sepsis and a localized infection, such as pneumonia or cellulitis, a code(s) for the underlying systemic infection should be assigned first and the code for the localized infection should be assigned as a secondary diagnosis. If the patient has severe sepsis, a code from subcategory R65.2 should also be assigned as a secondary diagnosis. If the patient is admitted with a localized infection, such as pneumonia, and sepsis/severe sepsis doesn't develop until after admission, the localized infection should be assigned first, followed by the appropriate sepsis/severe sepsis codes.

SEPSIS DUE TO A POSTPROCEDURAL INFECTION

Documentation of causal relationship
As with all postprocedural complications, code assignment is based on the provider's documentation of the relationship between the infection and the procedure.

Sepsis due to a postprocedural infection
For such cases, the postprocedural infection code, such as, T80.2, Infections following infusion, transfusion, and therapeutic injection, T81.4, Infection following a procedure, or T88.0, Infection following immunization followed by the code for the specific infection. If the patient has severe sepsis the appropriate code from subcategory R65.2 should also be assigned with the additional code(s) for any acute organ dysfunction.

Postprocedural infection and postprocedural septic shock
In cases where a postprocedural infection has occurred and has resulted in severe sepsis the code for the precipitating complication such as code T81.4, Infection following a procedure, should be coded first followed by code R65.20, Severe sepsis without septic shock. A code for the systemic infection should also be assigned. If a postprocedural infection has resulted in postprocedural septic shock, the code for the precipitating complication such as code T81.4, Infection following a procedure should be coded first followed by code T81.12-, Postprocedural septic shock. A code for the systemic infection should also be assigned.

SEPSIS AND SEVERE SEPSIS ASSOCIATED WITH A NONINFECTIOUS PROCESS (CONDITION)
In some cases a noninfectious process (condition), such as trauma, may lead to an infection which can result in sepsis or severe sepsis. If sepsis or severe sepsis is documented as associated with a noninfectious condition, such as a burn or serious injury, and this condition meets the definition for principal diagnosis, the code for the noninfectious condition should be sequenced first, followed by the code for the resulting infection. If severe sepsis, is present a code from subcategory R65.2 should also be assigned with any associated organ dysfunction(s) codes. It is not necessary to assign a code from subcategory R65.1, SIRS of non-infectious origin, for these cases.

If the infection meets the definition of principal diagnosis it should be sequenced before the non-infectious condition. When both the associated non-infectious condition and the infection meet the definition of principal diagnosis either may be assigned as principal diagnosis.

Only one code from category R65, Symptoms and signs specifically associated with systemic inflammation and infection, should be assigned. Therefore, when a non-infectious condition leads to an infection resulting in severe sepsis, assign the appropriate code from subcategory R65.2, Severe sepsis. Do not additionally assign a code from subcategory R65.1, SIRS of non-infectious origin.

Includes: diseases generally recognized as communicable or transmissible
Use additional code to identify resistance to antimicrobial drugs (Z16.-)
Excludes1: certain localized infections—see body system-related chapters
Excludes2: carrier or suspected carrier of infectious disease (Z22.-)
    infectious and parasitic diseases specific to the perinatal period (P35–P39)
    influenza and other acute respiratory infections (J00–J22)

(A00–A09) INTESTINAL INFECTIOUS DISEASES

A02 **OTHER SALMONELLA INFECTIONS**
`4th`   *Includes:* infection or foodborne intoxication due to any Salmonella species other than S. typhi and S. paratyphi
    A02.0 **Salmonella enteritis**
      Salmonellosis
    A02.1 **Salmonella sepsis**
    A02.2 **Localized salmonella infections**
    `5th`   **A02.20** **Localized salmonella infection, unspecified**
        A02.21 **Salmonella meningitis**
        A02.22 **Salmonella pneumonia**
        A02.23 **Salmonella arthritis**
        A02.24 **Salmonella osteomyelitis**
        A02.25 **Salmonella pyelonephritis**
          Salmonella tubulo-interstitial nephropathy
        A02.29 **Salmonella with other localized infection**
    A02.8 **Other specified salmonella infections**
    A02.9 **Salmonella infection, unspecified**

 `4th` `5th` `6th` `7th`   Additional Character Required   ✔   3-character code

●=New Code
▲=Revised Code

Excludes1—Not coded here, do not use together
Excludes2—Not included here

A03 SHIGELLOSIS

4th

A03.0 Shigellosis due to Shigella dysenteriae
Group A shigellosis [Shiga-Kruse dysentery]

A03.1 Shigellosis due to Shigella flexneri
Group B shigellosis

A03.2 Shigellosis due to Shigella boydii
Group C shigellosis

A03.3 Shigellosis due to Shigella sonnei
Group D shigellosis

A03.8 Other shigellosis

A03.9 Shigellosis, unspecified
Bacillary dysentery NOS

A04 OTHER BACTERIAL INTESTINAL INFECTIONS

4th

Excludes1: bacterial foodborne intoxications, NEC (A05.-)
tuberculous enteritis (A18.32)

A04.0 Enteropathogenic E. coli infection

A04.1 Enterotoxigenic E. coli infection

A04.2 Enteroinvasive E. coli infection

A04.3 Enterohemorrhagic E. coli infection

A04.4 Other intestinal E. coli infections
E. coli enteritis NOS

A04.5 Campylobacter enteritis

A04.6 Enteritis due to Yersinia enterocolitica
Excludes1: extraintestinal yersiniosis (A28.2)

A04.7 Enterocolitis due to Clostridium difficile
Foodborne intoxication by Clostridium difficile
Pseudomembraneous colitis

A04.8 Other specified bacterial intestinal infections
H. pylori

A04.9 Bacterial intestinal infection, unspecified
Bacterial enteritis NOS

A05 OTHER BACTERIAL FOODBORNE INTOXICATIONS, NOT ELSEWHERE CLASSIFIED

4th

Excludes1: Clostridium difficile foodborne intoxication and infection (A04.7)
E. coli infection (A04.0–A04.4)
listeriosis (A32.-)
salmonella foodborne intoxication and infection (A02.-)
toxic effect of noxious foodstuffs (T61–T62)

A05.0 Foodborne staphylococcal intoxication

A05.1 Botulism food poisoning
Botulism NOS
Classical foodborne intoxication due to Clostridium botulinum
Excludes1: infant botulism (A48.51)
wound botulism (A48.52)

A05.2 Foodborne Clostridium perfringens [Clostridium welchii] intoxication
Enteritis necroticans
Pig-bel

A05.3 Foodborne Vibrio parahaemolyticus intoxication

A05.4 Foodborne Bacillus cereus intoxication

A05.5 Foodborne Vibrio vulnificus intoxication

A05.8 Other specified bacterial foodborne intoxications

A05.9 Bacterial foodborne intoxication, unspecified

A06 AMEBIASIS

4th

Includes: infection due to Entamoeba histolytica
Excludes1: other protozoal intestinal diseases (A07.-)
Excludes2: acanthamebiasis (B60.1-)
Naegleriasis (B60.2)

A06.0 Acute amebic dysentery
Acute amebiasis
Intestinal amebiasis NOS

A07 OTHER PROTOZOAL INTESTINAL DISEASES

4th

A07.1 Giardiasis [lambliasis]

A08 VIRAL AND OTHER SPECIFIED INTESTINAL INFECTIONS

4th

Excludes1: influenza with involvement of gastrointestinal tract (J09.X3, J10.2, J11.2)

A08.0 Rotaviral enteritis

A08.3 Other viral enteritis

5th

A08.39 Other viral enteritis
Coxsackie virus enteritis
Echovirus enteritis
Enterovirus enteritis NEC
Torovirus enteritis

A08.4 Viral intestinal infection, unspecified
Viral enteritis NOS
Viral gastroenteritis NOS
Viral gastroenteropathy NOS

A08.8 Other specified intestinal infections

A09 INFECTIOUS GASTROENTERITIS AND COLITIS, UNSPECIFIED

✓

Infectious colitis NOS
Infectious enteritis NOS
Infectious gastroenteritis NOS
Excludes1: colitis NOS (K52.9)
diarrhea NOS (R19.7)
enteritis NOS (K52.9)
gastroenteritis NOS (K52.9)
noninfective gastroenteritis and colitis, unspecified (K52.9)

(A15–A19) TUBERCULOSIS

Includes: infections due to Mycobacterium tuberculosis and Mycobacterium bovis
Excludes1: congenital tuberculosis (P37.0)
nonspecific reaction to test for tuberculosis without active tuberculosis (R76.1-)
pneumoconiosis associated with tuberculosis, any type in A15 (J65)
positive PPD (R76.11)
positive tuberculin skin test without active tuberculosis (R76.11)
sequelae of tuberculosis (B90.-)
silicotuberculosis (J65)

A15 RESPIRATORY TUBERCULOSIS

4th

A15.0 Tuberculosis of lung
Tuberculous bronchiectasis
Tuberculous fibrosis of lung
Tuberculous pneumonia
Tuberculous pneumothorax

A15.4 Tuberculosis of intrathoracic lymph nodes
Tuberculosis of hilar lymph nodes
Tuberculosis of mediastinal lymph nodes
Tuberculosis of tracheobronchial lymph nodes
Excludes1: tuberculosis specified as primary (A15.7)

A15.5 Tuberculosis of larynx, trachea and bronchus
Tuberculosis of bronchus
Tuberculosis of glottis
Tuberculosis of larynx
Tuberculosis of trachea

A15.6 Tuberculous pleurisy
Tuberculosis of pleura Tuberculous empyema
Excludes1: primary respiratory tuberculosis (A15.7)

A15.7 Primary respiratory tuberculosis

A15.8 Other respiratory tuberculosis
Mediastinal tuberculosis
Nasopharyngeal tuberculosis
Tuberculosis of nose
Tuberculosis of sinus [any nasal]

A15.9 Respiratory tuberculosis unspecified

A17 TUBERCULOSIS OF NERVOUS SYSTEM

4th

A17.0 Tuberculous meningitis
Tuberculosis of meninges (cerebral)(spinal)
Tuberculous leptomeningitis
Excludes1: tuberculous meningoencephalitis (A17.82)

A17.1 Meningeal tuberculoma
Tuberculoma of meninges (cerebral) (spinal)
Excludes2: tuberculoma of brain and spinal cord (A17.81)

4th **5th** **6th** **7th** Additional Character Required ✓ 3-character code

•=New Code
▲=Revised Code

Excludes1—Not coded here, do not use together
Excludes2—Not included here

A17.8   **Other tuberculosis of nervous system**

> **5th**   **A17.81**   **Tuberculoma of brain and spinal cord**
> Tuberculous abscess of brain and spinal cord
>
> **A17.82**   **Tuberculous meningoencephalitis**
> Tuberculous myelitis
>
> **A17.83**   **Tuberculous neuritis**
> Tuberculous mononeuropathy
>
> **A17.89**   **Other tuberculosis of nervous system**
> Tuberculous polyneuropathy

A17.9   **Tuberculosis of nervous system, unspecified**

A18   TUBERCULOSIS OF OTHER ORGANS

4th

A18.0   **Tuberculosis of bones and joints**

> **5th**   **A18.01**   **Tuberculosis of spine**
> Pott's disease or curvature of spine
> Tuberculous arthritis
> Tuberculous osteomyelitis of spine
> Tuberculous spondylitis
>
> **A18.02**   **Tuberculous arthritis of other joints**
> Tuberculosis of hip (joint)
> Tuberculosis of knee (joint)
>
> **A18.03**   **Tuberculosis of other bones**
> Tuberculous mastoiditis
> Tuberculous osteomyelitis
>
> **A18.09**   **Other musculoskeletal tuberculosis**
> Tuberculous myositis
> Tuberculous synovitis
> Tuberculous tenosynovitis

A18.2   **Tuberculous peripheral lymphadenopathy**
Tuberculous adenitis
Excludes2: tuberculosis of bronchial and mediastinal lymph nodes
     (A15.4)
     tuberculosis of mesenteric and retroperitoneal lymph nodes
     (A18.39)
     tuberculous tracheobronchial adenopathy (A15.4)

A18.3   **Tuberculosis of intestines, peritoneum and mesenteric glands**

> **5th**   **A18.31**   **Tuberculous peritonitis**
> Tuberculous ascites
>
> **A18.32**   **Tuberculous enteritis**
> Tuberculosis of anus and rectum
> Tuberculosis of intestine (large) (small)

A18.4   **Tuberculosis of skin and subcutaneous tissue**
Erythema induratum, tuberculous
Lupus excedens
Lupus vulgaris NOS
Lupus vulgaris of eyelid
Scrofuloderma
Tuberculosis of external ear
Excludes2: lupus erythematosus (L93.-)
     lupus NOS (M32.9)
     systemic (M32.-)

A18.6   **Tuberculosis of (inner) (middle) ear**
Tuberculous otitis media
Excludes2: tuberculosis of external ear (A18.4)
     tuberculous mastoiditis (A18.03)

A18.8   **Tuberculosis of other specified organs**

> **5th**   **A18.85**   **Tuberculosis of spleen**
>
> **A18.89**   **Tuberculosis of other sites**
> Tuberculosis of muscle
> Tuberculous cerebral arteritis

A19   MILIARY TUBERCULOSIS

4th

Includes: disseminated tuberculosis
     generalized tuberculosis
     tuberculous polyserositis

A19.0   **Acute miliary tuberculosis of a single specified site**

A19.1   **Acute miliary tuberculosis of multiple sites**

A19.2   **Acute miliary tuberculosis, unspecified**

A19.8   **Other miliary tuberculosis**

A19.9   **Miliary tuberculosis, unspecified**

(A20–A28) CERTAIN ZOONOTIC BACTERIAL DISEASES

A22   ANTHRAX

4th

Includes: infection due to Bacillus anthracis

A22.0   **Cutaneous anthrax**
Malignant carbuncle
Malignant pustule

A22.1   **Pulmonary anthrax**
Inhalation anthrax
Rag picker's disease
Wool sorter's disease

A22.2   **Gastrointestinal anthrax**

A22.9   **Anthrax, unspecified**

A25   RAT-BITE FEVERS

4th

A25.0   **Spirillosis**

A25.1   **Streptobacillosis**

A25.9   **Rat-bite fever, unspecified**

A26   ERYSIPELOID

4th

A26.0   **Cutaneous erysipeloid**

A26.7   **Erysipelothrix sepsis**

A26.8   **Other forms of erysipeloid**

A26.9   **Erysipeloid, unspecified**

A27   LEPTOSPIROSIS

4th

A27.0   **Leptospirosis icterohemorrhagica**

A27.8   **Other forms of leptospirosis**

> **5th**   **A27.81**   **Aseptic meningitis in leptospirosis**
>
> **A27.89**   **Other forms of leptospirosis**

A27.9   **Leptospirosis, unspecified**

A28   OTHER ZOONOTIC BACTERIAL DISEASES, NEC

4th

A28.0   **Pasteurellosis**

A28.1   **Cat-scratch disease**
Cat-scratch fever

(A30–A49) OTHER BACTERIAL DISEASES

A31   INFECTION DUE TO OTHER MYCOBACTERIA

4th

Excludes2: tuberculosis (A15–A19)

A31.0   **Pulmonary mycobacterial infection**

A31.1   **Cutaneous mycobacterial infection**

A31.2   **Disseminated mycobacterium avium-intracellulare complex (DMAC)**

A31.8   **Other mycobacterial infections**

A31.9   **Mycobacterial infection, unspecified**

A32   LISTERIOSIS

4th

Includes: listerial foodborne infection
Excludes1: neonatal (disseminated) listeriosis (P37.2)

A32.0   **Cutaneous listeriosis**

A32.1   **Listerial meningitis and meningoencephalitis**

> **5th**   **A32.11**   **Listerial meningitis**
>
> **A32.12**   **Listerial meningoencephalitis**

A32.7   **listeriosis   Listerial sepsis**

A32.8   **Other forms of listeriosis**

> **5th**   **A32.81**   **Oculoglandular listeriosis**
>
> **A32.82**   **Listerial endocarditis**
>
> **A32.89**   **Other forms of listeriosis**
> Listerial cerebral arteritis

A32.9   **Listeriosis, unspecified**

A35   OTHER TETANUS

✔

A36   DIPHTHERIA

4th

A36.0   **Pharyngeal diphtheria**

A36.1   **Nasopharyngeal diphtheria**

A36.2   **Laryngeal diphtheria**

A36.8   **Other diphtheria**

> **5th**   **A36.89**   **Other diphtheritic complications**

A36.9   **Diphtheria, unspecified**

CHAPTER 1. CERTAIN INFECTIOUS AND PARASITIC DISEASES   (A17.8–A36.9)

4th **5th** **6th** **7th**	Additional Character Required	✔	3-character code	•=New Code	*Excludes1*—Not coded here, do not use together
				▲=Revised Code	*Excludes2*—Not included here

A37 WHOOPING COUGH
A37.0 Whooping cough due to Bordetella pertussis;
- **A37.00 without pneumonia**
- **A37.01 with pneumonia**

A37.1 Whooping cough due to Bordetella parapertussis;
- **A37.10 without pneumonia**
- **A37.11 with pneumonia**

A37.8 Whooping cough due to other Bordetella species;
- **A37.80 without pneumonia**
- **A37.81 with pneumonia**

A37.9 Whooping cough, unspecified species;
- **A37.90 without pneumonia**
- **A37.91 with pneumonia**

A38 SCARLET FEVER
Includes: scarlatina
Excludes2: streptococcal sore throat (J02.0)
A38.0 Scarlet fever with otitis media
A38.1 Scarlet fever with myocarditis
A38.8 Scarlet fever with other complications
A38.9 Scarlet fever, uncomplicated
  Scarlet fever, NOS

A39 MENINGOCOCCAL INFECTION
A39.0 Meningococcal meningitis
A39.1 Waterhouse-Friderichsen syndrome
  Meningococcal hemorrhagic adrenalitis
  Meningococcic adrenal syndrome
A39.2 Acute meningococcemia
A39.3 Chronic meningococcemia
A39.4 Meningococcemia, unspecified
A39.5 Meningococcal heart disease
- **A39.50 Meningococcal carditis, unspecified**
- **A39.51 Meningococcal endocarditis**
- **A39.52 Meningococcal myocarditis**
- **A39.53 Meningococcal pericarditis**
A39.8 Other meningococcal infections
- **A39.89 Other meningococcal infections**
  Meningococcal conjunctivitis
A39.9 Meningococcal infection, unspecified
  Meningococcal disease NOS

A40 STREPTOCOCCAL SEPSIS
GUIDELINES
Refer to Chapter 1 guidelines for sepsis guidelines.
Code first: postprocedural streptococcal sepsis (T81.4-)
  streptococcal sepsis following immunization (T88.0)
  streptococcal sepsis following infusion, transfusion or therapeutic injection (T80.2-)
Excludes1: neonatal (P36.0–P36.1)
  sepsis due to Streptococcus, group D (A41.81)
A40.0 Sepsis due to streptococcus, group A
A40.1 Sepsis due to streptococcus, group B
A40.3 Sepsis due to Streptococcus pneumoniae
  Pneumococcal sepsis
A40.8 Other streptococcal sepsis
A40.9 Streptococcal sepsis, unspecified

A41 OTHER SEPSIS
GUIDELINES
Refer to Chapter 1 guidelines for sepsis guidelines.
Code first: postprocedural sepsis (T81.4-)
  sepsis following immunization (T88.0)
  sepsis following infusion, transfusion or therapeutic injection (T80.2-)
Excludes1: bacteremia NOS (R78.81)
  neonatal (P36.-)
  puerperal sepsis (O85)
  streptococcal sepsis (A40.-)

Excludes2: sepsis (due to) (in) actinomycotic (A42.7)
  sepsis (due to) (in) anthrax (A22.7)
  sepsis (due to) (in) candidal (B37.7)
  sepsis (due to) (in) Erysipelothrix (A26.7)
  sepsis (due to) (in) extraintestinal yersiniosis (A28.2)
  sepsis (due to) (in) gonococcal (A54.86)
  sepsis (due to) (in) herpesviral (B00.7)
  sepsis (due to) (in) listerial (A32.7)
  sepsis (due to) (in) melioidosis (A24.1)
  sepsis (due to) (in) meningococcal (A39.2–A39.4)
  sepsis (due to) (in) plague (A20.7)
  sepsis (due to) (in) tularemia (A21.7)
  toxic shock syndrome (A48.3)
A41.0 Sepsis due to Staphylococcus aureus
- **A41.01 Sepsis due to**
  MSSA
  MSSA sepsis
  Staphylococcus aureus sepsis NOS
- **A41.02 Sepsis due to MRSA**
A41.1 Sepsis due to other specified staphylococcus
  Coagulase negative staphylococcus sepsis
A41.2 Sepsis due to unspecified staphylococcus
A41.3 Sepsis due to H. influenzae
A41.4 Sepsis due to anaerobes
  Excludes1: gas gangrene (A48.0)
A41.5 Sepsis due to other Gram-negative organisms
- **A41.50 Gram-negative sepsis, unspecified**
  Gram-negative sepsis NOS
- **A41.51 Sepsis due to E. coli**
- **A41.52 Sepsis due to Pseudomonas**
  Pseudomonas aeroginosa
- **A41.53 Sepsis due to Serratia**
- **A41.59 Other Gram-negative sepsis**
A41.8 Other specified sepsis
- **A41.81 Sepsis due to Enterococcus**
- **A41.89 Other specified sepsis**
  If the type of infection or causal organism is not further specified for sepsis, assign code A41.9
A41.9 Sepsis, unspecified organism
  Septicemia NOS

A42 ACTINOMYCOSIS
Excludes1: actinomycetoma (B47.1)
A42.0 Pulmonary actinomycosis
A42.1 Abdominal actinomycosis
A42.2 Cervicofacial actinomycosis
A42.7 Actinomycotic sepsis
A42.8 Other forms of actinomycosis
- **A42.81 Actinomycotic meningitis**
- **A42.82 Actinomycotic encephalitis**
- **A42.89 Other forms of actinomycosis**
A42.9 Actinomycosis, unspecified

A43 NOCARDIOSIS
A43.0 Pulmonary nocardiosis
A43.1 Cutaneous nocardiosis
A43.8 Other forms of nocardiosis
A43.9 Nocardiosis, unspecified

A44 BARTONELLOSIS
A44.0 Systemic bartonellosis
A44.1 Cutaneous and mucocutaneous bartonellosis
A44.8 Other forms of bartonellosis
A44.9 Bartonellosis, unspecified

A46 ERYSIPELAS
Excludes1: postpartum or puerperal erysipelas (O86.89)

   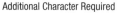 Additional Character Required   3-character code

•=New Code
▲=Revised Code

Excludes1—Not coded here, do not use together
Excludes2—Not included here

A48   OTHER BACTERIAL DISEASES, NOT ELSEWHERE CLASSIFIED
`4th`

Excludes1: actinomycetoma (B47.1)

A48.1   Legionnaires' disease

A48.2   Nonpneumonic Legionnaires' disease [Pontiac fever]

A48.3   Toxic shock syndrome
Use additional code to identify the organism (B95, B96)
Excludes1: endotoxic shock NOS (R57.8)
       sepsis NOS (A41.9)

A48.5   Other specified botulism
`5th`
Non-foodborne intoxication due to toxins of Clostridium botulinum [C. botulinum]
Excludes1: food poisoning due to toxins of Clostridium botulinum (A05.1)

     A48.51   Infant botulism

     A48.52   Wound botulism
         Non-foodborne botulism NOS
         Use additional code for associated wound

A48.8   Other specified bacterial diseases

A49   BACTERIAL INFECTION OF UNSPECIFIED SITE
`4th`

Excludes1: bacterial agents as the cause of diseases classified elsewhere (B95–B96)
     chlamydial infection NOS (A74.9)
     meningococcal infection NOS (A39.9)
     rickettsial infection NOS (A79.9)
     spirochetal infection NOS (A69.9)

A49.0   Staphylococcal infection, unspecified site

`5th` **GUIDELINES**

The condition or state of being colonized or carrying MSSA or MRSA is called colonization or carriage, while an individual person is described as being colonized or being a carrier. Colonization means that MSSA or MSRA is present on or in the body without necessarily causing illness. A positive MRSA colonization test might be documented by the provider as "MRSA screen positive" or "MRSA nasal swab positive". Assign code Z22.322, Carrier or suspected carrier of MRSA, for patients documented as having MRSA colonization. Assign code Z22.321, Carrier or suspected carrier of MSSA, for patient documented as having MSSA colonization. Colonization is not necessarily indicative of a disease process or as the cause of a specific condition the patient may have unless documented as such by the provider. If a patient is documented as having both MRSA colonization and infection during a hospital admission, code Z22.322, and a code for the MRSA infection may both be assigned.

     A49.01   MSSA infection, unspecified site
         MSSA infection
         Staphylococcus aureus infection NOS

     A49.02   MRSA infection, unspecified site
         MRSA infection

A49.1   Streptococcal infection, unspecified site

A49.2   H. influenzae infection, unspecified site

A49.3   Mycoplasma infection, unspecified site

A49.8   Other bacterial infections of unspecified site

A49.9   Bacterial infection, unspecified
Excludes1: bacteremia NOS (R78.81)

(A50–A64) INFECTIONS WITH A PREDOMINANTLY SEXUAL MODE OF TRANSMISSION

Excludes1: HIV disease (B20)
     nonspecific and nongonococcal urethritis (N34.1)
     Reiter's disease (M02.3-)

A50   CONGENITAL SYPHILIS
`4th`

A50.0   Early congenital syphilis, symptomatic
`5th`
Any congenital syphilitic condition specified as early or manifest less than two years after birth.

     A50.01   Early congenital syphilitic; oculopathy

     A50.02   osteochondropathy

     A50.03   pharyngitis
         Early congenital syphilitic laryngitis

     A50.04   pneumonia

     A50.05   rhinitis

     A50.06   Early cutaneous congenital syphilis

     A50.07   Early mucocutaneous congenital syphilis

     A50.08   Early visceral congenital syphilis

     A50.09   Other early congenital syphilis, symptomatic

A50.1   Early congenital syphilis, latent
Congenital syphilis without clinical manifestations, with positive serological reaction and negative spinal fluid test, less than two years after birth.

A50.2   Early congenital syphilis, unspecified
Congenital syphilis NOS less than two years after birth.

A50.3   Late congenital syphilitic oculopathy
`5th`
Excludes1: Hutchinson's triad (A50.53)

     A50.30   Late congenital syphilitic oculopathy, unspecified

     A50.31   Late congenital syphilitic interstitial keratitis

     A50.32   Late congenital syphilitic chorioretinitis

     A50.39   Other late congenital syphilitic oculopathy

A50.4   Late congenital neurosyphilis [juvenile neurosyphilis]
`5th`
Use additional code to identify any associated mental disorder
Excludes1: Hutchinson's triad (A50.53)

     A50.40   Late congenital neurosyphilis, unspecified
         Juvenile neurosyphilis NOS

     A50.41   Late congenital syphilitic meningitis

     A50.42   Late congenital syphilitic encephalitis

     A50.43   Late congenital syphilitic polyneuropathy

     A50.44   Late congenital syphilitic optic nerve atrophy

     A50.45   Juvenile general paresis
         Dementia paralytica juvenilis
         Juvenile tabetoparetic neurosyphilis

     A50.49   Other late congenital neurosyphilis
         Juvenile tabes dorsalis

A50.5   Other late congenital syphilis, symptomatic
`5th`
Any congenital syphilitic condition specified as late or manifest two years or more after birth.

     A50.51   Clutton's joints

     A50.52   Hutchinson's teeth

     A50.53   Hutchinson's triad

     A50.54   Late congenital cardiovascular syphilis

     A50.55   Late congenital syphilitic arthropathy

     A50.56   Late congenital syphilitic osteochondropathy

     A50.57   Syphilitic saddle nose

     A50.59   Other late congenital syphilis, symptomatic

A50.6   Late congenital syphilis, latent
Congenital syphilis without clinical manifestations, with positive serological reaction and negative spinal fluid test, two years or more after birth.

A50.7   Late congenital syphilis, unspecified
Congenital syphilis NOS two years or more after birth.

A50.9   Congenital syphilis, unspecified

A51   EARLY SYPHILIS
`4th`

A51.0   Primary genital syphilis
Syphilitic chancre NOS

A51.1   Primary anal syphilis

A51.2   Primary syphilis of other sites

A51.3   Secondary syphilis of skin and mucous membranes
`5th`
     A51.31   Condyloma latum

     A51.32   Syphilitic alopecia

     A51.39   Other secondary syphilis of skin

A51.5   Early syphilis, latent
Syphilis (acquired) without clinical manifestations, with positive serological reaction and negative spinal fluid test, less than two years after infection.

A51.9   Early syphilis, unspecified

A52   LATE SYPHILIS
`4th`

A52.7   Other symptomatic late syphilis
`5th`
     A52.76   Other genitourinary symptomatic late syphilis

     A52.79   Other symptomatic late syphilis

A52.8   Late syphilis, latent
Syphilis (acquired) without clinical manifestations, with positive serological reaction and negative spinal fluid test, two years or more after infection

A52.9   Late syphilis, unspecified

      Additional Character Required   3-character code

•=New Code   *Excludes1*—Not coded here, do not use together
▲=Revised Code   *Excludes2*—Not included here

A53 **OTHER AND UNSPECIFIED SYPHILIS**

A53.0 **Latent syphilis, unspecified as early or late**
Latent syphilis NOS
Positive serological reaction for syphilis

A53.9 **Syphilis, unspecified**
Infection due to Treponema pallidum NOS
Syphilis (acquired) NOS
Excludes1: syphilis NOS under two years of age (A50.2)

A54 **GONOCOCCAL INFECTION**

A54.0 **Gonococcal infection of lower genitourinary tract without periurethral or accessory gland abscess**
Excludes1: gonococcal infection with genitourinary gland abscess (A54.1)
gonococcal infection with periurethral abscess (A54.1)

  A54.00 **Gonococcal infection of lower genitourinary tract, unspecified**

  A54.01 **Gonococcal cystitis and urethritis, unspecified**

  A54.02 **Gonococcal vulvovaginitis, unspecified**

  A54.03 **Gonococcal cervicitis, unspecified**

  A54.09 **Other gonococcal infection of lower genitourinary tract**

A54.1 **Gonococcal infection of lower genitourinary tract with periurethral and accessory gland abscess**
Gonococcal Bartholin's gland abscess

A54.2 **Gonococcal pelviperitonitis and other gonococcal genitourinary infection**

  A54.21 **Gonococcal infection of kidney and ureter**

  A54.22 **Gonococcal prostatitis**

  A54.23 **Gonococcal infection of other male genital organs**
Gonococcal epididymitis
Gonococcal orchitis

  A54.24 **Gonococcal female pelvic inflammatory disease**
Gonococcal pelviperitonitis
Excludes1: gonococcal peritonitis (A54.85)

  A54.29 **Other gonococcal genitourinary infections**

A54.3 **Gonococcal infection of eye**

  A54.30 **Gonococcal infection of eye, unspecified**

  A54.31 **Gonococcal conjunctivitis**
Ophthalmia neonatorum due to gonococcus

  A54.32 **Gonococcal iridocyclitis**

  A54.33 **Gonococcal keratitis**

  A54.39 **Other gonococcal eye infection**
Gonococcal endophthalmia

A54.4 **Gonococcal infection of musculoskeletal system**

  A54.40 **Gonococcal infection of musculoskeletal system, unspecified**

  A54.41 **Gonococcal spondylopathy**
Excludes2: gonococcal infection of spine (A54.41)

  A54.49 **Gonococcal infection of other musculoskeletal tissue**
Gonococcal bursitis
Gonococcal myositis
Gonococcal synovitis
Gonococcal tenosynovitis

A54.5 **Gonococcal pharyngitis**

A54.6 **Gonococcal infection of anus and rectum**

A54.8 **Other gonococcal infections**

  A54.84 **Gonococcal pneumonia**

  A54.85 **Gonococcal peritonitis**
Excludes1: gonococcal pelviperitonitis (A54.24)

  A54.86 **Gonococcal sepsis**

  A54.89 **Other gonococcal infections**
Gonococcal keratoderma
Gonococcal lymphadenitis

A54.9 **Gonococcal infection, unspecified**

A56 **OTHER SEXUALLY TRANSMITTED CHLAMYDIAL DISEASES**
Includes: sexually transmitted diseases due to Chlamydia trachomatis
Excludes1: neonatal chlamydial conjunctivitis (P39.1)
neonatal chlamydial pneumonia (P23.1)
Excludes2: chlamydial lymphogranuloma (A55)
conditions classified to A74.-

A56.0 **Chlamydial infection of lower genitourinary tract**

  A56.00 **Chlamydial infection of lower genitourinary tract, unspecified**

  A56.01 **Chlamydial cystitis and urethritis**

  A56.02 **Chlamydial vulvovaginitis**

  A56.09 **Other chlamydial infection of lower genitourinary tract**
Chlamydial cervicitis

A56.1 **Chlamydial infection of pelviperitoneum and other genitourinary organs**

  A56.11 **Chlamydial female pelvic inflammatory disease**

  A56.19 **Other chlamydial genitourinary infection**
Chlamydial epididymitis
Chlamydial orchitis

A56.2 **Chlamydial infection of genitourinary tract, unspecified**

A56.3 **Chlamydial infection of anus and rectum**

A56.4 **Chlamydial infection of pharynx**

A56.8 **Sexually transmitted chlamydial infection of other sites**

A59 **TRICHOMONIASIS**
Excludes2: intestinal trichomoniasis (A07.8)

A59.0 **Urogenital trichomoniasis**

  A59.00 **Urogenital trichomoniasis, unspecified**
Fluor (vaginalis) due to Trichomonas
Leukorrhea (vaginalis) due to Trichomonas

  A59.01 **Trichomonal vulvovaginitis**

  A59.02 **Trichomonal prostatitis**

  A59.03 **Trichomonal cystitis and urethritis**

  A59.09 **Other urogenital trichomoniasis**
Trichomonas cervicitis

A59.8 **Trichomoniasis of other sites**

A59.9 **Trichomoniasis, unspecified**

A60 **ANOGENITAL HERPESVIRAL [HERPES SIMPLEX] INFECTIONS**

A60.0 **Herpesviral infection of genitalia and urogenital tract**

  A60.00 **Herpesviral infection of urogenital system, unspecified**

  A60.01 **Herpesviral infection of penis**

  A60.02 **Herpesviral infection of other male genital organs**

  A60.03 **Herpesviral cervicitis**

  A60.04 **Herpesviral vulvovaginitis**
Herpesviral [herpes simplex] ulceration
Herpesviral [herpes simplex] vaginitis
Herpesviral [herpes simplex] vulvitis

  A60.09 **Herpesviral infection of other urogenital tract**

A60.1 **Herpesviral infection of perianal skin and rectum**

A60.9 **Anogenital herpesviral infection, unspecified**

A63 **OTHER PREDOMINANTLY SEXUALLY TRANSMITTED DISEASES, NEC**
Excludes2: molluscum contagiosum (B08.1)
papilloma of cervix (D26.0)

A63.0 **Anogenital (venereal) warts**
Anogenital warts due to (human) papillomavirus [HPV]
Condyloma acuminatum

A63.8 **Other specified predominantly sexually transmitted diseases**

A64 **UNSPECIFIED SEXUALLY TRANSMITTED DISEASE**
Other spirochetal diseases (A65–A69)
Excludes2: leptospirosis (A27.-)
syphilis (A50–A53)

(A65–A69) OTHER SPIROCHETAL DISEASES

A68 **RELAPSING FEVERS**
Includes: recurrent fever
Excludes2: Lyme disease (A69.2-)

A68.0 **Louse-borne relapsing fever**
Relapsing fever due to Borrelia recurrentis

A68.1 **Tick-borne relapsing fever**
Relapsing fever due to any Borrelia species other than Borrelia recurrentis

A68.9 **Relapsing fever, unspecified**

   Additional Character Required   3-character code

•=New Code
▲=Revised Code

Excludes1—Not coded here, do not use together
Excludes2—Not included here

A69 OTHER SPIROCHETAL INFECTIONS

 A69.2 Lyme disease
Erythema chronicum migrans due to Borrelia burgdorferi
A69.20 Lyme disease, unspecified
A69.21 Meningitis due to Lyme disease
A69.22 Other neurologic disorders in Lyme disease
Cranial neuritis
Meningoencephalitis
Polyneuropathy
A69.23 Arthritis due to Lyme disease
A69.29 Other conditions associated with Lyme disease
Myopericarditis due to Lyme disease
A69.8 Other specified spirochetal infections
A69.9 Spirochetal infection, unspecified
Other diseases caused by chlamydiae (A70–A74)
Excludes1: sexually transmitted chlamydial diseases (A55–A56)

(A70–A74) OTHER DISEASES CAUSED BY CHLAMYDIAE

A71 TRACHOMA

 A71.0 Initial stage of trachoma
Trachoma dubium
A71.1 Active stage of trachoma
Granular conjunctivitis (trachomatous)
Trachomatous follicular conjunctivitis
Trachomatous pannus
A71.9 Trachoma, unspecified

A74 OTHER DISEASES CAUSED BY CHLAMYDIAE

 Excludes1: neonatal chlamydial conjunctivitis (P39.1)
neonatal chlamydial pneumonia (P23.1)
Reiter's disease (M02.3-)
sexually transmitted chlamydial diseases (A55–A56)
Excludes2: chlamydial pneumonia (J16.0)
A74.0 Chlamydial conjunctivitis
Paratrachoma
A74.8 Other chlamydial diseases
A74.81 Chlamydial peritonitis
A74.89 Other chlamydial diseases
A74.9 Chlamydial infection, unspecified
Chlamydiosis NOS

(A75–A79) RICKETTSIOSES

A77 SPOTTED FEVER [TICK-BORNE RICKETTSIOSES]

A77.0 Spotted fever due to Rickettsia rickettsii
Rocky Mountain spotted fever
Sao Paulo fever
A77.4 Ehrlichiosis
Excludes1: Rickettsiosis due to Ehrlichia sennetsu (A79.81)
A77.40 Ehrlichiosis, unspecified
A77.41 Ehrlichiosis chafeensis [E. chafeensis]
A77.49 Other ehrlichiosis
A77.8 Other spotted fevers
A77.9 Spotted fever, unspecified
Tick-borne typhus NOS

A79 OTHER RICKETTSIOSES

A79.1 Rickettsialpox due to Rickettsia akari
Kew Garden fever
Vesicular rickettsiosis
A79.8 Other specified rickettsioses
A79.89 Other specified rickettsioses

A79.9 Rickettsiosis, unspecified
Rickettsial infection NOS

(A80–A89) VIRAL AND PRION INFECTIONS OF THE CENTRAL NERVOUS SYSTEM

Excludes1: postpolio syndrome (G14)
sequelae of poliomyelitis (B91)
sequelae of viral encephalitis (B94.1)

A80 ACUTE POLIOMYELITIS

 A80.1 Acute paralytic poliomyelitis, wild virus, imported
A80.2 Acute paralytic poliomyelitis, wild virus, indigenous
A80.3 Acute paralytic poliomyelitis, other and unspecified
A80.30 Acute paralytic poliomyelitis, unspecified
A80.39 Other acute paralytic poliomyelitis
A80.9 Acute poliomyelitis, unspecified

A82 RABIES

 A82.0 Sylvatic rabies
A82.1 Urban rabies
A82.9 Rabies, unspecified

A83 MOSQUITO-BORNE VIRAL ENCEPHALITIS

Includes: mosquito-borne viral meningoencephalitis
Excludes2: Venezuelan equine encephalitis (A92.2)
West Nile fever (A92.3-)
West Nile virus (A92.3-)
A83.2 Eastern equine encephalitis
A83.3 St Louis encephalitis
A83.5 California encephalitis
California meningoencephalitis
La Crosse encephalitis
A83.8 Other mosquito-borne viral encephalitis
A83.9 Mosquito-borne viral encephalitis, unspecified

A84 TICK-BORNE VIRAL ENCEPHALITIS

Includes: tick-borne viral meningoencephalitis
A84.8 Other tick-borne viral encephalitis
Louping ill
Powassan virus disease
A84.9 Tick-borne viral encephalitis, unspecified

A85 OTHER VIRAL ENCEPHALITIS, NEC

Includes: specified viral encephalomyelitis NEC
specified viral meningoencephalitis NEC
Excludes1: benign myalgic encephalomyelitis (G93.3)
encephalitis due to cytomegalovirus (B25.8)
encephalitis due to herpesvirus NEC (B10.0-)
encephalitis due to herpesvirus [herpes simplex] (B00.4)
encephalitis due to measles virus (B05.0)
encephalitis due to mumps virus (B26.2)
encephalitis due to poliomyelitis virus (A80.-)
encephalitis due to zoster (B02.0)
lymphocytic choriomeningitis (A87.2)
A85.0 Enteroviral encephalitis
Enteroviral encephalomyelitis
A85.1 Adenoviral encephalitis
Adenoviral meningoencephalitis
A85.8 Other specified viral encephalitis
Encephalitis lethargica
Von Economo-Cruchet disease

A86 UNSPECIFIED VIRAL ENCEPHALITIS

 Viral encephalomyelitis NOS
Viral meningoencephalitis NOS

A87 VIRAL MENINGITIS

 Excludes1: meningitis due to herpesvirus [herpes simplex] (B00.3)
meningitis due to herpesvirus [herpes simplex] (B00.3)
meningitis due to measles virus (B05.1)
meningitis due to mumps virus (B26.1)
meningitis due to poliomyelitis virus (A80.-)
meningitis due to zoster (B02.1)
A87.0 Enteroviral meningitis
Coxsackievirus meningitis
Echovirus meningitis
A87.1 Adenoviral meningitis
A87.8 Other viral meningitis
A87.9 Viral meningitis, unspecified

  Additional Character Required | ✓ 3-character code

•=New Code
▲=Revised Code

Excludes1—Not coded here, do not use together
Excludes2—Not included here

CHAPTER 1. CERTAIN INFECTIOUS AND PARASITIC DISEASES   (A88–B01.9)

A88 **OTHER VIRAL INFECTIONS OF CENTRAL NERVOUS SYSTEM, NEC**
Excludes1: viral encephalitis NOS (A86)
viral meningitis NOS (A87.9)
  A88.0 Enteroviral exanthematous fever [Boston exanthem]
  A88.1 Epidemic vertigo
  A88.8 Other specified viral infections of central nervous system

A89 ✔ **UNSPECIFIED VIRAL INFECTION OF CENTRAL NERVOUS SYSTEM**

(A90–A99) ARTHROPOD-BORNE VIRAL FEVERS AND VIRAL HEMORRHAGIC FEVERS

A92 4th **OTHER MOSQUITO-BORNE VIRAL FEVERS**
Excludes1: Ross River disease (B33.1)
  A92.3 West Nile virus infection
    5th West Nile fever
      A92.30 West Nile virus infection, unspecified
        West Nile fever NOS
        West Nile fever without complications
        West Nile virus NOS
      A92.31 West Nile virus infection with encephalitis
        West Nile encephalitis
        West Nile encephalomyelitis
      A92.32 West Nile virus infection with other neurologic manifestation
        Use additional code to specify the neurologic manifestation
      A92.39 West Nile virus infection with other complications
        Use additional code to specify the other conditions
  •**A92.5** Zika virus disease
    Zika virus fever
    Zika virus infection
    Zika, NOS
  A92.8 Other specified mosquito-borne viral fevers
  A92.9 Mosquito-borne viral fever, unspecified

A93 4th **OTHER ARTHROPOD-BORNE VIRAL FEVERS, NOT ELSEWHERE CLASSIFIED**
  A93.0 Oropouche virus disease
    Oropouche fever
  A93.1 Sandfly fever
    Pappataci fever
    Phlebotomus fever
  A93.2 Colorado tick fever
  A93.8 Other specified arthropod-borne viral fevers
    Piry virus disease
    Vesicular stomatitis virus disease [Indiana fever]

A94 **UNSPECIFIED ARTHROPOD-BORNE VIRAL FEVER**
Arboviral fever NOS
Arbovirus infection NOS

A95 **YELLOW FEVER**
  A95.0 Sylvatic yellow fever
    Jungle yellow fever
  A95.1 Urban yellow fever
  A95.9 Yellow fever, unspecified

A96 4th **ARENAVIRAL HEMORRHAGIC FEVER**
  A96.0 Junin hemorrhagic fever
    Argentinian hemorrhagic fever
  A96.1 Machupo hemorrhagic fever
    Bolivian hemorrhagic fever
  A96.2 Lassa fever
  A96.8 Other arenaviral hemorrhagic fevers
  A96.9 Arenaviral hemorrhagic fever, unspecified

A98 **OTHER VIRAL HEMORRHAGIC FEVERS, NOT ELSEWHERE CLASSIFIED**
Excludes1: chikungunya hemorrhagic fever (A92.0)
dengue hemorrhagic fever (A91)
  A98.4 Ebola virus disease

  A98.5 Hemorrhagic fever with renal syndrome
    Epidemic hemorrhagic fever
    Korean hemorrhagic fever
    Russian hemorrhagic fever
    Hantaan virus disease
    Hantavirus disease with renal manifestations
    Nephropathia epidemica
    Songo fever
    Excludes1: hantavirus (cardio)-pulmonary syndrome (B33.4)
  A98.8 Other specified viral hemorrhagic fevers

A99 **UNSPECIFIED VIRAL HEMORRHAGIC FEVER**

(B00–B09) VIRAL INFECTIONS CHARACTERIZED BY SKIN AND MUCOUS MEMBRANE LESIONS

B00 **HERPESVIRAL [HERPES SIMPLEX] INFECTIONS**
Excludes1: congenital herpesviral infections (P35.2)
Excludes2: anogenital herpesviral infection (A60.-)
gammaherpesviral mononucleosis (B27.0-)
herpangina (B08.5)
  B00.0 Eczema herpeticum
    Kaposi's varicelliform eruption
  B00.1 Herpesviral vesicular dermatitis
    Herpes simplex facialis
    Herpes simplex labialis
    Herpes simplex otitis externa
    Vesicular dermatitis of ear
    Vesicular dermatitis of lip
  B00.2 Herpesviral gingivostomatitis and pharyngotonsillitis
    Herpesviral pharyngitis
  B00.3 Herpesviral meningitis
  B00.4 Herpesviral encephalitis
    Herpesviral meningoencephalitis
    Simian B disease
    Excludes1: herpesviral encephalitis due to herpesvirus 6 and 7 (B10.01, B10.09)
    non-simplex herpesviral encephalitis (B10.0-)
  B00.5 Herpesviral ocular disease
    5th **B00.50** Herpesviral ocular disease, unspecified
      B00.51 Herpesviral iridocyclitis
        Herpesviral iritis
        Herpesviral uveitis, anterior
      B00.52 Herpesviral keratitis
        Herpesviral keratoconjunctivitis
      B00.53 Herpesviral conjunctivitis
      B00.59 Other herpesviral disease of eye
        Herpesviral dermatitis of eyelid
  B00.8 Other forms of herpesviral infections
    5th **B00.81** Herpesviral hepatitis
      B00.82 Herpes simplex myelitis
      B00.89 Other herpesviral infection
        Herpesviral whitlow
  B00.9 Herpesviral infection, unspecified
    Herpes simplex infection NOS

B01 4th **VARICELLA [CHICKENPOX]**
  B01.0 Varicella meningitis
  B01.1 Varicella encephalitis, myelitis and encephalomyelitis
    5th Postchickenpox encephalitis, myelitis and encephalomyelitis
      B01.11 Varicella encephalitis and encephalomyelitis
        Postchickenpox encephalitis and encephalomyelitis
      B01.12 Varicella myelitis
        Postchickenpox myelitis
  B01.2 Varicella pneumonia
  B01.8 Varicella with other complications
    5th **B01.81** Varicella keratitis
      B01.89 Other varicella complications
  B01.9 Varicella without complication
    Varicella NOS

  6th 7th   Additional Character Required   3-character code

•=New Code   *Excludes1*—Not coded here, do not use together
▲=Revised Code   *Excludes2*—Not included here

B05 MEASLES

Includes: morbilli

Excludes1: subacute sclerosing panencephalitis (A81.1)

B05.0 Measles complicated by encephalitis
Postmeasles encephalitis

B05.1 Measles complicated by meningitis
Postmeasles meningitis

B05.2 Measles complicated by pneumonia
Postmeasles pneumonia

B05.3 Measles complicated by otitis media
Postmeasles otitis media

B05.4 Measles with intestinal complications

B05.8 Measles with other complications

> **B05.81 Measles keratitis and keratoconjunctivitis**
> **B05.89 Other measles complications**

B05.9 Measles without complication
Measles NOS

B06 RUBELLA [GERMAN MEASLES]

Excludes1: congenital rubella (P35.0)

B06.9 Rubella without complication
Rubella NOS

B07 VIRAL WARTS

Includes: verruca simplex
verruca vulgaris
viral warts due to human papillomavirus

Excludes2: anogenital (venereal) warts (A63.0)
papilloma of bladder (D41.4)
papilloma of cervix (D26.0)
papilloma larynx (D14.1)

B07.0 Plantar wart
Verruca plantaris

B07.8 Other viral warts
Common wart
Flat wart
Verruca plana

B07.9 Viral wart, unspecified

B08 OTHER VIRAL INFECTIONS CHARACTERIZED BY SKIN AND MUCOUS MEMBRANE LESIONS, NEC

Excludes1: vesicular stomatitis virus disease (A93.8)

B08.1 Molluscum contagiosum

B08.2 Exanthema subitum [sixth disease]
Roseola infantum

> **B08.20 Exanthema subitum [sixth disease], unspecified**
> Roseola infantum, unspecified
> **B08.21 Exanthema subitum [sixth disease] due to human herpesvirus 6**
> Roseola infantum due to human herpesvirus 6
> **B08.22 Exanthema subitum [sixth disease] due to human herpesvirus 7**
> Roseola infantum due to human herpesvirus 7

B08.3 Erythema infectiosum [fifth disease]

B08.4 Enteroviral vesicular stomatitis with exanthem
Hand, foot and mouth disease

B08.5 Enteroviral vesicular pharyngitis
Herpangina

B08.8 Other specified viral infections characterized by skin and mucous membrane lesions
Enteroviral lymphonodular pharyngitis
Foot-and-mouth disease
Poxvirus NEC

B09 UNSPECIFIED VIRAL INFECTION CHARACTERIZED BY SKIN AND MUCOUS MEMBRANE LESIONS
Viral enanthema NOS
Viral exanthema NOS

(B10) OTHER HUMAN HERPESVIRUSES

B10 OTHER HUMAN HERPESVIRUSES

Excludes2: cytomegalovirus (B25.9)
Epstein-Barr virus (B27.0-)
herpes NOS (B00.9)
herpes simplex (B00.-)
herpes zoster (B02.-)
human herpesvirus NOS (B00.-)
human herpesvirus 1 and 2 (B00.-)
human herpesvirus 3 (B01.-, B02.-)
human herpesvirus 4 (B27.0-)
human herpesvirus 5 (B25.-)
varicella (B01.-)
zoster (B02.-)

B10.0 Other human herpesvirus encephalitis

> *Excludes2:* herpes encephalitis NOS (B00.4)
> herpes simplex encephalitis (B00.4)
> human herpesvirus encephalitis (B00.4)
> simian B herpes virus encephalitis (B00.4)
>
> **B10.01 Human herpesvirus 6 encephalitis**
> **B10.09 Other human herpesvirus encephalitis**
> Human herpesvirus 7 encephalitis

B10.8 Other human herpesvirus infection

> **B10.81 Human herpesvirus 6 infection**
> **B10.82 Human herpesvirus 7 infection**
> **B10.89 Other human herpesvirus infection**
> Human herpesvirus 8 infection
> Kaposi's sarcoma-associated herpesvirus infection

(B15–B19) VIRAL HEPATITIS

Excludes1: sequelae of viral hepatitis (B94.2)
Excludes2: cytomegaloviral hepatitis (B25.1)
herpesviral [herpes simplex] hepatitis (B00.81)

B15 ACUTE HEPATITIS A

B15.9 Hepatitis A without hepatic coma
Hepatitis A (acute)(viral) NOS

B16 ACUTE HEPATITIS B

B16.9 Acute hepatitis B without delta-agent and without hepatic coma
Hepatitis B (acute) (viral) NOS

B17 OTHER ACUTE VIRAL HEPATITIS

B17.1 Acute hepatitis C

> **B17.10 Acute hepatitis C without hepatic coma**
> Acute hepatitis C NOS

B17.9 Acute viral hepatitis, unspecified
Acute infectious hepatitis NOS

B18 CHRONIC VIRAL HEPATITIS

Includes: Carrier of viral hepatitis

B18.1 Chronic viral hepatitis B without delta-agent
Carrier of viral hepatits B

B18.2 Chronic viral hepatitis C
Carrier of viral hepatitis C

B18.8 Other chronic viral hepatitis
Carrier of other viral hepatitis

B18.9 Chronic viral hepatitis, unspecified
Carrier of unspecified viral hepatitis

B19 UNSPECIFIED VIRAL HEPATITIS

B19.1 Unspecified viral hepatitis B

> **B19.10 Unspecified viral hepatitis B without hepatic coma**
> Unspecified viral hepatitis B NOS

B19.2 Unspecified viral hepatitis C

> **B19.20 Unspecified viral hepatitis C without hepatic coma**
> Viral hepatitis C NOS

B19.9 Unspecified viral hepatitis without hepatic coma
Viral hepatitis NOS

CHAPTER 1. CERTAIN INFECTIOUS AND PARASITIC DISEASES   (B20–B34.9)

(B20) HIV DISEASE

GUIDELINES

Code only confirmed cases of HIV infection/illness.

In this context, "confirmation" does not require documentation of positive serology or culture for HIV; the provider's diagnostic statement that the patient is HIV positive, or has an HIV-related illness is sufficient.

Asymptomatic HIV

Z21, Asymptomatic HIV infection status, is to be applied when the patient without any documentation of symptoms is listed as being "HIV positive," "known HIV," "HIV test positive," or similar terminology. Do not use this code if the term "AIDS" is used or if the patient is treated for any HIV-related illness or is described as having any condition(s) resulting from his/her HIV positive status; use B20 in these cases.

Patients with inconclusive HIV serology

Patients with inconclusive HIV serology, but no definitive diagnosis or manifestations of the illness, may be assigned code R75, Inconclusive laboratory evidence of HIV.

B20   HIV DISEASE

   Includes: acquired immune deficiency syndrome [AIDS]
       AIDS-related complex [ARC]
       HIV infection, symptomatic
   Use additional code(s) to identify all manifestations of HIV infection
   Excludes1: asymptomatic HIV infection status (Z21)
       exposure to HIV virus (Z20.6)
       inconclusive serologic evidence of HIV (R75)
       Other viral diseases (B25–B34)

(B25–B34) OTHER VIRAL DISEASES

B25   CYTOMEGALOVIRAL DISEASE
   Excludes1: congenital cytomegalovirus infection (P35.1)
       cytomegaloviral mononucleosis (B27.1-)
   B25.9   Cytomegaloviral disease, unspecified

B26   MUMPS
   Includes: epidemic parotitis
       infectious parotitis
   B26.0   Mumps orchitis
   B26.1   Mumps meningitis
   B26.2   Mumps encephalitis
   B26.8   Mumps with other complications
      B26.89   Other mumps complications

   B26.9   Mumps without complication
       Mumps NOS
       Mumps parotitis NOS

B27   INFECTIOUS MONONUCLEOSIS
   Includes: glandular fever
       monocytic angina
       Pfeiffer's disease
   B27.0   Gammaherpesviral mononucleosis
       Mononucleosis due to Epstein-Barr virus
      B27.00   Gammaherpesviral mononucleosis without complication
      B27.01   Gammaherpesviral mononucleosis with polyneuropathy
      B27.02   Gammaherpesviral mononucleosis with meningitis
      B27.09   Gammaherpesviral mononucleosis with other complications
          Hepatomegaly in gammaherpesviral mononucleosis
   B27.1   Cytomegaloviral mononucleosis
      B27.10   Cytomegaloviral mononucleosis without complications
      B27.11   Cytomegaloviral mononucleosis with polyneuropathy
      B27.12   Cytomegaloviral mononucleosis with meningitis

      B27.19   Cytomegaloviral mononucleosis with other complication
          Hepatomegaly in cytomegaloviral mononucleosis
   B27.8   Other infectious mononucleosis
      B27.80   Other infectious mononucleosis without complication
      B27.81   Other infectious mononucleosis with polyneuropathy
      B27.82   Other infectious mononucleosis with meningitis
      B27.89   Other infectious mononucleosis with other complication
          Hepatomegaly in other infectious mononucleosis
   B27.9   Infectious mononucleosis, unspecified
      B27.90   Infectious mononucleosis, unspecified without complication
      B27.91   Infectious mononucleosis, unspecified with polyneuropathy
      B27.92   Infectious mononucleosis, unspecified with meningitis
      B27.99   Infectious mononucleosis, unspecified with other complication
          Hepatomegaly in unspecified infectious mononucleosis

B30   VIRAL CONJUNCTIVITIS
   Excludes1: herpesviral [herpes simplex] ocular disease (B00.5)
       ocular zoster (B02.3)
   B30.0   Keratoconjunctivitis due to adenovirus
       Epidemic keratoconjunctivitis
       Shipyard eye
   B30.1   Conjunctivitis due to adenovirus
       Acute adenoviral follicular conjunctivitis
       Swimming-pool conjunctivitis
   B30.2   Viral pharyngoconjunctivitis
   B30.3   Acute epidemic hemorrhagic conjunctivitis (enteroviral)
       Conjunctivitis due to coxsackievirus 24
       Conjunctivitis due to enterovirus 70
       Hemorrhagic conjunctivitis (acute)(epidemic)
   B30.8   Other viral conjunctivitis
       Newcastle conjunctivitis
   B30.9   Viral conjunctivitis, unspecified

B33   OTHER VIRAL DISEASES, NEC
   B33.2   Viral carditis
       Coxsackie (virus) carditis
      B33.20   Viral carditis, unspecified
      B33.21   Viral endocarditis
      B33.22   Viral myocarditis
      B33.23   Viral pericarditis
      B33.24   Viral cardiomyopathy
   B33.3   Retrovirus infections, NEC
       Retrovirus infection NOS
   B33.8   Other specified viral diseases
      Excludes1: anogenital human papillomavirus infection (A63.0)
          viral warts due to human papillomavirus infection (B07)

B34   VIRAL INFECTION OF UNSPECIFIED SITE
   Excludes1: anogenital human papillomavirus infection (A63.0)
       cytomegaloviral disease NOS (B25.9)
       herpesvirus [herpes simplex] infection NOS (B00.9)
       retrovirus infection NOS (B33.3)
       viral agents as the cause of diseases classified elsewhere (B97.-)
       viral warts due to human papillomavirus infection (B07)
   B34.0   Adenovirus infection, unspecified
   B34.1   Enterovirus infection, unspecified
       Coxsackievirus infection NOS
       Echovirus infection NOS
   B34.2   Coronavirus infection, unspecified
      Excludes1: pneumonia due to SARS-associated coronavirus (J12.81)
   B34.3   Parvovirus infection, unspecified
   B34.4   Papovavirus infection, unspecified
   B34.8   Other viral infections of unspecified site
   B34.9   Viral infection, unspecified
       Viremia NOS

   Additional Character Required   3-character code

◦=New Code   ***Excludes1***—Not coded here, do not use together
▲=Revised Code   ***Excludes2***—Not included here

(B35–B49) MYCOSES

Excludes2: hypersensitivity pneumonitis due to organic dust (J67.-)
mycosis fungoides (C84.0-)

B35   **DERMATOPHYTOSIS**

     Includes: favus
     infections due to species of Epidermophyton, Micro-sporum and Trichophyton
     tinea, any type except those in B36.-

     B35.0   **Tinea barbae and tinea capitis**
        Beard ringworm
        Kerion
        Scalp ringworm
        Sycosis, mycotic

     B35.1   **Tinea unguium**
        Dermatophytic onychia
        Dermatophytosis of nail
        Onychomycosis
        Ringworm of nails

     B35.2   **Tinea manuum**
        Dermatophytosis of hand
        Hand ringworm

     B35.3   **Tinea pedis**
        Athlete's foot
        Dermatophytosis of foot
        Foot ringworm

     B35.4   **Tinea corporis**
        Ringworm of the body

     B35.6   **Tinea cruris**
        Dhobi itch
        Groin ringworm
        Jock itch

     B35.9   **Dermatophytosis, unspecified**
        Ringworm NOS

B36   **OTHER SUPERFICIAL MYCOSES**

     B36.0   **Pityriasis versicolor**
        Tinea flava
        Tinea versicolor

     B36.9   **Superficial mycosis, unspecified**

B37   **CANDIDIASIS**

     Includes: candidosis
        moniliasis
     Excludes1: neonatal candidiasis (P37.5)

     B37.0   **Candidal stomatitis**
        Oral thrush

     B37.1   **Pulmonary candidiasis**
        Candidal bronchitis
        Candidal pneumonia

     B37.2   **Candidiasis of skin and nail**
        Candidal onychia
        Candidal paronychia
        Excludes2: diaper dermatitis (L22)

     B37.3   **Candidiasis of vulva and vagina**
        Candidal vulvovaginitis
        Monilial vulvovaginitis
        Vaginal thrush

     B37.4   **Candidiasis of other urogenital sites**
        B37.41   **Candidal cystitis and urethritis**
        B37.42   **Candidal balanitis**
        B37.49   **Other urogenital candidiasis**
          Candidal pyelonephritis

     B37.5   **Candidal meningitis**

     B37.6   **Candidal endocarditis**

     B37.7   **Candidal sepsis**
        Disseminated candidiasis
        Systemic candidiasis

     B37.8   **Candidiasis of other sites**
        B37.81   **Candidal esophagitis**
        B37.82   **Candidal enteritis**
          Candidal proctitis

        B37.83   **Candidal cheilitis**
        B37.84   **Candidal otitis externa**
        B37.89   **Other sites of candidiasis**
          Candidal osteomyelitis

     B37.9   **Candidiasis, unspecified**
        Thrush NOS

B39   **HISTOPLASMOSIS**

     Code first associated AIDS (B20)
     Use additional code for any associated manifestations, such as:
        endocarditis (I39)
        meningitis (G02)
        pericarditis (I32)
        retinititis (H32)

     B39.0   **Acute pulmonary histoplasmosis capsulati**
     B39.1   **Chronic pulmonary histoplasmosis capsulati**
     B39.2   **Pulmonary histoplasmosis capsulati, unspecified**
     B39.3   **Disseminated histoplasmosis capsulati**
        Generalized histoplasmosis capsulati
     B39.4   **Histoplasmosis capsulati, unspecified**
        American histoplasmosis
     B39.9   **Histoplasmosis, unspecified**

B40   **BLASTOMYCOSIS**

     Excludes1: Brazilian blastomycosis (B41.-)
        keloidal blastomycosis (B48.0)

     B40.0   **Acute pulmonary blastomycosis**
     B40.1   **Chronic pulmonary blastomycosis**
     B40.2   **Pulmonary blastomycosis, unspecified**
     B40.3   **Cutaneous blastomycosis**
     B40.7   **Disseminated blastomycosis**
        Generalized blastomycosis
     B40.8   **Other forms of blastomycosis**
        B40.81   **Blastomycotic meningoencephalitis**
          Meningomyelitis due to blastomycosis
        B40.89   **Other forms of blastomycosis**
     B40.9   **Blastomycosis, unspecified**

B49   **UNSPECIFIED MYCOSIS**

     Fungemia NOS

(B50–B64) PROTOZOAL DISEASES

Excludes1: amebiasis (A06.-)
other protozoal intestinal diseases (A07.-)

B54   **UNSPECIFIED MALARIA**

B58   **TOXOPLASMOSIS**

     Includes: infection due to Toxoplasma gondii
     Excludes1: congenital toxoplasmosis (P37.1)
     B58.0   **Toxoplasma oculopathy**
        B58.00   **Toxoplasma oculopathy, unspecified**
        B58.01   **Toxoplasma chorioretinitis**
        B58.09   **Other toxoplasma oculopathy**
          Toxoplasma uveitis
     B58.9   **Toxoplasmosis, unspecified**

B60   **OTHER PROTOZOAL DISEASES, NOT ELSEWHERE CLASSIFIED**

     Excludes1: cryptosporidiosis (A07.2)
        intestinal microsporidiosis (A07.8)
        isosporiasis (A07.3)

     B60.0   **Babesiosis**
        Piroplasmosis
     B60.1   **Acanthamebiasis**

B64   **UNSPECIFIED PROTOZOAL DISEASE**

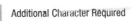   Additional Character Required   3-character code

•=New Code
▲=Revised Code

Excludes1—Not coded here, do not use together
Excludes2—Not included here

(B65–B83) HELMINTHIASES

B65 **SCHISTOSOMIASIS [BILHARZIASIS]**

Includes: snail fever
B65.3 **Cercarial dermatitis**
Swimmer's itch
B65.8 **Other schistosomiasis**
Infection due to Schistosoma intercalatum
Infection due to Schistosoma mattheei
Infection due to Schistosoma mekongi
B65.9 **Schistosomiasis, unspecified**

B66 **OTHER FLUKE INFECTIONS**
B66.8 **Other specified fluke infections**
Echinostomiasis
Heterophyiasis
Metagonimiasis
Nanophyetiasis
Watsoniasis
B66.9 **Fluke infection, unspecified**

B69 **CYSTICERCOSIS**
Includes: cysticerciasis infection due to larval form of Taenia solium
B69.0 **Cysticercosis of central nervous system**
B69.8 **Cysticercosis of other sites**
B69.89 **Cysticercosis of other sites**
B69.9 **Cysticercosis, unspecified**

B71 **OTHER CESTODE INFECTIONS**
B71.0 **Hymenolepiasis**
Dwarf tapeworm infection
Rat tapeworm (infection)
B71.8 **Other specified cestode infections**
Coenurosis
B71.9 **Cestode infection, unspecified**
Tapeworm (infection) NOS

B79 **TRICHURIASIS**

Includes: trichocephaliasis
whipworm (disease)(infection)

B80 **ENTEROBIASIS**

Includes: oxyuriasis
pinworm infection
threadworm infection

B82 **UNSPECIFIED INTESTINAL PARASITISM**
B82.0 **Intestinal helminthiasis, unspecified**
B82.9 **Intestinal parasitism, unspecified**

(B85–B89) PEDICULOSIS, ACARIASIS AND OTHER INFESTATIONS

B85 **PEDICULOSIS AND PHTHIRIASIS**
B85.0 **Pediculosis due to Pediculus humanus capitis**
Head-louse infestation
B85.1 **Pediculosis due to Pediculus humanus corporis**
Body-louse infestation
B85.2 **Pediculosis, unspecified**
B85.3 **Phthiriasis**
Infestation by crab-louse
Infestation by Phthirus pubis
B85.4 **Mixed pediculosis and phthiriasis**
Infestation classifiable to more than one of the categories B85.0–B85.3

B86 **SCABIES**

Sarcoptic itch

B88 **OTHER INFESTATIONS**

B88.0 **Other acariasis**
Acarine dermatitis
Dermatitis due to Demodex species
Dermatitis due to Dermanyssus gallinae
Dermatitis due to Liponyssoides sanguineus
Trombiculosis
Excludes2: scabies (B86)
B88.9 **Infestation, unspecified**
Infestation (skin) NOS
Infestation by mites NOS
Skin parasites NOS

B89 **UNSPECIFIED PARASITIC DISEASE**

(B90–B94) SEQUELAE OF INFECTIOUS AND PARASITIC DISEASES

Note: Categories B90–B94 are to be used to indicate conditions in categories A00–B89 as the cause of sequelae, which are themselves classified elsewhere. The 'sequelae' include conditions specified as such; they also include residuals of diseases classifiable to the above categories if there is evidence that the disease itself is no longer present. Codes from these categories are not to be used for chronic infections. Code chronic current infections to active infectious disease as appropriate.
Code first condition resulting from (sequela) the infectious or parasitic disease

B90 **SEQUELAE OF TUBERCULOSIS**
B90.0 **Sequelae of central nervous system tuberculosis**
B90.1 **Sequelae of genitourinary tuberculosis**
B90.2 **Sequelae of tuberculosis of bones and joints**
B90.8 **Sequelae of tuberculosis of other organs**
Excludes2: sequelae of respiratory tuberculosis (B90.9)
B90.9 **Sequelae of respiratory and unspecified tuberculosis**
Sequelae of tuberculosis NOS

B94 **SEQUELAE OF OTHER AND UNSPECIFIED INFECTIOUS AND PARASITIC DISEASES**
B94.1 **Sequelae of viral encephalitis**
B94.2 **Sequelae of viral hepatitis**
B94.8 **Sequelae of other specified infectious and parasitic diseases**
B94.9 **Sequelae of unspecified infectious and parasitic disease**

(B95–B97) BACTERIAL AND VIRAL INFECTIOUS AGENTS

Note: These categories are provided for use as supplementary or additional codes to identify the infectious agent(s) in diseases classified elsewhere.

B95 **STREPTOCOCCUS, STAPHYLOCOCCUS, AND ENTEROCOCCUS AS THE CAUSE OF DISEASES CLASSIFIED ELSEWHERE**
B95.0 **Streptococcus, group A, as the cause of diseases classified elsewhere**
B95.1 **Streptococcus, group B, as the cause of diseases classified elsewhere**
B95.2 **Enterococcus as the cause of diseases classified elsewhere**
B95.3 **Streptococcus pneumoniae as the cause of diseases classified elsewhere**
B95.4 **Other streptococcus as the cause of diseases classified elsewhere**
B95.5 **Unspecified streptococcus as the cause of diseases classified elsewhere**
B95.6 **Staphylococcus aureus as the cause of diseases classified elsewhere**
B95.61 **MSSA infection as the cause of diseases classified elsewhere**
MSSA infection as the cause of diseases classified elsewhere
Staphylococcus aureus infection NOS as the cause of diseases classified elsewhere
B95.62 **MRSA infection as the cause of diseases classified elsewhere**
MRSA infection as the cause of diseases classified elsewhere

  Additional Character Required 3-character code

•=New Code
▲=Revised Code

Excludes1—Not coded here, do not use together
Excludes2—Not included here

126 PEDIATRIC ICD-10-CM 2017: A MANUAL FOR PROVIDER-BASED CODING

B95.7   Other staphylococcus as the cause of diseases classified elsewhere

B95.8   Unspecified staphylococcus as the cause of diseases classified elsewhere

B96   **OTHER BACTERIAL AGENTS AS THE CAUSE OF DISEASES CLASSIFIED ELSEWHERE**

`4th`

B96.0   M. pneumoniae as the cause of diseases classified elsewhere
Pleuro-pneumonia-like-organism [PPLO]

B96.1   K. pneumoniae as the cause of diseases classified elsewhere

B96.2   E. coli as the cause of diseases classified elsewhere

`5th`

    B96.20   Unspecified E. coli as the cause of diseases classified elsewhere
E. coli NOS

    B96.21   STEC O157 as the cause of diseases classified elsewhere
E. coli O157:H- (nonmotile) with confirmation of Shiga toxin
E. coli O157 with confirmation of Shiga toxin when H antigen is unknown, or is not H7
O157:H7 E. coli with or without confirmation of Shiga toxin-production
STEC O157:H7 with or without confirmation of Shiga toxin-production
STEC O157:H7 with or without confirmation of Shiga toxin-production

    B96.22   Other specified STEC as the cause of diseases classified elsewhere
Non-O157 STEC
Non-O157 STEC with known O group

    B96.23   STEC as the cause of diseases classified elsewhere
STEC with unspecified O group
STEC NOS

    B96.29   Other E. coli as the cause of diseases classified elsewhere
Non-STEC

B96.3   H. influenzae as the cause of diseases classified elsewhere

B96.4   Proteus (mirabilis) (morganii) as the cause of diseases classified elsewhere

B96.5   Pseudomonas (aeruginosa) (mallei) (pseudomallei) as the cause of diseases classified elsewhere

B96.8   Other specified bacterial agents as the cause of diseases classified elsewhere

`5th`   **B96.81**   H. pylori as the cause of diseases classified elsewhere

B97   **VIRAL AGENTS AS THE CAUSE OF DISEASES CLASSIFIED ELSEWHERE**

`4th`

B97.0   Adenovirus as the cause of diseases classified elsewhere

B97.1   Enterovirus as the cause of diseases classified elsewhere

`5th`

    B97.10   Unspecified enterovirus as the cause of diseases classified elsewhere

    B97.11   Coxsackievirus as the cause of diseases classified elsewhere

    B97.12   Echovirus as the cause of diseases classified elsewhere

    B97.19   Other enterovirus as the cause of diseases classified elsewhere

B97.2   Coronavirus as the cause of diseases classified elsewhere

`5th`   **B97.21**   SARS-associated coronavirus as the cause of diseases classified elsewhere
Excludes1: pneumonia due to SARS-associated coronavirus (J12.81)

    B97.29   Other coronavirus as the cause of diseases classified elsewhere

B97.8   Other viral agents as the cause of diseases classified elsewhere

`5th`   **B97.89**   Other viral agents as the cause of diseases classified elsewhere

---

(B99) OTHER INFECTIOUS DISEASES

B99   **OTHER AND UNSPECIFIED INFECTIOUS DISEASES**

`4th`

B99.8   Other infectious disease

B99.9   Unspecified infectious disease

CHAPTER 1. CERTAIN INFECTIOUS AND PARASITIC DISEASES (B95.7–B99.9)

   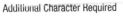 Additional Character Required   3-character code

•=New Code
▲=Revised Code

Excludes1—Not coded here, do not use together
Excludes2—Not included here

Chapter 2. Neoplasms (C00–D49)

GUIDELINES

Chapter 2 of the *ICD-10-CM* contains the codes for most benign and all malignant neoplasms. Certain benign neoplasms, such as prostatic adenomas, may be found in the specific body system chapters. To properly code a neoplasm it is necessary to determine from the record if the neoplasm is benign, in-situ, malignant, or of uncertain histologic behavior. If malignant, any secondary (metastatic) sites should also be determined.

Primary malignant neoplasms overlapping site boundaries

A primary malignant neoplasm that overlaps two or more contiguous (next to each other) sites should be classified to the subcategory/code .8 ('overlapping lesion'), unless the combination is specifically indexed elsewhere. For multiple neoplasms of the same site that are not contiguous such as tumors in different quadrants of the same breast, codes for each site should be assigned.

Malignant neoplasm of ectopic tissue

Malignant neoplasms of ectopic tissue are to be coded to the site of origin mentioned, e.g., ectopic pancreatic malignant neoplasms involving the stomach are coded to pancreas, unspecified (C25.9).

The neoplasm table in the Alphabetic Index should be referenced first. However, if the histological term is documented, that term should be referenced first, rather than going immediately to the Neoplasm Table, in order to determine which column in the Neoplasm Table is appropriate. For example, if the documentation indicates "adenoma," refer to the term in the Alphabetic Index to review the entries under this term and the instructional note to "see also neoplasm, by site, benign." The table provides the proper code based on the type of neoplasm and the site. It is important to select the proper column in the table that corresponds to the type of neoplasm. The Tabular List should then be referenced to verify that the correct code has been selected from the table and that a more specific site code does not exist.

Refer to the *ICD-10-CM* manual for information regarding Z15.0, codes for genetic susceptibility to cancer.

TREATMENT DIRECTED AT THE MALIGNANCY

If the treatment is directed at the malignancy, designate the malignancy as the principal diagnosis.

The only exception to this guideline is if a patient admission/encounter is solely for the administration of chemotherapy, immunotherapy or radiation therapy, assign the appropriate Z51.- code as the first-listed or principal diagnosis, and the diagnosis or problem for which the service is being performed as a secondary diagnosis.

TREATMENT OF SECONDARY SITE

When a patient is admitted because of a primary neoplasm with metastasis and treatment is directed toward the secondary site only, the secondary neoplasm is designated as the principal diagnosis even though the primary malignancy is still present.

CODING AND SEQUENCING OF COMPLICATIONS

Coding and sequencing of complications associated with the malignancies or with the therapy thereof are subject to the following guidelines:

Anemia associated with malignancy

When admission/encounter is for management of an anemia associated with the malignancy, and the treatment is only for anemia, the appropriate code for the malignancy is sequenced as the principal or first-listed diagnosis followed by the appropriate code for the anemia (such as code D63.0, Anemia in neoplastic disease).

Anemia associated with chemotherapy, immunotherapy and radiation therapy

When the admission/encounter is for management of an anemia associated with an adverse effect of the administration of chemotherapy or immunotherapy and the only treatment is for the anemia, the anemia code is sequenced first followed by the appropriate codes for the neoplasm and the adverse effect (T45.1X5, Adverse effect of antineoplastic and immunosuppressive drugs).

When the admission/encounter is for management of an anemia associated with an adverse effect of radiotherapy, the anemia code should be sequenced first, followed by the appropriate neoplasm code and code Y84.2, Radiological procedure and radiotherapy as the cause of abnormal reaction of the patient, or of later complication, without mention of misadventure at the time of the procedure.

Management of dehydration due to the malignancy

When the admission/encounter is for management of dehydration due to the malignancy and only the dehydration is being treated (intravenous rehydration), the dehydration is sequenced first, followed by the code(s) for the malignancy.

Treatment of a complication resulting from a surgical procedure

When the admission/encounter is for treatment of a complication resulting from a surgical procedure, designate the complication as the principal or first-listed diagnosis if treatment is directed at resolving the complication.

PRIMARY MALIGNANCY PREVIOUSLY EXCISED

When a primary malignancy has been previously excised or eradicated from its site and there is no further treatment directed to that site and there is no evidence of any existing primary malignancy, a code from category Z85, Personal history of malignant neoplasm, should be used to indicate the former site of the malignancy. Any mention of extension, invasion, or metastasis to another site is coded as a secondary malignant neoplasm to that site. The secondary site may be the principal or first-listed with the Z85 code used as a secondary code.

ADMISSIONS/ENCOUNTERS INVOLVING CHEMOTHERAPY, IMMUNOTHERAPY AND RADIATION THERAPY

Episode of care involves surgical removal of neoplasm

When an episode of care involves the surgical removal of a neoplasm, primary or secondary site, followed by adjunct chemotherapy or radiation treatment during the same episode of care, the code for the neoplasm should be assigned as principal or first-listed diagnosis.

Patient admission/encounter solely for administration of chemotherapy, immunotherapy and radiation therapy

If a patient admission/encounter is solely for the administration of chemotherapy, immunotherapy or radiation therapy assign code Z51.0, Encounter for antineoplastic radiation therapy, or Z51.11, Encounter for antineoplastic chemotherapy, or Z51.12, Encounter for antineoplastic immunotherapy as the first-listed or principal diagnosis. If a patient receives more than one of these therapies during the same admission more than one of these codes may be assigned, in any sequence.

Patient admitted for radiation therapy, chemotherapy or immunotherapy and develops complications

When a patient is admitted for the purpose of radiotherapy, immunotherapy or chemotherapy and develops complications such as uncontrolled nausea and vomiting or dehydration, the principal or first-listed diagnosis is Z51.0, Encounter for antineoplastic radiation therapy, or Z51.11, Encounter for antineoplastic chemotherapy, or Z51.12, Encounter for antineoplastic immunotherapy followed by any codes for the complications.

ADMISSION/ENCOUNTER TO DETERMINE EXTENT OF MALIGNANCY

When the reason for admission/encounter is to determine the extent of the malignancy, or for a procedure such as paracentesis or thoracentesis, the primary malignancy or appropriate metastatic site is designated as the principal or first-listed diagnosis, even though chemotherapy or radiotherapy is administered.

SYMPTOMS, SIGNS, AND ABNORMAL FINDINGS LISTED IN CHAPTER 18 ASSOCIATED WITH NEOPLASMS

Symptoms, signs, and ill-defined conditions listed in Chapter 18 characteristic of, or associated with, an existing primary or secondary site malignancy cannot be used to replace the malignancy as principal or first-listed diagnosis, regardless of the number of admissions or encounters for treatment and care of the neoplasm.

ADMISSION/ENCOUNTER FOR PAIN CONTROL/MANAGEMENT

Refer to category G89 for information on coding admission/encounter for pain control/management.

MALIGNANCY IN TWO OR MORE NONCONTIGUOUS SITES

A patient may have more than one malignant tumor in the same organ. These tumors may represent different primaries or metastatic disease, depending on the site. Should the documentation be unclear as to the status of each tumor so that the correct codes can be assigned, the provider should be queried.

DISSEMINATED MALIGNANT NEOPLASM, UNSPECIFIED

See code C80.0.

MALIGNANT NEOPLASM WITHOUT SPECIFICATION OF SITE

See code C80.1.

  Additional Character Required 3-character code | Unspecified laterality codes were excluded here. | °=New Code ▲=Revised Code | *Excludes1*—Not coded here, do not use together *Excludes2*—Not included here

SEQUENCING OF NEOPLASM CODES

Encounter for treatment of primary malignancy
If the reason for the encounter is for treatment of a primary malignancy, assign the malignancy as the principal/first-listed diagnosis. The primary site is to be sequenced first, followed by any metastatic sites.

Encounter for treatment of secondary malignancy
When an encounter is for a primary malignancy with metastasis and treatment is directed toward the metastatic (secondary) site(s) only, the metastatic site(s) is designated as the principal/first-listed diagnosis. The primary malignancy is coded as an additional code.

Encounter for complication associated with a neoplasm
When an encounter is for management of a complication associated with a neoplasm, such as dehydration, and the treatment is only for the complication, the complication is coded first, followed by the appropriate code(s) for the neoplasm.

    The exception to this guideline is anemia. When the admission/encounter is for management of an anemia associated with the malignancy, and the treatment is only for anemia, the appropriate code for the malignancy is sequenced as the principal or first-listed diagnosis followed by code D63.0, Anemia in neoplastic disease.

Complication from surgical procedure for treatment of a neoplasm
When an encounter is for treatment of a complication resulting from a surgical procedure performed for the treatment of the neoplasm, designate the complication as the principal/first-listed diagnosis. See guideline regarding the coding of a current malignancy versus personal history to determine if the code for the neoplasm should also be assigned.

Pathologic fracture due to a neoplasm
When an encounter is for a pathological fracture due to a neoplasm, and the focus of treatment is the fracture, a code from subcategory M84.5, should be sequenced first, followed by the code for the neoplasm.

    If the focus of treatment is the neoplasm with an associated pathological fracture, the neoplasm code should be sequenced first, followed by a code from M84.5 for the pathological fracture.

CURRENT MALIGNANCY VERSUS PERSONAL HISTORY OF MALIGNANCY
When a primary malignancy has been excised but further treatment, such as an dditional surgery for the malignancy, radiation therapy or chemotherapy is directed to that site, the primary malignancy code should be used until treatment is completed.

    When a primary malignancy has been previously excised or eradicated from its site, there is no further treatment (of the malignancy) directed to that site, and there is no evidence of any existing primary malignancy, a code from category Z85, Personal history of malignant neoplasm, should be used to indicate the former site of the malignancy.

    Refer to Chapter 21, Factors influencing health status and contact with health services, History (of)

LEUKEMIA, MULTIPLE MYELOMA, AND MALIGNANT PLASMA CELL NEOPLASMS IN REMISSION VERSUS PERSONAL HISTORY
The categories for leukemia, and category C90, have codes indicating whether or not the leukemia has achieved remission. There are also codes Z85.6, Personal history of leukemia, and Z85.79, Personal history of other malignant neoplasms of lymphoid, hematopoietic and related tissues. If the documentation is unclear, as to whether the leukemia has achieved remission, the provider should be queried.

    Refer to Chapter 21, Factors influencing health status and contact with health services, History (of)

AFTERCARE FOLLOWING SURGERY FOR NEOPLASM
Refer to Chapter 21, Factors influencing health status and contact with health services, Aftercare

FOLLOW-UP CARE FOR COMPLETED TREATMENT OF A MALIGNANCY
Refer to Chapter 21, Factors influencing health status and contact with health services, Follow-up

PROPHYLACTIC ORGAN REMOVAL FOR PREVENTION OF MALIGNANCY
Refer to Chapter 21, Factors influencing health

MALIGNANT NEOPLASM ASSOCIATED WITH TRANSPLANTED ORGAN
A malignant neoplasm of a transplanted organ should be coded as a transplant complication. Assign first the appropriate code from category T86.-, Complications of transplanted organs and tissue, followed by code C80.2, Malignant neoplasm associated with transplanted organ. Use an additional code for the specific malignancy.

NEOPLASMS (C00–D49)

Note: Functional activity
All neoplasms are classified in this chapter, whether they are functionally active or not. An additional code from Chapter 4 may be used, to identify functional activity associated with any neoplasm.

Morphology [Histology]
Chapter 2 classifies neoplasms primarily by site (topography), with broad groupings for behavior, malignant, in situ, benign, etc. The Table of Neoplasms should be used to identify the correct topography code. In a few cases, such as for malignant melanoma and certain neuroendocrine tumors, the morphology (histologic type) is included in the category and codes.

Primary malignant neoplasms overlapping site boundaries
A primary malignant neoplasm that overlaps two or more contiguous (next to each other) sites should be classified to the subcategory/code .8 ('overlapping lesion'), unless the combination is specifically indexed elsewhere. For multiple neoplasms of the same site that are not contiguous, such as tumors in different quadrants of the same breast, codes for each site should be assigned.

Malignant neoplasm of ectopic tissue
Malignant neoplasms of ectopic tissue are to be coded to the site mentioned, e.g., ectopic pancreatic malignant neoplasms are coded to pancreas, unspecified (C25.9).

(C00–C96) MALIGNANT NEOPLASMS

Includes: Malignant neoplasms, stated or presumed to be primary (of specified sites), and certain specified histologies, except neuroendocrine, and of lymphoid, hematopoietic and related tissue (C00–C75)

(C00–C14) MALIGNANT NEOPLASMS OF LIP, ORAL CAVITY AND PHARYNX

(C15–C26) MALIGNANT NEOPLASMS OF DIGESTIVE ORGANS

Excludes1: Kaposi's sarcoma of gastrointestinal sites (C46.4)

(C30–C39) MALIGNANT NEOPLASMS OF RESPIRATORY AND INTRATHORACIC ORGANS

Includes: malignant neoplasm of middle ear
Excludes1: mesothelioma (C45.-)

(C40–C41) MALIGNANT NEOPLASMS OF BONE AND ARTICULAR CARTILAGE

Includes: malignant neoplasm of cartilage (articular) (joint)
    malignant neoplasm of periosteum
Excludes1: malignant neoplasm of bone marrow NOS (C96.9)
    malignant neoplasm of synovia (C49.-)

C40   **MALIGNANT NEOPLASM OF BONE AND ARTICULAR CARTILAGE OF LIMBS**
(4th)   Use additional code to identify major osseous defect, if applicable (M89.7-)
    C40.0   **Malignant neoplasm of scapula and long bones of upper limb**
    (5th)   **C40.01**   Malignant neoplasm of scapula and long bones of right upper limb
        C40.02   Malignant neoplasm of scapula and long bones of left upper limb
    C40.1   **Malignant neoplasm of short bones of; upper limb**
    (5th)   **C40.11**   right upper limb
        C40.12   left upper limb
    C40.2   **Malignant neoplasm of long bones of; lower limb**
    (5th)   **C40.21**   right lower limb
        C40.22   left lower limb
    C40.3   **Malignant neoplasm of short bones of; lower limb**
    (5th)   **C40.31**   right lower limb
        C40.32   left lower limb
    C40.8   **Malignant neoplasm of overlapping sites of bone and articular cartilage of; limb**
    (5th)   **C40.81**   right limb
        C40.82   left limb

   Additional Character Required   3-character code

Unspecified laterality codes were excluded here.   •=New Code   ▲=Revised Code

Excludes1—Not coded here, do not use together
Excludes2—Not included here

C40.9 Malignant neoplasm of unspecified bones and articular
cartilage of; limb
[5th]
C40.91 right limb
C40.92 left limb

(C43–C44) MELANOMA AND OTHER MALIGNANT NEOPLASMS OF SKIN

(C45–C49) MALIGNANT NEOPLASMS OF MESOTHELIAL AND SOFT TISSUE

(C50) MALIGNANT NEOPLASMS OF BREAST

(C51–C58) MALIGNANT NEOPLASMS OF FEMALE GENITAL ORGANS

Includes: malignant neoplasm of skin of female genital organs

(C60–C63) MALIGNANT NEOPLASMS OF MALE GENITAL ORGANS

Includes: malignant neoplasm of skin of male genital organs

(C64–C68) MALIGNANT NEOPLASMS OF URINARY TRACT

C64 **MALIGNANT NEOPLASM OF KIDNEY, EXCEPT RENAL PELVIS**
[4th]
Excludes1: malignant carcinoid tumor of the kidney (C7A.093)
malignant neoplasm of renal calyces (C65.-)
malignant neoplasm of renal pelvis (C65.-)
C64.1 **Malignant neoplasm of right kidney, except renal pelvis**
C64.2 **Malignant neoplasm of left kidney, except renal pelvis**

(C69–C72) MALIGNANT NEOPLASMS OF EYE, BRAIN AND OTHER PARTS OF CENTRAL NERVOUS SYSTEM

C69 **MALIGNANT NEOPLASM OF EYE AND ADNEXA**
[4th]
Excludes1: malignant neoplasm of connective tissue of eyelid (C49.0)
malignant neoplasm of eyelid (skin) (C43.1-, C44.1-)
malignant neoplasm of optic nerve (C72.3-)
C69.2 **Malignant neoplasm of retina**
[5th]
Excludes1: dark area on retina (D49.81)
neoplasm of unspecified behavior of retina and choroid (D49.81)
retinal freckle (D49.81)
C69.21 Malignant neoplasm of right retina
C69.22 Malignant neoplasm of left retina

C71 **MALIGNANT NEOPLASM OF BRAIN**
[4th]
Excludes1: malignant neoplasm of cranial nerves (C72.2–C72.5)
retrobulbar malignant neoplasm (C69.6-)
C71.0 **Malignant neoplasm of; cerebrum, except lobes and ventricles**
Malignant neoplasm of supratentorial NOS
C71.1 **frontal lobe**
C71.2 **temporal lobe**
C71.3 **parietal lobe**
C71.4 **occipital lobe**
C71.5 **cerebral ventricle**
Excludes1: malignant neoplasm of fourth cerebral ventricle (C71.7)
C71.6 **cerebellum**
C71.7 **brain stem**
Malignant neoplasm of fourth cerebral ventricle
Infratentorial malignant neoplasm NOS
C71.8 **overlapping sites of brain**
C71.9 **brain, unspecified**

(C73–C75) MALIGNANT NEOPLASMS OF THYROID AND OTHER ENDOCRINE GLANDS

C74 **MALIGNANT NEOPLASM OF ADRENAL GLAND**
[4th]
C74.0 **Malignant neoplasm of cortex of; adrenal gland**
[5th]
C74.01 right adrenal gland
C74.02 left adrenal gland
C74.1 **Malignant neoplasm of medulla of; adrenal gland**
[5th]
C74.11 right adrenal gland
C74.12 left adrenal gland
C74.9 **Malignant neoplasm of unspecified part of; adrenal gland**
[5th]
C74.91 right adrenal gland
C74.92 left adrenal gland

(C7A) MALIGNANT NEUROENDOCRINE TUMORS

(C7B) SECONDARY NEUROENDOCRINE TUMORS

(C76–C80) MALIGNANT NEOPLASMS OF ILL-DEFINED, OTHER SECONDARY AND UNSPECIFIED SITES

C80 **MALIGNANT NEOPLASM WITHOUT SPECIFICATION OF SITE**
[4th]
Excludes1: malignant carcinoid tumor of unspecified site (C7A.00)
malignant neoplasm of specified multiple sites- code to each site
C80.0 **Disseminated malignant neoplasm, unspecified**
Use only in those cases where the patient has advanced metastatic disease and no known primary or secondary sites are specified. It should not be used in place of assigning codes for the primary site and all known secondary sites.
Carcinomatosis NOS
Generalized cancer, unspecified site (primary) (secondary)
Generalized malignancy, unspecified site (primary) (secondary)
C80.1 **Malignant (primary) neoplasm, unspecified**
Use only be used when no determination can be made as to the primary site of a malignancy.
Cancer NOS
Cancer unspecified site (primary)
Carcinoma unspecified site (primary)
Malignancy unspecified site (primary)
Excludes1: secondary malignant neoplasm of unspecified site (C79.9)
C80.2 **Malignant neoplasm associated with transplanted organ**
Code first complication of transplanted organ (T86.-)
Use additional code to identify the specific malignancy

(C81–C96) MALIGNANT NEOPLASMS OF LYMPHOID, HEMATOPOIETIC AND RELATED TISSUE

Excludes2: Kaposi's sarcoma of lymph nodes (C46.3)
secondary and unspecified neoplasm of lymph nodes (C77.-)
secondary neoplasm of bone marrow (C79.52)
secondary neoplasm of spleen (C78.89)

C81 **HODGKIN LYMPHOMA**
[4th]
Excludes1: personal history of Hodgkin lymphoma (Z85.71)
C81.9 **Hodgkin lymphoma, unspecified**
[5th]
C81.91 Hodgkin lymphoma, unspecified; lymph nodes of head, face, and neck
C81.92 intrathoracic lymph nodes
C81.93 intra-abdominal lymph nodes
C81.94 lymph nodes of axilla and upper limb
C81.95 lymph nodes of inguinal region and lower limb
C81.96 intrapelvic lymph nodes
C81.97 spleen
C81.98 lymph nodes of multiple sites
C81.99 extranodal and solid organ sites

CHAPTER 2. NEOPLASMS (C40.9–C81.99)

   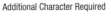   Additional Character Required [✓] 3-character code | Unspecified laterality codes were excluded here. | •=New Code ▲=Revised Code | *Excludes1*—Not coded here, do not use together *Excludes2*—Not included here

CHAPTER 2. NEOPLASMS   (C83–C93.1)

C83 NON-FOLLICULAR LYMPHOMA
Excludes1: personal history of non-Hodgkin lymphoma (Z85.72)
    C83.3 Diffuse large B-cell lymphoma
      Anaplastic diffuse large B-cell lymphoma
      CD30-positive diffuse large B-cell lymphoma
      Centroblastic diffuse large B-cell lymphoma
      Diffuse large B-cell lymphoma, subtype not specified
      Immunoblastic diffuse large B-cell lymphoma
      Plasmablastic diffuse large B-cell lymphoma
      Diffuse large B-cell lymphoma, subtype not specified
      T-cell rich diffuse large B-cell lymphoma
      Excludes1: mediastinal (thymic) large B-cell lymphoma (C85.2-)
        mature T/NK-cell lymphomas (C84.-)
      C83.30 Diffuse large B-cell lymphoma; unspecified site
      C83.31 lymph nodes of head, face, and neck
      C83.32 intrathoracic lymph nodes
      C83.33 intra-abdominal lymph nodes
      C83.34 lymph nodes of axilla and upper limb
      C83.35 lymph nodes of inguinal region and lower limb
      C83.36 intrapelvic lymph nodes
      C83.37 spleen
      C83.38 lymph nodes of multiple sites
      C83.39 extranodal and solid organ sites

C84 MATURE T/NK-CELL LYMPHOMAS
Excludes1: personal history of non-Hodgkin lymphoma (Z85.72)
    C84.4 Peripheral T-cell lymphoma, not classified
      Lennert's lymphoma
      Lymphoepithelioid lymphoma
      Mature T-cell lymphoma, not elsewhere classified
      C84.41 Peripheral T-cell lymphoma, not classified; lymph nodes of head, face, and neck
      C84.42 intrathoracic lymph nodes
      C84.43 intra-abdominal lymph nodes
      C84.44 lymph nodes of axilla and upper limb
      C84.45 lymph nodes of inguinal region and lower limb
      C84.46 intrapelvic lymph nodes
      C84.47 spleen
      C84.48 lymph nodes of multiple sites
      C84.49 extranodal and solid organ sites

C85 OTHER SPECIFIED AND UNSPECIFIED TYPES OF NON-HODGKIN LYMPHOMA
Excludes1: other specified types of T/NK-cell lymphoma (C86.-)
    personal history of non-Hodgkin lymphoma (Z85.72)
    C85.9 Non-Hodgkin lymphoma, unspecified
      Lymphoma NOS
      Malignant lymphoma NOS
      Non-Hodgkin lymphoma NOS
      C85.91 Non-Hodgkin lymphoma, unspecified; lymph nodes of head, face, and neck
      C85.92 intrathoracic lymph nodes
      C85.93 intra-abdominal lymph nodes
      C85.94 lymph nodes of axilla and upper limb
      C85.95 lymph nodes of inguinal region and lower limb
      C85.96 intrapelvic lymph nodes
      C85.97 spleen
      C85.98 lymph nodes of multiple sites
      C85.99 extranodal and solid organ sites

C91 LYMPHOID LEUKEMIA
Excludes1: personal history of leukemia (Z85.6)
    C91.0 ALL
      Note: Code C91.0 should only be used for T-cell and B-cell precursor leukemia
      C91.00 ALL; not having achieved remission
        ALL with failed remission
        ALL NOS
      C91.01 ALL, in remission
      C91.02 ALL, in relapse
    C91.9 Lymphoid leukemia, unspecified
      C91.90 Lymphoid leukemia, unspecified; not having achieved remission
        Lymphoid leukemia with failed remission
        Lymphoid leukemia NOS

      C91.91 in remission
      C91.92 in relapse

C92 MYELOID LEUKEMIA
Includes: granulocytic leukemia
myelogenous leukemia
Excludes1: personal history of leukemia (Z85.6)
    C92.0 Acute myeloblastic leukemia
      Acute myeloblastic leukemia, minimal differentiation
      Acute myeloblastic leukemia (with maturation)
      Acute myeloblastic leukemia 1/ETO
      Acute myeloblastic leukemia M0 or M1 or M2
      Acute myeloblastic leukemia with t(8;21)
      Acute myeloblastic leukemia (without a FAB classification) NOS
      Refractory anemia with excess blasts in transformation [RAEB T]
      Excludes1: acute exacerbation of chronic myeloid leukemia (C92.10)
        refractory anemia with excess of blasts not in transformation (D46.2-)
      C92.00 Acute myeloblastic leukemia; not having achieved remission
        Acute myeloblastic leukemia with failed remission
        Acute myeloblastic leukemia NOS
      C92.01 in remission
      C92.02 in relapse
    C92.1 Chronic myeloid leukemia, BCR/ABL-positive
      Chronic myelogenous leukemia, Philadelphia chromosome (Ph1) positive
      Chronic myelogenous leukemia, t(9;22) (q34;q11)
      Chronic myelogenous leukemia with crisis of blast cells
      Excludes1: atypical chronic myeloid leukemia BCR/ABL-negative (C92.2-)
        CMML (C93.1-)
        chronic myeloproliferative disease (D47.1)
      C92.10 Chronic myeloid leukemia, BCR/ABL-positive; not having achieved remission
        Chronic myeloid leukemia, BCR/ABL-positive with failed remission
        Chronic myeloid leukemia, BCR/ABL-positive NOS
      C92.11 in remission
      C92.12 in relapse
    C92.2 Atypical chronic myeloid leukemia, BCR/ABL-negative
      C92.20 Atypical chronic myeloid leukemia, BCR/ABL-negative; not having achieved remission
        Atypical chronic myeloid leukemia, BCR/ABL-negative with failed remission
        Atypical chronic myeloid leukemia, BCR/ABL-negative NOS
      C92.21 in remission
      C92.22 in relapse
    C92.9 Myeloid leukemia, unspecified
      C92.90 Myeloid leukemia, unspecified; not having achieved remission
        Myeloid leukemia, unspecified with failed remission
        Myeloid leukemia, unspecified NOS
      C92.91 in remission
      C92.92 unspecified in relapse

C93 MONOCYTIC LEUKEMIA
Includes: monocytoid leukemia
Excludes1: personal history of leukemia (Z85.6)
    C93.0 Acute monoblastic/monocytic leukemia
      AML M5 or AML M5a or AML M5b
      C93.00 Acute monoblastic/monocytic leukemia; not having achieved remission
        Acute monoblastic/monocytic leukemia with failed remission
        Acute monoblastic/monocytic leukemia NOS
      C93.01 in remission
      C93.02 in relapse
    C93.1 CMML
      Chronic monocytic leukemia
      CMML-1 or CMML-2
      CMML with eosinophilia

| 4th | 5th | 6th | 7th | Additional Character Required | ✓ 3-character code | Unspecified laterality codes were excluded here. | •=New Code ▲=Revised Code | *Excludes1*—Not coded here, do not use together *Excludes2*—Not included here |

C93.10 **CMML; not having achieved remission**
CMML with failed remission
CMML NOS
C93.11   **in remission**
C93.12   **in relapse**
C93.3 **Juvenile myelomonocytic leukemia**
C93.30 **Juvenile myelomonocytic leukemia; not having achieved remission**
Juvenile myelomonocytic leukemia with failed remission
Juvenile myelomonocytic leukemia NOS
C93.31   **in remission**
C93.32   **in relapse**
C93.Z **Other monocytic leukemia**
C93.Z0 **Other monocytic leukemia; not having achieved remission**
Other monocytic leukemia NOS
C93.Z1   **in remission**
C93.Z2   **in relapse**
C93.9 **Monocytic leukemia, unspecified**
C93.90 **Monocytic leukemia, unspecified; not having achieved remission**
Monocytic leukemia, unspecified with failed remission
leukemia, unspecified NOS
C93.91   **in remission**
C93.92   **in relapse**

(D00–D09) IN SITU NEOPLASMS

Includes: Bowen's disease
erythroplasia
grade III intraepithelial neoplasia
Queyrat's erythroplasia

(D10–D36) BENIGN NEOPLASMS, EXCEPT BENIGN NEUROENDOCRINE TUMORS

D12   **BENIGN NEOPLASM OF COLON, RECTUM, ANUS AND ANAL CANAL**
Excludes1: benign carcinoid tumors of the large intestine, and rectum (D3A.02-)
D12.0   **Benign neoplasm of; cecum**
Benign neoplasm of ileocecal valve
D12.1   **appendix**
Excludes1: benign carcinoid tumor of the appendix (D3A.020)
D12.2   **ascending colon**
D12.3   **transverse colon**
Benign neoplasm of hepatic flexure or splenic flexure
D12.4   **descending colon**
D12.5   **sigmoid colon**
D12.6   **colon, unspecified**
Adenomatosis of colon
Benign neoplasm of large intestine NOS
Polyposis (hereditary) of colon
Excludes1: inflammatory polyp of colon (K51.4-)
polyp of colon NOS (K63.5)
D12.7   **rectosigmoid junction**
D12.8   **rectum**
Excludes1: benign carcinoid tumor of the rectum (D3A.026)
D12.9   **Benign neoplasm of anus and anal canal**
Benign neoplasm of anus NOS
Excludes1: benign neoplasm of anal margin (D22.5, D23.5)
benign neoplasm of anal skin (D22.5, D23.5)
benign neoplasm of perianal skin (D22.5, D23.5)

D15   **BENIGN NEOPLASM OF OTHER AND UNSPECIFIED INTRATHORACIC ORGANS**
Excludes1: benign neoplasm of mesothelial tissue (D19.-)
D15.1   **Benign neoplasm of heart**
Excludes1: benign neoplasm of great vessels (D21.3)

D17   **BENIGN LIPOMATOUS NEOPLASM**
D17.0   **Benign lipomatous neoplasm of skin and subcutaneous tissue of; head, face and neck**
D17.1   **trunk**

D17.2   **Benign lipomatous neoplasm of skin and subcutaneous tissue of; limb**
D17.21   **right arm**
D17.22   **left arm**
D17.23   **right leg**
D17.24   **left leg**
D17.3   **Benign lipomatous neoplasm of skin and subcutaneous tissue of; other and unspecified sites**
D17.30   **unspecified sites**
D17.39   **other sites**
D17.4   **Benign lipomatous neoplasm of intrathoracic organs**
D17.5   **Benign lipomatous neoplasm of intra-abdominal organs**
Excludes1: benign lipomatous neoplasm of peritoneum and retroperitoneum (D17.79)
D17.6   **Benign lipomatous neoplasm of spermatic cord**
D17.7   **Benign lipomatous neoplasm of other sites**
D17.71 **Benign lipomatous neoplasm of; kidney**
D17.72   **other genitourinary organ**
D17.79   **other sites**
Benign lipomatous neoplasm of peritoneum or retroperitoneum
D17.9   **Benign lipomatous neoplasm, unspecified**
Lipoma NOS

D18   **HEMANGIOMA AND LYMPHANGIOMA, ANY SITE**
Excludes1: benign neoplasm of glomus jugulare (D35.6)
blue or pigmented nevus (D22.-)
nevus NOS (D22.-)
vascular nevus (Q82.5)
D18.0   **Hemangioma**
Angioma NOS
Cavernous nevus
D18.00 **Hemangioma unspecified site**
D18.01 **Hemangioma of skin and subcutaneous tissue**
D18.02 **Hemangioma of intracranial structures**
D18.03 **Hemangioma of intra-abdominal structures**
D18.09 **Hemangioma of other sites**
D18.1   **Lymphangioma, any site**

D23   **OTHER BENIGN NEOPLASMS OF SKIN**
Includes: benign neoplasm of hair follicles or sebaceous glands or sweat glands
Excludes1: benign lipomatous neoplasms of skin (D17.0-D17.3)
melanocytic nevi (D22.-)
D23.0   **Other benign neoplasm of skin of lip**
Excludes1: benign neoplasm of vermilion border of lip (D10.0)
D23.1   **Other benign neoplasm of skin of; eyelid, including canthus**
D23.11   **right eyelid, including canthus**
D23.12   **left eyelid, including canthus**
D23.2   **Other benign neoplasm of skin of; ear and external auricular canal**
D23.21   **right ear and external auricular canal**
D23.22   **left ear and external auricular canal**
D23.3   **Other benign neoplasm of skin of; other and unspecified parts of face**
D23.30   **unspecified part of face**
D23.39   **other parts of face**
D23.4   **Other benign neoplasm of skin of scalp and neck**
D23.5   **Other benign neoplasm of skin of trunk**
Other benign neoplasm of anal margin or anal skin or perianal skin
Other benign neoplasm of skin of breast
Excludes1: benign neoplasm of anus NOS (D12.9)
D23.6   **Other benign neoplasm of skin of; upper limb, including shoulder**
D23.61   **right upper limb, including shoulder**
D23.62   **left upper limb, including shoulder**
D23.7   **Other benign neoplasm of skin of; lower limb, including hip**
D23.71   **right lower limb, including hip**
D23.72   **left lower limb, including hip**
D23.9   **Other benign neoplasm of skin, unspecified**

(D3A) BENIGN NEUROENDOCRINE TUMORS

4th **5th** **6th** **7th**   Additional Character Required   ✔   3-character code   Unspecified laterality codes were excluded here.   ●=New Code   ▲=Revised Code   ***Excludes1***—Not coded here, do not use together   ***Excludes2***—Not included here

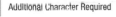

PEDIATRIC ICD-10-CM 2017: A MANUAL FOR PROVIDER-BASED CODING   133

(D37–D48) NEOPLASMS OF UNCERTAIN BEHAVIOR, POLYCY-THEMIA VERA AND MYELODYSPLASTIC SYNDROMES

Note: Categories D37–D44, and D48 classify by site neoplasms of uncertain behavior, i.e., histologic confirmation whether the neoplasm is malignant or benign cannot be made.

Excludes1: neoplasms of unspecified behavior (D49.-)

D47   **OTHER NEOPLASMS OF UNCERTAIN BEHAVIOR OF LYMPHOID, HEMATOPOIETIC AND RELATED TISSUE**
4th
    D47.3   **Essential (hemorrhagic) thrombocythemia**
         Essential thrombocytosis
         Idiopathic hemorrhagic thrombocythemia
    D47.Z   **Other specified neoplasms of uncertain behavior of lymphoid, hematopoietic and related tissue**
    5th
       D47.Z1   **Post-transplant lymphoproliferative disorder (PTLD)**
           Code first complications of transplanted organs and tissue (T86.-)
       D47.Z9   **Other specified neoplasms of uncertain behavior of lymphoid, hematopoietic and related tissue**
           Histiocytic tumors of uncertain behavior
    D47.9   **Neoplasm of uncertain behavior of lymphoid, hematopoietic and related tissue, unspecified**
         Lymphoproliferative disease NOS

(D49) NEOPLASMS OF UNSPECIFIED BEHAVIOR

D49   **NEOPLASMS OF UNSPECIFIED BEHAVIOR**
4th
   Note: Category D49 classifies by site neoplasms of unspecified morphology and behavior. *The term 'mass', unless otherwise stated, is not to be regarded as a neoplastic growth.*
   Includes: 'growth' NOS or neoplasm NOS or new growth NOS or tumor NOS
   Excludes1: neoplasms of uncertain behavior (D37–D44, D48)
   D49.0   **Neoplasm of unspecified behavior of; digestive system**
       Excludes1: neoplasm of unspecified behavior of margin of anus or perianal skin or skin of anus (D49.2)
   D49.1   **respiratory system**
   D49.2   **bone, soft tissue, and skin**
       Excludes1: neoplasm of unspecified behavior of anal canal or anus NOS (D49.0)
          bone marrow (D49.89)
          cartilage of larynx or nose (D49.1)
          connective tissue of breast (D49.3)
          skin of genital organs (D49.59)
          vermilion border of lip (D49.0)
   D49.3   **breast**
       Excludes1: neoplasm of unspecified behavior of skin of breast (D49.2)
   D49.4   **bladder**
   D49.5   **other genitourinary organs**
   5th   **D49.51**   **Neoplasm of unspecified behavior of kidney**
      6th   **D49.511**   **right kidney**
            D49.512   **left kidney**
       D49.59   **Neoplasm unspecified behavior of other genitourinary organ**
   D49.6   **brain**
       Excludes1: neoplasm of unspecified behavior of cerebral meninges (D49.7)
         neoplasm of unspecified behavior of cranial nerves (D49.7)
   D49.7   **endocrine glands and other parts of nervous system**
       Excludes1: neoplasm of unspecified behavior of peripheral, sympathetic, and parasympathetic nerves and ganglia (D49.2)
   D49.8   **other specified sites**
       Excludes1: neoplasm of unspecified behavior of eyelid (skin) (D49.2)
   D49.9   **unspecified site**

   7th   Additional Character Required   3-character code   Unspecified laterality codes were excluded here.   •=New Code   ▲=Revised Code   ***Excludes1***—Not coded here, do not use together   ***Excludes2***—Not included here

CHAPTER 2. NEOPLASMS   (D37 – D49.9)

Chapter 3. Diseases of the blood and blood-forming organs and certain disorders involving the immune mechanism (D50–D89)

GUIDELINES

None currently. Reserved for future guideline expansion.

Excludes2: autoimmune disease (systemic) NOS (M35.9)
    certain conditions originating in the perinatal period (P00–P96)
    complications of pregnancy, childbirth and the puerperium (O00–O9A)
    congenital malformations, deformations and chromosomal abnormalities
      (Q00–Q99)
    endocrine, nutritional and metabolic diseases (E00–E88)
    HIV disease (B20)
    injury, poisoning and certain other consequences of external causes (S00–T88)
    neoplasms (C00–D49)
    symptoms, signs and abnormal clinical and laboratory findings, NEC (R00–R94)

(D50–D53) NUTRITIONAL ANEMIAS

D50   **IRON DEFICIENCY ANEMIA**
   [4th]   ***Includes:*** asiderotic anemia
      hypochromic anemia
   D50.0   **Iron deficiency anemia secondary to blood loss (chronic)**
      Posthemorrhagic anemia (chronic)
      Excludes1: acute posthemorrhagic anemia (D62)
        congenital anemia from fetal blood loss (P61.3)
   D50.1   **Sideropenic dysphagia**
      Kelly-Paterson syndrome
      Plummer-Vinson syndrome
   D50.8   **Other iron deficiency anemias**
      Iron deficiency anemia due to inadequate dietary iron intake
   D50.9   **Iron deficiency anemia, unspecified**

D51   **VITAMIN B12 DEFICIENCY ANEMIA**
   [4th]   ***Excludes1:*** vitamin B12 deficiency (E53.8)
   D51.0   **Vitamin B12 deficiency anemia due to intrinsic factor**
      deficiency
      Addison anemia
      Biermer anemia
      Pernicious (congenital) anemia
      Congenital intrinsic factor deficiency
   D51.1   **Vitamin B12 deficiency anemia due to selective vitamin B12**
      malabsorption with proteinuria
      Imerslund (Gräsbeck) syndrome
      Megaloblastic hereditary anemia
   D51.2   **Transcobalamin II deficiency**
   D51.3   **Other dietary vitamin B12 deficiency anemia**
      Vegan anemia
   D51.8   **Other vitamin B12 deficiency anemias**
   D51.9   **Vitamin B12 deficiency anemia, unspecified**

D52   **FOLATE DEFICIENCY ANEMIA**
   [4th]   ***Excludes1:*** folate deficiency without anemia (E53.8)
   D52.0   **Dietary folate deficiency anemia**
      Nutritional megaloblastic anemia
   D52.1   **Drug-induced folate deficiency anemia**
      Use additional code for adverse effect, if applicable, to identify
        drug (T36–T50 with fifth or sixth character 5)
   D52.8   **Other folate deficiency anemias**
   D52.9   **Folate deficiency anemia, unspecified**
      Folic acid deficiency anemia NOS

D53   **OTHER NUTRITIONAL ANEMIAS**
   [4th]   ***Includes:*** megaloblastic anemia unresponsive to vitamin B12 or folate
      therapy
   D53.0   **Protein deficiency anemia**
      Amino-acid deficiency anemia
      Orotaciduric anemia
      Excludes1: Lesch-Nyhan syndrome (E79.1)
   D53.1   **Other megaloblastic anemias, NEC**
      Megaloblastic anemia NOS
      Excludes1: Di Guglielmo's disease (C94.0)
   D53.2   **Scorbutic anemia**
      Excludes1: scurvy (E54)

   D53.8   **Other specified nutritional anemias**
      Anemia associated with deficiency of copper
      Anemia associated with deficiency of molybdenum
      Anemia associated with deficiency of zinc
      Excludes1: nutritional deficiencies without anemia, such as:
        copper deficiency NOS (E61.0)
        molybdenum deficiency NOS (E61.5)
        zinc deficiency NOS (E60)
   D53.9   **Nutritional anemia, unspecified**
      Simple chronic anemia
      Excludes1: anemia NOS (D64.9)

(D55–D59) HEMOLYTIC ANEMIAS

D55   **ANEMIA DUE TO ENZYME DISORDERS**
   [4th]   ***Excludes1:*** drug-induced enzyme deficiency anemia (D59.2)
   D55.0   **Anemia due to glucose-6-phosphate dehydrogenase [G6PD]**
      deficiency
      Favism
      G6PD deficiency anemia
   D55.1   **Anemia due to other disorders of glutathione metabolism**
      Anemia (due to) enzyme deficiencies, except G6PD, related to the
        hexose monophosphate [HMP] shunt pathway
      Anemia (due to) hemolytic nonspherocytic (hereditary), type I
   D55.2   **Anemia due to disorders of glycolytic enzymes**
      Hemolytic nonspherocytic (hereditary) anemia, type II
      Hexokinase deficiency anemia
      Pyruvate kinase [PK] deficiency anemia
      Triose-phosphate isomerase deficiency anemia
      Excludes1: disorders of glycolysis not associated with anemia
        (E74.8)
   D55.3   **Anemia due to disorders of nucleotide metabolism**
   D55.8   **Other anemias due to enzyme disorders**
   D55.9   **Anemia due to enzyme disorder, unspecified**

D56   **THALASSEMIA**
   [4th]   ***Excludes1:*** sickle-cell thalassemia (D57.4-)
   D56.0   **Alpha thalassemia**
      Alpha thalassemia major
      Hemoglobin H Constant Spring
      Hemoglobin H disease
      Hydrops fetalis due to alpha thalassemia
      Severe alpha thalassemia
      Triple gene defect alpha thalassemia
      Use additional code, if applicable, for hydrops fetalis due to alpha
        thalassemia (P56.99)
      Excludes1: alpha thalassemia trait or minor (D56.3)
        asymptomatic alpha thalassemia (D56.3)
        hydrops fetalis due to isoimmunization (P56.0)
        hydrops fetalis not due to immune hemolysis (P83.2)
   D56.1   **Beta thalassemia**
      Beta thalassemia major
      Cooley's anemia
      Homozygous beta thalassemia
      Severe beta thalassemia
      Thalassemia intermedia
      Thalassemia major
      Excludes1: beta thalassemia minor (D56.3)
        beta thalassemia trait (D56.3)
        delta-beta thalassemia (D56.2)
        hemoglobin E-beta thalassemia (D56.5)
        sickle-cell beta thalassemia (D57.4-)
   D56.2   **Delta-beta thalassemia**
      Homozygous delta-beta thalassemia
      Excludes1: delta-beta thalassemia minor (D56.3)
        delta-beta thalassemia trait (D56.3)

  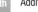   Additional Character Required   3-character code   •=New Code   ***Excludes1***—Not coded here, do not use together
                                        ▲=Revised Code   ***Excludes2***—Not included here

D56.3 Thalassemia minor
Alpha thalassemia minor
Alpha thalassemia silent carrier
Alpha thalassemia trait
Beta thalassemia minor
Beta thalassemia trait
Delta-beta thalassemia minor
Delta-beta thalassemia trait
Thalassemia trait NOS
Excludes1: alpha thalassemia (D56.0)
   beta thalassemia (D56.1)
   delta-beta thalassemia (D56.2)
   hemoglobin E-beta thalassemia (D56.5)
   sickle-cell trait (D57.3)

D56.4 Hereditary persistence of fetal hemoglobin [HPFH]

D56.5 Hemoglobin E-beta thalassemia
Excludes1: beta thalassemia (D56.1)
   beta thalassemia minor (D56.3)
   beta thalassemia trait (D56.3)
   delta-beta thalassemia (D56.2)
   delta-beta thalassemia trait (D56.3)
   hemoglobin E disease (D58.2)
   other hemoglobinopathies (D58.2)
   sickle-cell beta thalassemia (D57.4-)

D56.8 Other thalassemias
Dominant thalassemia
Hemoglobin C thalassemia
Mixed thalassemia
Thalassemia with other hemoglobinopathy
Excludes1: hemoglobin C disease (D58.2)
   hemoglobin E disease (D58.2)
   other hemoglobinopathies (D58.2)
   sickle-cell anemia (D57.-)
   sickle-cell thalassemia (D57.4)

D56.9 Thalassemia, unspecified
Mediterranean anemia (with other hemoglobinopathy)

D57 SICKLE-CELL DISORDERS
Use additional code for any associated fever (R50.81)
Excludes1: other hemoglobinopathies (D58.-)

D57.0 Hb-SS disease with crisis
Sickle-cell disease NOS with crisis
Hb-SS disease with vaso-occlusive pain
  D57.00 Hb-SS disease with crisis, unspecified
  D57.01 Hb-SS disease with acute chest syndrome
  D57.02 Hb-SS disease with splenic sequestration

D57.1 Sickle-cell disease without crisis
Hb-SS disease without crisis
Sickle-cell anemia NOS
Sickle-cell disease NOS
Sickle-cell disorder NOS

D57.2 Sickle-cell/Hb-C disease
Hb-SC disease
Hb-S/Hb-C disease
  D57.20 Sickle-cell/Hb-C disease without crisis
  D57.21 Sickle-cell/Hb-C disease with crisis
    D57.211 Sickle-cell/Hb-C disease with acute chest syndrome
    D57.212 Sickle-cell/Hb-C disease with splenic sequestration
    D57.219 Sickle-cell/Hb-C disease with crisis, unspecified
    Sickle-cell/Hb-C disease with crisis NOS

D57.3 Sickle-cell trait
Hb-S trait
Heterozygous hemoglobin S

D57.4 Sickle-cell thalassemia
Sickle-cell beta thalassemia
Thalassemia Hb-S disease
  D57.40 Sickle-cell thalassemia without crisis
  Microdrepanocytosis
  Sickle-cell thalassemia NOS

D57.41 Sickle-cell thalassemia with crisis
Sickle-cell thalassemia with vaso-occlusive pain
  D57.411 Sickle-cell thalassemia with acute chest syndrome
  D57.412 Sickle-cell thalassemia with splenic sequestration
  D57.419 Sickle-cell thalassemia with crisis, unspecified
  Sickle-cell thalassemia with crisis NOS

D57.8 Other sickle-cell disorders
Hb-SD disease
Hb-SE disease
  D57.80 Other sickle-cell disorders without crisis
  D57.81 Other sickle-cell disorders with crisis
    D57.811 Other sickle-cell disorders with acute chest syndrome
    D57.812 Other sickle-cell disorders with splenic sequestration
    D57.819 Other sickle-cell disorders with crisis, unspecified
    Other sickle-cell disorders with crisis NOS

D58 OTHER HEREDITARY HEMOLYTIC ANEMIAS
Excludes1: hemolytic anemia of the newborn (P55.-)
D58.0 Hereditary spherocytosis
Acholuric (familial) jaundice
Congenital (spherocytic) hemolytic icterus
Minkowski-Chauffard syndrome

D58.1 Hereditary elliptocytosis
Elliptocytosis (congenital)
Ovalocytosis (congenital) (hereditary)

D58.2 Other hemoglobinopathies
Abnormal hemoglobin NOS
Congenital Heinz body anemia
Hb-C disease
Hb-D disease
Hb-E disease
Hemoglobinopathy NOS
Unstable hemoglobin hemolytic disease
Excludes1: familial polycythemia (D75.0)
   Hb-M disease (D74.0)
   hemoglobin E-beta thalassemia (D56.5)
   hereditary persistence of fetal hemoglobin [HPFH] (D56.4)
   high-altitude polycythemia (D75.1)
   methemoglobinemia (D74.-)
   other hemoglobinopathies with thalassemia (D56.8)

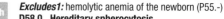
(D60–D64) APLASTIC AND OTHER ANEMIAS AND OTHER BONE MARROW FAILURE SYNDROMES

D60 ACQUIRED PURE RED CELL APLASIA [ERYTHROBLASTOPENIA]
Includes: red cell aplasia (acquired) (adult) (with thymoma)
Excludes1: congenital red cell aplasia (D61.01)
D60.9 Acquired pure red cell aplasia, unspecified

D61 OTHER APLASTIC ANEMIAS AND OTHER BONE MARROW FAILURE SYNDROMES
Excludes1: neutropenia (D70.-)
D61.0 Constitutional aplastic anemia
  D61.01 Constitutional (pure) red blood cell aplasia
  Blackfan-Diamond syndrome
  Congenital (pure) red cell aplasia
  Familial hypoplastic anemia
  Primary (pure) red cell aplasia
  Red cell (pure) aplasia of infants
  Excludes1: acquired red cell aplasia (D60.9)
  D61.09 Other constitutional aplastic anemia
  Fanconi's anemia
  Pancytopenia with malformations

D61.1 Drug-induced aplastic anemia
Use additional code for adverse effect, if applicable, to identify drug (T36–T50 with fifth or sixth character 5)

   Additional Character Required   3-character code

•=New Code   *Excludes1*—Not coded here, do not use together
▲=Revised Code   *Excludes2*—Not included here

D61.2 Aplastic anemia due to other external agents
Code first, if applicable, toxic effects of substances chiefly nonmedicinal as to source (T51–T65)

D61.3 Idiopathic aplastic anemia

D61.8 Other specified aplastic anemias and other bone marrow failure syndromes

 5th

> **D61.81 Pancytopenia**
>
> **6th**
>
> > **Excludes1:** pancytopenia (due to) (with) aplastic anemia (D61.9)
> >
> > pancytopenia (due to) (with) bone marrow infiltration (D61.82)
> >
> > pancytopenia (due to) (with) congenital (pure) red cell aplasia (D61.01)
> >
> > pancytopenia (due to) (with) hairy cell leukemia (C91.4-)
> >
> > pancytopenia (due to) (with) HIV disease (B20.-)
> >
> > pancytopenia (due to) (with) leukoerythroblastic anemia (D61.82)
> >
> > pancytopenia (due to) (with) myeloproliferative disease (D47.1)
> >
> > **Excludes2:** pancytopenia (due to) (with) myelodysplastic syndromes (D46.-)
> >
> > **D61.810 Antineoplastic chemotherapy induced pancytopenia**
> > > **Excludes2:** aplastic anemia due to antineoplastic chemotherapy (D61.1)
> >
> > **D61.811 Other drug-induced pancytopenia**
> > > **Excludes2:** aplastic anemia due to drugs (D61.1)
> >
> > **D61.818 Other pancytopenia**
>
> **D61.82 Myelophthisis**
> Leukoerythroblastic anemia
> Myelophthisic anemia
> Panmyelophthisis
> **Code also** the underlying disorder, such as: malignant neoplasm of breast (C50.-)
> tuberculosis (A15.-)
> **Excludes1:** idiopathic myelofibrosis (D47.1)
> myelofibrosis NOS (D75.81)
> myelofibrosis with myeloid metaplasia (D47.4)
> primary myelofibrosis (D47.1)
> secondary myelofibrosis (D75.81)
>
> **D61.89 Other specified aplastic anemias and other bone marrow failure syndromes**

D61.9 Aplastic anemia, unspecified
Hypoplastic anemia NOS
Medullary hypoplasia

D62 ACUTE POSTHEMORRHAGIC ANEMIA

Excludes1: anemia due to chronic blood loss (D50.0)
blood loss anemia NOS (D50.0)
congenital anemia from fetal blood loss (P61.3)

D63 ANEMIA IN CHRONIC DISEASES CLASSIFIED ELSEWHERE

4th

D63.0 Anemia in neoplastic disease
Code first neoplasm (C00–D49)
Excludes1: anemia due to antineoplastic chemotherapy (D64.81)
aplastic anemia due to antineoplastic chemotherapy (D61.1)

D64 OTHER ANEMIAS

4th

Excludes1: refractory anemia (D46.-)
refractory anemia with excess blasts in transformation [RAEB T] (C92.0-)

D64.8 Other specified anemias

> **5th**
>
> **D64.81 Anemia due to antineoplastic chemotherapy**
> Antineoplastic chemotherapy induced anemia
> **Excludes1:** aplastic anemia due to antineoplastic chemotherapy (D61.1)
> **Excludes2:** anemia in neoplastic disease (D63.0)
>
> **D64.89 Other specified anemias**
> Infantile pseudoleukemia

➤ D64.9 Anemia, unspecified

(D65–D69) COAGULATION DEFECTS, PURPURA AND OTHER HEMORRHAGIC CONDITIONS

D65 DISSEMINATED INTRAVASCULAR COAGULATION [DEFIBRINATION SYNDROME]

Afibrinogenemia, acquired
Consumption coagulopathy
Diffuse or disseminated intravascular coagulation [DIC]
Fibrinolytic hemorrhage, acquired
Fibrinolytic purpura
Purpura fulminans
Excludes1: disseminated intravascular coagulation (complicating):
abortion or ectopic or molar pregnancy (O00–O07, O08.1)
in newborn (P60)
pregnancy, childbirth and the puerperium (O45.0, O46.0, O67.0, O72.3)

D66 HEREDITARY FACTOR VIII DEFICIENCY

Classical hemophilia
Deficiency factor VIII (with functional defect)
Hemophilia NOS
Hemophilia A
Excludes1: factor VIII deficiency with vascular defect (D68.0)

D67 HEREDITARY FACTOR IX DEFICIENCY

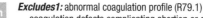

Christmas disease
Factor IX deficiency (with functional defect)
Hemophilia B
Plasma thromboplastin component [PTC] deficiency

D68 OTHER COAGULATION DEFECTS

4th

Excludes1: abnormal coagulation profile (R79.1)
coagulation defects complicating abortion or ectopic or molar pregnancy (O00–O07, O08.1)
coagulation defects complicating pregnancy, childbirth and the puerperium (O45.0, O46.0, O67.0, O72.3)

D68.2 Hereditary deficiency of other clotting factors
AC globulin deficiency
Congenital afibrinogenemia
Deficiency of factor I [fibrinogen]
Deficiency of factor II [prothrombin]
Deficiency of factor V [labile]
Deficiency of factor VII [stable]
Deficiency of factor X [Stuart-Prower]
Deficiency of factor XII [Hageman]
Deficiency of factor XIII [fibrin stabilizing]
Dysfibrinogenemia (congenital)
Hypoproconvertinemia
Owren's disease
Proaccelerin deficiency

D68.3 Hemorrhagic disorder due to circulating anticoagulants

> **5th**
>
> **D68.31 Hemorrhagic disorder due to intrinsic circulating anticoagulants, antibodies, or inhibitors**
>
> **6th**
>
> > **D68.311 Acquired hemophilia**
> > Autoimmune hemophilia
> > Autoimmune inhibitors to clotting factors
> > Secondary hemophilia
> >
> > **D68.312 Antiphospholipid antibody with hemorrhagic disorder**
> > LAC with hemorrhagic disorder
> > SLE inhibitor with hemorrhagic disorder
> > **Excludes1:** antiphospholipid antibody, finding without diagnosis (R76.0)
> > antiphospholipid antibody syndrome (D68.61)
> > antiphospholipid antibody with hypercoagulable state (D68.61)
> > LAC finding without diagnosis (R76.0)
> > LAC with hypercoagulable state (D68.62)
> > SLE inhibitor finding without diagnosis (R76.0)
> > SLE inhibitor with hypercoagulable state (D68.62)

 4th   **5th**   **6th** **7th**   Additional Character Required   3-character code

●=Now Code
▲=Revised Code

Excludes1—Not coded here, do not use together
Excludes2—Not included here

D68.318 **Other hemorrhagic disorder due to intrinsic circulating anticoagulants, antibodies, or inhibitors**
Antithromboplastinemia
Antithromboplastinogenemia
Hemorrhagic disorder due to intrinsic increase in antithrombin
Hemorrhagic disorder due to intrinsic increase in anti-VIIIa
Hemorrhagic disorder due to intrinsic increase in anti-IXa
Hemorrhagic disorder due to intrinsic increase in anti-XIa

D68.4 **Acquired coagulation factor deficiency**
Deficiency of coagulation factor due to liver disease
Deficiency of coagulation factor due to vitamin K deficiency
Excludes1: vitamin K deficiency of newborn (P53)

D68.5 **Primary thrombophilia**
Primary hypercoagulable states
Excludes1: antiphospholipid syndrome (D68.61)
LAC (D68.62)
secondary activated protein C resistance (D68.69)
secondary antiphospholipid antibody syndrome (D68.69)
secondary LAC with hypercoagulable state (D68.69)
SLE inhibitor with hypercoagulable state (D68.69)
SLE inhibitor finding without diagnosis (R76.0)
SLE inhibitor with hemorrhagic disorder (D68.312)
thrombotic thrombocytopenic purpura (M31.1)

D68.51 **Activated protein C resistance**
Factor V Leiden mutation
D68.52 **Prothrombin gene mutation**
D68.59 **Other primary thrombophilia**
Antithrombin III deficiency
Hypercoagulable state NOS
Primary hypercoagulable state NEC
Primary thrombophilia NEC
Protein C deficiency
Protein S deficiency
Thrombophilia NOS

D68.6 **Other thrombophilia**
Other hypercoagulable states
Excludes1: diffuse or disseminated intravascular coagulation [DIC] (D65)
heparin induced thrombocytopenia (HIT) (D75.82)
hyperhomocysteinemia (E72.11)

D68.61 **Antiphospholipid syndrome**
Anticardiolipin syndrome
Antiphospholipid antibody syndrome
Excludes1: anti-phospholipid antibody, finding without diagnosis (R76.0)
anti-phospholipid antibody with hemorrhagic disorder (D68.312)
LAC syndrome (D68.62)

D68.62 **LAC syndrome**
LAC
Presence of SLE inhibitor
Excludes1: anticardiolipin syndrome (D68.61)
antiphospholipid syndrome (D68.61)
LAC finding without diagnosis (R76.0)
LAC with hemorrhagic disorder (D68.312)

D68.69 **Other thrombophilia**
Hypercoagulable states NEC
Secondary hypercoagulable state NOS

D68.8 **Other specified coagulation defects**
Excludes1: hemorrhagic disease of newborn (P53)

D68.9 **Coagulation defect, unspecified**

D69 PURPURA AND OTHER HEMORRHAGIC CONDITIONS
Excludes1: benign hypergammaglobulinemic purpura (D89.0)
cryoglobulinemic purpura (D89.1)
essential (hemorrhagic) thrombocythemia (D47.3)
hemorrhagic thrombocythemia (D47.3)
purpura fulminans (D65)
thrombotic thrombocytopenic purpura (M31.1)
Waldenström hypergammaglobulinemic purpura (D89.0)

D69.0 **Allergic purpura**
Allergic vasculitis
Nonthrombocytopenic hemorrhagic purpura
Nonthrombocytopenic idiopathic purpura
Purpura anaphylactoid
Purpura Henoch(-Schönlein)
Purpura rheumatica
Vascular purpura
Excludes1: thrombocytopenic hemorrhagic purpura (D69.3)

D69.2 **Other nonthrombocytopenic purpura**
Purpura NOS
Purpura simplex
Senile purpura

D69.3 **Immune thrombocytopenic purpura**
Hemorrhagic (thrombocytopenic) purpura
Idiopathic thrombocytopenic purpura
Tidal platelet dysgenesis

D69.4 **Other primary thrombocytopenia**
Excludes1: transient neonatal thrombocytopenia (P61.0)
Wiskott-Aldrich syndrome (D82.0)
D69.41 **Evans syndrome**
D69.42 **Congenital and hereditary thrombocytopenia purpura**
Congenital thrombocytopenia
Hereditary thrombocytopenia
Code first congenital or hereditary disorder, such as:
TAR syndrome (Q87.2)
D69.49 **Other primary thrombocytopenia**
Megakaryocytic hypoplasia
Primary thrombocytopenia NOS

D69.5 **Secondary thrombocytopenia**
Excludes1: heparin induced thrombocytopenia (HIT) (D75.82)
transient thrombocytopenia of newborn (P61.0)
D69.51 **Posttransfusion purpura**
Posttransfusion purpura from whole blood (fresh) or blood products
PTP
D69.59 **Other secondary thrombocytopenia**

(D70–D77) OTHER DISORDERS OF BLOOD AND BLOOD-FORMING ORGANS

D70 NEUTROPENIA
Includes: agranulocytosis
decreased absolute neutrophil count (ANC)
Use additional code for any associated: fever (R50.81)
mucositis (J34.81, K12.3-, K92.81, N76.81)
Excludes1: neutropenic splenomegaly (D73.81)
transient neonatal neutropenia (P61.5)

D70.0 **Congenital agranulocytosis**
Congenital neutropenia
Infantile genetic agranulocytosis
Kostmann's disease

D70.1 **Agranulocytosis secondary to cancer chemotherapy**
Use additional code for adverse effect, if applicable, to identify drug (T45.1X5)
Code also underlying neoplasm

D70.2 **Other drug-induced agranulocytosis**
Use additional code for adverse effect, if applicable, to identify drug (T36–T50 with fifth or sixth character 5)

D70.3 **Neutropenia due to infection**
D70.4 **Cyclic neutropenia**
Cyclic hematopoiesis
Periodic neutropenia
D70.8 **Other neutropenia**
D70.9 **Neutropenia, unspecified**

   Additional Character Required   3-character code

•=New Code
▲=Revised Code
Excludes1—Not coded here, do not use together
Excludes2—Not included here

138   PEDIATRIC ICD-10-CM 2017: A MANUAL FOR PROVIDER-BASED CODING

D71 **FUNCTIONAL DISORDERS OF POLYMORPHONUCLEAR NEUTROPHILS**
Cell membrane receptor complex [CR3] defect
Chronic (childhood) granulomatous disease
Congenital dysphagocytosis
Progressive septic granulomatosis

D72 **OTHER DISORDERS OF WHITE BLOOD CELLS**
4th *Excludes1:* basophilia (D72.824)
immunity disorders (D80–D89)
neutropenia (D70)
preleukemia (syndrome) (D46.9)

D72.1 **Eosinophilia**
Allergic eosinophilia
Hereditary eosinophilia
Excludes1: Löffler's syndrome (J82)
pulmonary eosinophilia (J82)

D72.8 **Other specified disorders of white blood cells**
5th *Excludes1:* leukemia (C91–C95)

D72.81 **Decreased white blood cell count**
6th *Excludes1:* neutropenia (D70.-)

D72.810 **Lymphocytopenia**
Decreased lymphocytes

D72.818 **Other decreased white blood cell count**
Basophilic leukopenia
Eosinophilic leukopenia
Monocytopenia
Other decreased leukocytes
Plasmacytopenia

D72.819 **Decreased white blood cell count, unspecified**
Decreased leukocytes, unspecified
Leukocytopenia, unspecified
Leukopenia
Excludes1: malignant leukopenia (D70.9)

D72.82 **Elevated white blood cell count**
6th *Excludes1:* eosinophilia (D72.1)

D72.820 **Lymphocytosis (symptomatic)**
Elevated lymphocytes

D72.821 **Monocytosis (symptomatic)**
Excludes1: infectious mononucleosis (B27.-)

D72.822 **Plasmacytosis**

D72.823 **Leukemoid reaction**
Basophilic leukemoid reaction
Leukemoid reaction NOS
Lymphocytic leukemoid reaction
Monocytic leukemoid reaction
Myelocytic leukemoid reaction
Neutrophilic leukemoid reaction

D72.824 **Basophilia**

D72.825 **Bandemia**
Bandemia without diagnosis of specific infection
Excludes1: confirmed infection—code to infection
leukemia (C91.-, C92.-, C93.-, C94.-, C95.-)

D72.828 **Other elevated white blood cell count**

D72.829 **Elevated white blood cell count, unspecified**
Elevated leukocytes, unspecified
Leukocytosis, unspecified

D72.89 **Other specified disorders of white blood cells**
Abnormality of white blood cells NEC

D73 **DISEASES OF SPLEEN**
4th **D73.0** **Hyposplenism**
Atrophy of spleen
Excludes1: asplenia (congenital) (Q89.01)
postsurgical absence of spleen (Z90.81)

D73.1 **Hypersplenism**
Excludes1: neutropenic splenomegaly (D73.81)
primary splenic neutropenia (D73.81)
splenitis, splenomegaly in late syphilis (A52.79)
splenitis, splenomegaly in tuberculosis (A18.85)

splenomegaly NOS (R16.1)
splenomegaly congenital (Q89.0)

D73.2 **Chronic congestive splenomegaly**
D73.3 **Abscess of spleen**
D73.4 **Cyst of spleen**
D73.5 **Infarction of spleen**
Splenic rupture, nontraumatic
Torsion of spleen
Excludes1: rupture of spleen due to Plasmodium vivax malaria (B51.0)
traumatic rupture of spleen (S36.03-)

D73.8 **Other diseases of spleen**
5th **D73.81** **Neutropenic splenomegaly**
Werner-Schultz disease

D74 **METHEMOGLOBINEMIA**
4th **D74.0** **Congenital methemoglobinemia**
Congenital NADH-methemoglobin reductase deficiency
Hemoglobin-M [Hb-M] disease
Methemoglobinemia, hereditary

D74.8 **Other methemoglobinemias**
Acquired methemoglobinemia (with sulfhemoglobinemia)
Toxic methemoglobinemia

D74.9 **Methemoglobinemia, unspecified**

D75 **OTHER AND UNSPECIFIED DISEASES OF BLOOD AND BLOOD-FORMING ORGANS**
4th *Excludes2:* acute lymphadenitis (L04.-)
chronic lymphadenitis (I88.1)
enlarged lymph nodes (R59.-)
hypergammaglobulinemia NOS (D89.2)
lymphadenitis NOS (I88.9)
mesenteric lymphadenitis (acute) (chronic) (I88.0)

D75.1 **Secondary polycythemia**
Acquired polycythemia
Emotional polycythemia
Erythrocytosis NOS
Hypoxemic polycythemia
Nephrogenous polycythemia
Polycythemia due to erythropoietin
Polycythemia due to fall in plasma volume
Polycythemia due to high altitude
Polycythemia due to stress
Polycythemia NOS
Relative polycythemia
Excludes1: polycythemia neonatorum (P61.1)
polycythemia vera (D45)

D76 **OTHER SPECIFIED DISEASES WITH PARTICIPATION OF LYMPHORETICULAR AND RETICULOHISTIOCYTIC TISSUE**
4th *Excludes1:* (Abt-) Letterer-Siwe disease (C96.0)
eosinophilic granuloma (C96.6)
Hand-Schüller-Christian disease (C96.5)
histiocytic medullary reticulosis (C96.9)
histiocytic sarcoma (C96.A)
histiocytosis X, multifocal (C96.5)
histiocytosis X, unifocal (C96.6)
Langerhans-cell histiocytosis, multifocal (C96.5)
Langerhans-cell histiocytosis NOS (C96.6)
Langerhans-cell histiocytosis, unifocal (C96.6)
leukemic reticuloendotheliosis (C91.4-)
lipomelanotic reticulosis (I89.8)
malignant histiocytosis (C96.A)
malignant reticulosis (C86.0)
nonlipid reticuloendotheliosis (C96.0)

D76.1 **Hemophagocytic lymphohistiocytosis**
Familial hemophagocytic reticulosis
Histiocytoses of mononuclear phagocytes

D76.2 **Hemophagocytic syndrome, infection-associated**
Use additional code to identify infectious agent or disease.

D76.3 **Other histiocytosis syndromes**
Reticulohistiocytoma (giant-cell)
Sinus histiocytosis with massive lymphadenopathy
Xanthogranuloma

    Additional Character Required   3-character code   •=New Code   *Excludes1*—Not coded here, do not use together
▲=Revised Code   *Excludes2*—Not included here

(D78) INTRAOPERATIVE AND POSTPROCEDURAL COMPLICATIONS OF THE SPLEEN

(D80–D89) CERTAIN DISORDERS INVOLVING THE IMMUNE MECHANISM

Includes: defects in the complement system
immunodeficiency disorders, except HIV disease
sarcoidosis

Excludes1: autoimmune disease (systemic) NOS (M35.9)
functional disorders of polymorphonuclear neutrophils (D71)
HIV disease (B20)

D80 **IMMUNODEFICIENCY WITH PREDOMINANTLY ANTIBODY DEFECTS**

D80.0 **Hereditary hypogammaglobulinemia**
Autosomal recessive agammaglobulinemia (Swiss type)
X-linked agammaglobulinemia [Bruton] (with growth hormone deficiency)

D80.1 **Nonfamilial hypogammaglobulinemia**
Agammaglobulinemia with immunoglobulin-bearing B-lymphocytes
Common variable immunodeficiency [CVAgamma]
Hypogammaglobulinemia NOS

D80.2 **Selective deficiency of immunoglobulin A [IgA]**

D80.3 **Selective deficiency of immunoglobulin G [IgG] subclasses**

D80.4 **Selective deficiency of immunoglobulin M [IgM]**

D80.5 **Immunodeficiency with increased immunoglobulin M [IgM]**

D80.6 **Antibody deficiency with near-normal immunoglobulins or with hypogammaglobulinemia**

D80.7 **Transient hypogammaglobulinemia of infancy**

D81 **COMBINED IMMUNODEFICIENCIES**

Excludes1: autosomal recessive agammaglobulinemia (Swiss type) (D80.0)

D81.0 **SCID with reticular dysgenesis**

D81.1 **SCID with low T- and B-cell numbers**

D81.2 **SCID with low or normal B-cell numbers**

D81.3 **Adenosine deaminase [ADA] deficiency**

D81.4 **Nezelof's syndrome**

D81.5 **Purine nucleoside phosphorylase [PNP] deficiency**

D81.6 **Major histocompatibility complex class I deficiency**
Bare lymphocyte syndrome

D81.7 **Major histocompatibility complex class II deficiency**

D81.8 **Other combined immunodeficiencies**

> **D81.81** **Biotin-dependent carboxylase deficiency**
> Multiple carboxylase deficiency
>
>> **Excludes1:** biotin-dependent carboxylase deficiency due to dietary deficiency of biotin (E53.8)
>>
>> **D81.810** **Biotinidase deficiency**
>> **D81.818** **Other biotin-dependent carboxylase deficiency**
>> Holocarboxylase synthetase deficiency
>> Other multiple carboxylase deficiency
>> **D81.819** **Biotin-dependent carboxylase deficiency, unspecified**
>> Multiple carboxylase deficiency, unspecified
>
> **D81.89** **Other combined immunodeficiencies**

D81.9 **Combined immunodeficiency, unspecified**
SCID NOS

D82 **IMMUNODEFICIENCY ASSOCIATED WITH OTHER MAJOR DEFECTS**

Excludes1: ataxia telangiectasia [Louis-Bar] (G11.3)

D82.0 **Wiskott-Aldrich syndrome**
Immunodeficiency with thrombocytopenia and eczema

D82.1 **Di George's syndrome**
Pharyngeal pouch syndrome
Thymic alymphoplasia
Thymic aplasia or hypoplasia with immunodeficiency

D82.2 **Immunodeficiency with short-limbed stature**

D82.4 **Hyperimmunoglobulin E [IgE] syndrome**

D82.9 **Immunodeficiency associated with major defect, unspecified**

D84 **OTHER IMMUNODEFICIENCIES**

D84.1 **Defects in the complement system**
C1 esterase inhibitor [C1-INH] deficiency

D84.8 **Other specified immunodeficiencies**

D84.9 **Immunodeficiency, unspecified**

D86 **SARCOIDOSIS**

D86.0 **Sarcoidosis of lung**

D86.1 **Sarcoidosis of lymph nodes**

D86.2 **Sarcoidosis of lung with sarcoidosis of lymph nodes**

D86.3 **Sarcoidosis of skin**

D86.8 **Sarcoidosis of other sites**

> **D86.81** **Sarcoid meningitis**
> **D86.82** **Multiple cranial nerve palsies in sarcoidosis**
> **D86.83** **Sarcoid iridocyclitis**
> **D86.84** **Sarcoid pyelonephritis**
> Tubulo-interstitial nephropathy in sarcoidosis
> **D86.85** **Sarcoid myocarditis**
> **D86.86** **Sarcoid arthropathy**
> Polyarthritis in sarcoidosis
> **D86.87** **Sarcoid myositis**
> **D86.89** **Sarcoidosis of other sites**
> Hepatic granuloma
> Uveoparotid fever [Heerfordt]

D86.9 **Sarcoidosis, unspecified**

D89 **OTHER DISORDERS INVOLVING THE IMMUNE MECHANISM, NEC**

Excludes1: hyperglobulinemia NOS (R77.1)
monoclonal gammopathy (of undetermined significance) (D47.2)

Excludes2: transplant failure and rejection (T86.-)

D89.0 **Polyclonal hypergammaglobulinemia**
Benign hypergammaglobulinemic purpura
Polyclonal gammopathy NOS

D89.1 **Cryoglobulinemia**
Cryoglobulinemic purpura
Cryoglobulinemic vasculitis
Essential cryoglobulinemia
Idiopathic cryoglobulinemia
Mixed cryoglobulinemia
Primary cryoglobulinemia
Secondary cryoglobulinemia

D89.2 **Hypergammaglobulinemia, unspecified**

• **D89.4** **Mast cell activation syndrome and related disorders**

> **Excludes1:** aggressive systemic mastocytosis (C96.2)
> cutaneous mastocytosis (Q82.2)
> indolent systemic mastocytosis (D47.0)
> malignant mastocytoma (C96.2)
> mast cell leukemia (C94.3-)
> mastocytoma (D47.0)
> systemic mastocytosis associated with a clonal hematologic non-mast cell lineage disease (SM -AHNMD) (D47.0)
>
> • **D89.40** **Mast cell activation disorder, unspecified or NOS**
> • **D89.41** **Monoclonal mast cell activation syndrome**
> • **D89.42** **Idiopathic mast cell activation syndrome**
> • **D89.43** **Secondary mast cell activation syndrome**
> Secondary mast cell activation syndrome
> **Code also** underlying etiology, if known
> • **D89.49** **Other mast cell activation disorder**

D89.8 **Other specified disorders involving the immune mechanism, NEC**

     Additional Character Required   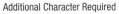 3-character code   •=New Code   **Excludes1**—Not coded here, do not use together
▲=Revised Code   **Excludes2**—Not included here

140   PEDIATRIC ICD-10-CM 2017: A MANUAL FOR PROVIDER-BASED CODING

D89.81   **Graft-versus-host disease**

Code first underlying cause, such as:
  complications of transplanted organs and tissue (T86.-)
  complications of blood transfusion (T80.89)

Use additional code to identify associated
  manifestations, such as:
  desquamative dermatitis (L30.8)
  diarrhea (R19.7)
  elevated bilirubin (R17)
  hair loss (L65.9)

D89.810   **Acute graft-versus-host disease**

D89.811   **Chronic graft-versus-host disease**

D89.812   **Acute on chronic graft-versus-host disease**

D89.813   **Graft-versus-host disease, unspecified**

D89.82   **Autoimmune lymphoproliferative syndrome [ALPS]**

D89.89   **Other specified disorders involving the immune mechanism, NEC**

Excludes1: HIV disease (B20)

D89.9   **Disorder involving the immune mechanism, unspecified**
Immune disease NOS

  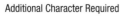   Additional Character Required   3-character code

•=New Code
▲=Revised Code

Excludes1—Not coded here, do not use together
Excludes2—Not included here

Chapter 4. Endocrine, nutritional and metabolic diseases (E00–E89)

GUIDELINES

Diabetes Mellitus (DM)

Refer to categories E08–E13 for guidelines.
Note: All neoplasms, whether functionally active or not, are classified in Chapter 2. Appropriate codes in this chapter (i.e. E05.8, E07.0, E16–E31, E34.-) may be used as additional codes to indicate either functional activity by neoplasms and ectopic endocrine tissue or hyperfunction and hypofunction of endocrine glands associated with neoplasms and other conditions classified elsewhere.
Excludes1: transitory endocrine and metabolic disorders specific to newborn (P70–P74)

(E00–E07) DISORDERS OF THYROID GLAND

E00   CONGENITAL IODINE-DEFICIENCY SYNDROME

`4th`   **Use additional code** (F70–F79) to identify associated intellectual disabilities.
Excludes1: subclinical iodine-deficiency hypothyroidism (E02)

E00.0   Congenital iodine-deficiency syndrome, neurological type
Endemic cretinism, neurological type

E00.1   Congenital iodine-deficiency syndrome, myxedematous type
Endemic hypothyroid cretinism
Endemic cretinism, myxedematous type

E00.2   Congenital iodine-deficiency syndrome, mixed type
Endemic cretinism, mixed type

E00.9   Congenital iodine-deficiency syndrome, unspecified
Congenital iodine-deficiency hypothyroidism NOS
Endemic cretinism NOS

E01   IODINE-DEFICIENCY RELATED THYROID DISORDERS AND ALLIED CONDITIONS

`4th`   ***Excludes1:*** congenital iodine-deficiency syndrome (E00.-)
subclinical iodine-deficiency hypothyroidism (E02)

E01.2   Iodine-deficiency related (endemic) goiter, unspecified
Endemic goiter NOS

E01.8   Other iodine-deficiency related thyroid disorders and allied conditions
Acquired iodine-deficiency hypothyroidism NOS

E03   OTHER HYPOTHYROIDISM

`4th`   ***Excludes1:*** iodine-deficiency related hypothyroidism (E00–E02)
postprocedural hypothyroidism (E89.0)

E03.0   Congenital hypothyroidism with diffuse goiter
Congenital parenchymatous goiter (nontoxic)
Congenital goiter (nontoxic) NOS
Excludes1: transitory congenital goiter with normal function (P72.0)

E03.1   Congenital hypothyroidism without goiter
Aplasia of thyroid (with myxedema)
Congenital atrophy of thyroid
Congenital hypothyroidism NOS

E03.2   Hypothyroidism due to medicines/drugs and other exogenous substances
Code first poisoning due to drug or toxin, if applicable (T36–T65 with fifth or sixth character 1–4 or 6)
Use additional code for adverse effect, if applicable, to identify drug (T36–T50 with fifth or sixth character 5)

E03.3   Postinfectious hypothyroidism

E03.4   Atrophy of thyroid (acquired)
Excludes1: congenital atrophy of thyroid (E03.1)

E03.8   Other specified hypothyroidism

E03.9   Hypothyroidism, unspecified
Myxedema NOS

E04   OTHER NONTOXIC GOITER

`4th`   ***Excludes1:*** congenital goiter (NOS) (diffuse) (parenchymatous) (E03.0)
iodine-deficiency related goiter (E00–E02)

E04.0   Nontoxic diffuse goiter
Diffuse (colloid) nontoxic goiter
Simple nontoxic goiter

E04.8   Other specified nontoxic goiter

E04.9   Nontoxic goiter, unspecified
Goiter NOS
Nodular goiter (nontoxic) NOS

E05   THYROTOXICOSIS [HYPERTHYROIDISM]

`4th`   ***Excludes1:*** chronic thyroiditis with transient thyrotoxicosis (E06.2)
neonatal thyrotoxicosis (P72.1)

E05.9   Thyrotoxicosis, unspecified

`5th`   Hyperthyroidism NOS

E05.90   Thyrotoxicosis, unspecified without thyrotoxic crisis or storm

E05.91   Thyrotoxicosis, unspecified with thyrotoxic crisis or storm

E06   THYROIDITIS

`4th`   ***Excludes1:*** postpartum thyroiditis (O90.5)

E06.0   Acute thyroiditis
Abscess of thyroid
Pyogenic thyroiditis
Suppurative thyroiditis
Use additional code (B95–B97) to identify infectious agent.

E06.9   Thyroiditis, unspecified

(E08–E13) DIABETES MELLITUS

GUIDELINES

The DM codes are combination codes that include the type of DM, the body system affected, and the complications affecting that body system. As many codes within a particular category as are necessary to describe all of the complications of the disease may be used. They should be sequenced based on the reason for a particular encounter. Assign as many codes from categories E08 – E13 as needed to identify all of the associated conditions that the patient has.

Type of diabetes

The age of a patient is not the sole determining factor, though most type 1 diabetics develop the condition before reaching puberty. For this reason type 1 DM is also referred to as juvenile diabetes.

Type of DM not documented

If the type of DM is not documented in the medical record the default is E11.-, Type 2 DM.

DM and the use of insulin

If the documentation in a medical record does not indicate the type of diabetes but does indicate that the patient uses insulin, code E11, Type 2 DM, should be assigned. Code Z79.4, Long-term (current) use of insulin, should also be assigned to indicate that the patient uses insulin. Code Z79.4 should not be assigned if insulin is given temporarily to bring a type 2 patient's blood sugar under control during an encounter.

Complications due to insulin pump malfunction

UNDERDOSE OF INSULIN DUE TO INSULIN PUMP FAILURE
An underdose of insulin due to an insulin pump failure should be assigned to a code from subcategory T85.6, Mechanical complication of other specified internal and external prosthetic devices, implants and grafts, that specifies the type of pump malfunction, as the principal or first-listed code, followed by code T38.3x6-, Underdosing of insulin and oral hypoglycemic [antidiabetic] drugs. Additional codes for the type of DM and any associated complications due to the underdosing should also be assigned.

OVERDOSE OF INSULIN DUE TO INSULIN PUMP FAILURE
The principal or first-listed code for an encounter due to an insulin pump malfunction resulting in an overdose of insulin, should also be T85.6-, Mechanical complication of other specified internal and external prosthetic devices, implants and grafts, followed by code T38.3x1-, Poisoning by insulin and oral hypoglycemic [antidiabetic] drugs, accidental (unintentional).

      Additional Character Required   3-character code   •=New Code   ▲=Revised Code   ***Excludes1***—Not coded here, do not use together   ***Excludes2***—Not included here

CHAPTER 4. ENDOCRINE, NUTRITIONAL AND METABOLIC DISEASES   (E08–E08.620)

Secondary DM

Codes under categories E08, DM due to underlying condition, E09, Drug or chemical induced DM, and E13, Other specified DM, identify complications/manifestations associated with secondary DM. Secondary diabetes is always caused by another condition or event (e.g., cystic fibrosis, malignant neoplasm of pancreas, pancreatectomy, adverse effect of drug, or poisoning).

SECONDARY DM AND THE USE OF INSULIN
For patients who routinely use insulin, code Z79.4, Long-term (current) use of insulin, should also be assigned. Code Z79.4 should not be assigned if insulin is given temporarily to bring a patient's blood sugar under control during an encounter.

ASSIGNING AND SEQUENCING SECONDARY DIABETES CODES AND ITS CAUSES
The sequencing of the secondary diabetes codes in relationship to codes for the cause of the diabetes is based on the Tabular List instructions for categories E08, E09 and E13.

Secondary DM due to pancreatectomy
For postpancreatectomy DM (lack of insulin due to the surgical removal of all or part of the pancreas), assign code E89.1, Postprocedural hypoinsulinemia. Assign a code from category E13 and a code from subcategory Z90.41-, Acquired absence of pancreas, as additional codes.

Secondary diabetes due to drugs
Secondary diabetes may be caused by an adverse effect of correctly administered medications, poisoning or sequela of poisoning.
     Refer to categories T36–T50 for coding of adverse effects and poisoning.
     Note for hyperglycemia not caused by DM or for transient hyperglycemia, refer to code R73.9, hyperglycemia, NOS

E08   **DM DUE TO UNDERLYING CONDITION**
Code first the underlying condition, such as:
     congenital rubella (P35.0)
     Cushing's syndrome (E24.-)
     cystic fibrosis (E84.-)
     malignant neoplasm (C00–C96)
     malnutrition (E40–E46)
     pancreatitis and other diseases of the pancreas (K85-K86.-)
Use additional code to identify control using:
     insulin (Z79.4)
     oral antidiabetic drugs (Z79.84)
     oral hypoglycemic drugs (Z79.84)
Excludes1: drug or chemical induced DM (E09.-)
     gestational diabetes (O24.4-)
     neonatal DM (transient) (P70.2)
     postpancreatectomy DM (E13.-)
     postprocedural DM (E13.-)
     secondary DM NEC (E13.-)
     type 1 DM (E10.-)
     type 2 DM (E11.-)

E08.0   **DM due to underlying condition with hyperosmolarity;**
     E08.00   **without NKHHC**
     E08.01   **with coma**

E08.1   **DM due to underlying condition with ketoacidosis;**
     E08.10   **without coma**
     E08.11   **with coma**

E08.2   **DM due to underlying condition with; kidney complications**
     E08.21   **diabetic nephropathy or intercapillary**
         glomerulosclerosis or intracapillary glomerulonephrosis or Kimmelstiel-Wilson disease
     E08.22   **diabetic CKD**
         Use additional code to identify stage of CKD (N18.1–N18.6)
     E08.29   **other diabetic kidney complication**
         Renal tubular degeneration in DM due to underlying condition

E08.3   **DM due to underlying condition with ophthalmic complications**

E08.31   **DM due to underlying condition with unspecified diabetic retinopathy;**
     E08.311   **with macular edema**
     E08.319   **without macular edema**

°7th characters for subcategories E08.31, E08.32, E08.33, E08.34, E08.35
1—left eye
2—right eye
3—bilateral

E08.32   **DM due to underlying condition with mild nonproliferative diabetic retinopathy (NOS);**
     E08.321   **with macular edema**
     E08.329   **without macular edema**

E08.33   **DM due to underlying condition with moderate nonproliferative diabetic retinopathy;**
     E08.331   **with macular edema**
     E08.339   **without macular edema**

E08.34   **DM due to underlying condition with severe nonproliferative diabetic retinopathy;**
     E08.341   **with macular edema**
     E08.349   **without macular edema**

E08.35   **DM due to underlying condition with proliferative diabetic retinopathy;**
     E08.351   **with macular edema**
     E08.359   **without macular edema**

E08.36   **DM due to underlying condition with diabetic cataract**

E08.39   **DM due to underlying condition with other diabetic ophthalmic complication**
     Use additional code to identify manifestation, such as: diabetic glaucoma (H40–H42)

E08.4   **DM due to underlying condition with; neurological complications**
     E08.40   **diabetic neuropathy, unspecified**
     E08.41   **diabetic mononeuropathy**
     E08.42   **diabetic polyneuropathy**
         diabetic neuralgia
     E08.43   **diabetic autonomic (poly)neuropathy**
         diabetic gastroparesis
     E08.44   **diabetic amyotrophy**
     E08.49   **other diabetic neurological complication**

E08.5   **DM due to underlying condition with; circulatory complications**
     E08.51   **diabetic peripheral angiopathy without gangrene**
     E08.52   **diabetic peripheral angiopathy with gangrene**
         diabetic gangrene
     E08.59   **other circulatory complications**

E08.6   **DM due to underlying condition with other specified complications**
     E08.61   **DM due to underlying condition with; diabetic arthropathy**
         E08.610   **diabetic neuropathic arthropathy**
             Charcôt's joints
         E08.618   **other diabetic arthropathy**
     E08.62   **DM due to underlying condition with; skin complications**
         E08.620   **diabetic dermatitis**
             diabetic necrobiosis lipoidica

site of ulcer

site of ulcer
9)

oglycemia;

erglycemia
er specified

on

ions

65 with

fy drug

ty
rosmolarity
rosmolarity
with coma

E09.1 | Drug or chemical induced DM with ketoacidosis;
5th | E09.10 | without coma
| E09.11 | with coma
E09.2 | Drug or chemical induced DM with; kidney complications
5th | E09.21 | diabetic nephropathy
| | Drug or chemical induced DM with intercapillary glomerulosclerosis or intracapillary glomerulonephrosis or Kimmelstiel-Wilson disease
| E09.22 | diabetic CKD
| | **Use additional code** to identify stage of CKD (N18.1–N18.6)
| E09.29 | other diabetic kidney complication
| | Drug or chemical induced DM with renal tubular degeneration
E09.3 | Drug or chemical induced DM with ophthalmic complications
5th | E09.31 | Drug or chemical induced DM with unspecified diabetic retinopathy;
6th | E09.311 | with macular edema
| E09.319 | without macular edema

E09.32 | Drug or chemical induced DM with mild nonproliferative diabetic retinopathy;
6th | Drug or chemical induced DM with nonproliferative diabetic retinopathy NOS

> °7th characters for subcategory E09.32
> 1—left eye
> 2—right eye
> 3—bilateral

▲ E09.321	with macular edema
7th	
▲ E09.329	without macular edema
7th	

E09.33 | Drug or chemical induced DM with moderate nonproliferative diabetic retinopathy;
6th | ▲ E09.331 | with macular edema
| 7th |
| ▲ E09.339 | without macular edema
| 7th |

> °7th characters for subcategory E09.33, E09.34, E09.35
> 1—left eye
> 2—right eye
> 3—bilateral

E09.34 | Drug or chemical induced DM with severe nonproliferative diabetic retinopathy;
6th | ▲ E09.341 | with macular edema
| 7th |
| ▲ E09.349 | without macular edema
| 7th |

E09.35 | Drug or chemical induced DM with proliferative diabetic retinopathy;
6th | ▲ E09.351 | with macular edema
| 7th |
| °E09.353 | with traction retinal detachment not involving the macula
| 7th |
| °E09.354 | with combined traction retinal detachment and rhegmatogenous retinal detachment
| 7th |
| °E09.355 | stable
| 7th |
| ▲ E09.359 | without macular edema
| 7th |

E09.36 | Drug or chemical induced DM with diabetic cataract
E09.39 | Drug or chemical induced DM with other diabetic ophthalmic complication
| **Use additional code** to identify manifestation, such as: diabetic glaucoma (H40–H42)

E09.4 | Drug or chemical induced DM with neurological complications;
5th | E09.40 | with diabetic neuropathy, unspecified
| E09.41 | with diabetic mononeuropathy
| E09.42 | with diabetic polyneuropathy
| | with diabetic neuralgia
| E09.43 | with diabetic autonomic (poly)neuropathy
| | with diabetic gastroparesis
| E09.44 | diabetic amyotrophy
| E09.49 | with other diabetic neurological complication
E09.5 | Drug or chemical induced DM with; circulatory complications
5th | E09.51 | diabetic peripheral angiopathy without gangrene
| E09.52 | diabetic peripheral angiopathy with gangrene
| | diabetic gangrene
| E09.59 | other circulatory complications
E09.6 | Drug or chemical induced DM with other specified complications
5th | E09.61 | Drug or chemical induced DM with; diabetic arthropathy
6th | E09.610 | diabetic neuropathic arthropathy
| | Charcôt's joints
| E09.618 | other diabetic arthropathy

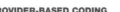

| 4th | 5th | 6th | 7th | Additional Character Required | ✔ | 3-character code |

°=New Code
▲=Revised Code

Excludes1—Not coded here, do not use together
Excludes2—Not included here

CHAPTER 4. ENDOCRINE, NUTRITIONAL AND METABOLIC DISEASES (E09.62–E10.9)

E09.62 **Drug or chemical induced DM with; skin complications** [6th]
    E09.620 **diabetic dermatitis**
        diabetic necrobiosis lipoidica
    E09.621 **foot ulcer**
        Use additional code to identify site of ulcer (L97.4-, L97.5-)
    E09.622 **other skin ulcer**
        Use additional code to identify site of ulcer (L97.1–L97.9, L98.41–L98.49)
    E09.628 **other skin complications**

E09.63 **Drug or chemical induced DM with; oral complications** [6th]
    E09.630 **periodontal disease**
    E09.638 **other oral complications**

E09.64 **Drug or chemical induced DM with hypoglycemia;** [6th]
    E09.641 **with coma**
    E09.649 **without coma**

E09.65 **Drug or chemical induced DM with hyperglycemia**

E09.69 **Drug or chemical induced DM with other specified complication**
    Use additional code to identify complication

E09.8 **Drug or chemical induced DM with unspecified complications**

E09.9 **Drug or chemical induced DM without complications**

E10 **TYPE 1 DM** [4th]
Refer to category E08 for guidelines
Includes: brittle diabetes (mellitus)
    diabetes (mellitus) due to autoimmune process
    diabetes (mellitus) due to immune mediated pancreatic islet beta-cell destruction
    idiopathic diabetes (mellitus)
    juvenile onset diabetes (mellitus)
    ketosis-prone diabetes (mellitus)
Excludes1: DM due to underlying condition (E08.-)
    drug or chemical induced DM (E09.-)
    gestational diabetes (O24.4-)
    hyperglycemia NOS (R73.9)
    neonatal DM (P70.2)
    postpancreatectomy DM (E13.-)
    postprocedural DM (E13.-)
    secondary DM NEC (E13.-)
    type 2 DM (E11.-)

E10.1 **Type 1 DM with ketoacidosis;** [5th]
    E10.10 **Type 1 DM with ketoacidosis without coma**
    E10.11 **Type 1 DM with ketoacidosis with coma**

E10.2 **Type 1 DM with kidney complications** [5th]
    E10.21 **Type 1 DM with diabetic nephropathy**
        Type 1 DM with intercapillary glomerulosclerosis or intracapillary glomerulonephrosis or Kimmelstiel-Wilson disease
    E10.22 **Type 1 DM with diabetic CKD**
        Use additional code to identify stage of CKD (N18.1–N18.6)
    E10.29 **Type 1 DM with other diabetic kidney complication**
        Type 1 DM with renal tubular degeneration

E10.3 **Type 1 DM with ophthalmic complications** [5th]
    E10.31 **Type 1 DM with unspecified diabetic retinopathy;** [6th]
        E10.311 **with macular edema**
        E10.319 **without macular edema**
    E10.32 **Type 1 DM with mild nonproliferative diabetic retinopathy;** [6th]
        diabetic retinopathy NOS
        ▴**E10.321** **with macular edema** [7th]

        ▴**E10.329** **without macular edema** [7th]

        | ∘7th characters for subcategory E10.32, E10.33 |
        | 1—left eye |
        | 2—right eye |
        | 3—bilateral |

    E10.33 **Type 1 DM with moderate nonproliferative diabetic retinopathy;** [6th]
        ▴**E10.331** **with macular edema** [7th]

        ▴**E10.339** **without macular edema** [7th]

    E10.34 **Type 1 DM with severe nonproliferative diabetic retinopathy;** [6th]
        ▴**E10.341** **with macular edema** [7th]

        ▴**E10.349** **without macular edema** [7th]

        | ∘7th characters for subcategory E10.34, E10.35 |
        | 1—left eye |
        | 2—right eye |
        | 3—bilateral |

    E10.35 **Type 1 DM with proliferative diabetic retinopathy;** [6th]
        ▴**E10.351** **with macular edema** [7th]

        ▴**E10.359** **without macular edema** [7th]

    E10.36 **Type 1 DM with diabetic cataract**
    E10.39 **Type 1 DM with other diabetic ophthalmic complication**
        Use additional code to identify manifestation, such as: diabetic glaucoma (H40–H42)

E10.4 **Type 1 DM with neurological complications** [5th]
    E10.40 **Type 1 DM with diabetic neuropathy, unspecified**
    E10.41 **Type 1 DM with diabetic mononeuropathy**
    E10.42 **Type 1 DM with diabetic polyneuropathy**
        Type 1 DM with diabetic neuralgia
    E10.43 **Type 1 DM with diabetic autonomic (poly)neuropathy**
    E10.44 **Type 1 DM with diabetic amyotrophy**
    E10.49 **Type 1 DM with other diabetic neurological complication**

E10.5 **Type 1 DM with circulatory complications** [5th]
    E10.51 **Type 1 DM with diabetic peripheral angiopathy without gangrene**
    E10.52 **Type 1 DM with diabetic peripheral angiopathy with gangrene**
        Type 1 DM with diabetic gangrene
    E10.59 **Type 1 DM with other circulatory complications**

E10.6 **Type 1 DM with other specified complications** [5th]
    E10.61 **Type 1 DM with diabetic arthropathy** [6th]
        E10.610 **Type 1 DM with diabetic neuropathic arthropathy**
            Type 1 DM with Charcôt's joints
        E10.618 **Type 1 DM with other diabetic arthropathy**
    E10.62 **Type 1 DM with skin complications** [6th]
        E10.620 **Type 1 DM with diabetic dermatitis**
            Type 1 DM with diabetic necrobiosis lipoidica
        E10.621 **Type 1 DM with foot ulcer**
            Use additional code to identify site of ulcer (L97.4-, L97.5-)
        E10.622 **Type 1 DM with other skin ulcer**
            Use additional code to identify site of ulcer (L97.1–L97.9, L98.41–L98.49)
        E10.628 **Type 1 DM with other skin complications**
    E10.63 **Type 1 DM with oral complications** [6th]
        E10.630 **Type 1 DM with periodontal disease**
        E10.638 **Type 1 DM with other oral complications**
    E10.64 **Type 1 DM with hypoglycemia** [6th]
        E10.641 **Type 1 DM with hypoglycemia with coma**
        E10.649 **Type 1 DM with hypoglycemia without coma**
    E10.65 **Type 1 DM with hyperglycemia**
    E10.69 **Type 1 DM with other specified complication**
        Use additional code to identify complication

E10.8 **Type 1 DM with unspecified complications**

E10.9 **Type 1 DM without complications**

   [4th] [5th] [6th] [7th] Additional Character Required   3-character code

∘=New Code   *Excludes1*—Not coded here, do not use together
▴=Revised Code   *Excludes2*—Not included here

E11 TYPE 2 DM

Refer to category E08 for guidelines

If the type of DM is not documented in the medical record the default is E11.-, Type 2 DM.

Includes: diabetes (mellitus) due to insulin secretory defect
diabetes NOS
insulin resistant diabetes (mellitus)

Use additional code to identify control using:
insulin (Z79.4)
oral antidiabetic drugs (Z79.84)
oral hypoglycemic drugs (Z79.84)

Excludes1: DM due to underlying condition (E08.-)
drug or chemical induced DM (E09.-)
gestational diabetes (O24.4-)
neonatal DM (P70.2)
postpancreatectomy DM (E13.-)
postprocedural DM (E13.-)
secondary DM NEC (E13.-)
type 1 DM (E10.-)

E11.0 Type 2 DM with hyperosmolarity;
5th
E11.00 **without NKHHC**
E11.01 **with coma**

E11.2 Type 2 DM with kidney complications
5th
E11.21 **Type 2 DM with diabetic nephropathy or intercapillary glomerulosclerosis or intracapillary glomerulonephrosis or Kimmelstiel-Wilson disease**
E11.22 **Type 2 DM with diabetic CKD**
Use additional code to identify stage of CKD (N18.1–N18.6)
E11.29 **Type 2 DM with other diabetic kidney complication**
Type 2 DM with renal tubular degeneration

E11.3 Type 2 DM with ophthalmic complications
5th
E11.31 **Type 2 DM with unspecified diabetic retinopathy;**
6th
E11.311 **with macular edema**
E11.319 **without macular edema**
E11.32 **Type 2 DM with mild nonproliferative diabetic retinopathy;**
6th
Type 2 DM with nonproliferative diabetic retinopathy NOS
▲ E11.321 **with macular edema**
7th
▲ E11.329 **without macular edema**
7th

E11.33 **Type 2 DM with moderate nonproliferative diabetic retinopathy;**
6th
▲ E11.331 **with macular edema**
7th
▲ E11.339 **without macular edema**
7th

E11.34 **Type 2 DM with severe nonproliferative diabetic retinopathy;**
6th
▲ E11.341 **with macular edema**
7th
▲ E11.349 **without macular edema**
7th

E11.35 **Type 2 DM with proliferative diabetic retinopathy;**
6th
▲ E11.351 **with macular edema**
7th
▲ E11.359 **without macular edema**
7th

E11.36 **Type 2 DM with diabetic cataract**

> • 7th character for subcategories E11.32, E11.33, E11.34, E11.35
>
> 1—right eye
> 2—left eye
> 3—bilateral

E11.39 **Type 2 DM with other diabetic ophthalmic complication**
Use additional code to identify manifestation, such as: diabetic glaucoma (H40–H42)

E11.4 Type 2 DM with neurological complications
5th
E11.40 **Type 2 DM with diabetic neuropathy, unspecified**
E11.41 **Type 2 DM with diabetic mononeuropathy**
E11.42 **Type 2 DM with diabetic polyneuropathy**
Type 2 DM with diabetic neuralgia
E11.43 **Type 2 DM with diabetic autonomic (poly)neuropathy**
Type 2 DM with diabetic gastroparesis
E11.44 **Type 2 DM with diabetic amyotrophy**
E11.49 **Type 2 DM with other diabetic neurological complication**

E11.5 Type 2 DM with circulatory complications
5th
E11.51 **Type 2 DM with diabetic peripheral angiopathy without gangrene**
E11.52 **Type 2 DM with diabetic peripheral angiopathy with gangrene**
Type 2 DM with diabetic gangrene
E11.59 **Type 2 DM with other circulatory complications**

E11.6 Type 2 DM with other specified complications
5th
E11.61 **Type 2 DM with diabetic arthropathy**
6th
E11.610 **Type 2 DM with diabetic neuropathic arthropathy**
Type 2 DM with Charcôt's joints
E11.618 **Type 2 DM with other diabetic arthropathy**
E11.62 **Type 2 DM with skin complications**
6th
E11.620 **Type 2 DM with diabetic dermatitis**
Type 2 DM with diabetic necrobiosis lipoidica
E11.621 **Type 2 DM with foot ulcer**
Use additional code to identify site of ulcer (L97.4-, L97.5-)
E11.622 **Type 2 DM with other skin ulcer**
Use additional code to identify site of ulcer (L97.1–L97.9, L98.41–L98.49)
E11.628 **Type 2 DM with other skin complications**
E11.63 **Type 2 DM with oral complications**
6th
E11.630 **Type 2 DM with periodontal disease**
E11.638 **Type 2 DM with other oral complications**
E11.64 **Type 2 DM with hypoglycemia**
6th
E11.641 **Type 2 DM with hypoglycemia with coma**
E11.649 **Type 2 DM with hypoglycemia without coma**
E11.65 **Type 2 DM with hyperglycemia**
E11.69 **Type 2 DM with other specified complication**
Use additional code to identify complication

E11.8 Type 2 DM with unspecified complications
E11.9 Type 2 DM without complications

(E15–E16) OTHER DISORDERS OF GLUCOSE REGULATION AND PANCREATIC INTERNAL SECRETION

E16 OTHER DISORDERS OF PANCREATIC INTERNAL SECRETION

E16.0 Drug-induced hypoglycemia without coma
Use additional code for adverse effect, if applicable, to identify drug (T36–T50 with fifth or sixth character 5)
Excludes 1: diabetes with hypoglycemia without coma (E09.692)

E16.1 Other hypoglycemia
Functional hyperinsulinism
Functional nonhyperinsulinemic hypoglycemia
Hyperinsulinism NOS
Hyperplasia of pancreatic islet beta cells NOS
Excludes1: diabetes with hypoglycemia (E08.649, E10.649, E11.649)
hypoglycemia in infant of diabetic mother (P70.1)
neonatal hypoglycemia (P70.4)

E16.2 Hypoglycemia, unspecified
Excludes 1: diabetes with hypoglycemia (E08.649, E10.649, E11.649)

    Additional Character Required   3-character code   •=New Code   ▲=Revised Code   ***Excludes1***—Not coded here, do not use together   ***Excludes2***—Not included here

CHAPTER 4. ENDOCRINE, NUTRITIONAL AND METABOLIC DISEASES   (E16.8–E34.3)

E16.8 Other specified disorders of pancreatic internal secretion
Increased secretion from endocrine pancreas of growth hormone-releasing hormone or pancreatic polypeptide or somatostatin or vasoactive-intestinal polypeptide

E16.9 Disorder of pancreatic internal secretion, unspecified
Islet-cell hyperplasia NOS
Pancreatic endocrine cell hyperplasia NOS

(E20–E35) DISORDERS OF OTHER ENDOCRINE GLANDS

Excludes1: galactorrhea (N64.3)
gynecomastia (N62)

E20 HYPOPARATHYROIDISM
Excludes1: Di George's syndrome (D82.1)
postprocedural hypoparathyroidism (E89.2)
tetany NOS (R29.0)
transitory neonatal hypoparathyroidism (P71.4)

E20.0 Idiopathic hypoparathyroidism
E20.1 Pseudohypoparathyroidism

E22 HYPERFUNCTION OF PITUITARY GLAND
Excludes1: Cushing's syndrome (E24.-)
Nelson's syndrome (E24.1)
overproduction of ACTH not associated with Cushing's disease (E27.0)
overproduction of pituitary ACTH (E24.0)
overproduction of thyroid-stimulating hormone (E05.8-)

E22.0 Acromegaly and pituitary gigantism
Overproduction of growth hormone
Excludes1: constitutional gigantism (E34.4)
constitutional tall stature (E34.4)
increased secretion from endocrine pancreas of growth hormone-releasing hormone (E16.8)

E22.2 Syndrome of inappropriate secretion of antidiuretic hormone
E22.8 Other hyperfunction of pituitary gland
Central precocious puberty
E22.9 Hyperfunction of pituitary gland, unspecified

E24 CUSHING'S SYNDROME
Excludes1: congenital adrenal hyperplasia (E25.0)
E24.0 Pituitary-dependent Cushing's disease
Overproduction of pituitary ACTH
Pituitary-dependent hypercorticalism
E24.2 Drug-induced Cushing's syndrome
Use additional code for adverse effect, if applicable, to identify drug (T36–T50 with fifth or sixth character 5)
E24.9 Cushing's syndrome, unspecified

E25 ADRENOGENITAL DISORDERS
Includes: adrenogenital syndromes, virilizing or feminizing, whether acquired or due to adrenal hyperplasia consequent on inborn enzyme defects in hormone synthesis
Female adrenal pseudohermaphroditism
Female heterosexual precocious pseudopuberty
Male isosexual precocious pseudopuberty
Male macrogenitosomia praecox
Male sexual precocity with adrenal hyperplasia
Male virilization (female)
Excludes1: indeterminate sex and pseudohermaphroditism (Q56)
chromosomal abnormalities (Q90–Q99)
E25.0 Congenital adrenogenital disorders associated with enzyme deficiency
Congenital adrenal hyperplasia
21-Hydroxylase deficiency
Salt-losing congenital adrenal hyperplasia
E25.8 Other adrenogenital disorders
Idiopathic adrenogenital disorder
Use additional code for adverse effect, if applicable, to identify drug (T36–T50 with fifth or sixth character 5)
E25.9 Adrenogenital disorder, unspecified
Adrenogenital syndrome NOS

E27 OTHER DISORDERS OF ADRENAL GLAND
Refer to code C74, Malignant neoplasm of adrenal gland, to report neuroblastomas

E27.0 Other adrenocortical overactivity
Overproduction of ACTH, not associated with Cushing's disease
Premature adrenarche
Excludes1: Cushing's syndrome (E24.-)
E27.1 Primary adrenocortical insufficiency
Addison's disease
Autoimmune adrenalitis
Excludes1: Addison only phenotype adrenoleukodystrophy (E71.528)
amyloidosis (E85.-)
tuberculous Addison's disease (A18.7)
Waterhouse-Friderichsen syndrome (A39.1)
E27.2 Addisonian crisis
Adrenal crisis
Adrenocortical crisis
E27.3 Drug-induced adrenocortical insufficiency
Use additional code for adverse effect, if applicable, to identify drug (T36–T50 with fifth or sixth character 5)
E27.4 Other and unspecified adrenocortical insufficiency
Excludes1: adrenoleukodystrophy [Addison-Schilder] (E71.528)
Waterhouse-Friderichsen syndrome (A39.1)
E27.40 Unspecified adrenocortical insufficiency
Adrenocortical insufficiency NOS
E27.49 Other adrenocortical insufficiency
Adrenal hemorrhage
Adrenal infarction

E28 OVARIAN DYSFUNCTION
Excludes1: isolated gonadotropin deficiency (E23.0)
postprocedural ovarian failure (E89.4-)
E28.0 Estrogen excess
Use additional code for adverse effect, if applicable, to identify drug (T36–T50 with fifth or sixth character 5)
E28.1 Androgen excess
Hypersecretion of ovarian androgens
Use additional code for adverse effect, if applicable, to identify drug (T36–T50 with fifth or sixth character 5)
E28.2 Polycystic ovarian syndrome
Sclerocystic ovary syndrome
Stein-Leventhal syndrome

E30 DISORDERS OF PUBERTY, NEC
E30.0 Delayed puberty
Constitutional delay of puberty
Delayed sexual development
E30.1 Precocious puberty
Precocious menstruation
Excludes1: Albright (-McCune) (-Sternberg) syndrome (Q78.1)
central precocious puberty (E22.8)
congenital adrenal hyperplasia (E25.0)
female heterosexual precocious pseudopuberty (E25.-)
male isosexual precocious pseudopuberty (E25.-)
E30.8 Other disorders of puberty
Premature thelarche
E30.9 Disorder of puberty, unspecified

E34 OTHER ENDOCRINE DISORDERS
Excludes1: pseudohypoparathyroidism (E20.1)
E34.0 Carcinoid syndrome
Note: May be used as an additional code to identify functional activity associated with a carcinoid tumor.
E34.3 Short stature due to endocrine disorder
Constitutional short stature
Laron-type short stature
Excludes1: achondroplastic short stature (Q77.4)
hypochondroplastic short stature (Q77.4)
nutritional short stature (E45)
pituitary short stature (E23.0)
progeria (E34.8)
renal short stature (N25.0)
Russell-Silver syndrome (Q87.1)
short-limbed stature with immunodeficiency (D82.2)
short stature in specific dysmorphic syndromes—**code to** syndrome—**see** Alphabetical Index
short stature NOS (R62.52)

| 4th | 5th | 6th | 7th | Additional Character Required | ✔ 3-character code | •=New Code | ***Excludes1***—Not coded here, do not use together |
| ▲=Revised Code | ***Excludes2***—Not included here |

E34.5 Androgen insensitivity syndrome

E34.50 Androgen insensitivity syndrome, unspecified
Androgen insensitivity NOS

E34.51 Complete androgen insensitivity syndrome
Complete androgen insensitivity
de Quervain syndrome
Goldberg-Maxwell syndrome

E34.52 Partial androgen insensitivity syndrome
Partial androgen insensitivity
Reifenstein syndrome

(E36) INTRAOPERATIVE COMPLICATIONS OF ENDOCRINE SYSTEM

(E40–E46) MALNUTRITION

E40 KWASHIORKOR

Severe malnutrition with nutritional edema with dyspigmentation of skin and hair
Excludes1: marasmic kwashiorkor (E42)

E46 UNSPECIFIED PROTEIN-CALORIE MALNUTRITION

Malnutrition NOS
Protein-calorie imbalance NOS
Excludes1: nutritional deficiency NOS (E63.9)

(E50–E64) OTHER NUTRITIONAL DEFICIENCIES

E55 VITAMIN D DEFICIENCY

Excludes1: adult osteomalacia (M83.-)
osteoporosis (M80.-)
sequelae of rickets (E64.3)

E55.0 Rickets, active
Infantile osteomalacia
Juvenile osteomalacia
Excludes1: celiac rickets (K90.0)
Crohn's rickets (K50.-)
hereditary vitamin D-dependent rickets (E83.32)
inactive rickets (E64.3)
renal rickets (N25.0)
sequelae of rickets (E64.3)
vitamin D-resistant rickets (E83.31)

E55.9 Vitamin D deficiency, unspecified
Avitaminosis D

E58 DIETARY CALCIUM DEFICIENCY

Excludes1: disorders of calcium metabolism (E83.5-)
sequelae of calcium deficiency (E64.8)

(E65–E68) OVERWEIGHT, OBESITY AND OTHER HYPERALIMENTATION

E66 OVERWEIGHT AND OBESITY

Use additional code to identify body mass index (BMI), if known (Z68.-)
Excludes1: adiposogenital dystrophy (E23.6)
lipomatosis NOS (E88.2)
lipomatosis dolorosa [Dercum] (E88.2)
Prader-Willi syndrome (Q87.1)

E66.0 Obesity due to excess calories
E66.01 Morbid (severe) obesity due to excess calories
Excludes1: morbid (severe) obesity with alveolar hypoventilation (E66.2)
E66.09 Other obesity due to excess calories

E66.1 Drug-induced obesity
Use additional code for adverse effect, if applicable, to identify drug (T36-T50 with fifth or sixth character 5)

E66.2 Morbid (severe) obesity with alveolar hypoventilation
obesity hypoventilation syndrome (OHS)
Use with Z68.30–Z68.45 (adults) or Z68.53 (pediatrics, 2–20 yrs)
Pickwickian syndrome

E66.3 Overweight
Use with Z68.25–Z68.29 (adults) or Z68.53 (pediatrics, 2–20 yrs)

E66.8 Other obesity
Use with Z68.30–Z68.45 (adults) or Z68.53 (pediatrics, 2–20 yrs)

E66.9 Obesity, unspecified
Use with Z68.30–Z68.45 (adults) or Z68.53 (pediatrics, 2–20 yrs)
Obesity NOS

(E70–E88) METABOLIC DISORDERS

Excludes1: androgen insensitivity syndrome (E34.5-)
congenital adrenal hyperplasia (E25.0)
Ehlers-Danlos syndrome (Q79.6)
hemolytic anemias attributable to enzyme disorders (D55.-)
Marfan's syndrome (Q87.4)
5-alpha-reductase deficiency (E29.1)

E70 DISORDERS OF AROMATIC AMINO-ACID METABOLISM

E70.0 Classical phenylketonuria

E71 DISORDERS OF BRANCHED-CHAIN AMINO-ACID METABOLISM AND FATTY-ACID METABOLISM
E71.0 Maple-syrup-urine disease
E71.1 Other disorders of branched-chain amino-acid metabolism
E71.11 Branched-chain organic acidurias
E71.110 Isovaleric acidemia
E71.111 3-methylglutaconic aciduria
E71.118 Other branched-chain organic acidurias
E71.12 Disorders of propionate metabolism
E71.120 Methylmalonic acidemia
E71.121 Propionic acidemia
E71.128 Other disorders of propionate metabolism
E71.19 Other disorders of branched-chain amino-acid metabolism
Hyperleucine-isoleucinemia
Hypervalinemia
E71.2 Disorder of branched-chain amino-acid metabolism, unspecified
E71.3 Disorders of fatty-acid metabolism
Excludes1: peroxisomal disorders (E71.5)
Refsum's disease (G60.1)
Schilder's disease (G37.0)
Excludes2: carnitine deficiency due to inborn error of metabolism (E71.42)
E71.30 Disorder of fatty-acid metabolism, unspecified
E71.31 Disorders of fatty-acid oxidation
E71.310 Long chain/very long chain acyl CoA dehydrogenase deficiency
LCAD
VLCAD
E71.311 Medium chain acyl CoA dehydrogenase deficiency
MCAD
E71.312 Short chain acyl CoA dehydrogenase deficiency
SCAD
E71.313 Glutaric aciduria type II
Glutaric aciduria type II A
Glutaric aciduria type II B
Glutaric aciduria type II C
Excludes1: glutaric aciduria (type 1) NOS (E72.3)
E71.314 Muscle carnitine palmitoyltransferase deficiency
E71.318 Other disorders of fatty-acid oxidation
E71.32 Disorders of ketone metabolism
E71.39 Other disorders of fatty-acid metabolism
E71.4 Disorders of carnitine metabolism
Excludes1: Muscle carnitine palmitoyltransferase deficiency (E71.314)
E71.40 Disorder of carnitine metabolism, unspecified
E71.41 Primary carnitine deficiency
E71.42 Carnitine deficiency due to inborn errors of metabolism
Code also associated inborn error or metabolism
E71.43 Iatrogenic carnitine deficiency
Carnitine deficiency due to hemodialysis
Carnitine deficiency due to Valproic acid therapy

  Additional Character Required   3-character code

●=New Code
▲=Revised Code

Excludes1—Not coded here, do not use together
Excludes2—Not included here

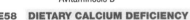

CHAPTER 4. ENDOCRINE, NUTRITIONAL AND METABOLIC DISEASES (E34.5-E71.43)

CHAPTER 4. ENDOCRINE, NUTRITIONAL AND METABOLIC DISEASES (E71.44–E78.1)

E71.44   **Other secondary carnitine deficiency**
      E71.440   **Ruvalcaba-Myhre-Smith syndrome**
      E71.448   **Other secondary carnitine deficiency**

E71.5   **Peroxisomal disorders**
   Excludes1: Schilder's disease (G37.0)
   E71.50   **Peroxisomal disorder, unspecified**
   E71.51   **Disorders of peroxisome biogenesis**
      Group 1 peroxisomal disorders
      Excludes1: Refsum's disease (G60.1)
      E71.510   **Zellweger syndrome**
      E71.511   **Neonatal adrenoleukodystrophy**
         Excludes1: X-linked adrenoleukodystrophy (E71.42-)
      E71.518   **Other disorders of peroxisome biogenesis**
   E71.52   **X-linked adrenoleukodystrophy**
      E71.520   **Childhood cerebral X-linked adrenoleukodystrophy**
      E71.521   **Adolescent X-linked adrenoleukodystrophy**
      E71.522   **Adrenomyeloneuropathy**
      E71.528   **Other X-linked adrenoleukodystrophy**
         Addison only phenotype adrenoleukodystrophy
         Addison-Schilder adrenoleukodystrophy
      E71.529   **X-linked adrenoleukodystrophy, unspecified type**
   E71.53   **Other group 2 peroxisomal disorders**
   E71.54   **Other peroxisomal disorders**
      E71.540   **Rhizomelic chondrodysplasia punctata**
         Excludes1: chondrodysplasia punctata NOS (Q77.3)
      E71.541   **Zellweger-like syndrome**
      E71.542   **Other group 3 peroxisomal disorders**
      E71.548   **Other peroxisomal disorders**

E72   OTHER DISORDERS OF AMINO-ACID METABOLISM
   Excludes1: disorders of aromatic amino-acid metabolism (E70.-)
      branched-chain amino-acid metabolism (E71.0–E71.2)
      fatty-acid metabolism (E71.3)
      purine and pyrimidine metabolism (E79.-)
      gout (M1A.-, M10.-)

E72.0   **Disorders of amino-acid transport**
   Excludes1: disorders of tryptophan metabolism (E70.5)
   E72.00   **Disorders of amino-acid transport, unspecified**
   E72.01   **Cystinuria**
   E72.02   **Hartnup's disease**
   E72.03   **Lowe's syndrome**
      Use additional code for associated glaucoma (H42)

E72.8   **Other specified disorders of amino-acid metabolism**
   Disorders of beta-amino-acid metabolism
   Disorders of gamma-glutamyl cycle

E72.9   **Disorder of amino-acid metabolism, unspecified**

E73   LACTOSE INTOLERANCE
E73.0   **Congenital lactase deficiency**
E73.1   **Secondary lactase deficiency**
E73.8   **Other lactose intolerance**
E73.9   **Lactose intolerance, unspecified**

E74   OTHER DISORDERS OF CARBOHYDRATE METABOLISM
   Excludes1: DM (E08–E13)
      hypoglycemia NOS (E16.2)
      increased secretion of glucagon (E16.3)
      mucopolysaccharidosis (E76.0–E76.3) E74.1

E74.1   **Disorders of fructose metabolism**
   Excludes1: muscle phosphofructokinase deficiency (E74.09)
   E74.10   **Disorder of fructose metabolism, unspecified**
   E74.11   **Essential fructosuria**
      Fructokinase deficiency
   E74.12   **Hereditary fructose intolerance**
      Fructosemia
   E74.19   **Other disorders of fructose metabolism**
      Fructose-1, 6-diphosphatase deficiency

E74.2   **Disorders of galactose metabolism**
   E74.20   **Disorders of galactose metabolism, unspecified**
   E74.21   **Galactosemia**
   E74.29   **Other disorders of galactose metabolism**
      Galactokinase deficiency

E74.3   **Other disorders of intestinal carbohydrate absorption**
   Excludes2: lactose intolerance (E73.-)
   E74.31   **Sucrase-isomaltase deficiency**
   E74.39   **Other disorders of intestinal carbohydrate absorption**
      Disorder of intestinal carbohydrate absorption NOS
      Glucose-galactose malabsorption
      Sucrase deficiency

E74.4   **Disorders of pyruvate metabolism and gluconeogenesis**
   Deficiency of phosphoenolpyruvate carboxykinase
   Deficiency of pyruvate carboxylase
   Deficiency of pyruvate dehydrogenase
   Excludes1: disorders of pyruvate metabolism and gluconeogenesis with anemia (D55.-)
      Leigh's syndrome (G31.82)

E75.0   **GM2 gangliosidosis**
   E75.02   **Tay-Sachs disease**

E76   DISORDERS OF GLYCOSAMINOGLYCAN METABOLISM
E76.0   **Mucopolysaccharidosis, type I**
   E76.01   **Hurler's syndrome**
   E76.02   **Hurler-Scheie syndrome**
   E76.03   **Scheie's syndrome**

E76.1   **Mucopolysaccharidosis, type II**
   Hunter's syndrome

E76.2   **Other mucopolysaccharidoses**
   E76.21   **Morquio mucopolysaccharidosis**
      E76.210   **Morquio A mucopolysaccharidoses**
         Classic Morquio syndrome
         Morquio syndrome A
         Mucopolysaccharidosis, type IVA
      E76.211   **Morquio B mucopolysaccharidoses**
         Morquio-like mucopolysaccharidoses
         Morquio-like syndrome
         Morquio syndrome B
         Mucopolysaccharidosis, type IVB
      E76.219   **Morquio mucopolysaccharidoses, unspecified**
         Morquio syndrome
         Mucopolysaccharidosis, type IV
   E76.22   **Sanfilippo mucopolysaccharidoses**
      Mucopolysaccharidosis, type III (A) (B) (C) (D)
      Sanfilippo A syndrome
      Sanfilippo B syndrome
      Sanfilippo C syndrome
      Sanfilippo D syndrome
   E76.29   **Other mucopolysaccharidoses**
      beta-Glucuronidase deficiency
      Maroteaux-Lamy (mild) (severe) syndrome
      Mucopolysaccharidosis, types VI, VII

E76.3   **Mucopolysaccharidosis, unspecified**
E76.8   **Other disorders of glucosaminoglycan metabolism**
E76.9   **Glucosaminoglycan metabolism disorder, unspecified**

E78   DISORDERS OF LIPOPROTEIN METABOLISM AND OTHER LIPIDEMIAS
   Excludes1: sphingolipidosis (E75.0–E75.3)
E78.0   **Pure hypercholesterolemia**
   •E78.00   **Pure hypercholesterolemia, unspecified**
      Fredrickson's hyperlipoproteinemia, type IIa
      Hyperbetalipoproteinemia
   •E78.01   **Familial hypercholesterolemia**

E78.1   **Pure hyperglyceridemia**
   Elevated fasting triglycerides
   Endogenous hyperglyceridemia
   Fredrickson's hyperlipoproteinemia, type IV
   Hyperlipidemia, group B
   Hyperprebetalipoproteinemia
   Very-low-density-lipoprotein-type [VLDL] hyperlipoproteinemia

---

   4th 5th 6th 7th Additional Character Required   3-character code

•=New Code   *Excludes1*—Not coded here, do not use together
▲=Revised Code   *Excludes2*—Not included here

E78.2 Mixed hyperlipidemia
Broad- or floating-betalipoproteinemia
Combined hyperlipidemia NOS
Elevated cholesterol with elevated triglycerides NEC
Fredrickson's hyperlipoproteinemia, type IIb or III
Hyperbetalipoproteinemia with prebetalipoproteinemia
Hypercholesteremia with endogenous hyperglyceridemia
Hyperlipidemia, group C
Tubo-eruptive xanthoma
Xanthoma tuberosum
Excludes1: cerebrotendinous cholesterosis [van Bogaert-Scherer-Epstein] (E75.5)
     familial combined hyperlipidemia (E78.4)

E78.3 Hyperchylomicronemia
Chylomicron retention disease
Fredrickson's hyperlipoproteinemia, type I or V
Hyperlipidemia, group D
Mixed hyperglyceridemia

E78.4 Other hyperlipidemia
Familial combined hyperlipidemia

E78.5 Hyperlipidemia, unspecified

E78.6 Lipoprotein deficiency
Abetalipoproteinemia
Depressed HDL cholesterol
High-density lipoprotein deficiency
Hypoalphalipoproteinemia
Hypobetalipoproteinemia (familial)
Lecithin cholesterol acyltransferase deficiency
Tangier disease

E78.7 Disorders of bile acid and cholesterol metabolism
Excludes1: Niemann-Pick disease type C (E75.242)
- **E78.70** Disorder of bile acid and cholesterol metabolism, unspecified
- **E78.71** Barth syndrome
- **E78.72** Smith-Lemli-Opitz syndrome
- **E78.79** Other disorders of bile acid and cholesterol metabolism

E78.8 Other disorders of lipoprotein metabolism
- **E78.81** Lipoid dermatoarthritis
- **E78.89** Other lipoprotein metabolism disorders

E78.9 Disorder of lipoprotein metabolism, unspecified

E80 DISORDERS OF PORPHYRIN AND BILIRUBIN METABOLISM
Includes: defects of catalase and peroxidase

E80.0 Hereditary erythropoietic porphyria
Congenital erythropoietic porphyria
Erythropoietic protoporphyria

E80.2 Other and unspecified porphyria
- **E80.20** Unspecified porphyria
  Porphyria NOS
- **E80.21** Acute intermittent (hepatic) porphyria
- **E80.29** Other porphyria
  Hereditary coproporphyria

E80.4 Gilbert syndrome

E80.5 Crigler-Najjar syndrome

E80.6 Other disorders of bilirubin metabolism
Dubin-Johnson syndrome
Rotor's syndrome

E83 DISORDERS OF MINERAL METABOLISM
Excludes1: dietary mineral deficiency (E58–E61)
     parathyroid disorders (E20–E21)
     vitamin D deficiency (E55.-)

E83.0 Disorders of copper metabolism
- **E83.00** Disorder of copper metabolism, unspecified
- **E83.01** Wilson's disease
  Code also associated Kayser Fleischer ring (H18.04-)
- **E83.09** Other disorders of copper metabolism
  Menkes' (kinky hair) (steely hair) disease

E83.1 Disorders of iron metabolism
Excludes1: iron deficiency anemia (D50.-)
     sideroblastic anemia (D64.0–D64.3)
- **E83.10** Disorder of iron metabolism, unspecified

- **E83.11** Hemochromatosis
  - **E83.110** Hereditary hemochromatosis
    Bronzed diabetes
    Pigmentary cirrhosis (of liver)
    Primary (hereditary) hemochromatosis
  - **E83.111** Hemochromatosis due to repeated red blood cell transfusions
    Iron overload due to repeated red blood cell transfusions
    Transfusion (red blood cell) associated hemochromatosis
  - **E83.118** Other hemochromatosis
  - **E83.119** Hemochromatosis, unspecified
- **E83.19** Other disorders of iron metabolism
  Use additional code, if applicable, for idiopathic pulmonary hemosiderosis (J84.03)

E83.2 Disorders of zinc metabolism
Acrodermatitis enteropathica

E83.3 Disorders of phosphorus metabolism and phosphatases
Excludes1: adult osteomalacia (M83.-)
     osteoporosis (M80.-)
- **E83.30** Disorder of phosphorus metabolism, unspecified
- **E83.31** Familial hypophosphatemia
  Vitamin D-resistant osteomalacia
  Vitamin D-resistant rickets
  Excludes1: vitamin D-deficiency rickets (E55.0)
- **E83.32** Hereditary vitamin D-dependent rickets (type 1) (type 2)
  25-hydroxyvitamin D 1-alpha-hydroxylase deficiency
  Pseudovitamin D deficiency
  Vitamin D receptor defect
- **E83.39** Other disorders of phosphorus metabolism
  Acid phosphatase deficiency
  Hyperphosphatemia
  Hypophosphatasia

E83.4 Disorders of magnesium metabolism
Use P71.8–P71.9 for transitory neonatal disorders of magnesium metabolism
- **E83.40** Disorders of magnesium metabolism, unspecified
- **E83.41** Hypermagnesemia
- **E83.42** Hypomagnesemia
- **E83.49** Other disorders of magnesium metabolism

E83.5 Disorders of calcium metabolism
Excludes1: chondrocalcinosis (M11.1–M11.2)
     hungry bone syndrome (E83.81)
     hyperparathyroidism (E21.0–E21.3)
- **E83.50** Unspecified disorder of calcium metabolism
- **E83.51** Hypocalcemia
  For associated tetany report R29.0
- **E83.52** Hypercalcemia
  Familial hypocalciuric hypercalcemia
- **E83.59** Other disorders of calcium metabolism
  Idiopathic hypercalciuria

E83.8 Other disorders of mineral metabolism
- **E83.81** Hungry bone syndrome
- **E83.89** Other disorders of mineral metabolism

E83.9 Disorder of mineral metabolism, unspecified

E84 CYSTIC FIBROSIS
Includes: mucoviscidosis
Code also exocrine pancreatic insufficiency (K86.81)

E84.0 Cystic fibrosis with pulmonary manifestations
Use additional code to identify any infectious organism present, such as: Pseudomonas (B96.5)

E84.1 Cystic fibrosis with intestinal manifestations
- **E84.11** Meconium ileus in cystic fibrosis
  Excludes1: meconium ileus not due to cystic fibrosis (P76.0)
- **E84.19** Cystic fibrosis with other intestinal manifestations
  Distal intestinal obstruction syndrome

E84.8 Cystic fibrosis with other manifestations

E84.9 Cystic fibrosis, unspecified

CHAPTER 4. ENDOCRINE, NUTRITIONAL AND METABOLIC DISEASES (E78.2–E84.9)

  Additional Character Required   3-character code

●=New Code
▲=Revised Code

Excludes1—Not coded here, do not use together
Excludes2—Not included here

E86 VOLUME DEPLETION

Use additional code(s) for any associated disorders of electrolyte and acid-base balance (E87.-)

Excludes1: dehydration of newborn (P74.1)
hypovolemic shock NOS (R57.1)
postprocedural hypovolemic shock (T81.19)
traumatic hypovolemic shock (T79.4)

E86.0 Dehydration

E86.1 Hypovolemia
Depletion of volume of plasma

E86.9 Volume depletion, unspecified

E87 OTHER DISORDERS OF FLUID, ELECTROLYTE AND ACID-BASE BALANCE

Excludes1: diabetes insipidus (E23.2)
electrolyte imbalance associated with hyperemesis gravidarum (O21.1)
electrolyte imbalance following ectopic or molar pregnancy (O08.5)
familial periodic paralysis (G72.3)

E87.0 Hyperosmolality and hypernatremia
Sodium [Na] excess
Sodium [Na] overload

E87.1 Hypo-osmolality and hyponatremia
Sodium [Na] deficiency
Excludes1: syndrome of inappropriate secretion of antidiuretic hormone (E22.2)

E87.2 Acidosis
Acidosis NOS
Lactic acidosis
Metabolic acidosis
Respiratory acidosis
Excludes1: diabetic acidosis—see categories E08–E10, E13 with ketoacidosis

E87.3 Alkalosis
Alkalosis NOS
Metabolic alkalosis
Respiratory alkalosis

E87.4 Mixed disorder of acid-base balance

E87.5 Hyperkalemia
Potassium [K] excess
Potassium [K] overload

E87.6 Hypokalemia
Potassium [K] deficiency

E87.7 Fluid overload

Excludes1: edema NOS (R60.9)
fluid retention (R60.9)

    E87.70 Fluid overload, unspecified

    E87.71 Transfusion associated circulatory overload
        Fluid overload due to transfusion (blood) (blood components)
        TACO

    E87.79 Other fluid overload

E87.8 Other disorders of electrolyte and fluid balance, NEC
Electrolyte imbalance NOS
Hyperchloremia
Hypochloremia

E88 OTHER AND UNSPECIFIED METABOLIC DISORDERS

Use additional codes for associated conditions

E88.0 Disorders of plasma-protein metabolism, NEC

    Excludes1: disorder of lipoprotein metabolism (E78.-)
    monoclonal gammopathy (of undetermined significance) (D47.2)
    polyclonal hypergammaglobulinemia (D89.0)
    Waldenström macroglobulinemia (C88.0)

    E88.01 Alpha-1-antitrypsin deficiency
        AAT deficiency

    E88.09 Other disorders of plasma-protein metabolism, NEC
        Bisalbuminemia

E88.1 Lipodystrophy, NEC
Lipodystrophy NOS

E88.2 Lipomatosis, NEC
Lipomatosis NOS
Lipomatosis (Check) dolorosa [Dercum]

E88.3 Tumor lysis syndrome
Tumor lysis syndrome (spontaneous)
Tumor lysis syndrome following antineoplastic drug chemotherapy
Use additional code for adverse effect, if applicable, to identify drug (T45.1X5)

E88.4 Mitochondrial metabolism disorders

    Excludes1: disorders of pyruvate metabolism (E74.4)
    Kearns-Sayre syndrome (H49.81)
    Leber's disease (H47.22)
    Leigh's encephalopathy (G31.82)
    Mitochondrial myopathy, NEC (G71.3)
    Reye's syndrome (G93.7)

    E88.40 Mitochondrial metabolism disorder, unspecified

    E88.41 MELAS syndrome
        Mitochondrial myopathy, encephalopathy, lactic acidosis and stroke-like episodes

    E88.42 MERRF syndrome
        Myoclonic epilepsy associated with ragged-red fibers
        Code also progressive myoclonic epilepsy (G40.3-)

    E88.49 Other mitochondrial metabolism disorders

E88.8 Other specified metabolic disorders

    E88.81 Metabolic syndrome
        Dysmetabolic syndrome X
        Use additional codes for associated manifestations, such as: obesity (E66.-)

    E88.89 Other specified metabolic disorders
        Launois-Bensaude adenolipomatosis
        Excludes1: adult pulmonary Langerhans cell histiocytosis (J84.82)

(E89) POSTPROCEDURAL ENDOCRINE AND METABOLIC COMPLICATIONS AND DISORDERS, NOT ELSEWHERE CLASSIFIED

  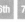

Chapter 5. Mental, behavioral and neurodevelopmental disorders (F01–F99)

Pain disorders related to psychological factors

Refer to category F45.

Mental and behavioral disorders due to psychoactive substance use

Refer to categories F10–F19
Includes: disorders of psychological development
Excludes2: symptoms, signs and abnormal clinical laboratory findings, not elsewhere classified (R00–R99)

(F01–F09) MENTAL DISORDERS DUE TO KNOWN PHYSIOLOGICAL CONDITIONS

Note: This block comprises a range of mental disorders grouped together on the basis of their having in common a demonstrable etiology in cerebral disease, brain injury, or other insult leading to cerebral dysfunction. The dysfunction may be primary, as in diseases, injuries, and insults that affect the brain directly and selectively; or secondary, as in systemic diseases and disorders that attack the brain only as one of the multiple organs or systems of the body that are involved.

F02 **DEMENTIA IN OTHER DISEASES CLASSIFIED ELSEWHERE**
`4th`
Code first the underlying physiological condition, such as:
cerebral lipidosis (E75.4)
Creutzfeldt-Jakob disease (A81.0-)
dementia with Lewy bodies (G31.83)
dementia with Parkinsonism (G31.83)
epilepsy and recurrent seizures (G40.-)
frontotemporal dementia (G31.09)
hepatolenticular degeneration (E83.0)
HIV disease (B20)
Huntington's disease (G10)
hypercalcemia (E83.52)
hypothyroidism, acquired (E00-E03.-)
intoxications (T36-T65)
Jakob-Creutzfeldt disease (A81.0-)
multiple sclerosis (G35)
neurosyphilis (A52.17)
niacin deficiency [pellagra] (E52)
Parkinson's disease (G20)
Pick's disease (G31.01)
polyarteritis nodosa (M30.0)
SLE (M32.-)
traumatic brain injury (S06.-)
trypanosomiasis (B56.-, B57.-)
vitamin B deficiency (E53.8)
Includes: major neurocognitive disorders in other diseases classified elsewhere
Excludes2: dementia in alcohol and psychoactive substance disorders (F10–F19, with .17, .27, .97)
vascular dementia (F01.5-)

F02.8 **Dementia in other diseases classified elsewhere**
`5th`
F02.80 **Dementia in other diseases classified elsewhere without behavioral disturbance**
Dementia in other diseases classified elsewhere NOS
Major neurocognitive disorder in other diseases classified elsewhere

F02.81 **Dementia in other diseases classified elsewhere with behavioral disturbance**
Use additional code, if applicable, to identify wandering in dementia in conditions classified elsewhere (Z91.83)
Dementia in other diseases classified elsewhere with aggressive behavior
Dementia in other diseases classified elsewhere with combative behavior
Dementia in other diseases classified elsewhere with violent behavior

Major neurocognitive disorder in other diseases classified elsewhere with aggressive behavior
Major neurocognitive disorder in other diseases classified elsewhere with combative behavior
Major neurocognitive disorder in other diseases classified elsewhere with violent behavior

F07 **PERSONALITY AND BEHAVIORAL DISORDERS DUE TO KNOWN PHYSIOLOGICAL CONDITION**
`4th`
Code first the underlying physiological condition

F07.8 **Other personality and behavioral disorders due to known physiological condition**
`5th`

F07.81 **Postconcussional syndrome**
Postcontusional syndrome (encephalopathy)
Post-traumatic brain syndrome, nonpsychotic
Use additional code to identify associated post-traumatic headache, if applicable (G44.3-)
Excludes1: current concussion (brain) (S06.0-)
postencephalitic syndrome (F07.89)

F07.89 **Other personality and behavioral disorders due to known physiological condition**
Postencephalitic syndrome
Right hemispheric organic affective disorder

F07.9 **Unspecified personality and behavioral disorder due to known physiological condition**
Organic p syndrome

(F10–F19) MENTAL AND BEHAVIORAL DISORDERS DUE TO PSYCHOACTIVE SUBSTANCE USE

Mental and behavioral disorders due to psychoactive substance use

IN REMISSION

Selection of codes for "in remission" for categories F10–F19, Mental and behavioral disorders due to psychoactive substance use (categories F10–F19 with -.21) requires the provider's clinical judgment. The appropriate codes for "in remission" are assigned only on the basis of provider documentation (as defined in the Official Guidelines for Coding and Reporting).

PSYCHOACTIVE SUBSTANCE USE, ABUSE AND DEPENDENCE

When the provider documentation refers to use, abuse and dependence of the same substance (e.g. alcohol, opioid, cannabis, etc.), only one code should be assigned to identify the pattern of use based on the following hierarchy:
- If both use and abuse are documented, assign only the code for abuse
- If both abuse and dependence are documented, assign only the code for dependence
- If use, abuse and dependence are all documented, assign only the code for dependence
- If both use and dependence are documented, assign only the code for dependence.

PSYCHOACTIVE SUBSTANCE USE

As with all other diagnoses, the codes for psychoactive substance use (F10.9-, F11.9-, F12.9-, F13.9-, F14.9-, F15.9-, F16.9-) should only be assigned based on provider documentation and when they meet the definition of a reportable diagnosis (see Section III, Reporting Additional Diagnoses). The codes are to be used only when the psychoactive substance use is associated with a mental or behavioral disorder, and such a relationship is documented by the provider.

F10 **ALCOHOL RELATED DISORDERS**
`4th`
Use additional code for blood alcohol level, if applicable (Y90.-)
F10.1 **Alcohol abuse**
`5th`
Excludes1: alcohol dependence (F10.2-)
alcohol use, unspecified (F10.9-)

F10.10 **Alcohol abuse, uncomplicated**
Alcohol use disorder, mild

`4th` `5th` `6th` `7th` Additional Character Required   ✔ 3-character code

●=New Code
▲=Revised Code

Excludes1—Not coded here, do not use together
Excludes2—Not included here

CHAPTER 5. MENTAL, BEHAVIORAL AND NEURODEVELOPMENTAL DISORDERS   **(F10.12–F15.222)**

F10.12   **Alcohol abuse with intoxication**
> **6th**
> **F10.120**   **Alcohol abuse with intoxication, uncomplicated**
> **F10.121**   **Alcohol abuse with intoxication delirium**
> **F10.129**   **Alcohol abuse with intoxication, unspecified**

F10.2   **Alcohol dependence**
> **5th**
> *Excludes1:* alcohol abuse (F10.1-)
> alcohol use, unspecified (F10.9-)
> *Excludes2:* toxic effect of alcohol (T51.0-)

> **F10.20**   **Alcohol dependence, uncomplicated**
> Alcohol use disorder, moderate
> Alcohol use disorder, severe

> **F10.21**   **Alcohol dependence, in remission**

> **F10.22**   **Alcohol dependence with intoxication**
> > **6th**
> > Acute drunkenness (in alcoholism)
> > *Excludes2:* alcohol dependence with withdrawal (F10.23-)
> > **F10.220**   **Alcohol dependence with intoxication, uncomplicated**
> > **F10.221**   **Alcohol dependence with intoxication delirium**
> > **F10.229**   **Alcohol dependence with intoxication, unspecified**

F10.9   **Alcohol use, unspecified**
> **5th**
> *Excludes1:* alcohol abuse (F10.1-)
> alcohol dependence (F10.2-)

> **F10.92**   **Alcohol use, unspecified with intoxication;**
> > **6th**
> > **F10.920**   **uncomplicated**
> > **F10.921**   **delirium**
> > **F10.929**   **unspecified**

F11   **OPIOD RELATED DISORDERS**
> **4th**
> **F11.1**   **Opioid abuse**
> > **5th**
> > *Excludes1:* opioid dependence (F11.2-)
> > opioid use, unspecified (F11.9-)
> > **F11.10**   **Opioid abuse, uncomplicated**
> > Opioid use disorder, mild

F12   **CANNABIS RELATED DISORDERS**
> **4th**
> *Includes:* marijuana
> **F12.1**   **Cannabis abuse**
> > **5th**
> > *Excludes1:* cannabis dependence (F12.2-)
> > cannabis use, unspecified (F12.9-)
> > **F12.10**   **Cannabis abuse, uncomplicated**
> > cannabis use disorder, mild

> **F12.2**   **Cannabis dependence**
> > **5th**
> > *Excludes1:* cannabis abuse (F12.1-)
> > cannabis use, unspecified (F12.9-)
> > *Excludes2:* cannabis poisoning (T40.7-)
> > **F12.20**   **Cannabis dependence, uncomplicated**
> > **F12.21**   **Cannabis dependence, in remission**
> > **F12.22**   **Cannabis dependence with intoxication;**
> > > **6th**
> > > **F12.220**   **uncomplicated**
> > > Cannabis use disorder, moderate
> > > Cannabis use disorder, severe
> > > **F12.221**   **delirium**
> > > **F12.222**   **with perceptual disturbance**
> > > **F12.229**   **unspecified**

> **F12.9**   **Cannabis use, unspecified**
> > **5th**
> > *Excludes1:* cannabis abuse (F12.1-)
> > cannabis dependence (F12.2-)
> > **F12.90**   **Cannabis use, unspecified, uncomplicated**

F14   **COCAINE RELATED DISORDERS**
> **4th**
> *Excludes2:* other stimulant-related disorders (F15.-)
> **F14.1**   **Cocaine abuse**
> > **5th**
> > *Excludes1:* cocaine dependence (F14.2-)
> > cocaine use, unspecified (F14.9-)
> > **F14.10**   **Cocaine abuse, uncomplicated**
> > Cocaine use disorder, mild

F14.12   **Cocaine abuse with intoxication;**
> **6th**
> **F14.120**   **uncomplicated**
> **F14.121**   **delirium**
> **F14.122**   **with perceptual disturbance**
> **F14.129**   **unspecified**

F14.2   **Cocaine dependence**
> **5th**
> *Excludes1:* cocaine abuse (F14.1-)
> cocaine use, unspecified (F14.9-)
> *Excludes2:* cocaine poisoning (T40.5-)

> **F14.20**   **Cocaine dependence, uncomplicated**
> Cocaine use disorder, moderate
> Cocaine use disorder, severe

> **F14.21**   **Cocaine dependence, in remission**

> **F14.22**   **Cocaine dependence with intoxication;**
> > **6th**
> > *Excludes1:* cocaine dependence with withdrawal (F14.23)
> > **F14.220**   **uncomplicated**
> > **F14.221**   **delirium**
> > **F14.222**   **with perceptual disturbance**
> > **F14.229**   **unspecified**

> **F14.23**   **Cocaine dependence with withdrawal**
> *Excludes1:* cocaine dependence with intoxication (F14.22-)

F14.9   **Cocaine use, unspecified**
> **5th**
> *Excludes1:* cocaine abuse (F14.1-)
> cocaine dependence (F14.2-)
> **F14.90**   **Cocaine use, unspecified, uncomplicated**
> **F14.92**   **Cocaine use, unspecified with intoxication;**
> > **6th**
> > **F14.920**   **uncomplicated**
> > **F14.921**   **delirium**
> > **F14.922**   **with perceptual disturbance**
> > **F14.929**   **unspecified**

F15   **OTHER STIMULANT RELATED DISORDERS**
> **4th**
> *Includes:* amphetamine-related disorders
> caffeine
> *Excludes2:* cocaine-related disorders (F14.-)
> **F15.1**   **Other stimulant abuse**
> > **5th**
> > *Excludes1:* other stimulant dependence (F15.2-)
> > other stimulant use, unspecified (F15.9-)
> > **F15.10**   **Other stimulant abuse, uncomplicated**
> > Amphetamine type substance use disorder, mild
> > Other or unspecified stimulant use disorder, mild
> > **F15.12**   **Other stimulant abuse with intoxication;**
> > > **6th**
> > > **F15.120**   **uncomplicated**
> > > **F15.121**   **delirium**
> > > **F15.122**   **perceptual disturbance**
> > > Amphetamine or other stimulant use disorder, mild, with amphetamine or other stimulant intoxication, with perceptual disturbances
> > > **F15.129**   **unspecified**
> > > Amphetamine or other stimulant use disorder, mild, with amphetamine or other stimulant intoxication, without perceptual disturbances

F15.2   **Other stimulant dependence**
> **5th**
> *Excludes1:* other stimulant abuse (F15.1-)
> other stimulant use, unspecified (F15.9-)
> **F15.20**   **Other stimulant dependence, uncomplicated**
> Amphetamine type substance use disorder, moderate
> Amphetamine type substance use disorder, severe
> Other or unspecified stimulant use disorder, moderate
> Other or unspecified stimulant use disorder, severe
> **F15.21**   **Other stimulant dependence, in remission**
> **F15.22**   **Other stimulant dependence with intoxication;**
> > **6th**
> > *Excludes1:* other stimulant dependence with withdrawal (F15.23)
> > **F15.220**   **uncomplicated**
> > **F15.221**   **delirium**
> > **F15.222**   **with perceptual disturbance**
> > Amphetamine or other stimulant use disorder, moderate, with amphetamine or other stimulant intoxication, with perceptual disturbances

---

     Additional Character Required   3-character code   •=New Code   *Excludes1*—Not coded here, do not use together

▲=Revised Code   *Excludes2*—Not included here

F15.229   unspecified
Amphetamine or other stimulant use disorder, severe, with amphetamine or other stimulant intoxication, with perceptual disturbances

F15.23   **Other stimulant dependence with withdrawal**
Amphetamine or other stimulant withdrawal
Excludes1: other stimulant dependence with intoxication (F15.22-)

F16 HALLUCINOGEN RELATED DISORDERS
`4th`

Includes: ecstasy
PCP
phencyclidine

F16.1   **Hallucinogen abuse**
`5th`
Excludes1: hallucinogen dependence (F16.2-)
hallucinogen use, unspecified (F16.9-)

    F16.10   **Hallucinogen abuse, uncomplicated**
        Other hallucinogen use disorder, mild
        Phencyclidine use disorder, mild

F16.2   **Hallucinogen dependence**
`5th`
Excludes1: hallucinogen abuse (F16.1-)
hallucinogen use, unspecified (F16.9-)

    F16.20   **Hallucinogen dependence, uncomplicated**
        Other hallucinogen use disorder, moderate
        Other hallucinogen use disorder, severe
        Phencyclidine use disorder, moderate
        Phencyclidine use disorder, severe

F17 NICOTINE DEPENDENCE
`4th`

Excludes1: history of tobacco dependence (Z87.891)
tobacco use NOS (Z72.0)
Excludes2: tobacco use (smoking) during pregnancy, childbirth and the puerperium (O99.33-)
toxic effect of nicotine (T65.2-)

F17.2   **Nicotine dependence**

    F17.20   **Nicotine dependence, unspecified**
`5th`
        F17.200   **Nicotine dependence, unspecified; uncomplicated**
`6th`
            Tobacco use disorder, mild
            Tobacco use disorder, moderate
            Tobacco use disorder, severe
        F17.201   **in remission**
        F17.203   **with withdrawal**
            Tobacco withdrawal
        F17.208   **with other nicotine-induced disorders**
        F17.209   **with unspecified nicotine-induced disorders**

    F17.21   **Nicotine dependence, cigarettes**
`6th`
        F17.210   **Nicotine dependence, cigarettes; uncomplicated**
        F17.211   **in remission**
        F17.213   **with withdrawal**
        F17.218   **with other nicotine-induced disorders**
        F17.219   **with unspecified nicotine-induced disorders**

    F17.22   **Nicotine dependence, chewing tobacco**
`6th`
        F17.220   **Nicotine dependence, chewing tobacco; uncomplicated**
        F17.221   **in remission**
        F17.223   **with withdrawal**
        F17.228   **with other nicotine-induced disorders**
        F17.229   **with unspecified nicotine-induced disorders**

    F17.29   **Nicotine dependence, other tobacco product**
`6th`
        F17.290   **Nicotine dependence, other tobacco product; uncomplicated**
        F17.291   **in remission**
        F17.293   **with withdrawal**
        F17.298   **with other nicotine-induced disorders**
        F17.299   **with unspecified nicotine-induced disorders**

F18 INHALANT RELATED DISORDERS
`4th`

Includes: volatile solvents

F18.1   **Inhalant abuse**
`5th`
Excludes1: inhalant dependence (F18.2-)
inhalant use, unspecified (F18.9-)

    F18.10   **Inhalant abuse, uncomplicated**
        Inhalant use disorder, mild
    F18.12   **Inhalant abuse with intoxication**
`6th`
        F18.120   **Inhalant abuse with intoxication; uncomplicated**
        F18.121   **delirium**
        F18.129   **unspecified**

F18.2   **Inhalant dependence**
`5th`
Excludes1: inhalant abuse (F18.1-)
inhalant use, unspecified (F18.9-)

    F18.20   **Inhalant dependence, uncomplicated**
        Inhalant use disorder, moderate
        Inhalant use disorder, severe
    F18.21   **Inhalant dependence, in remission**
    F18.22   **Inhalant dependence with intoxication**
`6th`
        F18.220   **Inhalant dependence with intoxication; uncomplicated**
        F18.221   **delirium**
        F18.229   **unspecified**

F18.9   **Inhalant use, unspecified**
`5th`
Excludes1: inhalant abuse (F18.1-)
inhalant dependence (F18.2-)

    F18.90   **Inhalant use, unspecified, uncomplicated**
    F18.92   **Inhalant use, unspecified with intoxication**
`6th`
        F18.920   **Inhalant use, unspecified with intoxication, uncomplicated**
        F18.921   **Inhalant use, unspecified with intoxication with delirium**
        F18.929   **Inhalant use, unspecified with intoxication, unspecified**

F19 OTHER PSYCHOACTIVE SUBSTANCE RELATED DISORDERS
`4th`

Includes: polysubstance drug use (indiscriminate drug use)

F19.1   **Other psychoactive substance abuse**
`5th`
Excludes1: other psychoactive substance dependence (F19.2-)
other psychoactive substance use, unspecified (F19.9-)

    F19.10   **Other psychoactive substance abuse, uncomplicated**
        Other (or unknown) substance use disorder, mild
    F19.12   **Other psychoactive substance abuse with intoxication**
`6th`
        F19.120   **Other psychoactive substance abuse with intoxication; uncomplicated**
        F19.121   **delirium**
        F19.122   **with perceptual disturbances**
        F19.129   **unspecified**

F19.2   **Other psychoactive substance dependence**
`5th`
Excludes1: other psychoactive substance abuse (F19.1-)
other psychoactive substance use, unspecified (F19.9-)

    F19.20   **Other psychoactive substance dependence, uncomplicated**
        Other (or unknown) substance use disorder, moderate
        Other (or unknown) substance use disorder, severe
    F19.21   **Other psychoactive substance dependence, in remission**
    F19.22   **Other psychoactive substance dependence with intoxication**
`6th`
        Excludes1: psychoactive other substance dependence with withdrawal (F19.23-)
        F19.220   **Other psychoactive substance dependence with intoxication; uncomplicated**
        F19.221   **delirium**
        F19.222   **with perceptual disturbance**
        F19.229   **unspecified**
    F19.23   **Other psychoactive substance dependence with withdrawal**
`6th`
        Excludes1: other psychoactive substance dependence with intoxication (F19.22-)

F19.230   **Other psychoactive substance dependence with withdrawal; uncomplicated**
F19.231   **delirium**
F19.232   **with perceptual disturbance**
F19.239   **unspecified**
F19.9   **Other psychoactive substance use, unspecified**
5th   *Excludes1:* other psychoactive substance abuse (F19.1-)
other psychoactive substance dependence (F19.2-)
F19.90   **Other psychoactive substance use, unspecified, uncomplicated**
F19.92   **Other psychoactive substance use, unspecified with intoxication**
6th   *Excludes1:* other psychoactive substance use, unspecified with withdrawal (F19.93)
F19.920   **Other psychoactive substance use, unspecified with intoxication; uncomplicated**
F19.921   **with delirium**
Other (or unknown) substance-induced delirium
F19.922   **with perceptual disturbance**
F19.929   **unspecified**

(F20–F29) SCHIZOPHRENIA, SCHIZOTYPAL, DELUSIONAL, AND OTHER NON-MOOD PSYCHOTIC DISORDERS

(F30–F39) MOOD [AFFECTIVE] DISORDERS

F32   **MAJOR DEPRESSIVE DISORDER, SINGLE EPISODE**
4th   *Includes:* single episode of agitated depression
single episode of depressive reaction
single episode of major depression
single episode of psychogenic depression
single episode of reactive depression
single episode of vital depression
Excludes1: bipolar disorder (F31.-)
manic episode (F30.-)
recurrent depressive disorder (F33.-)
Excludes2: adjustment disorder (F43.2)
F32.0   **Major depressive disorder, single episode, mild**
F32.1   **Major depressive disorder, single episode, moderate**
F32.2   **Major depressive disorder, single episode, severe without psychotic features**
F32.3   **Major depressive disorder, single episode, severe with psychotic features**
Single episode of major depression with mood-congruent psychotic symptoms
Single episode of major depression with mood-incongruent psychotic symptoms
Single episode of major depression with psychotic symptoms
Single episode of psychogenic depressive psychosis
Single episode of psychotic depression
Single episode of reactive depressive psychosis
F32.4   **Major depressive disorder, single episode, in partial remission**
F32.5   **Major depressive disorder, single episode, in full remission**
F32.8   **Other depressive episodes**
5th   •F32.81   **Premenstrual dysphoric disorder**
Excludes1: premenstrual tension syndrome (N94.3)
•F32.89   **Other specified depressive episodes**
Atypical depression
Post-schizophrenic depression
Single episode of 'masked' depression NOS
F32.9   **Major depressive disorder, single episode, unspecified**
Depression NOS
Depressive disorder NOS
Major depression NOS

F33   **MAJOR DEPRESSIVE DISORDER, RECURRENT**
4th   *Includes:* recurrent episodes of depressive reaction
recurrent episodes of endogenous depression
recurrent episodes of major depression
recurrent episodes of psychogenic depression
recurrent episodes of reactive depression

recurrent episodes of seasonal depressive disorder
recurrent episodes of vital depression
Excludes1: bipolar disorder (F31.-)
manic episode (F30.-)
F33.0   **Major depressive disorder, recurrent, mild**
F33.1   **Major depressive disorder, recurrent, moderate**
F33.2   **Major depressive disorder, recurrent severe without psychotic features**
F33.3   **Major depressive disorder, recurrent, severe with psychotic symptoms**
Endogenous depression with psychotic symptoms
Recurrent severe episodes of major depression with mood-congruent psychotic symptoms
Recurrent severe episodes of major depression with mood-incongruent psychotic symptoms
Recurrent severe episodes of major depression with psychotic symptoms
Recurrent severe episodes of psychogenic depressive psychosis
Recurrent severe episodes of psychotic depression
Recurrent severe episodes of reactive depressive psychosis
F33.4   **Major depressive disorder, recurrent, in remission**
5th   F33.40   **Major depressive disorder, recurrent, in remission, unspecified**
F33.41   **Major depressive disorder, recurrent, in partial remission**
F33.42   **Major depressive disorder, recurrent, in full remission**
F33.8   **Other recurrent depressive disorders**
Recurrent brief depressive episodes
F33.9   **Major depressive disorder, recurrent, unspecified**
Monopolar depression NOS

F39   **UNSPECIFIED MOOD [AFFECTIVE] DISORDER**
✓   Affective psychosis NOS

(F40–F48) ANXIETY, DISSOCIATIVE, STRESS-RELATED, SOMATOFORM AND OTHER NONPSYCHOTIC MENTAL DISORDERS

F40   **PHOBIC ANXIETY DISORDERS**
4th   F40.0   **Agoraphobia**
5th   F40.00   **Agoraphobia, unspecified**
F40.01   **Agoraphobia with panic disorder**
Panic disorder with agoraphobia
Excludes1: panic disorder without agoraphobia (F41.0)
F40.02   **Agoraphobia without panic disorder**
F40.8   **Other phobic anxiety disorders**
Phobic anxiety disorder of childhood
F40.9   **Phobic anxiety disorder, unspecified**
Phobia NOS
Phobic state NOS

F41   **OTHER ANXIETY DISORDERS**
4th   *Excludes2:* anxiety in: acute stress reaction (F43.0)
transient adjustment reaction (F43.2)
neurasthenia (F48.8)
psychophysiologic disorders (F45.-)
separation anxiety (F93.0)
F41.0   **Panic disorder [episodic paroxysmal anxiety] without agoraphobia**
Panic attack
Panic state
Excludes1: panic disorder with agoraphobia (F40.01)
F41.1   **Generalized anxiety disorder**
Anxiety neurosis
Anxiety reaction
Anxiety state
Overanxious disorder
Excludes2: neurasthenia (F48.8)
F41.3   **Other mixed anxiety disorders**
F41.8   **Other specified anxiety disorders**
Anxiety depression (mild or not persistent)
Anxiety hysteria
Mixed anxiety and depressive disorder

4th 5th 6th 7th   Additional Character Required   **✓**   3-character code   •=New Code   *Excludes1*—Not coded here, do not use together
▲=Revised Code   *Excludes2*—Not included here

F42   OBSESSIVE-COMPULSIVE DISORDER

4th

Excludes2: obsessive-compulsive personality (disorder) (F60.5)
    obsessive-compulsive symptoms occurring in depression (F32–F33)
    obsessive-compulsive symptoms occurring in schizophrenia (F20.-)

- • **F42.2   Mixed obsessional thoughts and acts**
- • **F42.3   Hoarding disorder**
- • **F42.4   Excoriation (skin-picking) disorder**
      Excludes1: factitial dermatitis (L98.1)
        other specified behavioral and emotional disorders with onset
          usually occurring in early childhood and adolescence
          (F98.8)
- • **F42.8   Other obsessive compulsive disorder**
      Anancastic neurosis
      Obsessive-compulsive neurosis
- • **F42.9   Obsessive-compulsive disorder, unspecified**

F43   REACTION TO SEVERE STRESS, AND ADJUSTMENT DISORDERS

4th

F43.0   Acute stress reaction
    Acute crisis reaction
    Acute reaction to stress
    Combat and operational stress reaction
    Combat fatigue
    Crisis state
    Psychic shock

F43.1   Post-traumatic stress disorder (PTSD)
5th   Traumatic neurosis
- **F43.10   Post-traumatic stress disorder, unspecified**
- **F43.11   Post-traumatic stress disorder, acute**
- **F43.12   Post-traumatic stress disorder, chronic**

F43.2   Adjustment disorders
5th
    Culture shock
    Grief reaction
    Hospitalism in children
    Excludes2: separation anxiety disorder of childhood (F93.0)
- **F43.20   Adjustment disorder, unspecified**
- **F43.21   Adjustment disorder with depressed mood**
- **F43.22   Adjustment disorder with anxiety**
- **F43.23   Adjustment disorder with mixed anxiety and depressed mood**
- **F43.24   Adjustment disorder with disturbance of conduct**
- **F43.25   Adjustment disorder with mixed disturbance of emotions and conduct**
- **F43.29   Adjustment disorder with other symptoms**

F43.8   Other reactions to severe stress
    Other specified trauma and stressor-related disorder

F43.9   Reaction to severe stress, unspecified
    Trauma and stressor-related disorder, NOS

F44   DISSOCIATIVE AND CONVERSION DISORDERS

4th

Includes: conversion hysteria
    conversion reaction
    hysteria
    hysterical psychosis
Excludes2: malingering [conscious simulation] (Z76.5)

F44.4   Conversion disorder with motor symptom or deficit
    Dissociative motor disorders
    Psychogenic aphonia
    Psychogenic dysphonia

F44.6   Conversion disorder with sensory symptom or deficit
    Dissociative anesthesia and sensory loss
    Psychogenic deafness

F44.8   Other dissociative and conversion disorders
5th
- **F44.81   Dissociative identity disorder**
      Multiple personality disorder
- **F44.89   Other dissociative and conversion disorders**
      Ganser's syndrome
      Psychogenic confusion
      Psychogenic twilight state
      Trance and possession disorders

F44.9   Dissociative and conversion disorder, unspecified
    Dissociative disorder NOS

F45   SOMATOFORM DISORDERS

4th

> **GUIDELINES**
>
> Pain disorders related to psychological factors
>   Assign code F45.41, for pain that is exclusively related to psychological disorders. As indicated by the *Excludes1* note under category G89, a code from category G89 should not be assigned with code F45.41
>   Code F45.42, Pain disorders with related psychological factors, should be used with a code from category G89, Pain, not elsewhere classified, if there is documentation of a psychological component for a patient with acute or chronic pain.
>   See Chapter 6 <pg xx>

Excludes2: dissociative and conversion disorders (F44.-)
    factitious disorders (F68.1-)
    hair-plucking (F63.3)
    lalling (F80.0)
    lisping (F80.0)
    malingering [conscious simulation] (Z76.5)
    nail-biting (F98.8)
    psychological or behavioral factors associated with disorders or diseases classified elsewhere (F54)
    sexual dysfunction, not due to a substance or known physiological condition (F52.-)
    thumb-sucking (F98.8)
    tic disorders (in childhood and adolescence) (F95.-)
    Tourette's syndrome (F95.2)
    trichotillomania (F63.3)

F45.0   Somatization disorder
    Briquet's disorder
    Multiple psychosomatic disorders

F45.1   Undifferentiated somatoform disorder
    Somatic symptom disorder
    Undifferentiated psychosomatic disorder

F45.2   Hypochondriacal disorders
5th
    Excludes2: delusional dysmorphophobia (F22)
      fixed delusions about bodily functions or shape (F22)
- **F45.20   Hypochondriacal disorder, unspecified**
- **F45.21   Hypochondriasis**
      Hypochondriacal neurosis
      Illness anxiety disorder
- **F45.22   Body dysmorphic disorder**
      Dysmorphophobia (nondelusional)
      Nosophobia
- **F45.29   Other hypochondriacal disorders**

F45.8   Other somatoform disorders
    Psychogenic dysmenorrhea
    Psychogenic dysphagia, including 'globus hystericus'
    Psychogenic pruritus
    Psychogenic torticollis
    Somatoform autonomic dysfunction
    Teeth grinding
    Excludes1: sleep related teeth grinding (G47.63)

F45.9   Somatoform disorder, unspecified
    Psychosomatic disorder NOS

F48   OTHER NONPSYCHOTIC MENTAL DISORDERS

4th

F48.8   Other specified nonpsychotic mental disorders
    Dhat syndrome
    Neurasthenia
    Occupational neurosis, including writer's cramp
    Psychasthenia
    Psychasthenic neurosis
    Psychogenic syncope

F48.9   Nonpsychotic mental disorder, unspecified
    Neurosis NOS

(F50–F59) BEHAVIORAL SYNDROMES ASSOCIATED WITH PHYSIOLOGICAL DISTURBANCES AND PHYSICAL FACTORS

4th   **5th**   **6th**   **7th**   Additional Character Required   ✓   3-character code   • =New Code   ▲ =Revised Code

Excludes1—Not coded here, do not use together
Excludes2—Not included here

F50 **EATING DISORDERS**
Excludes1: anorexia NOS (R63.0)
  feeding difficulties (R63.3)
  polyphagia (R63.2)
Excludes2: feeding disorder in infancy or childhood (F98.2-)

F50.0 Anorexia nervosa
 Excludes1: loss of appetite (R63.0)
  psychogenic loss of appetite (F50.89)
  F50.00   Anorexia nervosa, unspecified
  F50.01   Anorexia nervosa, restricting type
  F50.02   Anorexia nervosa, binge eating/purging type
      Excludes1: bulimia nervosa (F50.2)

F50.2 Bulimia nervosa
  Bulimia NOS
  Hyperorexia nervosa
  Excludes1: anorexia nervosa, binge eating/purging type (F50.02)

F50.8 Other eating disorders
  F50.81   Binge eating disorder
  F50.89   Other specified eating disorder
      Pica in adults
      Psychogenic loss of appetite
      Excludes2: pica of infancy and childhood (F98.3)

F50.9 Eating disorder, unspecified
  Atypical anorexia nervosa
  Atypical bulimia nervosa

F51 **SLEEP DISORDERS NOT DUE TO A SUBSTANCE OR KNOWN PHYSIOLOGICAL CONDITION**
Excludes2: organic sleep disorders (G47.-)
F51.3 Sleepwalking [somnambulism]
F51.4 Sleep terrors [night terrors]
F51.5 Nightmare disorder
  Dream anxiety disorder
F51.8 Other sleep disorders not due to a substance or known physiological condition
F51.9 Sleep disorder not due to a substance or known physiological condition, unspecified
  Emotional sleep disorder NOS

(F60–F69) DISORDERS OF ADULT PERSONALITY AND BEHAVIOR

F60 **SPECIFIC PERSONALITY DISORDERS**
F60.9 Personality disorder, unspecified
  Character disorder NOS
  Character neurosis NOS
  Pathological personality NOS

F63 **IMPULSE DISORDERS**
Excludes2: habitual excessive use of alcohol or psychoactive substances (F10–F19)
  impulse disorders involving sexual behavior (F65.-)
F63.0 Pathological gambling
  Compulsive gambling
  Excludes1: gambling and betting NOS (Z72.6)
  Excludes2: excessive gambling by manic patients (F30, F31)
    gambling in antisocial personality disorder (F60.2)
F63.1 Pyromania
  Pathological fire-setting
  Excludes2: fire-setting (by) (in):
    adult with antisocial personality disorder (F60.2)
    alcohol or psychoactive substance intoxication (F10–F19)
    conduct disorders (F91.-)
    mental disorders due to known physiological condition (F01–F09)
    schizophrenia (F20.-)
F63.2 Kleptomania
  Pathological stealing
  Excludes1: shoplifting as the reason for observation for suspected mental disorder (Z03.8)
  Excludes2: depressive disorder with stealing (F31–F33)
    stealing due to underlying mental condition-code to mental condition
    stealing in mental disorders due to known physiological condition (F01–F09)

F63.3 Trichotillomania
  Hair plucking
  Excludes2: other stereotyped movement disorder (F98.4)
F63.8 Other impulse disorders
  F63.81   Intermittent explosive disorder
  F63.89   Other impulse disorders
F63.9 Impulse disorder, unspecified
  Impulse control disorder NOS

F64 **GENDER IDENTITY DISORDERS**
 •**F64.0 Transsexualism**
  Gender identity disorder in adolescence and adulthood
  Gender dysphoria in adolescents and adults
▲**F64.1 Dual role transvestism**
  Use additional code to identify sex reassignment status (Z87.890)
  Excludes1: gender identity disorder in childhood (F64.2)
  Excludes2: fetishistic transvestism (F65.1)
F64.2 Gender identity disorder of childhood
  Gender dysphoria in children
  Excludes1: gender identity disorder in adolescence and adulthood (F64.0)
  Excludes2: sexual maturation disorder (F66)
F64.8 Other gender identity disorders
F64.9 Gender identity disorder, unspecified
  Gender-role disorder NOS

(F70–F79) INTELLECTUAL DISABILITIES

Code first any associated physical or developmental disorders
Excludes1: borderline intellectual functioning, IQ above 70 to 84 (R41.83)

F70 **MILD INTELLECTUAL DISABILITIES**
  IQ level 50–55 to approximately 70
  Mild mental subnormality

F71 **MODERATE INTELLECTUAL DISABILITIES**
  IQ level 35–40 to 50–55
  Moderate mental subnormality

F72 **SEVERE INTELLECTUAL DISABILITIES**
  IQ 20–25 to 35–40
  Severe mental subnormality

F73 **PROFOUND INTELLECTUAL DISABILITIES**
  IQ level below 20–25
  Profound mental subnormality

F78 **OTHER INTELLECTUAL DISABILITIES**

F79 **UNSPECIFIED INTELLECTUAL DISABILITIES**
  Mental deficiency NOS
  Mental subnormality NOS

(F80–F89) PERVASIVE AND SPECIFIC DEVELOPMENTAL DISORDERS

F80 **SPECIFIC DEVELOPMENTAL DISORDERS OF SPEECH AND LANGUAGE**
F80.0 Phonological disorder
  Dyslalia
  Functional speech articulation disorder
  Lalling
  Lisping
  Phonological developmental disorder
  Speech articulation developmental disorder
  Speech-sound disorder
  Excludes1: speech articulation impairment due to aphasia NOS (R47.01)
    speech articulation impairment due to apraxia (R48.2)
  Excludes2: speech articulation impairment due to hearing loss (F80.4)
    speech articulation impairment due to intellectual disabilities (F70–F79)
    speech articulation impairment with expressive language developmental disorder (F80.1)

   Additional Character Required   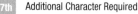 3-character code   •=New Code   *Excludes1*—Not coded here, do not use together
▲=Revised Code   *Excludes2*—Not included here

speech articulation impairment with mixed receptive expressive language developmental disorder (F80.2)

F80.1 Expressive language disorder
Developmental dysphasia or aphasia, expressive type
Excludes1: mixed receptive-expressive language disorder (F80.2)
dysphasia and aphasia NOS (R47.-)
Excludes2: acquired aphasia with epilepsy [Landau-Kleffner] (G40.80-)
selective mutism (F94.0)
intellectual disabilities (F70–F79)
pervasive developmental disorders (F84.-)

F80.2 Mixed receptive-expressive language disorder
Developmental dysphasia or aphasia, receptive type
Developmental Wernicke's aphasia
Excludes1: central auditory processing disorder (H93.25)
dysphasia or aphasia NOS (R47.-)
expressive language disorder (F80.1)
expressive type dysphasia or aphasia (F80.1)
word deafness (H93.25)
Excludes2: acquired aphasia with epilepsy [Landau-Kleffner] (G40.80-)
pervasive developmental disorders (F84.-)
selective mutism (F94.0)
intellectual disabilities (F70–F79)

F80.4 Speech and language development delay due to hearing loss
Code also type of hearing loss (H90.-, H91.-)

F80.8 Other developmental disorders of speech and language

5th   **F80.81 Childhood onset fluency disorder**
Cluttering NOS
Stuttering NOS
Excludes1: adult onset fluency disorder (F98.5)
fluency disorder in conditions classified elsewhere (R47.82)
fluency disorder (stuttering) following cerebrovascular disease (I69. with final characters -23)

   •**F80.82 Social pragmatic communication disorder**
Excludes1: Asperger's syndrome (F84.5)
autistic disorder (F84.0)

   F80.89 Other developmental disorders of speech and language

F80.9 Developmental disorder of speech and language, unspecified
Communication disorder NOS
Language disorder NOS

F81 SPECIFIC DEVELOPMENTAL DISORDERS OF SCHOLASTIC SKILLS
4th

F81.0 Specific reading disorder
'Backward reading'
Developmental dyslexia
Specific reading retardation
Excludes1: alexia NOS (R48.0)
dyslexia NOS (R48.0)

F81.2 Mathematics disorder
Developmental acalculia
Developmental arithmetical disorder
Developmental Gerstmann's syndrome
Excludes1: acalculia NOS (R48.8)
Excludes2: arithmetical difficulties associated with a reading disorder (F81.0)
arithmetical difficulties associated with a spelling disorder (F81.81)
arithmetical difficulties due to inadequate teaching (Z55.8)

F81.8 Other developmental disorders of scholastic skills

5th   **F81.81 Disorder of written expression**
Specific spelling disorder

   F81.89 Other developmental disorders of scholastic skills

F81.9 Developmental disorder of scholastic skills, unspecified
Knowledge acquisition disability NOS
Learning disability NOS
Learning disorder NOS

F82 SPECIFIC DEVELOPMENTAL DISORDER OF MOTOR FUNCTION

Clumsy child syndrome
Developmental coordination disorder
Developmental dyspraxia
Excludes1: abnormalities of gait and mobility (R26.-)
lack of coordination (R27.-)
Excludes2: lack of coordination secondary to intellectual disabilities (F70–F79)

F84 PERVASIVE DEVELOPMENTAL DISORDERS
4th   **Use additional code** to identify any associated medical condition and intellectual disabilities.

F84.0 Autistic disorder
Autism spectrum disorder
Infantile autism
Infantile psychosis
Kanner's syndrome
Excludes1: Asperger's syndrome (F84.5)

F84.2 Rett's syndrome
Excludes1: Asperger's syndrome (F84.5)
Autistic disorder (F84.0)
Other childhood disintegrative disorder (F84.3)

F84.3 Other childhood disintegrative disorder
Dementia infantilis
Disintegrative psychosis
Heller's syndrome
Symbiotic psychosis
Use additional code to identify any associated neurological condition.
Excludes1: Asperger's syndrome (F84.5)
Autistic disorder (F84.0)
Rett's syndrome (F84.2)

F84.5 Asperger's syndrome
Asperger's disorder
Autistic psychopathy
Schizoid disorder of childhood

F84.8 Other pervasive developmental disorders
Overactive disorder associated with intellectual disabilities and stereotyped movements

F84.9 Pervasive developmental disorder, unspecified
Atypical autism

F88 OTHER DISORDERS OF PSYCHOLOGICAL DEVELOPMENT

Developmental agnosia
Global developmental delay
Other specified neurodevelopmental disorder

F89 UNSPECIFIED DISORDER OF PSYCHOLOGICAL DEVELOPMENT
Developmental disorder NOS
Neurodevelopmental disorder NOS

(F90–F98) BEHAVIORAL AND EMOTIONAL DISORDERS WITH ONSET USUALLY OCCURRING IN CHILDHOOD AND ADOLESCENCE

Note: Codes within categories F90–F98 may be used regardless of the age of a patient. These disorders generally have onset within the childhood or adolescent years, but may continue throughout life or not be diagnosed until adulthood

F90 ATTENTION-DEFICIT HYPERACTIVITY DISORDERS
4th   ***Includes:*** attention deficit disorder with hyperactivity
attention deficit syndrome with hyperactivity
Excludes2: anxiety disorders (F40.-, F41.-)
mood [affective] disorders (F30–F39)
pervasive developmental disorders (F84.-)
schizophrenia (F20.-)

F90.0 Attention-deficit hyperactivity disorder, predominantly inattentive type
ADD without hyperactivity

F90.1 Attention-deficit hyperactivity disorder, predominantly hyperactive type

F90.2 Attention-deficit hyperactivity disorder, combined type

F90.8 Attention-deficit hyperactivity disorder, other type

 Additional Character Required   3 character code   •=New Code   ***Excludes1***—Not coded here, do not use together
▲=Revised Code   ***Excludes2***—Not included here

F90.9 Attention-deficit hyperactivity disorder, unspecified type
Attention-deficit hyperactivity disorder of childhood or adolescence NOS
Attention-deficit hyperactivity disorder NOS

F91 CONDUCT DISORDERS

4th

Excludes1: antisocial behavior (Z72.81-)
   antisocial personality disorder (F60.2)
Excludes2: conduct problems associated with attention-deficit
   hyperactivity disorder (F90.-)
   mood [affective] disorders (F30–F39)
   pervasive developmental disorders (F84.-)
   schizophrenia (F20.-)

F91.0 Conduct disorder confined to family context

F91.1 Conduct disorder, childhood-onset type
Unsocialized conduct disorder
Conduct disorder, solitary aggressive type
Unsocialized aggressive disorder

F91.2 Conduct disorder, adolescent-onset type
Socialized conduct disorder
Conduct disorder, group type

F91.3 Oppositional defiant disorder

F91.8 Other conduct disorders
Other specified conduct disorder
Other specified disruptive disorder

F91.9 Conduct disorder, unspecified
Behavioral disorder NOS
Conduct disorder NOS
Disruptive behavior disorder NOS

F93 EMOTIONAL DISORDERS WITH ONSET SPECIFIC TO CHILDHOOD

4th

F93.0 Separation anxiety disorder of childhood
Excludes2: mood [affective] disorders (F30–F39)
   nonpsychotic mental disorders (F40–F48)
   phobic anxiety disorder of childhood (F40.8)
   social phobia (F40.1)

F93.8 Other childhood emotional disorders
Identity disorder
Excludes2: gender identity disorder of childhood (F64.2)

F93.9 Childhood emotional disorder, unspecified

F94 DISORDERS OF SOCIAL FUNCTIONING WITH ONSET SPECIFIC TO CHILDHOOD AND ADOLESCENCE

4th

F94.0 Selective mutism
Elective mutism
Excludes2: pervasive developmental disorders (F84.-)
   schizophrenia (F20.-)
   specific developmental disorders of speech and language (F80.-)
   transient mutism as part of separation anxiety in young children (F93.0)

F94.1 Reactive attachment disorder of childhood
Use additional code to identify any associated failure to thrive or growth retardation
Excludes1: disinhibited attachment disorder of childhood (F94.2)
   normal variation in pattern of selective attachment
Excludes2: Asperger's syndrome (F84.5)
   maltreatment syndromes (T74.-)
   sexual or physical abuse in childhood, resulting in psychosocial problems (Z62.81-)

F94.2 Disinhibited attachment disorder of childhood
Affectionless psychopathy
Institutional syndrome
Excludes1: reactive attachment disorder of childhood (F94.1)
Excludes2: Asperger's syndrome (F84.5)
   attention-deficit hyperactivity disorders (F90.-)
   hospitalism in children (F43.2-)

F94.8 Other childhood disorders of social functioning

F94.9 Childhood disorder of social functioning, unspecified

F95 TIC DISORDER

4th

F95.0 Transient tic disorder
Provisional tic disorder

F95.1 Chronic motor or vocal tic disorder

F95.2 Tourette's disorder
Combined vocal and multiple motor tic disorder [de la Tourette]
Tourette's syndrome

F95.8 Other tic disorders

F95.9 Tic disorder, unspecified
Tic NOS

F98 OTHER BEHAVIORAL AND EMOTIONAL DISORDERS WITH ONSET USUALLY OCCURRING IN CHILDHOOD AND ADOLESCENCE

4th

Excludes2: breath-holding spells (R06.89)
   gender identity disorder of childhood (F64.2)
   Kleine-Levin syndrome (G47.13)
   obsessive-compulsive disorder (F42.-)
   sleep disorders not due to a substance or known physiological condition (F51.-)

F98.0 Enuresis not due to a substance or known physiological condition
Enuresis (primary) (secondary) of nonorganic origin
Functional enuresis
Psychogenic enuresis
Urinary incontinence of nonorganic origin
Excludes1: enuresis NOS (R32)

F98.1 Encopresis not due to a substance or known physiological condition
Functional encopresis
Incontinence of feces of nonorganic origin
Psychogenic encopresis
Use additional code to identify the cause of any coexisting constipation.
Excludes1: encopresis NOS (R15.-)

F98.2 Other feeding disorders of infancy and childhood

5th

Excludes1: feeding difficulties (R63.3)
Excludes2: anorexia nervosa and other eating disorders (F50.-)
   feeding problems of newborn (P92.-)
   pica of infancy or childhood (F98.3)

   F98.21 Rumination disorder of infancy
   F98.29 Other feeding disorders of infancy and early childhood

F98.3 Pica of infancy and childhood

F98.4 Stereotyped movement disorders
Stereotype/habit disorder
Excludes1: abnormal involuntary movements (R25.-)
Excludes2: compulsions in obsessive-compulsive disorder (F42-)
   hair plucking (F63.3)
   movement disorders of organic origin (G20–G25)
   nail-biting (F98.8)
   nose-picking (F98.8)
   stereotypies that are part of a broader psychiatric condition (F01–F95)
   thumb-sucking (F98.8)
   tic disorders (F95.-)
   trichotillomania (F63.3)

F98.8 Other specified behavioral and emotional disorders with onset usually occurring in childhood and adolescence
Excessive masturbation
Nail-biting
Nose-picking
Thumb-sucking

F98.9 Unspecified behavioral and emotional disorders with onset usually occurring in childhood and adolescence

(F99) UNSPECIFIED MENTAL DISORDER

F99 MENTAL DISORDER, NOT OTHERWISE SPECIFIED

 Mental illness NOS
Excludes1: unspecified mental disorder due to known physiological condition (F09)

      Additional Character Required   3-character code   •=New Code   *Excludes1*—Not coded here, do not use together
                                                ▲=Revised Code   *Excludes2*—Not included here

Chapter 6. Diseases of the nervous system (G00–G99)

GUIDELINES

Dominant/nondominant side

Refer to category G81 and subcategories G83.1 and G83.2.

Pain

Refer to category G89.
Excludes2: certain conditions originating in the perinatal period (P04–P96)
certain infectious and parasitic diseases (A00–B99)
complications of pregnancy, childbirth and the puerperium (O00–O9A)
congenital malformations, deformations, and chromosomal abnormalities (Q00–Q99)
endocrine, nutritional and metabolic diseases (E00–E88)
injury, poisoning and certain other consequences of external causes (S00–T88)
neoplasms (C00–D49)
symptoms, signs and abnormal clinical and laboratory findings, not elsewhere classified (R00–R94)

(G00–G09) INFLAMMATORY DISEASES OF THE CENTRAL NERVOUS SYSTEM

G00 BACTERIAL MENINGITIS, NOT ELSEWHERE CLASSIFIED
`4th`
Includes: bacterial arachnoiditis
bacterial leptomeningitis
bacterial meningitis
bacterial pachymeningitis
Excludes1: bacterial: meningoencephalitis (G04.2)
meningomyelitis (G04.2)
G00.0 Hemophilus meningitis
Meningitis due to H. influenzae
G00.1 Pneumococcal meningitis
Meningitis due to streptococcus pneumoniae
G00.2 Streptococcal meningitis
Use additional code to further identify organism (B95.0–B95.5)
G00.3 Staphylococcal meningitis
Use additional code to further identify organism (B95.61–B95.8)
G00.8 Other bacterial meningitis
Meningitis due to E. coli
Meningitis due to Friedländer's bacillus
Meningitis due to Klebsiella
Use additional code to further identify organism (B96.-)
G00.9 Bacterial meningitis, unspecified
Meningitis due to gram-negative bacteria, unspecified
Purulent meningitis NOS
Pyogenic meningitis NOS
Suppurative meningitis NOS

G01 MENINGITIS IN BACTERIAL DISEASES CLASSIFIED ELSEWHERE
✔
Code first underlying disease
Excludes1: meningitis (in): gonococcal (A54.81)
leptospirosis (A27.81)
listeriosis (A32.11)
Lyme disease (A69.21)
meningococcal (A39.0)
neurosyphilis (A52.13)
tuberculosis (A17.0)
meningoencephalitis and meningomyelitis in bacterial diseases classified elsewhere (G05)

G02 MENINGITIS IN OTHER INFECTIOUS AND PARASITIC DISEASES CLASSIFIED ELSEWHERE
✔
Code first underlying disease, such as: African trypanosomiasis (B56.-)
poliovirus infection (A80.-)
Excludes1: candidal meningitis (B37.5)
coccidioidomycosis meningitis (B38.4)
cryptococcal meningitis (B45.1)
herpesviral [herpes simplex] meningitis (B00.3)
infectious mononucleosis complicated by meningitis (B27.- with 4th character 2)

measles complicated by meningitis (B05.1)
meningoencephalitis and meningomyelitis in other infectious and parasitic diseases classified elsewhere (G05)
mumps meningitis (B26.1)
rubella meningitis (B06.02)
varicella [chickenpox] meningitis (B01.0)
zoster meningitis (B02.1)

G03 MENINGITIS DUE TO OTHER AND UNSPECIFIED CAUSES
`4th`
Includes: arachnoiditis NOS
leptomeningitis NOS
meningitis NOS
pachymeningitis NOS
Excludes1: meningoencephalitis (G04.-)
meningomyelitis (G04.-)
G03.0 Nonpyogenic meningitis
Aseptic meningitis
Nonbacterial meningitis
G03.1 Chronic meningitis
G03.2 Benign recurrent meningitis [Mollaret]
G03.8 Meningitis due to other specified causes
G03.9 Meningitis, unspecified
Arachnoiditis (spinal) NOS

G04 ENCEPHALITIS, MYELITIS AND ENCEPHALOMYELITIS
`4th`
Includes: acute ascending myelitis
meningoencephalitis
meningomyelitis
Excludes1: encephalopathy NOS (G93.40)
Excludes2: acute transverse myelitis (G37.3-)
alcoholic encephalopathy (G31.2)
benign myalgic encephalomyelitis (G93.3)
multiple sclerosis (G35)
subacute necrotizing myelitis (G37.4)
toxic encephalitis (G92)
toxic encephalopathy (G92)
G04.0 Acute disseminated encephalitis and encephalomyelitis (ADEM)
`5th`
Excludes1: acute necrotizing hemorrhagic encephalopathy (G04.3-)
other noninfectious acute disseminated encephalomyelitis (noninfectious ADEM) (G04.81)
G04.00 Acute disseminated encephalitis and encephalomyelitis, unspecified
G04.01 Postinfectious acute disseminated encephalitis and encephalomyelitis (postinfectious ADEM)
Excludes1: post chickenpox encephalitis (B01.1)
post measles encephalitis (B05.0)
post measles myelitis (B05.1)
G04.02 Postimmunization acute disseminated encephalitis, myelitis and encephalomyelitis
Encephalitis, post immunization
Encephalomyelitis, post immunization
Use additional code to identify the vaccine (T50.A-, T50.B-, T50.Z-)
G04.3 Acute necrotizing hemorrhagic encephalopathy
`5th`
Excludes1: acute disseminated encephalitis and encephalomyelitis (G04.0-)
G04.30 Acute necrotizing hemorrhagic encephalopathy, unspecified
G04.8 Other encephalitis, myelitis and encephalomyelitis
`5th`
Code also any associated seizure (G40.-, R56.9)
G04.81 Other encephalitis and encephalomyelitis
Noninfectious acute disseminated encephalomyelitis (noninfectious ADEM)
G04.89 Other myelitis
G04.9 Encephalitis, myelitis and encephalomyelitis, unspecified
`5th`
G04.90 Encephalitis and encephalomyelitis, unspecified
Ventriculitis (cerebral) NOS
G04.91 Myelitis, unspecified

`4th` `5th` `6th` `7th` Additional Character Required ✔ 3-character code

°=New Code
▲=Revised Code

Excludes1—Not coded here, do not use together
Excludes2—Not included here

PEDIATRIC ICD-10-CM 2017: A MANUAL FOR PROVIDER-BASED CODING | 161

G05 ENCEPHALITIS, MYELITIS AND ENCEPHALOMYELITIS IN DISEASES CLASSIFIED ELSEWHERE
4th

Code first underlying disease, such as:
- HIV disease (B20)
- poliovirus (A80.-)
- suppurative otitis media (H66.01–H66.4)
- trichinellosis (B75)

Excludes1:
- adenoviral encephalitis, myelitis and encephalomyelitis (A85.1)
- congenital toxoplasmosis encephalitis, myelitis and encephalomyelitis (P37.1)
- cytomegaloviral encephalitis, myelitis and encephalomyelitis (B25.8)
- encephalitis, myelitis and encephalomyelitis (in) measles (B05.0)
- encephalitis, myelitis and encephalomyelitis (in) SLE (M32.19)
- enteroviral encephalitis, myelitis and encephalomyelitis (A85.0)
- eosinophilic meningoencephalitis (B83.2)
- herpesviral [herpes simplex] encephalitis, myelitis and encephalomyelitis (B00.4)
- listerial encephalitis, myelitis and encephalomyelitis (A32.12)
- meningococcal encephalitis, myelitis and encephalomyelitis (A39.81)
- mumps encephalitis, myelitis and encephalomyelitis (B26.2)
- postchickenpox encephalitis, myelitis and encephalomyelitis (B01.1-)
- rubella encephalitis, myelitis and encephalomyelitis (B06.01)
- toxoplasmosis encephalitis, myelitis and encephalomyelitis (B58.2)
- zoster encephalitis, myelitis and encephalomyelitis (B02.0)

G05.3 Encephalitis and encephalomyelitis in diseases classified elsewhere
Meningoencephalitis in diseases classified elsewhere

G05.4 Myelitis in diseases classified elsewhere
Meningomyelitis in diseases classified elsewhere

G06 INTRACRANIAL AND INTRASPINAL ABSCESS AND GRANULOMA
4th

Use additional code (B95–B97) to identify infectious agent.

G06.0 Intracranial abscess and granuloma
Brain [any part] abscess (embolic)
Cerebellar abscess (embolic)
Cerebral abscess (embolic)
Intracranial epidural abscess or granuloma
Intracranial extradural abscess or granuloma
Intracranial subdural abscess or granuloma
Otogenic abscess (embolic)
Excludes1: tuberculous intracranial abscess and granuloma (A17.81)

(G10–G14) SYSTEMIC ATROPHIES PRIMARILY AFFECTING THE CENTRAL NERVOUS SYSTEM

G11 HEREDITARY ATAXIA
4th

Excludes2: cerebral palsy (G80.-)
hereditary and idiopathic neuropathy (G60.-)
metabolic disorders (E70–E88)

G11.0 Congenital nonprogressive ataxia
G11.1 Early-onset cerebellar ataxia
Early-onset cerebellar ataxia with essential tremor
Early-onset cerebellar ataxia with myoclonus [Hunt's ataxia]
Early-onset cerebellar ataxia with retained tendon reflexes
Friedreich's ataxia (autosomal recessive)
X-linked recessive spinocerebellar ataxia
G11.2 Late-onset cerebellar ataxia
G11.3 Cerebellar ataxia with defective DNA repair
Ataxia telangiectasia [Louis-Bar]
Excludes2: Cockayne's syndrome (Q87.1)
other disorders of purine and pyrimidine metabolism (E79.-)
xeroderma pigmentosum (Q82.1)

G12 SPINAL MUSCULAR ATROPHY AND RELATED SYNDROMES
4th

G12.0 Infantile spinal muscular atrophy, type I [Werdnig-Hoffman]

(G20–G26) EXTRAPYRAMIDAL AND MOVEMENT DISORDERS

G25 OTHER EXTRAPYRAMIDAL AND MOVEMENT DISORDERS
4th

Excludes2: sleep related movement disorders (G47.6-)

G25.3 Myoclonus
Drug-induced myoclonus
Palatal myoclonus
Use additional code for adverse effect, if applicable, to identify drug (T36–T50 with fifth or sixth character 5)
Excludes1: facial myokymia (G51.4)
myoclonic epilepsy (G40.-)

(G30–G32) OTHER DEGENERATIVE DISEASES OF THE NERVOUS SYSTEM

G31 OTHER DEGENERATIVE DISEASES OF NERVOUS SYSTEM, NOT ELSEWHERE CLASSIFIED
4th

Use additional code to identify:
dementia with behavioral disturbance (F02.81)
dementia without behavioral disturbance (F02.80)
Excludes2: Reye's syndrome (G93.7)

G31.8 Other specified degenerative diseases of nervous system
5th   **G31.89 Other specified degenerative diseases of nervous system**

(G35–G37) DEMYELINATING DISEASES OF THE CENTRAL NERVOUS SYSTEM

(G40–G47) EPISODIC AND PAROXYSMAL DISORDERS

G40 EPILEPSY AND RECURRENT SEIZURES
4th

Note: the following terms are to be considered equivalent to intractable: pharmacoresistant (pharmacologically resistant), treatment resistant, refractory (medically) and poorly controlled

Excludes1: conversion disorder with seizures (F44.5)
convulsions NOS (R56.9)
post traumatic seizures (R56.1)
seizure (convulsive) NOS (R56.9)
seizure of newborn (P90)
Excludes2: hippocampal sclerosis (G93.81)
mesial temporal sclerosis (G93.81)
temporal sclerosis (G93.81)
Todd's paralysis (G83.8)

> G40.0-, G40.1-, G40.2-, G40.3-, G40.A-, G40.B-, G40.91- Codes require a 6th character:
> 1—with status epilepticus
> 9—without status epilepticus or NOS

G40.0 Localization-related (focal) (partial) idiopathic epilepsy and epileptic syndromes with seizures of localized onset
5th
Benign childhood epilepsy with centrotemporal EEG spikes
Childhood epilepsy with occipital EEG paroxysms
Excludes1: adult onset localization-related epilepsy (G40.1-, G40.2-)

   G40.00 Localization-related (focal) (partial) idiopathic epilepsy and epileptic syndromes with seizures of localized onset, not intractable (without intractability)
6th

   G40.01 Localization-related (focal) (partial) idiopathic epilepsy and epileptic syndromes with seizures of localized onset, intractable
6th

G40.1 Localization-related (focal) (partial) symptomatic epilepsy and epileptic syndromes with simple partial seizures
5th
Attacks without alteration of consciousness
Epilepsia partialis continua [Kozhevnikof]
Simple partial seizures developing into secondarily generalized seizures

   G40.10 Localization-related (focal) (partial) symptomatic epilepsy and epileptic syndromes with simple partial seizures, not intractable (without intractability)
6th

   G40.11 Localization-related (focal) (partial) symptomatic epilepsy and epileptic syndromes with simple partial seizures, intractable
6th

4th **5th** **6th** **7th**   Additional Character Required   3-character code   •=New Code   ▲=Revised Code   ***Excludes1***—Not coded here, do not use together   ***Excludes2***—Not included here

162   PEDIATRIC ICD-10-CM 2017: A MANUAL FOR PROVIDER-BASED CODING

G40.2 **Localization-related (focal) (partial) symptomatic epilepsy and epileptic syndromes with complex partial seizures**
`5th`
Attacks with alteration of consciousness, often with automatisms
Complex partial seizures developing into secondarily generalized seizures

     G40.20 **Localization-related (focal) (partial) symptomatic epilepsy and epileptic syndromes with complex partial seizures, not intractable (without intractability)**
`6th`

> G40.2-, G40.3-, G40.A-, G40.B-, G40.91- Codes require a 6th character:
> 1—with status epilepticus
> 9—without status epilepticus or NOS

     G40.21 **Localization-related (focal) (partial) symptomatic epilepsy and epileptic syndromes with complex partial seizures, intractable**
`6th`

G40.3 **Generalized idiopathic epilepsy and epileptic syndromes**
`5th`
Code also MERRF syndrome, if applicable (E88.42)

     G40.30 **Generalized idiopathic epilepsy and epileptic syndromes, not intractable (without intractability)**
`6th`

     G40.31 **Generalized idiopathic epilepsy and epileptic syndromes, intractable**
`6th`

G40.A **Absence epileptic syndrome**
`5th`
Childhood absence epilepsy [pyknolepsy]
Juvenile absence epilepsy
Absence epileptic syndrome, NOS

     G40.A0 **Absence epileptic syndrome, not intractable**
`6th`

     G40.A1 **Absence epileptic syndrome, intractable**
`6th`

G40.B **Juvenile myoclonic epilepsy [impulsive petit mal]**
`5th`
     G40.B0 **Juvenile myoclonic epilepsy, not intractable**
`6th`

     G40.B1 **Juvenile myoclonic epilepsy, intractable**
`6th`

G40.8 **Other epilepsy and recurrent seizures**
`5th`
Epilepsies and epileptic syndromes undetermined as to whether they are focal or generalized
Landau-Kleffner syndrome

     G40.82 **Epileptic spasms**
`6th`
Infantile spasms
Salaam attacks
West's syndrome

         G40.821 **Epileptic spasms, not intractable, with status epilepticus**
         G40.822 **Epileptic spasms, not intractable, without status epilepticus**
         G40.823 **Epileptic spasms, intractable, with status epilepticus**
         G40.824 **Epileptic spasms, intractable, without status epilepticus**

     G40.89 **Other seizures**
         Excludes1: post traumatic seizures (R56.1)
             recurrent seizures NOS (G40.909)
             seizure NOS (R56.9)

G40.9 **Epilepsy, unspecified**
`5th`
     G40.90 **Epilepsy, unspecified, not intractable**
`6th`
Epilepsy, unspecified, without intractability

         G40.901 **Epilepsy, unspecified, not intractable, with status epilepticus**
         G40.909 **Epilepsy, unspecified, not intractable, without status epilepticus**
             Epilepsy NOS
             Epileptic convulsions NOS
             Epileptic fits NOS
             Epileptic seizures NOS
             Recurrent seizures NOS
             Seizure disorder NOS

     G40.91 **Epilepsy, unspecified, intractable**
`6th`
Intractable seizure disorder NOS

G43 **MIGRAINE**
`4th`
Note: the following terms are to be considered equivalent to intractable: pharmacoresistant (pharmacologically resistant), treatment resistant, refractory (medically) and poorly controlled
Use additional code for adverse effect, if applicable, to identify drug (T36–T50 with fifth or sixth character 5)
Excludes1: headache NOS (R51)
             lower half migraine (G44.00)
Excludes2: headache syndromes (G44.-)

G43.0 **Migraine without aura**
`5th`
Common migraine
Excludes1: chronic migraine without aura (G43.7-)

     G43.00 **Migraine without aura, not intractable**
`6th`
Migraine without aura without mention of refractory migraine

         G43.001 **Migraine without aura, not intractable, with status migrainosus**
         G43.009 **Migraine without aura, not intractable, without status migrainosus**
             Migraine without aura NOS

     G43.01 **Migraine without aura, intractable**
`6th`
Migraine without aura with refractory migraine

         G43.011 **Migraine without aura, intractable, with status migrainosus**
         G43.019 **Migraine without aura, intractable, without status migrainosus**

G43.1 **Migraine with aura**
`5th`
Basilar migraine
Classical migraine
Migraine equivalents
Migraine preceded or accompanied by transient focal neurological phenomena
Migraine triggered seizures
Migraine with acute-onset aura
Migraine with aura without headache (migraine equivalents)
Migraine with prolonged aura
Migraine with typical aura
Retinal migraine
Code also any associated seizure (G40.-, R56.9)
Excludes1: persistent migraine aura (G43.5-, G43.6-)

     G43.10 **Migraine with aura, not intractable**
`6th`
Migraine with aura without mention of refractory migraine
         G43.101 **Migraine with aura, not intractable, with status migrainosus**
         G43.109 **Migraine with aura, not intractable, without status migrainosus**
             Migraine with aura NOS

     G43.11 **Migraine with aura, intractable**
`6th`
Migraine with aura with refractory migraine
         G43.111 **Migraine with aura, intractable, with status migrainosus**
         G43.119 **Migraine with aura, intractable, without status migrainosus**

G43.A **Cyclical vomiting**
`5th`
     G43.A0 **Cyclical vomiting, not intractable**
Cyclical vomiting, without refractory migraine
     G43.A1 **Cyclical vomiting, intractable**
Cyclical vomiting, with refractory migraine

G43.C **Periodic headache syndromes in child or adult**
`5th`
     G43.C0 **Periodic headache syndromes in child or adult, not intractable**
Periodic headache syndromes in child or adult, without refractory migraine
     G43.C1 **Periodic headache syndromes in child or adult, intractable**
Periodic headache syndromes in child or adult, with refractory migraine

---

      Additional Character Required   3 character code

•=New Code
▲=Revised Code

Excludes1—Not coded here, do not use together
Excludes2—Not included here

CHAPTER 6. DISEASES OF THE NERVOUS SYSTEM   (G44–G71.11)

G44   OTHER HEADACHE SYNDROMES

Excludes1: headache NOS (R51)
Excludes2: atypical facial pain (G50.1)
     headache due to lumbar puncture (G97.1)
     migraines (G43.-)
     trigeminal neuralgia (G50.0)

G44.0   Cluster headaches and other trigeminal autonomic cephalgias (TAC)

     G44.00   Cluster headache syndrome, unspecified
         Ciliary neuralgia
         Cluster headache NOS
         Histamine cephalgia
         Lower half migraine
         Migrainous neuralgia
         G44.001   Cluster headache syndrome, unspecified, intractable
         G44.009   Cluster headache syndrome, unspecified, not intractable
             Cluster headache syndrome NOS

G44.2   Tension-type headache

     G44.20   Tension-type headache, unspecified
         G44.201   Tension-type headache, unspecified, intractable
         G44.209   Tension-type headache, unspecified, not intractable
             Tension headache NOS

     G44.21   Episodic tension-type headache
         G44.211   Episodic tension-type headache, intractable
         G44.219   Episodic tension-type headache, not intractable
             Episodic tension-type headache NOS

     G44.22   Chronic tension-type headache
         G44.221   Chronic tension-type headache, intractable
         G44.229   Chronic tension-type headache, not intractable
             Chronic tension-type headache NOS

G45   TRANSIENT CEREBRAL ISCHEMIC ATTACKS AND RELATED SYNDROMES

Excludes1: neonatal cerebral ischemia (P91.0)
     transient retinal artery occlusion (H34.0-)

G45.9   Transient cerebral ischemic attack, unspecified
     Spasm of cerebral artery
     TIA
     Transient cerebral ischemia NOS

G47   SLEEP DISORDERS

Excludes2: nightmares (F51.5)
     nonorganic sleep disorders (F51.-)
     sleep terrors (F51.4)
     sleepwalking (F51.3)

G47.3   Sleep apnea
     Code also any associated underlying condition
     Excludes1: apnea NOS (R06.81)
         Cheyne-Stokes breathing (R06.3)
         pickwickian syndrome (E66.2)
         sleep apnea of newborn (P28.3)
     G47.30   Sleep apnea, unspecified
         Sleep apnea NOS
     G47.31   Primary central sleep apnea
     G47.32   High altitude periodic breathing
     G47.33   Obstructive sleep apnea (adult) (pediatric)
         Excludes1: obstructive sleep apnea of newborn (P28.3)

G47.9   Sleep disorder, unspecified
     Sleep disorder NOS

(G50–G59) NERVE, NERVE ROOT AND PLEXUS DISORDERS

Excludes1: current traumatic nerve, nerve root and plexus disorders—see Injury, nerve by body region
     neuralgia NOS (M79.2)
     neuritis NOS (M79.2)
     peripheral neuritis in pregnancy (O26.82-)
     radiculitis NOS (M54.1-)

G51   FACIAL NERVE DISORDERS

Includes: disorders of 7th cranial nerve

G51.0   Bell's palsy
     Facial palsy
G51.8   Other disorders of facial nerve
G51.9   Disorder of facial nerve, unspecified

G52   DISORDERS OF OTHER CRANIAL NERVES

Excludes2: disorders of acoustic [8th] nerve (H93.3)
     disorders of optic [2nd] nerve (H46, H47.0)
     paralytic strabismus due to nerve palsy (H49.0–H49.2)

G52.7   Disorders of multiple cranial nerves
     Polyneuritis cranialis

(G60–G65) POLYNEUROPATHIES AND OTHER DISORDERS OF THE PERIPHERAL NERVOUS SYSTEM

Excludes1: neuralgia NOS (M79.2)
     neuritis NOS (M79.2)
     peripheral neuritis in pregnancy (O26.82-)
     radiculitis NOS (M54.10)

G60   HEREDITARY AND IDIOPATHIC NEUROPATHY

G60.8   Other hereditary and idiopathic neuropathies
     Dominantly inherited sensory neuropathy
     Morvan's disease
     Nelaton's syndrome
     Recessively inherited sensory neuropathy
G60.9   Hereditary and idiopathic neuropathy, unspecified

G61   INFLAMMATORY POLYNEUROPATHY

G61.0   Guillain-Barre syndrome
     Acute (post-) infective polyneuritis
     Miller Fisher Syndrome

(G70–G73) DISEASES OF MYONEURAL JUNCTION AND MUSCLE

G70   MYASTHENIA GRAVIS AND OTHER MYONEURAL DISORDERS

Excludes1: botulism (A05.1, A48.51–A48.52)
     transient neonatal myasthenia gravis (P94.0)

G70.0   Myasthenia gravis
     G70.00   Myasthenia gravis without (acute) exacerbation
         Myasthenia gravis NOS
     G70.01   Myasthenia gravis with (acute) exacerbation
         Myasthenia gravis in crisis
G70.9   Myoneural disorder, unspecified

G71   PRIMARY DISORDERS OF MUSCLES

Excludes2: arthrogryposis multiplex congenita (Q74.3)
     metabolic disorders (E70–E88)
     myositis (M60.-)

G71.0   Muscular dystrophy
     Autosomal recessive, childhood type, muscular dystrophy resembling Duchenne or Becker muscular dystrophy
     Benign [Becker] muscular dystrophy
     Benign scapuloperoneal muscular dystrophy with early contractures [Emery-Dreifuss]
     Congenital muscular dystrophy NOS
     Congenital muscular dystrophy with specific morphological abnormalities of the muscle fiber
     Distal muscular dystrophy
     Facioscapulohumeral muscular dystrophy
     Limb-girdle muscular dystrophy
     Ocular muscular dystrophy
     Oculopharyngeal muscular dystrophy
     Scapuloperoneal muscular dystrophy
     Severe [Duchenne] muscular dystrophy

G71.1   Myotonic disorders
     G71.11   Myotonic muscular dystrophy
         Dystrophia myotonica [Steinert]
         Myotonia atrophica

 4th **5th** **6th** **7th**   Additional Character Required   ✓   3-character code   •=New Code   ▲=Revised Code   ***Excludes1***—Not coded here, do not use together   ***Excludes2***—Not included here

G71.12　Myotonia congenita
　　Acetazolamide responsive myotonia congenita
　　Dominant myotonia congenita [Thomsen disease]
　　Myotonia levior
　　Recessive myotonia congenita [Becker disease]

G71.2　Congenital myopathies
　　Central core disease
　　Fiber-type disproportion
　　Minicore disease
　　Multicore disease
　　Myotubular (centronuclear) myopathy
　　Nemaline myopathy
　　Excludes1: arthrogryposis multiplex congenita (Q74.3)

(G80–G83) CEREBRAL PALSY AND OTHER PARALYTIC SYNDROMES

G80　CEREBRAL PALSY

 4th

Excludes1: hereditary spastic paraplegia (G11.4)

G80.0　Spastic quadriplegic cerebral palsy
　　Congenital spastic paralysis (cerebral)

G80.1　Spastic diplegic cerebral palsy
　　Spastic cerebral palsy NOS

G80.2　Spastic hemiplegic cerebral palsy

G80.3　Athetoid cerebral palsy
　　Double athetosis (syndrome)
　　Dyskinetic cerebral palsy
　　Dystonic cerebral palsy
　　Vogt disease

G80.4　Ataxic cerebral palsy

G80.8　Other cerebral palsy
　　Mixed cerebral palsy syndromes

G80.9　Cerebral palsy, unspecified
　　Cerebral palsy NOS

G81　HEMIPLEGIA AND HEMIPARESIS

4th

GUIDELINES

Codes from category G81, identify whether the dominant or nondominant side is affected. Should the affected side be documented, but not specified as dominant or nondominant, and the classification system does not indicate a default, code selection is as follows:
For ambidextrous patients, the default should be dominant.
If the left side is affected, the default is non-dominant.
If the right side is affected, the default is dominant.
　Note: This category is to be used only when hemiplegia (complete) (incomplete) is reported without further specification, or is stated to be old or longstanding but of unspecified cause. The category is also for use in multiple coding to identify these types of hemiplegia resulting from any cause.
Excludes1: congenital cerebral palsy (G80.-)
　hemiplegia and hemiparesis due to sequela of cerebrovascular disease (I69.05-, I69.15-, I69.25-, I69.35-, I69.85-, I69.95-)

G81.0　Flaccid hemiplegia
　5th
　　G81.01　Flaccid hemiplegia affecting right dominant side
　　G81.02　Flaccid hemiplegia affecting left dominant side
　　G81.03　Flaccid hemiplegia affecting right nondominant side
　　G81.04　Flaccid hemiplegia affecting left nondominant side

G81.1　Spastic hemiplegia
　5th
　　G81.11　Spastic hemiplegia affecting right dominant side
　　G81.12　Spastic hemiplegia affecting left dominant side
　　G81.13　Spastic hemiplegia affecting right nondominant side
　　G81.14　Spastic hemiplegia affecting left nondominant side

G81.9　Hemiplegia, unspecified
　5th
　　G81.91　Hemiplegia, unspecified affecting right dominant side
　　G81.92　Hemiplegia, unspecified affecting left dominant side
　　G81.93　Hemiplegia, unspecified affecting right nondominant side
　　G81.94　Hemiplegia, unspecified affecting left nondominant side

G82　PARAPLEGIA (PARAPARESIS) AND QUADRIPLEGIA (QUADRIPARESIS)

 4th

Note: This category is to be used only when the listed conditions are reported without further specification, or are stated to be old or longstanding but of unspecified cause. The category is also for use in multiple coding to identify these conditions resulting from any cause
Excludes1: congenital cerebral palsy (G80.-)
　functional quadriplegia (R53.2)
　hysterical paralysis (F44.4)

G82.2　Paraplegia
　5th
　　Paralysis of both lower limbs NOS
　　Paraparesis (lower) NOS
　　Paraplegia (lower) NOS
　　G82.20　Paraplegia, unspecified
　　G82.21　Paraplegia, complete
　　G82.22　Paraplegia, incomplete

G82.5　Quadriplegia
　5th
　　G82.50　Quadriplegia, unspecified
　　G82.51　Quadriplegia, C1-C4 complete
　　G82.52　Quadriplegia, C1-C4 incomplete
　　G82.53　Quadriplegia, C5-C7 complete
　　G82.54　Quadriplegia, C5-C7 incomplete

G83　OTHER PARALYTIC SYNDROMES

 4th

GUIDELINES

Codes from subcategories, G83.1, G83.2, and G83.3, identify whether the dominant or nondominant side is affected. Should the affected side be documented, but not specified as dominant or nondominant, and the classification system does not indicate a default, code selection is as follows:
For ambidextrous patients, the default should be dominant.
If the left side is affected, the default is non-dominant.
If the right side is affected, the default is dominant.
　Note: This category is to be used only when the listed conditions are reported without further specification, or are stated to be old or longstanding but of unspecified cause. The category is also for use in multiple coding to identify these conditions resulting from any cause.
Includes: paralysis (complete) (incomplete), except as in G80–G82

G83.0　Diplegia of upper limbs
　　Diplegia (upper)
　　Paralysis of both upper limbs

G83.1　Monoplegia of lower limb
　5th
　　Paralysis of lower limb
　　Excludes1: monoplegia of lower limbs due to sequela of cerebrovascular disease (I69.04-, I69.14-, I69.24-, I69.34-, I69.84-, I69.94-)
　　G83.10　Monoplegia of lower limb affecting; unspecified side
　　G83.11　　right dominant side
　　G83.12　　left dominant side
　　G83.13　　right nondominant side
　　G83.14　　left nondominant side

G83.2　Monoplegia of upper limb
　5th
　　Paralysis of upper limb
　　Excludes1: monoplegia of upper limbs due to sequela of cerebrovascular disease (I69.03-, I69.13-, I69.23-, I69.33-, I69.83-, I69.93-)
　　G83.21　Monoplegia of upper limb affecting; right dominant side
　　G83.22　　left dominant side
　　G83.23　　right nondominant side
　　G83.24　　left nondominant side

G83.3　Monoplegia, unspecified
　5th
　　G83.31　Monoplegia, unspecified affecting; right dominant side
　　G83.32　　left dominant side
　　G83.33　　right nondominant side
　　G83.34　　left nondominant side

G83.9　Paralytic syndrome, unspecified

4th　5th　6th　7th　Additional Character Required　　　✓　　3 character code

　•＝New Code　　***Excludes1***—Not coded here, do not use together
　▲＝Revised Code　　***Excludes2***—Not included here

CHAPTER 6. DISEASES OF THE NERVOUS SYSTEM   (G89–G99)

(G89–G99) OTHER DISORDERS OF THE NERVOUS SYSTEM

G89   **PAIN, NOT ELSEWHERE CLASSIFIED**

4th   GUIDELINES

General coding information

Codes in category G89, Pain, not elsewhere classified, may be used in conjunction with codes from other categories and chapters to provide more detail about acute or chronic pain and neoplasm-related pain, unless otherwise indicated below.

If the pain is not specified as acute or chronic, post-thoracotomy, postprocedural, or neoplasm-related, do not assign codes from category G89.

A code from category G89 should not be assigned if the underlying (definitive) diagnosis is known, unless the reason for the encounter is pain control/ management and not management of the underlying condition.

When an admission or encounter is for a procedure aimed at treating the underlying condition (e.g., spinal fusion, kyphoplasty), a code for the underlying condition (e.g., vertebral fracture, spinal stenosis) should be assigned as the principal diagnosis. No code from category G89 should be assigned.

CATEGORY G89 CODES AS PRINCIPAL OR FIRST-LISTED DIAGNOSIS

Category G89 codes are acceptable as principal diagnosis or the first-listed code:

- When pain control or pain management is the reason for the admission/ encounter. The underlying cause of the pain should be reported as an additional diagnosis, if known.
- When a patient is admitted for the insertion of a neurostimulator for pain control. When an admission or encounter is for a procedure aimed at treating the underlying condition and a neurostimulator is inserted for pain control during the same admission/encounter, a code for the underlying condition should be assigned as the principal diagnosis and the appropriate pain code should be assigned as a secondary diagnosis.

USE OF CATEGORY G89 CODES IN CONJUNCTION WITH SITE SPECIFIC PAIN CODES

Assigning Category G89 and Site-Specific Pain Codes

Codes from category G89 may be used in conjunction with codes that identify the site of pain (including codes from chapter 18) if the category G89 code provides additional information. For example, if the code describes the site of the pain, but does not fully describe whether the pain is acute or chronic, then both codes should be assigned.

Sequencing of Category G89 Codes with Site-Specific Pain Codes

The sequencing of category G89 codes with site-specific pain codes (including chapter 18 codes), is dependent on the circumstances of the encounter/admission as follows:

- If the encounter is for pain control or pain management, assign the code from category G89 followed by the code identifying the specific site of pain (e.g., encounter for pain management for acute neck pain from trauma is assigned code G89.11, Acute pain due to trauma, followed by code M54.2, Cervicalgia, to identify the site of pain).
- If the encounter is for any other reason except pain control or pain management, and a related definitive diagnosis has not been established (confirmed) by the provider, assign the code for the specific site of pain first, followed by the appropriate code from category G89.

Pain due to devices, implants and grafts

Refer to Chapter 19 for pain due to medical devices.

Postoperative Pain

The provider's documentation should be used to guide the coding of postoperative pain, as well as Section IV. Diagnostic Coding and Reporting in the Outpatient Setting (page xvi).

The default for post-thoracotomy and other postoperative pain not specified as acute or chronic is the code for the acute form.

Routine or expected postoperative pain immediately after surgery should not be coded.

- Postoperative pain not associated with a specific postoperative complication is assigned to the appropriate postoperative pain code in category G89.
- Postoperative pain associated with a specific postoperative complication (such as painful wire sutures) is assigned to the appropriate code(s) found in Chapter 19. If appropriate, use additional code(s) from category G89 to identify acute or chronic pain (G89.18 or G89.28).

Chronic pain

Chronic pain is classified to subcategory G89.2. There is no time frame defining when pain becomes chronic pain. The provider's documentation should be used to guide use of these codes.

Neoplasm Related Pain

Code G89.3 is assigned to pain documented as being related, associated or due to cancer, primary or secondary malignancy, or tumor. This code is assigned regardless of whether the pain is acute or chronic. This code may be assigned as the principal or first-listed code when the stated reason for the admission/encounter is documented as pain control/pain management. The underlying neoplasm should be reported as an additional diagnosis.

When the reason for the admission/encounter is management of the neoplasm and the pain associated with the neoplasm is also documented, code G89.3 may be assigned as an additional diagnosis. It is not necessary to assign an additional code for the site of the pain.

Refer to Chapter 2 for instructions on the sequencing of neoplasms for all other stated reasons for the admission/encounter (except for pain control/pain management).

Chronic Pain Syndrome

Central pain syndrome (G89.0) and chronic pain syndrome (G89.4) are different than the term "chronic pain," and therefore codes should only be used when the provider has specifically documented this condition.

See Chapter 5 for pain disorders related to psychological factors
Code also related psychological factors associated with pain (F45.42)
Excludes1: generalized pain NOS (R52)
     pain disorders exclusively related to psychological factors (F45.41)
     pain NOS (R52)
Excludes2: atypical face pain (G50.1)
     headache syndromes (G44.-)
     localized pain, unspecified type—code to pain by site, such as:
     abdomen pain (R10.-)
     back pain (M54.9)
     breast pain (N64.4)
     chest pain (R07.1–R07.9)
     ear pain (H92.0-)
     eye pain (H57.1)
     headache (R51)
     joint pain (M25.5-)
     limb pain (M79.6-)
     lumbar region pain (M54.5)
     painful urination (R30.9)
     pelvic and perineal pain (R10.2)
     shoulder pain (M25.51-)
     spine pain (M54.-)
     throat pain (R07.0)
     tongue pain (K14.6)
     tooth pain (K08.8)
     renal colic (N23)
     migraines (G43.-)
     myalgia (M79.1)
     pain from prosthetic devices, implants, and grafts (T82.84, T83.84, T84.84, T85.84-)
     phantom limb syndrome with pain (G54.6)
     vulvar vestibulitis (N94.810)
     vulvodynia (N94.81-)

   4th   5th   6th   7th   Additional Character Required   3-character code

•=New Code   ***Excludes1***—Not coded here, do not use together
▲=Revised Code   ***Excludes2***—Not included here

G89.1 Acute pain, not elsewhere classified
> **G89.11 Acute pain due to trauma**
> **G89.12 Acute post-thoracotomy pain**
> Post-thoracotomy pain NOS
> **G89.18 Other acute postprocedural pain**
> Postoperative pain NOS
> Postprocedural pain NOS

G89.2 Chronic pain, NEC
> *Excludes1:* causalgia, lower limb (G57.7-)
> causalgia, upper limb (G56.4-)
> central pain syndrome (G89.0)
> chronic pain syndrome (G89.4)
> complex regional pain syndrome II, lower limb (G57.7-)
> complex regional pain syndrome II, upper limb (G56.4-)
> neoplasm related chronic pain (G89.3)
> reflex sympathetic dystrophy (G90.5-)
> **G89.21 Chronic pain due to trauma**
> **G89.22 Chronic post-thoracotomy pain**
> **G89.28 Other chronic postprocedural pain**
> Other chronic postoperative pain

G89.3 Neoplasm related pain (acute) (chronic)
> Cancer associated pain
> Pain due to malignancy (primary) (secondary)
> Tumor associated pain

G90 DISORDERS OF AUTONOMIC NERVOUS SYSTEM
Excludes1: dysfunction of the autonomic nervous system due to alcohol (G31.2)

G90.5 Complex regional pain syndrome I (CRPS I)
> Reflex sympathetic dystrophy
> *Excludes1:* causalgia of lower limb (G57.7-)
> causalgia of upper limb (G56.4-)
> complex regional pain syndrome II of lower limb (G57.7-)
> complex regional pain syndrome II of upper limb (G56.4-)
> **G90.51 Complex regional pain syndrome I of upper limb**
> > **G90.511 Complex regional pain syndrome I of; right upper limb**
> > **G90.512 left upper limb**
> > **G90.513 bilateral**
> > **G90.519 unspecified upper limb**
> **G90.52 Complex regional pain syndrome I of lower limb**
> > **G90.521 Complex regional pain syndrome I of; right lower limb**
> > **G90.522 left lower limb**
> > **G90.523 bilateral**
> > **G90.529 unspecified lower limb**
> **G90.59 Complex regional pain syndrome I of other specified site**

G90.8 Other disorders of autonomic nervous system
G90.9 Disorder of the autonomic nervous system, unspecified

G91 HYDROCEPHALUS
Includes: acquired hydrocephalus
Excludes1: Arnold-Chiari syndrome with hydrocephalus (Q07.-)
> congenital hydrocephalus (Q03.-)
> spina bifida with hydrocephalus (Q05.-)
G91.0 Communicating hydrocephalus
> Secondary normal pressure hydrocephalus
G91.1 Obstructive hydrocephalus
G91.2 (Idiopathic) normal pressure hydrocephalus
> Normal pressure hydrocephalus NOS

G92 TOXIC ENCEPHALOPATHY
Toxic encephalitis
Toxic metabolic encephalopathy
Code first (T51–T65) to identify toxic agent

G93 OTHER DISORDERS OF BRAIN
G93.1 Anoxic brain damage, not elsewhere classified
> *Excludes1:* cerebral anoxia due to anesthesia during labor and delivery (O74.3)
> cerebral anoxia due to anesthesia during the puerperium (O89.2)
> neonatal anoxia (P84)
G93.2 Benign intracranial hypertension
> *Excludes1:* hypertensive encephalopathy (I67.4)
G93.4 Other and unspecified encephalopathy
> *Excludes1:* alcoholic encephalopathy (G31.2)
> encephalopathy in diseases classified elsewhere (G94)
> hypertensive encephalopathy (I67.4)
> toxic (metabolic) encephalopathy (G92)
> **G93.40 Encephalopathy, unspecified**
> **G93.49 Other encephalopathy**
> Encephalopathy NEC
G93.6 Cerebral edema
> *Excludes1:* cerebral edema due to birth injury (P11.0)
> traumatic cerebral edema (S06.1-)
G93.8 Other specified disorders of brain
> **G93.81 Temporal sclerosis**
> Hippocampal sclerosis
> Mesial temporal sclerosis
> **G93.82 Brain death**
> **G93.89 Other specified disorders of brain**
> Post-radiation encephalopathy
G93.9 Disorder of brain, unspecified

4th 5th 6th 7th Additional Character Required ✓ 3-character code
•=New Code ▲=Revised Code
Excludes1—Not coded here, do not use together
Excludes2—Not included here

PEDIATRIC ICD-10-CM 2017: A MANUAL FOR PROVIDER-BASED CODING 167

Chapter 7. Diseases of the eye and adnexa (H00–H59)

GUIDELINES

Refer to ICD-10-CM Official Guidelines for Coding and Reporting for reporting adult glaucoma

Note: Use an external cause code following the code for the eye condition, if applicable, to identify the cause of the eye condition

Excludes2: certain conditions originating in the perinatal period (P04–P96)
    certain infectious and parasitic diseases (A00–B99)
    complications of pregnancy, childbirth and the puerperium (O00–O9A)
    congenital malformations, deformations, and chromosomal abnormalities (Q00–Q99)
    DM related eye conditions (E09.3-, E10.3-, E11.3-, E13.3-)
    endocrine, nutritional and metabolic diseases (E00–E88)
    injury (trauma) of eye and orbit (S05.-)
    injury, poisoning and certain other consequences of external causes (S00–T88)
    neoplasms (C00–D49)
    symptoms, signs and abnormal clinical and laboratory findings, not elsewhere classified (R00–R94)
    syphilis related eye disorders (A50.01, A50.3-, A51.43, A52.71)

(H00–H05) DISORDERS OF EYELID, LACRIMAL SYSTEM AND ORBIT

H00 HORDEOLUM AND CHALAZION
[4th] H00.0 Hordeolum (externum) (internum) of eyelid
    [5th] H00.01 Hordeolum externum
      [6th] Hordeolum NOS
      Stye
      H00.011 Hordeolum externum right upper eyelid
      H00.012 Hordeolum externum right lower eyelid
      H00.013 Hordeolum externum right eye, unspecified eyelid
      H00.014 Hordeolum externum left upper eyelid
      H00.015 Hordeolum externum left lower eyelid
      H00.016 Hordeolum externum left eye, unspecified eyelid
    H00.03 Abscess of eyelid
      [6th] Furuncle of eyelid
      H00.031 Abscess of right upper eyelid
      H00.032 Abscess of right lower eyelid
      H00.033 Abscess of eyelid right eye, unspecified eyelid
      H00.034 Abscess of left upper eyelid
      H00.035 Abscess of left lower eyelid
      H00.036 Abscess of eyelid left eye, unspecified eyelid
[5th] H00.1 Chalazion
    Meibomian (gland) cyst
    Excludes2: infected meibomian gland (H00.02-)
    H00.11 Chalazion right upper eyelid
    H00.12 Chalazion right lower eyelid
    H00.13 Chalazion right eye, unspecified eyelid
    H00.14 Chalazion left upper eyelid
    H00.15 Chalazion left lower eyelid
    H00.16 Chalazion left eye, unspecified eyelid

H01 OTHER INFLAMMATION OF EYELID
[4th] H01.0 Blepharitis
    Excludes1: blepharoconjunctivitis (H10.5-)
    [5th] H01.00 Unspecified blepharitis
      [6th] H01.001 Unspecified blepharitis right upper eyelid
      H01.002 Unspecified blepharitis right lower eyelid
      H01.003 Unspecified blepharitis right eye, unspecified eyelid
      H01.004 Unspecified blepharitis left upper eyelid
      H01.005 Unspecified blepharitis left lower eyelid
      H01.006 Unspecified blepharitis left eye, unspecified eyelid

H02 OTHER DISORDERS OF EYELID
[4th] ***Excludes1:*** congenital malformations of eyelid (Q10.0–Q10.3)
H02.4 Ptosis of eyelid
    [5th] H02.40 Unspecified ptosis of eyelid
      [6th] H02.401 Unspecified ptosis of right eyelid
      H02.402 Unspecified ptosis of left eyelid
      H02.403 Unspecified ptosis of bilateral eyelids
      H02.409 Unspecified ptosis of unspecified eyelid
H02.8 Other specified disorders of eyelid
    [5th] H02.82 Cysts of eyelid
      [6th] Sebaceous cyst of eyelid
      H02.821 Cysts of right upper eyelid
      H02.822 Cysts of right lower eyelid
      H02.823 Cysts of right eye, unspecified eyelid
      H02.824 Cysts of left upper eyelid
      H02.825 Cysts of left lower eyelid
      H02.826 Cysts of left eye, unspecified eyelid
H04.5 Stenosis and insufficiency of lacrimal passages
    [5th] H04.53 Neonatal obstruction of nasolacrimal duct
      [6th] ***Excludes1:*** congenital stenosis and stricture of lacrimal duct (Q10.5)
      H04.531 Neonatal obstruction of right nasolacrimal duct
      H04.532 Neonatal obstruction of left nasolacrimal duct
      H04.533 Neonatal obstruction of bilateral nasolacrimal duct

H05 DISORDERS OF ORBIT
[4th] ***Excludes1:*** congenital malformation of orbit (Q10.7)
H05.0 Acute inflammation of orbit
    [5th] H05.00 Unspecified acute inflammation of orbit
    H05.01 Cellulitis of orbit
      [6th] Abscess of orbit
      H05.011 Cellulitis of right orbit
      H05.012 Cellulitis of left orbit
      H05.013 Cellulitis of bilateral orbits

(H10–H11) DISORDERS OF CONJUNCTIVA

H10 CONJUNCTIVITIS
[4th] ***Excludes1:*** keratoconjunctivitis (H16.2-)
H10.0 Mucopurulent conjunctivitis
    [5th] H10.01 Acute follicular conjunctivitis
      [6th] H10.011 Acute follicular conjunctivitis, right eye
      H10.012 Acute follicular conjunctivitis, left eye
      H10.013 Acute follicular conjunctivitis, bilateral
    H10.02 Other mucopurulent conjunctivitis
      [6th] H10.021 Other mucopurulent conjunctivitis, right eye
      H10.022 Other mucopurulent conjunctivitis, left eye
      H10.023 Other mucopurulent conjunctivitis, bilateral
H10.1 Acute atopic conjunctivitis
    [5th] Acute papillary conjunctivitis
    H10.11 Acute atopic conjunctivitis, right eye
    H10.12 Acute atopic conjunctivitis, left eye
    H10.13 Acute atopic conjunctivitis, bilateral
H10.2 Other acute conjunctivitis
    [5th] H10.21 Acute toxic conjunctivitis
      [6th] Acute chemical conjunctivitis
      Code first (T51–T65) to identify chemical and intent
      Excludes1: burn and corrosion of eye and adnexa (T26.-)
      H10.211 Acute toxic conjunctivitis, right eye
      H10.212 Acute toxic conjunctivitis, left eye
      H10.213 Acute toxic conjunctivitis, bilateral
    H10.22 Pseudomembranous conjunctivitis
      [6th] H10.221 Pseudomembranous conjunctivitis, right eye
      H10.222 Pseudomembranous conjunctivitis, left eye
      H10.223 Pseudomembranous conjunctivitis, bilateral

[4th] [5th] [6th] [7th] Additional Character Required   3-character code   Unspecified laterality codes were excluded here.   •=New Code   ▲=Revised Code   ***Excludes1***—Not coded here, do not use together   ***Excludes2***—Not included here

H10.23   Serous conjunctivitis, except viral
> **6th**   *Excludes1:* viral conjunctivitis (B30.-)
>> **H10.231**   Serous conjunctivitis, except viral, right eye
>> **H10.232**   Serous conjunctivitis, except viral, left eye
>> **H10.233**   Serous conjunctivitis, except viral, bilateral
>> **H10.239**   Serous conjunctivitis, except viral, unspecified eye

H10.3   Unspecified acute conjunctivitis
> **5th**   *Excludes1:* ophthalmia neonatorum NOS (P39.1)
> **H10.31**   Unspecified acute conjunctivitis, right eye
> **H10.32**   Unspecified acute conjunctivitis, left eye
> **H10.33**   Unspecified acute conjunctivitis, bilateral

H10.5   Blepharoconjunctivitis
> **5th**   **H10.50**   Unspecified blepharoconjunctivitis
>> **6th**   **H10.501**   Unspecified blepharoconjunctivitis, right eye
>> **H10.502**   Unspecified blepharoconjunctivitis, left eye
>> **H10.503**   Unspecified blepharoconjunctivitis, bilateral

H11   OTHER DISORDERS OF CONJUNCTIVA

4th   *Excludes1:* keratoconjunctivitis (H16.2-)

H11.3   Conjunctival hemorrhage
> **5th**   Subconjunctival hemorrhage
> **H11.31**   Conjunctival hemorrhage, right eye
> **H11.32**   Conjunctival hemorrhage, left eye
> **H11.33**   Conjunctival hemorrhage, bilateral

H11.4   Other conjunctival vascular disorders and cysts
> **5th**   **H11.42**   Conjunctival edema
>> **6th**   **H11.421**   Conjunctival edema, right eye
>> **H11.422**   Conjunctival edema, left eye
>> **H11.423**   Conjunctival edema, bilateral

(H15–H22) DISORDERS OF SCLERA, CORNEA, IRIS AND CILIARY BODY

H18   OTHER DISORDERS OF CORNEA
4th   **H18.8**   Other specified disorders of cornea
> **5th**   **H18.82**   Corneal disorder due to contact lens
>> **6th**   *Excludes2:* corneal edema due to contact lens (H18.21-)
>> **H18.821**   Corneal disorder due to contact lens, right eye
>> **H18.822**   Corneal disorder due to contact lens, left eye
>> **H18.823**   Corneal disorder due to contact lens, bilateral

(H25–H28) DISORDERS OF LENS

H26   OTHER CATARACT

4th   *Excludes1:* congenital cataract (Q12.0)

H26.0   Infantile and juvenile cataract
> **5th**   **H26.00**   Unspecified infantile and juvenile cataract
>> **6th**   **H26.001**   Unspecified infantile and juvenile cataract, right eye
>> **H26.002**   Unspecified infantile and juvenile cataract, left eye
>> **H26.003**   Unspecified infantile and juvenile cataract, bilateral
>
> **H26.01**   Infantile and juvenile cortical, lamellar, or zonular cataract
>> **6th**   **H26.011**   Infantile and juvenile cortical, lamellar, or zonular cataract, right eye
>> **H26.012**   Infantile and juvenile cortical, lamellar, or zonular cataract, left eye
>> **H26.013**   Infantile and juvenile cortical, lamellar, or zonular cataract, bilateral

H26.03   Infantile and juvenile nuclear cataract
> **6th**   **H26.031**   Infantile and juvenile nuclear cataract, right eye
> **H26.032**   Infantile and juvenile nuclear cataract, left eye
> **H26.033**   Infantile and juvenile nuclear cataract, bilateral

H26.04   Anterior subcapsular polar infantile and juvenile cataract
> **6th**   **H26.041**   Anterior subcapsular polar infantile and juvenile cataract, right eye
> **H26.042**   Anterior subcapsular polar infantile and juvenile cataract, left eye
> **H26.043**   Anterior subcapsular polar infantile and juvenile cataract, bilateral

H26.05   Posterior subcapsular polar infantile and juvenile cataract
> **6th**   **H26.051**   Posterior subcapsular polar infantile and juvenile cataract, right eye
> **H26.052**   Posterior subcapsular polar infantile and juvenile cataract, left eye
> **H26.053**   Posterior subcapsular polar infantile and juvenile cataract, bilateral

H26.06   Combined forms of infantile and juvenile cataract
> **6th**   **H26.061**   Combined forms of infantile and juvenile cataract, right eye
> **H26.062**   Combined forms of infantile and juvenile cataract, left eye
> **H26.063**   Combined forms of infantile and juvenile cataract, bilateral

H26.09   Other infantile and juvenile cataract

(H30–H36) DISORDERS OF CHOROID AND RETINA

H35   OTHER RETINAL DISORDERS

4th   *Excludes2:* diabetic retinal disorders (E08.311–E08.359, E09.311–E09.359, E10.311–E10.359, E11.311–E11.359, E13.311–E13.359)

H35.1   Retinopathy of prematurity
> **5th**   **H35.10**   Retinopathy of prematurity, unspecified
>> **6th**   Retinopathy of prematurity NOS
>> **H35.101**   Retinopathy of prematurity, unspecified, right eye
>> **H35.102**   Retinopathy of prematurity, unspecified, left eye
>> **H35.103**   Retinopathy of prematurity, unspecified, bilateral
>
> **H35.11**   Retinopathy of prematurity, stage 0
>> **6th**   **H35.111**   Retinopathy of prematurity, stage 0, right eye
>> **H35.112**   Retinopathy of prematurity, stage 0, left eye
>> **H35.113**   Retinopathy of prematurity, stage 0, bilateral
>
> **H35.12**   Retinopathy of prematurity, stage 1
>> **6th**   **H35.121**   Retinopathy of prematurity, stage 1, right eye
>> **H35.122**   Retinopathy of prematurity, stage 1, left eye
>> **H35.123**   Retinopathy of prematurity, stage 1, bilateral
>
> **H35.13**   Retinopathy of prematurity, stage 2
>> **6th**   **H35.131**   Retinopathy of prematurity, stage 2, right eye
>> **H35.132**   Retinopathy of prematurity, stage 2, left eye
>> **H35.133**   Retinopathy of prematurity, stage 2, bilateral

  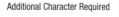   Additional Character Required   ✓   3-character code   Unspecified laterality codes were excluded here.   •=New Code   ▲=Revised Code   *Excludes1*—Not coded here, do not use together   *Excludes2*—Not included here

170   **PEDIATRIC ICD-10-CM 2017: A MANUAL FOR PROVIDER-BASED CODING**

H35.14 Retinopathy of prematurity, stage 3
- **H35.141** Retinopathy of prematurity, stage 3, right eye
- **H35.142** Retinopathy of prematurity, stage 3, left eye
- **H35.143** Retinopathy of prematurity, stage 3, bilateral

H35.15 Retinopathy of prematurity, stage 4
- **H35.151** Retinopathy of prematurity, stage 4, right eye
- **H35.152** Retinopathy of prematurity, stage 4, left eye
- **H35.153** Retinopathy of prematurity, stage 4, bilateral

H35.16 Retinopathy of prematurity, stage 5
- **H35.161** Retinopathy of prematurity, stage 5, right eye
- **H35.162** Retinopathy of prematurity, stage 5, left eye
- **H35.163** Retinopathy of prematurity, stage 5, bilateral

H35.17 Retrolental fibroplasia
- **H35.171** Retrolental fibroplasia, right eye
- **H35.172** Retrolental fibroplasia, left eye
- **H35.173** Retrolental fibroplasia, bilateral
- **H35.179** Retrolental fibroplasia, unspecified eye

H35.5 Hereditary retinal dystrophy
Excludes1: dystrophies primarily involving Bruch's membrane (H31.1-)
- **H35.50** Unspecified hereditary retinal dystrophy
- **H35.51** Vitreoretinal dystrophy
- **H35.52** Pigmentary retinal dystrophy
  Albipunctate retinal dystrophy
  Retinitis pigmentosa
  Tapetoretinal dystrophy
- **H35.53** Other dystrophies primarily involving the sensory retina
  Stargardt's disease
- **H35.54** Dystrophies primarily involving the retinal pigment epithelium
  Vitelliform retinal dystrophy

(H40–H42) GLAUCOMA

H40 GLAUCOMA

Excludes1: absolute glaucoma (H44.51-)
  congenital glaucoma (Q15.0)
  traumatic glaucoma due to birth injury (P15.3)

H40.3 Glaucoma secondary to eye trauma
  Code also underlying condition
- **H40.31X** Glaucoma secondary to eye trauma, right eye
  - **H40.31X0** Glaucoma secondary to eye trauma, right eye; stage unspecified
  - **H40.31X1** mild stage
  - **H40.31X2** moderate stage
  - **H40.31X3** severe stage
  - **H40.31X4** indeterminate stage
- **H40.32X** Glaucoma secondary to eye trauma, left eye
  - **H40.32X0** Glaucoma secondary to eye trauma, left eye; stage unspecified
  - **H40.32X1** mild stage
  - **H40.32X2** moderate stage
  - **H40.32X3** severe stage
  - **H40.32X4** indeterminate stage

- **H40.33X** Glaucoma secondary to eye trauma, bilateral
  - **H40.33X0** Glaucoma secondary to eye trauma, bilateral; stage unspecified
  - **H40.33X1** mild stage
  - **H40.33X2** moderate stage
  - **H40.33X3** severe stage
  - **H40.33X4** indeterminate stage

H42 GLAUCOMA IN DISEASES CLASSIFIED ELSEWHERE

Code first underlying condition, such as: amyloidosis (E85.-)
  aniridia (Q13.1)
  Lowe's syndrome (E72.03)
  Reiger's anomaly (Q13.81)
  specified metabolic disorder (E70–E88)
Excludes1: glaucoma (in):
  onchocerciasis (B73.02)
  syphilis (A52.71)
  tuberculous (A18.59)
Excludes2: DM (E08.39, E09.39, E10.39, E11.39, E13.39)

(H43–H44) DISORDERS OF VITREOUS BODY AND GLOBE

(H46–H47) DISORDERS OF OPTIC NERVE AND VISUAL PATHWAYS

H47 OTHER DISORDERS OF OPTIC [2ND] NERVE AND VISUAL PATHWAYS
H47.0 Disorders of optic nerve, not elsewhere classified
- **H47.03** Optic nerve hypoplasia
  - **H47.031** Optic nerve hypoplasia, right eye
  - **H47.032** Optic nerve hypoplasia, left eye
  - **H47.033** Optic nerve hypoplasia, bilateral
  - **H47.039** Optic nerve hypoplasia, unspecified eye

H47.1 Papilledema
- **H47.10** Unspecified papilledema
- **H47.11** Papilledema associated with increased intracranial pressure
- **H47.12** Papilledema associated with decreased ocular pressure
- **H47.13** Papilledema associated with retinal disorder

(H49–H52) DISORDERS OF OCULAR MUSCLES, BINOCULAR MOVEMENT, ACCOMMODATION AND REFRACTION

H50 OTHER STRABISMUS
H50.0 Esotropia
  Convergent concomitant strabismus
  Excludes1: intermittent esotropia (H50.31-, H50.32)
- **H50.00** Unspecified esotropia
- **H50.01** Monocular esotropia
  - **H50.011** Monocular esotropia, right eye
  - **H50.012** Monocular esotropia, left eye
- **H50.02** Monocular esotropia with A pattern
  - **H50.021** Monocular esotropia with A pattern, right eye
  - **H50.022** Monocular esotropia with A pattern, left eye
- **H50.03** Monocular esotropia with V pattern
  - **H50.031** Monocular esotropia with V pattern, right eye
  - **H50.032** Monocular esotropia with V pattern, left eye
- **H50.04** Monocular esotropia with other noncomitancies
  - **H50.041** Monocular esotropia with other noncomitancies, right eye
  - **H50.042** Monocular esotropia with other noncomitancies, left eye
- **H50.05** Alternating esotropia
- **H50.06** Alternating esotropia with A pattern
- **H50.07** Alternating esotropia with V pattern
- **H50.08** Alternating esotropia with other noncomitancies

    Additional Character Required   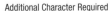 3-character code   Unspecified laterality codes were excluded here.   •=New Code ▲=Revised Code   *Excludes1*—Not coded here, do not use together *Excludes2*—Not included here

PEDIATRIC ICD-10-CM 2017: A MANUAL FOR PROVIDER-BASED CODING   171

CHAPTER 7. DISEASES OF THE EYE AND ADNEXA (H35.14–H50.08)

CHAPTER 7. DISEASES OF THE EYE AND ADNEXA (H50.1–H53.9)

H50.1 **Exotropia**
`5th` Divergent concomitant strabismus
Excludes1: intermittent exotropia (H50.33-, H50.34)
  H50.10 **Unspecified exotropia**
  H50.11 **Monocular exotropia**
    `6th` **H50.111** **Monocular exotropia, right eye**
    H50.112 **Monocular exotropia, left eye**
  H50.12 **Monocular exotropia with A pattern**
    `6th` **H50.121** **Monocular exotropia with A pattern, right eye**
    H50.122 **Monocular exotropia with A pattern, left eye**
  H50.13 **Monocular exotropia with V pattern**
    `6th` **H50.131** **Monocular exotropia with V pattern, right eye**
    H50.132 **Monocular exotropia with V pattern, left eye**
  H50.14 **Monocular exotropia with other noncomitancies**
    `6th` **H50.141** **Monocular exotropia with other noncomitancies, right eye**
    H50.142 **Monocular exotropia with other noncomitancies, left eye**
  H50.15 **Alternating exotropia**
  H50.16 **Alternating exotropia with A pattern**
  H50.17 **Alternating exotropia with V pattern**
  H50.18 **Alternating exotropia with other noncomitancies**
H50.2 **Vertical strabismus**
`5th` Hypertropia
  H50.21 **Vertical strabismus, right eye**
  H50.22 **Vertical strabismus, left eye**
H50.3 **Intermittent heterotropia**
`5th` **H50.30** **Unspecified intermittent heterotropia**
  H50.31 **Intermittent monocular esotropia**
    `6th` **H50.311** **Intermittent monocular esotropia, right eye**
    H50.312 **Intermittent monocular esotropia, left eye**
  H50.32 **Intermittent alternating esotropia**
  H50.33 **Intermittent monocular exotropia**
    `6th` **H50.331** **Intermittent monocular exotropia, right eye**
    H50.332 **Intermittent monocular exotropia, left eye**
  H50.34 **Intermittent alternating exotropia**
H50.4 **Other and unspecified heterotropia**
`5th` **H50.40** **Unspecified heterotropia**
  H50.41 **Cyclotropia**
    `6th` **H50.411** **Cyclotropia, right eye**
    H50.412 **Cyclotropia, left eye**
  H50.42 **Monofixation syndrome**
  H50.43 **Accommodative component in esotropia**
H50.5 **Heterophoria**
`5th` **H50.50** **Unspecified heterophoria**
  H50.51 **Esophoria**
  H50.52 **Exophoria**
  H50.53 **Vertical heterophoria**
  H50.54 **Cyclophoria**
  H50.55 **Alternating heterophoria**
H50.6 **Mechanical strabismus**
`5th` **H50.60** **Mechanical strabismus, unspecified**
  H50.61 **Brown's sheath syndrome**
    `6th` **H50.611** **Brown's sheath syndrome, right eye**
    H50.612 **Brown's sheath syndrome, left eye**
  H50.69 **Other mechanical strabismus**
    Strabismus due to adhesions
    Traumatic limitation of duction of eye muscle
H50.8 **Other specified strabismus**
`5th` **H50.81** **Duane's syndrome**
    `6th` **H50.811** **Duane's syndrome, right eye**
    H50.812 **Duane's syndrome, left eye**
  H50.89 **Other specified strabismus**
H50.9 **Unspecified strabismus**

H52 **DISORDERS OF REFRACTION AND ACCOMMODATION**
`4th` **H52.0** **Hypermetropia**
  `5th` **H52.01** **Hypermetropia, right eye**
  H52.02 **Hypermetropia, left eye**
  H52.03 **Hypermetropia, bilateral**
H52.1 **Myopia**
`5th` *Excludes1:* degenerative myopia (H44.2-)
  H52.11 **Myopia, right eye**
  H52.12 **Myopia, left eye**
  H52.13 **Myopia, bilateral**
H52.2 **Astigmatism**
`5th` **H52.20** **Unspecified astigmatism**
    `6th` **H52.201** **Unspecified astigmatism, right eye**
    H52.202 **Unspecified astigmatism, left eye**
    H52.203 **Unspecified astigmatism, bilateral**
  H52.21 **Irregular astigmatism**
    `6th` **H52.211** **Irregular astigmatism, right eye**
    H52.212 **Irregular astigmatism, left eye**
    H52.213 **Irregular astigmatism, bilateral**
  H52.22 **Regular astigmatism**
    `6th` **H52.221** **Regular astigmatism, right eye**
    H52.222 **Regular astigmatism, left eye**
    H52.223 **Regular astigmatism, bilateral**
H52.3 **Anisometropia and aniseikonia**
`5th` **H52.31** **Anisometropia**
  H52.32 **Aniseikonia**
H52.4 **Presbyopia**
H52.5 **Disorders of accommodation**
`5th` **H52.51** **Internal ophthalmoplegia (complete) (total)**
    `6th` **H52.511** **Internal ophthalmoplegia (complete) (total), right eye**
    H52.512 **Internal ophthalmoplegia (complete) (total), left eye**
    H52.513 **Internal ophthalmoplegia (complete) (total), bilateral**
  H52.52 **Paresis of accommodation**
    `6th` **H52.521** **Paresis of accommodation, right eye**
    H52.522 **Paresis of accommodation, left eye**
    H52.523 **Paresis of accommodation, bilateral**
  H52.53 **Spasm of accommodation**
    `6th` **H52.531** **Spasm of accommodation, right eye**
    H52.532 **Spasm of accommodation, left eye**
    H52.533 **Spasm of accommodation, bilateral**
H52.6 **Other disorders of refraction**
H52.7 **Unspecified disorder of refraction**

(H53–H54) VISUAL DISTURBANCES AND BLINDNESS

H53 **VISUAL DISTURBANCES**
`4th` **H53.0** **Amblyopia ex anopsia**
`5th` *Excludes1:* amblyopia due to vitamin A deficiency (E50.5)
  H53.00 **Unspecified amblyopia**
    `6th` **H53.001** **Unspecified amblyopia, right eye**
    H53.002 **Unspecified amblyopia, left eye**
    H53.003 **Unspecified amblyopia, bilateral**
  H53.01 **Deprivation amblyopia**
    `6th` **H53.011** **Deprivation amblyopia, right eye**
    H53.012 **Deprivation amblyopia, left eye**
    H53.013 **Deprivation amblyopia, bilateral**
  H53.02 **Refractive amblyopia**
    `6th` **H53.021** **Refractive amblyopia, right eye**
    H53.022 **Refractive amblyopia, left eye**
    H53.023 **Refractive amblyopia, bilateral**
  •**H53.04** **Amblyopia suspect**
    `6th` •**H53.041** **Amblyopia suspect, right eye**
    •**H53.042** **Amblyopia suspect, left eye**
    •**H53.043** **Amblyopia suspect, bilateral eye**
H53.8 **Other visual disturbances**
H53.9 **Unspecified visual disturbance**

   Additional Character Required   3-character code   Unspecified laterality codes were excluded here.   •=New Code   ▲=Revised Code   *Excludes1*—Not coded here, do not use together   *Excludes2*—Not included here

H54 BLINDNESS AND LOW VISION

 4th

Note: For definition of visual impairment categories see table below

Code first any associated underlying cause of the blindness

Excludes1: amaurosis fugax (G45.3)

H54.0 Blindness, both eyes
Visual impairment categories 3, 4, 5 in both eyes.

H54.1 Blindness, one eye, low vision other eye

5th Visual impairment categories 3, 4, 5 in one eye, with categories 1 or 2 in the other eye.

    H54.11 Blindness, right eye, low vision left eye
    H54.12 Blindness, left eye, low vision right eye

H54.2 Low vision, both eyes
Visual impairment categories 1 or 2 in both eyes.

H54.3 Unqualified visual loss, both eyes
Visual impairment category 9 in both eyes.

H54.4 Blindness, one eye

5th Visual impairment categories 3, 4, 5 in one eye [normal vision in other eye]

    H54.41 Blindness, right eye, normal vision left eye
    H54.42 Blindness, left eye, normal vision right eye

H54.5 Low vision, one eye

5th Visual impairment categories 1 or 2 in one eye [normal vision in other eye].

    H54.51 Low vision, right eye, normal vision left eye
    H54.52 Low vision, left eye, normal vision right eye

H54.6 Unqualified visual loss, one eye

5th Visual impairment category 9 in one eye [normal vision in other eye].

    H54.61 Unqualified visual loss, right eye, normal vision left eye
    H54.62 Unqualified visual loss, left eye, normal vision right eye

H54.7 Unspecified visual loss
Visual impairment category 9 NOS

H54.8 Legal blindness, as defined in USA
Blindness NOS according to USA definition

Excludes1: legal blindness with specification of impairment level (H54.0–H54.7)

Note: The term 'low vision' in category H54 comprises categories 1 and 2 of the table, the term 'blindness' categories 3, 4 and 5, and the term 'unqualified visual loss' category 9.

If the extent of the visual field is taken into account, patients with a field no greater than 10 but greater than 5 around central fixation should be placed in category 3 and patients with a field no greater than 5around central fixation should be placed in category 4, even if the central acuity is not impaired.

Category of visual impairment	Visual acuity with best possible correction	
	Maximum less than:	Minimum equal to or better than
	6/18	6/60
3/10 (0.3)	1/10 (0.1)	
20/70	20/200	
	6/60	3/60
1/10 (0.1)	1/20 (0.05)	
20/200	20/400	
	3/60	1/60 (finger counting at one meter)
1/20 (0.05)	1/50 (0.02)	
20/400	5/300 (20/1200)	
	1/60 (finer counting at one meter)	Light perception
1/50 (0.02)		
5/300		
	No light perception	
	Undetermined or unspecified	

(H55–H57) OTHER DISORDERS OF EYE AND ADNEXA

H55 NYSTAGMUS AND OTHER IRREGULAR EYE MOVEMENTS

4th **H55.0 Nystagmus**

5th   **H55.00 Unspecified nystagmus**
  H55.01 Congenital nystagmus
  H55.02 Latent nystagmus
  H55.03 Visual deprivation nystagmus
  H55.04 Dissociated nystagmus
  H55.09 Other forms of nystagmus

(H59) INTRAOPERATIVE AND POSTPROCEDURAL COMPLICATIONS AND DISORDERS OF EYE AND ADNEXA, NOT ELSEWHERE CLASSIFIED

   Additional Character Required **3-character code**

Unspecified laterality codes were excluded here.

•=New Code
▲=Revised Code

Excludes1—Not coded here, do not use together
Excludes2—Not included here

Chapter 8. Diseases of the ear and mastoid process (H60–H95)

GUIDELINES

Note: Use an external cause code following the code for the ear condition, if applicable, to identify the cause of the ear condition

Excludes2: certain conditions originating in the perinatal period (P04–P96)
    certain infectious and parasitic diseases (A00–B99)
    complications of pregnancy, childbirth and the puerperium (O00–O9A)
    congenital malformations, deformations and chromosomal abnormalities (Q00–Q99)
    endocrine, nutritional and metabolic diseases (E00–E88)
    injury, poisoning and certain other consequences of external causes (S00–T88)
    neoplasms (C00–D49)
    symptoms, signs and abnormal clinical and laboratory findings, not elsewhere classified (R00–R94)

(H60–H62) DISEASES OF EXTERNAL EAR

H60 **OTITIS EXTERNA** `4th`
H60.0 **Abscess of external ear** `5th`
  Boil of external ear
  Carbuncle of auricle or external auditory canal
  Furuncle of external ear
  H60.01 **Abscess of right external ear**
  H60.02 **Abscess of left external ear**
  H60.03 **Abscess of external ear, bilateral**
H60.1 **Cellulitis of external ear** `5th`
  Cellulitis of auricle
  Cellulitis of external auditory canal
  H60.11 **Cellulitis of right external ear**
  H60.12 **Cellulitis of left external ear**
  H60.13 **Cellulitis of external ear, bilateral**
H60.3 **Other infective otitis externa**
  H60.31 **Diffuse otitis externa** `5th`
    H60.311 **Diffuse otitis externa, right ear** `6th`
    H60.312 **Diffuse otitis externa, left ear**
    H60.313 **Diffuse otitis externa, bilateral**
  H60.32 **Hemorrhagic otitis externa**
    H60.321 **Hemorrhagic otitis externa, right ear** `6th`
    H60.322 **Hemorrhagic otitis externa, left ear**
    H60.323 **Hemorrhagic otitis externa, bilateral**
  H60.33 **Swimmer's ear**
    H60.331 **Swimmer's ear, right ear** `6th`
    H60.332 **Swimmer's ear, left ear**
    H60.333 **Swimmer's ear, bilateral**
  H60.39 **Other infective otitis externa**
    H60.391 **Other infective otitis externa, right ear** `6th`
    H60.392 **Other infective otitis externa, left ear**
    H60.393 **Other infective otitis externa, bilateral**
H60.5 **Acute noninfective otitis externa**
  H60.50 **Unspecified acute noninfective otitis externa** `5th`
    Acute otitis externa NOS
    H60.501 **Unspecified acute noninfective otitis externa, right ear** `6th`
    H60.502 **Unspecified acute noninfective otitis externa, left ear**
    H60.503 **Unspecified acute noninfective otitis externa, bilateral**
H60.9 **Unspecified otitis externa**
  H60.91 **Unspecified otitis externa, right ear** `5th`
  H60.92 **Unspecified otitis externa, left ear**
  H60.93 **Unspecified otitis externa, bilateral**

H61 **OTHER DISORDERS OF EXTERNAL EAR** `4th`
H61.1 **Noninfective disorders of pinna** `5th`
  Excludes2: cauliflower ear (M95.1-)
    gouty tophi of ear (M1A.-)
  H61.10 **Unspecified noninfective disorders of pinna**
    Disorder of pinna NOS `6th`
    H61.101 **Unspecified noninfective disorders of pinna, right ear**
    H61.102 **Unspecified noninfective disorders of pinna, left ear**
    H61.103 **Unspecified noninfective disorders of pinna, bilateral**

H61.11 **Acquired deformity of pinna**
  Acquired deformity of auricle `6th`
  Excludes2: cauliflower ear (M95.1-)
  H61.111 **Acquired deformity of pinna, right ear**
  H61.112 **Acquired deformity of pinna, left ear**
  H61.113 **Acquired deformity of pinna, bilateral**
H61.12 **Hematoma of pinna**
  Hematoma of auricle `6th`
  H61.121 **Hematoma of pinna, right ear**
  H61.122 **Hematoma of pinna, left ear**
  H61.123 **Hematoma of pinna, bilateral**
H61.19 **Other noninfective disorders of pinna**
  H61.191 **Noninfective disorders of pinna, right ear** `6th`
  H61.192 **Noninfective disorders of pinna, left ear**
  H61.193 **Noninfective disorders of pinna, bilateral**
H61.2 **Impacted cerumen** `5th`
  Wax in ear
  H61.21 **Impacted cerumen, right ear**
  H61.22 **Impacted cerumen, left ear**
  H61.23 **Impacted cerumen, bilateral**

H62 **DISORDERS OF EXTERNAL EAR IN DISEASES CLASSIFIED ELSEWHERE** `4th`
H62.4 **Otitis externa in other diseases classified elsewhere** `5th`
  Code first underlying disease, such as: erysipelas (A46)
    impetigo (L01.0)
  Excludes1: otitis externa (in):
    candidiasis (B37.84)
    herpes viral [herpes simplex] (B00.1)
    herpes zoster (B02.8)
  H62.41 **Otitis externa in other diseases classified elsewhere, right ear**
  H62.42 **Otitis externa in other diseases classified elsewhere, left ear**
  H62.43 **Otitis externa in other diseases classified elsewhere, bilateral**

(H65–H75) DISEASES OF MIDDLE EAR AND MASTOID

H65 **NONSUPPURATIVE OTITIS MEDIA** `4th`
  Includes: nonsuppurative otitis media with myringitis
  Use additional code for any associated perforated tympanic membrane (H72.-)
  Use additional code to identify:
    exposure to environmental tobacco smoke (Z77.22)
    exposure to tobacco smoke in the perinatal period (P96.81)
    history of tobacco dependence (Z87.891)
    occupational exposure to environmental tobacco smoke (Z57.31)
    tobacco dependence (F17.-)
    tobacco use (Z72.0)
H65.0 **Acute serous otitis media** `5th`
  Acute and subacute secretory otitis
  H65.01 **Acute serous otitis media, right ear**
  H65.02 **Acute serous otitis media, left ear**
  H65.03 **Acute serous otitis media, bilateral**
  H65.04 **Acute serous otitis media, recurrent, right ear**
  H65.05 **Acute serous otitis media, recurrent, left ear**
  H65.06 **Acute serous otitis media, recurrent, bilateral**
H65.2 **Chronic serous otitis media** `5th`
  Chronic tubotympanal catarrh
  H65.21 **Chronic serous otitis media, right ear**
  H65.22 **Chronic serous otitis media, left ear**
  H65.23 **Chronic serous otitis media, bilateral**
H65.9 **Unspecified nonsuppurative otitis media** `5th`
  Allergic otitis media NOS
  Catarrhal otitis media NOS
  Exudative otitis media NOS
  Mucoid otitis media NOS
  Otitis media with effusion (nonpurulent) NOS
  Secretory otitis media NOS
  Seromucinous otitis media NOS
  Serous otitis media NOS
  Transudative otitis media NOS

`4th` `5th` `6th` `7th` Additional Character Required   ✓ 3-character code   Unspecified laterality codes were excluded here.   •=New Code   ▲=Revised Code   *Excludes1*—Not coded here, do not use together   *Excludes2*—Not included here

CHAPTER 8. DISEASES OF THE EAR AND MASTOID PROCESS   (H65.91–H83.09)

H65.91   Unspecified nonsuppurative otitis media, right ear
H65.92   Unspecified nonsuppurative otitis media, left ear
H65.93   Unspecified nonsuppurative otitis media, bilateral

H66 **SUPPURATIVE AND UNSPECIFIED OTITIS MEDIA**

Includes: suppurative and unspecified otitis media with myringitis
Use additional code to identify: exposure to environmental tobacco smoke (Z77.22)
    exposure to tobacco smoke in the perinatal period (P96.81)
    history of tobacco dependence (Z87.891)
    occupational exposure to environmental tobacco smoke (Z57.31)
    tobacco dependence (F17.-)
    tobacco use (Z72.0)

H66.0   **Acute suppurative otitis media**
   H66.00   **Acute suppurative otitis media without spontaneous rupture of; ear drum**
       H66.001   right ear drum
       H66.002   left ear drum
       H66.003   bilateral ear drums
       H66.004   recurrent, right ear drum
       H66.005   recurrent, left ear drum
       H66.006   recurrent, bilateral ear drums
    H66.01   **Acute suppurative otitis media with spontaneous rupture of; ear drum**
       H66.011   right ear drum
       H66.012   left ear drum
       H66.013   bilateral ear drums
       H66.014   recurrent, right ear drum
       H66.015   recurrent, left ear drum
       H66.016   recurrent, bilateral ear drums

H66.3   **Other chronic suppurative otitis media**
   Chronic suppurative otitis media NOS
Use additional code for any associated perforated tympanic membrane (H72.-)
Excludes1: tuberculous otitis media (A18.6)
    H66.3X   **Other chronic suppurative otitis media**
       H66.3X1 Other chronic suppurative otitis media, right ear
       H66.3X2 Other chronic suppurative otitis media, left ear
       H66.3X3 Other chronic suppurative otitis media, bilateral

H66.4   **Suppurative otitis media, unspecified**
   Purulent otitis media NOS
Use additional code for any associated perforated tympanic membrane (H72.-)
    H66.41   Suppurative otitis media, unspecified, right ear
    H66.42   Suppurative otitis media, unspecified, left ear
    H66.43   Suppurative otitis media, unspecified, bilateral

H66.9   **Otitis media, unspecified**
   Otitis media NOS
Acute otitis media NOS
Chronic otitis media NOS
Use additional code for any associated perforated tympanic membrane (H72.-)
    H66.91   Otitis media, unspecified, right ear
    H66.92   Otitis media, unspecified, left ear
    H66.93   Otitis media, unspecified, bilateral

H67 **OTITIS MEDIA IN DISEASES CLASSIFIED ELSEWHERE**

Code first underlying disease, such as:
    viral disease NEC (B00–B34)
Use additional code for any associated perforated tympanic membrane (H72.-)
Excludes1: otitis media in: influenza (J09.X9, J10.83, J11.83)
    measles (B05.3)
    scarlet fever (A38.0)
    tuberculosis (A18.6)
H67.1   Otitis media in diseases classified elsewhere, right ear
H67.2   Otitis media in diseases classified elsewhere, left ear
H67.3   Otitis media in diseases classified elsewhere, bilateral

H69 **OTHER AND UNSPECIFIED DISORDERS OF EUSTACHIAN TUBE**

H69.9   **Unspecified Eustachian tube disorder**
    H69.91   Unspecified Eustachian tube disorder, right ear
    H69.92   Unspecified Eustachian tube disorder, left ear
    H69.93   Unspecified Eustachian tube disorder, bilateral

H72   **PERFORATION OF TYMPANIC MEMBRANE**

Includes: persistent post-traumatic perforation of ear drum
    postinflammatory perforation of ear drum
Code first any associated otitis media (H65.-, H66.1-, H66.2-, H66.3-, H66.4-, H66.9-, H67.-)
Excludes1: acute suppurative otitis media with rupture of the tympanic membrane (H66.01-)
    traumatic rupture of ear drum (S09.2-)

H72.0   **Central perforation of tympanic membrane**
   H72.01   Central perforation of tympanic membrane, right ear
    H72.02   Central perforation of tympanic membrane, left ear
    H72.03   Central perforation of tympanic membrane, bilateral

H72.1   **Attic perforation of tympanic membrane**
    Perforation of pars flaccida
    H72.11   Attic perforation of tympanic membrane, right ear
    H72.12   Attic perforation of tympanic membrane, left ear
    H72.13   Attic perforation of tympanic membrane, bilateral

H72.2   **Other marginal perforations of tympanic membrane**
   H72.2X   **Other marginal perforations of tympanic membrane**
       H72.2X1   Other marginal perforations of tympanic membrane, right ear
       H72.2X2   Other marginal perforations of tympanic membrane, left ear
       H72.2X3   Other marginal perforations of tympanic membrane, bilateral

H72.8   **Other perforations of tympanic membrane**
   H72.81   **Multiple perforations of tympanic membrane**
       H72.811   Multiple perforations of tympanic membrane, right ear
       H72.812   Multiple perforations of tympanic membrane, left ear
       H72.813   Multiple perforations of tympanic membrane, bilateral
    H72.82   **Total perforations of tympanic membrane**
       H72.821   Total perforations of tympanic membrane, right ear
       H72.822   Total perforations of tympanic membrane, left ear
       H72.823   Total perforations of tympanic membrane, bilateral

H72.9   **Unspecified perforation of tympanic membrane**
   H72.91   Unspecified perforation of tympanic membrane, right ear
    H72.92   Unspecified perforation of tympanic membrane, left ear
    H72.93   Unspecified perforation of tympanic membrane, bilateral

H73   **OTHER DISORDERS OF TYMPANIC MEMBRANE**

H73.0   **Acute myringitis**
Excludes1: acute myringitis with otitis media (H65, H66)
   H73.01   Bullous myringitis
       H73.011   Bullous myringitis, right ear
       H73.012   Bullous myringitis, left ear
       H73.013   Bullous myringitis, bilateral

(H80–H83) DISEASES OF INNER EAR

H83   **OTHER DISEASES OF INNER EAR**

H83.0   **Labyrinthitis**
    H83.01   Labyrinthitis, right ear
    H83.02   Labyrinthitis, left ear
    H83.03   Labyrinthitis, bilateral
    H83.09   Labyrinthitis, unspecified ear

  Additional Character Required   ✔ 3-character code   Unspecified laterality codes were excluded here.   •=New Code   ▲=Revised Code   *Excludes1*—Not coded here, do not use together   *Excludes2*—Not included here

(H90–H94) OTHER DISORDERS OF EAR

H90   **CONDUCTIVE AND SENSORINEURAL HEARING LOSS**

`4th`

    Excludes1: deaf nonspeaking NEC (H91.3)
      deafness NOS (H91.9-)
      hearing loss NOS (H91.9-)
      noise-induced hearing loss (H83.3-)
      ototoxic hearing loss (H91.0-)
      sudden (idiopathic) hearing loss (H91.2-)

H90.0   Conductive hearing loss, bilateral

H90.1   Conductive hearing loss, unilateral with unrestricted hearing on the contralateral side

`5th`

    H90.11   Conductive hearing loss, unilateral, right ear, with unrestricted hearing on the contralateral side
    H90.12   Conductive hearing loss, unilateral, left ear, with unrestricted hearing on the contralateral side

H90.2   Conductive hearing loss, unspecified
    Conductive deafness NOS

H90.3   Sensorineural hearing loss, bilateral

H90.4   Sensorineural hearing loss, unilateral with unrestricted hearing on the contralateral side

`5th`

    H90.41   Sensorineural hearing loss, unilateral, right ear, with unrestricted hearing on the contralateral side
    H90.42   Sensorineural hearing loss, unilateral, left ear, with unrestricted hearing on the contralateral side

H90.5   Unspecified sensorineural hearing loss
    Central hearing loss NOS
    Congenital deafness NOS
    Neural hearing loss NOS
    Perceptive hearing loss NOS
    Sensorineural deafness NOS
    Sensory hearing loss NOS
    Excludes1: abnormal auditory perception (H93.2-)
      psychogenic deafness (F44.6)

H90.6   Mixed conductive and sensorineural hearing loss, bilateral

H90.7   Mixed conductive and sensorineural hearing loss, unilateral with unrestricted hearing on the contralateral side

`5th`

    H90.71   Mixed conductive and sensorineural hearing loss, unilateral, right ear, with unrestricted hearing on the contralateral side
    H90.72   Mixed conductive and sensorineural hearing loss, unilateral, left ear, with unrestricted hearing on the contralateral side

• **H90.A**   Hearing loss, unilateral, with restricted hearing on the contralateral side

`5th`

    • **H90.A1**   Conductive hearing loss, unilateral, with restricted hearing on the contralateral side

    `6th`

      • **H90.A11**   Conductive hearing loss, unilateral, right ear with restricted hearing on the contralateral side
      • **H90.A12**   Conductive hearing loss, unilateral, left ear with restricted hearing on the contralateral side

    • **H90.A2**   Sensorineural hearing loss, unilateral, with restricted hearing on the contralateral side

    `6th`

      • **H90.A21**   Sensorineural hearing loss, unilateral, right ear, with restricted hearing on the contralateral side
      • **H90.A22**   Sensorineural hearing loss, unilateral, left ear, with restricted hearing on the contralateral side

    • **H90.A3**   Mixed conductive and sensorineural hearing loss, unilateral, with restricted hearing on the contralateral side

    `6th`

      • **H90.A31**   Mixed conductive and sensorineural hearing loss, unilateral, right ear with restricted hearing on the contralateral side
      • **H90.A32**   Mixed conductive and sensorineural hearing, unilateral, left ear with restricted hearing on the contralateral side

H90.8   Mixed conductive and sensorineural hearing loss, unspecified

H91   **OTHER AND UNSPECIFIED HEARING LOSS**

`4th`

    Excludes1: abnormal auditory perception (H93.2-)
      hearing loss as classified in H90.-
      impacted cerumen (H61.2-)
      noise-induced hearing loss (H83.3-)
      psychogenic deafness (F44.6)
      transient ischemic deafness (H93.01-)

H91.2   Sudden idiopathic hearing loss
    Sudden hearing loss NOS

`5th`

    H91.21   Sudden idiopathic hearing loss, right ear
    H91.22   Sudden idiopathic hearing loss, left ear
    H91.23   Sudden idiopathic hearing loss, bilateral

H91.3   Deaf nonspeaking, not elsewhere classified

H91.8   Other specified hearing loss

    H91.8X Other specified hearing loss

`5th`

    `6th`

      H91.8X1   Other specified hearing loss, right ear
      H91.8X2   Other specified hearing loss, left ear
      H91.8X3   Other specified hearing loss, bilateral

H91.9   Unspecified hearing loss
    Deafness NOS

`5th`

    High frequency deafness
    Low frequency deafness
    H91.91   Unspecified hearing loss, right ear
    H91.92   Unspecified hearing loss, left ear
    H91.93   Unspecified hearing loss, bilateral

H92   **OTALGIA AND EFFUSION OF EAR**

`4th`

H92.0   Otalgia

`5th`

    H92.01   Otalgia, right ear
    H92.02   Otalgia, left ear
    H92.03   Otalgia, bilateral

H92.1   Otorrhea

`5th`

    Excludes1: leakage of cerebrospinal fluid through ear (G96.0)
    H92.11   Otorrhea, right ear
    H92.12   Otorrhea, left ear
    H92.13   Otorrhea, bilateral

H93   **OTHER DISORDERS OF EAR, NOT ELSEWHERE CLASSIFIED**

`4th`

H93.1   Tinnitus

`5th`

    H93.11   Tinnitus, right ear
    H93.12   Tinnitus, left ear
    H93.13   Tinnitus, bilateral

• **H93.A**   Pulsatile tinnitus

`5th`

    • **H93.A1**   Pulsatile tinnitus, right ear
    • **H93.A2**   Pulsatile tinnitus, left ear
    • **H93.A3**   Pulsatile tinnitus, bilateral

H93.2   Other abnormal auditory perceptions

`5th`

    Excludes2: auditory hallucinations (R44.0)
    H93.25   Central auditory processing disorder
      Congenital auditory imperception
      Word deafness
    H93.29   Other abnormal auditory perceptions

    `6th`

      H93.291   Other abnormal auditory perceptions, right ear
      H93.292   Other abnormal auditory perceptions, left ear
      H93.293   Other abnormal auditory perceptions, bilateral

(H95) INTRAOPERATIVE AND POSTPROCEDURAL COMPLICATIONS AND DISORDERS OF EAR AND MASTOID PROCESS, NOT ELSEWHERE CLASSIFIED

CHAPTER 8. DISEASES OF THE EAR AND MASTOID PROCESS   (H90–H95)

   `4th` `5th` `6th` `7th`   Additional Character Required   3-character code   Unspecified laterality codes were excluded here.   •=New Code   ▲=Revised Code   ***Excludes1***—Not coded here, do not use together   ***Excludes2***—Not included here

Chapter 9. Diseases of the circulatory system (I00–I99)

GUIDELINES

Refer to ICD-10-CM Official Guidelines for Coding and Reporting for instructions for reporting hypertensive diseases, atherosclerotic coronary artery disease, cerebrovascular accident, and/or myocardial infarction

Excludes2:
certain conditions originating in the perinatal period (P04 – P96)
certain infectious and parasitic diseases (A00 – B99)
complications of pregnancy, childbirth and the puerperium (O00 – O9A)
congenital malformations, deformations, and chromosomal abnormalities (Q00 – Q99)
endocrine, nutritional and metabolic diseases (E00 – E88)
injury, poisoning and certain other consequences of external causes (S00 – T88)
neoplasms (C00 – D49)
symptoms, signs and abnormal clinical and laboratory findings, not elsewhere classified (R00 – R94)
systemic connective tissue disorders (M30 – M36)
transient cerebral ischemic attacks and related syndromes (G45.-)

(I00–I02) ACUTE RHEUMATIC FEVER

I00 — RHEUMATIC FEVER WITHOUT HEART INVOLVEMENT
Includes: arthritis, rheumatic, acute or subacute
Excludes1: rheumatic fever with heart involvement (I01.0 – I01.9)

I01 — RHEUMATIC FEVER WITH HEART INVOLVEMENT `4th`
Excludes1: chronic diseases of rheumatic origin (I05 – I09) unless rheumatic fever is also present or there is evidence of reactivation or activity of the rheumatic process.

I01.0 Acute rheumatic pericarditis
Any condition in I00 with pericarditis
Rheumatic pericarditis (acute)
Excludes1: acute pericarditis not specified as rheumatic (I30.-)

I01.1 Acute rheumatic endocarditis
Any condition in I00 with endocarditis or valvulitis
Acute rheumatic valvulitis

I01.2 Acute rheumatic myocarditis
Any condition in I00 with myocarditis

I01.8 Other acute rheumatic heart disease
Any condition in I00 with other or multiple types of heart involvement
Acute rheumatic pancarditis

I01.9 Acute rheumatic heart disease, unspecified
Any condition in I00 with unspecified type of heart involvement
Rheumatic carditis, acute
Rheumatic heart disease, active or acute

(I05–I09) CHRONIC RHEUMATIC HEART DISEASES

I05 — RHEUMATIC MITRAL VALVE DISEASES `4th`
Includes: conditions classifiable to both I05.0 and I05.2 – I05.9, whether specified as rheumatic or not
Excludes1: mitral valve disease specified as nonrheumatic (I34.-)
mitral valve disease with aortic and/or tricuspid valve involvement (I08.-)

I05.0 Rheumatic mitral stenosis
Mitral (valve) obstruction (rheumatic)

I05.1 Rheumatic mitral insufficiency
Rheumatic mitral incompetence
Rheumatic mitral regurgitation
Excludes1: mitral insufficiency not specified as rheumatic (I34.0)

I05.2 Rheumatic mitral stenosis with insufficiency
Rheumatic mitral stenosis with incompetence or regurgitation

I05.8 Other rheumatic mitral valve diseases
Rheumatic mitral (valve) failure

I05.9 Rheumatic mitral valve disease, unspecified
Rheumatic mitral (valve) disorder (chronic) NOS

I06 — RHEUMATIC AORTIC VALVE DISEASES `4th`
Excludes1: aortic valve disease not specified as rheumatic (I35.-)
aortic valve disease with mitral and/or tricuspid valve involvement (I08.-)

I06.0 Rheumatic aortic stenosis
Rheumatic aortic (valve) obstruction

I06.1 Rheumatic aortic insufficiency
Rheumatic aortic incompetence
Rheumatic aortic regurgitation

I06.2 Rheumatic aortic stenosis with insufficiency
Rheumatic aortic stenosis with incompetence or regurgitation

I06.8 Other rheumatic aortic valve diseases

I06.9 Rheumatic aortic valve disease, unspecified
Rheumatic aortic (valve) disease NOS

I07 — RHEUMATIC TRICUSPID VALVE DISEASES `4th`
Includes: rheumatic tricuspid valve diseases specified as rheumatic or unspecified
Excludes1: tricuspid valve disease specified as nonrheumatic (I36.-)
tricuspid valve disease with aortic and/or mitral valve involvement (I08.-)

I07.0 Rheumatic tricuspid stenosis
Tricuspid (valve) stenosis (rheumatic)

I07.1 Rheumatic tricuspid insufficiency
Tricuspid (valve) insufficiency (rheumatic)

I07.2 Rheumatic tricuspid stenosis and insufficiency

I07.8 Other rheumatic tricuspid valve diseases

I07.9 Rheumatic tricuspid valve disease, unspecified
Rheumatic tricuspid valve disorder NOS

(I10–I16) HYPERTENSIVE DISEASES

Use additional code to identify: exposure to environmental tobacco smoke (Z77.22)
history of tobacco dependence (Z87.891)
occupational exposure to environmental tobacco smoke (Z57.31)
tobacco dependence (F17.-)
tobacco use (Z72.0)
Excludes1: neonatal hypertension (P29.2)
primary pulmonary hypertension (I27.0)
Excludes2: hypertensive disease complicating pregnancy, childbirth and the puerperium (O10 – O11, O13 – O16)

I10 — ESSENTIAL (PRIMARY) HYPERTENSION
Includes: high blood pressure
hypertension (arterial) (benign) (essential) (malignant) (primary) (systemic)
Excludes1: hypertensive disease complicating pregnancy, childbirth and the puerperium (O10 – O11, O13 – O16)
Excludes2: essential (primary) hypertension involving vessels of brain (I60 – I69)
essential (primary) hypertension involving vessels of eye (H35.0-)

•I16 — HYPERTENSIVE CRISIS `4th`
Code also any identified hypertensive disease (I10–I15)
•I16.0 Hypertensive urgency
•I16.1 Hypertensive emergency
•I16.9 Hypertensive crisis, unspecified

(I20–I25) ISCHEMIC HEART DISEASES

Use additional code to identify presence of hypertension (I10–I16)
Please see full ICD-10-CM manual for cardiovascular disease with symptoms or infarction

I25 — CHRONIC ISCHEMIC HEART DISEASE `4th`
Use additional history of tobacco dependence (Z87.891)

I25.1 Atherosclerotic cardiovascular disease `5th`
Coronary (artery) atheroma
Coronary (artery) atherosclerosis
Coronary (artery) disease
Coronary (artery) sclerosis

I25.10 Atherosclerotic heart disease of native coronary artery without angina pectoris
Atherosclerotic heart disease NOS

   Additional Character Required   3-character code

•=New Code
▲=Revised Code

Excludes1—Not coded here, do not use together
Excludes2—Not included here

CHAPTER 9. DISEASES OF THE CIRCULATORY SYSTEM (I26–I37.0)

(I26–I28) PULMONARY HEART DISEASE AND DISEASES OF PULMONARY CIRCULATION

I27 OTHER PULMONARY HEART DISEASES

I27.0 Primary pulmonary hypertension
Excludes1: pulmonary hypertension NOS (I27.2)
secondary pulmonary hypertension (I27.2)

I27.1 Kyphoscoliotic heart disease

I27.2 Other secondary pulmonary hypertension
Pulmonary hypertension NOS
Code also associated underlying condition

I27.8 Other specified pulmonary heart diseases

    I27.81 Cor pulmonale (chronic)
Cor pulmonale NOS
Excludes1: acute cor pulmonale (I26.0-)

    I27.82 Chronic pulmonary embolism
Use additional code, if applicable, for associated long-term (current) use of anticoagulants (Z79.01)
Excludes1: personal history of pulmonary embolism (Z86.711)

    I27.89 Other specified pulmonary heart diseases
Eisenmenger's complex
Eisenmenger's syndrome
Excludes1: Eisenmenger's defect (Q21.8)

I27.9 Pulmonary heart disease, unspecified
Chronic cardiopulmonary disease

(I30–I52) OTHER FORMS OF HEART DISEASE

I30 ACUTE PERICARDITIS

Includes: acute mediastinopericarditis
acute myopericarditis
acute pericardial effusion
acute pleuropericarditis
acute pneumopericarditis
Excludes1: Dressler's syndrome (I24.1)
rheumatic pericarditis (acute) (I01.0)

I30.0 Acute nonspecific idiopathic pericarditis

I30.1 Infective pericarditis
Pneumococcal pericarditis
Pneumopyopericardium
Purulent pericarditis
Pyopericarditis
Pyopericardium
Pyopneumopericardium
Staphylococcal pericarditis
Streptococcal pericarditis
Suppurative pericarditis
Viral pericarditis
Use additional code (B95–B97) to identify infectious agent

I30.8 Other forms of acute pericarditis

I30.9 Acute pericarditis, unspecified

I31 OTHER DISEASES OF PERICARDIUM

Excludes1: diseases of pericardium specified as rheumatic (I09.2)
postcardiotomy syndrome (I97.0)
traumatic injury to pericardium (S26.-)

I31.0 Chronic adhesive pericarditis
Accretio cordis
Adherent pericardium
Adhesive mediastinopericarditis

I31.1 Chronic constrictive pericarditis
Concretio cordis
Pericardial calcification

I31.2 Hemopericardium, not elsewhere classified
Excludes1: hemopericardium as current complication following acute myocardial infarction (I23.0)

I31.3 Pericardial effusion (noninflammatory)
Chylopericardium
Excludes1: acute pericardial effusion (I30.9)

I31.4 Cardiac tamponade
Code first underlying cause

I31.8 Other specified diseases of pericardium
Epicardial plaques
Focal pericardial adhesions

I31.9 Disease of pericardium, unspecified
Pericarditis (chronic) NOS

I33 ACUTE AND SUBACUTE ENDOCARDITIS

Excludes1: acute rheumatic endocarditis (I01.1)
endocarditis NOS (I38)

I33.0 Acute and subacute infective endocarditis
Bacterial endocarditis (acute) (subacute)
Infective endocarditis (acute) (subacute) NOS
Endocarditis lenta (acute) (subacute)
Malignant endocarditis (acute) (subacute)
Purulent endocarditis (acute) (subacute)
Septic endocarditis (acute) (subacute)
Ulcerative endocarditis (acute) (subacute)
Vegetative endocarditis (acute) (subacute)
Use additional code (B95–B97) to identify infectious agent

I33.9 Acute and subacute endocarditis, unspecified
Acute endocarditis NOS
Acute myoendocarditis NOS
Acute periendocarditis NOS
Subacute endocarditis NOS
Subacute myoendocarditis NOS
Subacute periendocarditis NOS

I34 NONRHEUMATIC MITRAL VALVE DISORDERS

Excludes1: mitral valve disease (I05.9)
mitral valve failure (I05.8)
mitral valve stenosis (I05.0)
mitral valve disorder of unspecified cause with diseases of aortic and/or tricuspid valve(s) (I08.-)
mitral valve disorder of unspecified cause with mitral stenosis or obstruction (I05.0)
mitral valve disorder specified as congenital (Q23.2, Q23.3)
mitral valve disorder specified as rheumatic (I05.-)

I34.0 Nonrheumatic mitral (valve) insufficiency
Nonrheumatic mitral (valve) incompetence NOS
Nonrheumatic mitral (valve) regurgitation NOS

I35 NONRHEUMATIC AORTIC VALVE DISORDERS

Excludes1: aortic valve disorder of unspecified cause but with diseases of mitral and/or tricuspid valve(s) (I08.-)
aortic valve disorder specified as congenital (Q23.0, Q23.1)
aortic valve disorder specified as rheumatic (I06.-)
hypertrophic subaortic stenosis (I42.1)

I35.0 Nonrheumatic aortic (valve) stenosis

I35.1 Nonrheumatic aortic (valve) insufficiency
Nonrheumatic aortic (valve) incompetence NOS
Nonrheumatic aortic (valve) regurgitation NOS

I35.2 Nonrheumatic aortic (valve) stenosis with insufficiency

I35.8 Other nonrheumatic aortic valve disorders

I35.9 Nonrheumatic aortic valve disorder, unspecified

I36 NONRHEUMATIC TRICUSPID VALVE DISORDERS

Excludes1: tricuspid valve disorders of unspecified cause (I07.-)
tricuspid valve disorders specified as congenital (Q22.4, Q22.8, Q22.9)
tricuspid valve disorders specified as rheumatic (I07.-)
tricuspid valve disorders with aortic and/or mitral valve involvement (I08.-)

I36.0 Nonrheumatic tricuspid (valve) stenosis

I36.1 Nonrheumatic tricuspid (valve) insufficiency
Nonrheumatic tricuspid (valve) incompetence
Nonrheumatic tricuspid (valve) regurgitation

I36.2 Nonrheumatic tricuspid (valve) stenosis with insufficiency

I36.8 Other nonrheumatic tricuspid valve disorders

I36.9 Nonrheumatic tricuspid valve disorder, unspecified

I37 NONRHEUMATIC PULMONARY VALVE DISORDERS

Excludes1: pulmonary valve disorder specified as congenital (Q22.1, Q22.2, Q22.3)
pulmonary valve disorder specified as rheumatic (I09.89)

I37.0 Nonrheumatic pulmonary valve stenosis

 Additional Character Required   3-character code

●=New Code
▲=Revised Code

Excludes1—Not coded here, do not use together
Excludes2—Not included here

I37.1 Nonrheumatic pulmonary valve insufficiency
Nonrheumatic pulmonary valve incompetence
Nonrheumatic pulmonary valve regurgitation
I37.2 Nonrheumatic pulmonary valve stenosis with insufficiency
I37.8 Other nonrheumatic pulmonary valve disorders
I37.9 Nonrheumatic pulmonary valve disorder, unspecified

I40 ACUTE MYOCARDITIS
4th
Includes: subacute myocarditis
Excludes1: acute rheumatic myocarditis (I01.2)
I40.0 Infective myocarditis
Septic myocarditis
Use additional code (B95–B97) to identify infectious agent
I40.8 Other acute myocarditis
I40.9 Acute myocarditis, unspecified

I42 CARDIOMYOPATHY
4th
Includes: myocardiopathy
Code first pre-existing cardiomyopathy complicating pregnancy and puerperium (O99.4)
Excludes2: ischemic cardiomyopathy (I25.5)
peripartum cardiomyopathy (O90.3)
ventricular hypertrophy (I51.7)
I42.1 Obstructive hypertrophic cardiomyopathy
Hypertrophic subaortic stenosis (idiopathic)
I42.2 Other hypertrophic cardiomyopathy
Nonobstructive hypertrophic cardiomyopathy
I42.5 Other restrictive cardiomyopathy
Constrictive cardiomyopathy NOS
I42.9 Cardiomyopathy, unspecified
Cardiomyopathy (primary) (secondary) NOS

I44 ATRIOVENTRICULAR AND LEFT BUNDLE-BRANCH BLOCK
4th
I44.0 Atrioventricular block, first degree
I44.1 Atrioventricular block, second degree
Atrioventricular block, type I and II
Möbitz block, type I and II
Second degree block, type I and II
Wenckebach's block
I44.2 Atrioventricular block, complete
Complete heart block NOS
Third degree block

I45 OTHER CONDUCTION DISORDERS
4th
I45.6 Pre-excitation syndrome
Accelerated atrioventricular conduction
Accessory atrioventricular conduction
Anomalous atrioventricular excitation
Lown-Ganong-Levine syndrome
Pre-excitation atrioventricular conduction
Wolff-Parkinson-White syndrome
I45.8 Other specified conduction disorders
5th   **I45.81 Long QT syndrome**
I45.9 Conduction disorder, unspecified
Heart block NOS
Stokes-Adams syndrome

I46 CARDIAC ARREST
4th
Excludes1: cardiogenic shock (R57.0)
I46.2 Cardiac arrest due to underlying cardiac condition
Code first underlying cardiac condition
I46.8 Cardiac arrest due to other underlying condition
Code first underlying condition
I46.9 Cardiac arrest, cause unspecified

I47 PAROXYSMAL TACHYCARDIA
4th
Code first tachycardia complicating: abortion or ectopic or molar pregnancy (O00–O07, O08.8)
obstetric surgery and procedures (O75.4)
Excludes1: tachycardia NOS (R00.0)
sinoauricular tachycardia NOS (R00.0)
sinus [sinusal] tachycardia NOS (R00.0)

I47.1 Supraventricular tachycardia
Atrial (paroxysmal) tachycardia
Atrioventricular [AV] (paroxysmal) tachycardia
Atrioventricular re-entrant (nodal) tachycardia [AVNRT] [AVRT]
Junctional (paroxysmal) tachycardia
Nodal (paroxysmal) tachycardia

I49 OTHER CARDIAC ARRHYTHMIAS
4th
Code first cardiac arrhythmia complicating: abortion or ectopic or molar pregnancy (O00–O07, O08.8)
obstetric surgery and procedures (O75.4)
Excludes1: bradycardia NOS (R00.1)
neonatal dysrhythmia (P29.1-)
sinoatrial bradycardia (R00.1)
sinus bradycardia (R00.1)
vagal bradycardia (R00.1)
I49.1 Atrial premature depolarization
Atrial premature beats
I49.5 Sick sinus syndrome
Tachycardia-bradycardia syndrome
I49.9 Cardiac arrhythmia, unspecified
Arrhythmia (cardiac) NOS

I50 HEART FAILURE
4th
Code first: heart failure complicating abortion or ectopic or molar pregnancy (O00–O07, O08.8)
heart failure due to hypertension (I11.0)
heart failure due to hypertension with CKD (I13.-)
heart failure following surgery (I97.13-)
obstetric surgery and procedures (O75.4)
rheumatic heart failure (I09.81)
Excludes1: neonatal cardiac failure (P29.0)
Excludes2: cardiac arrest (I46.-)
I50.4 Combined systolic (congestive) and diastolic (congestive) heart failure
5th
   I50.41 Acute combined systolic (congestive) and diastolic (congestive) heart failure
   I50.42 Chronic combined systolic (congestive) and diastolic (congestive) heart failure
   I50.43 Acute on chronic combined systolic (congestive) and diastolic (congestive) heart failure
I50.9 Heart failure, unspecified
Biventricular (heart) failure NOS
Cardiac, heart or myocardial failure NOS
Congestive heart disease
Congestive heart failure NOS
Right ventricular failure (secondary to left heart failure)
Excludes2: fluid overload (E87.70)

I51 COMPLICATIONS AND ILL-DEFINED DESCRIPTIONS OF HEART DISEASE
4th
Excludes1: any condition in I51.4–I51.9 due to hypertension (I11.-)
any condition in I51.4–I51.9 due to hypertension and CKD (I13.-)
heart disease specified as rheumatic (I00–I09)
I51.7 Cardiomegaly
Cardiac dilatation
Cardiac hypertrophy
Ventricular dilatation

(I60–I69) CEREBROVASCULAR DISEASES

Use additional code to identify presence of: alcohol abuse and dependence (F10.-)
exposure to environmental tobacco smoke (Z77.22)
history of tobacco dependence (Z87.891)
hypertension (I10–I15)
occupational exposure to environmental tobacco smoke (Z57.31)
tobacco dependence (F17.-)
tobacco use (Z72.0)
Excludes1: transient cerebral ischemic attacks and related syndromes (G45.-)
traumatic intracranial hemorrhage (S06.-)

 CHAPTER 9. DISEASES OF THE CIRCULATORY SYSTEM (I37.1–I69)

  4th 5th 6th 7th Additional Character Required   3-character code

•=New Code
▲=Revised Code

Excludes1—Not coded here, do not use together
Excludes2—Not included here

I60 NONTRAUMATIC SUBARACHNOID HEMORRHAGE

`4th`

Includes: ruptured cerebral aneurysm

Excludes1: syphilitic ruptured cerebral aneurysm (A52.05)

Excludes2: sequelae of subarachnoid hemorrhage (I69.0-)

I60.0 Nontraumatic subarachnoid hemorrhage from; carotid siphon and bifurcation

`5th`

    I60.00 unspecified carotid siphon and bifurcation

    I60.01 right carotid siphon and bifurcation

    I60.02 left carotid siphon and bifurcation

I60.1 Nontraumatic subarachnoid hemorrhage from; middle cerebral artery

I60.2 Nontraumatic subarachnoid hemorrhage from; anterior communicating artery

I60.3 Nontraumatic subarachnoid hemorrhage from; posterior communicating artery

`5th`

    I60.30 unspecified posterior communicating artery

    I60.31 right posterior communicating artery

    I60.32 left posterior communicating artery

I60.4 Nontraumatic subarachnoid hemorrhage from basilar artery

I60.5 Nontraumatic subarachnoid hemorrhage from; vertebral artery

`5th`

    I60.50 unspecified vertebral artery

    I60.51 from right vertebral artery

    I60.52 from left vertebral artery

I60.6 Nontraumatic subarachnoid hemorrhage from other intracranial arteries

I60.7 Nontraumatic subarachnoid hemorrhage from unspecified intracranial artery

    Ruptured (congenital) berry aneurysm

    Ruptured (congenital) cerebral aneurysm

    Subarachnoid hemorrhage (nontraumatic) from cerebral artery NOS

    Subarachnoid hemorrhage (nontraumatic) from communicating artery NOS

    Excludes1: berry aneurysm, nonruptured (I67.1)

I60.8 Other nontraumatic subarachnoid hemorrhage

    Meningeal hemorrhage

    Rupture of cerebral arteriovenous malformation

I60.9 Nontraumatic subarachnoid hemorrhage, unspecified

I61 NONTRAUMATIC INTRACEREBRAL HEMORRHAGE

`4th`

Excludes2: sequelae of intracerebral hemorrhage (I69.1-)

I61.0 Nontraumatic intracerebral hemorrhage in hemisphere, subcortical

    Deep intracerebral hemorrhage (nontraumatic)

I61.1 Nontraumatic intracerebral hemorrhage; in hemisphere, cortical

    Cerebral lobe hemorrhage (nontraumatic)

    Superficial intracerebral hemorrhage (nontraumatic)

I61.2 in hemisphere, unspecified

I61.3 in brain stem

I61.4 in cerebellum

I61.5 intraventricular

I61.6 multiple localized

I61.8 Other nontraumatic intracerebral hemorrhage

I61.9 Nontraumatic intracerebral hemorrhage, unspecified

I62 OTHER AND UNSPECIFIED NONTRAUMATIC INTRACRANIAL HEMORRHAGE

`4th`

Excludes2: sequelae of intracranial hemorrhage (I69.2)

I62.0 Nontraumatic subdural hemorrhage

`5th`

    I62.00 Nontraumatic subdural hemorrhage, unspecified

    I62.01 Nontraumatic acute subdural hemorrhage

    I62.02 Nontraumatic subacute subdural hemorrhage

    I62.03 Nontraumatic chronic subdural hemorrhage

I62.1 Nontraumatic extradural hemorrhage

    Nontraumatic epidural hemorrhage

I62.9 Nontraumatic intracranial hemorrhage, unspecified

I67 OTHER CEREBROVASCULAR DISEASES

`4th`

Excludes2: sequelae of the listed conditions (I69.8)

I67.4 Hypertensive encephalopathy

(I70–I79) DISEASES OF ARTERIES, ARTERIOLES AND CAPILLARIES

I73 OTHER PERIPHERAL VASCULAR DISEASES

`4th`

Excludes2: chilblains (T69.1)

    frostbite (T33–T34)

    immersion hand or foot (T69.0-)

    spasm of cerebral artery (G45.9)

I73.8 Other specified peripheral vascular diseases

`5th`

    Excludes1: diabetic (peripheral) angiopathy (E08–E13 with .51–.52)

    I73.89 Other specified peripheral vascular diseases

        Acrocyanosis

        Erythrocyanosis

        Simple acroparesthesia [Schultze's type]

        Vasomotor acroparesthesia [Nothnagel's type]

I74 ARTERIAL EMBOLISM AND THROMBOSIS

`4th`

Includes: embolic infarction

    embolic occlusion

    thrombotic infarction

    thrombotic occlusion

Code first embolism and thrombosis complicating abortion or ectopic or molar pregnancy (O00–O07, O08.2)

    embolism and thrombosis complicating pregnancy, childbirth and the puerperium (O88.-)

Excludes2: atheroembolism (I75.-)

    basilar embolism and thrombosis (I63.0–I63.2, I65.1)

    carotid embolism and thrombosis (I63.0–I63.2, I65.2)

    cerebral embolism and thrombosis (I63.3–I63.5, I66.-)

    coronary embolism and thrombosis (I21–I25)

    mesenteric embolism and thrombosis (K55.0-)

    ophthalmic embolism and thrombosis (H34.-)

    precerebral embolism and thrombosis NOS (I63.0–I63.2, I65.9)

    pulmonary embolism and thrombosis (I26.-)

    renal embolism and thrombosis (N28.0)

    retinal embolism and thrombosis (H34.-)

    septic embolism and thrombosis (I76)

    vertebral embolism and thrombosis (I63.0–I63.2, I65.0)

I74.9 Embolism and thrombosis of unspecified artery

I77 OTHER DISORDERS OF ARTERIES AND ARTERIOLES

`4th`

Excludes2: collagen (vascular) diseases (M30–M36)

    hypersensitivity angiitis (M31.0)

    pulmonary artery (I28.-)

I77.6 Arteritis, unspecified

    Aortitis NOS

    Endarteritis NOS

    Excludes1: arteritis or endarteritis:

        aortic arch (M31.4)

        cerebral NEC (I67.7)

        coronary (I25.89)

        deformans (I70.-)

        giant cell (M31.5., M31.6)

        obliterans (I70.-)

        senile (I70.-)

I78 DISEASES OF CAPILLARIES

`4th`

I78.0 Hereditary hemorrhagic telangiectasia

    Rendu-Osler-Weber disease

I78.1 Nevus, non-neoplastic

    Araneus nevus

    Senile nevus

    Spider nevus

    Stellar nevus

    Excludes1: nevus NOS (D22.-)

        vascular NOS (Q82.5)

    Excludes2: blue nevus (D22.-)

        flammeus nevus (Q82.5)

        hairy nevus (D22.-)

        melanocytic nevus (D22.-)

        pigmented nevus (D22.-)

        portwine nevus (Q82.5)

        sanguineous nevus (Q82.5)

        strawberry nevus (Q82.5)

        verrucous nevus (Q82.5)

`4th` `5th` `6th` `7th` Additional Character Required   3-character code

■=New Code   **Excludes1**—Not coded here, do not use together

▲=Revised Code   **Excludes2**—Not included here

(I80–I89) DISEASES OF VEINS, LYMPHATIC VESSELS AND LYMPH NODES, NOT ELSEWHERE CLASSIFIED

I80 `4th` **PHLEBITIS AND THROMBOPHLEBITIS**
Includes: endophlebitis
   inflammation, vein
   periphlebitis
   suppurative phlebitis
Code first phlebitis and thrombophlebitis complicating abortion, ectopic or molar pregnancy (O00–O07, O08.7)\phlebitis and thrombophlebitis complicating pregnancy, childbirth and the puerperium (O22.-, O87.-)
Excludes1: venous embolism and thrombosis of lower extremities (I82.4-, I82.5-, I82.81-)

I80.0 `5th` **Phlebitis and thrombophlebitis of superficial vessels of; lower extremities**
   Phlebitis and thrombophlebitis of femoropopliteal vein
   I80.00   **unspecified lower extremity**
   I80.01   **right lower extremity**
   I80.02   **left lower extremity**
   I80.03   **lower extremities, bilateral**

I80.1 `5th` **Phlebitis and thrombophlebitis of; femoral vein**
   I80.10   **unspecified femoral vein**
   I80.11   **right femoral vein**
   I80.12   **left femoral vein**
   I80.13   **femoral vein, bilateral**

I80.2 `5th` **Phlebitis and thrombophlebitis of other and unspecified deep vessels of lower extremities**
   I80.20 `6th` **Phlebitis and thrombophlebitis of unspecified deep vessels of; lower extremities**
      I80.201   **right lower extremity**
      I80.202   **left lower extremity**
      I80.203   **lower extremities, bilateral**
      I80.209   **unspecified lower extremity**
   I80.21 `6th` **Phlebitis and thrombophlebitis of; iliac vein**
      I80.211   **right iliac vein**
      I80.212   **left iliac vein**
      I80.213   **iliac vein, bilateral**
      I80.219   **unspecified iliac vein**
   I80.22 `6th` **Phlebitis and thrombophlebitis of; popliteal vein**
      I80.221   **right popliteal vein**
      I80.222   **left popliteal vein**
      I80.223   **popliteal vein, bilateral**
      I80.229   **unspecified popliteal vein**
   I80.23 `6th` **Phlebitis and thrombophlebitis of; tibial vein**
      I80.231   **right tibial vein**
      I80.232   **left tibial vein**
      I80.233   **tibial vein, bilateral**
      I80.239   **unspecified tibial vein**
   I80.29 `6th` **Phlebitis and thrombophlebitis of other deep vessels of; lower extremities**
      I80.291   **right lower extremity**
      I80.292   **left lower extremity**
      I80.293   **lower extremity, bilateral**
      I80.299   **unspecified lower extremity**

I80.3   **Phlebitis and thrombophlebitis of lower extremities, unspecified**
I80.8   **Phlebitis and thrombophlebitis of other sites**
I80.9   **Phlebitis and thrombophlebitis of unspecified site**

I81 `✓` **PORTAL VEIN THROMBOSIS**
Portal (vein) obstruction
Excludes2: hepatic vein thrombosis (I82.0)
   phlebitis of portal vein (K75.1)

I82 `4th` **OTHER VENOUS EMBOLISM AND THROMBOSIS**
Code first venous embolism and thrombosis complicating:
   abortion, ectopic or molar pregnancy (O00–O07, O08.7)
   pregnancy, childbirth and the puerperium (O22.-, O87.-)
Excludes2: venous embolism and thrombosis (of):
   cerebral (I63.6, I67.6)
   coronary (I21–I25)
   intracranial and intraspinal, septic or NOS (G08)
   intracranial, nonpyogenic (I67.6)
   intraspinal, nonpyogenic (G95.1)
   mesenteric (K55.0-)
   portal (I81)
   pulmonary (I26.-)
I82.3   **Embolism and thrombosis of renal vein**

I85 `4th` **ESOPHAGEAL VARICES**
Use additional code to identify:
   alcohol abuse and dependence (F10.-)
I85.0 `5th` **Esophageal varices**
   Idiopathic esophageal varices
   Primary esophageal varices
   I85.00   **Esophageal varices without bleeding**
      Esophageal varices NOS
   I85.01   **Esophageal varices with bleeding**

I86 `4th` **VARICOSE VEINS OF OTHER SITES**
Excludes1: varicose veins of unspecified site (I83.9-)
Excludes2: retinal varices (H35.0-)
I86.1   **Scrotal varices**
   Varicocele

I88 `4th` **NONSPECIFIC LYMPHADENITIS**
Excludes1: acute lymphadenitis, except mesenteric (L04.-)
   enlarged lymph nodes NOS (R59.-)
   HIV disease resulting in generalized lymphadenopathy (B20)
I88.0   **Nonspecific mesenteric lymphadenitis**
   Mesenteric lymphadenitis (acute)(chronic)
I88.1   **Chronic lymphadenitis, except mesenteric**
   Adenitis
   Lymphadenitis
I88.8   **Other nonspecific lymphadenitis**
I88.9   **Nonspecific lymphadenitis, unspecified**
   Lymphadenitis NOS

(I95–I99) OTHER AND UNSPECIFIED DISORDERS OF THE CIRCULATORY SYSTEM

I95 `4th` **HYPOTENSION**
Excludes1: cardiovascular collapse (R57.9)
   maternal hypotension syndrome (O26.5-)
   nonspecific low blood pressure reading NOS (R03.1)
I95.1   **Orthostatic hypotension**
   Hypotension, postural
   Excludes1: neurogenic orthostatic hypotension [Shy-Drager] (G90.3)
      orthostatic hypotension due to drugs (I95.2)
I95.9   **Hypotension, unspecified**

I97 `4th` **INTRAOPERATIVE AND POSTPROCEDURAL COMPLICATIONS AND DISORDERS OF CIRCULATORY SYSTEM, NOT ELSEWHERE CLASSIFIED**
Excludes2: postprocedural shock (T81.1-)
I97.0   **Postcardiotomy syndrome**
I97.1 `5th` **Other postprocedural cardiac functional disturbances**
   Excludes2: acute pulmonary insufficiency following thoracic surgery (J95.1)
      intraoperative cardiac functional disturbances (I97.7-)
   I97.11   **Postprocedural cardiac insufficiency**
     `6th` **I97.110**   **Postprocedural cardiac insufficiency following cardiac surgery**
      I97.111   **Postprocedural cardiac insufficiency following other surgery**
   I97.12   **Postprocedural cardiac arrest**
     `6th` **I97.120**   **Postprocedural cardiac arrest following cardiac surgery**
      I97.121   **Postprocedural cardiac arrest following other surgery**
   I97.13   **Postprocedural heart failure**
     `6th` **Use additional code** to identify the heart failure (I50.-)
     I97.130   **Postprocedural heart failure following cardiac surgery**
      I97.131   **Postprocedural heart failure following other surgery**

`4th` `5th` `6th` `7th` Additional Character Required   3-character code   •=New Code   *Excludes1*—Not coded here, do not use together
   ▲=Revised Code   *Excludes2*—Not included here

I97.19 **Other postprocedural cardiac functional disturbances**

6th

Use additional code, if applicable, to further specify disorder

    I97.190 **Other postprocedural cardiac functional disturbances following cardiac surgery**

    I97.191 **Other postprocedural cardiac functional disturbances following other surgery**

I99 **OTHER AND UNSPECIFIED DISORDERS OF CIRCULATORY SYSTEM**

4th

I99.8 **Other disorder of circulatory system**

I99.9 **Unspecified disorder of circulatory system**

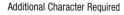 Additional Character Required   3-character code   • =New Code   *Excludes1*—Not coded here, do not use together
▲=Revised Code   *Excludes2*—Not included here

 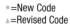

Chapter 10. Diseases of the respiratory system (J00–J99)

GUIDELINES

Acute Respiratory Failure

ACUTE RESPIRATORY FAILURE AS PRINCIPAL DIAGNOSIS
Refer to category J96 for guidelines.

ACUTE RESPIRATORY FAILURE AS SECONDARY DIAGNOSIS
Respiratory failure may be listed as a secondary diagnosis if it occurs after admission, or if it is present on admission, but does not meet the definition of principal diagnosis.

SEQUENCING OF ACUTE RESPIRATORY FAILURE AND ANOTHER ACUTE CONDITION
When a patient is admitted with respiratory failure and another acute condition, (e.g., myocardial infarction, cerebrovascular accident, aspiration pneumonia), the principal diagnosis will not be the same in every situation. This applies whether the other acute condition is a respiratory or nonrespiratory condition. Selection of the principal diagnosis will be dependent on the circumstances of admission. If both the respiratory failure and the other acute condition are equally responsible for occasioning the admission to the hospital, and there are no chapter-specific sequencing rules, the guideline regarding two or more diagnoses that equally meet the definition for principal diagnosis may be applied in these situations.

Influenza due to certain identified influenza viruses
See categories J09–J18 for guidelines.

Ventilator associated Pneumonia

DOCUMENTATION OF VENTILATOR ASSOCIATED PNEUMONIA
Refer to category J95 for guidelines.

VENTILATOR ASSOCIATED PNEUMONIA DEVELOPS AFTER ADMISSION
Refer to category J95 for guidelines.

Note: When a respiratory condition is described as occurring in more than one site and is not specifically indexed, it should be classified to the lower anatomic site (e.g. tracheobronchitis to bronchitis in J40).

Use additional code, where applicable, to identify:
exposure to environmental tobacco smoke (Z77.22)
exposure to tobacco smoke in the perinatal period (P96.81)
history of tobacco dependence (Z87.891)
occupational exposure to environmental tobacco smoke (Z57.31)
tobacco dependence (F17.-)
tobacco use (Z72.0)
Excludes2: certain conditions originating in the perinatal period (P04–P96)
certain infectious and parasitic diseases (A00–B99)
complications of pregnancy, childbirth and the puerperium (O00–O9A)
congenital malformations, deformations and chromosomal abnormalities (Q00–Q99)
endocrine, nutritional and metabolic diseases (E00–E88)
injury, poisoning and certain other consequences of external causes (S00–T88)
neoplasms (C00–D49)
smoke inhalation (T59.81-)
symptoms, signs and abnormal clinical and laboratory findings, NEC (R00–R94)

(J00–J06) ACUTE UPPER RESPIRATORY INFECTIONS

Excludes1: COPD with acute lower respiratory
infection (J44.0)
influenza virus with other respiratory manifestations (J09.X2, J10.1, J11.1)

J00   ACUTE NASOPHARYNGITIS [COMMON COLD]

Acute rhinitis
Coryza (acute)
Infective nasopharyngitis NOS
Infective rhinitis
Nasal catarrh, acute
Nasopharyngitis NOS

Excludes1: acute pharyngitis (J02.-)
acute sore throat NOS (J02.9)
pharyngitis NOS (J02.9)
rhinitis NOS (J31.0)
sore throat NOS (J02.9)
Excludes2: allergic rhinitis (J30.1–J30.9)
chronic pharyngitis (J31.2)
chronic rhinitis (J31.0)
chronic sore throat (J31.2)
nasopharyngitis, chronic (J31.1)
vasomotor rhinitis (J30.0)

J01   ACUTE SINUSITIS
4th
Includes: acute abscess of sinus
acute empyema of sinus
acute infection of sinus
acute inflammation of sinus
acute suppuration of sinus
Use additional code (B95–B97) to identify infectious agent.
Excludes1: sinusitis NOS (J32.9)
Excludes2: chronic sinusitis (J32.0–J32.8)
J01.0   Acute maxillary sinusitis
5th   Acute antritis
     J01.00   Acute maxillary sinusitis, unspecified
     J01.01   Acute recurrent maxillary sinusitis
J01.1   Acute frontal sinusitis
5th   **J01.10   Acute frontal sinusitis, unspecified**
     J01.11   Acute recurrent frontal sinusitis
J01.2   Acute ethmoidal sinusitis
5th   **J01.20   Acute ethmoidal sinusitis, unspecified**
     J01.21   Acute recurrent ethmoidal sinusitis
J01.3   Acute sphenoidal sinusitis
5th   **J01.30   Acute sphenoidal sinusitis, unspecified**
     J01.31   Acute recurrent sphenoidal sinusitis
J01.4   Acute pansinusitis
5th   **J01.40   Acute pansinusitis, unspecified**
     J01.41   Acute recurrent pansinusitis
J01.8   Other acute sinusitis
5th   **J01.80   Other acute sinusitis**
       Acute sinusitis involving more than one sinus but not pansinusitis
     J01.81   Other acute recurrent sinusitis
       Acute recurrent sinusitis involving more than one sinus but not pansinusitis
J01.9   Acute sinusitis, unspecified
5th   **J01.90   Acute sinusitis, unspecified**
     J01.91   Acute recurrent sinusitis, unspecified

J02   ACUTE PHARYNGITIS
4th
Includes: acute sore throat
Excludes1: acute laryngopharyngitis (J06.0)
peritonsillar abscess (J36)
pharyngeal abscess (J39.1)
retropharyngeal abscess (J39.0)
Excludes2: chronic pharyngitis (J31.2)
J02.0   Streptococcal pharyngitis
     Septic pharyngitis
     Streptococcal sore throat
     Excludes2: scarlet fever (A38.-)
J02.8   Acute pharyngitis due to other specified organisms
     Use additional code (B95–B97) to identify infectious agent
     Excludes1: acute pharyngitis due to coxsackie virus (B08.5)
       acute pharyngitis due to gonococcus (A54.5)
       acute pharyngitis due to herpes [simplex] virus (B00.2)
       acute pharyngitis due to infectious mononucleosis (B27.-)
       enteroviral vesicular pharyngitis (B08.5)
J02.9   Acute pharyngitis, unspecified
     Gangrenous pharyngitis (acute)
     Infective pharyngitis (acute) NOS
     Pharyngitis (acute) NOS
     Sore throat (acute) NOS
     Suppurative pharyngitis (acute)
     Ulcerative pharyngitis (acute)

4th   **5th**   **6th**   **7th**   Additional Character Required   3-character code

•=New Code
▲=Revised Code

Excludes1—Not coded here, do not use together
Excludes2—Not included here

J03 ACUTE TONSILLITIS

Excludes1: acute sore throat (J02.-)
    hypertrophy of tonsils (J35.1)
    peritonsillar abscess (J36)
    sore throat NOS (J02.9)
    streptococcal sore throat (J02.0)
Excludes2: chronic tonsillitis (J35.0)

J03.0 Streptococcal tonsillitis
    J03.00 Acute streptococcal tonsillitis, unspecified
    J03.01 Acute recurrent streptococcal tonsillitis

J03.8 Acute tonsillitis due to other specified organisms
    Use additional code (B95–B97) to identify infectious agent.
    Excludes1: diphtheritic tonsillitis (A36.0)
       herpesviral pharyngotonsillitis (B00.2)
       streptococcal tonsillitis (J03.0)
       tuberculous tonsillitis (A15.8)
       Vincent's tonsillitis (A69.1)
    J03.80 Acute tonsillitis due to other specified organisms
    J03.81 Acute recurrent tonsillitis due to other specified organisms

J03.9 Acute tonsillitis, unspecified
    Follicular tonsillitis (acute)
    Gangrenous tonsillitis (acute)
    Infective tonsillitis (acute)
    Tonsillitis (acute) NOS
    Ulcerative tonsillitis (acute)
    J03.90 Acute tonsillitis, unspecified
    J03.91 Acute recurrent tonsillitis, unspecified

J04 ACUTE LARYNGITIS AND TRACHEITIS

Use additional code (B95–B97) to identify infectious agent.
Excludes1: acute obstructive laryngitis [croup] and epiglottitis (J05.-)
Excludes2: laryngismus (stridulus) (J38.5)

J04.0 Acute laryngitis
    Edematous laryngitis (acute)
    Laryngitis (acute) NOS
    Subglottic laryngitis (acute)
    Suppurative laryngitis (acute)
    Ulcerative laryngitis (acute)
    Excludes1: acute obstructive laryngitis (J05.0)
    Excludes2: chronic laryngitis (J37.0)

J04.1 Acute tracheitis
    Acute viral tracheitis
    Catarrhal tracheitis (acute)
    Tracheitis (acute) NOS
    Excludes2: chronic tracheitis (J42)
    J04.10 Acute tracheitis without obstruction
    J04.11 Acute tracheitis with obstruction

J04.2 Acute laryngotracheitis
    Laryngotracheitis NOS
    Tracheitis (acute) with laryngitis (acute)
    Excludes1: acute obstructive laryngotracheitis (J05.0)
    Excludes2: chronic laryngotracheitis (J37.1)

J04.3 Supraglottitis, unspecified
    J04.30 Supraglottitis, unspecified, without obstruction
    J04.31 Supraglottitis, unspecified, with obstruction

J05 ACUTE OBSTRUCTIVE LARYNGITIS [CROUP] AND EPIGLOTTITIS

Use additional code (B95–B97) to identify infectious agent.

J05.0 Acute obstructive laryngitis [croup]
    Obstructive laryngitis (acute) NOS
    Obstructive laryngotracheitis NOS

J05.1 Acute epiglottitis
    Excludes2: epiglottitis, chronic (J37.0)
    J05.10 Acute epiglottitis without obstruction
       Epiglottitis NOS
    J05.11 Acute epiglottitis with obstruction

J06 ACUTE UPPER RESPIRATORY INFECTIONS OF MULTIPLE AND UNSPECIFIED SITES

Excludes1: acute respiratory infection NOS (J22)
    streptococcal pharyngitis (J02.0)

J06.0 Acute laryngopharyngitis
J06.9 Acute upper respiratory infection, unspecified
    Upper respiratory disease, acute
    Upper respiratory infection NOS

(J09–J18) INFLUENZA AND PNEUMONIA

GUIDELINES

Code only confirmed cases of influenza due to certain identified influenza viruses (category J09), and due to other identified influenza virus (category J10). This is an exception to the hospital inpatient guideline Section II, H. (Uncertain Diagnosis).

In this context, "confirmation" does not require documentation of positive laboratory testing specific for avian or other novel influenza A or other identified influenza virus. However, coding should be based on the provider's diagnostic statement that the patient has avian influenza, or other novel influenza A, for category J09, or has another particular identified strain of influenza, such as H1N1 or H3N2, but not identified as novel or variant, for category J10.

If the provider records "suspected" or "possible" or "probable" avian influenza, or novel influenza, or other identified influenza, then the appropriate influenza code from category J11, Influenza due to unidentified influenza virus, should be assigned. A code from category J09, Influenza due to certain identified influenza viruses, should not be assigned nor should a code from category J10, Influenza due to other identified influenza virus.

Excludes2: allergic or eosinophilic pneumonia (J82)
    aspiration pneumonia NOS (J69.0)
    meconium pneumonia (P24.01)
    neonatal aspiration pneumonia (P24.-)
    pneumonia due to solids and liquids (J69.-)
    congenital pneumonia (P23.9)
    lipid pneumonia (J69.1)
    rheumatic pneumonia (I00)
    ventilator associated pneumonia (J95.851)

J09 INFLUENZA DUE TO CERTAIN IDENTIFIED INFLUENZA VIRUSES

Excludes1: influenza due to other identified influenza virus (J10.-)
    influenza due to unidentified influenza virus (J11.-)
    seasonal influenza due to other identified influenza virus (J10.-)
    seasonal influenza due to unidentified influenza virus (J11.-)

J09.X Influenza due to identified novel influenza A virus

    Avian influenza
    Bird influenza
    Influenza A/H5N1
    Influenza of other animal origin, not bird or swine
    Swine influenza virus (viruses that normally cause infections in pigs)
    J09.X1 Influenza due to identified novel influenza A virus with pneumonia
       Code also, if applicable, associated: lung abscess (J85.1) other specified type of pneumonia
    J09.X2 Influenza due to identified novel influenza A virus with other respiratory manifestations
       Influenza due to identified novel influenza A virus NOS
       Influenza due to identified novel influenza A virus with laryngitis
       Influenza due to identified novel influenza A virus with pharyngitis
       Influenza due to identified novel influenza A virus with upper respiratory symptoms
       Use additional code, if applicable, for associated: pleural effusion (J91.8) sinusitis (J01.-)
    J09.X3 Influenza due to identified novel influenza A virus with gastrointestinal manifestations
       Influenza due to identified novel influenza A virus gastroenteritis
       Excludes1: 'intestinal flu' [viral gastroenteritis] (A08.-)

 Additional Character Required   3-character code

●=New Code
▲=Revised Code

Excludes1—Not coded here, do not use together
Excludes2—Not included here

PEDIATRIC ICD-10-CM 2017: A MANUAL FOR PROVIDER-BASED CODING

J09.X9 Influenza due to identified novel influenza A virus with other manifestations
Influenza due to identified novel influenza A virus with encephalopathy
Influenza due to identified novel influenza A virus with myocarditis
Influenza due to identified novel influenza A virus with otitis media
Use additional code to identify manifestation

J10 INFLUENZA DUE TO OTHER IDENTIFIED INFLUENZA VIRUS
Excludes1: influenza due to avian influenza virus (J09.X-)
influenza due to swine flu (J09.X-)
influenza due to unidentified influenza virus (J11.-)

J10.0 Influenza due to other identified influenza virus with pneumonia
Code also associated lung abscess, if applicable (J85.1)
J10.00 Influenza due to other identified influenza virus with unspecified type of pneumonia
J10.01 Influenza due to other identified influenza virus with the same other identified influenza virus pneumonia
J10.08 Influenza due to other identified influenza virus with other specified pneumonia
Code also other specified type of pneumonia

J10.1 Influenza due to other identified influenza virus with other respiratory manifestations
Influenza due to other identified influenza virus NOS
Influenza due to other identified influenza virus with laryngitis
Influenza due to other identified influenza virus with pharyngitis
Influenza due to other identified influenza virus with upper respiratory symptoms
Use additional code for associated pleural effusion, if applicable (J91.8)
Use additional code for associated sinusitis, if applicable (J01.-)

J10.2 Influenza due to other identified influenza virus with gastrointestinal manifestations
Influenza due to other identified influenza virus gastroenteritis
Excludes1: 'intestinal flu' [viral gastroenteritis] (A08.-)

J10.8 Influenza due to other identified influenza virus with other manifestations
J10.81 Influenza due to other identified influenza virus with encephalopathy
J10.82 Influenza due to other identified influenza virus with myocarditis
J10.83 Influenza due to other identified influenza virus with otitis media
Use additional code for any associated perforated tympanic membrane (H72.-)
J10.89 Influenza due to other identified influenza virus with other manifestations
Use additional codes to identify the manifestations

J11 INFLUENZA DUE TO UNIDENTIFIED INFLUENZA VIRUS
J11.0 Influenza due to unidentified influenza virus with pneumonia
Code also associated lung abscess, if applicable (J85.1)
J11.00 Influenza due to unidentified influenza virus with unspecified type of pneumonia
Influenza with pneumonia NOS
J11.08 Influenza due to unidentified influenza virus with specified pneumonia
Code also other specified type of pneumonia

J11.1 Influenza due to unidentified influenza virus with other respiratory manifestations
Influenza NOS
Influenzal laryngitis NOS
Influenzal pharyngitis NOS
Influenza with upper respiratory symptoms NOS
Use additional code for associated pleural effusion, if applicable (J91.8)
Use additional code for associated sinusitis, if applicable (J01.-)

J11.2 Influenza due to unidentified influenza virus with gastrointestinal manifestations
Influenza gastroenteritis NOS
Excludes1: 'intestinal flu' [viral gastroenteritis] (A08.-)

J11.8 Influenza due to unidentified influenza virus with other manifestations
J11.81 Influenza due to unidentified influenza virus with encephalopathy
Influenzal encephalopathy NOS
J11.82 Influenza due to unidentified influenza virus with myocarditis
Influenzal myocarditis NOS
J11.83 Influenza due to unidentified influenza virus with otitis media
Influenzal otitis media NOS
Use additional code for any associated perforated tympanic membrane (H72.-)
J11.89 Influenza due to unidentified influenza virus with other manifestations
Use additional codes to identify the manifestations

J12 VIRAL PNEUMONIA, NEC
Includes: bronchopneumonia due to viruses other than influenza viruses
Code first associated influenza, if applicable (J09.X1, J10.0-, J11.0-)
Code also associated abscess, if applicable (J85.1)
Excludes1: aspiration pneumonia due to solids and liquids (J69.-)
aspiration pneumonia NOS (J69.0)
congenital pneumonia (P23.0)
congenital rubella pneumonitis (P35.0)
interstitial pneumonia NOS (J84.9)
lipid pneumonia (J69.1)
neonatal aspiration pneumonia (P24.-)

J12.0 Adenoviral pneumonia
J12.1 Respiratory syncytial virus pneumonia
J12.2 Parainfluenza virus pneumonia
J12.3 Human metapneumovirus pneumonia
J12.8 Other viral pneumonia
J12.81 Pneumonia due to SARS-associated coronavirus
SARS NOS
J12.89 Other viral pneumonia
J12.9 Viral pneumonia, unspecified

J13 PNEUMONIA DUE TO STREPTOCOCCUS PNEUMONIAE
Bronchopneumonia due to S. pneumoniae
Code first associated influenza, if applicable (J09.X1, J10.0-, J11.0-)
Code also associated abscess, if applicable (J85.1)
Excludes1: congenital pneumonia due to S. pneumoniae (P23.6)
lobar pneumonia, unspecified organism (J18.1)
pneumonia due to other streptococci (J15.3-J15.4)

J14 PNEUMONIA DUE TO H. INFLUENZAE
Bronchopneumonia due to H. influenzae
Code first associated influenza, if applicable (J09.X1, J10.0-, J11.0-)
Code also associated abscess, if applicable (J85.1)
Excludes1: congenital pneumonia due to H. influenzae (P23.6)

J15 BACTERIAL PNEUMONIA, NEC
Includes: bronchopneumonia due to bacteria other than S. pneumoniae and H. influenzae
Code first associated influenza, if applicable (J09.X1, J10.0-, J11.0-)
Code also associated abscess, if applicable (J85.1)
Excludes1: chlamydial pneumonia (J16.0)
congenital pneumonia (P23.-)
Legionnaires' disease (A48.1)
spirochetal pneumonia (A69.8)

J15.0 Pneumonia due to K. pneumoniae
J15.1 Pneumonia due to Pseudomonas
J15.2 Pneumonia due to staphylococcus
J15.20 Pneumonia due to staphylococcus, unspecified
J15.21 Pneumonia due to staphylococcus aureus
J15.211 Pneumonia due to MSSA
MSSA pneumonia
Pneumonia due to Staphylococcus aureus NOS
J15.212 Pneumonia due to MRSA
J15.29 Pneumonia due to other staphylococcus

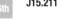

J15.3 Pneumonia due to streptococcus, group B

J15.4 Pneumonia due to other streptococci
Excludes1: pneumonia due to streptococcus, group B (J15.3)
    pneumonia due to Streptococcus pneumoniae (J13)

J15.5 Pneumonia due to E. coli

J15.6 Pneumonia due to other aerobic Gram-negative bacteria
Pneumonia due to Serratia marcescens

J15.7 Pneumonia due to M. pneumoniae

J15.8 Pneumonia due to other specified bacteria

J15.9 Unspecified bacterial pneumonia
Pneumonia due to gram-positive bacteria

J16 PNEUMONIA DUE TO OTHER INFECTIOUS ORGANISMS, NEC
Code first associated influenza, if applicable (J09.X1, J10.0-, J11.0-)
Code also associated abscess, if applicable (J85.1)
Excludes1: congenital pneumonia (P23.-)
    ornithosis (A70)
    pneumocystosis (B59)
    pneumonia NOS (J18.9)

J16.0 Chlamydial pneumonia

J16.8 Pneumonia due to other specified infectious organisms

J17 PNEUMONIA IN DISEASES CLASSIFIED ELSEWHERE
Code first underlying disease, such as:
Q fever (A78)
rheumatic fever (I00)
schistosomiasis (B65.0–B65.9)
Excludes1: candidial pneumonia (B37.1)
    chlamydial pneumonia (J16.0)
    gonorrheal pneumonia (A54.84)
    histoplasmosis pneumonia (B39.0–B39.2)
    measles pneumonia (B05.2)
    nocardiosis pneumonia (A43.0)
    pneumocystosis (B59)
    pneumonia due to Pneumocystis carinii (B59)
    pneumonia due to Pneumocystis jiroveci (B59)
    pneumonia in actinomycosis (A42.0)
    pneumonia in anthrax (A22.1)
    pneumonia in ascariasis (B77.81)
    pneumonia in aspergillosis (B44.0–B44.1)
    pneumonia in coccidioidomycosis (B38.0–B38.2)
    pneumonia in cytomegalovirus disease (B25.0)
    pneumonia in toxoplasmosis (B58.3)
    rubella pneumonia (B06.81)
    salmonella pneumonia (A02.22)
    spirochetal infection NEC with pneumonia (A69.8)
    tularemia pneumonia (A21.2)
    typhoid fever with pneumonia (A01.03)
    varicella pneumonia (B01.2)
    whooping cough with pneumonia (A37 with fifth-character 1)

J18 PNEUMONIA, UNSPECIFIED ORGANISM
Code first associated influenza, if applicable (J09.X1, J10.0-, J11.0-)
Excludes1: abscess of lung with pneumonia (J85.1)
    aspiration pneumonia due to solids and liquids (J69.-)
    aspiration pneumonia NOS (J69.0)
    congenital pneumonia (P23.0)
    drug-induced interstitial lung disorder (J70.2–J70.4)
    interstitial pneumonia NOS (J84.9)
    lipid pneumonia (J69.1)
    neonatal aspiration pneumonia (P24.-)
    pneumonitis due to external agents (J67–J70)
    pneumonitis due to fumes and vapors (J68.0)
    usual interstitial pneumonia (J84.17)

J18.0 Bronchopneumonia, unspecified organism
Excludes1: hypostatic bronchopneumonia (J18.2)
    lipid pneumonia (J69.1)
Excludes2: acute bronchiolitis (J21.-)
    chronic bronchiolitis (J44.9)

J18.1 Lobar pneumonia, unspecified organism

J18.8 Other pneumonia, unspecified organism

J18.9 Pneumonia, unspecified organism

(J20–J22) OTHER ACUTE LOWER RESPIRATORY INFECTIONS

Excludes2: COPD with acute lower respiratory infection (J44.0)

J20 ACUTE BRONCHITIS
Includes: acute and subacute bronchitis (with) bronchospasm
acute and subacute bronchitis (with) tracheitis
acute and subacute bronchitis (with) tracheobronchitis, acute
acute and subacute fibrinous bronchitis
acute and subacute membranous bronchitis
acute and subacute purulent bronchitis
acute and subacute septic bronchitis
Excludes1: bronchitis NOS (J40)
    tracheobronchitis NOS
Excludes2: acute bronchitis with bronchiectasis (J47.0)
    acute bronchitis with chronic obstructive asthma (J44.0)
    acute bronchitis with COPD (J44.0)
    allergic bronchitis NOS (J45.909-)
    bronchitis due to chemicals, fumes and vapors (J68.0)
    chronic bronchitis NOS (J42)
    chronic mucopurulent bronchitis (J41.1)
    chronic obstructive bronchitis (J44.-)
    chronic obstructive tracheobronchitis (J44.-)
    chronic simple bronchitis (J41.0)
    chronic tracheobronchitis (J42)

J20.0 Acute bronchitis due to M. pneumoniae

J20.1 Acute bronchitis due to H. influenzae

J20.2 Acute bronchitis due to streptococcus

J20.3 Acute bronchitis due to coxsackievirus

J20.4 Acute bronchitis due to parainfluenza virus

J20.5 Acute bronchitis due to respiratory syncytial virus

J20.6 Acute bronchitis due to rhinovirus

J20.7 Acute bronchitis due to echovirus

J20.8 Acute bronchitis due to other specified organisms

J20.9 Acute bronchitis, unspecified

J21 ACUTE BRONCHIOLITIS
Includes: acute bronchiolitis with bronchospasm
Excludes2: respiratory bronchiolitis interstitial lung disease (J84.115)

J21.0 Acute bronchiolitis due to respiratory syncytial virus

J21.1 Acute bronchiolitis due to human metapneumovirus

J21.8 Acute bronchiolitis due to other specified organisms

J21.9 Acute bronchiolitis, unspecified
Bronchiolitis (acute)
Excludes1: chronic bronchiolitis (J44.-)

(J30–J39) OTHER DISEASES OF UPPER RESPIRATORY TRACT

J30 VASOMOTOR AND ALLERGIC RHINITIS
Includes: spasmodic rhinorrhea
Excludes1: allergic rhinitis with asthma (bronchial) (J45.909)
    rhinitis NOS (J31.0)

J30.1 Allergic rhinitis due to pollen
Allergy NOS due to pollen
Hay fever
Pollinosis

J30.2 Other seasonal allergic rhinitis

J30.5 Allergic rhinitis due to food

J30.8 Other allergic rhinitis

    J30.81 Allergic rhinitis due to animal (cat) (dog) hair and dander

    J30.89 Other allergic rhinitis
    Perennial allergic rhinitis

J30.9 Allergic rhinitis, unspecified

   7th Additional Character Required   3-character code   •=New Code   ▲=Revised Code   *Excludes1*—Not coded here, do not use together   *Excludes2*—Not included here

J31   **CHRONIC RHINITIS, NASOPHARYNGITIS AND PHARYNGITIS**

`4th`

Use additional code to identify: (Refer to Chapter 10 guidelines for codes) {Refer to the main chapter guidelines}

J31.0   **Chronic rhinitis**
Atrophic rhinitis (chronic)
Granulomatous rhinitis (chronic)
Hypertrophic rhinitis (chronic)
Obstructive rhinitis (chronic)
Ozena
Purulent rhinitis (chronic)
Rhinitis (chronic) NOS
Ulcerative rhinitis (chronic)
Excludes1: allergic rhinitis (J30.1–J30.9)
    vasomotor rhinitis (J30.0)

J31.2   **Chronic pharyngitis**
Chronic sore throat
Atrophic pharyngitis (chronic)
Granular pharyngitis (chronic)
Hypertrophic pharyngitis (chronic)
Excludes2 acute pharyngitis (J02.9)

J32   **CHRONIC SINUSITIS**

`4th`

Includes: sinus abscess
sinus empyema
sinus infection
sinus suppuration

Use additional code to identify: (Refer to Chapter 10 guidelines for codes) {Refer to main chapter guidelines}

Excludes2: acute sinusitis (J01.-)

J32.0   **Chronic maxillary sinusitis**
Antritis (chronic)
Maxillary sinusitis NOS

J32.1   **Chronic frontal sinusitis**
Frontal sinusitis NOS

J32.2   **Chronic ethmoidal sinusitis**
Ethmoidal sinusitis NOS
Excludes1: Woakes' ethmoiditis (J33.1)

J32.3   **Chronic sphenoidal sinusitis**
Sphenoidal sinusitis NOS

J32.4   **Chronic pansinusitis**
Pansinusitis NOS

J32.8   **Other chronic sinusitis**
Sinusitis (chronic) involving more than one sinus but not pansinusitis

J32.9   **Chronic sinusitis, unspecified**
Sinusitis (chronic) NOS

J33   **NASAL POLYP**

`4th`

Use additional code to identify: (Refer to Chapter 10 guidelines for codes) {Refer to main chapter guidelines}

Excludes1: adenomatous polyps (D14.0)

J33.0   **Polyp of nasal cavity**
Choanal polyp
Nasopharyngeal polyp

J33.8   **Other polyp of sinus**
Accessory polyp of sinus
Ethmoidal polyp of sinus
Maxillary polyp of sinus
Sphenoidal polyp of sinus

J33.9   **Nasal polyp, unspecified**

J34   **OTHER AND UNSPECIFIED DISORDERS OF NOSE AND NASAL SINUSES**

`4th`

Excludes2: varicose ulcer of nasal septum (I86.8)

J34.2   **Deviated nasal septum**
Deflection or deviation of septum (nasal) (acquired)
Excludes1: congenital deviated nasal septum (Q67.4)

J34.8   **Other specified disorders of nose and nasal sinuses**

J34.81   **Nasal mucositis (ulcerative)**
`5th`
Code also type of associated therapy, such as:
antineoplastic and immunosuppressive drugs (T45.1X-)
radiological procedure and radiotherapy (Y84.2)
Excludes2: gastrointestinal mucositis (ulcerative) (K92.81)
    mucositis (ulcerative) of vagina and vulva (N76.81)
    oral mucositis (ulcerative) (K12.3-)

J34.89   **Other specified disorders of nose and nasal sinuses**
Perforation of nasal septum NOS
Rhinolith

J34.9   **Unspecified disorder of nose and nasal sinuses**

J35   **CHRONIC DISEASES OF TONSILS AND ADENOIDS**

`4th`

Use additional code to identify: (Refer to Chapter 10 guidelines for codes) {Refer to main chapter guidelines}

J35.0   **Chronic tonsillitis and adenoiditis**
`5th`
Excludes2: acute tonsillitis (J03.-)

J35.01   **Chronic tonsillitis**

J35.02   **Chronic adenoiditis**

J35.03   **Chronic tonsillitis and adenoiditis**

J35.1   **Hypertrophy of tonsils**
Enlargement of tonsils
Excludes1: hypertrophy of tonsils with tonsillitis (J35.0-)

J35.2   **Hypertrophy of adenoids**
Enlargement of adenoids
Excludes1: hypertrophy of adenoids with adenoiditis (J35.0-)

J35.3   **Hypertrophy of tonsils with hypertrophy of adenoids**
Excludes1: hypertrophy of tonsils and adenoids with tonsillitis and adenoiditis (J35.03)

J35.8   **Other chronic diseases of tonsils and adenoids**
Adenoid vegetations
Amygdalolith
Calculus, tonsil
Cicatrix of tonsil (and adenoid)
Tonsillar tag
Ulcer of tonsil

J35.9   **Chronic disease of tonsils and adenoids, unspecified**
Disease (chronic) of tonsils and adenoids NOS

J36   **PERITONSILLAR ABSCESS**

`✓`

Includes: abscess of tonsil
peritonsillar cellulitis
quinsy

Use additional code (B95-B97) to identify infectious agent.
Excludes1: acute tonsillitis (J03.-)
chronic tonsillitis (J35.0)
retropharyngeal abscess (J39.0)
tonsillitis NOS (J03.9-)

J37   **CHRONIC LARYNGITIS AND LARYNGOTRACHEITIS**

`4th`

Use additional code to identify: (Refer to Chapter 10 guidelines for codes) {Refer to main chapter guidelines}

J37.0   **Chronic laryngitis**
Catarrhal laryngitis
Hypertrophic laryngitis
Sicca laryngitis
Excludes2: acute laryngitis (J04.0)
obstructive (acute) laryngitis (J05.0)

J37.1   **Chronic laryngotracheitis**
Laryngitis, chronic, with tracheitis (chronic)
Tracheitis, chronic, with laryngitis
Excludes1: chronic tracheitis (J42)
Excludes2: acute laryngotracheitis (J04.2)
acute tracheitis (J04.1)

CHAPTER 10. DISEASES OF THE RESPIRATORY SYSTEM   (J31–J37.1)

`4th` `5th` `6th` `7th`   Additional Character Required   `✓`   3-character code

•=New Code
▲=Revised Code

Excludes1—Not coded here, do not use together
Excludes2—Not included here

CHAPTER 10. DISEASES OF THE RESPIRATORY SYSTEM   (J38–J80)

J38 DISEASES OF VOCAL CORDS AND LARYNX, NEC

 4th

Use additional code to identify: (Refer to Chapter 10 guidelines for codes)
{Refer to main chapter guidelines}

Excludes1: congenital laryngeal stridor (P28.89)
obstructive laryngitis (acute) (J05.0)
postprocedural subglottic stenosis (J95.5)
stridor (R06.1)
ulcerative laryngitis (J04.0)

J38.0 Paralysis of vocal cords and larynx

5th   Laryngoplegia
Paralysis of glottis

    J38.00 Paralysis of vocal cords and larynx, unspecified
    J38.01 Paralysis of vocal cords and larynx, unilateral
    J38.02 Paralysis of vocal cords and larynx, bilateral

J38.4 Edema of larynx
Edema (of) glottis
Subglottic edema
Supraglottic edema
Excludes1: acute obstructive laryngitis [croup] (J05.0)
edematous laryngitis (J04.0)

J39 OTHER DISEASES OF UPPER RESPIRATORY TRACT

 4th

Excludes1: acute respiratory infection NOS (J22)
acute upper respiratory infection (J06.9)
upper respiratory inflammation due to chemicals, gases, fumes or vapors (J68.2)

J39.0 Retropharyngeal and parapharyngeal abscess
Peripharyngeal abscess
Excludes1: peritonsillar abscess (J36)

(J40–J47) CHRONIC LOWER RESPIRATORY DISEASES

Excludes1: bronchitis due to chemicals, gases, fumes and vapors (J68.0)
Excludes2: cystic fibrosis (E84.-)

J40 BRONCHITIS, NOT SPECIFIED AS ACUTE OR CHRONIC

   Bronchitis NOS
Bronchitis with tracheitis NOS
Catarrhal bronchitis
Tracheobronchitis NOS
Use additional code to identify: (Refer to Chapter 10 guidelines for codes)
{Refer to main chapter guidelines}
Excludes1: acute bronchitis (J20.-)
allergic bronchitis NOS (J45.909-)
asthmatic bronchitis NOS (J45.9-)
bronchitis due to chemicals, gases, fumes and vapors (J68.0)

J45 ASTHMA

4th

Includes: allergic (predominantly) asthma
allergic bronchitis NOS
allergic rhinitis with asthma
atopic asthma
extrinsic allergic asthma
hay fever with asthma
idiosyncratic asthma
intrinsic nonallergic asthma
nonallergic asthma
Use additional code to identify: (Refer to Chapter 10 guidelines for codes)
{Refer to main chapter guidelines}
Excludes1: detergent asthma (J69.8)
eosinophilic asthma (J82)
lung diseases due to external agents (J60-J70)
miner's asthma (J60)
wheezing NOS (R06.2)
wood asthma (J67.8)
Excludes2: asthma with COPD (J44.9)
chronic asthmatic (obstructive) bronchitis (J44.9)
chronic obstructive asthma (J44.9)

J45.2 Mild intermittent asthma

5th   **J45.20 Mild intermittent asthma, uncomplicated**
Mild intermittent asthma NOS
    J45.21 Mild intermittent asthma with (acute) exacerbation
    J45.22 Mild intermittent asthma with status asthmaticus

J45.3 Mild persistent asthma

 5th

J45.30 Mild persistent asthma, uncomplicated
Mild persistent asthma NOS
J45.31 Mild persistent asthma with (acute) exacerbation
J45.32 Mild persistent asthma with status asthmaticus

J45.4 Moderate persistent asthma

 5th   **J45.40 Moderate persistent asthma, uncomplicated**
Moderate persistent asthma NOS
    J45.41 Moderate persistent asthma with (acute) exacerbation
    J45.42 Moderate persistent asthma with status asthmaticus

J45.5 Severe persistent asthma

5th   **J45.50 Severe persistent asthma, uncomplicated**
Severe persistent asthma NOS
    J45.51 Severe persistent asthma with (acute) exacerbation
    J45.52 Severe persistent asthma with status asthmaticus

J45.9 Other and unspecified asthma

5th   **J45.90 Unspecified asthma**

6th   Asthmatic bronchitis NOS
Childhood asthma NOS
Late onset asthma

    J45.901 Unspecified asthma with (acute) exacerbation
    J45.902 Unspecified asthma with status asthmaticus
    J45.909 Unspecified asthma, uncomplicated
Asthma NOS

J45.99 Other asthma

6th   **J45.990 Exercise induced bronchospasm**
    J45.991 Cough variant asthma
    J45.998 Other asthma

(J60–J70) LUNG DISEASES DUE TO EXTERNAL AGENTS

Excludes2: asthma (J45.-)
malignant neoplasm of bronchus and lung (C34.-)

J69 PNEUMONITIS DUE TO SOLIDS AND LIQUIDS

 4th

Excludes1: neonatal aspiration syndromes (P24.-)
postprocedural pneumonitis (J95.4)

J69.0 Pneumonitis due to inhalation of food and vomit
Aspiration pneumonia NOS
Aspiration pneumonia (due to) food (regurgitated)
Aspiration pneumonia (due to) gastric secretions
Aspiration pneumonia (due to) milk
Aspiration pneumonia (due to) vomit
Code also any associated FB in respiratory tract (T17.-)
Excludes1: chemical pneumonitis due to anesthesia (J95.4)

J69.1 Pneumonitis due to inhalation of oils and essences
Exogenous lipoid pneumonia
Lipid pneumonia NOS
Code first (T51-T65) to identify substance
Excludes1: endogenous lipoid pneumonia (J84.89)

J69.8 Pneumonitis due to inhalation of other solids and liquids
Pneumonitis due to aspiration of blood
Pneumonitis due to aspiration of detergent
Code first (T51-T65) to identify substance

J70 RESPIRATORY CONDITIONS DUE TO OTHER EXTERNAL AGENTS

 4th

J70.5 Respiratory conditions due to smoke inhalation
Smoke inhalation NOS
Excludes1: smoke inhalation due to chemicals, gases, fumes and vapors (J68.9)

J70.9 Respiratory conditions due to unspecified external agent
Code first (T51-T65) to identify the external agent

(J80–J84) OTHER RESPIRATORY DISEASES PRINCIPALLY AFFECTING THE INTERSTITIUM

J80 ACUTE RESPIRATORY DISTRESS SYNDROME

Acute respiratory distress syndrome in adult or child
Adult hyaline membrane disease
Excludes1: respiratory distress syndrome in newborn (perinatal) (P22.0)

    Additional Character Required   **3-character code**   •=New Code   ▲=Revised Code   ***Excludes1***—Not coded here, do not use together   ***Excludes2***—Not included here

J81   **PULMONARY EDEMA**

`4th` **Use additional code** to identify: (Refer to Chapter 10 guidelines for codes) {Refer to main chapter guidelines}

Excludes1: chemical (acute) pulmonary edema (J68.1)
    hypostatic pneumonia (J18.2)
    passive pneumonia (J18.2)
    pulmonary edema due to external agents (J60-J70)
    pulmonary edema with heart disease NOS (I50.1)
    pulmonary edema with heart failure (I50.1)

J81.0   **Acute pulmonary edema**
    Acute edema of lung

J84   **OTHER INTERSTITIAL PULMONARY DISEASES**

`4th` *Excludes1:* drug-induced interstitial lung disorders (J70.2-J70.4)
    interstitial emphysema (J98.2)
    lung diseases due to external agents (J60-J70)

J84.0   **Alveolar and parieto-alveolar conditions**

`5th` **J84.01**   **Alveolar proteinosis**

J84.02   **Pulmonary alveolar microlithiasis**

J84.03   **Idiopathic pulmonary hemosiderosis**
    Essential brown induration of lung
    Code first underlying disease, such as:
    disorders of iron metabolism (E83.1-)
    Excludes1: acute idiopathic pulmonary hemorrhage in
      infants [AIPHI] (R04.81)

J84.09   **Other alveolar and parieto-alveolar conditions**

J84.8   **Other specified interstitial pulmonary diseases**

`5th` *Excludes1:* exogenous or unspecified lipoid pneumonia (J69.1)

J84.83   **Surfactant mutations of the lung**

J84.84   **Other interstitial lung diseases of childhood**

`6th` **J84.841**   **Neuroendocrine cell hyperplasia of infancy**

J84.842   **Pulmonary interstitial glycogenosis**

J84.843   **Alveolar capillary dysplasia with vein misalignment**

J84.848   **Other interstitial lung diseases of childhood**

J84.89   **Other specified interstitial pulmonary disease**

J84.9   **Interstitial pulmonary disease, unspecified**
    Interstitial pneumonia NOS

(J85–J86) SUPPURATIVE AND NECROTIC CONDITIONS OF THE LOWER RESPIRATORY TRACT

J86   **PYOTHORAX**

`4th` **Use additional code** (B95–B97) to identify infectious agent.
Excludes1: abscess of lung (J85.-)
    pyothorax due to tuberculosis (A15.6)

J86.0   **Pyothorax with fistula**
    Bronchocutaneous fistula
    Bronchopleural fistula
    Hepatopleural fistula
    Mediastinal fistula
    Pleural fistula
    Thoracic fistula
    Any condition classifiable to J86.9 with fistula

J86.9   **Pyothorax without fistula**
    Abscess of pleura
    Abscess of thorax
    Empyema (chest) (lung) (pleura)
    Fibrinopurulent pleurisy
    Purulent pleurisy
    Pyopneumothorax
    Septic pleurisy
    Seropurulent pleurisy
    Suppurative pleurisy

(J90–J94) OTHER DISEASES OF THE PLEURA

J90   **PLEURAL EFFUSION, NEC**

`✓` Encysted pleurisy
Pleural effusion NOS
Pleurisy with effusion (exudative) (serous)
Excludes1: chylous (pleural) effusion (J94.0)
    malignant pleural effusion (J91.0))
    pleurisy NOS (R09.1)
    tuberculous pleural effusion (A15.6)

J91   **PLEURAL EFFUSION IN CONDITIONS CLASSIFIED ELSEWHERE**

`4th` *Excludes2:* pleural effusion in heart failure (I50.-)
    pleural effusion in SLE (M32.13)

J91.0   **Malignant pleural effusion**
    Code first underlying neoplasm

J91.8   **Pleural effusion in other conditions classified elsewhere**
    Code first underlying disease, such as:
    filariasis (B74.0-B74.9)
    influenza (J09.X2, J10.1, J11.1)

J93   **PNEUMOTHORAX AND AIR LEAK**

`4th` *Excludes1:* congenital or perinatal pneumothorax (P25.1)
    postprocedural air leak (J95.812)
    postprocedural pneumothorax (J95.811)
    traumatic pneumothorax (S27.0)
    tuberculous (current disease) pneumothorax (A15.-)
    pyopneumothorax (J86.-)

J93.0   **Spontaneous tension pneumothorax**

J93.1   **Other spontaneous pneumothorax**

`5th` **J93.11**   **Primary spontaneous pneumothorax**

J93.12   **Secondary spontaneous pneumothorax**
    Code first underlying condition, such as:
    catamenial pneumothorax due to endometriosis (N80.8)
    cystic fibrosis (E84.-)
    eosinophilic pneumonia (J82)
    lymphangioleiomyomatosis (J84.81)
    malignant neoplasm of bronchus and lung (C34.-)
    Marfan's syndrome (Q87.4)
    pneumonia due to Pneumocystis carinii (B59)
    secondary malignant neoplasm of lung (C78.0-)
    spontaneous rupture of the esophagus (K22.3)

J93.8   **Other pneumothorax and air leak**

`5th` **J93.81**   **Chronic pneumothorax**

J93.82   **Other air leak**
    Persistent air leak

J93.83   **Other pneumothorax**
    Acute pneumothorax
    Spontaneous pneumothorax NOS

J93.9   **Pneumothorax, unspecified**
    Pneumothorax NOS

(J95) INTRAOPERATIVE AND POSTPROCEDURAL COMPLICATIONS AND DISORDERS OF RESPIRATORY SYSTEM, NEC

GUIDELINES

As with all procedural or postprocedural complications, code assignment is based on the provider's documentation of the relationship between the condition and the procedure.

Code J95.851, Ventilator associated pneumonia(VAP), should be assigned only when the provider has documented VAP. An additional code to identify the organism (e.g., Pseudomonas aeruginosa, code B96.5) should also be assigned. Do not assign an additional code from categories J12-J18 to identify the type of pneumonia.

Code J95.851 should not be assigned for cases where the patient has pneumonia and is on a mechanical ventilator and the provider has not specifically stated that the pneumonia is ventilator-associated pneumonia. If the documentation is unclear as to whether the patient has a pneumonia that is a complication attributable to the mechanical ventilator, query the provider.

`4th` `5th` `6th` `7th`   Additional Character Required   `✓`   3-character code   •=New Code   ▲=Revised Code   *Excludes1*—Not coded here, do not use together   *Excludes2*—Not included here

A patient may be admitted with one type of pneumonia (e.g., code J13, Pneumonia due to Streptococcus pneumonia) and subsequently develop VAP. In this instance, the principal diagnosis would be the appropriate code from categories J12-J18 for the pneumonia diagnosed at the time of admission. Code J95.851, Ventilator associated pneumonia, would be assigned as an additional diagnosis when the provider has also documented the presence of ventilator associated pneumonia.

J95 INTRAOPERATIVE AND POSTPROCEDURAL COMPLICATIONS AND DISORDERS OF RESPIRATORY SYSTEM, NEC

> **Excludes2:** aspiration pneumonia (J69.-)
> emphysema (subcutaneous) resulting from a procedure (T81.82)
> hypostatic pneumonia (J18.2)
> pulmonary manifestations due to radiation (J70.0-J70.1)

J95.8 Other intraoperative and postprocedural complications and disorders of respiratory system, NEC

J95.81 Postprocedural pneumothorax and air leak

J95.811 Postprocedural pneumothorax
J95.812 Postprocedural air leak

J95.82 Postprocedural respiratory failure

> **Excludes1:** Respiratory failure in other conditions (J96.-)

J95.821 Acute postprocedural respiratory failure
Postprocedural respiratory failure NOS
J95.822 Acute and chronic post–procedural respiratory failure

J95.83 Postprocedural hemorrhage of a respiratory system organ or structure; following a procedure

J95.830 following a respiratory system procedure
J95.831 following other procedure

J95.84 Transfusion-related acute lung injury (TRALI)

J95.85 Complication of respirator [ventilator]

J95.850 Mechanical complication of respirator
> **Excludes1:** encounter for respirator [ventilator] dependence during power failure (Z99.12)
J95.851 Ventilator associated pneumonia
Ventilator associated pneumonitis
Use additional code to identify organism, if known (B95.-, B96.-, B97.-)
> **Excludes1:** ventilator lung in newborn (P27.8)
J95.859 Other complication of respirator [ventilator]

J95.86 Postprocedural hematoma and seroma of a respiratory system organ or structure following a procedure

J95.860 Postprocedural hematoma of a respiratory system organ or structure following a respiratory system procedure
J95.861 Postprocedural hematoma of a respiratory system organ or structure following other procedure
J95.862 Postprocedural seroma of a respiratory system organ or structure following a respiratory system procedure
J95.863 Postprocedural seroma of a respiratory system organ or structure following other procedure

J95.88 Other intraoperative complications of respiratory system, NEC

J95.89 Other postprocedural complications and disorders of respiratory system, NEC

Use additional code to identify disorder, such as:
aspiration pneumonia (J69.-)
bacterial or viral pneumonia (J12-J18)
> **Excludes2:** acute pulmonary insufficiency following thoracic surgery (J95.1)
> postprocedural subglottic stenosis (J95.5)

J96 RESPIRATORY FAILURE, NEC

> **GUIDELINES**

Acute Respiratory Failure

AS PRINCIPLE DIAGNOSIS

A code from subcategory J96.0, Acute respiratory failure, or subcategory J96.2, Acute and chronic respiratory failure, may be assigned as a principal diagnosis when it is the condition established after study to be chiefly responsible for occasioning the admission to the hospital, and the selection is supported by the Alphabetic Index and Tabular List. However, chapter-specific coding guidelines (such as obstetrics, poisoning, HIV, newborn) that provide sequencing direction take precedence.

AS SECONDARY DIAGNOSIS

Respiratory failure may be listed as a secondary diagnosis if it occurs after admission, or if it is present on admission, but does not meet the definition of principal diagnosis.

SEQUENCING OF ACUTE RESPIRATORY FAILURE AND ANOTHER ACUTE CONDITION

When a patient is admitted with respiratory failure and another acute condition, (eg, myocardial infarction, cerebrovascular accident, aspiration pneumonia), the principal diagnosis will not be the same in every situation. This applies whether the other acute condition is a respiratory or nonrespiratory condition. Selection of the principal diagnosis will be dependent on the circumstances of admission. If both the respiratory failure and the other acute condition are equally responsible for occasioning the admission to the hospital, and there are no chapter-specific sequencing rules, the guideline regarding two or more diagnoses that equally meet the definition for principal diagnosis may be applied in these situations.

> **Excludes1:** acute respiratory distress syndrome (J80)
> cardiorespiratory failure (R09.2)
> newborn respiratory distress syndrome (P22.0)
> postprocedural respiratory failure (J95.82-)
> respiratory arrest (R09.2)
> respiratory arrest of newborn (P28.81)
> respiratory failure of newborn (P28.5)

J96.0 Acute respiratory failure

J96.00 Acute respiratory failure, unspecified whether with hypoxia or hypercapnia
J96.01 Acute respiratory failure with hypoxia

J96.1 Chronic respiratory failure

J96.10 Chronic respiratory failure, unspecified whether with hypoxia or hypercapnia
J96.11 Chronic respiratory failure with hypoxia
J96.12 Chronic respiratory failure with hypercapnia

J96.2 Acute and chronic respiratory failure

Acute on chronic respiratory failure
J96.20 Acute and chronic respiratory failure, unspecified whether with hypoxia or hypercapnia
J96.21 Acute and chronic respiratory failure with hypoxia
J96.22 Acute and chronic respiratory failure with hypercapnia

J96.9 Respiratory failure, unspecified

J96.90 Respiratory failure, unspecified, unspecified whether with hypoxia or hypercapnia
J96.91 Respiratory failure, unspecified with hypoxia
J96.92 Respiratory failure, unspecified with hypercapnia

J98 OTHER RESPIRATORY DISORDERS

Use additional code to identify (Refer to Chapter 10 guidelines for codes) {Refer to main chapter guidelines}
> **Excludes1:** newborn apnea (P28.4)
> newborn sleep apnea (P28.3)
> **Excludes2:** apnea NOS (R06.81)
> sleep apnea (G47.3-)

   Additional Character Required   3-character code

*=New Code
▲=Revised Code

Excludes1—Not coded here, do not use together
Excludes2—Not included here

J98.0   **Diseases of bronchus, NEC**

> **J98.01**   **Acute bronchospasm**
> *5th*
> > ***Excludes1:*** acute bronchiolitis with bronchospasm (J21.-)
> > acute bronchitis with bronchospasm (J20.-)
> > asthma (J45.-)
> > exercise induced bronchospasm (J45.990)

J98.1   **Pulmonary collapse**

> ***Excludes1:*** therapeutic collapse of lung status (Z98.3)
> *5th*
> **J98.11**   **Atelectasis**
> > ***Excludes1:*** newborn atelectasis
> > tuberculous atelectasis (current disease) (A15)

J98.2   **Interstitial emphysema**

> Mediastinal emphysema
> ***Excludes1:*** emphysema NOS (J43.9)
> > emphysema in newborn (P25.0)
> > surgical emphysema (subcutaneous) (T81.82)
> > traumatic subcutaneous emphysema (T79.7)

J98.6   **Disorders of diaphragm**

> Diaphragmatitis
> Paralysis of diaphragm
> Relaxation of diaphragm
> ***Excludes1:*** congenital malformation of diaphragm NEC (Q79.1)
> > congenital diaphragmatic hernia (Q79.0)
> ***Excludes2:*** diaphragmatic hernia (K44.-)

J98.8   **Other specified respiratory disorders**

J98.9   **Respiratory disorder, unspecified**

> Respiratory disease (chronic) NOS

J99   **RESPIRATORY DISORDERS IN DISEASES CLASSIFIED ELSEWHERE**
✓

Code first underlying disease, such as:

> amyloidosis (E85.-)
> ankylosing spondylitis (M45)
> congenital syphilis (A50.5)
> cryoglobulinemia (D89.1)
> early congenital syphilis (A50.0)
> schistosomiasis (B65.0-B65.9)

Excludes1: respiratory disorders in:

> amebiasis (A06.5)
> blastomycosis (B40.0-B40.2)
> candidiasis (B37.1)
> coccidioidomycosis (B38.0-B38.2)
> cystic fibrosis with pulmonary manifestations (E84.0)
> dermatomyositis (M33.01, M33.11)
> histoplasmosis (B39.0-B39.2)
> late syphilis (A52.72, A52.73)
> polymyositis (M33.21)
> sicca syndrome (M35.02)
> SLE (M32.13)
> systemic sclerosis (M34.81)
> Wegener's granulomatosis (M31.30-M31.31)

CHAPTER 10. DISEASES OF THE RESPIRATORY SYSTEM   (J98.0–J99)

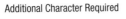 Additional Character Required   ✓   3-character code

•=New Code
▲=Revised Code

Excludes1—Not coded here, do not use together
Excludes2—Not included here

Chapter 11. Diseases of the digestive system (K00–K95)

GUIDELINES

Reserved for future guideline expansion

Excludes2: certain conditions originating in the perinatal period (P04–P96)
certain infectious and parasitic diseases (A00–B99)
complications of pregnancy, childbirth and the puerperium (O00–O9A)
congenital malformations, deformations and chromosomal abnormalities (Q00–Q99)
endocrine, nutritional and metabolic diseases (E00–E88)
injury, poisoning and certain other consequences of external causes (S00–T88)
neoplasms (C00–D49)
symptoms, signs and abnormal clinical and laboratory findings, NEC (R00–R94)

(K00–K14) DISEASES OF ORAL CAVITY AND SALIVARY GLANDS

K00 DISORDERS OF TOOTH DEVELOPMENT AND ERUPTION
4th

Excludes2: embedded and impacted teeth (K01.-)

K00.0 Anodontia
Hypodontia
Oligodontia
Excludes1: acquired absence of teeth (K08.1-)

K00.1 Supernumerary teeth
Distomolar
Fourth molar
Mesiodens
Paramolar
Supplementary teeth
Excludes2: supernumerary roots (K00.2)

K00.6 Disturbances in tooth eruption
Dentia praecox
Natal tooth
Neonatal tooth
Premature eruption of tooth
Premature shedding of primary [deciduous] tooth
Prenatal teeth
Retained [persistent] primary tooth
Excludes2: embedded and impacted teeth (K01.-)

K00.7 Teething syndrome

K00.8 Other disorders of tooth development
Color changes during tooth formation
Intrinsic staining of teeth NOS
Excludes2: posteruptive color changes (K03.7)

K00.9 Disorder of tooth development, unspecified
Disorder of odontogenesis NOS

K02 DENTAL CARIES
4th

Includes: caries of dentine
early childhood caries
pre-eruptive caries
ecurrent caries (dentino enamel junction) (enamel) (to the pulp)
dental cavities
tooth decay

K02.9 Dental caries, unspecified

K03 OTHER DISEASES OF HARD TISSUES OF TEETH
4th

Excludes2: bruxism (F45.8)
dental caries (K02.-)
teeth-grinding NOS (F45.8)

K03.8 Other specified diseases of hard tissues of teeth
5th **K03.81 Cracked tooth**
Excludes1: broken or fractured tooth due to trauma (S02.5)
K03.89 Other specified diseases of hard tissues of teeth
K03.9 Disease of hard tissues of teeth, unspecified

K04 DISEASES OF PULP AND PERIAPICAL TISSUES
4th

K04.7 Periapical abscess without sinus
Dental abscess without sinus
Dentoalveolar abscess without sinus
Periapical abscess without sinus

K05 GINGIVITIS AND PERIODONTAL DISEASES
4th

Use additional code to identify:
alcohol abuse and dependence (F10.-)
exposure to environmental tobacco smoke (Z77.22)
exposure to tobacco smoke in the perinatal period (P96.81)
history of tobacco dependence (Z87.891)
occupational exposure to environmental tobacco smoke (Z57.31)
tobacco dependence (F17.-)
tobacco use (Z72.0)

K05.0 Acute gingivitis
5th **Excludes1:** acute necrotizing ulcerative gingivitis (A69.1)
herpesviral [herpes simplex] gingivostomatitis (B00.2)
K05.00 Acute gingivitis, plaque induced
Acute gingivitis NOS
Plaque induced gingival disease

K06 OTHER DISORDERS OF GINGIVA AND EDENTULOUS ALVEOLAR RIDGE
4th

Excludes2: acute gingivitis (K05.0)
atrophy of edentulous alveolar ridge (K08.2)
chronic gingivitis (K05.1)
gingivitis NOS (K05.1)

K06.1 Gingival enlargement
Gingival fibromatosis

K08 OTHER DISORDERS OF TEETH AND SUPPORTING STRUCTURES
4th

Excludes2: dentofacial anomalies [including malocclusion] (M26.-)
disorders of jaw (M27.-)

K08.1 Complete loss of teeth
5th Acquired loss of teeth, complete
Excludes1: congenital absence of teeth (K00.0)
exfoliation of teeth due to systemic causes (K08.0)
partial loss of teeth (K08.4-)
K08.10 Complete loss of teeth, unspecified cause
6th **K08.101 Complete loss of teeth, unspecified cause; class I**
K08.102 class II
K08.103 class III
K08.104 class IV
K08.109 unspecified class
Edentulism NOS
K08.11 Complete loss of teeth due to trauma
6th **K08.111 Complete loss of teeth due to trauma; class I**
K08.112 class II
K08.113 class III
K08.114 class IV
K08.119 unspecified class
K08.12 Complete loss of teeth due to periodontal diseases
6th **K08.129 Complete loss of teeth due to periodontal diseases, unspecified class**
K08.13 Complete loss of teeth due to caries
6th **K08.131 Complete loss of teeth due to caries; class I**
K08.132 class II
K08.133 class III
K08.134 class IV
K08.139 unspecified class

K08.4 Partial loss of teeth
5th Acquired loss of teeth, partial
Excludes1: complete loss of teeth (K08.1-)
congenital absence of teeth (K00.0)
Excludes2: exfoliation of teeth due to systemic causes (K08.0)
K08.40 Partial loss of teeth, unspecified cause
6th **K08.401 Partial loss of teeth, unspecified cause; class I**
K08.402 class II
K08.403 class III
K08.404 class IV
K08.409 unspecified class
Tooth extraction status NOS

●=New Code
▲=Revised Code

4th **5th** **6th** **7th** Additional Character Required   ✓ 3-character code

Excludes1—Not coded here, do not use together
Excludes2—Not included here

K08.41 Partial loss of teeth due to trauma

6th
- **K08.411 Partial loss of teeth due to trauma; class I**
- **K08.412 class II**
- **K08.413 class III**
- **K08.414 class IV**
- **K08.419 unspecified class**

K08.42 Partial loss of teeth due to periodontal diseases

6th
- **K08.429 Partial loss of teeth due to periodontal diseases, unspecified class**

K08.43 Partial loss of teeth due to caries

6th
- **K08.431 Partial loss of teeth due to caries; class I**
- **K08.432 class II**
- **K08.433 class III**
- **K08.434 class IV**
- **K08.439 unspecified class**

K08.8 Other specified disorders of teeth and supporting structures

5th
- • **K08.81 Primary occlusal trauma**
- • **K08.82 Secondary occlusal trauma**
- • **K08.89 Other specified disorders of teeth and supporting structures**
  - Enlargement of alveolar ridge NOS
  - Insufficient anatomic crown height
  - Insufficient clinical crown length
  - Irregular alveolar process
  - Toothache NOS

K09 CYSTS OF ORAL REGION, NEC

4th
Includes: lesions showing histological features both of aneurysmal cyst and of another fibro-osseous lesion
Excludes2: cysts of jaw (M27.0-, M27.4-)
     radicular cyst (K04.8)

K09.0 Developmental odontogenic cysts
- Dentigerous cyst
- Eruption cyst
- Follicular cyst
- Gingival cyst
- Lateral periodontal cyst
- Primordial cyst
- *Excludes2:* keratocysts (D16.4, D16.5)
  - odontogenic keratocystic tumors (D16.4, D16.5)

K09.1 Developmental (nonodontogenic) cysts of oral region
- Cyst (of) incisive canal or palatine of papilla
- Globulomaxillary cyst
- Median palatal cyst
- Nasoalveolar cyst
- Nasolabial cyst
- Nasopalatine duct cyst

K09.8 Other cysts of oral region, NEC
- Dermoid cyst
- Epidermoid cyst
- Lymphoepithelial cyst
- Epstein's pearl

K09.9 Cyst of oral region, unspecified

K11 DISEASES OF SALIVARY GLANDS

4th
Use additional code to identify:
- alcohol abuse and dependence (F10.-)
- exposure to environmental tobacco smoke (Z77.22)
- exposure to tobacco smoke in the perinatal period (P96.81)
- history of tobacco dependence (Z87.891)
- occupational exposure to environmental tobacco smoke (Z57.31)
- tobacco dependence (F17.-)
- tobacco use (Z72.0)

K11.2 Sialoadenitis

5th
Parotitis
Excludes1: epidemic parotitis (B26.-)
     mumps (B26.-)
     uveoparotid fever [Heerfordt] (D86.89)

- **K11.20 Sialoadenitis, unspecified**
- **K11.21 Acute sialoadenitis**
  - *Excludes1:* acute recurrent sialoadenitis (K11.22)
- **K11.22 Acute recurrent sialoadenitis**
- **K11.23 Chronic sialoadenitis**

K12 STOMATITIS AND RELATED LESIONS

4th
Use additional code to identify: alcohol abuse and dependence (F10.-)
- exposure to environmental tobacco smoke (Z77.22)
- exposure to tobacco smoke in the perinatal period (P96.81)
- history of tobacco dependence (Z87.891)
- occupational exposure to environmental tobacco smoke (Z57.31)
- tobacco dependence (F17.-)
- tobacco use (Z72.0)

Excludes1: cancrum oris (A69.0)
- cheilitis (K13.0)
- gangrenous stomatitis (A69.0)
- herpesviral [herpes simplex] gingivostomatitis (B00.2)
- noma (A69.0)

K12.0 Recurrent oral aphthae
- Aphthous stomatitis (major) (minor)
- Bednar's aphthae
- Periadenitis mucosa necrotica recurrens
- Recurrent aphthous ulcer
- Stomatitis herpetiformis

K12.1 Other forms of stomatitis
- Stomatitis NOS
- Denture stomatitis
- Ulcerative stomatitis
- Vesicular stomatitis
- *Excludes1:* acute necrotizing ulcerative stomatitis (A69.1)

K12.2 Cellulitis and abscess of mouth
- Cellulitis of mouth (floor)
- Submandibular abscess
- *Excludes2:* abscess of salivary gland (K11.3)
  - abscess of tongue (K14.0)
  - periapical abscess (K04.6–K04.7)
  - periodontal abscess (K05.21)
  - peritonsillar abscess (J36)

K13 OTHER DISEASES OF LIP AND ORAL MUCOSA

4th
Includes: epithelial disturbances of tongue
Use additional code to identify:
- alcohol abuse and dependence (F10.-)
- exposure to environmental tobacco smoke (Z77.22)
- exposure to tobacco smoke in the perinatal period (P96.81)
- history of tobacco dependence (Z87.891)
- occupational exposure to environmental tobacco smoke (Z57.31)
- tobacco dependence (F17.-)
- tobacco use (Z72.0)

Excludes2: certain disorders of gingiva and edentulous alveolar ridge (K05–K06)
- cysts of oral region (K09.-)
- diseases of tongue (K14.-)
- stomatitis and related lesions (K12.-)

K13.0 Diseases of lips
- Abscess of lips
- Angular cheilitis
- Cellulitis of lips
- Cheilitis NOS
- Cheilodynia
- Cheilosis
- Exfoliative cheilitis
- Fistula of lips
- Glandular cheilitis
- Hypertrophy of lips
- Perlèche NEC
- *Excludes1:* ariboflavinosis (E53.0)
  - cheilitis due to radiation-related disorders (L55–L59)
  - congenital fistula of lips (Q38.0)
  - congenital hypertrophy of lips (Q18.6)
  - Perlèche due to candidiasis (B37.83)
  - Perlèche due to riboflavin deficiency (E53.0)

K13.7 Other and unspecified lesions of oral mucosa

5th
- **K13.70 Unspecified lesions of oral mucosa**
- **K13.79 Other lesions of oral mucosa**
  - Focal oral mucinosis

       Additional Character Required   ✓   3-character code

•=New Code
▲=Revised Code

Excludes1—Not coded here, do not use together
Excludes2—Not included here

K14 DISEASES OF TONGUE

Use additional code to identify: alcohol abuse and dependence (F10.-)
exposure to environmental tobacco smoke (Z77.22)
history of tobacco dependence (Z87.891)
occupational exposure to environmental tobacco smoke (Z57.31)
tobacco dependence (F17.-)
tobacco use (Z72.0)
Excludes2: erythroplakia (K13.29)
focal epithelial hyperplasia (K13.29)
leukedema of tongue (K13.29)
leukoplakia of tongue (K13.21)
hairy leukoplakia (K13.3)
macroglossia (congenital) (Q38.2)
submucous fibrosis of tongue (K13.5)

K14.0 Glossitis
Abscess of tongue
Ulceration (traumatic) of tongue
Excludes1: atrophic glossitis (K14.4)

K14.1 Geographic tongue
Benign migratory glossitis
Glossitis areata exfoliativa

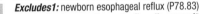
(K20–K31) DISEASES OF ESOPHAGUS, STOMACH AND DUODENUM

Excludes2: hiatus hernia (K44.-)

K20 ESOPHAGITIS

Use additional code to identify: alcohol abuse and dependence (F10.-)
Excludes1: erosion of esophagus (K22.1-)
esophagitis with gastro-esophageal reflux disease (K21.0)
reflux esophagitis (K21.0)
ulcerative esophagitis (K22.1-)
Excludes2: eosinophilic gastritis or gastroenteritis (K52.81)

K20.0 Eosinophilic esophagitis
K20.8 Other esophagitis
Abscess of esophagus
K20.9 Esophagitis, unspecified
Esophagitis NOS

K21 GASTRO-ESOPHAGEAL REFLUX DISEASE
Excludes1: newborn esophageal reflux (P78.83)
K21.0 Gastro-esophageal reflux disease with esophagitis
Reflux esophagitis
K21.9 Gastro-esophageal reflux disease without esophagitis
Esophageal reflux NOS

K25 GASTRIC ULCER
Includes: erosion (acute) of stomach
pylorus ulcer (peptic)
stomach ulcer (peptic)
Use additional code to identify: alcohol abuse and dependence (F10.-)
Excludes1: acute gastritis (K29.0-)
peptic ulcer NOS (K27.-)
K25.0 Acute gastric ulcer; with hemorrhage
K25.1   with perforation
K25.2   with both hemorrhage and perforation
K25.3   without hemorrhage or perforation
K25.4 Chronic or unspecified gastric ulcer; with hemorrhage
K25.5   with perforation
K25.6   with both hemorrhage and perforation
K25.7   without hemorrhage or perforation
K25.9 Gastric ulcer, unspecified as acute or chronic, without hemorrhage or perforation

K26 DUODENAL ULCER
Includes: erosion (acute) of duodenum
duodenum ulcer (peptic)
postpyloric ulcer (peptic)
Use additional code to identify: alcohol abuse and dependence (F10.-)
Excludes1: peptic ulcer NOS (K27.-)
K26.0 Acute duodenal ulcer; with hemorrhage
K26.1   with perforation
K26.2   with both hemorrhage and perforation
K26.3   without hemorrhage or perforation
K26.4 Chronic or unspecified duodenal ulcer; with hemorrhage

K26.5   with perforation
K26.6   with both hemorrhage and perforation
K26.7   without hemorrhage or perforation
K26.9 Duodenal ulcer, unspecified as acute or chronic, without hemorrhage or perforation

K27 PEPTIC ULCER, SITE UNSPECIFIED
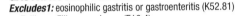
Includes: gastroduodenal ulcer NOS
peptic ulcer NOS
Use additional code to identify: alcohol abuse and dependence (F10.-)
Excludes1: peptic ulcer of newborn (P78.82)
K27.0 Acute peptic ulcer, site unspecified; with hemorrhage
K27.1   with perforation
K27.2   with both hemorrhage and perforation
K27.3   without hemorrhage or perforation
K27.4 Chronic or unspecified peptic ulcer, site unspecified; with hemorrhage
K27.5   with perforation
K27.6   with both hemorrhage and perforation
K27.7   without hemorrhage or perforation
K27.9 Peptic ulcer, site unspecified, unspecified as acute or chronic, without hemorrhage or perforation

K29 GASTRITIS AND DUODENITIS
Excludes1: eosinophilic gastritis or gastroenteritis (K52.81)
Zollinger-Ellison syndrome (E16.4)
K29.0 Acute gastritis

Use additional code to identify: alcohol abuse and dependence (F10.-)
Excludes1: erosion (acute) of stomach (K25.-)
K29.00   Acute gastritis without bleeding
K29.01   Acute gastritis with bleeding
K29.7 Gastritis, unspecified
K29.70   Gastritis, unspecified, without bleeding
K29.71   Gastritis, unspecified, with bleeding
K29.8 Duodenitis
K29.80   Duodenitis without bleeding
K29.81   Duodenitis with bleeding
K29.9 Gastroduodenitis, unspecified
K29.90   Gastroduodenitis, unspecified, without bleeding
K29.91   Gastroduodenitis, unspecified, with bleeding

K30 FUNCTIONAL DYSPEPSIA

Indigestion
Excludes1: dyspepsia NOS (R10.13)
heartburn (R12)
nervous dyspepsia (F45.8)
neurotic dyspepsia (F45.8)
psychogenic dyspepsia (F45.8)

K31 OTHER DISEASES OF STOMACH AND DUODENUM
Includes: functional disorders of stomach
Excludes2: diabetic gastroparesis (E08.43, E09.43, E10.43, E11.43, E13.43)
diverticulum of duodenum (K57.00–K57.13)
K31.3 Pylorospasm, NEC
Excludes1: congenital or infantile pylorospasm (Q40.0)
neurotic pylorospasm (F45.8)
psychogenic pylorospasm (F45.8)
K31.5 Obstruction of duodenum
Constriction of duodenum
Duodenal ileus (chronic)
Stenosis of duodenum
Stricture of duodenum
Volvulus of duodenum
Excludes 1: congenital stenosis of duodenum (Q41.0)

(K35–K38) DISEASES OF APPENDIX

K35 ACUTE APPENDICITIS
K35.2 Acute appendicitis with generalized peritonitis
Appendicitis (acute) with generalized (diffuse) peritonitis following rupture or perforation of appendix
Perforated or Ruptured appendix NOS

 Additional Character Required   3-character code

•=New Code
▲=Revised Code

Excludes1—Not coded here, do not use together
Excludes2—Not included here

K35.3 Acute appendicitis with localized peritonitis
Acute appendicitis with or without perforation or rupture with peritonitis NOS
Acute appendicitis with or without perforation or rupture with localized peritonitis
Acute appendicitis with peritoneal abscess

K35.8 Other and unspecified acute appendicitis
 K35.80 Unspecified acute appendicitis
Acute appendicitis NOS
Acute appendicitis without (localized) (generalized) peritonitis

K35.89 Other acute appendicitis

(K40–K46) HERNIA

Note: Hernia with both gangrene and obstruction is classified to hernia with gangrene.
Includes: acquired hernia
congenital [except diaphragmatic or hiatus] hernia
recurrent hernia

K40 INGUINAL HERNIA
 Includes: bubonocele
direct inguinal hernia
double inguinal hernia
indirect inguinal hernia
inguinal hernia NOS
oblique inguinal hernia
scrotal hernia

K40.0 Bilateral inguinal hernia, with obstruction, without gangrene
Inguinal hernia (bilateral) causing obstruction without gangrene
Incarcerated or Irreducible or Strangulated inguinal hernia (bilateral) without gangrene

K40.00 Bilateral inguinal hernia, with obstruction, without gangrene, not specified as recurrent
Bilateral inguinal hernia, with obstruction, without gangrene NOS

K40.01 Bilateral inguinal hernia, with obstruction, without gangrene, recurrent

K40.1 Bilateral inguinal hernia, with gangrene
K40.10 Bilateral inguinal hernia, with gangrene, not specified as recurrent
Bilateral inguinal hernia, with gangrene NOS

K40.11 Bilateral inguinal hernia, with gangrene, recurrent

K40.2 Bilateral inguinal hernia, without obstruction or gangrene
K40.20 Bilateral inguinal hernia, without obstruction or gangrene, not specified as recurrent
Bilateral inguinal hernia NOS

K40.21 Bilateral inguinal hernia, without obstruction or gangrene, recurrent

K40.3 Unilateral inguinal hernia, with obstruction, without gangrene
Inguinal hernia (unilateral) causing obstruction without gangrene
Incarcerated or Irreducible or Strangulated inguinal hernia (unilateral) without gangrene

K40.30 Unilateral inguinal hernia, with obstruction, without gangrene, not specified as recurrent
Inguinal hernia, with obstruction NOS
Unilateral inguinal hernia, with obstruction, without gangrene NOS

K40.31 Unilateral inguinal hernia, with obstruction, without gangrene, recurrent

K40.4 Unilateral inguinal hernia, with gangrene
K40.40 Unilateral inguinal hernia, with gangrene, not specified as recurrent
Inguinal hernia with gangrene NOS
Unilateral inguinal hernia with gangrene NOS

K40.41 Unilateral inguinal hernia, with gangrene, recurrent

K40.9 Unilateral inguinal hernia, without obstruction or gangrene
K40.90 Unilateral inguinal hernia, without obstruction or gangrene, not specified as recurrent
Inguinal hernia NOS
Unilateral inguinal hernia NOS

K40.91 Unilateral inguinal hernia, without obstruction or gangrene, recurrent

K42 UMBILICAL HERNIA
 Includes: paraumbilical hernia
Excludes1: omphalocele (Q79.2)
K42.0 Umbilical hernia with obstruction, without gangrene
Umbilical hernia causing obstruction, without gangrene
Incarcerated or Irreducible or Strangulated umbilical hernia, without gangrene

K42.1 Umbilical hernia with gangrene
Gangrenous umbilical hernia

K42.9 Umbilical hernia without obstruction or gangrene
Umbilical hernia NOS

K43 VENTRAL HERNIA
 K43.0 Incisional hernia with obstruction, without gangrene
Incisional hernia causing obstruction, without gangrene
Incarcerated or Irreducible or Strangulated incisional hernia, without gangrene

K43.1 Incisional hernia with gangrene
Gangrenous incisional hernia

K43.2 Incisional hernia without obstruction or gangrene
Incisional hernia NOS

K43.9 Ventral hernia without obstruction or gangrene
Epigastric hernia
Ventral hernia NOS

K44 DIAPHRAGMATIC HERNIA
 Includes: hiatus hernia (esophageal) (sliding)
paraesophageal hernia
Excludes1: congenital diaphragmatic hernia (Q79.0)
congenital hiatus hernia (Q40.1)
K44.0 Diaphragmatic hernia with obstruction, without gangrene
Diaphragmatic hernia causing obstruction
Incarcerated or Irreducible or Strangulated diaphragmatic hernia

K44.1 Diaphragmatic hernia with gangrene
Gangrenous diaphragmatic hernia

K44.9 Diaphragmatic hernia without obstruction or gangrene
Diaphragmatic hernia NOS

(K50–K52) NONINFECTIVE ENTERITIS AND COLITIS

Includes: noninfective inflammatory bowel disease
Excludes1: irritable bowel syndrome (K58.-)
megacolon (K59.3-)

K50 CROHN'S DISEASE [REGIONAL ENTERITIS]
 Includes: granulomatous enteritis
Use additional code to identify manifestations, such as: pyoderma gangrenosum (L88)
Excludes1: ulcerative colitis (K51.-)
K50.0 Crohn's disease of small intestine
 Crohn's disease [regional enteritis] of duodenum or ileum or jejunum
Regional ileitis
Terminal ileitis
Excludes1: Crohn's disease of both small and large intestine (K50.8-)

K50.00 Crohn's disease of small intestine without complications

K50.01 Crohn's disease of small intestine with complications
 K50.011 Crohn's disease of small intestine; with rectal bleeding
K50.012 with intestinal obstruction
K50.013 with fistula
K50.014 with abscess
K50.018 with other complication
K50.019 with unspecified complications

K50.1 Crohn's disease of large intestine
 Crohn's disease [regional enteritis] of colon or large bowel or rectum
Granulomatous colitis
Regional colitis
Excludes1: Crohn's disease of both small and large intestine (K50.8)

●=New Code
▲=Revised Code

Excludes1—Not coded here, do not use together
Excludes2—Not included here

K50.10   Crohn's disease of large intestine without complications
K50.11   Crohn's disease of large intestine with complications
    6th   K50.111   Crohn's disease of large intestine; with rectal bleeding
    K50.112   with intestinal obstruction
    K50.113   with fistula
    K50.114   with abscess
    K50.118   with other complication
    K50.119   with unspecified complications

K50.8   Crohn's disease of both small and large intestine
    5th   K50.80   Crohn's disease of both small and large intestine without complications
    K50.81   Crohn's disease of both small and large intestine with complications
    6th   K50.811   Crohn's disease of both small and large intestine; with rectal bleeding
    K50.812   with intestinal obstruction
    K50.813   with fistula
    K50.814   with abscess
    K50.818   with other complication
    K50.819   with unspecified complications

K50.9   Crohn's disease, unspecified
    5th   K50.90   Crohn's disease, unspecified, without complications
     Crohn's disease NOS
     Regional enteritis NOS
    K50.91   Crohn's disease, unspecified, with complications
    6th   K50.911   Crohn's disease, unspecified; with rectal bleeding
    K50.912   with intestinal obstruction
    K50.913   with fistula
    K50.914   with abscess
    K50.918   with other complication
    K50.919   with unspecified complications

K51   ULCERATIVE COLITIS
    4th   **Use additional code** to identify manifestations, such as: pyoderma gangrenosum (L88)
    Excludes1: Crohn's disease [regional enteritis] (K50.-)

K51.0   Ulcerative (chronic) pancolitis
    5th   Backwash ileitis
    K51.00   Ulcerative (chronic) pancolitis without complications
     Ulcerative (chronic) pancolitis NOS
    K51.01   Ulcerative (chronic) pancolitis with complications
    6th   K51.011   Ulcerative (chronic) pancolitis; with rectal bleeding
    K51.012   with intestinal obstruction
    K51.013   with fistula
    K51.014   with abscess
    K51.018   with other complication
    K51.019   with unspecified complications

K51.2   Ulcerative (chronic) proctitis
    5th   K51.20   Ulcerative (chronic) proctitis without complications
     Ulcerative (chronic) proctitis NOS
    K51.21   Ulcerative (chronic) proctitis with complications
    6th   K51.211   Ulcerative (chronic) proctitis; with rectal bleeding
    K51.212   with intestinal obstruction
    K51.213   with fistula
    K51.214   with abscess
    K51.218   with other complication
    K51.219   with unspecified complications

K51.3   Ulcerative (chronic) rectosigmoiditis
    5th   K51.30   Ulcerative (chronic) rectosigmoiditis without complications
     Ulcerative (chronic) rectosigmoiditis NOS
    K51.31   Ulcerative (chronic) rectosigmoiditis with complications
    6th   K51.311   Ulcerative (chronic) rectosigmoiditis; with rectal bleeding
    K51.312   with intestinal obstruction
    K51.313   with fistula
    K51.314   with abscess

    K51.318   with other complication
    K51.319   with unspecified complications

K51.4   Inflammatory polyps of colon
    5th   *Excludes1:* adenomatous polyp of colon (D12.6)
     polyposis of colon (D12.6)
     polyps of colon NOS (K63.5)
    K51.40   Inflammatory polyps of colon without complications
     Inflammatory polyps of colon NOS
    K51.41   Inflammatory polyps of colon with complications
    6th   K51.411   Inflammatory polyps of colon; with rectal bleeding
    K51.412   with intestinal obstruction
    K51.413   with fistula
    K51.414   with abscess
    K51.418   with other complication
    K51.419   with unspecified complications

K51.5   Left sided colitis
    5th   Left hemicolitis
    K51.50   Left sided colitis without complications
     Left sided colitis NOS
    K51.51   Left sided colitis with complications
    6th   K51.511   Left sided colitis; with rectal bleeding
    K51.512   with intestinal obstruction
    K51.513   with fistula
    K51.514   with abscess
    K51.518   with other complication
    K51.519   with unspecified complications

K51.8   Other ulcerative colitis
    5th   K51.80   Other ulcerative colitis without complications
    K51.81   Other ulcerative colitis with complications
    6th   K51.811   Other ulcerative colitis; with rectal bleeding
    K51.812   with intestinal obstruction
    K51.813   with fistula
    K51.814   with abscess
    K51.818   with other complication
    K51.819   with unspecified complications

K51.9   Ulcerative colitis, unspecified
    5th   K51.90   Ulcerative colitis, unspecified, without complications
    K51.91   Ulcerative colitis, unspecified, with complications
    6th   K51.911   Ulcerative colitis, unspecified; with rectal bleeding
    K51.912   with intestinal obstruction
    K51.913   with fistula
    K51.914   with abscess
    K51.918   with other complication
    K51.919   with unspecified complications

K52   OTHER AND UNSPECIFIED NONINFECTIVE GASTROENTERITIS AND COLITIS
    4th   **K52.2   Allergic and dietetic gastroenteritis and colitis**
    5th   Food hypersensitivity gastroenteritis or colitis
    Use additional code to identify type of food allergy (Z91.01-, Z91.02-)
    Excludes2: allergic eosinophilic colitis (K52.82)
     allergic eosinophilic esophagitis (K20.0)
     allergic eosinophilic gastritis (K52.81)
     allergic eosinophilic gastroenteritis (K52.81)
     food protein-induced proctocolitis (K52.82)
    • K52.21   Food protein-induced enterocolitis syndrome
     Use additional code for hypovolemic shock, if present (R57.1)
    • K52.22   Food protein-induced enteropathy
    • K52.29   Other allergic and dietetic gastroenteritis and colitis
     Food hypersensitivity gastroenteritis or colitis
     Immediate gastrointestinal hypersensitivity

    • **K52.3   Indeterminate colitis**
     Colonic inflammatory bowel disease unclassified (IBDU)
     Excludes1: unspecified colitis (K52.9)

    K52.8   Other specified noninfective gastroenteritis and colitis
    5th   K52.81   Eosinophilic gastritis or gastroenteritis
     Eosinophilic enteritis
     Excludes2: eosinophilic esophagitis (K20.0)

     Additional Character Required   ✔ 3-character code   •=New Code   ▲=Revised Code   *Excludes1*—Not coded here, do not use together   *Excludes2*—Not included here

CHAPTER 11. DISEASES OF THE DIGESTIVE SYSTEM   (K52.82–K58.9)

K52.82   **Eosinophilic colitis**
Allergic proctocolitis
Food-induced eosinophilic proctocolitis
Food protein-induced proctocolitis
Milk protein-induced proctocolitis

K52.83   **Microscopic colitis**
- °**K52.831**   **Collagenous colitis**
- °**K52.832**   **Lymphocytic colitis**
- °**K52.838**   **Other microscopic colitis**
- °**K52.839**   **Microscopic colitis, unspecified**

K52.89   **Other specified noninfective gastroenteritis and colitis**

K52.9   **Noninfective gastroenteritis and colitis, unspecified**
Colitis or Enteritis or Gastroenteritis NOS
Ileitis or Jejunitis or Sigmoiditis NOS
Excludes1: diarrhea NOS (R19.7)
functional diarrhea (K59.1)
infectious gastroenteritis and colitis NOS (A09)
neonatal diarrhea (noninfective) (P78.3)
psychogenic diarrhea (F45.8)

(K55–K64) OTHER DISEASES OF INTESTINES

K55   **VASCULAR DISORDERS OF INTESTINES**
K55.0   **Acute vascular disorders of intestine**
Infarction of appendices epiploicae
Mesenteric (artery) (vein) embolism
Mesenteric (artery) (vein) infarction
Mesenteric (artery) (vein) thrombosis

K55.01   **Ischemia of small intestines**
- °**K55.011**   **Focal (segmental) acute (reversible) ischemia of small intestine**
- °**K55.012**   **Diffuse acute (reversible) ischemia of small intestine**
- °**K55.019**   **Acute (reversible) ischemia of small intestine, extent unspecified**

K55.02   **Infarction of small intestines**
Gangrene or necrosis of small intestine
- °**K55.021**   **Focal (segmental) acute infarction of small intestine**
- °**K55.022**   **Diffuse acute infarction of small intestine**
- °**K55.029**   **Acute infarction of small intestine, extent unspecified**

K55.03   **Ischemia of small intestine**
Acute fulminant ischemic colitis
Subacute ischemic colitis
- °**K55.031**   **Focal (segmental) acute (reversible) ischemia of large intestine**
- °**K55.032**   **Diffuse acute (reversible) ischemia of large intestine**
- °**K55.039**   **Acute (reversible) ischemia of large intestine, extent unspecified**

K55.04   **Infarction of intestine, part unspecified**
Gangrene or necrosis of large intestine
- °**K55.041**   **Focal (segmental) acute infarction of large intestine**
- °**K55.042**   **Diffuse acute infarction of large intestine**
- °**K55.049**   **Acute infarction of large intestine, extent unspecified**

K55.05   **Ischemia of intestine, part unspecified**
- °**K55.051**   **Focal (segmental) acute (reversible) ischemia of intestine, part unspecified**
- °**K55.052**   **Diffuse acute (reversible) ischemia of intestine, part unspecified**
- °**K55.059**   **Acute (reversible) ischemia of intestine, part and extent unspecified**

K55.06   **Infarction of intestine, part unspecified**
- °**K55.061**   **Focal (segmental) acute infarction of intestine, part unspecified**
- °**K55.062**   **Diffuse acute infarction of intestine, part unspecified**
- °**K55.069**   **Acute infarction of intestine, part and extent unspecified**

K55.1   **Chronic vascular disorders of intestine**
Chronic ischemic colitis
Chronic ischemic enteritis
Chronic ischemic enterocolitis
Ischemic stricture of intestine
Mesenteric atherosclerosis
Mesenteric vascular insufficiency

°**K55.3**   **Necrotizing enterocolitis**
Excludes1: necrotizing enterocolitis of newborn (P77.-)
- °**K55.30**   **Necrotizing enterocolitis, unspecified**
Necrotizing enterocolitis, NOS
- °**K55.31**   **Stage 1 necrotizing enterocolitis**
Necrotizing enterocolitis without pneumonia or perforation
- °**K55.32**   **Stage 2 necrotizing enterocolitis**
Necrotizing enterocolitis with pneumonia, without perforation
- °**K55.33**   **Stage 3 necrotizing enterocolitis**
Necrotizing enterocolitis with perforation
Necrotizing enterocolitis with pneumatosis and perforation

K56   **PARALYTIC ILEUS AND INTESTINAL OBSTRUCTION WITHOUT HERNIA**
Excludes1: congenital stricture or stenosis of intestine (Q41–Q42)
cystic fibrosis with meconium ileus (E84.11)
ischemic stricture of intestine (K55.1)
meconium ileus NOS (P76.0)
neonatal intestinal obstructions classifiable to P76.-
obstruction of duodenum (K31.5)
postprocedural intestinal obstruction (K91.3)
stenosis of anus or rectum (K62.4)
intestinal obstruction with hernia (K40–K46)

K56.0   **Paralytic ileus**
Paralysis of bowel or colon or intestine
Excludes1: gallstone ileus (K56.3)
ileus NOS (K56.7)
obstructive ileus NOS (K56.69)

K56.1   **Intussusception**
Intussusception or invagination of bowel or colon or intestine or rectum
Excludes2: intussusception of appendix (K38.8)

K56.2   **Volvulus**
Strangulation of colon or intestine
Torsion or Twist of colon or intestine
Excludes2: volvulus of duodenum (K31.5)

K56.4   **Other impaction of intestine**
K56.41   **Fecal impaction**
Excludes1: constipation (K59.0-)
incomplete defecation (R15.0)
K56.49   **Other impaction of intestine**

K56.6   **Other and unspecified intestinal obstruction**
K56.60   **Unspecified intestinal obstruction**
Intestinal obstruction NOS
Excludes1: intestinal obstruction due to specified condition-code to condition
K56.69   **Other intestinal obstruction**
Enterostenosis NOS
Obstructive ileus NOS
Occlusion or Stenosis or Stricture of colon or intestine NOS
Excludes1: intestinal obstruction due to specified condition-code to condition

K58   **IRRITABLE BOWEL SYNDROME**
Includes: irritable colon
spastic colon
K58.0   **Irritable bowel syndrome with diarrhea**
°**K58.1**   **Irritable bowel syndrome with constipation**
°**K58.2**   **Mixed irritable bowel syndrome**
°**K58.8**   **Other Irritable bowel syndrome**
K58.9   **Irritable bowel syndrome without diarrhea**
Irritable bowel syndrome NOS

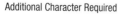 Additional Character Required   3-character code   °=New Code   △=Revised Code   ***Excludes1***—Not coded here, do not use together   ***Excludes2***—Not included here

K59 **OTHER FUNCTIONAL INTESTINAL DISORDERS**
`4th`
> *Excludes1:* change in bowel habit NOS (R19.4)
> intestinal malabsorption (K90.-)
> psychogenic intestinal disorders (F45.8)
>
> *Excludes2:* functional disorders of stomach (K31.-)

K59.0 **Constipation**
`5th`
> *Excludes1:* fecal impaction (K56.41)
> incomplete defecation (R15.0)

    K59.00 **Constipation, unspecified**

    K59.01 **Slow transit constipation**

    K59.02 **Outlet dysfunction constipation**

    •**K59.03** **Drug induced constipation**
        Use additional code for adverse effect, if applicable, to identify drug (T36–T50) with fifth or sixth character 5

    •**K59.04** **Chronic Idiopathic constipation**
        Functional constipation

    K59.09 **Other constipation**
        Chronic constipation

K59.3 **Megacolon, NEC**
`5th`
> Dilatation of colon
> *Excludes1:* congenital megacolon (aganglionic) (Q43.1)
> megacolon (due to) (in) Chagas' disease (B57.32)
> megacolon (due to) (in) Clostridium difficile (A04.7)
> megacolon (due to) (in) Hirschsprung's disease (Q43.1)

    •**K59.31** **Toxic megacolon**
        Code first (T51–T65) to identify toxic agent, if applicable

    •**K59.39** **Other megacolon**
        Megacolon NOS

K59.9 **Functional intestinal disorder, unspecified**

K60 **FISSURE AND FISTULA OF ANAL AND RECTAL REGIONS**
`4th`
> *Excludes1:* fissure and fistula of anal and rectal regions with abscess or cellulitis (K61.-)
> *Excludes2:* anal sphincter tear (healed) (nontraumatic) (old) (K62.81)

K60.0 **Acute anal fissure**

K60.1 **Chronic anal fissure**

K60.2 **Anal fissure, unspecified**

K61 **ABSCESS OF ANAL AND RECTAL REGIONS**
`4th`
> *Includes:* abscess of anal and rectal regions
> cellulitis of anal and rectal regions

K61.0 **Anal abscess**
> Perianal abscess
> *Excludes1:* intrasphincteric abscess (K61.4)

K62 **OTHER DISEASES OF ANUS AND RECTUM**
`4th`
> *Includes:* anal canal
> *Excludes2:* colostomy and enterostomy malfunction (K94.0-, K94.1-)
> fecal incontinence (R15.-)
> hemorrhoids (K64.-)

K62.0 **Anal polyp**

K62.1 **Rectal polyp**
> *Excludes1:* adenomatous polyp (D12.8)

K62.2 **Anal prolapse**
> Prolapse of anal canal

K62.3 **Rectal prolapse**
> Prolapse of rectal mucosa

K62.4 **Stenosis of anus and rectum**
> Stricture of anus (sphincter)

K62.5 **Hemorrhage of anus and rectum**
> *Excludes1:* gastrointestinal bleeding NOS (K92.2)
> melena (K92.1)
> neonatal rectal hemorrhage (P54.2)

K62.6 **Ulcer of anus and rectum**
> Solitary ulcer of anus and rectum
> Stercoral ulcer of anus and rectum

K62.8 **Other specified diseases of anus and rectum**
`5th`
> *Excludes2:* ulcerative proctitis (K51.2)

    K62.81 **Anal sphincter tear (healed) (nontraumatic) (old)**
        Tear of anus, nontraumatic
        Use additional code for any associated fecal incontinence (R15.-)

> *Excludes2:* anal fissure (K60.-)
> anal sphincter tear (healed) (old) complicating delivery (O34.7-)
> traumatic tear of anal sphincter (S31.831)

    K62.82 **Dysplasia of anus**
        Anal intraepithelial neoplasia I and II (AIN I and II) (histologically confirmed)
        Dysplasia of anus NOS
        Mild and moderate dysplasia of anus (histologically confirmed)
        Excludes1: abnormal results from anal cytologic examination without histologic confirmation (R85.61-)
        anal intraepithelial neoplasia III (D01.3)
        carcinoma in situ of anus (D01.3)
        HGSIL of anus (R85.613)
        severe dysplasia of anus (D01.3)

    K62.89 **Other specified diseases of anus and rectum**
        Proctitis NOS
        Use additional code for any associated fecal incontinence (R15.-)

K62.9 **Disease of anus and rectum, unspecified**

K64 **HEMORRHOIDS AND PERIANAL VENOUS THROMBOSIS**
`4th`
> *Includes:* piles
> *Excludes1:* hemorrhoids complicating childbirth and the puerperium (O87.2)
> hemorrhoids complicating pregnancy (O22.4)

K64.0 **First degree hemorrhoids**
> Grade/stage I hemorrhoids
> Hemorrhoids (bleeding) without prolapse outside of anal canal

K64.1 **Second degree hemorrhoids**
> Grade/stage II hemorrhoids
> Hemorrhoids (bleeding) that prolapse with straining, but retract spontaneously

K64.2 **Third degree hemorrhoids**
> Grade/stage III hemorrhoids
> Hemorrhoids (bleeding) that prolapse with straining and require manual replacement back inside anal canal

K64.3 **Fourth degree hemorrhoids**
> Grade/stage IV hemorrhoids
> Hemorrhoids (bleeding) with prolapsed tissue that cannot be manually replaced

K64.4 **Residual hemorrhoidal skin tags**
> External hemorrhoids, NOS
> Skin tags of anus

K64.8 **Other hemorrhoids**
> Internal hemorrhoids, without mention of degree
> Prolapsed hemorrhoids, degree not specified

K64.9 **Unspecified hemorrhoids**
> Hemorrhoids (bleeding) NOS
> Hemorrhoids (bleeding) without mention of degree

(K65–K68) DISEASES OF PERITONEUM AND RETROPERITONEUM

K65 **PERITONITIS**
`4th`
> **Use additional code** (B95–B97), to identify infectious agent
> *Excludes1:* acute appendicitis with generalized peritonitis (K35.2)
> aseptic peritonitis (T81.6)
> benign paroxysmal peritonitis (E85.0)
> chemical peritonitis (T81.6)
> diverticulitis of both small and large intestine with peritonitis (K57.4-)
> diverticulitis of colon with peritonitis (K57.2-)
> diverticulitis of intestine, NOS, with peritonitis (K57.8-)
> diverticulitis of small intestine with peritonitis (K57.0-)
> gonococcal peritonitis (A54.85)
> neonatal peritonitis (P78.0–P78.1)
> pelvic peritonitis, female (N73.3–N73.5)
> periodic familial peritonitis (E85.0)
> peritonitis due to talc or other foreign substance (T81.6)
> peritonitis in chlamydia (A74.81) or in diphtheria (A36.89) or syphilis (late) (A52.74)
> peritonitis in tuberculosis (A18.31)

     Additional Character Required   3-character code

•=New Code   *Excludes1*—Not coded here, do not use together
▲=Revised Code   *Excludes2*—Not included here

peritonitis with or following abortion or ectopic or molar pregnancy (O00–O07, O08.0)
peritonitis with or following appendicitis (K35.-)
peritonitis with or following diverticular disease of intestine (K57.-)
puerperal peritonitis (O85)
retroperitoneal infections (K68.-)

K65.0   **Generalized (acute) peritonitis**
Pelvic peritonitis (acute), male
Subphrenic peritonitis (acute)
Suppurative peritonitis (acute)

(K70–K77) DISEASES OF LIVER

Excludes1: jaundice NOS (R17)
Excludes2: hemochromatosis (E83.11-)
Reye's syndrome (G93.7)
viral hepatitis (B15–B19)
Wilson's disease (E83.0)

K73   **CHRONIC HEPATITIS, NEC**
[4th]
Excludes1: alcoholic hepatitis (chronic) (K70.1-)
drug-induced hepatitis (chronic) (K71.-)
granulomatous hepatitis (chronic) NEC (K75.3)
reactive, nonspecific hepatitis (chronic) (K75.2)
viral hepatitis (chronic) (B15–B19)
K73.0   **Chronic persistent hepatitis, NEC**
K73.1   **Chronic lobular hepatitis, NEC**
K73.2   **Chronic active hepatitis, NEC**
K73.8   **Other chronic hepatitis, NEC**
K73.9   **Chronic hepatitis, unspecified**

K76   **OTHER DISEASES OF LIVER**
[4th]
Excludes2: alcoholic liver disease (K70.-)
amyloid degeneration of liver (E85.-)
cystic disease of liver (congenital) (Q44.6)
hepatic vein thrombosis (I82.0)
hepatomegaly NOS (R16.0)
pigmentary cirrhosis (of liver) (E83.110)
portal vein thrombosis (I81)
toxic liver disease (K71.-)
K76.8   **Other specified diseases of liver**
    K76.81   **Hepatopulmonary syndrome**
       Code first underlying liver disease, such as:
       alcoholic cirrhosis of liver (K70.3-)
       cirrhosis of liver without mention of alcohol (K74.6-)
    K76.89   **Other specified diseases of liver**
       Cyst (simple) of liver
       Focal nodular hyperplasia of liver
       Hepatoptosis
K76.9   **Liver disease, unspecified**

K77   **LIVER DISORDERS IN DISEASES CLASSIFIED ELSEWHERE**

Code first underlying disease, such as: amyloidosis (E85.-)
congenital syphilis (A50.0, A50.5)
congenital toxoplasmosis (P37.1)
schistosomiasis (B65.0–B65.9)
Excludes1: alcoholic hepatitis (K70.1-)
alcoholic liver disease (K70.-)
cytomegaloviral hepatitis (B25.1)
herpesviral [herpes simplex] hepatitis (B00.81)
infectious mononucleosis with liver disease (B27.0–B27.9 with .9)
mumps hepatitis (B26.81)
sarcoidosis with liver disease (D86.89)
secondary syphilis with liver disease (A51.45)
syphilis (late) with liver disease (A52.74)
toxoplasmosis (acquired) hepatitis (B58.1)
tuberculosis with liver disease (A18.83)

(K80–K87) DISORDERS OF GALLBLADDER, BILIARY TRACT AND PANCREAS

K80   **CHOLELITHIASIS**
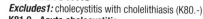
Excludes1: retained cholelithiasis following cholecystectomy (K91.86)
K80.0   **Calculus of gallbladder with acute cholecystitis**
   Any condition listed in K80.2 with acute cholecystitis
    K80.00   **Calculus of gallbladder with acute cholecystitis without obstruction**
    K80.01   **Calculus of gallbladder with acute cholecystitis with obstruction**
K80.1   **Calculus of gallbladder; with other cholecystitis**
    K80.10   **with chronic cholecystitis without obstruction**
       Cholelithiasis with cholecystitis NOS
    K80.11   **with chronic cholecystitis with obstruction**
    K80.12   **with acute and chronic cholecystitis without obstruction**
    K80.13   **with acute and chronic cholecystitis with obstruction**
    K80.18   **with other cholecystitis without obstruction**
    K80.19   **with other cholecystitis with obstruction**
K80.2   **Calculus of gallbladder without cholecystitis**
   Cholecystolithiasis with cholecystitis
   Cholelithiasis (without cholecystitis)
   Colic (recurrent) of gallbladder (without cholecystitis)
   Gallstone (impacted) of cystic duct (without cholecystitis)
   Gallstone (impacted) of gallbladder (without cholecystitis)
    K80.20   **Calculus of gallbladder without cholecystitis without obstruction**
    K80.21   **Calculus of gallbladder without cholecystitis with obstruction**

K81   **CHOLECYSTITIS**
[4th]
Excludes1: cholecystitis with cholelithiasis (K80.-)
K81.0   **Acute cholecystitis**
   Abscess of gallbladder
   Angiocholecystitis
   Emphysematous (acute) cholecystitis
   Empyema of gallbladder
   Gangrene of gallbladder
   Gangrenous cholecystitis
   Suppurative cholecystitis
K81.1   **Chronic cholecystitis**
K81.2   **Acute cholecystitis with chronic cholecystitis**
K81.9   **Cholecystitis, unspecified**

K85   **ACUTE PANCREATITIS**
[4th]
Includes: acute (recurrent) pancreatitis
   subacute pancreatitis
K85.0   **Idiopathic acute pancreatitis**
    •**K85.00**   **Idiopathic acute pancreatitis without necrosis or infection**
    •**K85.01**   **Idiopathic acute pancreatitis with uninfected necrosis**
    •**K85.02**   **Idiopathic acute pancreatitis with infected necrosis**
K85.9   **Acute pancreatitis, unspecified**
   Pancreatitis NOS
    •**K85.90**   **Acute pancreatitis without necrosis or infection, unspecified**
    •**K85.91**   **Acute pancreatitis with uninfected necrosis, unspecified**
    •**K85.92**   **Acute pancreatitis with infected necrosis, unspecified**

   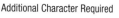

(K90–K95) OTHER DISEASES OF THE DIGESTIVE SYSTEM

K90   INTESTINAL MALABSORPTION

4th

Excludes1: intestinal malabsorption following gastrointestinal surgery (K91.2)

K90.0   Celiac disease
Celiac disease with steatorrhea
Gluten-sensitive enteropathy
Nontropical sprue
Code also exocrine pancreatic insufficiency (K86.81)
Use additional code for associated disorders including: dermatitis herpetiformis (L13.0)
gluten ataxia (G32.81)

K90.4   Other malabsorption due to intolerance
5th
Excludes2: gluten-sensitive enteropathy (K90.0)
lactose intolerance (E73.-)

• **K90.41   Non-celiac gluten sensitivity**
Gluten sensitivity NOS
Non-celiac gluten sensitive enteropathy

• **K40.49   Malabsorption due to intolerance, NEC**
Malabsorption due to intolerance to carbohydrate or fat or protein or starch

K90.8   Other intestinal malabsorption
5th
K90.81   Whipple's disease
K90.89   Other intestinal malabsorption

K90.9   Intestinal malabsorption, unspecified

K91   INTRAOPERATIVE AND POSTPROCEDURAL COMPLICATIONS AND DISORDERS OF DIGESTIVE SYSTEM, NEC

4th

Excludes2: complications of artificial opening of digestive system (K94.-)
complications of bariatric procedures (K95.-)
gastrojejunal ulcer (K28.-)
postprocedural (radiation) retroperitoneal abscess (K68.11)
radiation colitis (K52.0)
radiation gastroenteritis (K52.0)
radiation proctitis (K62.7)

K91.2   Postsurgical malabsorption, NEC
Postsurgical blind loop syndrome
Excludes1: malabsorption osteomalacia in adults (M83.2)
malabsorption osteoporosis, postsurgical (M80.8-, M81.8)

K92   OTHER DISEASES OF DIGESTIVE SYSTEM

4th

Excludes1: neonatal gastrointestinal hemorrhage (P54.0–P54.3)

K92.0   Hematemesis

K92.1   Melena
Excludes1: occult blood in feces (R19.5)

K92.2   Gastrointestinal hemorrhage, unspecified
Gastric hemorrhage NOS
Intestinal hemorrhage NOS
Excludes1: acute hemorrhagic gastritis (K29.01)
hemorrhage of anus and rectum (K62.5)
angiodysplasia of stomach with hemorrhage (K31.811)
diverticular disease with hemorrhage (K57.-)
gastritis and duodenitis with hemorrhage (K29.-)
peptic ulcer with hemorrhage (K25–K28)

K94   COMPLICATIONS OF ARTIFICIAL OPENINGS OF THE DIGESTIVE SYSTEM

4th

K94.2   Gastrostomy complications
5th
K94.20   Gastrostomy complication, unspecified
K94.21   Gastrostomy hemorrhage
K94.22   Gastrostomy infection
Use additional code to specify type of infection, such as: sepsis (A40.-, A41.-)
cellulitis of abdominal wall (L03.311)
K94.23   Gastrostomy malfunction
Mechanical complication of gastrostomy
K94.29   Other complications of gastrostomy

4th **5th** **6th** **7th**   Additional Character Required   ✔ 3-character code

•=New Code
▲=Revised Code

Excludes1—Not coded here, do not use together
Excludes2—Not included here

Chapter 12. Diseases of the skin and subcutaneous tissue (L00–L99)

GUIDELINES

Pressure ulcer stages
Refer to category L89.
Excludes2: certain conditions originating in the perinatal period (P04–P96)
    certain infectious and parasitic diseases (A00–B99)
    complications of pregnancy, childbirth and the puerperium (O00–O9A)
    congenital malformations, deformations, and chromosomal abnormalities
      (Q00–Q99)
    endocrine, nutritional and metabolic diseases (E00–E88)
    lipomelanotic reticulosis (I89.8)
    neoplasms (C00–D49)
    symptoms, signs and abnormal clinical and laboratory findings, NEC (R00–R94)
    systemic connective tissue disorders (M30–M36)
    viral warts (B07.-)

(L00–L08) INFECTIONS OF THE SKIN AND SUBCUTANEOUS TISSUE

Use additional code (B95–B97) to identify infectious agent.
Excludes2: hordeolum (H00.0)
    infective dermatitis (L30.3)
    local infections of skin classified in Chapter 1
    lupus panniculitis (L93.2)
    panniculitis NOS (M79.3)
    panniculitis of neck and back (M54.0-)
    Perlèche NOS (K13.0)
    Perlèche due to candidiasis (B37.0)
    Perlèche due to riboflavin deficiency (E53.0)
    pyogenic granuloma (L98.0)
    relapsing panniculitis [Weber-Christian] (M35.6)
    viral warts (B07.-)
    zoster (B02.-)

L00 STAPHYLOCOCCAL SCALDED SKIN SYNDROME
    Ritter's disease
    Use additional code to identify percentage of skin exfoliation (L49.-)
    Excludes1: bullous impetigo (L01.03)
      pemphigus neonatorum (L01.03)
      toxic epidermal necrolysis [Lyell] (L51.2)

L01 IMPETIGO
    Excludes1: impetigo herpetiformis (L40.1)
    L01.0 Impetigo
      Impetigo contagiosa
      Impetigo vulgaris
        L01.00 Impetigo, unspecified
          Impetigo NOS
        L01.01 Non-bullous impetigo
        L01.02 Bockhart's impetigo
          Impetigo follicularis
          Perifolliculitis NOS
          Superficial pustular perifolliculitis
        L01.03 Bullous impetigo
          Impetigo neonatorum
          Pemphigus neonatorum
        L01.09 Other impetigo
          Ulcerative impetigo
    L01.1 Impetiginization of other dermatoses

L02 CUTANEOUS ABSCESS, FURUNCLE AND CARBUNCLE
    Use additional code to identify organism (B95–B96)
    Excludes2: abscess of anus and rectal regions (K61.-)
      abscess of female genital organs (external) (N76.4)
      abscess of male genital organs (external) (N48.2, N49.-)

L02.0 Cutaneous abscess, furuncle and carbuncle of face
    Excludes2: abscess of ear, external (H60.0)
      abscess of eyelid (H00.0)
      abscess of head [any part, except face] (L02.8)
      abscess of lacrimal gland (H04.0)
      abscess of lacrimal passages (H04.3)
      abscess of mouth (K12.2)
      abscess of nose (J34.0)
      abscess of orbit (H05.0)
      submandibular abscess (K12.2)
    L02.01 Cutaneous abscess of face
    L02.02 Furuncle of face
      Boil of face
      Folliculitis of face
    L02.03 Carbuncle of face
L02.1 Cutaneous abscess, furuncle and carbuncle of neck
    L02.11 Cutaneous abscess of neck
    L02.12 Furuncle of neck
      Boil of neck
      Folliculitis of neck
    L02.13 Carbuncle of neck
L02.2 Cutaneous abscess, furuncle and carbuncle of trunk
    Excludes1: non-newborn omphalitis (L08.82)
      omphalitis of newborn (P38.-)
    Excludes2: abscess of breast (N61.1)
      abscess of buttocks (L02.3)
      abscess of female external genital organs (N76.4)
      abscess of male external genital organs (N48.2, N49.-)
      abscess of hip (L02.4)
    L02.21 Cutaneous abscess of trunk
        L02.211 Cutaneous abscess of; abdominal wall
        L02.212   back [any part, except buttock]
        L02.213   chest wall
        L02.214   groin
        L02.215   perineum
        L02.216   umbilicus
        L02.219   trunk, unspecified
    L02.22 Furuncle of trunk
      Boil of trunk
      Folliculitis of trunk
        L02.221 Furuncle of; abdominal wall
        L02.222   back [any part, except buttock]
        L02.223   chest wall
        L02.224   groin
        L02.225   perineum
        L02.226   umbilicus
        L02.229   trunk, unspecified
    L02.23 Carbuncle of trunk
        L02.231 Carbuncle of; abdominal wall
        L02.232   back [any part, except buttock]
        L02.233   chest wall
        L02.234   groin
        L02.235   perineum
        L02.236   umbilicus
        L02.239   trunk, unspecified
L02.3 Cutaneous abscess, furuncle and carbuncle of buttock
    Excludes1: pilonidal cyst with abscess (L05.01)
    L02.31 Cutaneous abscess of buttock
      Cutaneous abscess of gluteal region
    L02.32 Furuncle of buttock
      Boil of buttock
      Folliculitis of buttock
      Furuncle of gluteal region
    L02.33 Carbuncle of buttock
      Carbuncle of gluteal region
L02.4 Cutaneous abscess, furuncle and carbuncle of limb
    Excludes2: Cutaneous abscess, furuncle and carbuncle of groin
      (L02.214, L02.224, L02.234)
      Cutaneous abscess, furuncle and carbuncle of hand (L02.5-)
      Cutaneous abscess, furuncle and carbuncle of foot (L02.6-)

  Additional Character Required   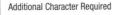 3-character code   Unspecified laterality codes were excluded here.   •=New Code   ▲=Revised Code   **Excludes1**—Not coded here, do not use together   **Excludes2**—Not included here

CHAPTER 12. DISEASES OF THE SKIN AND SUBCUTANEOUS TISSUE (L02.41–L03.222)

L02.41 Cutaneous abscess of; limb
- [6th] L02.411 right axilla
- L02.412 left axilla
- L02.413 right upper limb
- L02.414 left upper limb
- L02.415 right lower limb
- L02.416 left lower limb

L02.42 Furuncle of; limb
- [6th] Boil of limb
- Folliculitis of limb
- L02.421 right axilla
- L02.422 left axilla
- L02.423 right upper limb
- L02.424 left upper limb
- L02.425 right lower limb
- L02.426 left lower limb

L02.43 Carbuncle of; limb
- [6th] L02.431 right axilla
- L02.432 left axilla
- L02.433 right upper limb
- L02.434 left upper limb
- L02.435 right lower limb
- L02.436 left lower limb

L02.5 Cutaneous abscess, furuncle and carbuncle of hand
- [5th] **L02.51 Cutaneous abscess of; hand**
  - [6th] L02.511 right hand
  - L02.512 left hand
- **L02.52 Furuncle; hand**
  - [6th] Boil of hand
  - Folliculitis of hand
  - L02.521 right hand
  - L02.522 left hand
- **L02.53 Carbuncle of; hand**
  - [6th] L02.531 right hand
  - L02.532 left hand

L02.6 Cutaneous abscess, furuncle and carbuncle of foot
- [5th] **L02.61 Cutaneous abscess of; foot**
  - [6th] L02.611 right foot
  - L02.612 left foot
- **L02.62 Furuncle of; foot**
  - [6th] Boil of foot
  - Folliculitis of foot
  - L02.621 right foot
  - L02.622 left foot
- **L02.63 Carbuncle of; foot**
  - [6th] L02.631 right foot
  - L02.632 left foot

L02.8 Cutaneous abscess, furuncle and carbuncle of other sites
- [5th] **L02.81 Cutaneous abscess of; other sites**
  - [6th] L02.811 head [any part, except face]
  - L02.818 other sites
- **L02.82 Furuncle of; other sites**
  - [6th] Boil of other sites
  - Folliculitis of other sites
  - L02.821 head [any part, except face]
  - L02.828 other sites
- **L02.83 Carbuncle of; other sites**
  - [6th] L02.831 head [any part, except face]
  - L02.838 other sites

L02.9 Cutaneous abscess, furuncle and carbuncle, unspecified
- [5th] **L02.91 Cutaneous abscess, unspecified**
- **L02.92 Furuncle, unspecified**
  - Boil NOS
  - Furunculosis NOS
- **L02.93 Carbuncle, unspecified**

L03 CELLULITIS AND ACUTE LYMPHANGITIS
[4th] *Excludes2:* cellulitis of anal and rectal region (K61.-)
- cellulitis of external auditory canal (H60.1)
- cellulitis of eyelid (H00.0)
- cellulitis of female external genital organs (N76.4)
- cellulitis of lacrimal apparatus (H04.3)
- cellulitis of male external genital organs (N48.2, N49.-)
- cellulitis of mouth (K12.2)
- cellulitis of nose (J34.0)
- eosinophilic cellulitis [Wells] (L98.3)
- febrile neutrophilic dermatosis [Sweet] (L98.2)
- lymphangitis (chronic) (subacute) (I89.1)

L03.0 Cellulitis and acute lymphangitis of finger and toe
- [5th] Infection of nail
- Onychia
- Paronychia
- Perionychia
- **L03.01 Cellulitis of; finger**
  - [6th] Felon
  - Whitlow
  - *Excludes1:* herpetic whitlow (B00.89)
  - L03.011 right finger
  - L03.012 left finger
- **L03.02 Acute lymphangitis of; finger**
  - [6th] Hangnail with lymphangitis of finger
  - L03.021 right finger
  - L03.022 left finger
- **L03.03 Cellulitis of; toe**
  - [6th] L03.031 right toe
  - L03.032 left toe
- **L03.04 Acute lymphangitis of; toe**
  - [6th] Hangnail with lymphangitis of toe
  - L03.041 right toe
  - L03.042 left toe

L03.1 Cellulitis and acute lymphangitis of other parts of limb
- [5th] **L03.11 Cellulitis of other parts of limb**
  - [6th] *Excludes2:* cellulitis of fingers (L03.01-)
    - cellulitis of toes (L03.03-)
    - groin (L03.314)
  - L03.111 Cellulitis of; right axilla
  - L03.112 left axilla
  - L03.113 right upper limb
  - L03.114 left upper limb
  - L03.115 right lower limb
  - L03.116 left lower limb
- **L03.12 Acute lymphangitis of other parts of limb**
  - [6th] *Excludes2:* acute lymphangitis of fingers (L03.2-)
    - acute lymphangitis of toes (L03.04-)
    - acute lymphangitis of groin (L03.324)
  - L03.121 Acute lymphangitis of; right axilla
  - L03.122 left axilla
  - L03.123 right upper limb
  - L03.124 left upper limb
  - L03.125 right lower limb
  - L03.126 left lower limb

L03.2 Cellulitis and acute lymphangitis of face and neck
- [5th] **L03.21 Cellulitis and acute lymphangitis of face**
  - [6th] L03.211 Cellulitis of face
  - *Excludes2:* abscess of orbit (H05.01-)
    - cellulitis of ear (H60.1-)
    - cellulitis of eyelid (H00.0-)
    - cellulitis of head or scalp (L03.81)
    - cellulitis of lacrimal apparatus (H04.3)
    - cellulitis of lip (K13.0)
    - cellulitis of mouth (K12.2)
    - cellulitis of nose (internal) (J34.0)
    - cellulitis of orbit (H05.01-)
  - L03.212 Acute lymphangitis of face
  - • L03.213 Periorbital cellulitis
    - Preseptal cellulitis
- **L03.22 Cellulitis and acute lymphangitis of neck**
  - [6th] L03.221 Cellulitis of neck
  - L03.222 Acute lymphangitis of neck

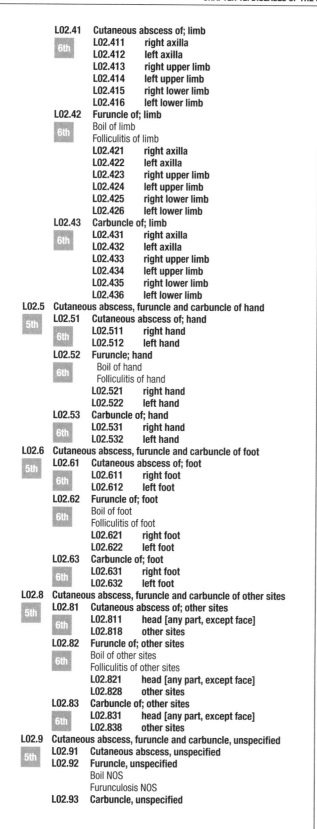

   Additional Character Required   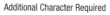 3-character code   Unspecified laterality codes were excluded here.   =New Code   ▲=Revised Code   *Excludes1*—Not coded here, do not use together   *Excludes2*—Not included here

L03.3   Cellulitis and acute lymphangitis of trunk
- **L03.31   Cellulitis of trunk** `5th`
  - `6th` ***Excludes2:*** cellulitis of anal and rectal regions (K61.-)
  - cellulitis of breast NOS (N61.0)
  - cellulitis of female external genital organs (N76.4)
  - cellulitis of male external genital organs (N48.2, N49.-)
  - omphalitis of newborn (P38.-)
  - puerperal cellulitis of breast (O91.2)
  - **L03.311   Cellulitis of; abdominal wall**
    - ***Excludes2:*** cellulitis of umbilicus (L03.316)
    - cellulitis of groin (L03.314)
  - **L03.312   back [any part except buttock]**
  - **L03.313   chest wall**
  - **L03.314   groin**
  - **L03.315   perineum**
  - **L03.316   umbilicus**
  - **L03.317   buttock**
  - **L03.319   trunk, unspecified** ✓
- **L03.32   Acute lymphangitis of; trunk**
  - `6th`
  - **L03.321   abdominal wall**
  - **L03.322   back [any part except buttock]**
  - **L03.323   chest wall**
  - **L03.324   groin**
  - **L03.325   perineum**
  - **L03.326   umbilicus**
  - **L03.327   buttock**
  - **L03.329   trunk, unspecified**

L03.8   Cellulitis and acute lymphangitis of other sites
- **L03.81   Cellulitis of; other sites** `5th`
  - `6th`
  - **L03.811   head [any part, except face]**
    - Cellulitis of scalp
    - ***Excludes2:*** cellulitis of face (L03.211)
  - **L03.818   other sites**
- **L03.89   Acute lymphangitis of; other sites**
  - `6th`
  - **L03.891   head [any part, except face]**
  - **L03.898   other sites**

L03.9   Cellulitis and acute lymphangitis, unspecified
- **L03.90   Cellulitis, unspecified** `5th`
- **L03.91   Acute lymphangitis, unspecified**
  - ***Excludes1:*** lymphangitis NOS (I89.1)

L04   ACUTE LYMPHADENITIS `4th`
- ***Includes:*** abscess (acute) of lymph nodes, except mesenteric
- acute lymphadenitis, except mesenteric
- ***Excludes1:*** chronic or subacute lymphadenitis, except mesenteric (I88.1)
- enlarged lymph nodes (R59.-)
- HIV disease resulting in generalized lymphadenopathy (B20)
- lymphadenitis NOS (I88.9)
- nonspecific mesenteric lymphadenitis (I88.0)
- **L04.0   Acute lymphadenitis of; face, head and neck**
- **L04.1   trunk**
- **L04.2   upper limb**
  - Acute lymphadenitis of axilla or shoulder
- **L04.3   lower limb**
  - Acute lymphadenitis of hip
  - ***Excludes2:*** acute lymphadenitis of groin (L04.1)
- **L04.8   other sites**
- **L04.9   unspecified**

L05   PILONIDAL CYST AND SINUS `4th`
- **L05.01   Pilonidal cyst with abscess**
  - Parasacral dimple with abscess
  - ***Excludes 2:*** congenital sacral dimple (Q82.6)
  - parasacral dimple (Q82.6)
- **L05.9   Pilonidal cyst and sinus without abscess**
  - **L05.91   Pilonidal cyst without abscess** `5th`
    - Parasacral or Pilonidal or Postanal dimple
    - Pilonidal cyst NOS
    - ***Excludes 2:*** congenital sacral dimple (Q82.6)
    - parasacral dimple (Q82.6)
  - **L05.92   Pilonidal sinus without abscess**
    - Coccygeal fistula
    - Coccygeal sinus without abscess
    - Pilonidal fistula

L08   OTHER LOCAL INFECTIONS OF SKIN AND SUBCUTANEOUS TISSUE `4th`
- **L08.0   Pyoderma**
  - Dermatitis gangrenosa
  - Purulent or Septic or Suppurative dermatitis
  - ***Excludes1:*** pyoderma gangrenosum (L88)
  - pyoderma vegetans (L08.81)
- **L08.9   Local infection of the skin and subcutaneous tissue, unspecified**

(L10–L14) BULLOUS DISORDERS

Excludes1: benign familial pemphigus [Hailey-Hailey] (Q82.8)
staphylococcal scalded skin syndrome (L00)
toxic epidermal necrolysis [Lyell] (L51.2)

(L20–L30) DERMATITIS AND ECZEMA

Note: In this block the terms dermatitis and eczema are used synonymously and interchangeably.
Excludes2: chronic (childhood) granulomatous disease (D71)
dermatitis gangrenosa (L08.0)
dermatitis herpetiformis (L13.0)
dry skin dermatitis (L85.3)
factitial dermatitis (L98.1)
perioral dermatitis (L71.0)
radiation-related disorders of the skin and subcutaneous tissue (L55–L59)
stasis dermatitis (I87.2)

L20   ATOPIC DERMATITIS `4th`
- **L20.0   Besnier's prurigo**
- **L20.8   Other atopic dermatitis**
  - `5th` ***Excludes2:*** circumscribed neurodermatitis (L28.0)
  - **L20.81   Atopic neurodermatitis**
    - Diffuse neurodermatitis
  - **L20.82   Flexural eczema**
  - **L20.83   Infantile (acute) (chronic) eczema**
  - **L20.84   Intrinsic (allergic) eczema**
  - **L20.89   Other atopic dermatitis**
- **L20.9   Atopic dermatitis, unspecified**

L21   SEBORRHEIC DERMATITIS `4th`
- ***Excludes2:*** infective dermatitis (L30.3)
- seborrheic keratosis (L82.-)
- **L21.0   Seborrhea capitis**
  - Cradle cap
- **L21.1   Seborrheic infantile dermatitis**
- **L21.8   Other seborrheic dermatitis**
- **L21.9   Seborrheic dermatitis, unspecified**
  - Seborrhea NOS

L22   DIAPER DERMATITIS `✓`
- Diaper erythema
- Diaper rash
- Psoriasiform diaper rash

L23   ALLERGIC CONTACT DERMATITIS `4th`
- ***Excludes1:*** allergy NOS (T78.40)
- contact dermatitis NOS (L25.9)
- dermatitis NOS (L30.9)
- ***Excludes2:*** dermatitis due to substances taken internally (L27.-)
- dermatitis of eyelid (H01.1-)
- diaper dermatitis (L22)
- eczema of external ear (H60.5-)
- irritant contact dermatitis (L24.-)
- perioral dermatitis (L71.0)
- radiation-related disorders of the skin and subcutaneous tissue (L55–L59)
- **L23.0   Allergic contact dermatitis due to; metals**
  - Allergic contact dermatitis due to chromium or nickel
- **L23.1   adhesives**
- **L23.2   cosmetics**

`4th` `5th` `6th` `7th`   Additional Character Required   ✓   3-character code   Unspecified laterality codes were excluded here.   •=New Code   ▲=Revised Code   ***Excludes1***—Not coded here, do not use together   ***Excludes2***—Not included here

PEDIATRIC ICD-10-CM 2017: A MANUAL FOR PROVIDER-BASED CODING   207

CHAPTER 12. DISEASES OF THE SKIN AND SUBCUTANEOUS TISSUE   (L03.3–L23.2)

L23.3   **drugs in contact with skin**
Use additional code for adverse effect, if applicable, to identify drug (T36–T50 with fifth or sixth character 5)
Excludes2: dermatitis due to ingested drugs and medicaments (L27.0–L27.1)

L23.4   **Allergic contact dermatitis due to; dyes**

L23.5   **other chemical products**
Allergic contact dermatitis due to cement or to insecticide

L23.6   **food in contact with the skin**
Excludes2: dermatitis due to ingested food (L27.2)

L23.7   **plants, except food**
Excludes2: allergy NOS due to pollen (J30.1)

L23.8   **Allergic contact dermatitis due to; other agents**
5th   **L23.81**   **animal (cat) (dog) dander or hair**
L23.89   **other agents**

L23.9   **Allergic contact dermatitis, unspecified cause**
Allergic contact eczema NOS

L27 DERMATITIS DUE TO SUBSTANCES TAKEN INTERNALLY
4th
Excludes1: allergy NOS (T78.40)
Excludes2: adverse food reaction, except dermatitis (T78.0–T78.1)
contact dermatitis (L23–L25)
drug photoallergic response (L56.1)
drug phototoxic response (L56.0)
urticaria (L50.-)

L27.0   **Generalized skin eruption due to drugs and medicaments taken internally**
Use additional code for adverse effect, if applicable, to identify drug (T36–T50 with fifth or sixth character 5)

L27.1   **Localized skin eruption due to drugs and medicaments taken internally**
Use additional code for adverse effect, if applicable, to identify drug (T36–T50 with fifth or sixth character 5)

L27.2   **Dermatitis due to ingested food**
Excludes2: dermatitis due to food in contact with skin (L23.6, L24.6, L25.4)

L27.8   **Dermatitis due to other substances taken internally**

L27.9   **Dermatitis due to unspecified substance taken internally**

L29 PRURITUS
4th
Excludes1: neurotic excoriation (L98.1)
psychogenic pruritus (F45.8)

L29.0   **Pruritus ani**
L29.1   **Pruritus scroti**
L29.2   **Pruritus vulvae**
L29.3   **Anogenital pruritus, unspecified**
L29.8   **Other pruritus**
L29.9   **Pruritus, unspecified**
Itch NOS

L30 OTHER AND UNSPECIFIED DERMATITIS
4th
Excludes2: contact dermatitis (L23–L25)
dry skin dermatitis (L85.3)
small plaque parapsoriasis (L41.3)
stasis dermatitis (I83.1–.2)

L30.1   **Dyshidrosis [pompholyx]**
L30.4   **Erythema intertrigo**

(L40–L45) PAPULOSQUAMOUS DISORDERS

L40 PSORIASIS
L40.5   **Arthropathic psoriasis**
5th   **L40.54**   **Psoriatic juvenile arthropathy**

L40.8   **Other psoriasis**
Flexural psoriasis
L40.9   **Psoriasis, unspecified**

L42 PITYRIASIS ROSEA

L44 OTHER PAPULOSQUAMOUS DISORDERS
4th
L44.0   **Pityriasis rubra pilaris**
L44.1   **Lichen nitidus**
L44.2   **Lichen striatus**
L44.3   **Lichen ruber moniliformis**
L44.4   **Infantile papular acrodermatitis [Gianotti-Crosti]**
L44.8   **Other specified papulosquamous disorders**
L44.9   **Papulosquamous disorder, unspecified**

(L49–L54) URTICARIA AND ERYTHEMA

Excludes1: Lyme disease (A69.2-)
rosacea (L71.-)

L50 URTICARIA
4th
Excludes1: allergic contact dermatitis (L23.-)
angioneurotic edema or giant urticarial or Quincke's edema (T78.3)
hereditary angio-edema (D84.1)
serum urticaria (T80.6-)
solar urticaria (L56.3)
urticaria neonatorum (P83.8)
urticaria papulosa (L28.2)
urticaria pigmentosa (Q82.2)

L50.0   **Allergic urticaria**
L50.8   **Other urticaria**
Chronic urticaria
Recurrent periodic urticaria
L50.9   **Urticaria, unspecified**

L51 ERYTHEMA MULTIFORME
4th
Use additional code for adverse effect, if applicable, to identify drug (T36–T50 with fifth or sixth character 5)
Use additional code to identify associated manifestations, such as:
arthropathy associated with dermatological disorders (M14.8-)
conjunctival edema (H11.42)
conjunctivitis (H10.22-)
corneal scars and opacities (H17.-)
corneal ulcer (H16.0-)
edema of eyelid (H02.84)
inflammation of eyelid (H01.8)
keratoconjunctivitis sicca (H16.22-)
mechanical lagophthalmos (H02.22-)
stomatitis (K12.-)
symblepharon (H11.23-)
Use additional code to identify percentage of skin exfoliation (L49.-)
Excludes1: staphylococcal scalded skin syndrome (L00)
Ritter's disease (L00)

L51.0   **Nonbullous erythema multiforme**
L51.1   **Stevens-Johnson syndrome**
L51.2   **Toxic epidermal necrolysis [Lyell]**
L51.3   **Stevens-Johnson syndrome-toxic epidermal necrolysis overlap syndrome**
SJS-TEN overlap syndrome
L51.8   **Other erythema multiforme**
L51.9   **Erythema multiforme, unspecified**
Erythema iris
Erythema multiforme major NOS
Erythema multiforme minor NOS
Herpes iris

L52 ERYTHEMA NODOSUM

Excludes1: tuberculous erythema nodosum (A18.4)

(L55–L59) RADIATION-RELATED DISORDERS OF THE SKIN AND SUBCUTANEOUS TISSUE

L55 SUNBURN
4th
L55.0   **Sunburn of first degree**
L55.1   **Sunburn of second degree**
L55.2   **Sunburn of third degree**
L55.9   **Sunburn, unspecified**

  4th 5th 6th 7th Additional Character Required   3-character code   Unspecified laterality codes were excluded here.   •=New Code   ▲=Revised Code   *Excludes1*—Not coded here, do not use together   *Excludes2*—Not included here

L56   OTHER ACUTE SKIN CHANGES DUE TO ULTRAVIOLET RADIATION
4th

Use additional code to identify the source of the ultraviolet radiation (W89, X32)

L56.8   Other specified acute skin changes due to ultraviolet radiation
L56.9   Acute skin change due to ultraviolet radiation, unspecified

(L60–L75) DISORDERS OF SKIN APPENDAGES

Excludes1: congenital malformations of integument (Q84.-)

L60   NAIL DISORDERS
4th

Excludes2: clubbing of nails (R68.3)
onychia and paronychia (L03.0-)

L60.0   Ingrowing nail
L60.1   Onycholysis
L60.8   Other nail disorders
L60.9   Nail disorder, unspecified

L65   OTHER NON-SCARRING HAIR LOSS
4th

Use additional code for adverse effect, if applicable, to identify drug (T36–T50 with fifth or sixth character 5)

Excludes1: trichotillomania (F63.3)

L65.8   Other specified non-scarring hair loss
L65.9   Non-scarring hair loss, unspecified
Alopecia NOS

L68   HYPERTRICHOSIS
4th

Includes: excess hair
Excludes1: congenital hypertrichosis (Q84.2)
persistent lanugo (Q84.2)

L68.0   Hirsutism

L70   ACNE
4th

Excludes2: acne keloid (L73.0)

L70.0   Acne vulgaris
L70.1   Acne conglobata
L70.2   Acne varioliformis
Acne necrotica miliaris
L70.3   Acne tropica
L70.4   Infantile acne
L70.5   Acné excoriée
Acné excoriée des jeunes filles
Picker's acne
L70.8   Other acne

L72   FOLLICULAR CYSTS OF SKIN AND SUBCUTANEOUS TISSUE
4th

L72.0   Epidermal cyst
L72.1   Pilar and trichodermal cyst
  5th   **L72.11**   Pilar cyst
       L72.12   Trichodermal cyst
         Trichilemmal (proliferating) cyst

L73   OTHER FOLLICULAR DISORDERS
4th

L73.2   Hidradenitis suppurativa
L73.8   Other specified follicular disorders
Sycosis barbae
L73.9   Follicular disorder, unspecified

L74   ECCRINE SWEAT DISORDERS
4th

Excludes2: generalized hyperhidrosis (R61)

L74.0   Miliaria rubra
L74.1   Miliaria crystallina

(L76) INTRAOPERATIVE AND POSTPROCEDURAL COMPLICATIONS OF SKIN AND SUBCUTANEOUS TISSUE

(L80–L99) OTHER DISORDERS OF THE SKIN AND SUBCUTANEOUS TISSUE

L80   VITILIGO
✓

Excludes2: vitiligo of eyelids (H02.73-)
vitiligo of vulva (N90.89)

L81   OTHER DISORDERS OF PIGMENTATION
4th

Excludes1: birthmark NOS (Q82.5)
Peutz-Jeghers syndrome (Q85.8)
Excludes2: nevus—see Alphabetical Index

L81.2   Freckles
L81.4   Other melanin hyperpigmentation
Lentigo
L81.8   Other specified disorders of pigmentation
Iron pigmentation
Tattoo pigmentation

L83   ACANTHOSIS NIGRICANS
✓

Confluent and reticulated papillomatosis

L84   CORNS AND CALLOSITIES
✓

Callus
Clavus

L88   PYODERMA GANGRENOSUM
✓

Phagedenic pyoderma
Excludes1: dermatitis gangrenosa (L08.0)

L89   PRESSURE ULCER
4th

GUIDELINES

Pressure ulcer stages
Codes from category L89, Pressure ulcer, are combination codes that identify the site of the pressure ulcer as well as the stage of the ulcer. The *ICD-10-CM* classifies pressure ulcer stages based on severity, which is designated by stages 1–4, unspecified stage and unstageable. Assign as many codes from category L89 as needed to identify all the pressure ulcers the patient has, if applicable.

Unstageable pressure ulcers
Refer to the ICD-10-CM manual.

Documented pressure ulcer stage
Assignment of the pressure ulcer stage code should be guided by clinical documentation of the stage or documentation of the terms found in the Alphabetic Index. For clinical terms describing the stage that are not found in the Alphabetic Index, and there is no documentation of the stage, the provider should be queried.

Patients admitted with pressure ulcers documented as healed
No code is assigned if the documentation states that the pressure ulcer is completely healed.

Patients admitted with pressure ulcers documented as healing
Refer to the ICD-10-CM manual.

Patient admitted with pressure ulcer evolving into another stage during the admission
Refer to the ICD-10-CM manual.
Includes: bed sore
decubitus ulcer
plaster ulcer
pressure area
pressure sore
Code first any associated gangrene (I96)

Stage 1—Pressure pre-ulcer skin changes limited to persistent focal edema
Stage 2—Pressure ulcer with abrasion, blister, partial thickness skin loss involving epidermis and/or dermis
Stage 3—Pressure ulcer with full thickness skin loss involving damage or necrosis of subcutaneous tissue
Stage 4—Pressure ulcer with necrosis of soft tissues through to underlying muscle, tendon, or bone

---

   Additional Character Required   3-character code | Unspecified laterality codes were excluded here. | •=New Code   ▲=Revised Code | **Excludes1**—Not coded here, do not use together
Excludes2—Not included here

Excludes2: decubitus (trophic) ulcer of cervix (uteri) (N86)
  diabetic ulcers (E08.621, E08.622, E09.621, E09.622, E10.621,
    E10.622, E11.621, E11.622, E13.621, E13.622)
  non-pressure chronic ulcer of skin (L97.-)
  skin infections (L00–L08)
  varicose ulcer (I83.0, I83.2)

L89.0   Pressure ulcer of elbow

5th

L89.01   Pressure ulcer of right elbow

6th   Healing pressure ulcer of right elbow
  L89.010   Pressure ulcer of right elbow; unstageable
  L89.011   stage 1
  L89.012   stage 2
  L89.013   stage 3
  L89.014   stage 4
  L89.019   unspecified stage
            Healing pressure right of elbow NOS

L89.02   Pressure ulcer of left elbow

6th   Healing pressure ulcer of left elbow
  L89.020   Pressure ulcer of left elbow; unstageable
  L89.021   stage 1
  L89.022   stage 2
  L89.023   stage 3
  L89.024   stage 4
  **L89.029   Pressure ulcer of left elbow, unspecified
                stage**
            Healing pressure ulcer of left of elbow NOS
            Healing pressure ulcer of unspecified elbow,
                unspecified stage

L89.1   Pressure ulcer of back

5th

L89.10   Pressure ulcer of unspecified part of back

6th   Healing pressure ulcer of unspecified part of back
  Pressure pre-ulcer skin changes limited to persistent
      focal edema, unspecified part of back
  **L89.100   Pressure ulcer of unspecified part of back;
                unstageable**
  L89.101   stage 1
  L89.102   stage 2
  L89.103   stage 3
  L89.104   stage 4
  L89.109   unspecified stage
            Healing pressure ulcer of unspecified part of
                back NOS

L89.11   Pressure ulcer of right upper back

6th   Pressure ulcer of right shoulder blade
  Healing pressure ulcer of right upper back
  **L89.110   Pressure ulcer of right upper back;
                unstageable**
  L89.111   stage 1
  L89.112   stage 2
  L89.113   stage 3
  L89.114   stage 4
  L89.119   unspecified stage
            Healing pressure ulcer of right upper back
                NOS

L89.12   Pressure ulcer of left upper back

6th   Healing pressure ulcer of left upper back,
  Pressure ulcer of left shoulder blade
  **L89.120   Pressure ulcer of left upper back;
                unstageable**
  L89.121   stage 1
  L89.122   stage 2
  L89.123   stage 3
  L89.124   stage 4
  L89.129   unspecified stage
            Healing pressure ulcer of left upper back NOS
            Healing pressure ulcer of left upper back,
                unspecified stage

L89.13   Pressure ulcer of right lower back

6th   Healing pressure ulcer of right lower back
  **L89.130   Pressure ulcer of right lower back;
                unstageable**
  L89.131   stage 1
  L89.132   stage 2
  L89.133   stage 3
  L89.134   stage 4
  L89.139   unspecified stage
            Healing pressure ulcer of right lower back
                NOS

L89.14   Pressure ulcer of left lower back

6th   Healing pressure ulcer of left lower back
  **L89.140   Pressure ulcer of left lower back;
                unstageable**
  L89.141   stage 1
  L89.142   stage 2
  L89.143   stage 3
  L89.144   stage 4
  L89.149   unspecified stage
            Healing pressure ulcer of left lower back
                NOS

L89.15   Pressure ulcer of sacral region

6th   Healing pressure ulcer of sacral region,
  Pressure ulcer of coccyx
  Pressure ulcer of tailbone
  **L89.150   Pressure ulcer of sacral region;
                unstageable**
  L89.151   stage 1
  L89.152   stage 2
  L89.153   stage 3
  L89.154   stage 4
  L89.159   unspecified stage
            Healing pressure ulcer of sacral region NOS

L89.2   Pressure ulcer of hip

5th

L89.21   Pressure ulcer of right hip

6th   Healing pressure ulcer of right hip
  L89.210   Pressure ulcer of right hip; unstageable
  L89.211   stage 1
  L89.212   stage 2
  L89.213   stage 3
  L89.214   stage 4
  L89.219   unspecified stage
            Healing pressure ulcer of right hip NOS

L89.22   Pressure ulcer of left hip

6th   Healing pressure ulcer of left hip back
  L89.220   Pressure ulcer of left hip; unstageable
  L89.221   stage 1
  L89.222   stage 2
  L89.223   stage 3
  L89.224   stage 4
  L89.229   unspecified stage
            Healing pressure ulcer of left hip NOS

L89.3   Pressure ulcer of buttock

5th

L89.31   Pressure ulcer of right buttock

6th   Healing pressure ulcer of right buttock
  **L89.310   Pressure ulcer of right buttock;
                unstageable**
  L89.311   stage 1
  L89.312   stage 2
  L89.313   stage 3
  L89.314   stage 4
  L89.319   unspecified stage
            Healing pressure ulcer of right buttock NOS

L89.32   Pressure ulcer of left buttock

6th   Healing pressure ulcer of left buttock
  L89.320   Pressure ulcer of left buttock; unstageable
  L89.321   stage 1
  L89.322   stage 2
  L89.323   stage 3
  L89.324   stage 4
  **L89.329   Pressure ulcer of left buttock, unspecified
                stage**
            Healing pressure ulcer of left buttock NOS

      Additional Character Required   3-character code   Unspecified laterality codes   •=New Code   **Excludes1**—Not coded here, do not use together
                                                    were excluded here.   ▲=Revised Code   **Excludes2**—Not included here

210   **PEDIATRIC ICD-10-CM 2017: A MANUAL FOR PROVIDER-BASED CODING**

L89.4   **Pressure ulcer of contiguous site of back, buttock and hip**
> [5th] Healing pressure ulcer of contiguous site of back, buttock and hip
>> **L89.40**   **Pressure ulcer of contiguous site of back, buttock and hip; unspecified stage**
>>> Healing pressure ulcer of contiguous site of back, buttock and hip NOS
>> **L89.41**   stage 1
>> **L89.42**   stage 2
>> **L89.43**   stage 3
>> **L89.44**   stage 4
>> **L89.45**   unstageable

L89.5   **Pressure ulcer of ankle**
> [5th]
>> **L89.51**   **Pressure ulcer of right ankle**
>>> [6th] Healing pressure ulcer of right ankle
>>> **L89.510**   **Pressure ulcer of right ankle; unstageable**
>>> **L89.511**   stage 1
>>> **L89.512**   stage 2
>>> **L89.513**   stage 3
>>> **L89.514**   stage 4
>>> **L89.519**   unspecified stage
>>>> Healing pressure ulcer of right ankle NOS
>> **L89.52**   **Pressure ulcer of left ankle**
>>> [6th] Healing pressure ulcer of left ankle
>>> **L89.520**   **Pressure ulcer of left ankle; unstageable**
>>> **L89.521**   stage 1
>>>> Pressure pre-ulcer skin changes limited to persistent focal edema, left ankle
>>> **L89.522**   stage 2
>>> **L89.523**   stage 3
>>> **L89.524**   stage 4
>>> **L89.529**   unspecified stage
>>>> Healing pressure ulcer of left ankle NOS

L89.6   **Pressure ulcer of heel**
> [5th]
>> **L89.61**   **Pressure ulcer of right heel**
>>> [6th] Healing pressure ulcer of right heel
>>> **L89.610**   **Pressure ulcer of right heel; unstageable**
>>> **L89.611**   stage 1
>>> **L89.612**   stage 2
>>> **L89.613**   stage 3
>>> **L89.614**   stage 4
>>> **L89.619**   unspecified stage
>>>> Healing pressure ulcer of right heel NOS
>> **L89.62**   **Pressure ulcer of left heel**
>>> [6th] Healing pressure ulcer of left heel
>>> **L89.620**   **Pressure ulcer of left heel; unstageable**
>>> **L89.621**   stage 1
>>> **L89.622**   stage 2
>>> **L89.623**   stage 3
>>> **L89.624**   stage 4
>>> **L89.629**   unspecified stage
>>>> Healing pressure ulcer of left heel NOS

L89.8   **Pressure ulcer of other site**
> [5th]
>> **L89.81**   **Pressure ulcer of head**
>>> [6th] Pressure ulcer of face
>>> Healing pressure ulcer of head
>>> **L89.810**   **Pressure ulcer of head; unstageable**
>>> **L89.811**   stage 1
>>> **L89.812**   stage 2
>>> **L89.813**   stage 3
>>> **L89.814**   stage 4
>>> **L89.819**   unspecified stage
>>>> Healing pressure ulcer of head NOS

L89.89   **Pressure ulcer of other site**
> [6th] Healing pressure ulcer of other site
>> **L89.890**   **Pressure ulcer of other site; unstageable**
>> **L89.891**   stage 1
>> **L89.892**   stage 2
>> **L89.893**   stage 3
>> **L89.894**   stage 4
>> **L89.899**   unspecified stage
>>> Healing pressure ulcer of other site NOS

L89.9   **Pressure ulcer of unspecified site**
> [5th] Healing pressure ulcer of unspecified site
>> **L89.90**   **Pressure ulcer of unspecified site; unspecified stage**
>> **L89.91**   stage 1
>> **L89.92**   stage 2
>> **L89.93**   stage 3
>> **L89.94**   stage 4
>> **L89.95**   unstageable

L90   **ATROPHIC DISORDERS OF SKIN**
> [4th]
> **L90.5**   **Scar conditions and fibrosis of skin**
>> Adherent scar (skin)
>> Cicatrix
>> Disfigurement of skin due to scar
>> Fibrosis of skin NOS

L91   **HYPERTROPHIC DISORDERS OF SKIN**
> [4th]
> **L91.0**   **Hypertrophic scar**
>> Keloid
>> Keloid scar
>> ***Excludes2:*** acne keloid (L73.0)
>>> scar NOS (L90.5)
> **L91.8**   **Other hypertrophic disorders of the skin**
> **L91.9**   **Hypertrophic disorder of the skin, unspecified**

L92   **GRANULOMATOUS DISORDERS OF SKIN AND SUBCUTANEOUS TISSUE**
> [4th]
> ***Excludes2:*** actinic granuloma (L57.5)
> **L92.3**   **FB granuloma of the skin and subcutaneous tissue**
>> **Use additional code** to identify the type of retained FB (Z18.-)

L94   **OTHER LOCALIZED CONNECTIVE TISSUE DISORDERS**
> [4th]
> ***Excludes1:*** systemic connective tissue disorders (M30–M36)
> **L94.2**   **Calcinosis cutis**

L98   **OTHER DISORDERS OF SKIN AND SUBCUTANEOUS TISSUE, NOT ELSEWHERE CLASSIFIED**
> [4th]
> **L98.0**   **Pyogenic granuloma**
>> ***Excludes2:*** pyogenic granuloma of gingiva (K06.8)
>>> pyogenic granuloma of maxillary alveolar ridge (K04.5)
>>> pyogenic granuloma of oral mucosa (K13.4)
> **L98.1**   **Factitial dermatitis**
>> Neurotic excoriation
>> ***Excludes1:*** excoriation (skin-picking) disorder (F42.4)
> •**L98.7**   **Excessive and redundant skin and subcutaneous tissue**
>> Loose or sagging skin following bariatric surgery weight loss
>> Loose or sagging skin following dietary weight loss
>> Loose or sagging skin, NOS
>> ***Excludes2:*** acquired excess or redundant skin of eyelid (H02.3-)
>>> congenital excess or redundant skin of eyelid (Q10.3)
>>> skin changes due to chronic exposure to nonionizing radiation (L57.-)
> **L98.8**   **Other specified disorders of the skin and subcutaneous tissue**
> **L98.9**   **Disorder of the skin and subcutaneous tissue, unspecified**

L99   **OTHER DISORDERS OF SKIN AND SUBCUTANEOUS TISSUE IN DISEASES CLASSIFIED ELSEWHERE**
> [✓]
> **Code first underlying** disease, such as:
>> amyloidosis (E85.-)
> ***Excludes1:*** skin disorders in diabetes (E08–E13 with .62)
>> skin disorders in gonorrhea (A54.89)
>> skin disorders in syphilis (A51.31, A52.79)

[4th] [5th] [6th] [7th]   Additional Character Required   [✓]   3-character code   Unspecified laterality codes were excluded here.   •=New Code   ▲=Revised Code   ***Excludes1***—Not coded here, do not use together   ***Excludes2***—Not included here

Chapter 13. Diseases of the musculoskeletal system and connective tissue (M00–M99)

GUIDELINES

Site and laterality

Most of the codes within Chapter 13 have site and laterality designations. The site represents the bone, joint or the muscle involved. For some conditions where more than one bone, joint or muscle is usually involved, such as osteoarthritis, there is a "multiple sites" code available. For categories where no multiple site code is provided and more than one bone, joint or muscle is involved, multiple codes should be used to indicate the different sites involved.

BONE VERSUS JOINT

For certain conditions, the bone may be affected at the upper or lower end. Though the portion of the bone affected may be at the joint, the site designation will be the bone, not the joint.

Acute traumatic versus chronic or recurrent musculoskeletal conditions

Many musculoskeletal conditions are a result of previous injury or trauma to a site, or are recurrent conditions. Bone, joint or muscle conditions that are the result of a healed injury are usually found in chapter 13. Recurrent bone, joint or muscle conditions are also usually found in chapter 13. Any current, acute injury should be coded to the appropriate injury code from chapter 19. Chronic or recurrent conditions should generally be coded with a code from chapter 13. If it is difficult to determine from the documentation in the record which code is best to describe a condition, query the provider.

Coding of Pathologic Fractures

Refer to category M84.

Note: Use an external cause code following the code for the musculoskeletal condition, if applicable, to identify the cause of the musculoskeletal condition

Excludes2: arthropathic psoriasis (L40.5-)
    certain conditions originating in the perinatal period (P04–P96)
    certain infectious and parasitic diseases (A00–B99)
    compartment syndrome (traumatic) (T79.A-)
    complications of pregnancy, childbirth and the puerperium (O00–O9A)
    congenital malformations, deformations, and chromosomal abnormalities (Q00–Q99)
    endocrine, nutritional and metabolic diseases (E00–E88)
    injury, poisoning and certain other consequences of external causes (S00–T88)
    neoplasms (C00–D49)
    symptoms, signs and abnormal clinical and laboratory findings, not elsewhere classified (R00–R94)

(M00–M25) ARTHROPATHIES

Includes: Disorders affecting predominantly peripheral (limb) joints

(M00–M02) INFECTIOUS ARTHROPATHIES

Note: This block comprises arthropathies due to microbiological agents. Distinction is made between the following types of etiological relationship:
a) direct infection of joint, where organisms invade synovial tissue and microbial antigen is present in the joint;
b) indirect infection, which may be of two types: a reactive arthropathy, where microbial infection of the body is established but neither organisms nor antigens can be identified in the joint, and a postinfective arthropathy, where microbial antigen is present but recovery of an organism is inconstant and evidence of local multiplication is lacking.

M00 PYOGENIC ARTHRITIS

   M00.0 Staphylococcal arthritis and polyarthritis
    Use additional code (B95.61–B95.8) to identify bacterial agent
    Excludes2: infection and inflammatory reaction due to internal joint prosthesis (T84.5-)
     M00.00 Staphylococcal arthritis, unspecified joint
     M00.01 Staphylococcal arthritis, shoulder
      M00.011 Staphylococcal arthritis, right shoulder
      M00.012 Staphylococcal arthritis, left shoulder

     M00.02 Staphylococcal arthritis, elbow
      M00.021 Staphylococcal arthritis, right elbow
      M00.022 Staphylococcal arthritis, left elbow
     M00.03 Staphylococcal arthritis, wrist
      Staphylococcal arthritis of carpal bones
      M00.031 Staphylococcal arthritis, right wrist
      M00.032 Staphylococcal arthritis, left wrist
     M00.04 Staphylococcal arthritis, hand
      Staphylococcal arthritis of metacarpus and phalanges
      M00.041 Staphylococcal arthritis, right hand
      M00.042 Staphylococcal arthritis, left hand
     M00.05 Staphylococcal arthritis, hip
      M00.051 Staphylococcal arthritis, right hip
      M00.052 Staphylococcal arthritis, left hip
     M00.06 Staphylococcal arthritis, knee
      M00.061 Staphylococcal arthritis, right knee
      M00.062 Staphylococcal arthritis, left knee
     M00.07 Staphylococcal arthritis, ankle and foot
      Staphylococcal arthritis, tarsus, metatarsus and phalanges
      M00.071 Staphylococcal arthritis, right ankle and foot
      M00.072 Staphylococcal arthritis, left ankle and foot
     M00.08 Staphylococcal arthritis, vertebrae
     M00.09 Staphylococcal polyarthritis
   M00.1 Pneumococcal arthritis and polyarthritis
     M00.10 Pneumococcal arthritis, unspecified joint
     M00.11 Pneumococcal arthritis, shoulder
      M00.111 Pneumococcal arthritis, right shoulder
      M00.112 Pneumococcal arthritis, left shoulder
     M00.12 Pneumococcal arthritis, elbow
      M00.121 Pneumococcal arthritis, right elbow
      M00.122 Pneumococcal arthritis, left elbow
     M00.13 Pneumococcal arthritis, wrist
      Pneumococcal arthritis of carpal bones
      M00.131 Pneumococcal arthritis, right wrist
      M00.132 Pneumococcal arthritis, left wrist
     M00.14 Pneumococcal arthritis, hand
      Pneumococcal arthritis of metacarpus and phalanges
      M00.141 Pneumococcal arthritis, right hand
      M00.142 Pneumococcal arthritis, left hand
     M00.15 Pneumococcal arthritis, hip
      M00.151 Pneumococcal arthritis, right hip
      M00.152 Pneumococcal arthritis, left hip
     M00.16 Pneumococcal arthritis, knee
      M00.161 Pneumococcal arthritis, right knee
      M00.162 Pneumococcal arthritis, left knee
     M00.17 Pneumococcal arthritis, ankle and foot
      Pneumococcal arthritis, tarsus, metatarsus and phalanges
      M00.171 Pneumococcal arthritis, right ankle and foot
      M00.172 Pneumococcal arthritis, left ankle and foot
      M00.172 Pneumococcal arthritis, left ankle and foot
     M00.18 Pneumococcal arthritis, vertebrae
     M00.19 Pneumococcal polyarthritis
   M00.2 Other streptococcal arthritis and polyarthritis
    Use additional code (B95.0–B95.2, B95.4–B95.5) to identify bacterial agent
     M00.20 Other streptococcal arthritis, unspecified joint
     M00.21 Other streptococcal arthritis, shoulder
      M00.211 Other streptococcal arthritis, right shoulder
      M00.212 Other streptococcal arthritis, left shoulder
     M00.22 Other streptococcal arthritis, elbow
      M00.221 Other streptococcal arthritis, right elbow
      M00.222 Other streptococcal arthritis, left elbow
     M00.23 Other streptococcal arthritis, wrist
      Other streptococcal arthritis of carpal bones
      M00.231 Other streptococcal arthritis, right wrist
      M00.232 Other streptococcal arthritis, left wrist
     M00.24 Other streptococcal arthritis, hand
      Other streptococcal arthritis metacarpus and phalanges
      M00.241 Other streptococcal arthritis, right hand
      M00.242 Other streptococcal arthritis, left hand

  Additional Character Required   3-character code   Unspecified laterality codes were excluded here.   •=New Code   ▲=Revised Code   *Excludes1*—Not coded here, do not use together   *Excludes2*—Not included here

CHAPTER 13. DISEASES OF THE MUSCULOSKELETAL SYSTEM AND CONNECTIVE TISSUE (M00.25–M08.922)

M00.25 Other streptococcal arthritis, hip
- **6th** M00.251 Other streptococcal arthritis, right hip
- M00.252 Other streptococcal arthritis, left hip

M00.26 Other streptococcal arthritis, knee
- **6th** M00.261 Other streptococcal arthritis, right knee
- M00.262 Other streptococcal arthritis, left knee

M00.27 Other streptococcal arthritis, ankle and foot
- **6th** Other streptococcal arthritis, tarsus, metatarsus and phalanges
  - M00.271 Other streptococcal arthritis, right ankle and foot
  - M00.272 Other streptococcal arthritis, left ankle and foot

M00.28 Other streptococcal arthritis, vertebrae

M00.29 Other streptococcal polyarthritis

M00.8 Arthritis and polyarthritis due to other bacteria
- **5th** Use additional code (B96) to identify bacteria

M00.80 Arthritis due to other bacteria, unspecified joint

M00.81 Arthritis due to other bacteria, shoulder
- **6th** M00.811 Arthritis due to other bacteria, right shoulder
- M00.812 Arthritis due to other bacteria, left shoulder

M00.82 Arthritis due to other bacteria, elbow
- **6th** M00.821 Arthritis due to other bacteria, right elbow
- M00.822 Arthritis due to other bacteria, left elbow

M00.83 Arthritis due to other bacteria, wrist
- **6th** Arthritis due to other bacteria, carpal bones
  - M00.831 Arthritis due to other bacteria, right wrist
  - M00.832 Arthritis due to other bacteria, left wrist

M00.84 Arthritis due to other bacteria, hand
- **6th** Arthritis due to other bacteria, metacarpus and phalanges
  - M00.841 Arthritis due to other bacteria, right hand
  - M00.842 Arthritis due to other bacteria, left hand

M00.85 Arthritis due to other bacteria, hip
- **6th** M00.851 Arthritis due to other bacteria, right hip
- M00.852 Arthritis due to other bacteria, left hip

M00.86 Arthritis due to other bacteria, knee
- **6th** M00.861 Arthritis due to other bacteria, right knee
- M00.862 Arthritis due to other bacteria, left knee

M00.87 Arthritis due to other bacteria, ankle and foot
- **6th** Arthritis due to other bacteria, tarsus, metatarsus, and phalanges
  - M00.871 Arthritis due to other bacteria, right ankle and foot
  - M00.872 Arthritis due to other bacteria, left ankle and foot

M00.88 Arthritis due to other bacteria, vertebrae

M00.89 Polyarthritis due to other bacteria

M00.9 Pyogenic arthritis, unspecified
Infective arthritis NOS
Autoinflammatory syndromes (M04)

(M04) AUTOINFLAMMATORY SYNDROMES

M04 AUTOINFLAMMATORY SYNDROMES
- **4th** *Excludes2:* Crohn's disease (K50.-)

- **M04.1 Periodic fever syndromes**
  Familial Mediterranean fever
  Hyperimmunoglobin D syndrome
  Mevalonate kinase deficiency
  Tumor necrosis factor receptor associated periodic syndrome [TRAPS]

- **M04.2 Cryopyrin-associated periodic syndromes**
  Chronic infantile neurological, cutaneous and articular syndrome [CINCA]
  Familial cold autoinflammatory syndrome
  Familial cold urticaria
  Muckle-Wells syndrome
  Neonatal onset multisystemic inflammatory disorder [NOMID]

- **M04.8 Other autoinflammatory syndromes**
  Blau syndrome
  Deficiency of interleukin 1 receptor antagonist [DIRA]
  Majeed syndrome
  Periodic fever, aphthous stomatitis, pharyngitis, and adenopathy syndrome [PFAPA]
  Pyogenic arthritis, pyoderma gangrenosum, and acne syndrome [PAPA]

- **M04.9 Autoinflammatory syndrome, unspecified**

(M05–M14) INFLAMMATORY POLYARTHROPATHIES

M08 JUVENILE ARTHRITIS
- **4th** Code also any associated underlying condition, such as: regional enteritis [Crohn's disease] (K50.-)
  ulcerative colitis (K51.-)
  Excludes1: arthropathy in Whipple's disease (M14.8)
  Felty's syndrome (M05.0)
  juvenile dermatomyositis (M33.0-)
  psoriatic juvenile arthropathy (L40.54)

M08.0 Unspecified juvenile rheumatoid arthritis
- **5th** Juvenile rheumatoid arthritis with or without rheumatoid factor

M08.00 Unspecified juvenile rheumatoid arthritis of unspecified site

M08.01 Unspecified juvenile rheumatoid arthritis, shoulder
- **6th** M08.011 Unspecified juvenile rheumatoid arthritis, right shoulder
- M08.012 Unspecified juvenile rheumatoid arthritis, left shoulder

M08.02 Unspecified juvenile rheumatoid arthritis of elbow
- **6th** M08.021 Unspecified juvenile rheumatoid arthritis, right elbow
- M08.022 Unspecified juvenile rheumatoid arthritis, left elbow

M08.03 Unspecified juvenile rheumatoid arthritis, wrist
- **6th** M08.031 Unspecified juvenile rheumatoid arthritis, right wrist
- M08.032 Unspecified juvenile rheumatoid arthritis, left wrist

M08.04 Unspecified juvenile rheumatoid arthritis, hand
- **6th** M08.041 Unspecified juvenile rheumatoid arthritis, right hand
- M08.042 Unspecified juvenile rheumatoid arthritis, left hand

M08.05 Unspecified juvenile rheumatoid arthritis, hip
- **6th** M08.051 Unspecified juvenile rheumatoid arthritis, right hip
- M08.052 Unspecified juvenile rheumatoid arthritis, left hip

M08.06 Unspecified juvenile rheumatoid arthritis, knee
- **6th** M08.061 Unspecified juvenile rheumatoid arthritis, right knee
- M08.062 Unspecified juvenile rheumatoid arthritis, left knee

M08.07 Unspecified juvenile rheumatoid arthritis, ankle and foot
- **6th** M08.071 Unspecified juvenile rheumatoid arthritis, right ankle and foot
- M08.072 Unspecified juvenile rheumatoid arthritis, left ankle and foot

M08.08 Unspecified juvenile rheumatoid arthritis, vertebrae

M08.09 Unspecified juvenile rheumatoid arthritis, multiple sites

M08.9 Juvenile arthritis, unspecified
- **5th** *Excludes1:* juvenile rheumatoid arthritis, unspecified (M08.0-)

M08.90 Juvenile arthritis, unspecified, unspecified site

M08.91 Juvenile arthritis, unspecified, shoulder
- **6th** M08.911 Juvenile arthritis, unspecified, right shoulder
- M08.912 Juvenile arthritis, unspecified, left shoulder

M08.92 Juvenile arthritis, unspecified, elbow
- **6th** M08.921 Juvenile arthritis, unspecified, right elbow
- M08.922 Juvenile arthritis, unspecified, left elbow

   Additional Character Required | 3-character code | Unspecified laterality codes were excluded here. | •=New Code ▲=Revised Code | ***Excludes1***—Not coded here, do not use together ***Excludes2***—Not included here

M08.93 **Juvenile arthritis, unspecified, wrist**
> M08.931 Juvenile arthritis, unspecified, right wrist
> M08.932 Juvenile arthritis, unspecified, left wrist

M08.94 **Juvenile arthritis, unspecified, hand**
> M08.941 Juvenile arthritis, unspecified, right hand
> M08.942 Juvenile arthritis, unspecified, left hand

M08.95 **Juvenile arthritis, unspecified, hip**
> M08.951 Juvenile arthritis, unspecified, right hip
> M08.952 Juvenile arthritis, unspecified, left hip

M08.96 **Juvenile arthritis, unspecified, knee**
> M08.961 Juvenile arthritis, unspecified, right knee
> M08.962 Juvenile arthritis, unspecified, left knee

M08.97 **Juvenile arthritis, unspecified, ankle and foot**
> M08.971 Juvenile arthritis, unspecified, right ankle and foot
> M08.972 Juvenile arthritis, unspecified, left ankle and foot

M08.98 **Juvenile arthritis, unspecified, vertebrae**
M08.99 **Juvenile arthritis, unspecified, multiple sites**

M12 OTHER AND UNSPECIFIED ARTHROPATHY
Excludes1: arthrosis (M15-M19)
> cricoarytenoid arthropathy (J38.7)

M12.5 **Traumatic arthropathy**
Excludes1: current injury-see Alphabetic Index
> post-traumatic osteoarthritis of first carpometacarpal joint (M18.2–M18.3)
> post-traumatic osteoarthritis of hip (M16.4–M16.5)
> post-traumatic osteoarthritis of knee (M17.2–M17.3)
> post-traumatic osteoarthritis NOS (M19.1-)
> post-traumatic osteoarthritis of other single joints (M19.1-)

M12.50 **Traumatic arthropathy, unspecified site**
M12.51 **Traumatic arthropathy, shoulder**
> M12.511 Traumatic arthropathy, right shoulder
> M12.512 Traumatic arthropathy, left shoulder

M12.52 **Traumatic arthropathy, elbow**
> M12.521 Traumatic arthropathy, right elbow
> M12.522 Traumatic arthropathy, left elbow

M12.53 **Traumatic arthropathy, wrist**
> M12.531 Traumatic arthropathy, right wrist
> M12.532 Traumatic arthropathy, left wrist

M12.54 **Traumatic arthropathy, hand**
> M12.541 Traumatic arthropathy, right hand
> M12.542 Traumatic arthropathy, left hand

M12.55 **Traumatic arthropathy, hip**
> M12.551 Traumatic arthropathy, right hip
> M12.552 Traumatic arthropathy, left hip

M12.56 **Traumatic arthropathy, knee**
> M12.561 Traumatic arthropathy, right knee
> M12.562 Traumatic arthropathy, left knee

M12.57 **Traumatic arthropathy, ankle and foot**
> M12.571 Traumatic arthropathy, right ankle and foot
> M12.572 Traumatic arthropathy, left ankle and foot

M12.58 **Traumatic arthropathy, other specified site**
> Traumatic arthropathy, vertebrae
M12.59 **Traumatic arthropathy, multiple sites**
M12.9 **Arthropathy, unspecified**

M14 ARTHROPATHIES IN OTHER DISEASES CLASSIFIED ELSEWHERE
Excludes1: arthropathy in:
> DM (E08-E13 with .61-)
> hematological disorders (M36.2-M36.3)
> hypersensitivity reactions (M36.4)
> neoplastic disease (M36.1)
> neurosyphillis (A52.16)
> sarcoidosis (D86.86)
> enteropathic arthropathies (M07.-)
> juvenile psoriatic arthropathy (L40.54)
> lipoid dermatoarthritis (E78.81)

M14.8 **Arthropathies in other specified diseases classified elsewhere**
Code first underlying disease, such as:
> amyloidosis (E85.-)
> erythema multiforme (L51.-)
> erythema nodosum (L52)
> hemochromatosis (E83.11-)
> hyperparathyroidism (E21.-)
> hypothyroidism (E00–E03)
> sickle-cell disorders (D57.-)
> thyrotoxicosis [hyperthyroidism] (E05.-)
> Whipple's disease (K90.81)

M14.80 **Arthropathies in other specified diseases classified elsewhere, unspecified site**
M14.81 **Arthropathies in other specified diseases classified elsewhere; shoulder**
> M14.811 right shoulder
> M14.812 left shoulder

M14.82 **Arthropathies in other specified diseases classified elsewhere; elbow**
> M14.821 right elbow
> M14.822 left elbow

M14.83 **Arthropathies in other specified diseases classified elsewhere; wrist**
> M14.831 right wrist
> M14.832 left wrist

M14.84 **Arthropathies in other specified diseases classified elsewhere; hand**
> M14.841 right hand
> M14.842 left hand

M14.85 **Arthropathies in other specified diseases classified elsewhere; hip**
> M14.851 right hip
> M14.852 left hip

M14.86 **Arthropathies in other specified diseases classified elsewhere; knee**
> M14.861 right knee
> M14.862 left knee

M14.87 **Arthropathies in other specified diseases classified elsewhere; ankle and foot**
> M14.871 right ankle and foot
> M14.872 left ankle and foot

M14.88 **Arthropathies in other specified diseases classified elsewhere, vertebrae**
M14.89 **Arthropathies in other specified diseases classified elsewhere, multiple sites**

(M15–M19) OSTEOARTHRITIS

Excludes2: osteoarthritis of spine (M47.-)

(M20–M25) OTHER JOINT DISORDERS

Excludes2: joints of the spine (M40–M54)

M20 ACQUIRED DEFORMITIES OF FINGERS AND TOES
Excludes1: acquired absence of fingers and toes (Z89.-)
> congenital absence of fingers and toes (Q71.3-, Q72.3-)
> congenital deformities and malformations of fingers and toes (Q66.-, Q68–Q70, Q74.-)

M20.0 **Deformity of finger(s)**
Excludes1: clubbing of fingers (R68.3)
> palmar fascial fibromatosis [Dupuytren] (M72.0)
> trigger finger (M65.3)

M20.00 **Unspecified deformity of finger(s)**
> M20.001 Unspecified deformity of right finger(s)
> M20.002 Unspecified deformity of left finger(s)

M20.01 **Mallet finger**
> M20.011 Mallet finger of right finger(s)
> M20.012 Mallet finger of left finger(s)

M20.09 **Other deformity of finger(s)**
> M20.091 Other deformity of right finger(s)
> M20.092 Other deformity of left finger(s)

   4th 5th 6th 7th Additional Character Required   ✔ 3-character code   Unspecified laterality codes were excluded here.   •=New Code   ▲=Revised Code   *Excludes1*—Not coded here, do not use together   *Excludes2*—Not included here

CHAPTER 13. DISEASES OF THE MUSCULOSKELETAL SYSTEM AND CONNECTIVE TISSUE   (M20.1–M25.48)

M20.1 Hallux valgus (acquired)
- *Excludes 2:* bunion (M21.6-)
- **M20.11 Hallux valgus (acquired), right foot**
- **M20.12 Hallux valgus (acquired), left foot**

M21 OTHER ACQUIRED DEFORMITIES OF LIMBS
- *Excludes1:* acquired absence of limb (Z89.-)
  - congenital absence of limbs (Q71–Q73)
  - congenital deformities and malformations of limbs (Q65–Q66, Q68–Q74)
- *Excludes2:* acquired deformities of fingers or toes (M20.-)
  - coxa plana (M91.2)
- **M21.0 Valgus deformity, NEC**
  - *Excludes1:* metatarsus valgus (Q66.6)
    - talipes calcaneovalgus (Q66.4)
  - **M21.06 Valgus deformity, NEC, knee**
    - Genu valgum
    - Knock knee
    - **M21.061 Valgus deformity, NEC, right knee**
    - **M21.062 Valgus deformity, NEC, left knee**
- **M21.1 Varus deformity, NEC**
  - *Excludes1:* metatarsus varus (Q66.22)
    - tibia vara (M92.5)
  - **M21.16 Varus deformity, NEC, knee**
    - Bow leg
    - Genu varum
    - **M21.161 Varus deformity, NEC, right knee**
    - **M21.162 Varus deformity, NEC, left knee**
- **M21.4 Flat foot [pes planus] (acquired)**
  - *Excludes1:* congenital pes planus (Q66.5-)
  - **M21.41 Flat foot [pes planus] (acquired), right foot**
  - **M21.42 Flat foot [pes planus] (acquired), left foot**
- **M21.8 Other specified acquired deformities of limbs**
  - *Excludes2:* coxa plana (M91.2)
  - **M21.80 Other specified acquired deformities of unspecified limb**
  - **M21.86 Other specified acquired deformities of lower leg**
    - **M21.861 Other specified acquired deformities of right lower leg**
    - **M21.862 Other specified acquired deformities of left lower leg**

M22 DISORDER OF PATELLA
- *Excludes1:* traumatic dislocation of patella (S83.0-)
- **M22.4 Chondromalacia patellae**
  - **M22.41 Chondromalacia patellae, right knee**
  - **M22.42 Chondromalacia patellae, left knee**

M25 OTHER JOINT DISORDER, NEC
- *Excludes2:* abnormality of gait and mobility (R26.-)
  - acquired deformities of limb (M20–M21)
  - calcification of bursa (M71.4-)
  - calcification of shoulder (joint) (M75.3)
  - calcification of tendon (M65.2-)
  - difficulty in walking (R26.2)
  - temporomandibular joint disorder (M26.6-)
- **M25.0 Hemarthrosis**
  - *Excludes1:* current injury—see injury of joint by body region
    - hemophilic arthropathy (M36.2)
  - **M25.00 Hemarthrosis, unspecified joint**
  - **M25.01 Hemarthrosis, shoulder**
    - **M25.011 Hemarthrosis, right shoulder**
    - **M25.012 Hemarthrosis, left shoulder**
  - **M25.02 Hemarthrosis, elbow**
    - **M25.021 Hemarthrosis, right elbow**
    - **M25.022 Hemarthrosis, left elbow**
  - **M25.03 Hemarthrosis, wrist**
    - **M25.031 Hemarthrosis, right wrist**
    - **M25.032 Hemarthrosis, left wrist**
  - **M25.04 Hemarthrosis, hand**
    - **M25.041 Hemarthrosis, right hand**
    - **M25.042 Hemarthrosis, left hand**

M25.05 Hemarthrosis, hip
- **M25.051 Hemarthrosis, right hip**
- **M25.052 Hemarthrosis, left hip**

M25.06 Hemarthrosis, knee
- **M25.061 Hemarthrosis, right knee**
- **M25.062 Hemarthrosis, left knee**

M25.07 Hemarthrosis, ankle and foot
- **M25.071 Hemarthrosis, right ankle**
- **M25.072 Hemarthrosis, left ankle**
- **M25.074 Hemarthrosis, right foot**
- **M25.075 Hemarthrosis, left foot**

M25.08 Hemarthrosis, other specified site
- Hemarthrosis, vertebrae

M25.3 Other instability of joint
- *Excludes1:* instability of joint secondary to old ligament injury (M24.2-)
  - instability of joint secondary to removal of joint prosthesis (M96.8-)
- *Excludes2:* spinal instabilities (M53.2-)
- **M25.30 Other instability, unspecified joint**
- **M25.31 Other instability, shoulder**
  - **M25.311 Other instability, right shoulder**
  - **M25.312 Other instability, left shoulder**
- **M25.32 Other instability, elbow**
  - **M25.321 Other instability, right elbow**
  - **M25.322 Other instability, left elbow**
- **M25.33 Other instability, wrist**
  - **M25.331 Other instability, right wrist**
  - **M25.332 Other instability, left wrist**
- **M25.34 Other instability, hand**
  - **M25.341 Other instability, right hand**
  - **M25.342 Other instability, left hand**
- **M25.35 Other instability, hip**
  - **M25.351 Other instability, right hip**
  - **M25.352 Other instability, left hip**
- **M25.36 Other instability, knee**
  - **M25.361 Other instability, right knee**
  - **M25.362 Other instability, left knee**
- **M25.37 Other instability, ankle and foot**
  - **M25.371 Other instability, right ankle**
  - **M25.372 Other instability, left ankle**
  - **M25.374 Other instability, right foot**
  - **M25.375 Other instability, left foot**

M25.4 Effusion of joint
- *Excludes1:* hydrarthrosis in yaws (A66.6)
  - intermittent hydrarthrosis (M12.4-)
  - other infective (teno)synovitis (M65.1-)
- **M25.40 Effusion, unspecified joint**
- **M25.41 Effusion, shoulder**
  - **M25.411 Effusion, right shoulder**
  - **M25.412 Effusion, left shoulder**
- **M25.42 Effusion, elbow**
  - **M25.421 Effusion, right elbow**
  - **M25.422 Effusion, left elbow**
- **M25.43 Effusion, wrist**
  - **M25.431 Effusion, right wrist**
  - **M25.432 Effusion, left wrist**
- **M25.44 Effusion, hand**
  - **M25.441 Effusion, right hand**
  - **M25.442 Effusion, left hand**
- **M25.45 Effusion, hip**
  - **M25.451 Effusion, right hip**
  - **M25.452 Effusion, left hip**
- **M25.46 Effusion, knee**
  - **M25.461 Effusion, right knee**
  - **M25.462 Effusion, left knee**
- **M25.47 Effusion, ankle and foot**
  - **M25.471 Effusion, right ankle**
  - **M25.472 Effusion, left ankle**
  - **M25.474 Effusion, right foot**
  - **M25.475 Effusion, left foot**
- **M25.48 Effusion, other site**

   Additional Character Required   3-character code   Unspecified laterality codes were excluded here.   •=New Code   ▲=Revised Code   *Excludes1*—Not coded here, do not use together   *Excludes2*—Not included here

M25.5 Pain in joint

Excludes2: pain in hand (M79.64-)
     pain in fingers (M79.64-)
     pain in foot (M79.67-)
     pain in limb (M79.6-)
     pain in toes (M79.67-)

M25.50 Pain in unspecified joint

M25.51 Pain in shoulder
     M25.511 Pain in right shoulder
     M25.512 Pain in left shoulder

M25.52 Pain in elbow
     M25.521 Pain in right elbow
     M25.522 Pain in left elbow

M25.53 Pain in wrist
     M25.531 Pain in right wrist
     M25.532 Pain in left wrist

•M25.54 Pain in hand joints
     •M25.541 Pain in joints of right hand
     •M25.542 Pain in joints of left hand

M25.55 Pain in hip
     M25.551 Pain in right hip
     M25.552 Pain in left hip

M25.56 Pain in knee
     M25.561 Pain in right knee
     M25.562 Pain in left knee

M25.57 Pain in ankle and joints of foot
     M25.571 Pain in right ankle and joints of right foot
     M25.572 Pain in left ankle and joints of left foot

M25.6 Stiffness of joint, NEC

Excludes1: ankylosis of joint (M24.6-)
     contracture of joint (M24.5-)

M25.60 Stiffness of unspecified joint, NEC

M25.61 Stiffness of shoulder, NEC
     M25.611 Stiffness of right shoulder, NEC
     M25.612 Stiffness of left shoulder, NEC

M25.62 Stiffness of elbow, NEC
     M25.621 Stiffness of right elbow, NEC
     M25.622 Stiffness of left elbow, NEC

M25.63 Stiffness of wrist, NEC
     M25.631 Stiffness of right wrist, NEC
     M25.632 Stiffness of left wrist, NEC

M25.64 Stiffness of hand, NEC
     M25.641 Stiffness of right hand, NEC
     M25.642 Stiffness of left hand, NEC

M25.65 Stiffness of hip, NEC
     M25.651 Stiffness of right hip, NEC
     M25.652 Stiffness of left hip, NEC

M25.66 Stiffness of knee, NEC
     M25.661 Stiffness of right knee, NEC
     M25.662 Stiffness of left knee, NEC

M25.67 Stiffness of ankle and foot, NEC
     M25.671 Stiffness of right ankle, NEC
     M25.672 Stiffness of left ankle, NEC
     M25.674 Stiffness of right foot, NEC
     M25.675 Stiffness of left foot, NEC

M25.7 Osteophyte

M25.70 Osteophyte, unspecified joint

M25.71 Osteophyte, shoulder
     M25.711 Osteophyte, right shoulder
     M25.712 Osteophyte, left shoulder

M25.72 Osteophyte, elbow
     M25.721 Osteophyte, right elbow
     M25.722 Osteophyte, left elbow

M25.73 Osteophyte, wrist
     M25.731 Osteophyte, right wrist
     M25.732 Osteophyte, left wrist

M25.74 Osteophyte, hand
     M25.741 Osteophyte, right hand
     M25.742 Osteophyte, left hand

M25.75 Osteophyte, hip
     M25.751 Osteophyte, right hip
     M25.752 Osteophyte, left hip

M25.76 Osteophyte, knee
     M25.761 Osteophyte, right knee
     M25.762 Osteophyte, left knee

M25.77 Osteophyte, ankle and foot
     M25.771 Osteophyte, right ankle
     M25.772 Osteophyte, left ankle
     M25.774 Osteophyte, right foot
     M25.775 Osteophyte, left foot

M25.78 Osteophyte, vertebrae

(M26–M27) DENTOFACIAL ANOMALIES [INCLUDING MALOCCLUSION] AND OTHER DISORDERS OF JAW

Excludes1: hemifacial atrophy or hypertrophy (Q67.4)
     unilateral condylar hyperplasia or hypoplasia (M27.8)

M26 DENTOFACIAL ANOMALIES [INCLUDING MALOCCLUSION]

M26.0 Major anomalies of jaw size

Excludes1: acromegaly (E22.0)
     Robin's syndrome (Q87.0)

M26.04 Mandibular hypoplasia

M26.4 Malocclusion, unspecified

M26.6 Temporomandibular joint disorders

Excludes2: current temporomandibular joint dislocation (S03.0)
     current temporomandibular joint sprain (S03.4)

M26.60 Temporomandibular joint disorder, unspecified
     •M26.601 Right temporomandibular joint disorder
     •M26.602 Left temporomandibular joint disorder
     •M26.603 Bilateral temporomandibular joint disorder

M26.61 Adhesions and ankylosis of temporomandibular joint
     •M26.611 Adhesions and ankylosis of right temporomandibular joint
     •M26.612 Adhesions and ankylosis of left temporomandibular joint
     •M26.613 Adhesions and ankylosis of bilateral temporomandibular joint

M26.62 Arthralgia of temporomandibular joint
     •M26.621 Arthralgia of right temporomandibular joint
     •M26.622 Arthralgia of left temporomandibular joint
     •M26.623 Arthralgia of bilateral temporomandibular joint

M26.63 Articular disc disorder of temporomandibular joint
     •M26.631 Articular disc disorder of right temporomandibular joint
     •M26.632 Articular disc disorder of left temporomandibular joint
     •M26.633 Articular disc disorder of bilateral temporomandibular joint

M26.69 Other specified disorders of temporomandibular joint

M27 OTHER DISEASES OF JAWS

M27.0 Developmental disorders of jaws
     Latent bone cyst of jaw
     Stafne's cyst
     Torus mandibularis
     Torus palatinus

M27.2 Inflammatory conditions of jaws
     Osteitis of jaw(s)
     Osteomyelitis (neonatal) jaw(s)
     Osteoradionecrosis jaw(s)
     Periostitis jaw(s)
     Sequestrum of jaw bone

Use additional code (W88–W90, X39.0) to identify radiation, if radiation-induced

Excludes2: osteonecrosis of jaw due to drug (M87.180)

M27.4 Other and unspecified cysts of jaw

Excludes1: cysts of oral region (K09.-)
     latent bone cyst of jaw (M27.0)
     Stafne's cyst (M27.0)

M27.40 Unspecified cyst of jaw
     Cyst of jaw NOS

   Additional Character Required   ✔ 3-character code   Unspecified laterality codes were excluded here.   •=New Code   ▲=Revised Code   *Excludes1*—Not coded here, do not use together   *Excludes2*—Not included here

M27.49 Other cysts of jaw
Aneurysmal cyst of jaw
Hemorrhagic cyst of jaw
Traumatic cyst of jaw

(M30–M36) SYSTEMIC CONNECTIVE TISSUE DISORDERS

Includes: autoimmune disease NOS
collagen (vascular) disease NOS
systemic autoimmune disease
systemic collagen (vascular) disease
Excludes1: autoimmune disease, single organ or single cell-type—**code to** relevant condition category

M30 POLYARTERITIS NODOSA AND RELATED CONDITIONS
`4th` **Excludes1:** microscopic polyarteritis (M31.7)
M30.2 Juvenile polyarteritis
M30.3 Mucocutaneous lymph node syndrome [Kawasaki]
M30.8 Other conditions related to polyarteritis nodosa
Polyangiitis overlap syndrome

M31 OTHER NECROTIZING VASCULOPATHIES
`4th` **M31.0 Hypersensitivity angiitis**
Goodpasture's syndrome
M31.3 Wegener's granulomatosis
Necrotizing respiratory granulomatosis
`5th`   **M31.30 Wegener's granulomatosis without renal involvement**
Wegener's granulomatosis NOS
M31.31 Wegener's granulomatosis with renal involvement
M31.4 Aortic arch syndrome [Takayasu]
M31.8 Other specified necrotizing vasculopathies
Hypocomplementemic vasculitis
Septic vasculitis
M31.9 Necrotizing vasculopathy, unspecified

M32 SLE
`4th` **Excludes1:** lupus erythematosus (discoid) (NOS) (L93.0)
M32.1 SLE with organ or system involvement
`5th`   **M32.10 SLE, organ or system involvement unspecified**
M32.11 Endocarditis in SLE
Libman-Sacks disease
M32.12 Pericarditis in SLE
Lupus pericarditis
M32.13 Lung involvement in SLE
Pleural effusion due to SLE
M32.14 Glomerular disease in SLE
Lupus renal disease NOS
M32.15 Tubulo-interstitial nephropathy in SLE
M32.19 Other organ or system involvement in SLE
M32.8 Other forms of SLE
M32.9 SLE, unspecified
SLE NOS
SLE NOS
SLE without organ involvement

M33 DERMATOPOLYMYOSITIS
`4th` **M33.0 Juvenile dermatopolymyositis**
`5th`   **M33.00 Juvenile dermatopolymyositis, organ involvement unspecified**
M33.01 Juvenile dermatopolymyositis with respiratory involvement
M33.02 Juvenile dermatopolymyositis with myopathy
M33.09 Juvenile dermatopolymyositis with other organ involvement
M33.9 Dermatopolymyositis, unspecified
`5th`   **M33.90 Dermatopolymyositis, unspecified, organ involvement unspecified**
M33.91 Dermatopolymyositis, unspecified with respiratory involvement
M33.92 Dermatopolymyositis, unspecified with myopathy
M33.99 Dermatopolymyositis, unspecified with other organ involvement

M35 OTHER SYSTEMIC INVOLVEMENT OF CONNECTIVE TISSUE
`4th` **Excludes1:** reactive perforating collagenosis (L87.1)
M35.8 Other specified systemic involvement of connective tissue
M35.9 Systemic involvement of connective tissue, unspecified
Autoimmune disease (systemic) NOS
Collagen (vascular) disease NOS

M36 SYSTEMIC DISORDERS OF CONNECTIVE TISSUE IN DISEASES CLASSIFIED ELSEWHERE
`4th` **Excludes2:** arthropathies in diseases classified elsewhere (M14.-)
M36.2 Hemophilic arthropathy
Hemarthrosis in hemophilic arthropathy
Code first underlying disease, such as: factor VIII deficiency (D66)
with vascular defect (D68.0)
factor IX deficiency (D67)
hemophilia (classical) (D66)
hemophilia B (D67)
hemophilia C (D68.1)
M36.3 Arthropathy in other blood disorders
M36.4 Arthropathy in hypersensitivity reactions classified elsewhere
Code first underlying disease, such as: Henoch (-Schönlein) purpura (D69.0)
serum sickness (T80.6-)

(M40–M54) DORSOPATHIES

(M40–M43) DEFORMING DORSOPATHIES

M40 KYPHOSIS AND LORDOSIS
`4th` **Excludes1:** congenital kyphosis and lordosis (Q76.4)
kyphoscoliosis (M41.-)
postprocedural kyphosis and lordosis (M96.-)
M40.2 Other and unspecified kyphosis
`5th`   **M40.20 Unspecified kyphosis**
 `6th`   **M40.202 Unspecified kyphosis, cervical region**
M40.203 Unspecified kyphosis, cervicothoracic region
M40.204 Unspecified kyphosis, thoracic region
M40.205 Unspecified kyphosis, thoracolumbar region
M40.209 Unspecified kyphosis, site unspecified
M40.29 Other kyphosis
`6th`   **M40.292 Other kyphosis, cervical region**
M40.293 Other kyphosis, cervicothoracic region
M40.294 Other kyphosis, thoracic region
M40.295 Other kyphosis, thoracolumbar region
M40.299 Other kyphosis, site unspecified
M40.4 Postural lordosis
`5th`   Acquired lordosis
M40.40 Postural lordosis, site unspecified
M40.45 Postural lordosis, thoracolumbar region
M40.46 Postural lordosis, lumbar region
M40.47 Postural lordosis, lumbosacral region
M40.5 Lordosis, unspecified
`5th`   **M40.50 Lordosis, unspecified, site unspecified**
M40.55 Lordosis, unspecified, thoracolumbar region
M40.56 Lordosis, unspecified, lumbar region
M40.57 Lordosis, unspecified, lumbosacral region

M41 SCOLIOSIS
`4th` **Includes:** kyphoscoliosis
Excludes1: congenital scoliosis NOS (Q67.5)
congenital scoliosis due to bony malformation (Q76.3)
postural congenital scoliosis (Q67.5)
kyphoscoliotic heart disease (I27.1)
postprocedural scoliosis (M96.-)
M41.0 Infantile idiopathic scoliosis
 `5th`   **M41.00 Infantile idiopathic scoliosis, site unspecified**
M41.02 Infantile idiopathic scoliosis, cervical region
M41.03 Infantile idiopathic scoliosis, cervicothoracic region
M41.04 Infantile idiopathic scoliosis, thoracic region
M41.05 Infantile idiopathic scoliosis, thoracolumbar region
M41.06 Infantile idiopathic scoliosis, lumbar region

 `4th` `5th` `6th` `7th` Additional Character Required   ✔ 3-character code   Unspecified laterality codes were excluded here.   •=New Code   ▲=Revised Code   **Excludes1**—Not coded here, do not use together   **Excludes2**—Not included here

218   **PEDIATRIC ICD-10-CM 2017: A MANUAL FOR PROVIDER-BASED CODING**

M41.07 **Infantile idiopathic scoliosis, lumbosacral region**
M41.08 **Infantile idiopathic scoliosis, sacral and sacrococcygeal region**

M41.1 **Juvenile and adolescent idiopathic scoliosis**

 M41.11 **Juvenile idiopathic scoliosis**
　　M41.112 **Juvenile idiopathic scoliosis, cervical region**
　　M41.113 **Juvenile idiopathic scoliosis, cervicothoracic region**
　　M41.114 **Juvenile idiopathic scoliosis, thoracic region**
　　M41.115 **Juvenile idiopathic scoliosis, thoracolumbar region**
　　M41.116 **Juvenile idiopathic scoliosis, lumbar region**
　　M41.117 **Juvenile idiopathic scoliosis, lumbosacral region**
　　M41.119 **Juvenile idiopathic scoliosis, site unspecified**

M41.12 **Adolescent scoliosis**
　　M41.122 **Adolescent idiopathic scoliosis, cervical region**
　　M41.123 **Adolescent idiopathic scoliosis, cervicothoracic region**
　　M41.124 **Adolescent idiopathic scoliosis, thoracic region**
　　M41.125 **Adolescent idiopathic scoliosis, thoracolumbar region**
　　M41.126 **Adolescent idiopathic scoliosis, lumbar region**
　　M41.127 **Adolescent idiopathic scoliosis, lumbosacral region**
　　M41.129 **Adolescent idiopathic scoliosis, site unspecified**

M41.9 **Scoliosis, unspecified**

M43　OTHER DEFORMING DORSOPATHIES
Excludes1: congenital spondylolysis and spondylolisthesis (Q76.2)
　　hemivertebra (Q76.3–Q76.4)
　　Klippel-Feil syndrome (Q76.1)
　　lumbarization and sacralization (Q76.4)
　　platyspondylisis (Q76.4)
　　spina bifida occulta (Q76.0)
　　spinal curvature in osteoporosis (M80.-)
　　spinal curvature in Paget's disease of bone [osteitis deformans] (M88.-)

M43.6 **Torticollis**
Excludes1: congenital (sternomastoid) torticollis (Q68.0)
　　current injury—*see Injury*, of spine, by body region
　　ocular torticollis (R29.891)
　　psychogenic torticollis (F45.8)
　　spasmodic torticollis (G24.3)
　　torticollis due to birth injury (P15.2)

(M45–M49) SPONDYLOPATHIES

M48　OTHER SPONDYLOPATHIES
M48.0 **Spinal stenosis**
Caudal stenosis
M48.00 **Spinal stenosis, site unspecified**
M48.01 **Spinal stenosis, occipito-atlanto-axial region**
M48.02 **Spinal stenosis, cervical region**
M48.03 **Spinal stenosis, cervicothoracic region**
M48.04 **Spinal stenosis, thoracic region**
M48.05 **Spinal stenosis, thoracolumbar region**
M48.06 **Spinal stenosis, lumbar region**
M48.07 **Spinal stenosis, lumbosacral region**
M48.08 **Spinal stenosis, sacral and sacrococcygeal region**

(M50–M54) OTHER DORSOPATHIES

Excludes1: current injury - **see** injury of spine by body region
discitis NOS (M46.4-)

M54　DORSALGIA
Excludes1: psychogenic dorsalgia (F45.41)
M54.2 **Cervicalgia**
Excludes1: cervicalgia due to intervertebral cervical disc disorder (M50.-)

M54.5 **Low back pain**
Loin pain
Lumbago NOS
Excludes1: low back strain (S39.012)
　　lumbago due to intervertebral disc displacement (M51.2-)
　　lumbago with sciatica (M54.4-)
M54.9 **Dorsalgia, unspecified**
Backache NOS
Back pain NOS

(M60–M79) Soft tissue disorders

(M60–M63) DISORDERS OF MUSCLES

M60　MYOSITIS
 Excludes2: inclusion body myositis [IBM] (G72.41)
M60.0 **Infective myositis**
Tropical pyomyositis
Use additional code (B95–B97) to identify infectious agent
M60.00 **Infective myositis, unspecified site**
　　M60.000 **Infective myositis, unspecified right arm**
　　　Infective myositis, right upper limb NOS
　　M60.001 **Infective myositis, unspecified left arm**
　　　Infective myositis, left upper limb NOS
　　M60.003 **Infective myositis, unspecified right leg**
　　　Infective myositis, right lower limb NOS
　　M60.004 **Infective myositis, unspecified left leg**
　　　Infective myositis, left lower limb NOS
　　M60.009 **Infective myositis, unspecified site**
M60.01 **Infective myositis, shoulder**
　　M60.011 **Infective myositis, right shoulder**
　　M60.012 **Infective myositis, left shoulder**
M60.02 **Infective myositis, upper arm**
　　M60.021 **Infective myositis, right upper arm**
　　M60.022 **Infective myositis, left upper arm**
M60.03 **Infective myositis, forearm**
　　M60.031 **Infective myositis, right forearm**
　　M60.032 **Infective myositis, left forearm**
M60.04 **Infective myositis, hand and fingers**
　　M60.041 **Infective myositis, right hand**
　　M60.042 **Infective myositis, left hand**
　　M60.044 **Infective myositis, right finger(s)**
　　M60.045 **Infective myositis, left finger(s)**
M60.05 **Infective myositis, thigh**
　　M60.051 **Infective myositis, right thigh**
　　M60.052 **Infective myositis, left thigh**
M60.06 **Infective myositis, lower leg**
　　M60.061 **Infective myositis, right lower leg**
　　M60.062 **Infective myositis, left lower leg**
M60.07 **Infective myositis, ankle, foot and toes**
　　M60.070 **Infective myositis, right ankle**
　　M60.071 **Infective myositis, left ankle**
　　M60.073 **Infective myositis, right foot**
　　M60.074 **Infective myositis, left foot**
　　M60.076 **Infective myositis, right toe(s)**
　　M60.077 **Infective myositis, left toe(s)**
M60.08 **Infective myositis, other site**
M60.09 **Infective myositis, multiple sites**
M60.1 **Interstitial myositis**
M60.10 **Interstitial myositis of unspecified site**
M60.11 **Interstitial myositis, shoulder**
　　M60.111 **Interstitial myositis, right shoulder**
　　M60.112 **Interstitial myositis, left shoulder**
M60.12 **Interstitial myositis, upper arm**
　　M60.121 **Interstitial myositis, right upper arm**
　　M60.122 **Interstitial myositis, left upper arm**
M60.13 **Interstitial myositis, forearm**
　　M60.131 **Interstitial myositis, right forearm**
　　M60.132 **Interstitial myositis, left forearm**
M60.14 **Interstitial myositis, hand**
　　M60.141 **Interstitial myositis, right hand**
　　M60.142 **Interstitial myositis, left hand**

   Additional Character Required　 3-character code

Unspecified laterality codes were excluded here.
•=New Code
▲=Revised Code

Excludes1—Not coded here, do not use together
Excludes2—Not included here

CHAPTER 13. DISEASES OF THE MUSCULOSKELETAL SYSTEM AND CONNECTIVE TISSUE (M41.07–M60.142)

CHAPTER 13. DISEASES OF THE MUSCULOSKELETAL SYSTEM AND CONNECTIVE TISSUE   (M60.15–M71.532)

M60.15   Interstitial myositis, thigh
- **6th**   M60.151   Interstitial myositis, right thigh
- M60.152   Interstitial myositis, left thigh

M60.16   Interstitial myositis, lower leg
- **6th**   M60.161   Interstitial myositis, right lower leg
- M60.162   Interstitial myositis, left lower leg

M60.9   Myositis, unspecified

M62   **OTHER DISORDERS OF MUSCLE**
4th

Excludes1: alcoholic myopathy (G72.1)
   cramp and spasm (R25.2)
   drug-induced myopathy (G72.0)
   myalgia (M79.1)
   stiff-man syndrome (G25.82)

Excludes2: nontraumatic hematoma of muscle (M79.81)

M62.4   Contracture of muscle
5th   Contracture of tendon (sheath)
Excludes1: contracture of joint (M24.5-)

M62.40   Contracture of muscle, unspecified site

M62.41   Contracture of muscle, shoulder
- **6th**   M62.411   Contracture of muscle, right shoulder
- M62.412   Contracture of muscle, left shoulder

M62.42   Contracture of muscle, upper arm
- **6th**   M62.421   Contracture of muscle, right upper arm
- M62.422   Contracture of muscle, left upper arm

M62.43   Contracture of muscle, forearm
- **6th**   M62.431   Contracture of muscle, right forearm
- M62.432   Contracture of muscle, left forearm

M62.44   Contracture of muscle, hand
- **6th**   M62.441   Contracture of muscle, right hand
- M62.442   Contracture of muscle, left hand

M62.45   Contracture of muscle, thigh
- **6th**   M62.451   Contracture of muscle, right thigh
- M62.452   Contracture of muscle, left thigh

M62.46   Contracture of muscle, lower leg
- **6th**   M62.461   Contracture of muscle, right lower leg
- M62.462   Contracture of muscle, left lower leg

M62.47   Contracture of muscle, ankle and foot
- **6th**   M62.471   Contracture of muscle, right ankle and foot
- M62.472   Contracture of muscle, left ankle and foot

M62.48   Contracture of muscle, other site

M62.49   Contracture of muscle, multiple sites

M62.8   Other specified disorders of muscle
5th   *Excludes2:* nontraumatic hematoma of muscle (M79.81)

M62.81   Muscle weakness (generalized)
Excludes 1: muscle weakness in sarcopenia (M62.84)

M62.82   Rhabdomyolysis
Excludes1: traumatic rhabdomyolysis (T79.6)

M62.83   Muscle spasm
- **6th**   M62.830   Muscle spasm of back
- M62.831   Muscle spasm of calf
    Charley-horse
- M62.838   Other muscle spasm

M62.89   Other specified disorders of muscle
   Muscle (sheath) hernia

M62.9   Disorder of muscle, unspecified

(M65–M67) DISORDERS OF SYNOVIUM AND TENDON

M65   **SYNOVITIS AND TENOSYNOVITIS**
4th

Excludes1: chronic crepitant synovitis of hand and wrist (M70.0-)
   current injury—see injury of ligament or tendon by body region
   soft tissue disorders related to use, overuse and pressure (M70.-)

M65.8   Other synovitis and tenosynovitis
5th   M65.80   Other synovitis and tenosynovitis, unspecified site
M65.81   Other synovitis and tenosynovitis; shoulder
- **6th**   M65.811   right shoulder
- M65.812   left shoulder

M65.82   Other synovitis and tenosynovitis; upper arm
- **6th**   M65.821   right upper arm
- M65.822   left upper arm

M65.83   Other synovitis and tenosynovitis; forearm
- **6th**   M65.831   right forearm
- M65.832   left forearm

M65.84   Other synovitis and tenosynovitis; hand
- **6th**   M65.841   right hand
- M65.842   left hand

M65.85   Other synovitis and tenosynovitis; thigh
- **6th**   M65.851   right thigh
- M65.852   left thigh

M65.86   Other synovitis and tenosynovitis; lower leg
- **6th**   M65.861   right lower leg
- M65.862   left lower leg

M65.87   Other synovitis and tenosynovitis; ankle and foot
- **6th**   M65.871   right ankle and foot
- M65.872   left ankle and foot

M65.88   Other synovitis and tenosynovitis, other site

M65.89   Other synovitis and tenosynovitis, multiple sites

M65.9   Synovitis and tenosynovitis, unspecified

M67   **OTHER DISORDERS OF SYNOVIUM AND TENDON**

Excludes1: palmar fascial fibromatosis [Dupuytren] (M72.0)
   tendinitis NOS (M77.9-)
   xanthomatosis localized to tendons (E78.2)

M67.0   Short Achilles tendon (acquired)
- **5th**   M67.01   Short Achilles tendon (acquired), right ankle
- M67.02   Short Achilles tendon (acquired), left ankle

M67.4   Ganglion
5th   Ganglion of joint or tendon (sheath)
Excludes1: ganglion in yaws (A66.6)
Excludes2: cyst of bursa (M71.2–M71.3)
   cyst of synovium (M71.2–M71.3)

M67.40   Ganglion, unspecified site

M67.41   Ganglion, shoulder
- **6th**   M67.411   Ganglion, right shoulder
- M67.412   Ganglion, left shoulder

M67.42   Ganglion, elbow
- **6th**   M67.421   Ganglion, right elbow
- M67.422   Ganglion, left elbow

M67.43   Ganglion, wrist
- **6th**   M67.431   Ganglion, right wrist
- M67.432   Ganglion, left wrist

M67.44   Ganglion, hand
- **6th**   M67.441   Ganglion, right hand
- M67.442   Ganglion, left hand

M67.45   Ganglion, hip
- **6th**   M67.451   Ganglion, right hip
- M67.452   Ganglion, left hip

M67.46   Ganglion, knee
- **6th**   M67.461   Ganglion, right knee
- M67.462   Ganglion, left knee

M67.47   Ganglion, ankle and foot
- **6th**   M67.471   Ganglion, right ankle and foot
- M67.472   Ganglion, left ankle and foot

M67.48   Ganglion, other site

M67.49   Ganglion, multiple sites

(M70–M79) OTHER SOFT TISSUE DISORDERS

M71   **OTHER BURSOPATHIES**
4th

Excludes1: bunion (M20.1)
   bursitis related to use, overuse or pressure (M70.-)
   enthesopathies (M76–M77)

M71.2   Synovial cyst of popliteal space [Baker]
5th   *Excludes1:* synovial cyst of popliteal space with rupture (M66.0)
M71.21   Synovial cyst of popliteal space [Baker], right knee
M71.22   Synovial cyst of popliteal space [Baker], left knee

M71.5   Other bursitis, NEC
5th   *Excludes1:* bursitis NOS (M71.9-)
Excludes2: bursitis of shoulder (M75.5)
   bursitis of tibial collateral [Pellegrini-Stieda] (M76.4-)

M71.50   Other bursitis, NEC, unspecified site

M71.52   Other bursitis, NEC, elbow
- **6th**   M71.521   Other bursitis, NEC, right elbow
- M71.522   Other bursitis, NEC, left elbow

M71.53   Other bursitis, NEC, wrist
- **6th**   M71.531   Other bursitis, NEC, right wrist
- M71.532   Other bursitis, NEC, left wrist

4th   **5th**   **6th**   **7th**   Additional Character Required   ✔   3-character code   Unspecified laterality codes were excluded here.   •=New Code   ▲=Revised Code   *Excludes1*—Not coded here, do not use together   *Excludes2*—Not included here

M71.54 **Other bursitis, NEC, hand**
6th
  M71.541 **Other bursitis, NEC, right hand**
  M71.542 **Other bursitis, NEC, left hand**
M71.55 **Other bursitis, NEC, hip**
6th
  M71.551 **Other bursitis, NEC, right hip**
  M71.552 **Other bursitis, NEC, left hip**
M71.56 **Other bursitis, NEC, knee**
6th
  M71.561 **Other bursitis, NEC, right knee**
  M71.562 **Other bursitis, NEC, left knee**
M71.57 **Other bursitis, NEC, ankle and foot**
6th
  M71.571 **Other bursitis, NEC, right ankle and foot**
  M71.572 **Other bursitis, NEC, left ankle and foot**
M71.58 **Other bursitis, NEC, other site**
M71.9 **Bursopathy, unspecified**
Bursitis NOS

M72 **FIBROBLASTIC DISORDERS**
4th
Excludes2: retroperitoneal fibromatosis (D48.3)
M72.6 **Necrotizing fasciitis**
Use additional code (B95.-, B96.-) to identify causative organism
M72.9 **Fibroblastic disorder, unspecified**
Fasciitis NOS
Fibromatosis NOS

M75 **SHOULDER LESIONS**
4th
M75.1 **Rotator cuff tear or rupture, not specified as traumatic**
5th
Rotator cuff syndrome
Supraspinatus tear or rupture, not specified as traumatic
Supraspinatus syndrome
Excludes1: tear of rotator cuff, traumatic (S46.01-)
Excludes2: shoulder-hand syndrome (M89.0-)
M75.10 **Unspecified rotator cuff tear or rupture, not specified as traumatic**
6th
  M75.101 **Unspecified rotator cuff tear or rupture of right shoulder, not specified as traumatic**
  M75.102 **Unspecified rotator cuff tear or rupture of left shoulder, not specified as traumatic**
M75.11 **Incomplete rotator cuff tear or rupture not specified as traumatic**
6th
  M75.111 **Incomplete rotator cuff tear or rupture of right shoulder, not specified as traumatic**
  M75.112 **Incomplete rotator cuff tear or rupture of left shoulder, not specified as traumatic**
M75.12 **Complete rotator cuff tear or rupture not specified as traumatic**
6th
  M75.121 **Complete rotator cuff tear or rupture of right shoulder, not specified as traumatic**
  M75.122 **Complete rotator cuff tear or rupture of left shoulder, not specified as traumatic**

M76 **ENTHESOPATHIES, LOWER LIMB, EXCLUDING FOOT**
4th
Excludes2: bursitis due to use, overuse and pressure (M70.-)
enthesopathies of ankle and foot (M77.5-)
M76.6 **Achilles tendinitis**
5th
Achilles bursitis
M76.61 **Achilles tendinitis, right leg**
M76.62 **Achilles tendinitis, left leg**

M79 **OTHER AND UNSPECIFIED SOFT TISSUE DISORDERS, NEC**
4th
Excludes1: psychogenic rheumatism (F45.8)
soft tissue pain, psychogenic (F45.41)
M79.1 **Myalgia**
Myofascial pain syndrome
Excludes1: fibromyalgia (M79.7)
myositis (M60.-)
M79.6 **Pain in limb, hand, foot, fingers and toes**
5th
Excludes2: pain in joint (M25.5-)
M79.60 **Pain in limb, unspecified**
6th
  M79.601 **Pain in right arm**
    Pain in right upper limb NOS
  M79.602 **Pain in left arm**
    Pain in left upper limb NOS
  M79.604 **Pain in right leg**
    Pain in right lower limb NOS

M79.605 **Pain in left leg**
  Pain in left lower limb NOS
M79.62 **Pain in upper arm**
6th
  Pain in axillary region
  M79.621 **Pain in right upper arm**
  M79.622 **Pain in left upper arm**
M79.63 **Pain in forearm**
6th
  M79.631 **Pain in right forearm**
  M79.632 **Pain in left forearm**
M79.64 **Pain in hand and fingers**
6th
  M79.641 **Pain in right hand**
  M79.642 **Pain in left hand**
  M79.644 **Pain in right finger(s)**
  M79.645 **Pain in left finger(s)**
M79.65 **Pain in thigh**
6th
  M79.651 **Pain in right thigh**
  M79.652 **Pain in left thigh**
M79.66 **Pain in lower leg**
6th
  M79.661 **Pain in right lower leg**
  M79.662 **Pain in left lower leg**
M79.67 **Pain in foot and toes**
6th
  M79.671 **Pain in right foot**
  M79.672 **Pain in left foot**
  M79.674 **Pain in right toe(s)**
  M79.675 **Pain in left toe(s)**
M79.8 **Other specified soft tissue disorders**
5th
M79.81 **Nontraumatic hematoma of soft tissue**
  Nontraumatic hematoma of muscle
  Nontraumatic seroma of muscle and soft tissue
M79.89 **Other specified soft tissue disorders**
  Polyalgia
M79.9 **Soft tissue disorder, unspecified**

(M80–M94) OSTEOPATHIES AND CHONDROPATHIES

(M80–M85) DISORDERS OF BONE DENSITY AND STRUCTURE

M84 **DISORDER OF CONTINUITY OF BONE**
4th
GUIDELINES

Coding of Pathologic Fractures

7th character A is for use as long as the patient is receiving active treatment for the fracture. Examples of active treatment are: surgical treatment, emergency department encounter, evaluation and continuing treatment by the same or a different physician. While the patient may be seen by a new or different provider over the course of treatment for a pathological fracture, assignment of the 7th character is based on whether the patient is undergoing active treatment and not whether the provider is seeing the patient for the first time. 7th character, D is to be used for encounters after the patient has completed active treatment. The other 7th characters, listed under each subcategory in the Tabular List, are to be used for subsequent encounters for treatment of problems associated with the healing, such as malunions, nonunions, and sequelae.
Care for complications of surgical treatment for fracture repairs during the healing or recovery phase should be coded with the appropriate complication codes.
Excludes2: traumatic fracture of bone-see fracture, by site
M84.3 **Stress fracture**
5th
Fatigue fracture
March fracture
Stress fracture NOS
Stress fracture reaction
Use additional external cause code(s) to identify the cause of the stress fracture
Excludes1: pathological fracture NOS (M84.4-)
pathological fracture due to osteoporosis (M80.-)
traumatic fracture (S12.-, S22.-, S32.-, S42.-, S52.-, S62.-, S72.-, S82.-, S92.-)

> M84 requires 7th character to identify the encounter type
> A—initial encounter for fracture care
> D—subsequent encounter with routine healing
> G—subsequent encounter for fracture with delayed healing
> K—subsequent encounter for fracture with nonunion
> P—subsequent encounter for fracture with malunion
> S—sequel

 4th 5th 6th 7th Additional Character Required   3-character code

Unspecified laterality codes were excluded here.

•=New Code
▲=Revised Code

Excludes1—Not coded here, do not use together
Excludes2—Not included here

Excludes2: personal history of (healed) stress (fatigue) fracture
(Z87.312)
stress fracture of vertebra (M48.4-)
M84.30X Stress fracture, unspecified site

`7th`

M84.31 Stress fracture, shoulder
`6th`
  **M84.311 Stress fracture,
  right shoulder**
  `7th`

  **M84.312 Stress fracture,
  left shoulder**
  `7th`

M84.32 Stress fracture, humerus
`6th`
  **M84.321 Stress fracture,
  right humerus**
  `7th`

  **M84.322 Stress fracture,
  left humerus**
  `7th`

> M84 requires 7th character to
> identify the encounter type
> A—initial encounter for fracture
> care
> D—subsequent encounter with
> routine healing
> G—subsequent encounter for
> fracture with delayed healing
> K—subsequent encounter for
> fracture with nonunion
> P—subsequent encounter for
> fracture with malunion
> S—sequel

M84.33 Stress fracture, ulna and radius
`6th`
  M84.331 Stress fracture, right ulna
  `7th`

  M84.332 Stress fracture, left ulna
  `7th`

  M84.333 Stress fracture, right radius
  `7th`

  M84.334 Stress fracture, left radius
  `7th`

M84.34 Stress fracture, hand and fingers
`6th`
  M84.341 Stress fracture, right hand
  `7th`

  M84.342 Stress fracture, left hand
  `7th`

  M84.344 Stress fracture, right finger(s)
  `7th`

  M84.345 Stress fracture, left finger(s)
  `7th`

M84.35 Stress fracture, pelvis and femur
`6th`
  Stress fracture, hip
  M84.350 Stress fracture, pelvis
  `7th`

  M84.351 Stress fracture, right femur
  `7th`

  M84.352 Stress fracture, left femur
  `7th`

M84.36 Stress fracture, tibia and fibula
`6th`
  M84.361 Stress fracture, right tibia
  `7th`

  M84.362 Stress fracture, left tibia
  `7th`

  M84.363 Stress fracture, right fibula
  `7th`

  M84.364 Stress fracture, left fibula
  `7th`

M84.37 Stress fracture, ankle, foot and toes
`6th`
  M84.371 Stress fracture, right ankle
  `7th`

M84.372 Stress fracture, left ankle
`7th`

M84.374 Stress fracture, right foot
`7th`

M84.375 Stress fracture, left foot
`7th`

M84.377 Stress fracture, right toe(s)
`7th`

M84.378 Stress fracture, left toe(s)
`7th`

M84.38X Stress fracture, other site
`7th`   *Excludes2:* stress fracture of vertebra (M48.4-)

M85   **OTHER DISORDERS OF BONE DENSITY AND STRUCTURE**
`4th`   *Excludes1:* osteogenesis imperfecta (Q78.0)
     osteopetrosis (Q78.2)
     osteopoikilosis (Q78.8)
     polyostotic fibrous dysplasia (Q78.1)
  M85.6 Other cyst of bone
  `5th`   *Excludes1:* cyst of jaw NEC (M27.4)
     osteitis fibrosa cystica generalisata [von Recklinghausen's
     disease of bone] (E21.0)
    M85.60 Other cyst of bone, unspecified site
    M85.61 Other cyst of bone, shoulder
    `6th`   **M85.611 Other cyst of bone, right shoulder**
       M85.612 Other cyst of bone, left shoulder
    M85.62 Other cyst of bone, upper arm
    `6th`   **M85.621 Other cyst of bone, right upper arm**
       M85.622 Other cyst of bone, left upper arm
    M85.63 Other cyst of bone, forearm
    `6th`   **M85.631 Other cyst of bone, right forearm**
       M85.632 Other cyst of bone, left forearm
    M85.64 Other cyst of bone, hand
    `6th`   **M85.641 Other cyst of bone, right hand**
       M85.642 Other cyst of bone, left hand
    M85.65 Other cyst of bone, thigh
    `6th`   **M85.651 Other cyst of bone, right thigh**
       M85.652 Other cyst of bone, left thigh
    M85.66 Other cyst of bone, lower leg
    `6th`   **M85.661 Other cyst of bone, right lower leg**
       M85.662 Other cyst of bone, left lower leg
    M85.67 Other cyst of bone, ankle and foot
    `6th`   **M85.671 Other cyst of bone, right ankle and foot**
       M85.672 Other cyst of bone, left ankle and foot
    M85.68 Other cyst of bone, other site
    M85.69 Other cyst of bone, multiple sites

(M86–M90) OTHER OSTEOPATHIES

Excludes1: postprocedural osteopathies (M96.-)

M86   **OSTEOMYELITIS**
`4th`   **Use additional code** (B95–B97) to identify infectious agent
   Use additional code to identify major osseous defect, if applicable
   (M89.7-)
   Excludes1: osteomyelitis due to:
     echinococcus (B67.2)
     gonococcus (A54.43)
     salmonella (A02.24)
   Excludes2: osteomyelitis of:
     orbit (H05.0-)
     petrous bone (H70.2-)
     vertebra (M46.2-)
  M86.1 Other acute osteomyelitis
  `5th`   **M86.10 Other acute osteomyelitis, unspecified site**
     M86.11 Other acute osteomyelitis, shoulder
    `6th`   **M86.111 Other acute osteomyelitis, right shoulder**
       M86.112 Other acute osteomyelitis, left shoulder

 `4th` `5th` `6th` `7th`   Additional Character Required   ✔   3-character code   Unspecified laterality codes
were excluded here.   •=New Code
▲=Revised Code   ***Excludes1***—Not coded here, do not use together
Excludes2—Not included here

M86.12 Other acute osteomyelitis, humerus
- **6th**   M86.121 Other acute osteomyelitis, right humerus
- M86.122 Other acute osteomyelitis, left humerus

M86.13 Other acute osteomyelitis, radius and ulna
- **6th**   M86.131 Other acute osteomyelitis, right radius and ulna
- M86.132 Other acute osteomyelitis, left radius and ulna

M86.14 Other acute osteomyelitis, hand
- **6th**   M86.141 Other acute osteomyelitis, right hand
- M86.142 Other acute osteomyelitis, left hand

M86.15 Other acute osteomyelitis, femur
- **6th**   M86.151 Other acute osteomyelitis, right femur
- M86.152 Other acute osteomyelitis, left femur

M86.16 Other acute osteomyelitis, tibia and fibula
- **6th**   M86.161 Other acute osteomyelitis, right tibia and fibula
- M86.162 Other acute osteomyelitis, left tibia and fibula

M86.17 Other acute osteomyelitis, ankle and foot
- **6th**   M86.171 Other acute osteomyelitis, right ankle and foot
- M86.172 Other acute osteomyelitis, left ankle and foot

M86.18 Other acute osteomyelitis, other site

M86.19 Other acute osteomyelitis, multiple sites

M86.9 Osteomyelitis, unspecified
Infection of bone NOS
Periostitis without osteomyelitis

M88 OSTEITIS DEFORMANS [PAGET'S DISEASE OF BONE]
4th   *Excludes1:* osteitis deformans in neoplastic disease (M90.6)

M88.0 Osteitis deformans of skull

M88.1 Osteitis deformans of vertebrae

M88.8 Osteitis deformans of other bones
- **5th**   M88.81 Osteitis deformans of shoulder
  - **6th**   M88.811 Osteitis deformans of right shoulder
  - M88.812 Osteitis deformans of left shoulder
- M88.82 Osteitis deformans of upper arm
  - **6th**   M88.821 Osteitis deformans of right upper arm
  - M88.822 Osteitis deformans of left upper arm
- M88.83 Osteitis deformans of forearm
  - **6th**   M88.831 Osteitis deformans of right forearm
  - M88.832 Osteitis deformans of left forearm
- M88.84 Osteitis deformans of hand
  - **6th**   M88.841 Osteitis deformans of right hand
  - M88.842 Osteitis deformans of left hand
- M88.85 Osteitis deformans of thigh
  - **6th**   M88.851 Osteitis deformans of right thigh
  - M88.852 Osteitis deformans of left thigh
- M88.86 Osteitis deformans of lower leg
  - **6th**   M88.861 Osteitis deformans of right lower leg
  - M88.862 Osteitis deformans of left lower leg
- M88.87 Osteitis deformans of ankle and foot
  - **6th**   M88.871 Osteitis deformans of right ankle and foot
  - M88.872 Osteitis deformans of left ankle and foot
- M88.88 Osteitis deformans of other bones
  - *Excludes2:* osteitis deformans of skull (M88.0)
    osteitis deformans of vertebrae (M88.1)
- M88.89 Osteitis deformans of multiple sites

M88.9 Osteitis deformans of unspecified bone

M89 OTHER DISORDERS OF BONE
4th

M89.1 Physeal arrest
- **5th**   Arrest of growth plate
  Epiphyseal arrest
  Growth plate arrest
- M89.12 Physeal arrest, humerus
  - **6th**   M89.121 Complete physeal arrest, right proximal humerus
  - M89.122 Complete physeal arrest, left proximal humerus
  - M89.123 Partial physeal arrest, right proximal humerus
  - M89.124 Partial physeal arrest, left proximal humerus

- M89.125 Complete physeal arrest, right distal humerus
- M89.126 Complete physeal arrest, left distal humerus
- M89.127 Partial physeal arrest, right distal humerus
- M89.128 Partial physeal arrest, left distal humerus
- M89.129 Physeal arrest, humerus, unspecified

M89.13 Physeal arrest, forearm
- **6th**   M89.131 Complete physeal arrest, right distal radius
- M89.132 Complete physeal arrest, left distal radius
- M89.133 Partial physeal arrest, right distal radius
- M89.134 Partial physeal arrest, left distal radius
- M89.138 Other physeal arrest of forearm
- M89.139 Physeal arrest, forearm, unspecified

M89.15 Physeal arrest, femur
- **6th**   M89.151 Complete physeal arrest, right proximal femur
- M89.152 Complete physeal arrest, left proximal femur
- M89.153 Partial physeal arrest, right proximal femur
- M89.154 Partial physeal arrest, left proximal femur
- M89.155 Complete physeal arrest, right distal femur
- M89.156 Complete physeal arrest, left distal femur
- M89.157 Partial physeal arrest, right distal femur
- M89.158 Partial physeal arrest, left distal femur
- M89.159 Physeal arrest, femur, unspecified

M89.16 Physeal arrest, lower leg
- **6th**   M89.160 Complete physeal arrest, right proximal tibia
- M89.161 Complete physeal arrest, left proximal tibia
- M89.162 Partial physeal arrest, right proximal tibia
- M89.163 Partial physeal arrest, left proximal tibia
- M89.164 Complete physeal arrest, right distal tibia
- M89.165 Complete physeal arrest, left distal tibia
- M89.166 Partial physeal arrest, right distal tibia
- M89.167 Partial physeal arrest, left distal tibia
- M89.168 Other physeal arrest of lower leg
- M89.169 Physeal arrest, lower leg, unspecified

M89.18 Physeal arrest, other site

M90 OSTEOPATHIES IN DISEASES CLASSIFIED ELSEWHERE
4th   *Excludes1:* osteochondritis, osteomyelitis, and osteopathy (in):
cryptococcosis (B45.3)
DM (E08–E13 with .69-)
gonococcal (A54.43)
neurogenic syphilis (A52.11)
renal osteodystrophy (N25.0)
salmonellosis (A02.24)
secondary syphilis (A51.46)
syphilis (late) (A52.77)

M90.5 Osteonecrosis in diseases classified elsewhere
- **5th**   **Code first** underlying disease, such as: caisson disease (T70.3)
  hemoglobinopathy (D50–D64)
- M90.50 Osteonecrosis in diseases classified elsewhere, unspecified site
- M90.51 Osteonecrosis in diseases classified elsewhere; shoulder
  - **6th**   M90.511   right shoulder
  - M90.512   left shoulder
- M90.52 Osteonecrosis in diseases classified elsewhere; upper arm
  - **6th**   M90.521   right upper arm
  - M90.522   left upper arm
- M90.53 Osteonecrosis in diseases classified elsewhere; forearm
  - **6th**   M90.531   right forearm
  - M90.532   left forearm
- M90.54 Osteonecrosis in diseases classified elsewhere; hand
  - **6th**   M90.541   right hand
  - M90.542   left hand
- M90.55 Osteonecrosis in diseases classified elsewhere; thigh
  - **6th**   M90.551   right thigh
  - M90.552   left thigh
- M90.56 Osteonecrosis in diseases classified elsewhere; lower leg
  - **6th**

  Additional Character Required   ✓   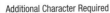 **3-character code**   Unspecified laterality codes were excluded here.   •=New Code   ▲=Revised Code   *Excludes1*—Not coded here, do not use together   *Excludes2*—Not included here

CHAPTER 13. DISEASES OF THE MUSCULOSKELETAL SYSTEM AND CONNECTIVE TISSUE   (M90.561–M95.2)

M90.561   right lower leg
M90.562   left lower leg
M90.57   Osteonecrosis in diseases classified elsewhere; **[6th]** ankle and foot
     M90.571   right ankle and foot
     M90.572   left ankle and foot
M90.58   Osteonecrosis in diseases classified elsewhere, other site
M90.59   Osteonecrosis in diseases classified elsewhere, multiple sites

(M91–M94) CHONDROPATHIES

Excludes1: postprocedural chondropathies (M96.-)

M91   JUVENILE OSTEOCHONDROSIS OF HIP AND PELVIS
[4th]   *Excludes1:* slipped upper femoral epiphysis (nontraumatic) (M93.0)
   M91.0   Juvenile osteochondrosis of pelvis
     Osteochondrosis (juvenile) of acetabulum
     Osteochondrosis (juvenile) of iliac crest [Buchanan]
     Osteochondrosis (juvenile) of ischiopubic synchondrosis [van Neck]
     Osteochondrosis (juvenile) of symphysis pubis [Pierson]
   M91.1   Juvenile osteochondrosis of head of femur [Legg-Calvé- **[5th]** Perthes]
     M91.11   Juvenile osteochondrosis of head of femur [Legg-Calvé-Perthes], right leg
     M91.12   Juvenile osteochondrosis of head of femur [Legg-Calvé-Perthes], left leg
   M91.2   Coxa plana
     [5th] Hip deformity due to previous juvenile osteochondrosis
     M91.21   Coxa plana, right hip
     M91.22   Coxa plana, left hip
   M91.3   Pseudocoxalgia
     [5th] M91.31   Pseudocoxalgia, right hip
     M91.32   Pseudocoxalgia, left hip
   M91.4   Coxa magna
     [5th] M91.41   Coxa magna, right hip
     M91.42   Coxa magna, left hip
   M91.8   Other juvenile osteochondrosis of hip and pelvis
     [5th] Juvenile osteochondrosis after reduction of congenital dislocation of hip
     M91.81   Other juvenile osteochondrosis of hip and pelvis, right leg
     M91.82   Other juvenile osteochondrosis of hip and pelvis, left leg
   M91.9   Juvenile osteochondrosis of hip and pelvis, unspecified
     [5th] M91.91   Juvenile osteochondrosis of hip and pelvis, unspecified, right leg
     M91.92   Juvenile osteochondrosis of hip and pelvis, unspecified, left leg

M92   OTHER JUVENILE OSTEOCHONDROSIS
[4th]   M92.0   Juvenile osteochondrosis of humerus
     [5th] Osteochondrosis (juvenile) of capitulum of humerus [Panner]
     Osteochondrosis (juvenile) of head of humerus [Haas]
     M92.01   Juvenile osteochondrosis of humerus, right arm
     M92.02   Juvenile osteochondrosis of humerus, left arm
   M92.1   Juvenile osteochondrosis of radius and ulna
     [5th] Osteochondrosis (juvenile) of lower ulna [Burns]
     Osteochondrosis (juvenile) of radial head [Brailsford]
     M92.11   Juvenile osteochondrosis of radius and ulna, right arm
     M92.12   Juvenile osteochondrosis of radius and ulna, left arm
   M92.2   Juvenile osteochondrosis, hand
     [5th] M92.20   Unspecified juvenile osteochondrosis; hand
       [6th] M92.201   right hand
       M92.202   left hand
     M92.21   Osteochondrosis (juvenile) of carpal lunate [Kienböck]; **[6th]**
       M92.211   right hand
       M92.212   left hand
     M92.22   Osteochondrosis (juvenile) of metacarpal heads [Mauclaire]; **[6th]**
       M92.221   right hand
       M92.222   left hand

M92.29 Other juvenile osteochondrosis; hand
   [6th] M92.291   right hand
     M92.292   left hand
M92.3   Other juvenile osteochondrosis; upper limb
   [5th] M92.31   right upper limb
     M92.32   left upper limb
M92.4   Juvenile osteochondrosis of patella;
   [5th] Osteochondrosis (juvenile) of primary patellar center [Köhler]
   Osteochondrosis (juvenile) of secondary patellar centre [Sinding Larsen]
   M92.41   right knee
   M92.42   left knee
M92.5   Juvenile osteochondrosis of tibia and fibula;
   [5th] Osteochondrosis (juvenile) of proximal tibia [Blount]
   Osteochondrosis (juvenile) of tibial tubercle [Osgood-Schlatter's]
   Tibia vara
   M92.51   right leg
   M92.52   left leg
M92.6   Juvenile osteochondrosis of tarsus;
   [5th] Osteochondrosis (juvenile) of calcaneum [Sever]
   Osteochondrosis (juvenile) of os tibiale externum [Haglund]
   Osteochondrosis (juvenile) of talus [Diaz]
   Osteochondrosis (juvenile) of tarsal navicular [Köhler]
   M92.61   right ankle
   M92.62   left ankle
M92.7   Juvenile osteochondrosis of metatarsus;
   [5th] Osteochondrosis (juvenile) of fifth metatarsus [Iselin]
   Osteochondrosis (juvenile) of second metatarsus [Freiberg]
   M92.71   right foot
   M92.72   left foot
M92.8   Other specified juvenile osteochondrosis
   Calcaneal apophysitis
M92.9   Juvenile osteochondrosis, unspecified
   Juvenile apophysitis NOS
   Juvenile epiphysitis NOS
   Juvenile osteochondritis NOS
   Juvenile osteochondrosis NOS
M93.0   Slipped upper femoral epiphysis (nontraumatic)
   [5th] Use additional code for associated chondrolysis (M94.3)
   M93.00   Unspecified slipped upper femoral epiphysis (nontraumatic); **[6th]**
     M93.001   right hip
     M93.002   left hip
   M93.01   Acute slipped upper femoral epiphysis (nontraumatic);
     [6th] M93.011   right hip
     M93.012   left hip
   M93.02   Chronic slipped upper femoral epiphysis (nontraumatic); **[6th]**
     M93.021   right hip
     M93.022   left hip
   M93.03   Acute on chronic slipped upper femoral epiphysis (nontraumatic); **[6th]**
     M93.031   right hip
     M93.032   left hip

M94   OTHER DISORDERS OF CARTILAGE
[4th]   M94.0   Chondrocostal junction syndrome [Tietze]
   Costochondritis

(M95) OTHER DISORDERS OF THE MUSCULOSKELETAL SYSTEM AND CONNECTIVE TISSUE

M95   OTHER ACQUIRED DEFORMITIES OF MUSCULOSKELETAL SYSTEM AND CONNECTIVE TISSUE
[4th]   *Excludes2:* acquired absence of limbs and organs (Z89–Z90)
   acquired deformities of limbs (M20–M21)
   congenital malformations and deformations of the musculoskeletal system (Q65–Q79)
   deforming dorsopathies (M40–M43)
   dentofacial anomalies [including malocclusion] (M26.-)
   postprocedural musculoskeletal disorders (M96.-)
   M95.2   Other acquired deformity of head

    Additional Character Required   ✓ 3-character code   Unspecified laterality codes were excluded here.   •=New Code   ▲=Revised Code   *Excludes1*—Not coded here, do not use together   *Excludes2*—Not included here

Chapter 14. Diseases of the genitourinary system (N00–N99)

GUIDELINES

Chronic kidney disease

STAGES OF CKD
Refer to category N18 for guidelines.

CKD AND KIDNEY TRANSPLANT STATUS
Refer to category N18 for guidelines.

CKD WITH OTHER CONDITIONS
Patients with CKD may also suffer from other serious conditions, most commonly DM and hypertension (in adults). The sequencing of the CKD code in relationship to codes for other contributing conditions is based on the conventions in the Tabular List.

> *Refer to Chapter 19.* CKD and kidney transplant complications.

Excludes2: certain conditions originating in the perinatal period (P04–P96)
certain infectious and parasitic diseases (A00–B99)
complications of pregnancy, childbirth and the puerperium (O00–O9A)
congenital malformations, deformations and chromosomal abnormalities (Q00–Q99)
endocrine, nutritional and metabolic diseases (E00–E88)
injury, poisoning and certain other consequences of external causes (S00–T88)
neoplasms (C00–D49)
symptoms, signs and abnormal clinical and laboratory findings, NEC (R00–R94)

(N00–N08) GLOMERULAR DISEASES

Code also any associated kidney failure (N17–N19).
Excludes1: hypertensive CKD (I12.-)

N00   **ACUTE NEPHRITIC SYNDROME**
Includes: acute glomerular disease
    acute glomerulonephritis
    acute nephritis
Excludes1: acute tubulo-interstitial nephritis (N10)
    nephritic syndrome NOS (N05.-)

N00.0   **Acute nephritic syndrome with; minor glomerular abnormality**
    Acute nephritic syndrome with minimal change lesion

N00.1   **focal and segmental glomerular lesions**
    Acute nephritic syndrome with focal and segmental hyalinosis or with focal and segmental sclerosis or with focal glomerulonephritis

N00.2   **diffuse membranous glomerulonephritis**

N00.3   **diffuse mesangial proliferative glomerulonephritis**

N00.4   **diffuse endocapillary proliferative glomerulonephritis**

N00.5   **diffuse mesangiocapillary glomerulonephritis**
    Acute nephritic syndrome with MPGN, types 1 and 3, or NOS

N00.6   **dense deposit disease**
    Acute nephritic syndrome with MPGN, type 2

N00.7   **diffuse crescentic glomerulonephritis**
    Acute nephritic syndrome with extracapillary glomerulonephritis

N00.8   **other morphologic changes**
    Acute nephritic syndrome with proliferative glomerulonephritis NOS

N00.9   **unspecified morphologic changes**

N01   **RAPIDLY PROGRESSIVE NEPHRITIC SYNDROME**
Includes: rapidly progressive glomerular disease
    rapidly progressive glomerulonephritis
    rapidly progressive nephritis
Excludes1: nephritic syndrome NOS (N05.-)

N01.0   **Rapidly progressive nephritic syndrome with; minor glomerular abnormality**
    Rapidly progressive nephritic syndrome with minimal change lesion

N01.1   **focal and segmental glomerular lesions**
    Rapidly progressive nephritic syndrome with focal and segmental hyalinosis or with focal and segmental sclerosis or with focal glomerulonephritis

N01.2   **diffuse membranous glomerulonephritis**

N01.3   **diffuse mesangial proliferative glomerulonephritis**

N01.4   **diffuse endocapillary proliferative glomerulonephritis**

N01.5   **diffuse mesangiocapillary glomerulonephritis**
    Rapidly progressive nephritic syndrome with MPGN, types 1 and 3, or NOS

N01.6   **dense deposit disease**
    Rapidly progressive nephritic syndrome with MPGN, type 2

N01.7   **diffuse crescentic glomerulonephritis**
    Rapidly progressive nephritic syndrome with extracapillary glomerulonephritis

N01.8   **other morphologic changes**
    Rapidly progressive nephritic syndrome with proliferative glomerulonephritis NOS

N01.9   **unspecified morphologic changes**

N03   **CHRONIC NEPHRITIC SYNDROME**
Includes: chronic glomerular disease
    chronic glomerulonephritis
    chronic nephritis
Excludes1: chronic tubulo-interstitial nephritis (N11.-)
    diffuse sclerosing glomerulonephritis (N05.8-)
    nephritic syndrome NOS (N05.-)

N03.0   **Chronic nephritic syndrome with; minor glomerular abnormality**
    Chronic nephritic syndrome with minimal change lesion

N03.1   **focal and segmental glomerular lesions**
    Chronic nephritic syndrome with focal and segmental hyalinosis or with focal and segmental sclerosis or with focal glomerulonephritis

N03.2   **diffuse membranous glomerulonephritis**

N03.3   **diffuse mesangial proliferative glomerulonephritis**

N03.4   **diffuse endocapillary proliferative glomerulonephritis**

N03.5   **diffuse mesangiocapillary glomerulonephritis**
    Chronic nephritic syndrome with MPGN, types 1 and 3, or NOS

N03.6   **dense deposit disease**
    Chronic nephritic syndrome with MPGN, type 2

N03.7   **diffuse crescentic glomerulonephritis**
    Chronic nephritic syndrome with extracapillary glomerulonephritis

N03.8   **other morphologic changes**
    Chronic nephritic syndrome with proliferative glomerulonephritis NOS

N03.9   **unspecified morphologic changes**

N04   **NEPHROTIC SYNDROME**
Includes: congenital nephrotic syndrome
    lipoid nephrosis

N04.0   **Nephrotic syndrome with; minor glomerular abnormality**
    Nephrotic syndrome with minimal change lesion

N04.1   **focal and segmental glomerular lesions**
    Nephrotic syndrome with focal and segmental hyalinosis or with focal and segmental sclerosis or with focal glomerulonephritis

N04.2   **diffuse membranous glomerulonephritis**

N04.3   **diffuse mesangial proliferative glomerulonephritis**

N04.4   **diffuse endocapillary proliferative glomerulonephritis**

N04.5   **diffuse mesangiocapillary glomerulonephritis**
    Nephrotic syndrome with MPGN, types 1 and 3, or NOS

N04.6   **dense deposit disease**
    Nephrotic syndrome with MPGN, type 2

N04.7   **diffuse crescentic glomerulonephritis**
    Nephrotic syndrome with extracapillary glomerulonephritis

N04.8   **other morphologic changes**
    Nephrotic syndrome with proliferative glomerulonephritis NOS

N04.9   **unspecified morphologic changes**

  Additional Character Required   3-character code

•=New Code
▲=Revised Code

Excludes1—Not coded here, do not use together
Excludes2—Not included here

CHAPTER 14. DISEASES OF THE GENITOURINARY SYSTEM   (N08–N18.9)

N08 GLOMERULAR DISORDERS IN DISEASES CLASSIFIED ELSEWHERE

Glomerulonephritis
Nephritis
Nephropathy

Please note the numerous exclusions below.

Code first underlying disease, such as: amyloidosis (E85.-)
    congenital syphilis (A50.5)
    cryoglobulinemia (D89.1)
    disseminated intravascular coagulation (D65)
    gout (M1A.-, M10.-)
    microscopic polyangiitis (M31.7)
    multiple myeloma (C90.0-)
    sepsis (A40.0–A41.9)
    sickle-cell disease (D57.0–D57.8)
Excludes1: glomerulonephritis, nephritis and nephropathy (in):
    antiglomerular basement membrane disease (M31.0)
    diabetes (E08–E13 with .21)
    gonococcal (A54.21)
    Goodpasture's syndrome (M31.0)
    hemolytic-uremic syndrome (D59.3)
    lupus (M32.14)
    mumps (B26.83)
    syphilis (A52.75)
    SLE (M32.14)
    Wegener's granulomatosis (M31.31)
    pyelonephritis in diseases classified elsewhere (N16)
    renal tubulo-interstitial disorders classified elsewhere (N16)

(N10–N16) RENAL TUBULO-INTERSTITIAL DISEASES

Includes: pyelonephritis
Excludes1: pyeloureteritis cystica (N28.85)

▲N10 ACUTE PYELONEPHRITIS

Acute infectious interstitial nephritis
Acute pyelitis
Hemoglobin nephrosis
Myoglobin nephrosis
Use additional code (B95–B97), to identify infectious agent.

N13 OBSTRUCTIVE AND REFLUX UROPATHY
Excludes2: calculus of kidney and ureter without hydronephrosis (N20.-)
    congenital obstructive defects of renal pelvis and ureter (Q62.0–Q62.3)
    hydronephrosis with ureteropelvic junction obstruction (Q62.1)
    obstructive pyelonephritis (N11.1)
- **N13.0 Hydronephrosis with ureteropelvic junction obstruction**
    Hydronephrosis due to acquired occlusion ureteropelvic junction
    Excludes2: hydronephrosis with ureteropelvic junction obstruction due to calculus (N13.2)
- **N13.1 Hydronephrosis with ureteral stricture, NEC**
    Excludes1: hydronephrosis with ureteral stricture with infection (N13.6)
- **N13.2 Hydronephrosis with renal and ureteral calculous obstruction**
    Excludes1: hydronephrosis with renal and ureteral calculous obstruction with infection (N13.6)
- **N13.3 Other and unspecified hydronephrosis**
    Excludes1: hydronephrosis with infection (N13.6)
    N13.30 Unspecified hydronephrosis
    N13.39 Other hydronephrosis
- **N13.7 Vesicoureteral-reflux**
    Excludes1: reflux-associated pyelonephritis (N11.0)
    N13.70 Vesicoureteral-reflux, unspecified
      Vesicoureteral-reflux NOS
    N13.71 Vesicoureteral-reflux without reflux nephropathy
- **N13.8 Other obstructive and reflux uropathy**
    Urinary tract obstruction due to specified cause
    Code first, if applicable, any causal condition, such as:
      enlarged prostate (N40.1)
- **N13.9 Obstructive and reflux uropathy, unspecified**
    Urinary tract obstruction NOS

(N17–N19) ACUTE KIDNEY FAILURE AND CKD

Excludes2: congenital renal failure (P96.0)
    drug- and heavy-metal-induced tubulo-interstitial and tubular conditions (N14.-)
    extrarenal uremia (R39.2)
    hemolytic-uremic syndrome (D59.3)
    hepatorenal syndrome (K76.7)
    postpartum hepatorenal syndrome (O90.4)
    posttraumatic renal failure (T79.5)
    prerenal uremia (R39.2)
    renal failure complicating abortion or ectopic or molar pregnancy (O00–O07, O08.4)
    renal failure following labor and delivery (O90.4)
    renal failure postprocedural (N99.0)

N17 ACUTE KIDNEY FAILURE
Code also associated underlying condition
Excludes1: posttraumatic renal failure (T79.5)
- **N17.0 Acute kidney failure with tubular necrosis**
    Acute tubular necrosis
    Renal tubular necrosis
    Tubular necrosis NOS
- **N17.1 Acute kidney failure with acute cortical necrosis**
    Acute cortical necrosis
    Cortical necrosis NOS
    Renal cortical necrosis
- **N17.2 Acute kidney failure with medullary necrosis**
    Medullary [papillary] necrosis NOS
    Acute medullary [papillary] necrosis
    Renal medullary [papillary] necrosis
- **N17.8 Other acute kidney failure**
- **N17.9 Acute kidney failure, unspecified**
    Acute kidney injury (nontraumatic)
    Excludes2: traumatic kidney injury (S37.0-)

N18 CHRONIC KIDNEY DISEASE (CKD)

GUIDELINES

Stages of CKD
The *ICD-10-CM* classifies CKD based on severity. The severity of CKD is designated by stages 1–5. Stage 2, code N18.2, equates to mild CKD; stage 3, code N18.3, equates to moderate CKD; and stage 4, code N18.4, equates to severe CKD. Code N18.6, ESRD, is assigned when the provider has documented ESRD.

If both a stage of CKD and ESRD are documented by the provider, only assign code N18.6 for ESRD (CKD requiring dialysis) only.

Patients who have undergone kidney transplant may still have some form of CKD because the kidney transplant may not fully restore kidney function. Therefore, the presence of CKD alone does not constitute a transplant complication. Assign the appropriate N18 code for the patient's stage of CKD and code Z94.0, Kidney transplant status. If a transplant complication such as failure or rejection or other transplant complication is documented, refer to code T86.1 for information on coding complications of a kidney transplant. If the documentation is unclear as to whether the patient has a complication of the transplant, query the provider.
Code first any associated: diabetic CKD (E08.22, E09.22, E10.22, E11.22, E13.22)
    hypertensive chronic kidney disease (I12.-, I13.-)
Use additional code to identify kidney transplant status, if applicable, (Z94.0)
- **N18.1 CKD stage 1**
- **N18.2 CKD stage 2 (mild)**
- **N18.3 CKD stage 3 (moderate)**
- **N18.4 CKD stage 4 (severe)**
- **N18.5 CKD stage 5**
    Excludes1: CKD, stage 5 requiring chronic dialysis (N18.6)
- **N18.6 ESRD**
    CKD requiring chronic dialysis
    Use additional code to identify dialysis status (Z99.2)
- **N18.9 CKD, unspecified**
    Chronic renal disease
    Chronic renal failure NOS
    Chronic renal insufficiency
    Chronic uremia

   Additional Character Required   ✓ 3-character code   •=New Code   ▲=Revised Code   **Excludes1**—Not coded here, do not use together   **Excludes2**—Not included here

(N20–N23) UROLITHIASIS

N20 **CALCULUS OF KIDNEY AND URETER**
[4th] Calculous pyelonephritis
Excludes1: nephrocalcinosis (E83.5)
    that with hydronephrosis (N13.2)
    N20.0 **Calculus of kidney**
        Nephrolithiasis NOS
        Renal calculus
        Renal stone
        Staghorn calculus
        Stone in kidney
    N20.1 **Calculus of ureter**
        Ureteric stone
    N20.2 **Calculus of kidney with calculus of ureter**
    N20.9 **Urinary calculus, unspecified**

N21 **CALCULUS OF LOWER URINARY TRACT**
[4th] *Includes:* calculus of lower urinary tract with cystitis and urethritis
    N21.0 **Calculus in bladder**
        Calculus in diverticulum of bladder
        Urinary bladder stone
        Excludes2: staghorn calculus (N20.0)
    N21.1 **Calculus in urethra**
        Excludes2: calculus of prostate (N42.0)

N23 **UNSPECIFIED RENAL COLIC**

(N25–N29) OTHER DISORDERS OF KIDNEY AND URETER

Excludes2: disorders of kidney and ureter with urolithiasis (N20–N23)

N27 **SMALL KIDNEY OF UNKNOWN CAUSE**
[4th] *Includes:* oligonephronia
    N27.0 **Small kidney, unilateral**
    N27.1 **Small kidney, bilateral**

N28 **OTHER DISORDERS OF KIDNEY AND URETER, NEC**
[4th] **N28.1** **Cyst of kidney, acquired**
        Cyst (multiple)(solitary) of kidney, acquired
        Excludes1: cystic kidney disease (congenital) (Q61.-)

(N30–N39) OTHER DISEASES OF THE URINARY SYSTEM

Excludes1: urinary infection (complicating): abortion or ectopic or molar pregnancy (O00–O07, O08.8)
    pregnancy, childbirth and the puerperium (O23.-, O75.3, O86.2-)

N30 **CYSTITIS**
[4th] **Use additional code** to identify infectious agent (B95–B97)
Excludes1: prostatocystitis (N41.3)
    N30.0 **Acute cystitis**
    [5th] *Excludes1:* irradiation cystitis (N30.4-)
        trigonitis (N30.3-)
        N30.00 **Acute cystitis without hematuria**
        N30.01 **Acute cystitis with hematuria**
    N30.4 **Irradiation cystitis**
    [5th]   **N30.40** **Irradiation cystitis without hematuria**
        N30.41 **Irradiation cystitis with hematuria**
    N30.8 **Other cystitis**
    [5th] Abscess of bladder
        N30.80 **Other cystitis without hematuria**
        N30.81 **Other cystitis with hematuria**
    N30.9 **Cystitis, unspecified**
    [5th]   **N30.90** **Cystitis, unspecified without hematuria**
        N30.91 **Cystitis, unspecified with hematuria**

N31 **NEUROMUSCULAR DYSFUNCTION OF BLADDER, NEC**
[4th] **Use additional code** to identify any associated urinary incontinence (N39.3–N39.4-)
Excludes1: cord bladder NOS (G95.89)
    neurogenic bladder due to cauda equina syndrome (G83.4)
    neuromuscular dysfunction due to spinal cord lesion (G95.89)
    N31.0 **Uninhibited neuropathic bladder, NEC**
    N31.1 **Reflex neuropathic bladder, NEC**

    N31.2 **Flaccid neuropathic bladder, NEC**
        Atonic (motor) (sensory) neuropathic bladder
        Autonomous neuropathic bladder
        Nonreflex neuropathic bladder
    N31.8 **Other neuromuscular dysfunction of bladder**
    N31.9 **Neuromuscular dysfunction of bladder, unspecified**
        Neurogenic bladder dysfunction NOS

N32 **OTHER DISORDERS OF BLADDER**
[4th] *Excludes2:* calculus of bladder (N21.0)
    cystocele (N81.1-)
    hernia or prolapse of bladder, female (N81.1-)
    N32.0 **Bladder-neck obstruction**
        Bladder-neck stenosis (acquired)
        Excludes1: congenital bladder-neck obstruction (Q64.3-)
    N32.1 **Vesicointestinal fistula**
        Vesicorectal fistula
    N32.2 **Vesical fistula, NEC**
        Excludes1: fistula between bladder and female genital tract (N82.0–N82.1)
    N32.3 **Diverticulum of bladder**
        Excludes1: congenital diverticulum of bladder (Q64.6)
        diverticulitis of bladder (N30.8-)
    N32.8 **Other specified disorders of bladder**
    [5th]   **N32.81** **Overactive bladder**
        Detrusor muscle hyperactivity
        Excludes1: frequent urination due to specified bladder condition—code to condition
        N32.89 **Other specified disorders of bladder**
            Bladder hemorrhage
            Bladder hypertrophy
            Calcified bladder
            Contracted bladder
    N32.9 **Bladder disorder, unspecified**

N34 **URETHRITIS AND URETHRAL SYNDROME**
[4th] **Use additional code** (B95–B97), to identify infectious agent.
Excludes2: Reiter's disease (M02.3-)
    urethritis in diseases with a predominantly sexual mode of transmission (A50–A64)
    urethrotrigonitis (N30.3-)
    N34.1 **Nonspecific urethritis**
        Nongonococcal urethritis
        Nonvenereal urethritis
    N34.2 **Other urethritis**
        Meatitis, urethral
        Postmenopausal urethritis
        Ulcer of urethra (meatus)
        Urethritis NOS
    N34.3 **Urethral syndrome, unspecified**

N35 **URETHRAL STRICTURE**
[4th] *Excludes1:* congenital urethral stricture (Q64.3-)
    postprocedural urethral stricture (N99.1-)
    N35.0 **Post-traumatic urethral stricture**
    [5th] Urethral stricture due to injury
        Excludes1: postprocedural urethral stricture (N99.1-)
        N35.01 **Post-traumatic urethral stricture, male**
        [6th]   **N35.010** **Post-traumatic urethral stricture, male, meatal**
            N35.011 **Post-traumatic bulbous urethral stricture**
            N35.012 **Post-traumatic membranous urethral stricture**
            N35.013 **Post-traumatic anterior urethral stricture**
            N35.014 **Post-traumatic urethral stricture, male, unspecified**
        N35.02 **Post-traumatic urethral stricture, female**
        [6th]   **N35.021** **Urethral stricture due to childbirth**
            N35.028 **Other post-traumatic urethral stricture, female**
    N35.1 **Postinfective urethral stricture, NEC**
    [5th] *Excludes1:* urethral stricture associated with schistosomiasis (B65.-, N29)
        gonococcal urethral stricture (A54.01)
        syphilitic urethral stricture (A52.76)

[4th] [5th] [6th] [7th]   Additional Character Required   ✓   3-character code

●=New Code   *Excludes1*—Not coded here, do not use together
▲=Revised Code   *Excludes2*—Not included here

N35.11   Postinfective urethral stricture, NEC, male

6th   **N35.111**   Postinfective urethral stricture, NEC, male, meatal

N35.112   Postinfective bulbous urethral stricture, NEC

N35.113   Postinfective membranous urethral stricture, NEC

N35.114   Postinfective anterior urethral stricture, NEC

N35.119   Postinfective urethral stricture, NEC, male, unspecified

N35.12   Postinfective urethral stricture, NEC, female

N35.8   **Other urethral stricture**
Excludes1: postprocedural urethral stricture (N99.1-)

N35.9   **Urethral stricture, unspecified**

N39   **OTHER DISORDERS OF URINARY SYSTEM**

Excludes2: hematuria NOS (R31.-)
    recurrent or persistent hematuria (N02.-)
    recurrent or persistent hematuria with specified morphological lesion (N02.-)
    proteinuria NOS (R80.-)

N39.0   **Urinary tract infection, site not specified**
Use additional code (B95–B97), to identify infectious agent.
Excludes1: candidiasis of urinary tract (B37.4-)
    neonatal urinary tract infection (P39.3)
    urinary tract infection of specified site, such as:
    cystitis (N30.-)
    urethritis (N34.-)

N39.4   **Other specified urinary incontinence**

Code also any associated overactive bladder (N32.81)
Excludes1: enuresis NOS (R32)
    functional urinary incontinence (R39.81)
    urinary incontinence associated with cognitive impairment (R39.81)
    urinary incontinence NOS (R32)
    urinary incontinence of nonorganic origin (F98.0)

N39.44   Nocturnal enuresis

N39.8   **Other specified disorders of urinary system**

N39.9   **Disorder of urinary system, unspecified**

(N40–N53) DISEASES OF MALE GENITAL ORGANS

N41   **INFLAMMATORY DISEASES OF PROSTATE**

Use additional code (B95–B97), to identify infectious agent.

N41.0   **Acute prostatitis**

N41.9   **Inflammatory disease of prostate, unspecified**
Prostatitis NOS

N43   **HYDROCELE AND SPERMATOCELE**
Includes: hydrocele of spermatic cord, testis or tunica vaginalis
Excludes1: congenital hydrocele (P83.5)

N43.0   **Encysted hydrocele**

N43.1   **Infected hydrocele**
Use additional code (B95–B97), to identify infectious agent

N43.2   **Other hydrocele**

N43.3   **Hydrocele, unspecified**

N43.4   **Spermatocele of epididymis**
Spermatic cyst

N43.40   Spermatocele of epididymis, unspecified

N43.41   Spermatocele of epididymis, single

N43.42   Spermatocele of epididymis, multiple

N44   **NONINFLAMMATORY DISORDERS OF TESTIS**

N44.0   **Torsion of testis**

N44.00   Torsion of testis, unspecified

N44.01   Extravaginal torsion of spermatic cord

N44.02   Intravaginal torsion of spermatic cord
Torsion of spermatic cord NOS

N44.03   Torsion of appendix testis

N44.04   Torsion of appendix epididymis

N44.1   **Cyst of tunica albuginea testis**

N44.2   **Benign cyst of testis**

N44.8   **Other noninflammatory disorders of the testis**

N45   **ORCHITIS AND EPIDIDYMITIS**
Use additional code (B95–B97), to identify infectious agent.

N45.1   **Epididymitis**

N45.2   **Orchitis**

N45.3   **Epididymo-orchitis**

N45.4   **Abscess of epididymis or testis**

N47   **DISORDERS OF PREPUCE**

N47.0   **Adherent prepuce, newborn**

N47.1   **Phimosis**

N47.2   **Paraphimosis**

N47.5   **Adhesions of prepuce and glans penis**

N47.6   **Balanoposthitis**

N47.8   **Other disorders of prepuce**
Use additional code (B95–B97), to identify infectious agent.
Excludes1: balanitis (N48.1)

N48   **OTHER DISORDERS OF PENIS**

N48.1   **Balanitis**
Use additional code (B95–B97), to identify infectious agent
Excludes1: amebic balanitis (A06.8)
    balanitis xerotica obliterans (N48.0)
    candidal balanitis (B37.42)
    gonococcal balanitis (A54.23)
    herpesviral [herpes simplex] balanitis (A60.01)

N48.3   **Priapism**
Painful erection
Code first underlying cause

N48.30   Priapism, unspecified

N48.31   Priapism due to trauma

N48.32   Priapism due to disease classified elsewhere

N48.33   Priapism, drug-induced

N48.39   Other priapism

N48.8   **Other specified disorders of penis**

N48.89   Other specified disorders of penis

N48.9   **Disorder of penis, unspecified**

N50   **OTHER AND UNSPECIFIED DISORDERS OF MALE GENITAL ORGANS**
Excludes2: torsion of testis (N44.0-)

N50.0   **Atrophy of testis**

N50.8   **Other specified disorders of male genital organs**

• **N50.81**   **Testicular pain**

 • **N50.811**   Right testicular pain

• **N50.812**   Left testicular pain

• **N50.82**   Scrotal pain

• **N50.89**   **Other specified disorders of the male genital organs**
Atrophy of scrotum, seminal vesicle, spermatic cord, tunica vaginalis and vas deferens
Edema of scrotum, seminal vesicle, spermatic cord, testis, tunica vaginalis and vas deferens
Hypertrophy of scrotum, seminal vesicle, spermatic cord, testis, tunica vaginalis and vas deferens
Ulcer of scrotum, seminal vesicle, spermatic cord, testis, and vas deferens
Chylocele, tunica vaginalis (nonfilarial) NOS
Urethroscrotal fistula
Stricture of spermatic cord, tunica vaginalis, and vas deferens

N50.9   **Disorder of male genital organs, unspecified**

(N60–N65) DISORDERS OF BREAST

Excludes1: disorders of breast associated with childbirth (O91–O92)

N60   **BENIGN MAMMARY DYSPLASIA**
Includes: fibrocystic mastopathy

N60.0   **Solitary cyst of breast**
Cyst of breast

N60.01   Solitary cyst of right breast

N60.02   Solitary cyst of left breast

N60.09   Solitary cyst of unspecified breast

     Additional Character Required   3-character code

•=New Code
▲=Revised Code

Excludes1—Not coded here, do not use together
Excludes2—Not included here

228

PEDIATRIC ICD-10-CM 2017: A MANUAL FOR PROVIDER-BASED CODING

N61 INFLAMMATORY DISORDERS OF BREAST
4th

Excludes1: inflammatory carcinoma of breast (C50.9)
  inflammatory disorder of breast associated with childbirth (O91.-)
  neonatal infective mastitis (P39.0)
  thrombophlebitis of breast [Mondor's disease] (I80.8)

- **N61.0 Mastitis without abscess**
  Infective mastitis (acute) (subacute) (nonpuerperal)
  Mastitis (acute) (subacute) (nonpuerperal) NOS
  Cellulitis (acute) (nonpuerperal) (subacute) of breast NOS
  Cellulitis (acute) (nonpuerperal) (subacute) of nipple NOS

- **N61.1 Abscess of the breast and nipple**
  Abscess (acute) (chronic) (nonpuerperal) of areola
  Abscess (acute) (chronic) (nonpuerperal) of breast
  Carbuncle of breast
  Mastitis with abscess

N62 HYPERTROPHY OF BREAST
✓

Gynecomastia
Hypertrophy of breast NOS
Massive pubertal hypertrophy of breast
Excludes1: breast engorgement of newborn (P83.4)
  disproportion of reconstructed breast (N65.1)

N63 UNSPECIFIED LUMP IN BREAST
✓

Nodule(s) NOS in breast

N64 OTHER DISORDERS OF BREAST
4th

Excludes2: mechanical complication of breast prosthesis and implant
  (T85.4-)

- **N64.3 Galactorrhea not associated with childbirth**
- **N64.4 Mastodynia**
- **N64.5 Other signs and symptoms in breast**
  5th *Excludes2:* abnormal findings on diagnostic imaging of breast
    (R92.-)
  - **N64.51 Induration of breast**
  - **N64.52 Nipple discharge**
    Excludes1: abnormal findings in nipple discharge
      (R89.-)
  - **N64.53 Retraction of nipple**
  - **N64.59 Other signs and symptoms in breast**

(N70–N77) INFLAMMATORY DISEASES OF FEMALE PELVIC ORGANS

Excludes1: inflammatory diseases of female pelvic organs complicating:
  abortion or ectopic or molar pregnancy (O00–O07, O08.0)
  pregnancy, childbirth and the puerperium (O23.-, O75.3, O85, O86.-)

N70 SALPINGITIS AND OOPHORITIS
4th

Includes: abscess (of) fallopian tube
  abscess (of) ovary
  pyosalpinx
  salpingo-oophoritis
  tubo-ovarian abscess
  tubo-ovarian inflammatory disease
Use additional code (B95–B97), to identify infectious agent
Excludes1: gonococcal infection (A54.24)
  tuberculous infection (A18.17)

- **N70.0 Acute salpingitis and oophoritis**
  5th
  - **N70.01 Acute salpingitis**
  - **N70.02 Acute oophoritis**
  - **N70.03 Acute salpingitis and oophoritis**
- **N70.1 Chronic salpingitis and oophoritis**
  5th Hydrosalpinx
  - **N70.11 Chronic salpingitis**
  - **N70.12 Chronic oophoritis**
  - **N70.13 Chronic salpingitis and oophoritis**
- **N70.9 Salpingitis and oophoritis, unspecified**
  5th
  - **N70.91 Salpingitis, unspecified**
  - **N70.92 Oophoritis, unspecified**
  - **N70.93 Salpingitis and oophoritis, unspecified**

N72 INFLAMMATORY DISEASE OF CERVIX UTERI
✓

Includes: cervicitis or endocervicitis or exocervicitis (all with or without
  erosion or ectropion)
Use additional code (B95–B97), to identify infectious agent
Excludes1: erosion and ectropion of cervix without cervicitis (N86)

N73 OTHER FEMALE PELVIC INFLAMMATORY DISEASES
4th

Use additional code (B95–B97), to identify infectious agent.
N73.9 Female pelvic inflammatory disease, unspecified
  Female pelvic infection or inflammation NOS

N75 DISEASES OF BARTHOLIN'S GLAND
4th

N75.0 Cyst of Bartholin's gland
N75.1 Abscess of Bartholin's gland

N76 OTHER INFLAMMATION OF VAGINA AND VULVA
4th

Use additional code (B95–B97), to identify infectious agent
Excludes2: vulvar vestibulitis (N94.810)
N76.0 Acute vaginitis
  Acute vulvovaginitis

(N80–N98) NONINFLAMMATORY DISORDERS OF FEMALE GENITAL TRACT

N83 NONINFLAMMATORY DISORDERS OF OVARY, FALLOPIAN TUBE AND BROAD LIGAMENT
4th

Excludes2: hydrosalpinx (N70.1-)
N83.0 Follicular cyst of ovary
  5th Cyst of graafian follicle
  Hemorrhagic follicular cyst (of ovary)
- **N83.00 Follicular cyst of ovary, unspecified side**
- **N83.01 Follicular cyst of right ovary**
- **N83.02 Follicular cyst of left ovary**
N83.1 Corpus luteum cyst
  5th Hemorrhagic corpus luteum cyst
- **N83.10 Corpus luteum cyst of ovary, unspecified side**
- **N83.11 Corpus luteum cyst of right ovary**
- **N83.12 Corpus luteum cyst of left ovary**
N83.2 Other and unspecified ovarian cysts
  5th *Excludes1:* developmental ovarian cyst (Q50.1)
  neoplastic ovarian cyst (D27.-)
  polycystic ovarian syndrome (E28.2)
  Stein-Leventhal syndrome (E28.2)
- **N83.20 Unspecified ovarian cysts**
  6th
  - **N83.201 Unspecified ovarian cyst, right side**
  - **N83.202 Unspecified ovarian cyst, left side**
  - **N83.209 Unspecified ovarian cyst, unspecified side**
- **N83.29 Other ovarian cysts**
  6th Retention cyst of ovary
  Simple cyst of ovary
  - **N83.291 Other ovarian cyst, right side**
  - **N83.292 Other ovarian cyst, left side**
  - **N83.299 Other ovarian cyst, unspecified side**

N89 OTHER NONINFLAMMATORY DISORDERS OF VAGINA
4th

Excludes1: abnormal results from vaginal cytologic examination without
  histologic confirmation (R87.62-)
  carcinoma in situ of vagina (D07.2)
  HGSIL of vagina (R87.623)
  inflammation of vagina (N76.-)
  senile (atrophic) vaginitis (N95.2)
  severe dysplasia of vagina (D07.2)
  trichomonal leukorrhea (A59.00)
  vaginal intraepithelial neoplasia [VAIN], grade III (D07.2)
N89.5 Stricture and atresia of vagina
  Vaginal adhesions
  Vaginal stenosis
  Excludes1: congenital atresia or stricture (Q52.4)
  postprocedural adhesions of vagina (N99.2)
N89.7 Hematocolpos
  Hematocolpos with hematometra or hematosalpinx

4th **5th** **6th** **7th**   Additional Character Required   ✓   3-character code

•=New Code
▲=Revised Code

Excludes1—Not coded here, do not use together
Excludes2—Not included here

N89.8   **Other specified noninflammatory disorders of vagina**
Leukorrhea NOS
Old vaginal laceration
Pessary ulcer of vagina
Excludes1: current obstetric trauma (O70.-, O71.4, O71.7–O71.8)
     old laceration involving muscles of pelvic floor (N81.8)

N89.9   **Noninflammatory disorder of vagina, unspecified**

N90 `4th` **OTHER NONINFLAMMATORY DISORDERS OF VULVA AND PERINEUM**
Excludes1: anogenital (venereal) warts (A63.0)
     carcinoma in situ of vulva (D07.1)
     condyloma acuminatum (A63.0)
     current obstetric trauma (O70.-, O71.7–O71.8)
     inflammation of vulva (N76.-)
     severe dysplasia of vulva (D07.1)
     vulvar intraepithelial neoplasm III [VIN III] (D07.1)

N90.0   **Mild vulvar dysplasia**
Vulvar intraepithelial neoplasia [VIN], grade I

N90.1   **Moderate vulvar dysplasia**
Vulvar intraepithelial neoplasia [VIN], grade II

N90.3   **Dysplasia of vulva, unspecified**

N90.4   **Leukoplakia of vulva**
Dystrophy of vulva
Kraurosis of vulva
Lichen sclerosus of external female genital organs

N90.5   **Atrophy of vulva**
Stenosis of vulva

N90.6   **Hypertrophy of vulva**
   `5th` •**N90.60**   **Unspecified hypertrophy of vulva**
       Unspecified hypertrophy of labia
     •**N90.61**   **Childhood asymmetric labium majus enlargement**
       CALME
     •**N90.69**   **Other specified hypertrophy of vulva**
       Other specified hypertrophy of labia

N90.7   **Vulvar cyst**

N90.8   **Other specified noninflammatory disorders of vulva and**
   `5th` **perineum**
     N90.81   **Female genital mutilation status**
       Female genital cutting status
       `6th` **N90.810**   **Female genital mutilation status, unspecified**
         Female genital cutting status, unspecified
         Female genital mutilation status NOS
       N90.811   **Female genital mutilation Type I status**
         Clitorectomy status
         Female genital cutting Type I status
       N90.812   **Female genital mutilation Type II status**
         Clitorectomy with excision of labia minora status
       N90.813   **Female genital mutilation Type III status**
         Female genital cutting Type III status
         Infibulation status
       N90.818   **Other female genital mutilation status**
         Female genital cutting or mutilation Type IV status
         Other female genital cutting status
     N90.89   **Other specified noninflammatory disorders of vulva and perineum**
       Adhesions of vulva
       Hypertrophy of clitoris

N90.9   **Noninflammatory disorder of vulva and perineum, unspecified**

N91 `4th` **ABSENT, SCANTY AND RARE MENSTRUATION**
Excludes1: ovarian dysfunction (E28.-)
N91.0   **Primary amenorrhea**
N91.1   **Secondary amenorrhea**
N91.2   **Amenorrhea, unspecified**

N92 `4th` **EXCESSIVE, FREQUENT AND IRREGULAR MENSTRUATION**
Excludes1: postmenopausal bleeding (N95.0)
     precocious puberty (menstruation) (E30.1)

N92.0   **Excessive and frequent menstruation with regular cycle**
Heavy periods NOS
Menorrhagia NOS
Polymenorrhea

N92.1   **Excessive and frequent menstruation with irregular cycle**
Irregular intermenstrual bleeding
Irregular, shortened intervals between menstrual bleeding
Menometrorrhagia
Metrorrhagia

N92.2   **Excessive menstruation at puberty**
Excessive bleeding associated with onset of menstrual periods
Pubertal menorrhagia
Puberty bleeding

N92.3   **Ovulation bleeding**
Regular intermenstrual bleeding

N92.5   **Other specified irregular menstruation**

N92.6   **Irregular menstruation, unspecified**
Irregular bleeding NOS
Irregular periods NOS
Excludes1: irregular menstruation with:
     lengthened intervals or scanty bleeding (N91.3–N91.5)
     shortened intervals or excessive bleeding (N92.1)

N93 `4th` **OTHER ABNORMAL UTERINE AND VAGINAL BLEEDING**
Excludes1: neonatal vaginal hemorrhage (P54.6)
     precocious puberty (menstruation) (E30.1)
     pseudomenses (P54.6)
•**N93.1**   **Pre-pubertal vaginal bleeding**
N93.8   **Other specified abnormal uterine and vaginal bleeding**
Dysfunctional or functional uterine or vaginal bleeding NOS
N93.9   **Abnormal uterine and vaginal bleeding, unspecified**

N94 `4th` **PAIN AND OTHER CONDITIONS ASSOCIATED WITH FEMALE GENITAL ORGANS AND MENSTRUAL CYCLE**
N94.0   **Mittelschmerz**
N94.1   **Dyspareunia**
   `5th` *Excludes1:* psychogenic dyspareunia (F52.6)
     •**N94.10**   **Unspecified dyspareunia**
     •**N94.11**   **Superficial (introital) dyspareunia**
     •**N94.12**   **Deep dyspareunia**
     •**N94.19**   **Other specified dyspareunia**
N94.2   **Vaginismus**
Excludes1: psychogenic vaginismus (F52.5)
N94.3   **Premenstrual tension syndrome**
Excludes 1: premenstrual dysphoric disorder (F32.81)
Code also associated menstrual migraine (G43.82-, G43.83-)
N94.4   **Primary dysmenorrhea**
N94.5   **Secondary dysmenorrhea**
N94.6   **Dysmenorrhea, unspecified**
Excludes1: psychogenic dysmenorrhea (F45.8)
N94.8   **Other specified conditions associated with female genital**
   `5th` **organs and menstrual cycle**
     N94.81   **Vulvodynia**
       `6th` **N94.810**   **Vulvar vestibulitis**
       N94.818   **Other vulvodynia**
       N94.819   **Vulvodynia, unspecified**
         Vulvodynia NOS
     N94.89   **Other specified conditions associated with female genital organs and menstrual cycle**
N94.9   **Unspecified condition associated with female genital organs and menstrual cycle**

N97 `4th` **FEMALE INFERTILITY**
Includes: inability to achieve a pregnancy
     sterility, female NOS
Excludes1: female infertility associated with:
     hypopituitarism (E23.0)
     Stein-Leventhal syndrome (E28.2)
Excludes2: incompetence of cervix uteri (N88.3)
N97.0   **Female infertility associated with anovulation**

`4th` `5th` `6th` `7th`   Additional Character Required   3-character code   •=New Code   *Excludes1*—Not coded here, do not use together
▲=Revised Code   *Excludes2*—Not included here

230   **PEDIATRIC ICD-10-CM 2017: A MANUAL FOR PROVIDER-BASED CODING**

Chapter 15. Pregnancy, childbirth and the puerperium (O00–O9A)

General Rules for Obstetric Cases

CODES FROM CHAPTER 15 AND SEQUENCING PRIORITY

Obstetric cases require codes from chapter 15, codes in the range O00–O9A, Pregnancy, Childbirth, and the Puerperium. Chapter 15 codes have sequencing priority over codes from other chapters. Additional codes from other chapters may be used in conjunction with chapter 15 codes to further specify conditions. Should the provider document that the pregnancy is incidental to the encounter, then code Z33.1, Pregnant state, incidental, should be used in place of any chapter 15 codes. It is the provider's responsibility to state that the condition being treated is not affecting the pregnancy.

CHAPTER 15 CODES USED ONLY ON THE MATERNAL RECORD

Chapter 15 codes are to be used only on the maternal record, never on the record of the newborn.

FINAL CHARACTER FOR TRIMESTER

The majority of codes in Chapter 15 have a final character indicating the trimester of pregnancy. The timeframes for the trimesters are indicated at the beginning of the chapter.

Assignment of the final character for trimester should be based on the provider's documentation of the trimester (or number of weeks) for the current admission/ encounter. This applies to the assignment of trimester for pre-existing conditions as well as those that develop during or are due to the pregnancy. The provider's documentation of the number of weeks may be used to assign the appropriate code identifying the trimester.

Refer to the *ICD-10-CM* manual for complete guidelines.

SELECTION OF TRIMESTER FOR INPATIENT ADMISSIONS THAT EN-COMPASS MORE THAN ONE TRIMESTER

In instances when a patient is admitted to a hospital for complications of pregnancy during one trimester and remains in the hospital into a subsequent trimester, the trimester character for the antepartum complication code should be assigned on the basis of the trimester when the complication developed, not the trimester of the discharge. If the condition developed prior to the current admission/encounter or represents a pre-existing condition, the trimester character for the trimester at the time of the admission/encounter should be assigned.

UNSPECIFIED TRIMESTER

The "unspecified trimester" code should rarely be used, such as when the documentation in the record is insufficient to determine the trimester and it is not possible to obtain clarification.

7TH CHARACTER FOR FETUS IDENTIFICATION

Refer to categories O31, O35, O36, O40, and O41.

Selection of OB Principal or First-listed Diagnosis

ROUTINE OUTPATIENT PRENATAL VISITS

Refer to the *ICD-10-CM* manual for complete guidelines.

PRENATAL OUTPATIENT VISITS FOR HIGH-RISK PATIENTS

For routine prenatal outpatient visits for patients with high-risk pregnancies, a code from category O09, Supervision of high-risk pregnancy, should be used as the first-listed diagnosis. Secondary chapter 15 codes may be used in conjunction with these codes if appropriate.

EPISODES WHEN NO DELIVERY OCCURS

Refer to the *ICD-10-CM* manual for complete guidelines.

WHEN A DELIVERY OCCURS

Refer to the *ICD-10-CM* manual for complete guidelines.

OUTCOME OF DELIVERY

A code from category Z37, Outcome of delivery, should be included on every maternal record when a delivery has occurred. These codes are not to be used on subsequent records or on the newborn record.

Pre-existing conditions versus conditions due to the pregnancy

Certain categories in Chapter 15 distinguish between conditions of the mother that existed prior to pregnancy (pre-existing) and those that are a direct result of pregnancy. When assigning codes from Chapter 15, it is important to assess if a condition was pre-existing prior to pregnancy or developed during or due to the pregnancy in order to assign the correct code.

Categories that do not distinguish between pre-existing and pregnancy-related conditions may be used for either. It is acceptable to use codes specifically for the puerperium with codes complicating pregnancy and childbirth if a condition arises postpartum during the delivery encounter.

Pre-existing hypertension in pregnancy

Refer to category O10.
Refer to Chapter 9, Hypertension.

Fetal Conditions Affecting the Management of the Mother

CODES FROM CATEGORIES O35 AND O36

Refer to categories O35 and O36.

IN UTERO SURGERY

Refer to category O35.

No code from Chapter 16, the perinatal codes, should be used on the mother's record to identify fetal conditions. Surgery performed in utero on a fetus is still to be coded as an obstetric encounter.

HIV Infection in Pregnancy, Childbirth and the Puerperium

During pregnancy, childbirth or the puerperium, a patient admitted because of an HIV-related illness should receive a principal diagnosis from subcategory O98.7-, HIV disease complicating pregnancy, childbirth and the puerperium, followed by the code(s) for the HIV-related illness(es).

Patients with asymptomatic HIV infection status admitted during pregnancy, childbirth, or the puerperium should receive codes of O98.7- and Z21, Asymptomatic HIV infection status.

DM in pregnancy

Diabetes mellitus is a significant complicating factor in pregnancy. Pregnant women who are diabetic should be assigned a code from category O24, DM in pregnancy, childbirth, and the puerperium, first, followed by the appropriate diabetes code(s) (E08–E13) from Chapter 4.

Long term use of insulin

Code Z79.4, Long-term (current) use of insulin, should also be assigned if the DM is being treated with insulin.

Gestational (pregnancy induced) diabetes

Gestational (pregnancy induced) diabetes can occur during the second and third trimester of pregnancy in women who were not diabetic prior to pregnancy. Gestational diabetes can cause complications in the pregnancy similar to those of pre-existing DM. It also puts the woman at greater risk of developing diabetes after the pregnancy. Codes for gestational diabetes are in subcategory O24.4, Gestational DM. No other code from category O24, DM in pregnancy, childbirth, and the puerperium, should be used with a code from O24.4

The codes under subcategory O24.4 include diet controlled and insulin controlled. *If a patient with gestational diabetes is treated with both diet and insulin, only the code for insulin-controlled is required.*

Refer to the *ICD-10-CM* manual for complete guidelines.

Refer to the *ICD-10-CM* manual for guidelines for normal delivery (O80); peripartum and postpartum periods; sequela of complication of pregnancy, childbirth, and the puerperium (O94); sepsis and septic shock complicating abortion, pregnancy, childbirth and the puerperium; puerperal sepsis.

    Additional Character Required   3-character code   •=New Code   ▲=Revised Code   *Excludes1* Not coded here, do not use together   *Excludes2*—Not included here

Termination of Pregnancy and Spontaneous abortions

Refer to the *ICD-10-CM* manual for complete guidelines.

Abuse in a pregnant patient

Refer to the *ICD-10-CM* manual for complete guidelines.
Refer to Chapter 19. Adult and child abuse, neglect and other maltreatment.

Note: CODES FROM THIS CHAPTER ARE FOR USE ONLY ON MATERNAL RECORDS, NEVER ON NEWBORN RECORDS.

Codes from this chapter are for use for conditions related to or aggravated by the pregnancy, childbirth, or by the puerperium (maternal causes or obstetric causes).

Use additional code from category Z3A, Weeks of gestation, to identify the specific week of the pregnancy, if known

Excludes1: supervision of normal pregnancy (Z34.-)

Excludes2: mental and behavioral disorders associated with the puerperium (F53)
obstetrical tetanus (A34)
postpartum necrosis of pituitary gland (E23.0)
puerperal osteomalacia (M83.0)

Trimesters are counted from the first day of the last menstrual period. They are defined as follows: 1st trimester—less than 14 weeks 0 days 2nd trimester—14 weeks 0 days to less than 28 weeks 0 days 3rd trimester—28 weeks 0 days until delivery

(O00–O08) PREGNANCY WITH ABORTIVE OUTCOME

O00 **ECTOPIC PREGNANCY**
Includes: ruptured ectopic pregnancy
Use additional code from category O08 to identify any associated complication

O00.0 Abdominal pregnancy
5th *Excludes1:* maternal care for viable fetus in abdominal pregnancy (O36.7-)
- **O00.00 Abdominal pregnancy without intrauterine pregnancy**
- **O00.01 Abdominal pregnancy with intrauterine pregnancy**

O00.1 Tubal pregnancy
5th Fallopian pregnancy
Rupture of (fallopian) tube due to pregnancy
Tubal abortion
- **O00.10 Tubal pregnancy without intrauterine pregnancy**
- **O00.11 Tubal pregnancy with intrauterine pregnancy**

O00.2 Ovarian pregnancy
5th
- **O00.20 Ovarian pregnancy without intrauterine pregnancy**
- **O00.21 Ovarian pregnancy with intrauterine pregnancy**

O00.8 Other ectopic pregnancy
5th Cervical pregnancy
Cornual pregnancy
Intraligamentous pregnancy
Mural pregnancy
- **O00.80 Other ectopic pregnancy without intrauterine pregnancy**
- **O00.81 Other ectopic pregnancy with intrauterine pregnancy**

O00.9 Ectopic pregnancy, unspecified
5th
- **O00.90 Unspecified ectopic pregnancy without intrauterine pregnancy**
- **O00.91 Unspecified ectopic pregnancy with intrauterine pregnancy**

O02 **OTHER ABNORMAL PRODUCTS OF CONCEPTION**
Use additional code from category O08 to identify any associated complication.
Excludes1: papyraceous fetus (O31.0-)

O02.1 Missed abortion
Early fetal death, before completion of 20 weeks of gestation, with retention of dead fetus
Excludes1: failed induced abortion (O07.-)
fetal death (intrauterine) (late) (O36.4)
missed abortion with blighted ovum (O02.0)
missed abortion with hydatidiform mole (O01.-)
missed abortion with nonhydatidiform (O02.0)
missed abortion with other abnormal products of conception (O02.8-)
missed delivery (O36.4)
stillbirth (P95)

O03 **SPONTANEOUS ABORTION**
Note: Incomplete abortion includes retained products of conception following spontaneous abortion
Includes: miscarriage
O03.4 Incomplete spontaneous abortion without complication
O03.9 Complete or unspecified spontaneous abortion without complication
Miscarriage NOS
Spontaneous abortion NOS

(O09) SUPERVISION OF HIGH RISK PREGNANCY

O09 **SUPERVISION OF HIGH RISK PREGNANCY**
4th **O09.6 Supervision of young primigravida and multigravida**
5th Supervision of pregnancy for a female <16 years old at expected date of delivery

O09.61 Supervision of young primigravida
6th

O09.62 Supervision of young multigravida
6th

Requires 6th character to identify trimester 1 first trimester 2 second trimester 3 third trimester 9 unspecified trimester

(O10–O16) EDEMA, PROTEINURIA AND HYPERTENSIVE DISORDERS IN PREGNANCY, CHILDBIRTH AND THE PUERPERIUM

Category O10, Pre-existing hypertension complicating pregnancy, childbirth and the puerperium, includes codes for hypertensive heart and hypertensive CKD. When assigning one of the O10 codes that includes hypertensive heart disease or hypertensive CKD, it is necessary to add a secondary code from the appropriate hypertension category to specify the type of heart failure or CKD.

O10 **PRE-EXISTING HYPERTENSION COMPLICATING PREGNANCY, CHILDBIRTH AND THE PUERPERIUM**
4th *Includes:* pre-existing hypertension with pre-existing proteinuria complicating pregnancy, childbirth and the puerperium
Excludes2: pre-existing hypertension with superimposed pre-eclampsia complicating pregnancy, childbirth and the puerperium (O11.-)

O10.0 Pre-existing essential hypertension complicating pregnancy, childbirth and the puerperium
5th Any condition in I10 specified as a reason for obstetric care during pregnancy, childbirth or the puerperium

O10.01 Pre-existing essential hypertension complicating pregnancy
6th

O10.02 Pre-existing essential hypertension complicating childbirth
6th

O10.03 Pre-existing essential hypertension complicating the puerperium
6th

Requires 6th character to identify trimester 1 first trimester 2 second trimester 3 third trimester 9 unspecified trimester

O10.1 Pre-existing hypertensive heart disease complicating pregnancy, childbirth and the puerperium
5th Any condition in I11 specified as a reason for obstetric care during pregnancy, childbirth or the puerperium
Use additional code from I11 to identify the type of hypertensive heart disease

Requires 6th character to identify trimester 1 first trimester 2 second trimester 3 third trimester 9 unspecified trimester

O10.11 Pre-existing hypertensive heart disease complicating pregnancy
6th

    Additional Character Required   ✓ 3-character code   •=New Code   ▲=Revised Code

Excludes1—Not coded here, do not use together
Excludes2—Not included here

O10.4   **Pre-existing secondary hypertension complicating pregnancy, childbirth and the puerperium**

5th   Any condition in I15 specified as a reason for obstetric care during pregnancy, childbirth or the puerperium

Use additional code from I15 to identify the type of secondary hypertension

Requires 6th character to identify trimester	
1 first trimester	
2 second trimester	
3 third trimester	
9 unspecified trimester	

O10.41   **Pre-existing secondary hypertension complicating pregnancy**
6th

O14   **PRE-ECLAMPSIA**

4th   **Excludes1:** pre-existing hypertension with pre-eclampsia (O11)

O14.0   **Mild to moderate pre-eclampsia**

5th

• O14 requires 5th character
4 complicating childbirth
5 complicating the puerperium

O14.2   **HELLP syndrome**

5th   Severe pre-eclampsia with hemolysis, elevated liver enzymes and low platelet count (HELLP)

(O20–O29) OTHER MATERNAL DISORDERS PREDOMINANTLY RELATED TO PREGNANCY

Excludes2: maternal care related to the fetus and amniotic cavity and possible delivery problems (O30–O48)

maternal diseases classifiable elsewhere but complicating pregnancy, labor and delivery, and the puerperium (O98–O99)

O20   **HEMORRHAGE IN EARLY PREGNANCY**

4th   **Includes:** hemorrhage before completion of 20 weeks gestation

Excludes1: pregnancy with abortive outcome (O00–O08)

O20.0   **Threatened abortion**
Hemorrhage specified as due to threatened abortion

O20.8   **Other hemorrhage in early pregnancy**

O20.9   **Hemorrhage in early pregnancy, unspecified**

O24   **DM IN PREGNANCY, CHILDBIRTH, AND THE PUERPERIUM**

4th

O24.0   **Pre-existing type 1 DM**

5th   Juvenile onset DM, in pregnancy, childbirth and the puerperium
Ketosis-prone DM in pregnancy, childbirth and the puerperium

Use additional code from category E10 to further identify any manifestations

O24.01 and O24.11 require 6th character to identify trimester	
1 first trimester	
2 second trimester	
3 third trimester	
9 unspecified trimester	

O24.01   **Pre-existing type 1 DM, in pregnancy**
6th

O24.1   **Pre-existing type 2 DM**

5th   Insulin-resistant DM

Use additional code (for): from category E11 to further identify any manifestations long-term (current) use of insulin (Z79.4)

O24.11   **Pre-existing type 2 DM, in pregnancy**
6th

O24.4   **Gestational DM**

5th   DM arising in pregnancy
Gestational diabetes mellitus NOS

O24.41   **Gestational DM in pregnancy**

O24.410   **Gestational DM in pregnancy, diet controlled**
6th

O24.414   **Gestational DM in pregnancy, insulin controlled**

• **O24.415**   **Gestational DM in pregnancy, controlled by oral hypoglycemic drugs**
Gestational diabetes mellitus in pregnancy, controlled by oral antidiabetic drugs

O28   **ABNORMAL FINDINGS ON ANTENATAL SCREENING OF MOTHER**

4th   **Excludes1:** diagnostic findings classified elsewhere—**see Alphabetical Index**

O28.0   **Abnormal hematological finding on antenatal screening of mother**

O28.1   **Abnormal biochemical finding on antenatal screening of mother**

O28.2   **Abnormal cytological finding on antenatal screening of mother**

O28.3   **Abnormal ultrasonic finding on antenatal screening of mother**

O28.4   **Abnormal radiological finding on antenatal screening of mother**

O28.5   **Abnormal chromosomal and genetic finding on antenatal screening of mother**

O28.8   **Other abnormal findings on antenatal screening of mother**

O28.9   **Unspecified abnormal findings on antenatal screening of mother**

(O30–O48) MATERNAL CARE RELATED TO THE FETUS AND AMNIOTIC CAVITY AND POSSIBLE DELIVERY PROBLEMS

O30   **MULTIPLE GESTATION**

4th   **Code also** any complications specific to multiple gestation

Requires 6th character to identify trimester	
1 first trimester	
2 second trimester	
3 third trimester	
9 unspecified trimester	

O30.0   **Twin pregnancy**

5th   **O30.00**   **Twin pregnancy, unspecified number of placenta and unspecified number of amniotic sacs**
6th

O30.01   **Twin pregnancy, monochorionic/monoamniotic**
6th   Twin pregnancy, one placenta, one amniotic sac
Excludes1: conjoined twins (O30.02-)

O30.02   **Conjoined twin pregnancy**
6th

O30.03   **Twin pregnancy, monochorionic/diamniotic**
6th   Twin pregnancy, one placenta, two amniotic sacs

O30.04   **Twin pregnancy, dichorionic/diamniotic**
6th   Twin pregnancy, two placentae, two amniotic sacs

O30.09   **Twin pregnancy, unable to determine number of placenta and number of amniotic sacs**
6th

O30.1   **Triplet pregnancy**

5th   **O30.10**   **Triplet pregnancy, unspecified number of placenta and unspecified number of amniotic sacs**
6th

O30.11   **Triplet pregnancy with two or more monochorionic fetuses**
6th

O30.12   **Triplet pregnancy with two or more monoamniotic fetuses**
6th

O30.19   **Triplet pregnancy, unable to determine number of placenta and number of amniotic sacs**
6th

   Additional Character Required   3-character code

•=New Code
▲=Revised Code

Excludes1—Not coded here, do not use together
Excludes2—Not included here

PEDIATRIC ICD-10-CM 2017: A MANUAL FOR PROVIDER-BASED CODING   233

O31 COMPLICATIONS SPECIFIC TO MULTIPLE GESTATION

4th

Assign a 7th to identify the fetus for which the complication code applies.

Assign 7th character "0" for either a single gestation or when the documentation is insufficient to determine the fetus affected and it is not possible to obtain clarification or when it is not possible to clinically determine which fetus is affected.

Requires 7th character to identify affected fetus
0 not applicable (ie, only one fetus) or unspecified
1 fetus 1
2 fetus 2
3 fetus 3
4 fetus 4
5 fetus 5
9 other fetus

Excludes2: delayed delivery of second twin, triplet, etc. (O63.2)
malpresentation of one fetus or more (O32.9)
placental transfusion syndromes (O43.0-)

Code also the appropriate code from category O30, Multiple gestation, when assigning a code from category O31 that has a 7th character of 1 through 9.

O31.8 Other complications specific to multiple gestation

5th O31.8X Other complications specific to multiple gestation

6th O31.8X1 Other complications specific to multiple gestation, first trimester
7th

O31.8X2 Other complications specific to multiple gestation, second trimester
7th

O31.8X3 Other complications specific to multiple gestation, third trimester
7th

O35 MATERNAL CARE FOR KNOWN OR SUSPECTED FETAL ABNORMALITY AND DAMAGE

4th

Assign only when the fetal condition is actually responsible for modifying the management of the mother, i.e., by requiring diagnostic studies, additional observation, special care, or termination of pregnancy. The fact that the fetal condition exists does not justify assigning a code from this series to the mother's record.

In cases when surgery is performed on the fetus, a diagnosis code from category O35, Maternal care for known or suspected fetal abnormality and damage, should be assigned identifying the fetal condition. Assign the appropriate procedure code for the procedure performed.

No code from Chapter 16, the perinatal codes, should be used on the mother's record to identify fetal conditions. Surgery performed in utero on a fetus is still to be coded as an obstetric encounter.

Assign a 7th to identify the fetus for which the complication code applies.

Assign 7th character "0" for either a single gestation or when the documentation is insufficient to determine the fetus affected and it is not possible to obtain clarification or when it is not possible to clinically determine which fetus is affected.

Requires 7th character to identify affected fetus
0 not applicable (ie, single gestation) or unspecified
1 fetus 1
2 fetus 2
3 fetus 3
4 fetus 4
5 fetus 5
9 other fetus

Includes: the listed conditions in the fetus as a reason for hospitalization or other obstetric care to the mother, or for termination of pregnancy

Code also any associated maternal condition

Excludes1: encounter for suspected maternal and fetal conditions ruled out (Z03.7-)

Code also the appropriate code from category O30, Multiple gestation, when assigning a code from category O35 that has a 7th character of 1 through 9.

Use placeholder X to complete the full code

O35.0XX Maternal care for (suspected) central nervous system malformation in fetus
7th
Maternal care for fetal anencephaly
Maternal care for fetal hydrocephalus
Maternal care for fetal spina bifida
Excludes2: chromosomal abnormality in fetus (O35.1)

O35.1XX Maternal care for (suspected) chromosomal abnormality in fetus
7th

O35.2XX Maternal care for (suspected) hereditary disease in fetus
7th
Excludes2: chromosomal abnormality in fetus (O35.1)

O35.3XX Maternal care for (suspected) damage to fetus from viral disease in mother
7th
Maternal care for damage to fetus from maternal cytomegalovirus infection
Maternal care for damage to fetus from maternal rubella

O35.4XX Maternal care for (suspected) damage to fetus from alcohol
7th

O35.5XX Maternal care for (suspected) damage to fetus by drugs
7th
Maternal care for damage to fetus from drug addiction

O35.6XX Maternal care for (suspected) damage to fetus by radiation
7th

O35.7XX Maternal care for (suspected) damage to fetus by other medical procedures
7th
Maternal care for damage to fetus by amniocentesis
Maternal care for damage to fetus by biopsy procedures
Maternal care for damage to fetus by hematological investigation
Maternal care for damage to fetus by intrauterine contraceptive device
Maternal care for damage to fetus by intrauterine surgery

O35.8XX Maternal care for other (suspected) fetal abnormality and damage
7th
Maternal care for other (suspected) fetal abnormality and damage
Maternal care for damage to fetus from maternal listeriosis
Maternal care for damage to fetus from maternal toxoplasmosis

O35.9XX Maternal care for (suspected) fetal abnormality and damage, unspecified
7th

O36 MATERNAL CARE FOR OTHER FETAL PROBLEMS

4th

Assign only when the fetal condition is actually responsible for modifying the management of the mother, i.e., by requiring diagnostic studies, additional observation, special care, or termination of pregnancy. The fact that the fetal condition exists does not justify assigning a code from this series to the mother's record.

No code from Chapter 16, the perinatal codes, should be used on the mother's record to identify fetal conditions. Surgery performed in utero on a fetus is still to be coded as an obstetric encounter.

Assign a 7th to identify the fetus for which the complication code applies.

Assign 7th character "0" for either a single gestation or when the documentation is insufficient to determine the fetus affected and it is not possible to obtain clarification or when it is not possible to clinically determine which fetus is affected.

Includes: the listed conditions in the fetus as a reason for hospitalization or other obstetric care of the mother, or for termination of pregnancy

Excludes1: encounter for suspected maternal and fetal conditions ruled out (Z03.7-)
placental transfusion syndromes (O43.0-)

Excludes2: labor and delivery complicated by fetal stress (O77.-)

Code also the appropriate code from category O30, Multiple gestation, when assigning a code from category O36 that has a 7th character of 1 through 9.

Requires 7th character to identify affected fetus
0 not applicable (ie, only one fetus) or unspecified
1 fetus 1
2 fetus 2
3 fetus 3
4 fetus 4
5 fetus 5
9 other fetus

O36.0 Maternal care for rhesus isoimmunization

5th Maternal care for Rh incompatibility (with hydrops fetalis)

| Additional Character Required | 3-character code | •=New Code ▲=Revised Code | **Excludes1**—Not coded here, do not use together **Excludes2**—Not included here |

O36.01 Maternal care for anti-D [Rh] antibodies

6th   **O36.011** Maternal care for anti-D [Rh] antibodies, first trimester

     7th

   O36.012 Maternal care for anti-D [Rh] antibodies, second trimester

     7th

   O36.013 Maternal care for anti-D [Rh] antibodies, third trimester

     7th

O36.09 Maternal care for other rhesus isoimmunization

6th   **O36.091** Maternal care for other rhesus isoimmunization, first trimester

     7th

   O36.092 Maternal care for other rhesus isoimmunization, second trimester

     7th

   O36.093 Maternal care for other rhesus isoimmunization, third trimester

     7th

O36.1 Maternal care for other isoimmunization

5th   Maternal care for ABO isoimmunization

O36.11 Maternal care for Anti-A sensitization

6th   Maternal care for isoimmunization NOS (with hydrops fetalis)

   O36.111 Maternal care for Anti-A sensitization, first trimester

     7th

   O36.112 Maternal care for Anti-A sensitization, second trimester

     7th

   O36.113 Maternal care for Anti-A sensitization, third trimester

     7th

O36.19 Maternal care for other isoimmunization

6th   Maternal care for Anti-B sensitization

   O36.191 Maternal care for other isoimmunization, first trimester

     7th

   O36.192 Maternal care for other isoimmunization, second trimester

     7th

   O36.193 Maternal care for other isoimmunization, third trimester

     7th

O36.2 Maternal care for hydrops fetalis

5th   Maternal care for hydrops fetalis NOS

Maternal care for hydrops fetalis not associated with isoimmunization

Excludes1: hydrops fetalis associated with ABO isoimmunization (O36.1-)

hydrops fetalis associated with rhesus isoimmunization (O36.0-)

   O36.21X Maternal care for hydrops fetalis, first trimester

     7th

   O36.22X Maternal care for hydrops fetalis, second trimester

     7th

   O36.23X Maternal care for hydrops fetalis, third trimester

     7th

O36.5 Maternal care for known or suspected poor fetal growth

5th **O36.51** Maternal care for known or suspected placental insufficiency

6th   **O36.511** Maternal care for known or suspected placental insufficiency, first trimester

     7th

   O36.512 Maternal care for known or suspected placental insufficiency, second trimester

     7th

   O36.513 Maternal care for known or suspected placental insufficiency, third trimester

     7th

O36.59 Maternal care for other known or suspected poor fetal growth

6th Maternal care for known or suspected light-for-dates NOS

Maternal care for known or suspected small-for-dates NOS

   O36.591 Maternal care for other known or suspected poor fetal growth, first trimester

     7th

   O36.592 Maternal care for other known or suspected poor fetal growth, second trimester

     7th

   O36.593 Maternal care for other known or suspected poor fetal growth, third trimester

     7th

O36.6 Maternal care for excessive fetal growth

5th Maternal care for known or suspected large-for-dates

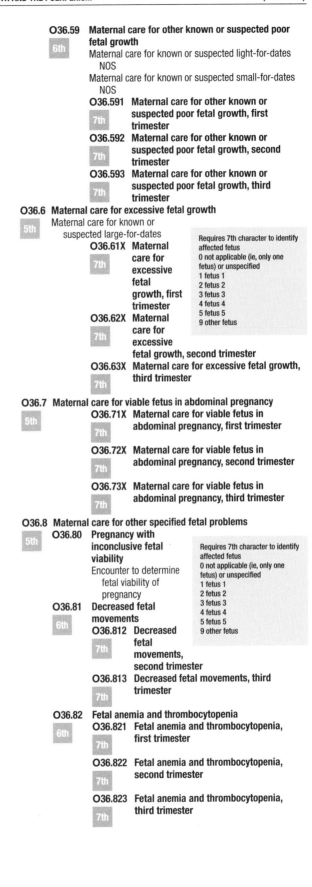

   O36.61X Maternal care for excessive fetal growth, first trimester

     7th

Requires 7th character to identify affected fetus
0 not applicable (ie, only one fetus) or unspecified
1 fetus 1
2 fetus 2
3 fetus 3
4 fetus 4
5 fetus 5
9 other fetus

   O36.62X Maternal care for excessive fetal growth, second trimester

     7th

   O36.63X Maternal care for excessive fetal growth, third trimester

     7th

O36.7 Maternal care for viable fetus in abdominal pregnancy

5th   **O36.71X** Maternal care for viable fetus in abdominal pregnancy, first trimester

     7th

   O36.72X Maternal care for viable fetus in abdominal pregnancy, second trimester

     7th

   O36.73X Maternal care for viable fetus in abdominal pregnancy, third trimester

     7th

O36.8 Maternal care for other specified fetal problems

5th **O36.80** Pregnancy with inconclusive fetal viability

Encounter to determine fetal viability of pregnancy

Requires 7th character to identify affected fetus
0 not applicable (ie, only one fetus) or unspecified
1 fetus 1
2 fetus 2
3 fetus 3
4 fetus 4
5 fetus 5
9 other fetus

O36.81 Decreased fetal movements

6th   **O36.812** Decreased fetal movements, second trimester

     7th

   O36.813 Decreased fetal movements, third trimester

     7th

O36.82 Fetal anemia and thrombocytopenia

6th   **O36.821** Fetal anemia and thrombocytopenia, first trimester

     7th

   O36.822 Fetal anemia and thrombocytopenia, second trimester

     7th

   O36.823 Fetal anemia and thrombocytopenia, third trimester

     7th

CHAPTER 15. PREGNANCY, CHILDBIRTH AND THE PUERPERIUM (O36.01–O36.823)

4th **5th** **6th** **7th**   Additional Character Required   ✔   3-character code

•=New Code
▲=Revised Code

Excludes1—Not coded here, do not use together
Excludes2—Not included here

O36.89 Maternal care for other specified fetal problems

6th   **O36.891 Maternal care for other specified fetal problems, first trimester**

7th

   O36.892 Maternal care for other specified fetal problems, second trimester

7th

   O36.893 Maternal care for other specified fetal problems, third trimester

7th

O40 POLYHYDRAMNIOS

4th Assign a 7th to identify the fetus for which the complication code applies. Assign 7th character "0" for either a single gestation or when the documentation is insufficient to determine the fetus affected and it is not possible to obtain clarification or when it is not possible to clinically determine which fetus is affected.

Includes: hydramnios

Excludes1: encounter for suspected maternal and fetal conditions ruled out (Z03.7-)

> Requires 7th character to identify affected fetus
> 0 not applicable (ie, only one fetus) or unspecified
> 1 fetus 1
> 2 fetus 2
> 3 fetus 3
> 4 fetus 4
> 5 fetus 5
> 9 other fetus

O40.1XX Polyhydramnios, first trimester

7th

O40.2XX Polyhydramnios, second trimester

7th

O40.3XX Polyhydramnios, third trimester

7th

O40.9XX Polyhydramnios, unspecified trimester

7th

O41 OTHER DISORDERS OF AMNIOTIC FLUID AND MEMBRANES

4th Assign a 7th to identify the fetus for which the complication code applies. Assign 7th character "0" for either a single gestation or when the documentation is insufficient to determine the fetus affected and it is not possible to obtain clarification or when it is not possible to clinically determine which fetus is affected.

Excludes1: encounter for suspected maternal and fetal conditions ruled out (Z03.7-)

Code also the appropriate code from category O30, Multiple gestation, when assigning a code from category O41 that has a 7th character of 1 through 9.

> Requires 7th character to identify affected fetus
> 0 not applicable (ie, only one fetus) or unspecified
> 1 fetus 1
> 2 fetus 2
> 3 fetus 3
> 4 fetus 4
> 5 fetus 5
> 9 other fetus

   O41.01X Oligohydramnios, first trimester, not applicable or unspecified

7th

   O41.02X Oligohydramnios, second trimester, not applicable or unspecified

7th

   O41.03X Oligohydramnios, third trimester, not applicable or unspecified

7th

O42 PREMATURE RUPTURE OF MEMBRANES

4th **O42.9 Premature rupture of membranes, unspecified as to length of time between rupture and onset of labor**

5th   **O42.91 Preterm premature rupture of membranes, unspecified as to length of time between rupture and onset of labor**

6th Premature rupture of membranes before 37 completed weeks of gestation

     O42.911 Preterm premature rupture of membranes, unspecified as to length of time between rupture and onset of labor; first trimester

     O42.912 second trimester

     O42.913 third trimester

O43 PLACENTAL DISORDERS

4th *Excludes2:* maternal care for poor fetal growth due to placental insufficiency (O36.5-)
placenta previa (O44.-)
placental polyp (O90.89)
placentitis (O41.14-)
premature separation of placenta [abruptio placentae] (O45.-)

O43.0 Placental transfusion syndromes

5th   **O43.01 Fetomaternal placental transfusion syndrome**

6th Maternofetal placental transfusion syndrome

     O43.011 Fetomaternal placental transfusion syndrome; first trimester

     O43.012 second trimester

     O43.013 third trimester

   O43.02 Fetus-to-fetus placental transfusion syndrome

6th   **O43.021 Fetus-to-fetus placental transfusion syndrome; first trimester**

     O43.022 second trimester

     O43.023 third trimester

(O60–O77) COMPLICATIONS OF LABOR AND DELIVERY

O60 PRETERM LABOR

4th *Includes:* onset (spontaneous) of labor before 37 completed weeks of gestation

Excludes1: false labor (O47.0-)
threatened labor NOS (O47.0-)

O60.0 Preterm labor without delivery

5th   **O60.02 Preterm labor without delivery, second trimester**

   O60.03 Preterm labor without delivery, third trimester

O75 OTHER COMPLICATIONS OF LABOR AND DELIVERY, NOT ELSEWHERE CLASSIFIED

4th *Excludes2:* puerperal (postpartum) infection (O86.-)
puerperal (postpartum) sepsis (O85)

O75.0 Maternal distress during labor and delivery

O75.1 Shock during or following labor and delivery
Obstetric shock following labor and delivery

O75.2 Pyrexia during labor, not elsewhere classified

O75.3 Other infection during labor
Sepsis during labor
Use additional code (B95–B97), to identify infectious agent

O75.4 Other complications of obstetric surgery and procedures
Cardiac arrest following obstetric surgery or procedures
Cardiac failure following obstetric surgery or procedures
Cerebral anoxia following obstetric surgery or procedures
Pulmonary edema following obstetric surgery or procedures
Use additional code to identify specific complication
Excludes2: complications of anesthesia during labor and delivery (O74.-)
disruption of obstetrical (surgical) wound (O90.0–O90.1)
hematoma of obstetrical (surgical) wound (O90.2)
infection of obstetrical (surgical) wound (O86.0)

O75.5 Delayed delivery after artificial rupture of membranes

O75.8 Other specified complications of labor and delivery

5th   **O75.81 Maternal exhaustion complicating labor and delivery**

   O75.82 Onset (spontaneous) of labor after 37 completed weeks of gestation but before 39 completed weeks gestation, with delivery by (planned) cesarean section
Delivery by (planned) cesarean section occurring after 37 completed weeks of gestation but before 39 completed weeks gestation due to (spontaneous) onset of labor
Code first to specify reason for planned cesarean section such as:
cephalopelvic disproportion (normally formed fetus) (O33.9)
previous cesarean delivery (O34.21)

   O75.89 Other specified complications of labor and delivery

O75.9 Complication of labor and delivery, unspecified

4th **5th** **6th** **7th**   Additional Character Required   ✓   3-character code   •=New Code   *Excludes1*—Not coded here, do not use together
▲=Revised Code   *Excludes2*—Not included here

236   PEDIATRIC ICD-10-CM 2017: A MANUAL FOR PROVIDER-BASED CODING

(O80–O82) ENCOUNTER FOR DELIVERY

(O85–O92) COMPLICATIONS PREDOMINANTLY RELATED TO THE PUERPERIUM

(O94–O9A) OTHER OBSTETRIC CONDITIONS, NOT ELSEWHERE CLASSIFIED

 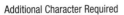 Additional Character Required   ✓   3-character code   •=New Code   ▲=Revised Code   *Excludes1*—Not coded here, do not use together   *Excludes2*—Not included here

Chapter 16. Certain conditions originating in the perinatal period (P00–P99)

GUIDELINES

For coding and reporting purposes the perinatal period is defined as before birth through the 28th day following birth. The following guidelines are provided for reporting purposes

General Perinatal Rules

Codes in this chapter are never for use on the maternal record. Codes from Chapter 15, the obstetric chapter, are never permitted on the newborn record. Chapter 16 codes may be used throughout the life of the patient if the condition is still present.

PRINCIPAL DIAGNOSIS FOR BIRTH RECORD

When coding the birth episode in a newborn record, assign a code from category Z38, Liveborn infants according to place of birth and type of delivery, as the principal diagnosis. Refer to code Z38 for further guidelines.

A code from category Z38 is used only on the newborn record, not on the mother's record.

USE OF CODES FROM OTHER CHAPTERS WITH CODES FROM CHAPTER 16

Codes from other chapters may be used with codes from chapter 16 if the codes from the other chapters provide more specific detail. Codes for signs and symptoms may be assigned when a definitive diagnosis has not been established. If the reason for the encounter is a perinatal condition, the code from chapter 16 should be sequenced first.

USE OF CHAPTER 16 CODES AFTER THE PERINATAL PERIOD

Should a condition originate in the perinatal period, and continue throughout the life of the patient, the perinatal code should continue to be used regardless of the patient's age.

BIRTH PROCESS OR COMMUNITY ACQUIRED CONDITIONS

If a newborn has a condition that may be either due to the birth process or community acquired and the documentation does not indicate which it is, the default is due to the birth process and the code from Chapter 16 should be used. If the condition is community-acquired, a code from Chapter 16 should not be assigned.

CODE ALL CLINICALLY SIGNIFICANT CONDITIONS

All clinically significant conditions noted on routine newborn examination should be coded. A condition is clinically significant if it requires:

- clinical evaluation; or
- therapeutic treatment; or
- diagnostic procedures; or
- extended length of hospital stay; or
- increased nursing care and/or monitoring; or
- has implications for future health care needs

Note: The perinatal guidelines listed above are the same as the general coding guidelines for "additional diagnoses", except for the final point regarding implications for future health care needs. Codes should be assigned for conditions that have been specified by the provider as having implications for future health care needs.

Coding Additional Perinatal Diagnoses

ASSIGNING CODES FOR CONDITIONS THAT REQUIRE TREATMENT

Assign codes for conditions that require treatment or further investigation, prolong the length of stay, or require resource utilization.

CODES FOR CONDITIONS SPECIFIED AS HAVING IMPLICATIONS FOR FUTURE HEALTH CARE NEEDS

Assign codes for conditions that have been specified by the provider as having implications for future health care needs.

Prematurity and Fetal Growth Retardation

Refer to categories P05–P07 for guidelines for prematurity and fetal growth retardation.

LBW and immaturity status

Refer to category P07, Disorders of newborn related to short gestation and LBW, not elsewhere classified, for associated guidelines.

Bacterial Sepsis of Newborn

Refer to category P36, Bacterial sepsis of newborn for guidelines for reporting newborn bacterial sepsis.

Stillbirth

Refer to code P95 for guidelines.

Note: Codes from this chapter are for use on newborn records only, never on maternal records

Includes: conditions that have their origin in the fetal or perinatal period (before birth through the first 28 days after birth) even if morbidity occurs later

Excludes2: congenital malformations, deformations and chromosomal abnormalities (Q00–Q99)
    endocrine, nutritional and metabolic diseases (E00–E88)
    injury, poisoning and certain other consequences of external causes (S00–T88)
    neoplasms (C00–D49)
    tetanus neonatorum (A33)

(P00–P04) NEWBORN AFFECTED BY MATERNAL FACTORS AND BY COMPLICATIONS OF PREGNANCY, LABOR, AND DELIVERY

Note: These codes are for use when the listed maternal conditions are specified as the cause of confirmed morbidity or potential morbidity which have their origin in the perinatal period (before birth through the first 28 days after birth). Codes from these categories are also for use for newborns who are suspected of having an abnormal condition resulting from exposure from the mother or the birth process.

⚐P00   **NEWBORN AFFECTED BY MATERNAL CONDITIONS THAT MAY BE UNRELATED TO PRESENT PREGNANCY**

   4th   **Code first** any current condition in newborn
    Excludes2: encounter for observation and evaluation of newborn for suspected diseases and conditions ruled out (Z05.-)
      newborn affected by maternal complications of pregnancy (P01.-)
      newborn affected by maternal endocrine and metabolic disorders (P70–P74)
      newborn affected by noxious substances transmitted via placenta or breast milk (P04.-)

⚐P00.0   **Newborn affected by maternal hypertensive disorders**
    Newborn affected by maternal conditions classifiable to O10–O11, O13–O16

⚐P00.1   **Newborn affected by maternal renal and urinary tract diseases**
    Newborn affected by maternal conditions classifiable to N00–N39

⚐P00.2   **Newborn affected by maternal infectious and parasitic diseases**
    Newborn affected by maternal infectious disease classifiable to A00–B99, J09 and J10
    Excludes1: infections specific to the perinatal period (P35–P39)
      maternal genital tract or other localized infections (P00.8)

⚐P00.3   **Newborn affected by other maternal circulatory and respiratory diseases**
    Newborn affected by maternal conditions classifiable to I00–I99, J00–J99, Q20–Q34 and not included in P00.0, P00.2

⚐P00.4   **Newborn affected by maternal nutritional disorders**
    Newborn affected by maternal disorders classifiable to E40–E64
    Maternal malnutrition NOS

⚐P00.5   **Newborn affected by maternal injury**
    Newborn affected by maternal conditions classifiable to O9A.2-

⚐P00.6   **Newborn affected by surgical procedure on mother**
    Newborn affected by amniocentesis
    Excludes1: cesarean delivery for present delivery (P03.4)
      damage to placenta from amniocentesis, Cesarean delivery or surgical induction (P02.1)
      previous surgery to uterus or pelvic organs (P03.89)
    Excludes2: newborn affected by complication of (fetal) intrauterine procedure (P96.5)

 4th **5th** **6th** **7th**   Additional Character Required   ✔   3-character code   •=New Code   ⚐=Revised Code   ***Excludes1***—Not coded here, do not use together   ***Excludes2***—Not included here

CHAPTER 16. CERTAIN CONDITIONS ORIGINATING IN THE PERINATAL PERIOD   (P00.7–P03.9)

▲**P00.7 Newborn affected by other medical procedures on mother, NEC**
Newborn affected by radiation to mother
Excludes1: damage to placenta from amniocentesis, cesarean delivery or surgical induction (P02.1)
newborn affected by other complications of labor and delivery (P03.-)

▲**P00.8 Newborn affected by other maternal conditions**
5th ▲**P00.81   Newborn affected by periodontal disease in mother**
▲**P00.89   Newborn affected by other maternal conditions**
Newborn affected by conditions classifiable to T80–T88
Newborn affected by maternal genital tract or other localized infections
Newborn affected by maternal SLE

▲**P00.9 Newborn affected by unspecified maternal condition**

▲**P01 NEWBORN AFFECTED BY MATERNAL COMPLICATIONS OF PREGNANCY**
4th
Code first any current condition in newborn
Excludes2: encounter for observation of newborn for suspected diseases and conditions ruled out (Z05.-)

▲**P01.0 Newborn affected by incompetent cervix**
▲**P01.1 Newborn affected by premature rupture of membranes**
▲**P01.2 Newborn affected by oligohydramnios**
Excludes1: oligohydramnios due to premature rupture of membranes (P01.1)

▲**P01.3 Newborn affected by polyhydramnios**
Newborn affected by hydramnios

▲**P01.4 Newborn affected by ectopic pregnancy**
Newborn affected by abdominal pregnancy

▲**P01.5 Newborn affected by multiple pregnancy**
Newborn affected by triplet (pregnancy)
Newborn affected by twin (pregnancy)

▲**P01.6 Newborn affected by maternal death**
▲**P01.7 Newborn affected by malpresentation before labor**
Newborn affected by breech presentation before labor
Newborn affected by external version before labor
Newborn affected by face presentation before labor
Newborn affected by transverse lie before labor
Newborn affected by unstable lie before labor

▲**P01.8 Newborn affected by other maternal complications of pregnancy**
▲**P01.9 Newborn affected by maternal complication of pregnancy, unspecified**

▲**P02 NEWBORN AFFECTED BY COMPLICATIONS OF PLACENTA, CORD AND MEMBRANES**
4th
Code first any current condition in newborn
Excludes2: encounter for observation of newborn for suspected diseases and conditions ruled out (Z05.-)

▲**P02.0 Newborn affected by placenta previa**
▲**P02.1 Newborn affected by other forms of placental separation and hemorrhage**
Newborn affected by abruptio placenta
Newborn affected by accidental hemorrhage
Newborn affected by antepartum hemorrhage
Newborn affected by damage to placenta from amniocentesis, cesarean delivery or surgical induction
Newborn affected by maternal blood loss
Newborn affected by premature separation of placenta

▲**P02.2 Newborn affected by other and unspecified morphological and functional abnormalities of placenta**
5th
▲**P02.20   Newborn affected by unspecified morphological and functional abnormalities of placenta**
▲**P02.29   Newborn affected by other morphological and functional abnormalities of placenta**
Newborn affected by placental dysfunction
Newborn affected by placental infarction
Newborn affected by placental insufficiency

▲**P02.3 Newborn affected by placental transfusion syndromes**
Newborn affected by placental and cord abnormalities resulting in twin-to-twin or other transplacental transfusion

▲**P02.4 Newborn affected by prolapsed cord**

▲**P02.5 Newborn affected by other compression of umbilical cord**
Newborn affected by umbilical cord (tightly) around neck
Newborn affected by entanglement of umbilical cord
Newborn affected by knot in umbilical cord

▲**P02.6 Newborn affected by other and unspecified conditions of umbilical cord**
5th
▲**P02.60   Newborn affected by unspecified conditions of umbilical cord**
▲**P02.69   Newborn affected by other conditions of umbilical cord**
Newborn affected by short umbilical cord
Newborn affected by vasa previa
Excludes1: newborn affected by single umbilical artery (Q27.0)

▲**P02.7 Newborn affected by chorioamnionitis**
Newborn affected by amnionitis
Newborn affected by membranitis
Newborn affected by placentitis

▲**P02.8 Newborn affected by other abnormalities of membranes**
▲**P02.9 Newborn affected by abnormality of membranes, unspecified**

▲**P03 NEWBORN AFFECTED BY OTHER COMPLICATIONS OF LABOR AND DELIVERY**
4th
Code first any current condition in newborn
Excludes2: encounter for observation of newborn for suspected diseases and conditions ruled out (Z05.-)

▲**P03.0 Newborn affected by breech delivery and extraction**
▲**P03.1 Newborn affected by other malpresentation, malposition and disproportion during labor and delivery**
Newborn affected by contracted pelvis
Newborn affected by conditions classifiable to O64–O66
Newborn affected by persistent occipitoposterior
Newborn affected by transverse lie

▲**P03.2 Newborn affected by forceps delivery**
▲**P03.3 Newborn affected by delivery by vacuum extractor [ventouse]**
▲**P03.4 Newborn affected by Cesarean delivery**
▲**P03.5 Newborn affected by precipitate delivery**
Newborn affected by rapid second stage

▲**P03.6 Newborn affected by abnormal uterine contractions**
Newborn affected by conditions classifiable to O62.-, except O62.3
Newborn affected by hypertonic labor
Newborn affected by uterine inertia

▲**P03.8 Newborn affected by other specified complications of labor and delivery**
5th
▲**P03.81   Newborn affected by abnormality in fetal (intrauterine) heart rate or rhythm**
6th
Excludes1: neonatal cardiac dysrhythmia (P29.1-)
▲**P03.810   Newborn affected by abnormality in fetal (intrauterine) heart rate or rhythm before the onset of labor**
▲**P03.811   Newborn affected by abnormality in fetal (intrauterine) heart rate or rhythm during labor**
▲**P03.819   Newborn affected by abnormality in fetal (intrauterine) heart rate or rhythm, unspecified as to time of onset**
▲**P03.82   Meconium passage during delivery**
Excludes1: meconium aspiration (P24.00, P24.01)
meconium staining (P96.83)
▲**P03.89   Newborn affected by other specified complications of labor and delivery**
Newborn affected by abnormality of maternal soft tissues
Newborn affected by conditions classifiable to O60–O75 and by procedures used in labor and delivery not included in P02.- and P03.0–P03.6
Newborn affected by induction of labor

▲**P03.9 Newborn affected by complication of labor and delivery, unspecified**

    Additional Character Required   3-character code   •=New Code   *Excludes1*—Not coded here, do not use together
▲=Revised Code   *Excludes2*—Not included here

240   PEDIATRIC ICD-10-CM 2017: A MANUAL FOR PROVIDER-BASED CODING

▲P04 NEWBORN AFFECTED BY NOXIOUS SUBSTANCES TRANSMITTED VIA PLACENTA OR BREAST MILK

4th

Includes: nonteratogenic effects of substances transmitted via placenta
Excludes2: congenital malformations (Q00–Q99)
    encounter for observation of newborn for suspected diseases and conditions ruled out (Z05.-)
    neonatal jaundice from excessive hemolysis due to drugs or toxins transmitted from mother (P58.4)
    newborn in contact with and (suspected) exposures hazardous to health not transmitted via placenta or breast milk (Z77.-)

▲**P04.0 Newborn affected by maternal anesthesia and analgesia in pregnancy, labor and delivery**
    Newborn affected by reactions and intoxications from maternal opiates and tranquilizers administered during labor and delivery

▲**P04.1 Newborn affected by other maternal medication**
    Newborn affected by cancer chemotherapy
    Newborn affected by cytotoxic drugs
    Excludes1: dysmorphism due to warfarin (Q86.2)
        fetal hydantoin syndrome (Q86.1)
        maternal use of drugs of addiction (P04.4-)

▲**P04.2 Newborn affected by maternal use of tobacco**
    Newborn affected by exposure in utero to tobacco smoke
    Excludes2: newborn exposure to environmental tobacco smoke (P96.81)

▲**P04.3 Newborn affected by maternal use of alcohol**
    Excludes1: fetal alcohol syndrome (Q86.0)

▲**P04.4 Newborn affected by maternal use of drugs of addiction**

5th   ▲**P04.41 Newborn affected by maternal use of cocaine**
        'Crack baby'

   ▲**P04.49 Newborn affected by maternal use of other drugs of addiction**
        Excludes2: newborn affected by maternal anesthesia and analgesia (P04.0)
            withdrawal symptoms from maternal use of drugs of addiction (P96.1)

▲**P04.5 Newborn affected by maternal use of nutritional chemical substances**

▲**P04.6 Newborn affected by maternal exposure to environmental chemical substances**

▲**P04.8 Newborn affected by other maternal noxious substances**

▲**P04.9 Newborn affected by maternal noxious substance, unspecified**

(P05–P08) DISORDERS OF NEWBORN RELATED TO LENGTH OF GESTATION AND FETAL GROWTH

Providers utilize different criteria in determining prematurity. A code for prematurity should not be assigned unless it is documented. Assignment of codes in categories P05, Disorders of newborn related to slow fetal growth and fetal malnutrition, and P07, Disorders of newborn related to short gestation and LBW, not elsewhere classified, should be based on the recorded birth weight and estimated gestational age. Codes from category P05 should not be assigned with codes from category P07.

P05 DISORDERS OF NEWBORN RELATED TO SLOW FETAL GROWTH AND FETAL MALNUTRITION

4th

P05.0 Newborn light for gestational age

5th   *Light-for-dates newborns are those who are smaller in size than normal for the gestational age, most commonly defined as weight below the 10th percentile but length above the 10th percentile for gestational age.*
    Newborn light-for-dates

   P05.00 Newborn light for gestational age, unspecified weight
   P05.01 Newborn light for gestational age, less than 500 g
   P05.02 Newborn light for gestational age, 500–749 g
   P05.03 Newborn light for gestational age, 750–999 g
   P05.04 Newborn light for gestational age, 1000–1249 g
   P05.05 Newborn light for gestational age, 1250–1499 g
   P05.06 Newborn light for gestational age, 1500–1749 g
   P05.07 Newborn light for gestational age, 1750–1999 g
   P05.08 Newborn light for gestational age, 2000–2499 g
   •**P05.09 Newborn light for gestational age, 2,500 g and over**

P05.1 Newborn small for gestational age

5th   *Small for gestational age newborns are those who are smaller in size than normal for the gestational age, most commonly defined as weight below the 10th percentile and length below 10th percentile for the gestational age.*
    Newborn small-and-light-for-dates
    Newborn small-for-dates

   P05.10 Newborn small for gestational age, unspecified weight
   P05.11 Newborn small for gestational age, less than 500 g
   P05.12 Newborn small for gestational age, 500–749 g
   P05.13 Newborn small for gestational age, 750–999 g
   P05.14 Newborn small for gestational age, 1000–1249 g
   P05.15 Newborn small for gestational age, 1250–1499 g
   P05.16 Newborn small for gestational age, 1500–1749 g
   P05.17 Newborn small for gestational age, 1750–1999 g
   P05.18 Newborn small for gestational age, 2000–2499 g
   •**P05.19 Newborn small for gestational age, other**
        Newborn small for gestational age, 2500 g and over

P05.2 Newborn affected by fetal (intrauterine) malnutrition not light or small for gestational age
    Infant, not light or small for gestational age, showing signs of fetal malnutrition, such as dry, peeling skin and loss of subcutaneous tissue
    Excludes1: newborn affected by fetal malnutrition with light for gestational age (P05.0-)
        newborn affected by fetal malnutrition with small for gestational age (P05.1-)

P05.9 Newborn affected by slow intrauterine growth, unspecified
    Newborn affected by fetal growth retardation NOS

P07 DISORDERS OF NEWBORN RELATED TO SHORT GESTATION AND LBW, NEC

4th

Note: When both birth weight and gestational age of the newborn are available, both should be coded with birth weight sequenced before gestational age

Includes: the listed conditions, without further specification, as the cause of morbidity or additional care, in newborn

P07.0 Extremely LBW newborn

5th   Newborn birth weight 999 g or less
    Excludes1: LBW due to slow fetal growth and fetal malnutrition (P05.-)

   P07.00 Extremely LBW newborn, unspecified weight
   P07.01 Extremely LBW newborn, less than 500 g
   P07.02 Extremely LBW newborn, 500–749 g
   P07.03 Extremely LBW newborn, 750–999 g

P07.1 Other LBW newborn

5th   Newborn birth weight 1000–2499 g.
    Excludes1: LBW due to slow fetal growth and fetal malnutrition (P05.-)

   P07.10 Other LBW newborn, unspecified weight
   P07.14 Other LBW newborn, 1000–1249 g
   P07.15 Other LBW newborn, 1250–1499 g
   P07.16 Other LBW newborn, 1500–1749 g
   P07.17 Other LBW newborn, 1750–1999 g
   P07.18 Other LBW newborn, 2000–2499 g

P07.2 Extreme immaturity of newborn

5th   Less than 28 completed weeks (less than 196 completed days) of gestation.

   P07.20 Extreme immaturity of newborn; unspecified weeks of gestation
        Gestational age less than 28 completed weeks NOS
   P07.21 gestational age less than 23 completed weeks
        gestational age less than 23 weeks, 0 days
   P07.22 gestational age 23 completed weeks
        gestational age 23 weeks, 0 days through 23 weeks, 6 days
   P07.23 gestational age 24 completed weeks
        gestational age 24 weeks, 0 days through 24 weeks, 6 days
   P07.24 gestational age 25 completed weeks
        gestational age 25 weeks, 0 days through 25 weeks, 6 days

   Additional Character Required   3-character code

•=New Code
▲=Revised Code

Excludes1—Not coded here, do not use together
Excludes2—Not included here

CHAPTER 16. CERTAIN CONDITIONS ORIGINATING IN THE PERINATAL PERIOD   (P07.25–P15.0)

P07.25 **gestational age 26 completed weeks**
gestational age 26 weeks, 0 days through 26 weeks, 6 days

P07.26 **gestational age 27 completed weeks**
gestational age 27 weeks, 0 days through 27 weeks, 6 days

P07.3 **Preterm [premature] newborn [other]**
 28 completed weeks or more but less than 37 completed weeks (196 completed days but less than 259 completed days) of gestation.
Prematurity NOS

P07.30 **Preterm newborn, unspecified weeks of gestation**

P07.31 **Preterm newborn, gestational age 28 completed weeks**
Preterm newborn, gestational age 28 weeks, 0 days through 28 weeks, 6 days

P07.32 **Preterm newborn, gestational age 29 completed weeks**
Preterm newborn, gestational age 29 weeks, 0 days through 29 weeks, 6 days

P07.33 **Preterm newborn, gestational age 30 completed weeks**
Preterm newborn, gestational age 30 weeks, 0 days through 30 weeks, 6 days

P07.34 **Preterm newborn, gestational age 31 completed weeks**
Preterm newborn, gestational age 31 weeks, 0 days through 31 weeks, 6 days

P07.35 **Preterm newborn, gestational age 32 completed weeks**
Preterm newborn, gestational age 32 weeks, 0 days through 32 weeks, 6 days

P07.36 **Preterm newborn, gestational age 33 completed weeks**
Preterm newborn, gestational age 33 weeks, 0 days through 33 weeks, 6 days

P07.37 **Preterm newborn, gestational age 34 completed weeks**
Preterm newborn, gestational age 34 weeks, 0 days through 34 weeks, 6 days

P07.38 **Preterm newborn, gestational age 35 completed weeks**
Preterm newborn, gestational age 35 weeks, 0 days through 35 weeks, 6 days

P07.39 **Preterm newborn, gestational age 36 completed weeks**
Preterm newborn, gestational age 36 weeks, 0 days through 36 weeks, 6 days

P08 DISORDERS OF NEWBORN RELATED TO LONG GESTATION AND HIGH BIRTH WEIGHT

Note: When both birth weight and gestational age of the newborn are available, priority of assignment should be given to birth weight
Includes: the listed conditions, without further specification, as causes of morbidity or additional care, in newborn

P08.0 **Exceptionally large newborn baby**
Usually implies a birth weight of 4500 g. or more
Excludes1: syndrome of infant of diabetic mother (P70.1)
syndrome of infant of mother with gestational diabetes (P70.0)

P08.1 **Other heavy for gestational age newborn**
Other newborn heavy- or large-for-dates regardless of period of gestation
Usually implies a birth weight of 4000 g. to 4499 g.
Excludes1: newborn with a birth weight of 4500 or more (P08.0)
syndrome of infant of diabetic mother (P70.1)
syndrome of infant of mother with gestational diabetes (P70.0).

P08.2 **Late newborn, not heavy for gestational age**

P08.21 **Post-term newborn**
Newborn with gestation period over 40 completed weeks to 42 completed weeks

P08.22 **Prolonged gestation of newborn**
Newborn with gestation period over 42 completed weeks (294 days or more), not heavy- or large-for-dates.
Postmaturity NOS

(P09) ABNORMAL FINDINGS ON NEONATAL SCREENING

P09 ABNORMAL FINDINGS ON NEONATAL SCREENING

Use additional code to identify signs, symptoms and conditions associated with the screening
Excludes2: nonspecific serologic evidence of HIV (R75)

(P10–P15) BIRTH TRAUMA

P10 INTRACRANIAL LACERATION AND HEMORRHAGE DUE TO BIRTH INJURY

Excludes1: intracranial hemorrhage of newborn NOS (P52.9)
intracranial hemorrhage of newborn due to anoxia or hypoxia (P52.-)
nontraumatic intracranial hemorrhage of newborn (P52.-)

P10.0 **Subdural hemorrhage due to birth injury**
Subdural hematoma (localized) due to birth injury

P10.1 **Cerebral hemorrhage due to birth injury**

P10.2 **Intraventricular hemorrhage due to birth injury**

P10.3 **Subarachnoid hemorrhage due to birth injury**

P10.4 **Tentorial tear due to birth injury**

P10.8 **Other intracranial lacerations and hemorrhages due to birth injury**

P10.9 **Unspecified intracranial laceration and hemorrhage due to birth injury**
Excludes1: subdural hemorrhage accompanying tentorial tear (P10.4)

P11 OTHER BIRTH INJURIES TO CENTRAL NERVOUS SYSTEM

P11.0 **Cerebral edema due to birth injury**

P11.1 **Other specified brain damage due to birth injury**

P11.2 **Unspecified brain damage due to birth injury**

P11.3 **Birth injury to facial nerve**
Facial palsy due to birth injury

P11.4 **Birth injury to other cranial nerves**

P11.5 **Birth injury to spine and spinal cord**
Fracture of spine due to birth injury

P11.9 **Birth injury to central nervous system, unspecified**

P12 BIRTH INJURY TO SCALP

P12.0 **Cephalhematoma due to birth injury**

P12.1 **Chignon (from vacuum extraction) due to birth injury**

P12.2 **Epicranial subaponeurotic hemorrhage due to birth injury**
Subgaleal hemorrhage

P12.3 **Bruising of scalp due to birth injury**

P12.4 **Injury of scalp of newborn due to monitoring equipment**
Sampling incision of scalp of newborn
Scalp clip (electrode) injury of newborn

P12.8 **Other birth injuries to scalp**
P12.81 **Caput succedaneum**
P12.89 **Other birth injuries to scalp**

P12.9 **Birth injury to scalp, unspecified**

P13 BIRTH INJURY TO SKELETON

Excludes2: birth injury to spine (P11.5)

P13.0 **Fracture of skull due to birth injury**

P13.1 **Other birth injuries to skull**
Excludes1: cephalhematoma (P12.0)

P13.2 **Birth injury to femur**

P13.3 **Birth injury to other long bones**

P13.4 **Fracture of clavicle due to birth injury**

P13.8 **Birth injuries to other parts of skeleton**

P13.9 **Birth injury to skeleton, unspecified**

P14 BIRTH INJURY TO PERIPHERAL NERVOUS SYSTEM

P14.0 **Erb's paralysis due to birth injury**

P14.1 **Klumpke's paralysis due to birth injury**

P14.2 **Phrenic nerve paralysis due to birth injury**

P14.3 **Other brachial plexus birth injuries**

P14.8 **Birth injuries to other parts of peripheral nervous system**

P14.9 **Birth injury to peripheral nervous system, unspecified**

P15 OTHER BIRTH INJURIES

P15.0 **Birth injury to liver**
Rupture of liver due to birth injury

   Additional Character Required   3-character code

•=New Code
▲=Revised Code

Excludes1—Not coded here, do not use together
Excludes2—Not included here

P15.1 Birth injury to spleen
Rupture of spleen due to birth injury
P15.2 Sternomastoid injury due to birth injury
P15.3 Birth injury to eye
Subconjunctival hemorrhage due to birth injury
Traumatic glaucoma due to birth injury
P15.4 Birth injury to face
Facial congestion due to birth injury
P15.5 Birth injury to external genitalia
P15.6 Subcutaneous fat necrosis due to birth injury
P15.8 Other specified birth injuries
P15.9 Birth injury, unspecified

(P19–P29) RESPIRATORY AND CARDIOVASCULAR DISORDERS SPECIFIC TO THE PERINATAL PERIOD

P19 METABOLIC ACIDEMIA IN NEWBORN
 Includes: metabolic acidemia in newborn
P19.0 Metabolic acidemia in newborn first noted before onset of labor
P19.1 Metabolic acidemia in newborn first noted during labor
P19.2 Metabolic acidemia noted at birth
P19.9 Metabolic acidemia, unspecified

P22 RESPIRATORY DISTRESS OF NEWBORN
Excludes1: respiratory arrest of newborn (P28.81)
respiratory failure of newborn NOS (P28.5)
P22.0 Respiratory distress syndrome of newborn
Cardiorespiratory distress syndrome of newborn
Hyaline membrane disease
Idiopathic respiratory distress syndrome [IRDS or RDS] of newborn
Pulmonary hypoperfusion syndrome
Respiratory distress syndrome, type I
P22.1 Transient tachypnea of newborn
Idiopathic tachypnea of newborn
Respiratory distress syndrome, type II
Wet lung syndrome

P23 CONGENITAL PNEUMONIA
Includes: infective pneumonia acquired in utero or during birth
Excludes1: neonatal pneumonia resulting from aspiration (P24.-)
P23.0 Congenital pneumonia; due to viral agent
Use additional code (B97) to identify organism
Excludes1: congenital rubella pneumonitis (P35.0)
P23.1 due to Chlamydia
P23.2 due to staphylococcus
P23.3 due to streptococcus, group B
P23.4 due to E. coli
P23.5 due to Pseudomonas
P23.6 due to other bacterial agents
due to H. influenzae
due to K. pneumoniae
due to Mycoplasma
due to Streptococcus, except group B
Use additional code (B95–B96) to identify organism
P23.8 due to other organisms
P23.9 unspecified

P24 NEONATAL ASPIRATION
 Includes: aspiration in utero and during delivery
P24.0 Meconium aspiration
Excludes1: meconium passage (without aspiration) during delivery (P03.82)
meconium staining (P96.83)
P24.00 Meconium aspiration without respiratory symptoms
Meconium aspiration NOS
P24.01 Meconium aspiration with respiratory symptoms
Meconium aspiration pneumonia
Meconium aspiration pneumonitis
Meconium aspiration syndrome NOS
Use additional code to identify any secondary pulmonary hypertension, if applicable (I27.2)
P24.1 Neonatal aspiration of (clear) amniotic fluid and mucus
Neonatal aspiration of liquor (amnii)

P24.10 Neonatal aspiration of (clear) amniotic fluid and mucus; without respiratory symptoms
Neonatal aspiration of amniotic fluid and mucus NOS
P24.11 with respiratory symptoms
with pneumonia
with pneumonitis
Use additional code to identify any secondary pulmonary hypertension, if applicable (I27.2)
P24.2 Neonatal aspiration of blood;
P24.20 without respiratory symptoms
Neonatal aspiration of blood NOS
P24.21 with respiratory symptoms
with pneumonia
with pneumonitis
Use additional code to identify any secondary pulmonary hypertension, if applicable (I27.2)
P24.3 Neonatal aspiration of milk and regurgitated food
Neonatal aspiration of stomach contents
P24.30 Neonatal aspiration of milk and regurgitated food; without respiratory symptoms
Neonatal aspiration of milk and regurgitated food NOS
P24.31 with respiratory symptoms
P24.8 Other neonatal aspiration;
P24.80 without respiratory symptoms
Neonatal aspiration NEC
P24.81 with respiratory symptoms
Neonatal aspiration pneumonia NEC
Neonatal aspiration with pneumonitis NEC
Neonatal aspiration with pneumonia NOS
Neonatal aspiration with pneumonitis NOS
Use additional code to identify any secondary pulmonary hypertension, if applicable (I27.2)
P24.9 Neonatal aspiration, unspecified

P25 INTERSTITIAL EMPHYSEMA AND RELATED CONDITIONS ORIGINATING IN THE PERINATAL PERIOD
 Do not report codes from P25 that do not originate in the perinatal period.
P25.0 Interstitial emphysema originating in the perinatal period
P25.1 Pneumothorax originating in the perinatal period
P25.2 Pneumomediastinum originating in the perinatal period
P25.3 Pneumopericardium originating in the perinatal period
P25.8 Other conditions related to interstitial emphysema originating in the perinatal period

P26 PULMONARY HEMORRHAGE ORIGINATING IN THE PERINATAL PERIOD
Do not report codes from P26 that do not originate in the perinatal period
Excludes1: acute idiopathic hemorrhage in infants over 28 days old (R04.81)
P26.0 Tracheobronchial hemorrhage
P26.1 Massive pulmonary hemorrhage
P26.8 Other pulmonary hemorrhages
P26.9 Unspecified pulmonary hemorrhage

P27 CHRONIC RESPIRATORY DISEASE ORIGINATING IN THE PERINATAL PERIOD
Do not report codes from P27 that do not originate in the perinatal period
Excludes1: respiratory distress of newborn (P22.0–P22.9)
P27.0 Wilson-Mikity syndrome
Pulmonary dysmaturity
P27.1 Bronchopulmonary dysplasia
P27.8 Other chronic respiratory diseases
Congenital pulmonary fibrosis
Ventilator lung in newborn
P27.9 Unspecified chronic respiratory disease

P28 OTHER RESPIRATORY CONDITIONS ORIGINATING IN THE PERINATAL PERIOD
Excludes1: congenital malformations of the respiratory system (Q30–Q34)
P28.0 Primary atelectasis of newborn
Primary failure to expand terminal respiratory units
Pulmonary hypoplasia associated with short gestation
Pulmonary immaturity NOS
P28.1 Other and unspecified atelectasis of newborn
P28.10 Unspecified atelectasis of newborn
Atelectasis of newborn NOS

  Additional Character Required 3-character code

•=New Code
▲=Revised Code

Excludes1—Not coded here, do not use together
Excludes2—Not included here

P28.11 Resorption atelectasis without respiratory distress syndrome
Excludes1: resorption atelectasis with respiratory distress syndrome (P22.0)

P28.19 Other atelectasis of newborn
Partial atelectasis of newborn
Secondary atelectasis of newborn

P28.2 Cyanotic attacks of newborn
Excludes1: apnea of newborn (P28.3–P28.4)

P28.3 Primary sleep apnea of newborn
Central sleep apnea of newborn
Obstructive sleep apnea of newborn
Sleep apnea of newborn NOS

P28.4 Other apnea of newborn
Apnea of prematurity
Obstructive apnea of newborn
Excludes1: obstructive sleep apnea of newborn (P28.3)

P28.5 Respiratory failure of newborn
Excludes1: respiratory arrest of newborn (P28.81)
respiratory distress of newborn (P22.0-)

P28.8 Other specified respiratory conditions of newborn
P28.81 Respiratory arrest of newborn
P28.89 Other specified respiratory conditions of newborn
Congenital laryngeal stridor
Sniffles in newborn
Snuffles in newborn
Excludes1: early congenital syphilitic rhinitis (A50.05)

P28.9 Respiratory condition of newborn, unspecified
Respiratory depression in newborn

P29 CARDIOVASCULAR DISORDERS ORIGINATING IN THE PERINATAL PERIOD
Excludes1: congenital malformations of the circulatory system (Q20–Q28)

P29.0 Neonatal cardiac failure
P29.1 Neonatal cardiac dysrhythmia
P29.11 Neonatal tachycardia
P29.12 Neonatal bradycardia
P29.2 Neonatal hypertension
P29.3 Persistent fetal circulation
Delayed closure of ductus arteriosus
(Persistent) pulmonary hypertension of newborn
P29.4 Transient myocardial ischemia in newborn
P29.8 Other cardiovascular disorders originating in the perinatal period
P29.81 Cardiac arrest of newborn
P29.89 Other cardiovascular disorders originating in the perinatal period
P29.9 Cardiovascular disorder originating in the perinatal period, unspecified

(P35–P39) INFECTIONS SPECIFIC TO THE PERINATAL PERIOD
Infections acquired in utero, during birth via the umbilicus, or during the first 28 days after birth
Excludes2: asymptomatic HIV infection status (Z21)
congenital gonococcal infection (A54.-)
congenital pneumonia (P23.-)
congenital syphilis (A50.-)
HIV disease (B20)
infant botulism (A48.51)
infectious diseases not specific to the perinatal period (A00–B99, J09, J10.-)
intestinal infectious disease (A00–A09)
laboratory evidence of HIV (R75)
tetanus neonatorum (A33)

P35 CONGENITAL VIRAL DISEASES
Includes: infections acquired in utero or during birth
P35.0 Congenital rubella syndrome
Congenital rubella pneumonitis
P35.1 Congenital cytomegalovirus infection
P35.2 Congenital herpesviral [herpes simplex] infection
P35.3 Congenital viral hepatitis
P35.8 Other congenital viral diseases
Congenital varicella [chickenpox]
P35.9 Congenital viral disease, unspecified

P36 BACTERIAL SEPSIS OF NEWBORN
GUIDELINES
Category P36, Bacterial sepsis of newborn, includes congenital sepsis. If a perinate is documented as having sepsis without documentation of congenital or community acquired, the default is congenital and a code from category P36 should be assigned. If the P36 code includes the causal organism, an additional code from category B95, Streptococcus, Staphylococcus, and Enterococcus as the cause of diseases classified elsewhere, or B96, Other bacterial agents as the cause of diseases classified elsewhere, should not be assigned. If the P36 code does not include the causal organism, assign an additional code from category B96. If applicable, use additional codes to identify severe sepsis (R65.2-) and any associated acute organ dysfunction.
Includes: congenital sepsis
Use additional code(s), if applicable, to identify severe sepsis (R65.2-) and associated acute organ dysfunction(s)

P36.0 Sepsis of newborn due to streptococcus, group B
P36.1 Sepsis of newborn due to other and unspecified streptococci
P36.10 Sepsis of newborn due to unspecified streptococci
P36.19 Sepsis of newborn due to other streptococci
P36.2 Sepsis of newborn due to Staphylococcus aureus
P36.3 Sepsis of newborn due to other and unspecified staphylococci
P36.30 Sepsis of newborn due to unspecified staphylococci
P36.39 Sepsis of newborn due to other staphylococci
P36.4 Sepsis of newborn due to E. coli
P36.5 Sepsis of newborn due to anaerobes
P36.8 Other bacterial sepsis of newborn
Use additional code from category B96 to identify organism
P36.9 Bacterial sepsis of newborn, unspecified

P37 OTHER CONGENITAL INFECTIOUS AND PARASITIC DISEASES
Excludes2: congenital syphilis (A50.-)
infectious neonatal diarrhea (A00–A09)
necrotizing enterocolitis in newborn (P77.-)
noninfectious neonatal diarrhea (P78.3)
ophthalmia neonatorum due to gonococcus (A54.31)
tetanus neonatorum (A33)

P37.0 Congenital tuberculosis
P37.1 Congenital toxoplasmosis
Hydrocephalus due to congenital toxoplasmosis
P37.2 Neonatal (disseminated) listeriosis
P37.3 Congenital falciparum malaria
P37.4 Other congenital malaria
P37.5 Neonatal candidiasis
P37.8 Other specified congenital infectious and parasitic diseases
P37.9 Congenital infectious or parasitic disease, unspecified

P38 OMPHALITIS OF NEWBORN
Excludes1: omphalitis not of newborn (L08.82)
tetanus omphalitis (A33)
umbilical hemorrhage of newborn (P51.-)

P38.1 Omphalitis with mild hemorrhage
P38.9 Omphalitis without hemorrhage
Omphalitis of newborn NOS

P39 OTHER INFECTIONS SPECIFIC TO THE PERINATAL PERIOD
Use additional code to identify organism or specific infection
P39.0 Neonatal infective mastitis
Excludes1: breast engorgement of newborn (P83.4)
noninfective mastitis of newborn (P83.4)
P39.1 Neonatal conjunctivitis and dacryocystitis
Neonatal chlamydial conjunctivitis
Ophthalmia neonatorum NOS
Excludes1: gonococcal conjunctivitis (A54.31)
P39.2 Intra-amniotic infection affecting newborn, NEC
P39.3 Neonatal urinary tract infection
P39.4 Neonatal skin infection
Neonatal pyoderma
Excludes1: pemphigus neonatorum (L00)
staphylococcal scalded skin syndrome (L00)
P39.8 Other specified infections specific to the perinatal period
P39.9 Infection specific to the perinatal period, unspecified

  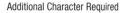

(P50–P61) HEMORRHAGIC AND HEMATOLOGICAL DISORDERS OF NEWBORN

Excludes1: congenital stenosis and stricture of bile ducts (Q44.3)
    Crigler-Najjar syndrome (E80.5)
    Dubin-Johnson syndrome (E80.6)
    Gilbert syndrome (E80.4)
    hereditary hemolytic anemias (D55–D58)

P50 `4th` **NEWBORN AFFECTED BY INTRAUTERINE (FETAL) BLOOD LOSS**
Excludes1: congenital anemia from intrauterine (fetal) blood loss (P61.3)
    P50.0 **Newborn affected by intrauterine (fetal) blood loss from vasa previa**
    P50.1 **Newborn affected by intrauterine (fetal) blood loss from ruptured cord**
    P50.2 **Newborn affected by intrauterine (fetal) blood loss from placenta**
    P50.3 **Newborn affected by hemorrhage into co-twin**
    P50.4 **Newborn affected by hemorrhage into maternal circulation**
    P50.5 **Newborn affected by intrauterine (fetal) blood loss from cut end of co-twin's cord**
    P50.8 **Newborn affected by other intrauterine (fetal) blood loss**
    P50.9 **Newborn affected by intrauterine (fetal) blood loss, unspecified**
        Newborn affected by fetal hemorrhage NOS

P51 `4th` **UMBILICAL HEMORRHAGE OF NEWBORN**
Excludes1: omphalitis with mild hemorrhage (P38.1)
    umbilical hemorrhage from cut end of co-twins cord (P50.5)
    P51.0 **Massive umbilical hemorrhage of newborn**
    P51.8 **Other umbilical hemorrhages of newborn**
        Slipped umbilical ligature NOS
    P51.9 **Umbilical hemorrhage of newborn, unspecified**

P52 `4th` **INTRACRANIAL NONTRAUMATIC HEMORRHAGE OF NEWBORN**
Includes: intracranial hemorrhage due to anoxia or hypoxia
Excludes1: intracranial hemorrhage due to birth injury (P10.-)
    intracranial hemorrhage due to other injury (S06.-)
    P52.0 **Intraventricular (nontraumatic) hemorrhage, grade 1, of newborn**
        Subependymal hemorrhage (without intraventricular extension)
        Bleeding into germinal matrix
    P52.1 **Intraventricular (nontraumatic) hemorrhage, grade 2, of newborn**
        Subependymal hemorrhage with intraventricular extension
        Bleeding into ventricle
    P52.2 **Intraventricular (nontraumatic) hemorrhage, grade 3 and grade 4, of newborn**
    `5th`
        P52.21 **Intraventricular (nontraumatic) hemorrhage, grade 3, of newborn**
            Subependymal hemorrhage with intraventricular extension with enlargement of ventricle
        P52.22 **Intraventricular (nontraumatic) hemorrhage, grade 4, of newborn**
            Bleeding into cerebral cortex
            Subependymal hemorrhage with intracerebral extension
    P52.3 **Unspecified intraventricular (nontraumatic) hemorrhage of newborn**

P53 ✔ **HEMORRHAGIC DISEASE OF NEWBORN**
Vitamin K deficiency of newborn

P54 `4th` **OTHER NEONATAL HEMORRHAGES**
Excludes1: newborn affected by (intrauterine) blood loss (P50.-)
    pulmonary hemorrhage originating in the perinatal period (P26.-)
    P54.5 **Neonatal cutaneous hemorrhage**
        Neonatal bruising
        Neonatal ecchymoses
        Neonatal petechiae
        Neonatal superficial hematomata
        Excludes2: bruising of scalp due to birth injury (P12.3)
            cephalhematoma due to birth injury (P12.0)

    P54.8 **Other specified neonatal hemorrhages**
    P54.9 **Neonatal hemorrhage, unspecified**

P55 `4th` **HEMOLYTIC DISEASE OF NEWBORN**
    P55.0 **Rh isoimmunization of newborn**
    P55.1 **ABO isoimmunization of newborn**
    P55.8 **Other hemolytic diseases of newborn**
    P55.9 **Hemolytic disease of newborn, unspecified**

P59 `4th` **NEONATAL JAUNDICE FROM OTHER AND UNSPECIFIED CAUSES**
Excludes1: jaundice due to inborn errors of metabolism (E70–E88)
    kernicterus (P57.-)
    P59.0 **Neonatal jaundice associated with preterm delivery**
        Hyperbilirubinemia of prematurity
        Jaundice due to delayed conjugation associated with preterm delivery
    P59.1 **Inspissated bile syndrome**
    P59.2 **Neonatal jaundice from other and unspecified hepatocellular damage**
    `5th`
        Excludes1: congenital viral hepatitis (P35.3)
        P59.20 **Neonatal jaundice from unspecified hepatocellular damage**
        P59.29 **Neonatal jaundice from other hepatocellular damage**
            Neonatal giant cell hepatitis
            Neonatal (idiopathic) hepatitis
    P59.3 **Neonatal jaundice from breast milk inhibitor**
    P59.8 **Neonatal jaundice from other specified causes**
    P59.9 **Neonatal jaundice, unspecified**
        Neonatal physiological jaundice (intense)(prolonged) NOS

P60 ✔ **DISSEMINATED INTRAVASCULAR COAGULATION OF NEWBORN**
Defibrination syndrome of newborn

P61 `4th` **OTHER PERINATAL HEMATOLOGICAL DISORDERS**
Excludes1: transient hypogammaglobulinemia of infancy (D80.7)
    P61.0 **Transient neonatal thrombocytopenia**
        Neonatal thrombocytopenia due to exchange transfusion
        Neonatal thrombocytopenia due to idiopathic maternal thrombocytopenia
        Neonatal thrombocytopenia due to isoimmunization
    P61.1 **Polycythemia neonatorum**
    P61.2 **Anemia of prematurity**
    P61.3 **Congenital anemia from fetal blood loss**
    P61.4 **Other congenital anemias, NEC**
        Congenital anemia NOS
    P61.5 **Transient neonatal neutropenia**
        Excludes1: congenital neutropenia (nontransient) (D70.0)
    P61.6 **Other transient neonatal disorders of coagulation**
    P61.8 **Other specified perinatal hematological disorders**
    P61.9 **Perinatal hematological disorder, unspecified**

(P70–P74) TRANSITORY ENDOCRINE AND METABOLIC DISORDERS SPECIFIC TO NEWBORN

Includes: transitory endocrine and metabolic disturbances caused by the infant's response to maternal endocrine and metabolic factors, or its adjustment to extrauterine environment

P70 `4th` **TRANSITORY DISORDERS OF CARBOHYDRATE METABOLISM SPECIFIC TO NEWBORN**
    P70.0 **Syndrome of infant of mother with gestational diabetes**
        Newborn (with hypoglycemia) affected by maternal gestational diabetes
        Excludes1: newborn (with hypoglycemia) affected by maternal (pre-existing) DM (P70.1)
            syndrome of infant of a diabetic mother (P70.1)
    P70.1 **Syndrome of infant of a diabetic mother**
        Newborn (with hypoglycemia) affected by maternal (pre-existing) DM
        Excludes1: newborn (with hypoglycemia) affected by maternal gestational diabetes (P70.0)
            syndrome of infant of mother with gestational diabetes (P70.0)

| `4th` `5th` `6th` `7th` | Additional Character Required | ✔ | 3-character code | •=New Code
 ▲=Revised Code | *Excludes1*—Not coded here, do not use together
 Excludes2—Not included here |

P70.2   **Neonatal DM**
P70.3   **Iatrogenic neonatal hypoglycemia**
P70.4   **Other neonatal hypoglycemia**
      Transitory neonatal hypoglycemia
P70.8   **Other transitory disorders of carbohydrate metabolism of newborn**

P71   TRANSITORY NEONATAL DISORDERS OF CALCIUM AND MAGNESIUM METABOLISM
`4th`
P71.0   **Cow's milk hypocalcemia in newborn**
P71.1   **Other neonatal hypocalcemia**
      Excludes1: neonatal hypoparathyroidism (P71.4)
P71.8   **Other transitory neonatal disorders of calcium and magnesium metabolism**
P71.9   **Transitory neonatal disorder of calcium and magnesium metabolism, unspecified**

P74   OTHER TRANSITORY NEONATAL ELECTROLYTE AND METABOLIC DISTURBANCES
`4th`
P74.0   **Late metabolic acidosis of newborn**
      Excludes1: (fetal) metabolic acidosis of newborn (P19)
P74.1   **Dehydration of newborn**
P74.2   **Disturbances of sodium balance of newborn**
P74.3   **Disturbances of potassium balance of newborn**
P74.4   **Other transitory electrolyte disturbances of newborn**
P74.5   **Transitory tyrosinemia of newborn**
P74.6   **Transitory hyperammonemia of newborn**
P74.8   **Other transitory metabolic disturbances of newborn**
      Amino-acid metabolic disorders described as transitory
P74.9   **Transitory metabolic disturbance of newborn, unspecified**

(P76–P78) DIGESTIVE SYSTEM DISORDERS OF NEWBORN

P76   OTHER INTESTINAL OBSTRUCTION OF NEWBORN
`4th`
P76.0   **Meconium plug syndrome**
      Meconium ileus NOS
      Excludes1: meconium ileus in cystic fibrosis (E84.11)

P77   NECROTIZING ENTEROCOLITIS OF NEWBORN
`4th`
P77.1   **Stage 1 necrotizing enterocolitis in newborn**
      Necrotizing enterocolitis without pneumatosis, without perforation

> For necrotizing enterocolitis that begins after the 28th day, see the alphabetic index for the appropriate reference (eg, necrotizing enterocolitis due to C. difficile A04.7).

P77.2   **Stage 2 necrotizing enterocolitis in newborn**
      Necrotizing enterocolitis with pneumatosis, without perforation
P77.3   **Stage 3 necrotizing enterocolitis in newborn**
      Necrotizing enterocolitis with perforation
      Necrotizing enterocolitis with pneumatosis and perforation
P77.9   **Necrotizing enterocolitis in newborn, unspecified**
      Necrotizing enterocolitis in newborn, NOS

P78   OTHER PERINATAL DIGESTIVE SYSTEM DISORDERS
`4th`
      Excludes1: cystic fibrosis (E84.0–E84.9)
      neonatal gastrointestinal hemorrhages (P54.0–P54.3)
P78.2   **Neonatal hematemesis and melena due to swallowed maternal blood**

(P80–P83) CONDITIONS INVOLVING THE INTEGUMENT AND TEMPERATURE REGULATION OF NEWBORN

P80   HYPOTHERMIA OF NEWBORN
`4th`
P80.0   **Cold injury syndrome**
      Severe and usually chronic hypothermia associated with a pink flushed appearance, edema and neurological and biochemical abnormalities.
      Excludes1: mild hypothermia of newborn (P80.8)
P80.8   **Other hypothermia of newborn**
      Mild hypothermia of newborn
P80.9   **Hypothermia of newborn, unspecified**

P81   OTHER DISTURBANCES OF TEMPERATURE REGULATION OF NEWBORN
`4th`
P81.0   **Environmental hyperthermia of newborn**
P81.8   **Other specified disturbances of temperature regulation of newborn**
P81.9   **Disturbance of temperature regulation of newborn, unspecified**
      Fever of newborn NOS

P83   OTHER CONDITIONS OF INTEGUMENT SPECIFIC TO NEWBORN
`4th`
      Excludes1: congenital malformations of skin and integument (Q80–Q84)
      hydrops fetalis due to hemolytic disease (P56.-)
      neonatal skin infection (P39.4)
      staphylococcal scalded skin syndrome (L00)
      Excludes2: cradle cap (L21.0)
      diaper [napkin] dermatitis (L22)
P83.0   **Sclerema neonatorum**
P83.1   **Neonatal erythema toxicum**
P83.4   **Breast engorgement of newborn**
      Noninfective mastitis of newborn
P83.5   **Congenital hydrocele**

(P84) OTHER PROBLEMS WITH NEWBORN

P84   OTHER PROBLEMS WITH NEWBORN
`✓`
      Acidemia of newborn
      Acidosis of newborn
      Anoxia of newborn NOS
      Asphyxia of newborn NOS
      Hypercapnia of newborn
      Hypoxemia of newborn
      Hypoxia of newborn NOS
      Mixed metabolic and respiratory acidosis of newborn
      Excludes1: intracranial hemorrhage due to anoxia or hypoxia (P52.-)
      hypoxic ischemic encephalopathy [HIE] (P91.6-)
      late metabolic acidosis of newborn (P74.0)

(P90–P96) OTHER DISORDERS ORIGINATING IN THE PERINATAL PERIOD

P90   CONVULSIONS OF NEWBORN
`✓`
      Excludes1: benign myoclonic epilepsy in infancy (G40.3-)
      benign neonatal convulsions (familial) (G40.3-)

P91   OTHER DISTURBANCES OF CEREBRAL STATUS OF NEWBORN
`4th`
P91.0   **Neonatal cerebral ischemia**
P91.2   **Neonatal cerebral leukomalacia**
      Periventricular leukomalacia
P91.4   **Neonatal cerebral depression**
P91.5   **Neonatal coma**
P91.6   **Hypoxic ischemic encephalopathy [HIE]**
`5th`   P91.60   **HIE, unspecified**
      P91.61   **Mild HIE**
      P91.62   **Moderate HIE**
      P91.63   **Severe HIE**
P91.9   **Disturbance of cerebral status of newborn, unspecified**

P92   FEEDING PROBLEMS OF NEWBORN
`4th`
      Excludes1: feeding problems in child over 28 days old (R63.3)
P92.0   **Vomiting of newborn**
      Excludes1: vomiting of child over 28 days old (R11.-)
`5th`   P92.01   **Bilious vomiting of newborn**
      Excludes1: bilious vomiting in child over 28 days old (R11.14)
      P92.09   **Other vomiting of newborn**
      Excludes1: regurgitation of food in newborn (P92.1)
P92.1   **Regurgitation and rumination of newborn**
P92.2   **Slow feeding of newborn**
P92.3   **Underfeeding of newborn**
P92.4   **Overfeeding of newborn**
P92.5   **Neonatal difficulty in feeding at breast**
P92.6   **Failure to thrive in newborn**
      Excludes1: failure to thrive in child over 28 days old (R62.51)

  `6th` `7th`   Additional Character Required   3-character code   ✱=New Code   ▲=Revised Code   ***Excludes1***—Not coded here, do not use together   ***Excludes2***—Not included here

P92.8   **Other feeding problems of newborn**

P92.9   **Feeding problem of newborn, unspecified**

P94   DISORDERS OF MUSCLE TONE OF NEWBORN

P94.0   **Transient neonatal myasthenia gravis**
myasthenia gravis (G70.0)

P94.1   **Congenital hypertonia**

P94.2   **Congenital hypotonia**
Floppy baby syndrome, unspecified

P94.8   **Other disorders of muscle tone of newborn**

P94.9   **Disorder of muscle tone of newborn, unspecified**

P95   STILLBIRTH

Deadborn fetus NOS
Fetal death of unspecified cause
Stillbirth NOS
Excludes1: maternal care for intrauterine death (O36.4)
     missed abortion (O02.1)
     outcome of delivery, stillbirth (Z37.1, Z37.3, Z37.4, Z37.7)
Code P95, Stillbirth, is only for use in institutions that maintain separate records for stillbirths. No other code should be used with P95. Code P95 should not be used on the mother's record.

P96   OTHER CONDITIONS ORIGINATING IN THE PERINATAL PERIOD

P96.1   **Neonatal withdrawal symptoms from maternal use of drugs of addiction**
Drug withdrawal syndrome in infant of dependent mother
Neonatal abstinence syndrome
Excludes1: reactions and intoxications from maternal opiates and tranquilizers administered during labor and delivery (P04.0)

P96.2   **Withdrawal symptoms from therapeutic use of drugs in newborn**

P96.3   **Wide cranial sutures of newborn**
Neonatal craniotabes

P96.5   **Complication to newborn due to (fetal) intrauterine procedure**
newborn affected by amniocentesis (P00.6)

P96.8   **Other specified conditions originating in the perinatal period**

P96.81   **Exposure to (parental) (environmental) tobacco smoke in the perinatal period**
Excludes2: newborn affected by in utero exposure to tobacco (P04.2)
     exposure to environmental tobacco smoke after the perinatal period (Z77.22)

P96.82   **Delayed separation of umbilical cord**

P96.83   **Meconium staining**
Excludes1: meconium aspiration (P24.00, P24.01)
     meconium passage during delivery (P03.82)

P96.89   **Other specified conditions originating in the perinatal period**
Use additional code to specify condition

P96.9   **Condition originating in the perinatal period, unspecified**
Congenital debility NOS

     Additional Character Required   3-character code   •=New Code   *Excludes1*—Not coded here, do not use together

▲=Revised Code   *Excludes2*—Not included here

Chapter 17. Congenital malformations, deformations and chromosomal abnormalities (Q00–Q99)

GUIDELINES

Assign an appropriate code(s) from categories Q00–Q99, Congenital malformations, deformations, and chromosomal abnormalities when a malformation/deformation or chromosomal abnormality is documented. A malformation/deformation/or chromosomal abnormality may be the principal/first-listed diagnosis on a record or a secondary diagnosis.

When a malformation/deformation/or chromosomal abnormality does not have a unique code assignment, assign additional code(s) for any manifestations that may be present.

When the code assignment specifically identifies the malformation/deformation/or chromosomal abnormality, manifestations that are an inherent component of the anomaly should not be coded separately. Additional codes should be assigned for manifestations that are not an inherent component.

Codes from Chapter 17 may be used throughout the life of the patient. If a congenital malformation or deformity has been corrected, a personal history code should be used to identify the history of the malformation or deformity. Although present at birth, malformation/deformation/or chromosomal abnormality may not be identified until later in life. Whenever the condition is diagnosed by the physician, it is appropriate to assign a code from codes Q00–Q99.For the birth admission, the appropriate code from category Z38, Liveborn infants, according to place of birth and type of delivery, should be sequenced as the principal diagnosis, followed by any congenital anomaly codes, Q00–Q99.

Note: Codes from this chapter are not for use on maternal or fetal records
Excludes2: inborn errors of metabolism (E70–E88)

(Q00–Q07) CONGENITAL MALFORMATIONS OF THE NERVOUS SYSTEM

Q02   MICROCEPHALY
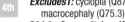
   Includes: hydromicrocephaly
   micrencephalon
   Excludes1: Meckel-Gruber syndrome (Q61.9)

Q03   CONGENITAL HYDROCEPHALUS
   Includes: hydrocephalus in newborn
   Excludes1: Arnold-Chiari syndrome, type II (Q07.0-)
     acquired hydrocephalus (G91.-)
     hydrocephalus due to congenital toxoplasmosis (P37.1)
     hydrocephalus with spina bifida (Q05.0–Q05.4)
   Q03.0   Malformations of aqueduct of Sylvius
     Anomaly of aqueduct of Sylvius
     Obstruction of aqueduct of Sylvius, congenital
     Stenosis of aqueduct of Sylvius
   Q03.1   Atresia of foramina of Magendie and Luschka
     Dandy-Walker syndrome
   Q03.8   Other congenital hydrocephalus
   Q03.9   Congenital hydrocephalus, unspecified

Q04   OTHER CONGENITAL MALFORMATIONS OF BRAIN
   Excludes1: cyclopia (Q87.0)
     macrocephaly (Q75.3)
   Q04.0   Congenital malformations of corpus callosum
     Agenesis of corpus callosum
   Q04.6   Congenital cerebral cysts
     Porencephaly
     Schizencephaly
     Excludes1: acquired porencephalic cyst (G93.0)

Q05   SPINA BIFIDA
   Includes: hydromeningocele (spinal)
     meningocele (spinal)
     meningomyelocele
     myelocele
     myelomeningocele
     rachischisis
     spina bifida (aperta) (cystica)
     syringomyelocele

> Lipomeningocele in spina bifida is also included in category Q05.

   Use additional code for any associated paraplegia (paraparesis) (G82.2-)
   Excludes1: Arnold-Chiari syndrome, type II (Q07.0-)
     spina bifida occulta (Q76.0)
   Q05.0   Cervical spina bifida with hydrocephalus

   Q05.1   Thoracic spina bifida with hydrocephalus
     Dorsal spina bifida with hydrocephalus
     Thoracolumbar spina bifida with hydrocephalus
   Q05.2   Lumbar spina bifida with hydrocephalus
     Lumbosacral spina bifida with hydrocephalus
   Q05.3   Sacral spina bifida with hydrocephalus
   Q05.4   Unspecified spina bifida with hydrocephalus
   Q05.5   Cervical spina bifida without hydrocephalus
   Q05.6   Thoracic spina bifida without hydrocephalus
     Dorsal spina bifida NOS
     Thoracolumbar spina bifida NOS
   Q05.7   Lumbar spina bifida without hydrocephalus
     Lumbosacral spina bifida NOS
   Q05.8   Sacral spina bifida without hydrocephalus
   Q05.9   Spina bifida, unspecified

Q07   OTHER CONGENITAL MALFORMATIONS OF NERVOUS SYSTEM

   Excludes2: congenital central alveolar hypoventilation syndrome (G47.35)
     familial dysautonomia [Riley-Day] (G90.1)
     neurofibromatosis (nonmalignant) (Q85.0-)
   Q07.0   Arnold-Chiari syndrome
     Arnold-Chiari syndrome, type II
     Excludes1: Arnold-Chiari syndrome, type III (Q01.-)
       Arnold-Chiari syndrome, type IV (Q04.8)
     Q07.00   without spina bifida or hydrocephalus
     Q07.01   with spina bifida
     Q07.02   with hydrocephalus
     Q07.03   with spina bifida and hydrocephalus
   Q07.9   Congenital malformation of nervous system, unspecified
     Congenital anomaly NOS of nervous system
     Congenital deformity NOS of nervous system
     Congenital disease or lesion NOS of nervous system

(Q10–Q18) CONGENITAL MALFORMATIONS OF EYE, EAR, FACE AND NECK

Excludes2: cleft lip and cleft palate (Q35–Q37)
   congenital malformation of cervical spine (Q05.0, Q05.5, Q67.5, Q76.0–Q76.4)
   congenital malformation of larynx (Q31.-)
   congenital malformation of lip NEC (Q38.0)
   congenital malformation of nose (Q30.-)
   congenital malformation of parathyroid gland (Q89.2)
   congenital malformation of thyroid gland (Q89.2)

Q10   CONGENITAL MALFORMATIONS OF EYELID, LACRIMAL APPARATUS AND ORBIT

   Excludes1: cryptophthalmos NOS (Q11.2)
     cryptophthalmos syndrome (Q87.0)
   Q10.0   Congenital ptosis

Q12   CONGENITAL LENS MALFORMATIONS

   Q12.0   Congenital cataract

Q13   CONGENITAL MALFORMATIONS OF ANTERIOR SEGMENT OF EYE
   Q13.0   Coloboma of iris
     Coloboma NOS

Q15   OTHER CONGENITAL MALFORMATIONS OF EYE
   Excludes1: congenital nystagmus (H55.01)
     ocular albinism (E70.31-)
     optic nerve hypoplasia (H47.03-)
     retinitis pigmentosa (H35.52)
   Q15.0   Congenital glaucoma
     Axenfeld's anomaly
     Buphthalmos
     Glaucoma of childhood
     Glaucoma of newborn
     Hydrophthalmos
     Keratoglobus, congenital, with glaucoma
     Macrocornea with glaucoma
     Macrophthalmos in congenital glaucoma
     Megalocornea with glaucoma

   Additional Character Required   3-character code

•=New Code
▲=Revised Code

Excludes1—Not coded here, do not use together
Excludes2—Not included here

CHAPTER 17. CONGENITAL MALFORMATIONS, DEFORMATIONS AND CHROMOSOMAL ABNORMALITIES   (Q15.9–Q26.2)

Q15.9   **Congenital malformation of eye, unspecified**
Congenital anomaly of eye
Congenital deformity of eye

Q17   OTHER CONGENITAL MALFORMATIONS OF EAR
 ***Excludes*1: co**ngenital malformations of ear with impairment of hearing (Q16.0–Q16.9)
preauricular sinus (Q18.1)

Q17.9   **Congenital malformation of ear, unspecified**
Congenital anomaly of ear NOS

Q18   OTHER CONGENITAL MALFORMATIONS OF FACE AND NECK
***Excludes*1:** cleft lip and cleft palate (Q35-Q37)
conditions classified to Q67.0-Q67.4
congenital malformations of skull and face bones (Q75.-)
cyclopia (Q87.0)
dentofacial anomalies [including malocclusion] (M26.-)
malformation syndromes affecting facial appearance (Q87.0)
persistent thyroglossal duct (Q89.2)

Q18.9   **Congenital malformation of face and neck, unspecified**
Congenital anomaly NOS of face and neck

(Q20–Q28) CONGENITAL MALFORMATIONS OF THE CIRCULATORY SYSTEM

Q20   CONGENITAL MALFORMATIONS OF CARDIAC CHAMBERS AND CONNECTIONS
***Excludes*1:** dextrocardia with situs inversus (Q89.3)
mirror-image atrial arrangement with situs inversus (Q89.3)

Q20.0   **Common arterial trunk**
Persistent truncus arteriosus
***Excludes*1:** aortic septal defect (Q21.4)

Q20.3   **Discordant ventriculoarterial connection**
Dextrotransposition of aorta
Transposition of great vessels (complete)

Q21   CONGENITAL MALFORMATIONS OF CARDIAC SEPTA
***Excludes*1:** acquired cardiac septal defect (I51.0)

Q21.0   **Ventricular septal defect**
Roger's disease

Q21.1   **Atrial septal defect**
Coronary sinus defect
Patent or persistent foramen ovale
Patent or persistent ostium secundum defect (type II)
Patent or persistent sinus venosus defect

Q21.2   **Atrioventricular septal defect**
Common atrioventricular canal
Endocardial cushion defect
Ostium primum atrial septal defect (type I)

Q21.3   **Tetralogy of Fallot**
Ventricular septal defect with pulmonary stenosis or atresia, dextroposition of aorta and hypertrophy of right ventricle

Q21.8   **Other congenital malformations of cardiac septa**
Eisenmenger's defect
Pentalogy of Fallot
***Excludes*1:** Eisenmenger's complex or syndrome (I27.8)

Q22   CONGENITAL MALFORMATIONS OF PULMONARY AND TRICUSPID VALVES
Q22.0   **Pulmonary valve atresia**
Q22.1   **Congenital pulmonary valve stenosis**
Q22.2   **Congenital pulmonary valve insufficiency**
Congenital pulmonary valve regurgitation
Q22.3   **Other congenital malformations of pulmonary valve**
Congenital malformation of pulmonary valve NOS
Supernumerary cusps of pulmonary valve
Q22.4   **Congenital tricuspid stenosis**
Congenital tricuspid atresia
Q22.5   **Ebstein's anomaly**
Q22.6   **Hypoplastic right heart syndrome**
Q22.8   **Other congenital malformations of tricuspid valve**
Q22.9   **Congenital malformation of tricuspid valve, unspecified**

Q23   CONGENITAL MALFORMATIONS OF AORTIC AND MITRAL VALVES
Q23.0   **Congenital stenosis of aortic valve**
Congenital aortic atresia
Congenital aortic stenosis NOS
***Excludes*1:** congenital stenosis of aortic valve in hypoplastic left heart syndrome (Q23.4)
congenital subaortic stenosis (Q24.4)
supravalvular aortic stenosis (congenital) (Q25.3)

Q23.1   **Congenital insufficiency of aortic valve**
Bicuspid aortic valve
Congenital aortic insufficiency

Q23.2   **Congenital mitral stenosis**
Congenital mitral atresia

Q23.3   **Congenital mitral insufficiency**
Q23.4   **Hypoplastic left heart syndrome**
Q23.8   **Other congenital malformations of aortic and mitral valves**
Q23.9   **Congenital malformation of aortic and mitral valves, unspecified**

Q24   OTHER CONGENITAL MALFORMATIONS OF HEART
***Excludes*1:** endocardial fibroelastosis (I42.4)

Q24.9   **Congenital malformation of heart, unspecified**
Congenital anomaly of heart
Congenital disease of heart

Q25   CONGENITAL MALFORMATIONS OF GREAT ARTERIES
Q25.0   **Patent ductus arteriosus**
Patent ductus Botallo
Persistent ductus arteriosus

Q25.1   **Coarctation of aorta**
Coarctation of aorta (preductal) (postductal)
Stenosis of aorta

Q25.2   **Atresia of aorta**
•Q25.21   **Interruption of aortic arch**
Atresia of aortic arch
•Q25.29   **Other atresia of aorta**
Atresia of aorta

Q25.4   **Other congenital malformations of aorta**
•Q25.40   **Congenital malformation of aorta unspecified**
•Q25.41   **Absence and aplasia of aorta**
•Q25.42   **Hypoplasia of aorta**
•Q25.43   **Congenital aneurysm of aorta**
Congenital aneurysm of aortic root
Congenital aneurysm of aortic sinus
•Q25.44   **Congenital dilation of aorta**
•Q25.45   **Double aortic arch**
Vascular ring of aorta
•Q25.46   **Tortuous aortic arch**
Persistent convolutions of aortic arch
•Q25.47   **Right aortic arch**
Persistent right aortic arch
•Q25.48   **Anomalous origin of subclavian artery**
•Q25.49   **Other congenital malformations of aorta**

Q25.5   **Atresia of pulmonary artery**
Q25.7   **Other congenital malformations of pulmonary artery**
Q25.71   **Coarctation of pulmonary artery**
Q25.72   **Congenital pulmonary arteriovenous malformation**
Congenital pulmonary arteriovenous aneurysm
Q25.79   **Other congenital malformations of pulmonary artery**
Aberrant pulmonary artery
Agenesis of pulmonary artery
Congenital aneurysm of pulmonary artery
Congenital anomaly of pulmonary artery
Hypoplasia of pulmonary artery

Q26   CONGENITAL MALFORMATIONS OF GREAT VEINS
Q26.2   **Total anomalous pulmonary venous connection**
TAPVR, subdiaphragmatic
TAPVR, supradiaphragmatic

   7th   Additional Character Required   3-character code   •=New Code   ***Excludes*1**—Not coded here, do not use together
▲=Revised Code   ***Excludes*2**—Not included here

250   **PEDIATRIC ICD-10-CM 2017: A MANUAL FOR PROVIDER-BASED CODING**

Q27 **OTHER CONGENITAL MALFORMATIONS OF PERIPHERAL VASCULAR SYSTEM**

4th

Excludes2: anomalies of cerebral and precerebral vessels (Q28.0–Q28.3)

anomalies of coronary vessels (Q24.5)

anomalies of pulmonary artery (Q25.5–Q25.7)

congenital retinal aneurysm (Q14.1)

hemangioma and lymphangioma (D18.-)

Q27.0 **Congenital absence and hypoplasia of umbilical artery**

Single umbilical artery

Q27.8 **Other specified congenital malformations of peripheral vascular system**

Absence of peripheral vascular system

Atresia of peripheral vascular system

Congenital aneurysm (peripheral)

Congenital stricture, artery

Congenital varix

Excludes1: arteriovenous malformation (Q27.3-)

Q27.9 **Congenital malformation of peripheral vascular system, unspecified**

Anomaly of artery or vein NOS

(Q30–Q34) CONGENITAL MALFORMATIONS OF THE RESPIRATORY SYSTEM

Q30 **CONGENITAL MALFORMATIONS OF NOSE**

4th

Excludes1: congenital deviation of nasal septum (Q67.4)

Q30.0 **Choanal atresia**

Atresia of nares (anterior) (posterior)

Congenital stenosis of nares (anterior) (posterior)

Q31 **CONGENITAL MALFORMATIONS OF LARYNX**

4th

Excludes1: congenital laryngeal stridor NOS (P28.89)

Q31.5 **Congenital laryngomalacia**

Q32 **CONGENITAL MALFORMATIONS OF TRACHEA AND BRONCHUS**

4th

Excludes1: congenital bronchiectasis (Q33.4)

For congenital tracheoesophageal fistula, see category Q39.

Q32.0 **Congenital tracheomalacia**

Q33 **CONGENITAL MALFORMATIONS OF LUNG**

4th

Excludes1: pulmonary hypoplasia associated with short gestation (P28.0)

Q33.6 **Congenital hypoplasia and dysplasia of lung**

Q34 **OTHER CONGENITAL MALFORMATIONS OF RESPIRATORY SYSTEM**

4th

Excludes2: congenital central alveolar hypoventilation syndrome (G47.35)

Q34.9 **Congenital malformation of respiratory system, unspecified**

Congenital absence of respiratory system

Congenital anomaly of respiratory system NOS

(Q35–Q37) CLEFT LIP AND CLEFT PALATE

Use additional code to identify associated malformation of the nose (Q30.2)

Excludes1: Robin's syndrome (Q87.0)

Q35 **CLEFT PALATE**

4th

Includes: fissure of palate

palatoschisis

Excludes1: cleft palate with cleft lip (Q37.-)

Q35.1 **Cleft hard palate**

Q35.3 **Cleft soft palate**

Q35.5 **Cleft hard palate with cleft soft palate**

Q35.7 **Cleft uvula**

Q35.9 **Cleft palate, unspecified**

Cleft palate NOS

Q36 **CLEFT LIP**

4th

Includes: cheiloschisis

congenital fissure of lip

harelip

labium leporinum

Excludes1: cleft lip with cleft palate (Q37.-)

Q36.0 **Cleft lip, bilateral**

Q36.1 **Cleft lip, median**

Q36.9 **Cleft lip, unilateral**

Cleft lip NOS

Q37 **CLEFT PALATE WITH CLEFT LIP**

4th

Includes: cheilopalatoschisis

Q37.0 **Cleft hard palate with bilateral cleft lip**

Q37.1 **Cleft hard palate with unilateral cleft lip**

Cleft hard palate with cleft lip NOS

Q37.2 **Cleft soft palate with bilateral cleft lip**

Q37.3 **Cleft soft palate with unilateral cleft lip**

Cleft soft palate with cleft lip NOS

Q37.4 **Cleft hard and soft palate with bilateral cleft lip**

Q37.5 **Cleft hard and soft palate with unilateral cleft lip**

Cleft hard and soft palate with cleft lip NOS

Q37.8 **Unspecified cleft palate with bilateral cleft lip**

Q37.9 **Unspecified cleft palate with unilateral cleft lip**

(Q38–Q45) OTHER CONGENITAL MALFORMATIONS OF THE DIGESTIVE SYSTEM

Q38 **OTHER CONGENITAL MALFORMATIONS OF TONGUE, MOUTH AND PHARYNX**

4th

Excludes1: dentofacial anomalies (M26.-)

macrostomia (Q18.4)

microstomia (Q18.5)

Q38.1 **Ankyloglossia**

Tongue tie

Q39 **CONGENITAL MALFORMATIONS OF ESOPHAGUS**

4th

Q39.1 **Atresia of esophagus with tracheo-esophageal fistula**

Atresia of esophagus with broncho-esophageal fistula

Code Q39.1 may be used to report congenital tracheo-esophageal fistula with atresia of esophagus.

Q40 **OTHER CONGENITAL MALFORMATIONS OF UPPER ALIMENTARY TRACT**

4th

Q40.0 **Congenital hypertrophic pyloric stenosis**

Congenital or infantile constriction

Congenital or infantile hypertrophy

Congenital or infantile spasm

Congenital or infantile stenosis

Congenital or infantile stricture

Q41 **CONGENITAL ABSENCE, ATRESIA AND STENOSIS OF SMALL INTESTINE**

4th

Includes: congenital obstruction, occlusion or stricture of small intestine or intestine NOS

Excludes1: cystic fibrosis with intestinal manifestation (E84.11)

meconium ileus NOS (without cystic fibrosis) (P76.0)

Q41.0 **Congenital absence, atresia and stenosis of duodenum**

Q41.1 **Congenital absence, atresia and stenosis of jejunum**

Apple peel syndrome

Imperforate jejunum

Q41.2 **Congenital absence, atresia and stenosis of ileum**

Q41.8 **Congenital absence, atresia and stenosis of other specified parts of small intestine**

Q41.9 **Congenital absence, atresia and stenosis of small intestine, part unspecified**

Congenital absence, atresia and stenosis of intestine NOS

Q42 **CONGENITAL ABSENCE, ATRESIA AND STENOSIS OF LARGE INTESTINE**

4th

Includes: congenital obstruction, occlusion and stricture of large intestine

Q42.0 **Congenital absence, atresia and stenosis of rectum with fistula**

Q42.1 **Congenital absence, atresia and stenosis of rectum without fistula**

Imperforate rectum

Q42.2 **Congenital absence, atresia and stenosis of anus with fistula**

Q42.3 **Congenital absence, atresia and stenosis of anus without fistula**

Imperforate anus

Q42.8 **Congenital absence, atresia and stenosis of other parts of large intestine**

Q42.9 **Congenital absence, atresia and stenosis of large intestine, part unspecified**

   4th 5th 6th 7th   Additional Character Required   3-character code

•=New Code

▲=Revised Code

Excludes1—Not coded here, do not use together

Excludes2—Not included here

CHAPTER 17. CONGENITAL MALFORMATIONS, DEFORMATIONS AND CHROMOSOMAL ABNORMALITIES   (Q43–Q56.4)

Q43 OTHER CONGENITAL MALFORMATIONS OF INTESTINE

 4th

Q43.0 Meckel's diverticulum (displaced) (hypertrophic)
Persistent omphalomesenteric duct
Persistent vitelline duct

Q43.1 Hirschsprung's disease
Aganglionosis
Congenital (aganglionic) megacolon

Q44 CONGENITAL MALFORMATIONS OF GALLBLADDER, BILE DUCTS AND LIVER

4th

Q44.0 Agenesis, aplasia and hypoplasia of gallbladder
Congenital absence of gallbladder

Q44.1 Other congenital malformations of gallbladder
Congenital malformation of gallbladder NOS
Intrahepatic gallbladder

Q44.2 Atresia of bile ducts

Q44.3 Congenital stenosis and stricture of bile ducts

Q44.4 Choledochal cyst

Q44.5 Other congenital malformations of bile ducts
Accessory hepatic duct
Biliary duct duplication
Congenital malformation of bile duct NOS
Cystic duct duplication

Q44.7 Other congenital malformations of liver
Accessory liver
Alagille's syndrome
Congenital absence of liver
Congenital hepatomegaly
Congenital malformation of liver NOS

Q45 OTHER CONGENITAL MALFORMATIONS OF DIGESTIVE SYSTEM

 4th

Excludes2: congenital diaphragmatic hernia (Q79.0)
congenital hiatus hernia (Q40.1)

Q45.8 Other specified congenital malformations of digestive system
Absence (complete) (partial) of alimentary tract NOS
Duplication of digestive system
Malposition, congenital of digestive system

Q45.9 Congenital malformation of digestive system, unspecified
Congenital anomaly of digestive system
Congenital deformity of digestive system

(Q50–Q56) CONGENITAL MALFORMATIONS OF GENITAL ORGANS

Excludes1: androgen insensitivity syndrome (E34.5-)
syndromes associated with anomalies in the number and form of chromosomes (Q90–Q99)

Q52 OTHER CONGENITAL MALFORMATIONS OF FEMALE GENITALIA

 4th

Q52.0 Congenital absence of vagina
Vaginal agenesis, total or partial

Q52.1 Doubling of vagina

 5th

Excludes1: doubling of vagina with doubling of uterus and cervix (Q51.1-)

Q52.10 Doubling of vagina, unspecified
Septate vagina NOS

Q52.11 Transverse vaginal septum

Q52.12 Longitudinal vaginal septum

6th

•**Q52.120 Longitudinal vaginal septum, nonobstructing**

•**Q52.121 Longitudinal vaginal septum, obstructing, right side**

•**Q52.122 Longitudinal vaginal septum, obstructing, left side**

•**Q52.123 Longitudinal vaginal septum, microperforate, right side**

•**Q52.124 Longitudinal vaginal septum, microperforate, left side**

•**Q52.129 Other and unspecified longitudinal vaginal septum**

Q52.2 Congenital rectovaginal fistula
Excludes1: cloaca (Q43.7)

Q52.3 Imperforate hymen

Q52.8 Other specified congenital malformations of female genitalia

Q52.9 Congenital malformation of female genitalia, unspecified

Q53 UNDESCENDED AND ECTOPIC TESTICLE

 4th

Q53.0 Ectopic testis

5th

Q53.00 Ectopic testis, unspecified

Q53.01 Ectopic testis, unilateral

Q53.02 Ectopic testes, bilateral

Q53.1 Undescended testicle, unilateral

5th

Q53.10 Unspecified undescended testicle, unilateral

Q53.11 Abdominal testis, unilateral

Q53.12 Ectopic perineal testis, unilateral

Q53.2 Undescended testicle, bilateral

5th

Q53.20 Undescended testicle, unspecified, bilateral

Q53.21 Abdominal testis, bilateral

Q53.22 Ectopic perineal testis, bilateral

Q53.9 Undescended testicle, unspecified
Cryptorchism NOS

Q54 HYPOSPADIAS

 4th

Excludes1: epispadias (Q64.0)

Q54.0 Hypospadias, balanic
Hypospadias, coronal
Hypospadias, glandular

Q54.1 Hypospadias, penile

Q54.2 Hypospadias, penoscrotal

Q54.3 Hypospadias, perineal

Q54.4 Congenital chordee
Chordee without hypospadias

Q54.8 Other hypospadias
Hypospadias with intersex state

Q54.9 Hypospadias, unspecified

Q55 OTHER CONGENITAL MALFORMATIONS OF MALE GENITAL ORGANS

 4th

Excludes1: congenital hydrocele (P83.5)
hypospadias (Q54.-)

Q55.0 Absence and aplasia of testis
Monorchism

Q55.2 Other and unspecified congenital malformations of testis and scrotum

5th

Q55.20 Unspecified congenital malformations of testis and scrotum
Congenital malformation of testis or scrotum NOS

Q55.21 Polyorchism

Q55.22 Retractile testis

Q55.23 Scrotal transposition

Q55.29 Other congenital malformations of testis and scrotum

Q55.6 Other congenital malformations of penis

5th

Q55.61 Curvature of penis (lateral)

Q55.62 Hypoplasia of penis
Micropenis

Q55.63 Congenital torsion of penis
Excludes1: acquired torsion of penis (N48.82)

Q55.64 Hidden penis
Buried penis
Concealed penis
Excludes1: acquired buried penis (N48.83)

Q55.69 Other congenital malformation of penis
Congenital malformation of penis NOS

Q55.9 Congenital malformation of male genital organ, unspecified
Congenital anomaly of male genital organ
Congenital deformity of male genital organ

Q56 INDETERMINATE SEX AND PSEUDOHERMAPHRODITISM

 4th

Excludes1: 46, XX true hermaphrodite (Q99.1)
androgen insensitivity syndrome (E34.5-)
chimera 46, XX/46, XY true hermaphrodite (Q99.0)
female pseudohermaphroditism with adrenocortical disorder (E25.-)
pseudohermaphroditism with specified chromosomal anomaly (Q96–Q99)
pure gonadal dysgenesis (Q99.1)

Q56.4 Indeterminate sex, unspecified
Ambiguous genitalia

4th **5th** **6th** **7th** Additional Character Required   ✓ 3-character code   •=New Code   ▲=Revised Code   ***Excludes1***—Not coded here, do not use together   ***Excludes2***—Not included here

252   PEDIATRIC ICD-10-CM 2017: A MANUAL FOR PROVIDER-BASED CODING

(Q60–Q64) CONGENITAL MALFORMATIONS OF THE URINARY SYSTEM

Q61   **CYSTIC KIDNEY DISEASE**
`4th`
Excludes1: acquired cyst of kidney (N28.1)
    Potter's syndrome (Q60.6)
   Q61.0   **Congenital renal cyst**
`5th`   **Q61.00**   **Congenital renal cyst, unspecified**
         Cyst of kidney NOS (congenital)
    Q61.01   **Congenital single renal cyst**
    Q61.02   **Congenital multiple renal cysts**
   Q61.1   **Polycystic kidney, infantile type**
     Polycystic kidney, autosomal recessive
`5th`   **Q61.11**   **Cystic dilatation of collecting ducts**
    Q61.19   **Other polycystic kidney, infantile type**
   Q61.2   **Polycystic kidney, adult type**
     Polycystic kidney, autosomal dominant
   Q61.3   **Polycystic kidney, unspecified**
   Q61.4   **Renal dysplasia**
     Multicystic dysplastic kidney
     Multicystic kidney (development)
     Multicystic kidney disease
     Multicystic renal dysplasia
     Excludes1: polycystic kidney disease (Q61.11–Q61.3)
   Q61.9   **Cystic kidney disease, unspecified**
     Meckel-Gruber syndrome

Q62   **CONGENITAL OBSTRUCTIVE DEFECTS OF RENAL PELVIS AND CONGENITAL MALFORMATIONS OF URETER**
`4th`
   Q62.0   **Congenital hydronephrosis**
   Q62.1   **Congenital occlusion of ureter**
     Atresia and stenosis of ureter
`5th`   **Q62.10**   **Congenital occlusion of ureter, unspecified**
    Q62.11   **Congenital occlusion of ureteropelvic junction**
    Q62.12   **Congenital occlusion of ureterovesical orifice**
   Q62.3   **Other obstructive defects of renal pelvis and ureter**
`5th`   **Q62.31**   **Congenital ureterocele, orthotopic**
    Q62.39   **Other obstructive defects of renal pelvis and ureter**
       Ureteropelvic junction obstruction NOS

Q64   **OTHER CONGENITAL MALFORMATIONS OF URINARY SYSTEM**
`4th`
   Q64.0   **Epispadias**
     Excludes1: hypospadias (Q54.-)
   Q64.1   **Exstrophy of urinary bladder**
`5th`   **Q64.10**   **Exstrophy of urinary bladder, unspecified**
       Ectopia vesicae
   Q64.2   **Congenital posterior urethral valves**
   Q64.9   **Congenital malformation of urinary system, unspecified**
     Congenital anomaly NOS of urinary system
     Congenital deformity NOS of urinary system

(Q65–Q79) CONGENITAL MALFORMATIONS AND DEFORMATIONS OF THE MUSCULOSKELETAL SYSTEM

Q65   **CONGENITAL DEFORMITIES OF HIP**
`4th`
Excludes1: clicking hip (R29.4)
   Q65.0   **Congenital dislocation of hip, unilateral**
`5th`   **Q65.00**   **Congenital dislocation of unspecified hip, unilateral**
    Q65.01   **Congenital dislocation of right hip, unilateral**
    Q65.02   **Congenital dislocation of left hip, unilateral**
   Q65.1   **Congenital dislocation of hip, bilateral**
   Q65.2   **Congenital dislocation of hip, unspecified**
   Q65.3   **Congenital partial dislocation of hip, unilateral**
`5th`   **Q65.30**   **Congenital partial dislocation of unspecified hip, unilateral**
    Q65.31   **Congenital partial dislocation of right hip, unilateral**
    Q65.32   **Congenital partial dislocation of left hip, unilateral**
   Q65.4   **Congenital partial dislocation of hip, bilateral**
   Q65.5   **Congenital partial dislocation of hip, unspecified**
   Q65.6   **Congenital unstable hip**
     Congenital dislocatable hip

   Q65.8   **Other congenital deformities of hip**
`5th`   **Q65.81**   **Congenital coxa valga**
    Q65.82   **Congenital coxa vara**
    Q65.89   **Other specified congenital deformities of hip**
       Anteversion of femoral neck
       Congenital acetabular dysplasia

Q66   **CONGENITAL DEFORMITIES OF FEET**
`4th`
Excludes1: reduction defects of feet (Q72.-)
    valgus deformities (acquired) (M21.0-)
    varus deformities (acquired) (M21.1-)
   Q66.0   **Congenital talipes equinovarus**
   Q66.1   **Congenital talipes calcaneovarus**
   Q66.2   **Congenital metatarsus deformities**
`5th`   •**Q66.21**   **Congenital metatarsus primus varus**
    •**Q66.22**   **Congenital metatarsus adductus**
       Congenital metatarsus varus
   Q66.3   **Other congenital varus deformities of feet**
     Hallux varus, congenital
   Q66.4   **Congenital talipes calcaneovalgus**
   Q66.5   **Congenital pes planus**
`5th`   Congenital flat foot
     Congenital rigid flat foot
     Congenital spastic (everted) flat foot
     Excludes1: pes planus, acquired (M21.4)
    Q66.50   **Congenital pes planus, unspecified foot**
    Q66.51   **Congenital pes planus, right foot**
    Q66.52   **Congenital pes planus, left foot**
   Q66.6   **Other congenital valgus deformities of feet**
     Congenital metatarsus valgus
   Q66.7   **Congenital pes cavus**
   Q66.8   **Other congenital deformities of feet**
`5th`   **Q66.80**   **Congenital vertical talus deformity, unspecified foot**
    Q66.81   **Congenital vertical talus deformity, right foot**
    Q66.82   **Congenital vertical talus deformity, left foot**
    Q66.89   **Other specified congenital deformities of feet**
       Congenital asymmetric talipes
       Congenital clubfoot NOS
       Congenital talipes NOS
       Congenital tarsal coalition
       Hammer toe, congenital
   Q66.9   **Congenital deformity of feet, unspecified**

Q67   **CONGENITAL MUSCULOSKELETAL DEFORMITIES OF HEAD, FACE, SPINE AND CHEST**
`4th`
Excludes1: congenital malformation syndromes classified to Q87.-
    Potter's syndrome (Q60.6)
   Q67.0   **Congenital facial asymmetry**
   Q67.1   **Congenital compression facies**
   Q67.2   **Dolichocephaly**
   Q67.3   **Plagiocephaly**
   Q67.4   **Other congenital deformities of skull, face and jaw**
     Congenital depressions in skull
     Congenital hemifacial atrophy or hypertrophy
     Deviation of nasal septum, congenital
     Squashed or bent nose, congenital
     Excludes1: dentofacial anomalies [including malocclusion] (M26.-)
       syphilitic saddle nose (A50.5)
   Q67.6   **Pectus excavatum**
     Congenital funnel chest
   Q67.7   **Pectus carinatum**
     Congenital pigeon chest
   Q67.8   **Other congenital deformities of chest**
     Congenital deformity of chest wall NOS

Q68   **OTHER CONGENITAL MUSCULOSKELETAL DEFORMITIES**
`4th`
Excludes1: reduction defects of limb(s) (Q71-Q73)
Excludes2: congenital myotonic chondrodystrophy (G71.13)
   Q68.0   **Congenital deformity of sternocleidomastoid muscle**
     Congenital contracture of sternocleidomastoid (muscle)
     Congenital (sternomastoid) torticollis
     Sternomastoid tumor (congenital)

   `4th` `5th` `6th` `7th`   Additional Character Required   3-character code

•=New Code   *Excludes1*—Not coded here, do not use together
▲=Revised Code   *Excludes2*—Not included here

CHAPTER 17. CONGENITAL MALFORMATIONS, DEFORMATIONS AND CHROMOSOMAL ABNORMALITIES (Q69–Q75.9)

Q69 POLYDACTYLY

[4th]

Q69.0 Accessory finger(s)

Q69.1 Accessory thumb(s)

Q69.2 Accessory toe(s)
Accessory hallux

Q69.9 Polydactyly, unspecified
Supernumerary digit(s) NOS

Q70 SYNDACTYLY

[4th]

Q70.0 Fused fingers
Complex syndactyly of fingers with synostosis

[5th]

    Q70.00 Fused fingers, unspecified hand
    Q70.01 Fused fingers, right hand
    Q70.02 Fused fingers, left hand
    Q70.03 Fused fingers, bilateral

Q70.1 Webbed fingers
Simple syndactyly of fingers without synostosis

[5th]

    Q70.10 Webbed fingers, unspecified hand
    Q70.11 Webbed fingers, right hand
    Q70.12 Webbed fingers, left hand
    Q70.13 Webbed fingers, bilateral

Q70.2 Fused toes
Complex syndactyly of toes with synostosis

[5th]

    Q70.20 Fused toes, unspecified foot
    Q70.21 Fused toes, right foot
    Q70.22 Fused toes, left foot
    Q70.23 Fused toes, bilateral

Q70.3 Webbed toes
Simple syndactyly of toes without synostosis

[5th]

    Q70.30 Webbed toes, unspecified foot
    Q70.31 Webbed toes, right foot
    Q70.32 Webbed toes, left foot
    Q70.33 Webbed toes, bilateral

Q70.4 Polysyndactyly, unspecified
Excludes1: specified syndactyly of hand and feet—code to
    specified conditions (Q70.0–Q70.3-)

Q70.9 Syndactyly, unspecified
Symphalangy NOS

Q71 REDUCTION DEFECTS OF UPPER LIMB

[4th]

Q71.4 Longitudinal reduction defect of radius
Clubhand (congenital)
Radial clubhand

[5th]

    Q71.40 Longitudinal reduction defect of unspecified radius
    Q71.41 Longitudinal reduction defect of right radius
    Q71.42 Longitudinal reduction defect of left radius
    Q71.43 Longitudinal reduction defect of radius, bilateral

Q71.5 Longitudinal reduction defect of ulna

[5th]

    Q71.50 Longitudinal reduction defect of unspecified ulna
    Q71.51 Longitudinal reduction defect of right ulna
    Q71.52 Longitudinal reduction defect of left ulna
    Q71.53 Longitudinal reduction defect of ulna, bilateral

Q71.6 Lobster-claw hand

[5th]

    Q71.61 Lobster-claw right hand
    Q71.62 Lobster-claw left hand
    Q71.63 Lobster-claw hand, bilateral

Q71.8 Other reduction defects of upper limb

[5th]

    Q71.81 Congenital shortening of upper limb

[6th]

        Q71.811 Congenital shortening of right upper limb
        Q71.812 Congenital shortening of left upper limb
        Q71.813 Congenital shortening of upper limb, bilateral
        Q71.819 Congenital shortening of unspecified upper limb

Q72 REDUCTION DEFECTS OF LOWER LIMB

[4th]

Q72.4 Longitudinal reduction defect of femur
Proximal femoral focal deficiency

[5th]

    Q72.40 Longitudinal reduction defect of unspecified femur
    Q72.41 Longitudinal reduction defect of right femur
    Q72.42 Longitudinal reduction defect of left femur
    Q72.43 Longitudinal reduction defect of femur, bilateral

Q72.5 Longitudinal reduction defect of tibia

[5th]

    Q72.50 Longitudinal reduction defect of unspecified tibia
    Q72.51 Longitudinal reduction defect of right tibia
    Q72.52 Longitudinal reduction defect of left tibia
    Q72.53 Longitudinal reduction defect of tibia, bilateral

Q72.6 Longitudinal reduction defect of fibula

[5th]

    Q72.60 Longitudinal reduction defect of unspecified fibula
    Q72.61 Longitudinal reduction defect of right fibula
    Q72.62 Longitudinal reduction defect of left fibula
    Q72.63 Longitudinal reduction defect of fibula, bilateral

Q72.7 Split foot

[5th]

    Q72.71 Split foot, right lower limb
    Q72.72 Split foot, left lower limb
    Q72.73 Split foot, bilateral

Q72.8 Other reduction defects of lower limb

[5th]

    Q72.81 Congenital shortening of lower limb

[6th]

        Q72.811 Congenital shortening of right lower limb
        Q72.812 Congenital shortening of left lower limb
        Q72.813 Congenital shortening of lower limb, bilateral
        Q72.819 Congenital shortening of unspecified lower limb

Q74 OTHER CONGENITAL MALFORMATIONS OF LIMB(S)

[4th]

Excludes1: polydactyly (Q69.-)
    reduction defect of limb (Q71–Q73)
    syndactyly (Q70.-)

Q74.2 Other congenital malformations of lower limb(s), including pelvic girdle
Congenital fusion of sacroiliac joint
Congenital malformation of ankle joint
Congenital malformation of sacroiliac joint
Excludes1: anteversion of femur (neck) (Q65.89)

Q74.3 Arthrogryposis multiplex congenita

Q74.9 Unspecified congenital malformation of limb(s)
Congenital anomaly of limb(s) NOS

Q75 OTHER CONGENITAL MALFORMATIONS OF SKULL AND FACE BONES

[4th]

Excludes1: congenital malformation of face NOS (Q18.-)
    congenital malformation syndromes classified to Q87.-
    dentofacial anomalies [including malocclusion] (M26.-)
    musculoskeletal deformities of head and face (Q67.0–Q67.4)
    skull defects associated with congenital anomalies of brain such as:
    anencephaly (Q00.0)
    encephalocele (Q01.-)
    hydrocephalus (Q03.-)
    microcephaly (Q02)

Q75.0 Craniosynostosis
Acrocephaly
Imperfect fusion of skull
Oxycephaly
Trigonocephaly

Q75.1 Craniofacial dysostosis
Crouzon's disease

Q75.2 Hypertelorism

Q75.3 Macrocephaly

Q75.4 Mandibulofacial dysostosis
Franceschetti syndrome
Treacher Collins syndrome

Q75.5 Oculomandibular dysostosis

Q75.8 Other specified congenital malformations of skull and face bones
Absence of skull bone, congenital
Congenital deformity of forehead
Platybasia

Q75.9 Congenital malformation of skull and face bones, unspecified
Congenital anomaly of face bones NOS
Congenital anomaly of skull NOS

[4th] [5th] [6th] [7th] Additional Character Required   ✔ 3-character code   •=New Code   ▲=Revised Code   *Excludes1*—Not coded here, do not use together   *Excludes2*—Not included here

Q76   CONGENITAL MALFORMATIONS OF SPINE AND BONY THORAX
4th
Excludes1: congenital musculoskeletal deformities of spine and chest (Q67.5–Q67.8)
Q76.2   Congenital spondylolisthesis
Congenital spondylolysis
Excludes1: spondylolisthesis (acquired) (M43.1-)

Q78   OTHER OSTEOCHONDRODYSPLASIAS
4th
Excludes2: congenital myotonic chondrodystrophy (G71.13)
Q78.0   Osteogenesis imperfecta
Fragilitas ossium
Osteopsathyrosis

Q79   CONGENITAL MALFORMATIONS OF MUSCULOSKELETAL SYSTEM, NEC
4th
Excludes2: congenital (sternomastoid) torticollis (Q68.0)
Q79.0   Congenital diaphragmatic hernia
Excludes1: congenital hiatus hernia (Q40.1)
Q79.2   Exomphalos
Omphalocele
Excludes1: umbilical hernia (K42.-)
Q79.3   Gastroschisis
Q79.4   Prune belly syndrome
Congenital prolapse of bladder mucosa
Eagle-Barrett syndrome
Q79.6   Ehlers-Danlos syndrome
Q79.9   Congenital malformation of musculoskeletal system, unspecified
Congenital anomaly of musculoskeletal system NOS
Congenital deformity of musculoskeletal system NOS

(Q80–Q89) OTHER CONGENITAL MALFORMATIONS

Q81   EPIDERMOLYSIS BULLOSA
4th
Q81.0   Epidermolysis bullosa simplex
Excludes1: Cockayne's syndrome (Q87.1)
Q81.1   Epidermolysis bullosa letalis
Herlitz' syndrome
Q81.2   Epidermolysis bullosa dystrophica
Q81.8   Other epidermolysis bullosa
Q81.9   Epidermolysis bullosa, unspecified

Q82   OTHER CONGENITAL MALFORMATIONS OF SKIN
4th
Excludes1: acrodermatitis enteropathica (E83.2)
congenital erythropoietic porphyria (E80.0)
pilonidal cyst or sinus (L05.-)
Sturge-Weber (-Dimitri) syndrome (Q85.8)
Q82.0   Hereditary lymphedema
Q82.1   Xeroderma pigmentosum
Q82.2   Mastocytosis
Urticaria pigmentosa
Excludes1: malignant mastocytosis (C96.2)
Q82.3   Incontinentia pigmenti
Q82.4   Ectodermal dysplasia (anhidrotic)
Excludes1: Ellis-van Creveld syndrome (Q77.6)
Q82.5   Congenital non-neoplastic nevus
Birthmark NOS
Flammeus Nevus
Portwine Nevus
Sanguineous Nevus
Strawberry Nevus
Vascular Nevus NOS
Verrucous Nevus
Excludes2: Café au lait spots (L81.3)
lentigo (L81.4)
nevus NOS (D22.-)
araneus nevus (I78.1)
melanocytic nevus (D22.-)
pigmented nevus (D22.-)
spider nevus (I78.1)
stellar nevus (I78.1)
∘Q82.6   Congenital sacral dimple
Parasacral dimple
Excludes2: pilonidal cyst with abscess (L05.01)
pilonidal cyst without abscess (L05.91)

Q82.8   Other specified congenital malformations of skin
Abnormal palmar creases
Accessory skin tags
Benign familial pemphigus [Hailey-Hailey]
Congenital poikiloderma
Cutis laxa (hyperelastica)
Dermatoglyphic anomalies
Inherited keratosis palmaris et plantaris
Keratosis follicularis *[Darier-White]*
Excludes1: Ehlers-Danlos syndrome (Q79.6)
Q82.9   Congenital malformation of skin, unspecified

Q83   CONGENITAL MALFORMATIONS OF BREAST
4th
Excludes2: absence of pectoral muscle (Q79.8)
hypoplasia of breast (N64.82)
micromastia (N64.82)
Q83.0   Congenital absence of breast with absent nipple
Q83.3   Accessory nipple
Supernumerary nipple

Q84   OTHER CONGENITAL MALFORMATIONS OF INTEGUMENT
4th
Q84.6   Other congenital malformations of nails
Congenital clubnail
Congenital koilonychia
Congenital malformation of nail NOS
Q84.8   Other specified congenital malformations of integument
Aplasia cutis congenita
Q84.9   Congenital malformation of integument, unspecified
Congenital anomaly of integument NOS
Congenital deformity of integument NOS

Q85   PHAKOMATOSES, NES
4th
Excludes1: ataxia telangiectasia [Louis-Bar] (G11.3)
familial dysautonomia [Riley-Day] (G90.1)
Q85.0   Neurofibromatosis (nonmalignant)
5th
Q85.00   Neurofibromatosis, unspecified
Q85.01   Neurofibromatosis, type 1
Von Recklinghausen disease
Q85.02   Neurofibromatosis, type 2
Acoustic neurofibromatosis
Q85.03   Schwannomatosis
Q85.09   Other neurofibromatosis
Q85.1   Tuberous sclerosis
Bourneville's disease
Epiloia
Q85.8   Other phakomatoses, NEC
Peutz-Jeghers Syndrome
Sturge-Weber (-Dimitri) syndrome
von Hippel-Lindau syndrome
Excludes1: Meckel-Gruber syndrome (Q61.9)
Q85.9   Phakomatosis, unspecified
Hamartosis NOS

Q86   CONGENITAL MALFORMATION SYNDROMES DUE TO KNOWN EXOGENOUS CAUSES, NEC
4th
Excludes2: iodine-deficiency-related hypothyroidism (E00–E02)
nonteratogenic effects of substances transmitted via placenta or breast milk (P04.-)
Q86.0   Fetal alcohol syndrome (dysmorphic)

Q87   OTHER SPECIFIED CONGENITAL MALFORMATION SYNDROMES AFFECTING MULTIPLE SYSTEMS
4th
Use additional code(s) to identify all associated manifestations
Q87.0   Congenital malformation syndromes predominantly affecting facial appearance
Acrocephalopolysyndactyly
Acrocephalosyndactyly [Apert]
Cryptophthalmos syndrome
Cyclopia
Goldenhar syndrome
Moebius syndrome
Oro-facial-digital syndrome
Robin syndrome
Whistling face

| 4th | 5th | 6th | 7th | Additional Character Required | ✓ 3-character code | •=New Code ▲=Revised Code | *Excludes1*—Not coded here, do not use together *Excludes2*—Not included here |

CHAPTER 17. CONGENITAL MALFORMATIONS, DEFORMATIONS AND CHROMOSOMAL ABNORMALITIES   (Q87.1–Q96.9)

Q87.1   Congenital malformation syndromes predominantly associated with short stature
Aarskog syndrome
Cockayne syndrome
De Lange syndrome
Dubowitz syndrome
Noonan syndrome
Prader-Willi syndrome
Robinow-Silverman-Smith syndrome
Russell-Silver syndrome
Seckel syndrome
Excludes1: Ellis-van Creveld syndrome (Q77.6)
Smith-Lemli-Opitz syndrome (E78.72)

Q87.2   Congenital malformation syndromes predominantly involving limbs
Holt-Oram syndrome
Klippel-Trenaunay-Weber syndrome
Nail patella syndrome
Rubinstein-Taybi syndrome
Sirenomelia syndrome
TAR syndrome
VATER syndrome

Q87.3   Congenital malformation syndromes involving early overgrowth
Beckwith-Wiedemann syndrome
Sotos syndrome
Weaver syndrome

Q87.4   Marfan's syndrome
5th   **Q87.40   Marfan's syndrome, unspecified**
Q87.41   Marfan's syndrome with cardiovascular
6th   **manifestations**
    Q87.410   Marfan's syndrome with aortic dilation
    Q87.418   Marfan's syndrome with other cardiovascular manifestations
Q87.42   Marfan's syndrome with ocular manifestations
Q87.43   Marfan's syndrome with skeletal manifestation

Q87.8   Other specified congenital malformation syndromes, NEC
5th   *Excludes1:* Zellweger syndrome (E71.510)
Q87.81   Alport syndrome
Use additional code to identify stage of CKD (N18.1–N18.6)
•**Q87.82   Arterial tortuosity syndrome**
Q87.89   Other specified congenital malformation syndromes, NEC
Laurence-Moon (-Bardet)-Biedl syndrome

Q89   OTHER CONGENITAL MALFORMATIONS, NEC
4th   **Q89.0   Congenital absence and malformations of spleen**
5th   *Excludes1:* isomerism of atrial appendages (with asplenia or polysplenia) (Q20.6)
Q89.01   Asplenia (congenital)
Q89.09   Congenital malformations of spleen
Congenital splenomegaly
Q89.1   Congenital malformations of adrenal gland
Excludes1: adrenogenital disorders (E25.-)
congenital adrenal hyperplasia (E25.0)
Q89.2   Congenital malformations of other endocrine glands
Congenital malformation of parathyroid or thyroid gland
Persistent thyroglossal duct
Thyroglossal cyst
Excludes1: congenital goiter (E03.0)
congenital hypothyroidism (E03.1)
Q89.3   Situs inversus
Dextrocardia with situs inversus
Mirror-image atrial arrangement with situs inversus
Situs inversus or transversus abdominalis
Situs inversus or transversus thoracis
Transposition of abdominal viscera
Transposition of thoracic viscera
Excludes1: dextrocardia NOS (Q24.0)

Q89.7   Multiple congenital malformations, NEC
Multiple congenital anomalies NOS
Multiple congenital deformities NOS
Excludes1: congenital malformation syndromes affecting multiple systems (Q87.-)
Q89.8   Other specified congenital malformations
Use additional code(s) to identify all associated manifestations

(Q90–Q99) CHROMOSOMAL ABNORMALITIES, NEC

Excludes2: mitochondrial metabolic disorders (E88.4-)

Q90   DOWN SYNDROME
4th   **Use additional code(s)** to identify any associated physical conditions and degree of intellectual disabilities (F70–F79)
Q90.0   Trisomy 21, nonmosaicism (meiotic nondisjunction)
Q90.1   Trisomy 21, mosaicism (mitotic nondisjunction)
Q90.2   Trisomy 21, translocation
Q90.9   Down syndrome, unspecified
Trisomy 21 NOS

Q91   TRISOMY 18 AND TRISOMY 13
4th   **Q91.0   Trisomy 18, nonmosaicism (meiotic nondisjunction)**
Q91.1   Trisomy 18, mosaicism (mitotic nondisjunction)
Q91.2   Trisomy 18, translocation
Q91.3   Trisomy 18, unspecified
Q91.4   Trisomy 13, nonmosaicism (meiotic nondisjunction)
Q91.5   Trisomy 13, mosaicism (mitotic nondisjunction)
Q91.6   Trisomy 13, translocation
Q91.7   Trisomy 13, unspecified

Q93   MONOSOMIES AND DELETIONS FROM THE AUTOSOMES, NEC
4th   **Q93.0   Whole chromosome monosomy, nonmosaicism (meiotic nondisjunction)**
Q93.1   Whole chromosome monosomy, mosaicism (mitotic nondisjunction)
Q93.2   Chromosome replaced with ring, dicentric or isochromosome
Q93.3   Deletion of short arm of chromosome 4
Wolff-Hirschorn syndrome
Q93.4   Deletion of short arm of chromosome 5
Cri-du-chat syndrome
Q93.5   Other deletions of part of a chromosome
Angelman syndrome
Q93.7   Deletions with other complex rearrangements
Deletions due to unbalanced translocations, inversions and insertions
Code also any associated duplications due to unbalanced translocations, inversions and insertions (Q92.5)
Q93.8   Other deletions from the autosomes
5th   **Q93.81   Velo-cardio-facial syndrome**
Deletion 22q11.2
Q93.88   Other microdeletions
Miller-Dieker syndrome
Smith-Magenis syndrome
Q93.89   Other deletions from the autosomes
Deletions identified by fluorescence in situ hybridization (FISH)
Deletions identified by in situ hybridization (ISH)
Deletions seen only at prometaphase
Q93.9   Deletion from autosomes, unspecified

Q96   TURNER'S SYNDROME
4th   *Excludes1:* Noonan syndrome (Q87.1)
Q96.0   Karyotype 45, X
Q96.1   Karyotype 46, X iso (Xq)
Karyotype 46, isochromosome Xq
Q96.2   Karyotype 46, X with abnormal sex chromosome, except iso (Xq)
Karyotype 46, X with abnormal sex chromosome, except isochromosome Xq
Q96.3   Mosaicism, 45, X/46, XX or XY
Q96.4   Mosaicism, 45, X/other cell line(s) with abnormal sex chromosome
Q96.8   Other variants of Turner's syndrome
Q96.9   Turner's syndrome, unspecified

  4th   5th   6th   7th   Additional Character Required   ✔ 3-character code

•=New Code   *Excludes1*—Not coded here, do not use together
▲=Revised Code   *Excludes2*—Not included here

Q97 OTHER SEX CHROMOSOME ABNORMALITIES, FEMALE
4th PHENOTYPE, NEC
Excludes1: Turner's syndrome (Q96.-)
Q97.0 Karyotype 47, XXX
Q97.9 Sex chromosome abnormality, female phenotype, unspecified

Q98 OTHER SEX CHROMOSOME ABNORMALITIES, MALE
4th PHENOTYPE, NEC
Q98.3 Other male with 46, XX karyotype
Q98.9 Sex chromosome abnormality, male phenotype, unspecified
Q98.4 Klinefelter syndrome, unspecified

Q99 OTHER CHROMOSOME ABNORMALITIES, NEC
4th Q99.2 Fragile X chromosome
Fragile X syndrome
Q99.8 Other specified chromosome abnormalities
Q99.9 Chromosomal abnormality, unspecified

CHAPTER 17. CONGENITAL MALFORMATIONS, DEFORMATIONS AND CHROMOSOMAL ABNORMALITIES　(Q97–Q99.9)

  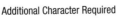 Additional Character Required 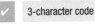 3-character code

＊=New Code
▲=Revised Code

Excludes1 Not coded here, do not use together
Excludes2—Not included here

PEDIATRIC ICD-10-CM 2017: A MANUAL FOR PROVIDER-BASED CODING

257

Chapter 18. Symptoms, signs, and abnormal clinical and laboratory findings, not elsewhere classified (R00–R99)

GUIDELINES

Chapter 18 includes symptoms, signs, abnormal results of clinical or other investigative procedures, and ill-defined conditions regarding which no diagnosis classifiable elsewhere is recorded. Signs and symptoms that point to a specific diagnosis have been assigned to a category in other chapters of the classification.

Use of symptom codes

Codes that describe symptoms and signs are acceptable for reporting purposes when a related definitive diagnosis has not been established (confirmed) by the provider.

Use of a symptom code with a definitive diagnosis code

Codes for signs and symptoms may be reported in addition to a related definitive diagnosis when the sign or symptom is not routinely associated with that diagnosis, such as the various signs and symptoms associated with complex syndromes. The definitive diagnosis code should be sequenced before the symptom code.

Signs or symptoms that are associated routinely with a disease process should not be assigned as additional codes, unless otherwise instructed by the classification.

Combination codes that include symptoms

ICD-10-CM contains a number of combination codes that identify both the definitive diagnosis and common symptoms of that diagnosis. When using one of these combination codes, an additional code should not be assigned for the symptom.

Repeated falls

Refer to the ICD-10-CM manual.

Coma scale

Refer to subcategory R40.2 for guidelines.

Functional quadriplegia

Refer to the *ICD-10-CM* manual

SIRS due to Non-Infectious Process

Refer to codes R65.10-R65.11

Death NOS

Refer to code R99

Note: This chapter includes symptoms, signs, abnormal results of clinical or other investigative procedures, and ill-defined conditions regarding which no diagnosis classifiable elsewhere is recorded.

Signs and symptoms that point rather definitely to a given diagnosis have been assigned to a category in other chapters of the classification. In general, categories in this chapter include the less well-defined conditions and symptoms that, without the necessary study of the case to establish a final diagnosis, point perhaps equally to two or more diseases or to two or more systems of the body. Practically all categories in the chapter could be designated 'not otherwise specified', 'unknown etiology' or 'transient'. The Alphabetical Index should be consulted to determine which symptoms and signs are to be allocated here and which to other chapters. The residual subcategories, numbered .8, are generally provided for other relevant symptoms that cannot be allocated elsewhere in the classification.

The conditions and signs or symptoms included in categories R00–R94 consist of:
a) cases for which no more specific diagnosis can be made even after all the facts bearing on the case have been investigated;
b) signs or symptoms existing at the time of initial encounter that proved to be transient and whose causes could not be determined;
c) provisional diagnosis in a patient who failed to return for further investigation or care;
d) cases referred elsewhere for investigation or treatment before the diagnosis was made;

e) cases in which a more precise diagnosis was not available for any other reason;
f) certain symptoms, for which supplementary information is provided, that represent important problems in medical care in their own right.

Excludes2: abnormal findings on antenatal screening of mother (O28.-)
certain conditions originating in the perinatal period (P04–P96)
signs and symptoms classified in the body system chapters signs and symptoms of breast (N63, N64.5)

(R00–R09) SYMPTOMS AND SIGNS INVOLVING THE CIRCULATORY AND RESPIRATORY SYSTEMS

R00   **ABNORMALITIES OF HEART BEAT**
(4th)   ***Excludes1:*** abnormalities originating in the perinatal period (P29.1-)
Excludes 2: specified arrhythmias (I47–I49)
   R00.0   **Tachycardia, unspecified**
     Rapid heart beat
     Sinoauricular tachycardia NOS
     Sinus [sinusal] tachycardia NOS
     Excludes1: neonatal tachycardia (P29.11)
       paroxysmal tachycardia (I47.-)
   R00.1   **Bradycardia, unspecified**
     Sinoatrial bradycardia
     Sinus bradycardia
     Slow heart beat
     Vagal bradycardia
     Use additional code for adverse effect, if applicable, to identify drug (T36–T50 with fifth or sixth character 5)
     Excludes1: neonatal bradycardia (P29.12)
   R00.2   **Palpitations**
     Awareness of heart beat
   R00.8   **Other abnormalities of heart beat**
   R00.9   **Unspecified abnormalities of heart beat**

R01   **CARDIAC MURMURS AND OTHER CARDIAC SOUNDS**
(4th)   ***Excludes1:*** cardiac murmurs and sounds originating in the perinatal period (P29.8)
   R01.0   **Benign and innocent cardiac murmurs**
     Functional cardiac murmur
   R01.1   **Cardiac murmur, unspecified**
     Cardiac bruit NOS
     Heart murmur NOS
     Systolic murmur NOS
   R01.2   **Other cardiac sounds**
     Cardiac dullness, increased or decreased
     Precordial friction

R03   **ABNORMAL BLOOD-PRESSURE READING, WITHOUT DIAGNOSIS**
(4th)   **R03.0**   **Elevated blood-pressure reading, without diagnosis of hypertension**
     Note: This category is to be used to record an episode of elevated blood pressure in a patient in whom no formal diagnosis of hypertension has been made, or as an isolated incidental finding.
   R03.1   **Nonspecific low blood-pressure reading**
     Excludes1: hypotension (I95.-)
       maternal hypotension syndrome (O26.5-)
       neurogenic orthostatic hypotension (G90.3)

R04   **HEMORRHAGE FROM RESPIRATORY PASSAGES**
(4th)   **R04.0**   **Epistaxis**
     Hemorrhage from nose
     Nosebleed
   R04.2   **Hemoptysis**
     Blood-stained sputum
     Cough with hemorrhage

  Additional Character Required   3-character code

•=New Code
▲=Revised Code

Excludes1—Not coded here, do not use together
Excludes2—Not included here

R04.8 Hemorrhage from other sites in respiratory passages

R04.81 Acute idiopathic pulmonary hemorrhage in infants *5th*
AIPHI
Acute idiopathic hemorrhage in infants over 28 days old
Excludes1: perinatal pulmonary hemorrhage (P26.-)
von Willebrand's disease (D68.0)

R04.89 Hemorrhage from other sites in respiratory passages
Pulmonary hemorrhage NOS

R04.9 Hemorrhage from respiratory passages, unspecified

R05 COUGH
Excludes1: cough with hemorrhage (R04.2)
smoker's cough (J41.0)

R06 ABNORMALITIES OF BREATHING *4th*
Excludes1: acute respiratory distress syndrome (J80)
respiratory arrest (R09.2)
respiratory arrest of newborn (P28.81)
respiratory distress syndrome of newborn (P22.-)
respiratory failure (J96.-)
respiratory failure of newborn (P28.5)

R06.0 Dyspnea *5th*
Excludes1: tachypnea NOS (R06.82)
transient tachypnea of newborn (P22.1)

R06.00 Dyspnea, unspecified
R06.01 Orthopnea
R06.02 Shortness of breath

R06.1 Stridor
Excludes1: congenital laryngeal stridor (P28.89)
laryngismus (stridulus) (J38.5)

R06.2 Wheezing
Excludes1: Asthma (J45.-)

R06.3 Periodic breathing
Cheyne-Stokes breathing

R06.4 Hyperventilation
Excludes1: psychogenic hyperventilation (F45.8)

R06.5 Mouth breathing
Excludes2: dry mouth NOS (R68.2)

R06.8 Other abnormalities of breathing *5th*

R06.81 Apnea, NEC
Apnea NOS
Excludes1: apnea (of) newborn (P28.4)
sleep apnea (G47.3-)
sleep apnea of newborn (primary) (P28.3)

R06.82 Tachypnea, NEC
Tachypnea NOS
Excludes1: transitory tachypnea of newborn (P22.1)

R06.83 Snoring
R06.89 Other abnormalities of breathing
Breath-holding (spells)
Sighing

R07 PAIN IN THROAT AND CHEST *4th*
Excludes1: epidemic myalgia (B33.0)
Excludes2: jaw pain R68.84
pain in breast (N64.4)

R07.0 Pain in throat
Excludes1: chronic sore throat (J31.2)
sore throat (acute) NOS (J02.9)
Excludes2: dysphagia (R13.1-)
pain in neck (M54.2)

R07.8 Other chest pain *5th*

R07.81 Pleurodynia
Pleurodynia NOS
Excludes1: epidemic pleurodynia (B33.0)

R07.82 Intercostal pain
R07.89 Other chest pain
Anterior chest-wall pain NOS

R07.9 Chest pain, unspecified

R09 OTHER SYMPTOMS AND SIGNS INVOLVING THE CIRCULATORY AND RESPIRATORY SYSTEM *4th*
Excludes1: acute respiratory distress syndrome (J80)
respiratory arrest of newborn (P28.81)
respiratory distress syndrome of newborn (P22.0)
respiratory failure (J96.-)
respiratory failure of newborn (P28.5)

R09.0 Asphyxia and hypoxemia *5th*
Excludes1: asphyxia due to carbon monoxide (T58.-)
asphyxia due to FB in respiratory tract (T17.-)
birth (intrauterine) asphyxia (P84)
hypercapnia (R06.4)
hyperventilation (R06.4)
traumatic asphyxia (T71.-)

R09.01 Asphyxia
R09.02 Hypoxemia

R09.1 Pleurisy
Excludes1: pleurisy with effusion (J90)

R09.2 Respiratory arrest
Cardiorespiratory failure
Excludes1: cardiac arrest (I46.-)
respiratory arrest of newborn (P28.81)
respiratory distress of newborn (P22.0)
respiratory failure (J96.-)
respiratory failure of newborn (P28.5)
respiratory insufficiency (R06.89)
respiratory insufficiency of newborn (P28.5)

R09.8 Other specified symptoms and signs involving the circulatory and respiratory systems *5th*
R09.81 Nasal congestion
R09.82 Postnasal drip
R09.89 Other specified symptoms and signs involving the circulatory and respiratory systems
Bruit (arterial)
Abnormal chest percussion
Feeling of FB in throat
Friction sounds in chest
Chest tympany
Choking sensation
Rales
Weak pulse
Excludes2: FB in throat (T17.2-)
wheezing (R06.2)

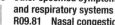
(R10–R19) SYMPTOMS AND SIGNS INVOLVING THE DIGESTIVE SYSTEM AND ABDOMEN

Excludes2: congenital or infantile pylorospasm (Q40.0)
gastrointestinal hemorrhage (K92.0–K92.2)
intestinal obstruction (K56.-)
newborn gastrointestinal hemorrhage (P54.0–P54.3)
newborn intestinal obstruction (P76.-)
pylorospasm (K31.3)
signs and symptoms involving the urinary system (R30–R39)
symptoms referable to female genital organs (N94.-)
symptoms referable to male genital organs male (N48–N50)

R10 ABDOMINAL AND PELVIC PAIN *4th*
Excludes1: renal colic (N23)
Excludes2: dorsalgia (M54.-)
flatulence and related conditions (R14.-)

R10.2 Pelvic and perineal pain
Excludes1: vulvodynia (N94.81)

R10.8 Other abdominal pain *5th*
R10.81 Abdominal tenderness *6th*
Abdominal tenderness NOS
R10.811 RUQ abdominal tenderness
R10.812 LUQ abdominal tenderness
R10.813 RLQ abdominal tenderness
R10.814 LLQ abdominal tenderness
R10.815 Periumbilic abdominal tenderness
R10.816 Epigastric abdominal tenderness
R10.817 Generalized abdominal tenderness
R10.819 Abdominal tenderness, unspecified site

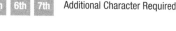 Additional Character Required 3-character code

•=New Code
▲=Revised Code

Excludes1—Not coded here, do not use together
Excludes2—Not included here

R10.82   **Rebound abdominal tenderness**
`6th`
     R10.821   **RUQ rebound abdominal tenderness**
     R10.822   **LUQ rebound abdominal tenderness**
     R10.823   **RLQ rebound abdominal tenderness**
     R10.824   **LLQ rebound abdominal tenderness**
     R10.825   **Periumbilic rebound abdominal tenderness**
     R10.826   **Epigastric rebound abdominal tenderness**
     R10.827   **Generalized rebound abdominal tenderness**
     R10.829   **Rebound abdominal tenderness, unspecified site**

R10.83   **Colic**
     Colic NOS
     Infantile colic
     Excludes1: colic in adult and child over 12 months old (R10.84)

R10.84   **Generalized abdominal pain**
     Excludes1: generalized abdominal pain associated with acute abdomen (R10.0)

R10.9   **Unspecified abdominal pain**

R11   **NAUSEA AND VOMITING**
`4th`
Excludes1: cyclical vomiting associated with migraine (G43.A-)
     excessive vomiting in pregnancy (O21.-)
     hematemesis (K92.0)
     neonatal hematemesis (P54.0)
     newborn vomiting (P92.0-)
     psychogenic vomiting (F50.89)
     vomiting associated with bulimia nervosa (F50.2)
     vomiting following gastrointestinal surgery (K91.0)

R11.0   **Nausea**
     Nausea NOS
     Nausea without vomiting

R11.1   **Vomiting**
`5th`
     R11.10   **Vomiting, unspecified**
       Vomiting NOS
     R11.11   **Vomiting without nausea**
     R11.12   **Projectile vomiting**
     R11.13   **Vomiting of fecal matter**
     R11.14   **Bilious vomiting**
       Bilious emesis

R11.2   **Nausea with vomiting, unspecified**
     Persistent nausea with vomiting NOS

R12   **HEARTBURN**
`✓`
Excludes1: dyspepsia NOS (R10.13)
     functional dyspepsia (K30)

R13   **APHAGIA AND DYSPHAGIA**
`4th`
R13.1   **Dysphagia**
`5th`
     Code first, if applicable, dysphagia following cerebrovascular disease (I69. with final characters -91)
     Excludes1: psychogenic dysphagia (F45.8)
     R13.10   **Dysphagia, unspecified**
       Difficulty in swallowing NOS
     R13.11   **Dysphagia, oral phase**
     R13.12   **Dysphagia, oropharyngeal phase**
     R13.13   **Dysphagia, pharyngeal phase**
     R13.14   **Dysphagia, pharyngoesophageal phase**
     R13.19   **Other dysphagia**
       Cervical dysphagia
       Neurogenic dysphagia

R14   **FLATULENCE AND RELATED CONDITIONS**
`4th`
Excludes1: psychogenic aerophagy (F45.8)
R14.0   **Abdominal distension (gaseous)**
     Bloating
     Tympanites (abdominal) (intestinal)

R15   **FECAL INCONTINENCE**
`4th`
Includes: encopresis NOS
Excludes1: fecal incontinence of nonorganic origin (F98.1)
R15.0   **Incomplete defecation**
     Excludes1: constipation (K59.0-)
       fecal impaction (K56.41)

R15.1   **Fecal smearing**
     Fecal soiling

R15.2   **Fecal urgency**

R15.9   **Full incontinence of feces**
     Fecal incontinence NOS

R16   **HEPATOMEGALY AND SPLENOMEGALY, NEC**
`4th`
R16.0   **Hepatomegaly, NEC**
     Hepatomegaly NOS

R16.1   **Splenomegaly, NEC**
     Splenomegaly NOS

R16.2   **Hepatomegaly with splenomegaly, NEC**
     Hepatosplenomegaly NOS

R17   **UNSPECIFIED JAUNDICE**
`✓`
Excludes1: neonatal jaundice (P55, P57–P59)

R18   **ASCITES**
`4th`
Includes: fluid in peritoneal cavity
Excludes1: ascites in alcoholic cirrhosis (K70.31)
     ascites in alcoholic hepatitis (K70.11)
     ascites in toxic liver disease with chronic active hepatitis (K71.51)

R18.0   **Malignant ascites**
     Code first malignancy, such as: malignant neoplasm of ovary (C56.-)
       secondary malignant neoplasm of retroperitoneum and peritoneum (C78.6)

R18.8   **Other ascites**
     Ascites NOS
     Peritoneal effusion (chronic)

R19   **OTHER SYMPTOMS AND SIGNS INVOLVING THE DIGESTIVE SYSTEM AND ABDOMEN**
`4th`
Excludes1: acute abdomen (R10.0)
R19.0   **Intra-abdominal and pelvic swelling, mass and lump**
`5th`
     Excludes1: abdominal distension (gaseous) (R14.-)
       ascites (R18.-)
     R19.00   **Intra-abdominal and pelvic swelling, mass and lump, unspecified site**
     R19.01   **RUQ abdominal swelling, mass and lump**
     R19.02   **LUQ abdominal swelling, mass and lump**
     R19.03   **RLQ abdominal swelling, mass and lump**
     R19.04   **LLQ abdominal swelling, mass and lump**
     R19.05   **Periumbilic swelling, mass or lump**
       Diffuse or generalized umbilical swelling or mass
     R19.06   **Epigastric swelling, mass or lump**
     R19.07   **Generalized intra-abdominal and pelvic swelling, mass and lump**
       Diffuse or generalized intra-abdominal swelling or mass NOS
       Diffuse or generalized pelvic swelling or mass NOS
     R19.09   **Other intra-abdominal and pelvic swelling, mass and lump**

R19.1   **Abnormal bowel sounds**
`5th`
     R19.11   **Absent bowel sounds**
     R19.12   **Hyperactive bowel sounds**
     R19.15   **Other abnormal bowel sounds**
       Abnormal bowel sounds NOS

R19.2   **Visible peristalsis**
     Hyperperistalsis

R19.3   **Abdominal rigidity**
`5th`
     Excludes1: abdominal rigidity with severe abdominal pain (R10.0)
     R19.30   **Abdominal rigidity, unspecified site**
     R19.31   **RUQ abdominal rigidity**
     R19.32   **LUQ abdominal rigidity**
     R19.33   **RLQ abdominal rigidity**
     R19.34   **LLQ abdominal rigidity**
     R19.35   **Periumbilic abdominal rigidity**
     R19.36   **Epigastric abdominal rigidity**
     R19.37   **Generalized abdominal rigidity**

R19.4   **Change in bowel habit**
     Excludes1: constipation (K59.0-)
       functional diarrhea (K59.1)

     Additional Character Required   3-character code   ∎ —New Code   ▲ =Revised Code   *Excludes1*—Not coded here, do not use together   *Excludes2*—Not included here

R19.5 Other fecal abnormalities
Abnormal stool color
Bulky stools
Mucus in stools
Occult blood in feces
Occult blood in stools
Excludes1: melena (K92.1)
    neonatal melena (P54.1)

R19.6 Halitosis

R19.7 Diarrhea, unspecified
Diarrhea NOS
Excludes1: functional diarrhea (K59.1)
    neonatal diarrhea (P78.3)
    psychogenic diarrhea (F45.8)

R19.8 Other specified symptoms and signs involving the digestive system and abdomen

(R20–R23) SYMPTOMS AND SIGNS INVOLVING THE SKIN AND SUBCUTANEOUS TISSUE

Excludes2: symptoms relating to breast (N64.4–N64.5)

R21 RASH AND OTHER NONSPECIFIC SKIN ERUPTION

Includes: rash NOS
Excludes1: specified type of rash—code to condition
    vesicular eruption (R23.8)

R22 LOCALIZED SWELLING, MASS AND LUMP OF SKIN AND SUBCUTANEOUS TISSUE
Includes: subcutaneous nodules (localized)(superficial)
Excludes1: abnormal findings on diagnostic imaging (R90–R93)
    edema (R60.-)
    enlarged lymph nodes (R59.-)
    localized adiposity (E65)
    swelling of joint (M25.4-)

R22.0 Localized swelling, mass and lump; head

R22.1   neck

R22.2   trunk
Excludes1: intra-abdominal or pelvic mass and lump (R19.0-)
    intra-abdominal or pelvic swelling (R19.0-)
Excludes2: breast mass and lump (N63)

R22.3 Localized swelling, mass and lump, upper limb
   R22.31 Localized swelling, mass and lump; right upper limb
   R22.32   left upper limb
   R22.33   upper limb, bilateral

R22.4 Localized swelling, mass and lump, lower limb
   R22.41 Localized swelling, mass and lump; right lower limb
   R22.42   left lower limb
   R22.43   lower limb, bilateral

R22.9 Localized swelling, mass and lump, unspecified

R23 OTHER SKIN CHANGES
R23.0 Cyanosis
Excludes1: acrocyanosis (I73.8)
    cyanotic attacks of newborn (P28.2)

R23.1 Pallor
Clammy skin

R23.3 Spontaneous ecchymoses
Petechiae
Excludes1: ecchymoses of newborn (P54.5)
    purpura (D69.-)

(R25–R29) SYMPTOMS AND SIGNS INVOLVING THE NERVOUS AND MUSCULOSKELETAL SYSTEMS

R25 ABNORMAL INVOLUNTARY MOVEMENTS
Excludes1: specific movement disorders (G20–G26)
    stereotyped movement disorders (F98.4)
    tic disorders (F95.-)
R25.1 Tremor, unspecified
Excludes1: chorea NOS (G25.5)
    essential tremor (G25.0)
    hysterical tremor (F44.4)
    intention tremor (G25.2)

R25.2 Cramp and spasm
Excludes2: carpopedal spasm (R29.0)
    charley-horse (M62.831)
    infantile spasms (G40.4-)
    muscle spasm of back (M62.830)
    muscle spasm of calf (M62.831)

R26 ABNORMALITIES OF GAIT AND MOBILITY
Excludes1: ataxia NOS (R27.0)
    hereditary ataxia (G11.-)
    locomotor (syphilitic) ataxia (A52.11)
    immobility syndrome (paraplegic) (M62.3)

R26.0 Ataxic gait
Staggering gait

R26.1 Paralytic gait
Spastic gait

R26.2 Difficulty in walking, NEC
Excludes1: falling (R29.6)
    unsteadiness on feet (R26.81)

R26.8 Other abnormalities of gait and mobility
   R26.81 Unsteadiness on feet
   R26.89 Other abnormalities of gait and mobility

R26.9 Unspecified abnormalities of gait and mobility

R27 OTHER LACK OF COORDINATION
Excludes1: ataxic gait (R26.0)
    hereditary ataxia (G11.-)
    vertigo NOS (R42)

R27.0 Ataxia, unspecified
Excludes1: ataxia following cerebrovascular disease (I69. with final characters -93)

R27.8 Other lack of coordination

R27.9 Unspecified lack of coordination

R29 OTHER SYMPTOMS AND SIGNS INVOLVING THE NERVOUS AND MUSCULOSKELETAL SYSTEMS
R29.1 Meningismus
R29.3 Abnormal posture
R29.4 Clicking hip
Excludes1: congenital deformities of hip (Q65.-)

R29.8 Other symptoms and signs involving the nervous and musculoskeletal systems
   R29.81 Other symptoms and signs involving the nervous system
     R29.810 Facial weakness
      Facial droop
     R29.818 Other symptoms and signs involving the nervous system
   R29.89 Other symptoms and signs involving the musculoskeletal system
     Excludes2: pain in limb (M79.6-)
     R29.891 Ocular torticollis
      Excludes1: congenital (sternomastoid) torticollis Q68.0
       psychogenic torticollis (F45.8)
       spasmodic torticollis (G24.3)
       torticollis due to birth injury (P15.8)
       torticollis NOS M43.6
     R29.898 Other symptoms and signs involving the musculoskeletal system

R29.9 Unspecified symptoms and signs involving the; nervous and musculoskeletal systems
   R29.90 nervous system
   R29.91 musculoskeletal system

(R30–R39) SYMPTOMS AND SIGNS INVOLVING THE GENITOURINARY SYSTEM

R30 PAIN ASSOCIATED WITH MICTURITION

Excludes1: psychogenic pain associated with micturition (F45.8)
R30.0 Dysuria
Strangury

 4th   5th   6th   7th   Additional Character Required   ✓ 3-character code   •=New Code   *Excludes1*—Not coded here, do not use together
▲=Revised Code   *Excludes2*—Not included here

R31   HEMATURIA

4th

Excludes1: hematuria included with underlying conditions, such as:
    acute cystitis with hematuria (N30.01)
    recurrent and persistent hematuria in glomerular diseases (N02.-)

R31.0   Gross hematuria
R31.1   Benign essential microscopic hematuria
R31.2   Other microscopic hematuria

5th
  •**R31.21**   Asymptomatic microscopic hematuria
  •**R31.29**   Other microscopic hematuria

R31.9   Hematuria, unspecified

R32   UNSPECIFIED URINARY INCONTINENCE

✓

Enuresis NOS

Excludes1: functional urinary incontinence (R39.81)
    nonorganic enuresis (F98.0)
    stress incontinence and other specified urinary incontinence
      (N39.3–N39.4-)
    urinary incontinence associated with cognitive impairment (R39.81)

R33   RETENTION OF URINE

4th

Excludes1: psychogenic retention of urine (F45.8)

R33.8   Other retention of urine
    Code first, if applicable, any causal condition, such as:
      enlarged prostate (N40.1)

R33.9   Retention of urine, unspecified

R34   ANURIA AND OLIGURIA

✓

Excludes1: anuria and oliguria complicating abortion or ectopic or
    molar pregnancy (O00–O07, O08.4)
    anuria and oliguria complicating pregnancy (O26.83–)

R35   POLYURIA

4th

Code first , if applicable, any causal condition, such as: enlarged
    prostate (N40.1)

Excludes1: psychogenic polyuria (F45.8)

R35.0   Frequency of micturition
R35.1   Nocturia
R35.8   Other polyuria
    Polyuria NOS

R36   URETHRAL DISCHARGE

4th

R36.0   Urethral discharge without blood
R36.1   Hematospermia
R36.9   Urethral discharge, unspecified
    Penile discharge NOS
    Urethrorrhea

R37   SEXUAL DYSFUNCTION, UNSPECIFIED

✓

R39   OTHER AND UNSPECIFIED SYMPTOMS AND SIGNS INVOLVING THE GENITOURINARY SYSTEM

4th

R39.0   Extravasation of urine
R39.1   Other difficulties with micturition

5th
    Code first, if applicable, any causal condition, such as:
      enlarged prostate (N40.1)

  R39.11   Hesitancy of micturition
  R39.12   Poor urinary stream
    Weak urinary steam
  R39.13   Splitting of urinary stream
  R39.14   Feeling of incomplete bladder emptying
  R39.15   Urgency of urination
    Excludes1: urge incontinence (N39.41, N39.46)
  R39.16   Straining to void
  R39.19   Other difficulties with micturition

6th
    •**R39.191**   Need to immediately re-void
    •**R39.192**   Position dependent micturition
    •**R39.198**   Other difficulties with micturition

R39.8   Other symptoms and signs involving the genitourinary system

5th
  R39.81   Functional urinary incontinence
  •**R39.82**   Chronic bladder pain
  R39.89   Other symptoms and signs involving the
    genitourinary system

R39.9   Unspecified symptoms and signs involving the
    genitourinary system

(R40–R46) SYMPTOMS AND SIGNS INVOLVING COGNITION, PERCEPTION, EMOTIONAL STATE AND BEHAVIOR

Excludes2: symptoms and signs constituting part of a pattern of mental disorder (F01–F99)

R40   SOMNOLENCE, STUPOR AND COMA

4th

Excludes1: neonatal coma (P91.5)
    somnolence, stupor and coma in diabetes (E08–E13)
    somnolence, stupor and coma in hepatic failure (K72.-)
    somnolence, stupor and coma in hypoglycemia (nondiabetic) (E15)

R40.1   Stupor
    Catatonic stupor
    Semicoma
    Excludes1: catatonic schizophrenia (F20.2)
      coma (R40.2-)
      depressive stupor (F31–F33)
      dissociative stupor (F44.2)
      manic stupor (F30.2)

R40.2   Coma

5th

GUIDELINES

The coma scale codes (R40.2-) can be used in conjunction with traumatic brain injury codes, acute cerebrovascular disease or sequelae of cerebrovascular disease codes. These codes are primarily for use by trauma registries, but they may be used in any setting where this information is collected. The coma scale codes should be sequenced after the diagnosis code(s).

These codes, one from each subcategory, are needed to complete the scale. The 7th character indicates when the scale was recorded. The 7th character should match for all three codes.

At a minimum, report the initial score documented on presentation at your facility. This may be a score from the emergency medicine technician (EMT) or in the emergency department. If desired, a facility may choose to capture multiple coma scale scores.

Assign code R40.24, Glasgow coma scale, total score, when only the total score is documented in the medical record and not the individual score(s).

Code first any associated: fracture of skull (S02.-)
    intracranial injury (S06.-)

Note: One code from each subcategory R40.21–R40.23 is required
    to complete the coma scale

R40.20   Unspecified coma
    Coma NOS
    Unconsciousness NOS

R40.21   Coma scale, eyes open

6th
  R40.211   Coma scale, eyes open, never

7th
    R40.2110   Coma scale, eyes open, never;
      unspecified time
    R40.2111   in the field [EMT or
      ambulance]
    R40.2112   at arrival to emergency
      department
    R40.2113   at hospital admission
    R40.2114   24 hours or more after
      hospital admission

  R40.212   Coma scale, eyes open, to pain

7th
    R40.2120   Coma scale, eyes open, to pain;
      unspecified time
    R40.2121   in the field [EMT or
      ambulance]
    R40.2122   at arrival to emergency
      department
    R40.2123   at hospital admission
    R40.2124   24 hours or more after
      hospital admission

4th   **5th**   **6th**   **7th**   Additional Character Required   ✓   3-character code   •=New Code   ▲=Revised Code   ***Excludes1***— Not coded here, do not use together   ***Excludes2***—Not included here

R40.213   Coma scale, eyes open, to sound

[7th]

R40.2130   Coma scale, eyes open, to sound; unspecified time

R40.2131   in the field [EMT or ambulance]

R40.2132   at arrival to emergency department

R40.2133   at hospital admission

R40.2134   24 hours or more after hospital admission

R40.214   Coma scale, eyes open, spontaneous

[7th]

R40.2140   Coma scale, eyes open, spontaneous; unspecified time

R40.2141   in the field [EMT or ambulance]

R40.2142   at arrival to emergency department

R40.2143   at hospital admission

R40.2144   24 hours or more after hospital admission

R40.3   Persistent vegetative state

R41   **OTHER SYMPTOMS AND SIGNS INVOLVING COGNITIVE FUNCTIONS AND AWARENESS**

[4th]

Excludes1: dissociative [conversion] disorders (F44.-)
    mild cognitive impairment, so stated (G31.84)

R41.8   **Other symptoms and signs involving cognitive functions and awareness**

[5th]

R41.82   **Altered mental status, unspecified**
    Change in mental status NOS
    Excludes1: altered level of consciousness (R40.-)
      altered mental status due to known condition—code to condition
      delirium NOS (R41.0)

R41.83   **Borderline intellectual functioning**
    IQ level 71 to 84
    Excludes1: intellectual disabilities (F70–F79)

R41.84   **Other specified cognitive deficit**

[6th]

    Excludes1: cognitive deficits as sequelae of cerebrovascular disease (I69.01-, I69.11-, I69.21-, I69.31-, I69.81-, I69.91-)

R41.840   **Attention and concentration deficit**
    Excludes1: attention-deficit hyperactivity disorders (F90.-)

R41.841   **Cognitive communication deficit**

R41.842   **Visuospatial deficit**

R41.843   **Psychomotor deficit**

R41.844   **Frontal lobe and executive function deficit**

R41.89   **Other symptoms and signs involving cognitive functions and awareness**
    Anosognosia

R41.9   **Unspecified symptoms and signs involving cognitive functions and awareness**

R42   **DIZZINESS AND GIDDINESS**

[✔]

Light-headedness
Vertigo NOS
Excludes1: vertiginous syndromes (H81.-)
    vertigo from infrasound (T75.23)

R44   **OTHER SYMPTOMS AND SIGNS INVOLVING GENERAL SENSATIONS AND PERCEPTIONS**

[4th]

Excludes1: alcoholic hallucinations (F1.5)
    hallucinations in drug psychosis (F11–F19 with .5)
    hallucinations in mood disorders with psychotic symptoms (F30.2, F31.5, F32.3, F33.3)
    hallucinations in schizophrenia, schizotypal and delusional disorders (F20–F29)
Excludes2: disturbances of skin sensation (R20.-)

R44.0   **Auditory hallucinations**

R44.1   **Visual hallucinations**

R44.2   **Other hallucinations**

R44.3   **Hallucinations, unspecified**

R44.8   **Other symptoms and signs involving general sensations and perceptions**

R44.9   **Unspecified symptoms and signs involving general sensations and perceptions**

R45   **SYMPTOMS AND SIGNS INVOLVING EMOTIONAL STATE**

[4th]

R45.0   **Nervousness**
    Nervous tension

R45.1   **Restlessness and agitation**

R45.2   **Unhappiness**

R45.3   **Demoralization and apathy**
    Excludes1: anhedonia (R45.84)

R45.4   **Irritability and anger**

R45.5   **Hostility**

R45.6   **Violent behavior**

R45.7   **State of emotional shock and stress, unspecified**

R45.8   **Other symptoms and signs involving emotional state**

[5th]

R45.81   **Low self-esteem**

R45.82   **Worries**

R45.83   **Excessive crying of child, adolescent or adult**
    Excludes1: excessive crying of infant (baby) R68.11

R45.84   **Anhedonia**

R45.85   **Homicidal and suicidal ideations**

R45.86   **Emotional lability**

R45.87   **Impulsiveness**

R45.89   **Other symptoms and signs involving emotional state**

R46   **SYMPTOMS AND SIGNS INVOLVING APPEARANCE AND BEHAVIOR**

[4th]

Excludes1: appearance and behavior in schizophrenia, schizotypal and delusional disorders (F20–F29)
    mental and behavioral disorders (F01–F99)

R46.0   **Very low level of personal hygiene**

R46.1   **Bizarre personal appearance**

R46.2   **Strange and inexplicable behavior**

R46.3   **Overactivity**

R46.4   **Slowness and poor responsiveness**
    Excludes 1: stupor (R40.1)

R46.5   **Suspiciousness and marked evasiveness**

R46.6   **Undue concern and preoccupation with stressful events**

R46.7   **Verbosity and circumstantial detail obscuring reason for contact**

R46.8   **Other symptoms and signs involving appearance and behavior**

[5th]

R46.81   **Obsessive-compulsive behavior**
    obsessive-compulsive disorder (F42-)

R46.89   **Other symptoms and signs involving appearance and behavior**

(R47–R49) SYMPTOMS AND SIGNS INVOLVING SPEECH AND VOICE

R47   **SPEECH DISTURBANCES, NEC**

[4th]

Excludes1: autism (F84.0)
    cluttering (F80.81)
    specific developmental disorders of speech and language (F80.-)
    stuttering (F80.81)

R47.1   **Dysarthria and anarthria**
    Excludes1: dysarthria following cerebrovascular disease (I69. with final characters -22)

R47.8   **Other speech disturbances**

[5th]

    Excludes1: dysarthria following cerebrovascular disease (I69. with final characters -28)

R47.81   **Slurred speech**

R47.82   **Fluency disorder in conditions classified elsewhere**
    Stuttering in conditions classified elsewhere
    Code first underlying disease or condition, such as: Parkinson's disease (G20)
    Excludes1: adult onset fluency disorder (F98.5)
      childhood onset fluency disorder (F80.81)
      fluency disorder (stuttering) following cerebrovascular disease (I69. with final characters -23)

R47.89   **Other speech disturbances**

R47.9   **Unspecified speech disturbances**

R48 DYSLEXIA AND OTHER SYMBOLIC DYSFUNCTIONS, NEC
4th **Excludes1:** specific developmental disorders of scholastic skills (F81.-)
R48.0 Dyslexia and alexia

R49 VOICE AND RESONANCE DISORDERS
4th **Excludes1:** psychogenic voice and resonance disorders (F44.4)
R49.0 Dysphonia
Hoarseness
R49.1 Aphonia
Loss of voice
R49.2 Hypernasality and hyponasality
5th **R49.21 Hypernasality**
R49.22 Hyponasality
R49.8 Other voice and resonance disorders
R49.9 Unspecified voice and resonance disorder
Change in voice NOS
Resonance disorder NOS

(R50–R69) GENERAL SYMPTOMS AND SIGNS

R50 FEVER OF OTHER AND UNKNOWN ORIGIN
4th **Excludes1:** chills without fever (R68.83)
febrile convulsions (R56.0-)
fever of unknown origin during labor (O75.2)
fever of unknown origin in newborn (P81.9)
hypothermia due to illness (R68.0)
malignant hyperthermia due to anesthesia (T88.3)
puerperal pyrexia NOS (O86.4)
R50.2 Drug induced fever
Use additional code for adverse effect, if applicable, to identify drug (T36–T50 with fifth or sixth character 5)
Excludes1: postvaccination (postimmunization) fever (R50.83)
R50.8 Other specified fever
5th **R50.81 Fever presenting with conditions classified elsewhere**   Do not use R50.81 with acute conditions
Code first underlying condition when associated fever is present, such as with: leukemia (C91–C95)
neutropenia (D70.-)
sickle-cell disease (D57.-)
R50.82 Postprocedural fever
Excludes1: postprocedural infection (T81.4-)
posttransfusion fever (R50.84)
postvaccination (postimmunization) fever (R50.83)
R50.83 Postvaccination fever
Postimmunization fever
R50.84 Febrile nonhemolytic transfusion reaction
FNHTR
Posttransfusion fever
R50.9 Fever, unspecified
Fever NOS
Fever of unknown origin [FUO]
Fever with chills
Fever with rigors
Hyperpyrexia NOS
Persistent fever

R51 HEADACHE
✓ Facial pain NOS
Excludes1: atypical face pain (G50.1)
migraine and other headache syndromes (G43–G44)
trigeminal neuralgia (G50.0)

R52 PAIN, UNSPECIFIED
✓ Acute pain NOS
Generalized pain NOS
Pain NOS
Excludes1: acute and chronic pain, NEC (G89.-)
localized pain, unspecified type—code to pain by site, such as:
abdomen pain (R10.-)
back pain (M54.9)
breast pain (N64.4)
chest pain (R07.1–R07.9)

ear pain (H92.0-)
eye pain (H57.1)
headache (R51)
joint pain (M25.5-)
limb pain (M79.6-)
lumbar region pain (M54.5)
pelvic and perineal pain (R10.2)
shoulder pain (M25.51-)
spine pain (M54.-)
throat pain (R07.0)
tongue pain (K14.6)
tooth pain (K08.8)
renal colic (N23)
pain disorders exclusively related to psychological factors (F45.41)

R53 MALAISE AND FATIGUE
R53.1 Weakness
4th Asthenia NOS
Excludes1: muscle weakness (M62.8-)
sarcopenia (M62.84)
R53.8 Other malaise and fatigue
5th **Excludes1:** combat exhaustion and fatigue (F43.0)
congenital debility (P96.9)
exhaustion and fatigue due to depressive episode (F32.-)
exhaustion and fatigue due to excessive exertion (T73.3)
exhaustion and fatigue due to exposure (T73.2)
exhaustion and fatigue due to heat (T67.-)
exhaustion and fatigue due to recurrent depressive episode (F33)
R53.81 Other malaise
Chronic debility
Debility NOS
General physical deterioration
Malaise NOS
Nervous debility
Excludes1: age-related physical debility (R54)
R53.82 Chronic fatigue, unspecified
Chronic fatigue syndrome NOS
Excludes1: postviral fatigue syndrome (G93.3)
R53.83 Other fatigue
Fatigue NOS
Lack of energy
Lethargy
Tiredness

R55 SYNCOPE AND COLLAPSE
✓ Blackout
Fainting
Vasovagal attack
Excludes1: cardiogenic shock (R57.0)
carotid sinus syncope (G90.01)
heat syncope (T67.1)
neurocirculatory asthenia (F45.8)
neurogenic orthostatic hypotension (G90.3)
orthostatic hypotension (I95.1)
postprocedural shock (T81.1-)
psychogenic syncope (F48.8)
shock NOS (R57.9)
shock complicating or following abortion or ectopic or molar pregnancy (O00–O07, O08.3)
Stokes-Adams attack (I45.9)
unconsciousness NOS (R40.2-)

R56 CONVULSIONS, NEC
4th **Excludes1:** dissociative convulsions and seizures (F44.5)
epileptic convulsions and seizures (G40.-)
newborn convulsions and seizures (P90)
R56.0 Febrile convulsions
5th **R56.00 Simple febrile convulsions**
Febrile convulsion NOS
Febrile seizure NOS

| **4th** **5th** **6th** **7th** | Additional Character Required | ✓ | 3-character code |

•=New Code   **Excludes1**—Not coded here, do not use together
▲=Revised Code   **Excludes2**—Not included here

CHAPTER 18. SYMPTOMS, SIGNS, AND ABNORMAL CLINICAL AND LABORATORY FINDINGS, NOT ELSEWHERE CLASSIFIED   (R56.01–R63.8)

R56.01   Complex febrile convulsions
Atypical febrile seizure
Complex febrile seizure
Complicated febrile seizure
Excludes1: status epilepticus (G40.901)

R56.1   Post traumatic seizures
Excludes1: post traumatic epilepsy (G40.-)

R56.9   Unspecified convulsions
Convulsion disorder
Fit NOS
Recurrent convulsions
Seizure(s) (convulsive) NOS

R57   SHOCK, NEC

Excludes1: anaphylactic shock NOS (T78.2)
anaphylactic reaction or shock due to adverse food reaction (T78.0-)
anaphylactic shock due to adverse effect of correct drug or medicament properly administered (T88.6)
anaphylactic shock due to serum (T80.5-)
anesthetic shock (T88.3)
electric shock (T75.4)
obstetric shock (O75.1)
postprocedural shock (T81.1-)
psychic shock (F43.0)
septic shock (R65.21)
shock complicating or following ectopic or molar pregnancy (O00–O07, O08.3)
shock due to lightning (T75.01)
traumatic shock (T79.4)
toxic shock syndrome (A48.3)

R57.0   Cardiogenic shock
R57.1   Hypovolemic shock
R57.8   Other shock
R57.9   Shock, unspecified
Failure of peripheral circulation NOS

R58   HEMORRHAGE, NEC

Hemorrhage NOS
Excludes1: hemorrhage included with underlying conditions, such as:
acute duodenal ulcer with hemorrhage (K26.0)
acute gastritis with bleeding (K29.01)
ulcerative enterocolitis with rectal bleeding (K51.01)

R59   ENLARGED LYMPH NODES

Includes: swollen glands
Excludes1: lymphadenitis NOS (I88.9)
acute lymphadenitis (L04.-)
chronic lymphadenitis (I88.1)
mesenteric (acute) (chronic) lymphadenitis (I88.0)

R59.0   Localized enlarged lymph nodes
R59.1   Generalized enlarged lymph nodes
Lymphadenopathy NOS
R59.9   Enlarged lymph nodes, unspecified

R60   EDEMA, NEC

Excludes1: angioneurotic edema (T78.3)
ascites (R18.-)
cerebral edema (G93.6)
cerebral edema due to birth injury (P11.0)
edema of larynx (J38.4)
edema of nasopharynx (J39.2)
edema of pharynx (J39.2)
gestational edema (O12.0-)
hereditary edema (Q82.0)
hydrops fetalis NOS (P83.2)
hydrothorax (J94.8)
nutritional edema (E40–E46)
hydrops fetalis NOS (P83.2)
newborn edema (P83.3)
pulmonary edema (J81.-)

R60.0   Localized edema
R60.1   Generalized edema
R60.9   Edema, unspecified
Fluid retention NOS

R61   GENERALIZED HYPERHIDROSIS

Excessive sweating
Night sweats
Secondary hyperhidrosis
Code first, if applicable, menopausal and female climacteric states (N95.1)
Excludes1: focal (primary) (secondary) hyperhidrosis (L74.5-)
Frey's syndrome (L74.52)
localized (primary) (secondary) hyperhidrosis (L74.5-)

R62   LACK OF EXPECTED NORMAL PHYSIOLOGICAL DEVELOPMENT IN CHILDHOOD AND ADULTS
Excludes1: delayed puberty (E30.0)
gonadal dysgenesis (Q99.1)
hypopituitarism (E23.0)

R62.0   Delayed milestone in childhood
Delayed attainment of expected physiological developmental stage
Late talker
Late walker

R62.5   Other and unspecified lack of expected normal physiological development in childhood
Excludes1: HIV disease resulting in failure to thrive (B20)
physical retardation due to malnutrition (E45)

R62.50   Unspecified lack of expected normal physiological development in childhood
Infantilism NOS

R62.51   Failure to thrive (child)
Failure to gain weight
Excludes1: failure to thrive in child under 28 days old (P92.6)

R62.52   Short stature (child)
Lack of growth
Physical retardation
Short stature NOS
Excludes1: short stature due to endocrine disorder (E34.3)

R62.59   Other lack of expected normal physiological development in childhood

R63   SYMPTOMS AND SIGNS CONCERNING FOOD AND FLUID INTAKE
Excludes1: bulimia NOS (F50.2)
eating disorders of nonorganic origin (F50.-)
malnutrition (E40–E46)

R63.0   Anorexia
Loss of appetite
Excludes1: anorexia nervosa (F50.0-)
loss of appetite of nonorganic origin (F50.89)

R63.1   Polydipsia
Excessive thirst

R63.2   Polyphagia
Excessive eating
Hyperalimentation NOS

R63.3   Feeding difficulties
Feeding problem (elderly) (infant) NOS
Excludes1: feeding problems of newborn (P92.-)
infant feeding disorder of nonorganic origin (F98.2-)

R63.4   Abnormal weight loss
R63.5   Abnormal weight gain
Excludes1: excessive weight gain in pregnancy (O26.0-)
obesity (E66.-)

R63.6   Underweight
Use additional code to identify body mass index (BMI), if known (Z68.-)
Excludes1: abnormal weight loss (R63.4)
anorexia nervosa (F50.0-)
malnutrition (E40–E46)

R63.8   Other symptoms and signs concerning food and fluid intake

---

  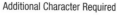 Additional Character Required   3-character code

*=New Code
▲=Revised Code

Excludes1—Not coded here, do not use together
Excludes2—Not included here

R65 SYMPTOMS AND SIGNS SPECIFICALLY ASSOCIATED WITH SYSTEMIC INFLAMMATION AND INFECTION

R65.1 SIRS of non-infectious origin

GUIDELINE

The SIRS can develop as a result of certain non-infectious disease processes, such as trauma, malignant neoplasm, or pancreatitis. When SIRS is documented with a noninfectious condition, and no subsequent infection is documented, the code for the underlying condition, such as an injury, should be assigned, followed by code R65.10 or code R65.11. If an associated acute organ dysfunction is documented, the appropriate code(s) for the specific type of organ dysfunction(s) should be assigned in addition to code R65.11. If acute organ dysfunction is documented, but it cannot be determined if the acute organ dysfunction is associated with SIRS or due to another condition (e.g., directly due to the trauma), the provider should be queried.

Code first underlying condition, such as: heatstroke (T67.0)
injury and trauma (S00–T88)

Excludes1: sepsis- code to infection
severe sepsis (R65.2)

R65.10 SIRS of non-infectious origin without acute organ dysfunction
SIRS NOS

R65.11 SIRS of non-infectious origin with acute organ dysfunction
Use additional code to identify specific acute organ dysfunction, such as:
acute kidney failure (N17.-)
cute respiratory failure (J96.0-)
critical illness myopathy (G72.81)
critical illness polyneuropathy (G62.81)
disseminated intravascular coagulopathy [DIC] (D65)
encephalopathy (metabolic) (septic) (G93.41)
hepatic failure (K72.0-)

R65.2 Severe sepsis
Infection with associated acute organ dysfunction
Sepsis with acute organ dysfunction
Sepsis with multiple organ dysfunction
SIRS due to infectious process with acute organ dysfunction
Code first underlying infection, such as: infection following a procedure (T81.4-)
infections following infusion, transfusion and therapeutic injection (T80.2-)
puerperal sepsis (O85)
sepsis following complete or unspecified spontaneous abortion (O03.87)
sepsis following ectopic and molar pregnancy (O08.82)
sepsis following incomplete spontaneous abortion (O03.37)
sepsis following (induced) termination of pregnancy (O04.87)
sepsis NOS (A41.9)
Use additional code to identify specific acute organ dysfunction, such as:
acute kidney failure (N17.-)
acute respiratory failure (J96.0-)
critical illness myopathy (G72.81)
critical illness polyneuropathy (G62.81)
disseminated intravascular coagulopathy [DIC] (D65)
encephalopathy (metabolic) (septic) (G93.41)
hepatic failure (K72.0-)

R65.20 Severe sepsis without septic shock
Severe sepsis NOS

R65.21 Severe sepsis with septic shock

R68 OTHER GENERAL SYMPTOMS AND SIGNS

R68.0 Hypothermia, not associated with low environmental temperature
Excludes1: hypothermia NOS (accidental) (T68)
hypothermia due to anesthesia (T88.51)
hypothermia due to low environmental temperature (T68)
newborn hypothermia (P80.-)

R68.1 Nonspecific symptoms peculiar to infancy

Excludes1: colic, infantile (R10.83)
neonatal cerebral irritability (P91.3)
teething syndrome (K00.7)

R68.11 Excessive crying of infant (baby)
Excludes1: excessive crying of child, adolescent, or adult (R45.83)

R68.12 Fussy infant (baby)
Irritable infant

R68.13 Apparent life threatening event in infant (ALTE)
Apparent life threatening event in newborn
Code first confirmed diagnosis, if known
Use additional code(s) for associated signs and symptoms if no confirmed diagnosis established, or if signs and symptoms are not associated routinely with confirmed diagnosis, or provide additional information for cause of ALTE

R68.19 Other nonspecific symptoms peculiar to infancy

R68.2 Dry mouth, unspecified
Excludes1: dry mouth due to dehydration (E86.0)
dry mouth due to sicca syndrome [Sjögren] (M35.0-)
salivary gland hyposecretion (K11.7)

R68.3 Clubbing of fingers
Clubbing of nails
Excludes1: congenital club finger (Q68.1)

R68.8 Other general symptoms and signs

R68.81 Early satiety

R68.83 Chills (without fever)
Chills NOS
Excludes1: chills with fever (R50.9)

R68.84 Jaw pain
Mandibular pain
Maxilla pain
Excludes1: temporomandibular joint arthralgia (M26.62-)

R68.89 Other general symptoms and signs

R69 ILLNESS, UNSPECIFIED

Unknown and unspecified cases of morbidity

(R70–R79) ABNORMAL FINDINGS ON EXAMINATION OF BLOOD, WITHOUT DIAGNOSIS

Excludes2: abnormalities (of) (on):
abnormal findings on antenatal screening of mother (O28.-)
coagulation hemorrhagic disorders (D65–D68)
lipids (E78.-)
platelets and thrombocytes (D69.-)
white blood cells classified elsewhere (D70–D72)
diagnostic abnormal findings classified elsewhere—see Alphabetical Index
hemorrhagic and hematological disorders of newborn (P50–P61)

R70 ELEVATED ERYTHROCYTE SEDIMENTATION RATE AND ABNORMALITY OF PLASMA VISCOSITY

R70.0 Elevated erythrocyte sedimentation rate

R71 ABNORMALITY OF RED BLOOD CELLS
Excludes1: anemias (D50–D64)
anemia of premature infant (P61.2)
benign (familial) polycythemia (D75.0)
congenital anemias (P61.2–P61.4)
newborn anemia due to isoimmunization (P55.-)
polycythemia neonatorum (P61.1)
polycythemia NOS (D75.1)
polycythemia vera (D45)
secondary polycythemia (D75.1)

R71.0 Precipitous drop in hematocrit
Drop (precipitous) in hemoglobin
Drop in hematocrit

R71.8 Other abnormality of red blood cells
Abnormal red-cell morphology NOS
Abnormal red-cell volume NOS
Anisocytosis
Poikilocytosis

   Additional Character Required   3-character code

•=New Code
▲=Revised Code

Excludes1 Not coded here, do not use together
Excludes2—Not included here

R73   ELEVATED BLOOD GLUCOSE LEVEL

Excludes1: DM (E08–E13)
DM in pregnancy, childbirth and the puerperium (O24.-)
neonatal disorders (P70.0–P70.2)
postsurgical hypoinsulinemia (E89.1)

> Do not report for hyperglycemia caused by DM

R73.0   Abnormal glucose

Excludes1: abnormal glucose in pregnancy (O99.81-)
DM (E08–E13)
dysmetabolic syndrome X (E88.81)
gestational diabetes (O24.4-)
glycosuria (R81)
hypoglycemia (E16.2)

R73.01   Impaired fasting glucose
Elevated fasting glucose

R73.02   Impaired glucose tolerance (oral)
Elevated glucose tolerance

•**R73.03   Prediabetes**
Latent diabetes

R73.09   Other abnormal glucose
Abnormal glucose NOS
Abnormal non-fasting glucose tolerance

R73.9   Hyperglycemia, unspecified

R75   INCONCLUSIVE LABORATORY EVIDENCE OF HIV

GUIDELINES

Patients with inconclusive HIV serology, but no definitive diagnosis or manifestations of the illness, may be assigned code R75, Inconclusive laboratory evidence of HIV.
Nonconclusive HIV-test finding in infants
Excludes1: asymptomatic HIV infection status (Z21)
HIV disease (B20)

R76   OTHER ABNORMAL IMMUNOLOGICAL FINDINGS IN SERUM

R76.0   Raised antibody titer
Excludes1: isoimmunization in pregnancy (O36.0–O36.1)
isoimmunization affecting newborn (P55.-)

R76.1   Nonspecific reaction to test for tuberculosis

R76.11   Nonspecific reaction to tuberculin skin test without active tuberculosis
Abnormal result of Mantoux test
PPD positive
Tuberculin (skin test) positive
Tuberculin (skin test) reactor
Excludes1: nonspecific reaction to cell mediated immunity measurement of gamma interferon antigen response without active tuberculosis (R76.12)

R76.12   Nonspecific reaction to cell mediated immunity measurement of gamma interferon antigen response without active tuberculosis
Nonspecific reaction to QFT without active tuberculosis
Excludes1: nonspecific reaction to tuberculin skin test without active tuberculosis (R76.11)
positive tuberculin skin test (R76.11)

R76.8   Other specified abnormal immunological findings in serum
Raised level of immunoglobulins NOS

R76.9   Abnormal immunological finding in serum, unspecified

R78   FINDINGS OF DRUGS AND OTHER SUBSTANCES, NOT NORMALLY FOUND IN BLOOD

Use additional code to identify the any retained FB, if applicable (Z18.-)
Excludes1: mental or behavioral disorders due to psychoactive substance use (F10–F19)

R78.0   Finding of alcohol in blood
Use additional external cause code (Y90.-), for detail regarding alcohol level.

R78.1   Finding of opiate drug in blood
R78.2   Finding of cocaine in blood
R78.3   Finding of hallucinogen in blood
R78.4   Finding of other drugs of addictive potential in blood
R78.5   Finding of other psychotropic drug in blood
R78.6   Finding of steroid agent in blood

R78.7   Finding of abnormal level of heavy metals in blood

R78.71   Abnormal lead level in blood
Excludes1: lead poisoning (T56.0-)

R78.79   Finding of abnormal level of heavy metals in blood

R78.8   Finding of other specified substances, not normally found in blood

R78.81   Bacteremia
Excludes1: sepsis-code to specified infection

R78.89   Finding of other specified substances, not normally found in blood
Finding of abnormal level of lithium in blood

R79   OTHER ABNORMAL FINDINGS OF BLOOD CHEMISTRY

Use additional code to identify any retained FB, if applicable (Z18.-)
Excludes1: abnormality of fluid, electrolyte or acid-base balance (E86–E87)
asymptomatic hyperuricemia (E79.0)
hyperglycemia NOS (R73.9)
hypoglycemia NOS (E16.2)
neonatal hypoglycemia (P70.3–P70.4)
specific findings indicating disorder of amino-acid metabolism (E70–E72)
specific findings indicating disorder of carbohydrate metabolism (E73–E74)
specific findings indicating disorder of lipid metabolism (E75.-)

R79.1   Abnormal coagulation profile
Abnormal or prolonged bleeding time
Abnormal or prolonged coagulation time
Abnormal or prolonged partial thromboplastin time [PTT]
Abnormal or prolonged prothrombin time [PT]
Excludes1: coagulation defects (D68.-)

R79.8   Other specified abnormal findings of blood chemistry

R79.81   Abnormal blood-gas level
R79.82   Elevated C-reactive protein (CRP)
R79.89   Other specified abnormal findings of blood chemistry

R79.9   Abnormal finding of blood chemistry, unspecified

(R80–R82) ABNORMAL FINDINGS ON EXAMINATION OF URINE, WITHOUT DIAGNOSIS

Excludes1: abnormal findings on antenatal screening of mother (O28.-)
diagnostic abnormal findings classified elsewhere—see Alphabetical Index
specific findings indicating disorder of amino-acid metabolism (E70–E72)
specific findings indicating disorder of carbohydrate metabolism (E73–E74)

R80   PROTEINURIA

Excludes1: gestational proteinuria (O12.1-)

R80.2   Orthostatic proteinuria, unspecified
Postural proteinuria

R80.9   Proteinuria, unspecified
Albuminuria NOS

R81   GLYCOSURIA

Excludes1: renal glycosuria (E74.8)

R82   OTHER AND UNSPECIFIED ABNORMAL FINDINGS IN URINE

Includes: chromoabnormalities in urine
Use additional code to identify any retained FB, if applicable (Z18.-)
Excludes2: hematuria (R31.-)

R82.0   Chyluria
Excludes1: filarial chyluria (B74.-)

R82.1   Myoglobinuria
R82.2   Biliuria
R82.3   Hemoglobinuria
Excludes1: hemoglobinuria due to hemolysis from external causes NEC (D59.6)
hemoglobinuria due to paroxysmal nocturnal [Marchiafava-Micheli] (D59.5)

R82.7   Abnormal findings on microbiological examination of urine
Excludes1: colonization status (Z22.-)

•**R82.71   Bacteriuria**
•**R82.79   Other abnormal findings on microbiological examination of urine**

     Additional Character Required   3-character code

•=New Code
▲=Revised Code

Excludes1—Not coded here, do not use together
Excludes2—Not included here

268   PEDIATRIC ICD-10-CM 2017: A MANUAL FOR PROVIDER-BASED CODING

R82.8 Abnormal findings on cytological and histological examination of urine

R82.9 Other and unspecified abnormal findings in urine

 R82.90 Unspecified abnormal findings in urine

R82.91 Other chromoabnormalities of urine
Chromoconversion (dipstick)
Idiopathic dipstick converts positive for blood with no cellular forms in sediment
Excludes1: hemoglobinuria (R82.3)
myoglobinuria (R82.1)

R82.99 Other abnormal findings in urine
Cells and casts in urine
Crystalluria
Melanuria

(R83–R89) ABNORMAL FINDINGS ON EXAMINATION OF OTHER BODY FLUIDS, SUBSTANCES AND TISSUES, WITHOUT DIAGNOSIS

Excludes1: abnormal findings on antenatal screening of mother (O28.-)
diagnostic abnormal findings classified elsewhere—see Alphabetical Index
Excludes2: abnormal findings on examination of blood, without diagnosis (R70–R79)
abnormal findings on examination of urine, without diagnosis (R80–R82)
abnormal tumor markers (R97.-)

R89 ABNORMAL FINDINGS IN SPECIMENS FROM OTHER ORGANS, SYSTEMS AND TISSUES
Includes: abnormal findings in nipple discharge
abnormal findings in synovial fluid
abnormal findings in wound secretions

R89.0 Abnormal level of enzymes in specimens from other organs, systems and tissues

R89.1 Abnormal level of hormones in specimens from other organs, systems and tissues

R89.2 Abnormal level of other drugs, medicaments and biological substances in specimens from other organs, systems and tissues

R89.3 Abnormal level of substances chiefly nonmedicinal as to source in specimens from other organs, systems and tissues

R89.4 Abnormal immunological findings in specimens from other organs, systems and tissues

R89.5 Abnormal microbiological findings in specimens from other organs, systems and tissues
Positive culture findings in specimens from other organs, systems and tissues
Excludes1: colonization status (Z22.-)

R89.6 Abnormal cytological findings in specimens from other organs, systems and tissues

R89.7 Abnormal histological findings in specimens from other organs, systems and tissues

R89.8 Other abnormal findings in specimens from other organs, systems and tissues
Abnormal chromosomal findings in specimens from other organs, systems and tissues

R89.9 Unspecified abnormal finding in specimens from other organs, systems and tissues

(R90–R94) ABNORMAL FINDINGS ON DIAGNOSTIC IMAGING AND IN FUNCTION STUDIES, WITHOUT DIAGNOSIS

Includes: nonspecific abnormal findings on diagnostic imaging by CAT scan
nonspecific abnormal findings on diagnostic imaging by MRI [NMR] or PET scan
nonspecific abnormal findings on diagnostic imaging by thermography
nonspecific abnormal findings on diagnostic imaging by ultrasound [echogram]
nonspecific abnormal findings on diagnostic imaging by X-ray examination
Excludes1: abnormal findings on antenatal screening of mother (O28.-)
diagnostic abnormal findings classified elsewhere—**see Alphabetical Index**

R91 ABNORMAL FINDINGS ON DIAGNOSTIC IMAGING OF LUNG

R91.8 Other nonspecific abnormal finding of lung field
Lung mass NOS found on diagnostic imaging of lung
Pulmonary infiltrate NOS
Shadow, lung

R93 ABNORMAL FINDINGS ON DIAGNOSTIC IMAGING OF OTHER BODY STRUCTURES

R93.0 Abnormal findings on diagnostic imaging of skull and head, NEC
Excludes1: intracranial space-occupying lesion found on diagnostic imaging (R90.0)

R93.1 Abnormal findings on diagnostic imaging of heart and coronary circulation
Abnormal echocardiogram NOS
Abnormal heart shadow

R93.4 Abnormal findings on diagnostic imaging of urinary organs
Excludes2: hypertrophy of kidney (N28.81)

• **R93.41 Abnormal radiologic findings on diagnostic imaging of renal pelvis, ureter, or bladder**
Filling defect of bladder found on diagnostic imaging
Filling defect of renal pelvis found on diagnostic imaging
Filling defect of ureter found on diagnostic imaging

• **R93.42 Abnormal radiologic findings on diagnostic imaging of kidney**

• **R93.421 Abnormal radiologic findings on diagnostic imaging of right kidney**

• **R93.422 Abnormal radiologic findings on diagnostic imaging of left kidney**

• **R93.429 Abnormal radiologic findings on diagnostic imaging of unspecified kidney**

• **R93.49 Abnormal radiologic findings on diagnostic imaging of other urinary organs**

R93.5 Abnormal findings on diagnostic imaging of other abdominal regions, including retroperitoneum

R93.7 Abnormal findings on diagnostic imaging of other parts of musculoskeletal system
Excludes2: abnormal findings on diagnostic imaging of skull (R93.0)

(R97) ABNORMAL TUMOR MARKERS

R97 ABNORMAL TUMOR MARKERS
Elevated tumor associated antigens [TAA]
Elevated tumor specific antigens [TSA]

R97.1 Elevated cancer antigen 125 [CA 125]

R97.8 Other abnormal tumor markers

(R99) ILL-DEFINED AND UNKNOWN CAUSE OF MORTALITY

R99 ILL-DEFINED AND UNKNOWN CAUSE OF MORTALITY
 Code R99, Ill-defined and unknown cause of mortality, is only for use in the very limited circumstance when a patient who has already died is brought into an emergency department or other healthcare facility and is pronounced dead upon arrival. It does not represent the discharge disposition of death.
Death (unexplained) NOS
Unspecified cause of mortality

   Additional Character Required   3-character code   •=New Code   *Excludes1* Not coded here, do not use together
▲=Revised Code   *Excludes2*—Not included here

PEDIATRIC ICD-10-CM 2017: A MANUAL FOR PROVIDER-BASED CODING   269

CHAPTER 18. SYMPTOMS, SIGNS, AND ABNORMAL CLINICAL AND LABORATORY FINDINGS, NOT ELSEWHERE CLASSIFIED (R82.8–R99)

Chapter 19. Injury, poisoning and certain other consequences of external causes (S00–T88)

GUIDELINES

Application of 7th Characters in Chapter 19

Most categories in chapter 19 have a 7th character requirement for each applicable code. Most categories in this chapter have three 7th character values (with the exception of fractures): A, initial encounter, D, subsequent encounter and S, sequela. Categories for traumatic fractures have additional 7th character values. While the patient may be seen by a new or different provider over the course of treatment for an injury, assignment of the 7th character is based on whether the patient is undergoing active treatment and not whether the provider is seeing the patient for the first time.

For complication codes, active treatment refers to treatment for the condition described by the code, even though it may be related to an earlier precipitating problem. For example, code T84.50XA, Infection and inflammatory reaction due to unspecified internal joint prosthesis, initial encounter, is used when active treatment is provided for the infection, even though the condition relates to the prosthetic device, implant or graft that was placed at a previous encounter.

7th character "A", initial encounter is used while the patient is receiving active treatment for the condition. Examples of active treatment are: surgical treatment, emergency department encounter, and evaluation and continuing treatment by the same or a different physician.

7th character "D" subsequent encounter is used for encounters after the patient has received active treatment of the condition and is receiving routine care for the condition during the healing or recovery phase. Examples of subsequent care are: cast change or removal, an x-ray to check healing status of fracture, removal of external or internal fixation device, medication adjustment, other aftercare and follow up visits following treatment of the injury or condition.

The aftercare Z codes should not be used for aftercare for conditions such as injuries or poisonings, where 7th characters are provided to identify subsequent care. For example, for aftercare of an injury, assign the acute injury code with the 7th character "D" (subsequent encounter).

7th character "S", sequela, is for use for complications or conditions that arise as a direct result of a condition, such as scar formation after a burn. The scars are sequelae of the burn. When using 7th character "S", it is necessary to use both the injury code that precipitated the sequela and the code for the sequela itself. The "S" is added only to the injury code, not the sequela code. The 7th character "S" identifies the injury responsible for the sequela. The specific type of sequela (e.g. scar) is sequenced first, followed by the injury code.

Coding of Injuries

When coding injuries, assign separate codes for each injury unless a combination code is provided, in which case the combination code is assigned. Code T07, Unspecified multiple injuries should not be assigned in the inpatient setting unless information for a more specific code is not available. Traumatic injury codes (S00–T14.9) are not to be used for normal, healing surgical wounds or to identify complications of surgical wounds.

The code for the most serious injury, as determined by the provider and the focus of treatment, is sequenced first.

SUPERFICIAL INJURIES

Superficial injuries such as abrasions or contusions are not coded when associated with more severe injuries of the same site.

PRIMARY INJURY WITH DAMAGE TO NERVES/BLOOD VESSELS

When a primary injury results in minor damage to peripheral nerves or blood vessels, the primary injury is sequenced first with additional code(s) for injuries to nerves and spinal cord (such as category S04), and/or injury to blood vessels (such as category S15). When the primary injury is to the blood vessels or nerves, that injury should be sequenced first.

Coding of Traumatic Fractures

The principles of multiple coding of injuries should be followed in coding fractures. Fractures of specified sites are coded individually by site in accordance with both the provisions within categories S02, S12, S22, S32, S42, S49, S52, S59, S62, S72, S79, S82, S89, S92 and the level of detail furnished by medical record content. A fracture not indicated as open or closed should be coded to closed. A fracture not indicated whether displaced or not displaced should be coded to displaced. More specific guidelines are as follows:

INITIAL VS. SUBSEQUENT ENCOUNTER FOR FRACTURES

Traumatic fractures are coded using the appropriate 7th character for initial encounter (A, B, C) while the patient is receiving active treatment for the fracture. Examples of active treatment are: surgical treatment, emergency department encounter, and evaluation and continuing (ongoing) treatment by the same or different physician. The appropriate 7th character for initial encounter should also be assigned for a patient who delayed seeking treatment for the fracture or nonunion. Fractures are coded using the appropriate 7th character for subsequent care for encounters after the patient has completed active treatment of the fracture and is receiving routine care for the fracture during the healing or recovery phase. Examples of fracture aftercare are: cast change or removal, an x-ray to check healing status of fracture, removal of external or internal fixation device, medication adjustment, and follow-up visits following fracture treatment.

Care for complications of surgical treatment for fracture repairs during the healing or recovery phase should be coded with the appropriate complication codes.

Care of complications of fractures, such as malunion and nonunion, should be reported with the appropriate 7th character for subsequent care with nonunion (K, M, N,) or subsequent care with malunion (P, Q, R).

Malunion/nonunion: The appropriate 7th character for initial encounter should also be assigned for a patient who delayed seeking treatment for the fracture or nonunion

A code from category M80, not a traumatic fracture code, should be used for any patient with known osteoporosis who suffers a fracture, even if the patient had a minor fall or trauma, if that fall or trauma would not usually break a normal, healthy bone.

The aftercare Z codes should not be used for aftercare for traumatic fractures. For aftercare of a traumatic fracture, assign the acute fracture code with the appropriate 7th character.

MULTIPLE FRACTURES SEQUENCING

Multiple fractures are sequenced in accordance with the severity of the fracture.

Coding of Burns and Corrosions

Refer to category T20 for guidelines.

Adverse Effects, Poisoning, Underdosing and Toxic Effects

Refer to category T36 for guidelines.

Adult and Child Abuse, Neglect and Other Maltreatment

Refer to category T74 for guidelines.

Complications of care

GENERAL GUIDELINES FOR COMPLICATIONS OF CARE

See Section I.B.16 (page XVI) for information on documentation of complications of care.

PAIN DUE TO MEDICAL DEVICES

Pain associated with devices, implants or grafts left in a surgical site (for example painful hip prosthesis) is assigned to the appropriate code(s) found in Chapter 19, Injury, poisoning, and certain other consequences of external causes. Specific codes for pain due to medical devices are found in the T code section of the *ICD-10-CM*. **Use additional code(s)** from category G89 to identify acute or chronic pain due to presence of the device, implant or graft (G89.18 or G89.28).

TRANSPLANT COMPLICATIONS

Transplant complications other than kidney
Please see category T86 for guidelines for complications of transplanted organs and tissue other than kidney.

Kidney transplant complications

Refer to code T86.1 for guidelines for complications of kidney transplant.

Additional Character Required	3-character code	Unspecified laterality codes were excluded here.	*=New Code ▲=Revised Code

| **Excludes1**—Not coded here, do not use together |
| **Excludes2**—Not included here |

CHAPTER 19. INJURY, POISONING AND CERTAIN OTHER CONSEQUENCES OF EXTERNAL CAUSES   (S00–S00.27)

COMPLICATION CODES THAT INCLUDE THE EXTERNAL CAUSE

As with certain other T codes, some of the complications of care codes have the external cause included in the code. The code includes the nature of the complication as well as the type of procedure that caused the complication. No external cause code indicating the type of procedure is necessary for these codes.

COMPLICATIONS OF CARE CODES WITHIN THE BODY SYSTEM CHAPTERS

Intraoperative and postprocedural complication codes are found within the body system chapters with codes specific to the organs and structures of that body system. These codes should be sequenced first, followed by a code(s) for the specific complication, if applicable.

Note: Use secondary code(s) from Chapter 20, External causes of morbidity, to indicate cause of injury. Codes within the T-section that include the external cause do not require an additional external cause code

    Use additional code to identify any retained FB, if applicable (Z18.-)
Excludes1: birth trauma (P10–P15)
    obstetric trauma (O70–O71)

Note: The chapter uses the S-section for coding different types of injuries related to single body regions and the T-section to cover injuries to unspecified body regions as well as poisoning and certain other consequences of external causes.

    Most codes in Chapter 19 require the addition of 7th characters to form complete codes. Descriptors for 7th characters are provided in text boxes throughout the chapter.

(S00–S09) INJURIES TO THE HEAD

Includes: Injuries of ear
    injuries of eye
    injuries of face [any part]
    injuries of gum
    injuries of jaw
    injuries of oral cavity
    injuries of palate
    injuries of periocular area
    injuries of scalp
    injuries of temporomandibular joint area
    injuries of tongue
    injuries of tooth
Code also for any associated infection
Excludes2: burns and corrosions (T20–T32)
    effects of FB in ear (T16)
    effects of FB in larynx (T17.3)
    effects of FB in mouth NOS (T18.0)
    effects of FB in nose (T17.0–T17.1)
    effects of FB in pharynx (T17.2)
    effects of FB on external eye (T15.-)
    frostbite (T33–T34)
    insect bite or sting, venomous (T63.4)

S00 `4th` **SUPERFICIAL INJURY OF HEAD**
Excludes1: diffuse cerebral contusion (S06.2-)
    focal cerebral contusion (S06.3-)
    injury of eye and orbit (S05.-)
    open wound of head (S01.-)

> **7th characters for category S00**
> A—initial encounter
> D—subsequent encounter
> S—sequela

S00.0 `5th` **Superficial injury of scalp**
    S00.00X `7th` Unspecified superficial injury of scalp
    S00.01X `7th` Abrasion of scalp
    S00.02X `7th` Blister (nonthermal) of scalp
    S00.03X `7th` Contusion of scalp
        Bruise of scalp
        Hematoma of scalp
    S00.04X `7th` External constriction of part of scalp
    S00.05X `7th` Superficial FB of scalp

        Splinter in the scalp
    S00.06X `7th` Insect bite (nonvenomous) of scalp
    S00.07X `7th` Other superficial bite of scalp
        Excludes1: open bite of scalp (S01.05)

S00.1 `5th` **Contusion of eyelid and periocular area**
Black eye
Excludes2: contusion of eyeball and orbital tissues (S05.1)
    S00.10X `7th` Contusion of unspecified eyelid and periocular area
    S00.11X `7th` Contusion of right eyelid and periocular area
    S00.12X `7th` Contusion of left eyelid and periocular area

S00.2 `5th` **Other and unspecified superficial injuries of eyelid and periocular area**
Excludes2: superficial injury of conjunctiva and cornea (S05.0-)
    S00.20 `6th` Unspecified superficial injury of eyelid and periocular area
        S00.201 `7th` Unspecified superficial injury of right eyelid and periocular area
        S00.202 `7th` Unspecified superficial injury of left eyelid and periocular area
    S00.21 `6th` Abrasion of eyelid and periocular area
        S00.211 `7th` Abrasion of right eyelid and periocular area
        S00.212 `7th` Abrasion of left eyelid and periocular area
    S00.22 `6th` Blister (nonthermal) of eyelid and periocular area
        S00.221 `7th` Blister (nonthermal) of right eyelid and periocular area
        S00.222 `7th` Blister (nonthermal) of left eyelid and periocular area
    S00.24 `6th` External constriction of eyelid and periocular area
        S00.241 `7th` External constriction of right eyelid and periocular area
        S00.242 `7th` External constriction of left eyelid and periocular area
    S00.25 `6th` Superficial FB of eyelid and periocular area
        Splinter of eyelid and periocular area
        Excludes2: retained FB in eyelid (H02.81-)
        S00.251 `7th` Superficial FB of right eyelid and periocular area
        S00.252 `7th` Superficial FB of left eyelid and periocular area
    S00.26 `6th` Insect bite (nonvenomous) of eyelid and periocular area
        S00.261 `7th` Insect bite (nonvenomous) of right eyelid and periocular area
        S00.262 `7th` Insect bite (nonvenomous) of left eyelid and periocular area
    S00.27 `6th` Other superficial bite of eyelid and periocular area
        Excludes1: open bite of eyelid and periocular area (S01.15)

   `7th`   Additional Character Required   ✔ 3-character code   Unspecified laterality codes were excluded here.   •=New Code   ▲=Revised Code   *Excludes1*—Not coded here, do not use together   *Excludes2*—Not included here

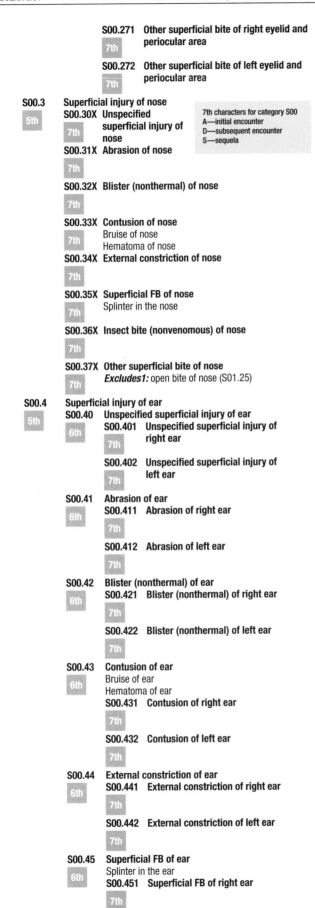

S00.271 [7th] Other superficial bite of right eyelid and periocular area

S00.272 [7th] Other superficial bite of left eyelid and periocular area

S00.3 [5th] **Superficial injury of nose**

S00.30X [7th] Unspecified superficial injury of nose

> 7th characters for category S00
> A—initial encounter
> D—subsequent encounter
> S—sequela

S00.31X [7th] Abrasion of nose

S00.32X [7th] Blister (nonthermal) of nose

S00.33X [7th] Contusion of nose
Bruise of nose
Hematoma of nose

S00.34X [7th] External constriction of nose

S00.35X [7th] Superficial FB of nose
Splinter in the nose

S00.36X [7th] Insect bite (nonvenomous) of nose

S00.37X [7th] Other superficial bite of nose
Excludes1: open bite of nose (S01.25)

S00.4 [5th] **Superficial injury of ear**

S00.40 [6th] Unspecified superficial injury of ear

S00.401 [7th] Unspecified superficial injury of right ear

S00.402 [7th] Unspecified superficial injury of left ear

S00.41 [6th] Abrasion of ear

S00.411 [7th] Abrasion of right ear

S00.412 [7th] Abrasion of left ear

S00.42 [6th] Blister (nonthermal) of ear

S00.421 [7th] Blister (nonthermal) of right ear

S00.422 [7th] Blister (nonthermal) of left ear

S00.43 [6th] Contusion of ear
Bruise of ear
Hematoma of ear

S00.431 [7th] Contusion of right ear

S00.432 [7th] Contusion of left ear

S00.44 [6th] External constriction of ear

S00.441 [7th] External constriction of right ear

S00.442 [7th] External constriction of left ear

S00.45 [6th] Superficial FB of ear
Splinter in the ear

S00.451 [7th] Superficial FB of right ear

S00.452 [7th] Superficial FB of left ear

S00.46 [6th] Insect bite (nonvenomous) of ear

S00.461 [7th] Insect bite (nonvenomous) of right ear

S00.462 [7th] Insect bite (nonvenomous) of left ear

S00.47 [6th] Other superficial bite of ear
Excludes1: open bite of ear (S01.35)

S00.471 [7th] Other superficial bite of right ear

S00.472 [7th] Other superficial bite of left ear

S00.5 [5th] **Superficial injury of lip and oral cavity**

S00.50 [6th] Unspecified superficial injury of lip and oral cavity

S00.501 [7th] Unspecified superficial injury of lip

S00.502 [7th] Unspecified superficial injury of oral cavity

S00.51 [6th] Abrasion of lip and oral cavity

S00.511 [7th] Abrasion of lip

S00.512 [7th] Abrasion of oral cavity

S00.52 [6th] Blister (nonthermal) of lip and oral cavity

S00.521 [7th] Blister (nonthermal) of lip

S00.522 [7th] Blister (nonthermal) of oral cavity

S00.53 [6th] Contusion of lip and oral cavity

S00.531 [7th] Contusion of lip
Bruise of lip
Hematoma of oral cavity

S00.532 [7th] Contusion of oral cavity
Bruise of lip
Hematoma of oral cavity

S00.54 [6th] External constriction of lip and oral cavity

S00.541 [7th] External constriction of lip

S00.542 [7th] External constriction of oral cavity

S00.55 [6th] Superficial FB of lip and oral cavity

S00.551 [7th] Superficial FB of lip
Splinter of lip and oral cavity

S00.552 [7th] Superficial FB of oral cavity
Splinter of lip and oral cavity

S00.56 [6th] Insect bite (nonvenomous) of lip and oral cavity

S00.561 [7th] Insect bite (nonvenomous) of lip

S00.562 [7th] Insect bite (nonvenomous) of oral cavity

S00.57 [6th] Other superficial bite of lip and oral cavity

S00.571 [7th] Other superficial bite of lip
Excludes1: open bite of lip (S01.551)

CHAPTER 19. INJURY, POISONING AND CERTAIN OTHER CONSEQUENCES OF EXTERNAL CAUSES   (S00.271–S00.571)

[4th] [5th] [6th] [7th] Additional Character Required ✓ 3-character code Unspecified laterality codes were excluded here. •=New Code ▲=Revised Code ***Excludes1***—Not coded here, do not use together ***Excludes2***—Not included here

 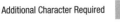

S00.572 Other superficial bite of oral cavity
> [7th]
> *Excludes1:* open bite of oral cavity (S01.552)

S00.8 Superficial injury of other parts of head
[5th]
Superficial injuries of face [any part]

S00.80X Unspecified superficial injury of other part of head
[7th]

7th characters for category S00
A—initial encounter
D—subsequent encounter
S—sequela

S00.81X Abrasion of other part of head
[7th]

S00.82X Blister (nonthermal) of other part of head
[7th]

S00.83X Contusion of other part of head
[7th]
Bruise of other part of head
Hematoma of other part of head

S00.84X External constriction of other part of head
[7th]

S00.85X Superficial FB of other part of head
[7th]
Splinter in other part of head

S00.86X Insect bite (nonvenomous) of other part of head
[7th]

S00.87X Other superficial bite of other part of head
[7th]
Excludes1: open bite of other part of head (S01.85)

S00.9 Superficial injury of unspecified part of head
[5th]

S00.90X Unspecified superficial injury of unspecified part of head
[7th]

S00.91X Abrasion of unspecified part of head
[7th]

S00.92X Blister (nonthermal) of unspecified part of head
[7th]

S00.93X Contusion of unspecified part of head
[7th]
Bruise of head
Hematoma of head

S00.94X External constriction of unspecified part of head
[7th]

S00.95X Superficial FB of unspecified part of head
[7th]
Splinter of head

S00.96X Insect bite (nonvenomous) of unspecified part of head
[7th]

S00.97X Other superficial bite of unspecified part of head
[7th]
Excludes1: open bite of head (S01.95)

S01 OPEN WOUND OF HEAD
[4th]

Code also any associated:
   injury of cranial nerve (S04.-)
   injury of muscle and tendon of head (S09.1-)
   intracranial injury (S06.-)
   wound infection

7th characters for category S01
A—initial encounter
D—subsequent encounter
S—sequela

Excludes1: open skull fracture (S02.- with 7th character)
Excludes2: injury of eye and orbit (S05.-)
   traumatic amputation of part of head (S08.-)

S01.0 Open wound of scalp
[5th]
Excludes1: avulsion of scalp (S08.0)

S01.01X Laceration without FB of scalp
[7th]

S01.02X Laceration with FB of scalp
[7th]

S01.03X Puncture wound without FB of scalp
[7th]

S01.04X Puncture wound with FB of scalp
[7th]

S01.05X Open bite of scalp
[7th]
Bite of scalp NOS
Excludes1: superficial bite of scalp (S00.06, S00.07-)

S01.1 Open wound of eyelid and periocular area
[5th]
Open wound of eyelid and periocular area with or without involvement of lacrimal passages

S01.11 Laceration without FB of eyelid and periocular area
[6th]
> **S01.111 Laceration without FB of right eyelid and periocular area**
> [7th]
>
> **S01.112 Laceration without FB of left eyelid and periocular area**
> [7th]

S01.12 Laceration with FB of eyelid and periocular area
[6th]
> **S01.121 Laceration with FB of right eyelid and periocular area**
> [7th]
>
> **S01.122 Laceration with FB of left eyelid and periocular area**
> [7th]

S01.13 Puncture wound without FB of eyelid and periocular area
[6th]
> **S01.131 Puncture wound without FB of right eyelid and periocular area**
> [7th]
>
> **S01.132 Puncture wound without FB of left eyelid and periocular area**
> [7th]

S01.14 Puncture wound with FB of eyelid and periocular area
[6th]
> **S01.141 Puncture wound with FB of right eyelid and periocular area**
> [7th]
>
> **S01.142 Puncture wound with FB of left eyelid and periocular area**
> [7th]

S01.15 Open bite of eyelid and periocular area
[6th]
Bite of eyelid and periocular area NOS
Excludes1: superficial bite of eyelid and periocular area (S00.26, S00.27)
> **S01.151 Open bite of right eyelid and periocular area**
> [7th]
>
> **S01.152 Open bite of left eyelid and periocular area**
> [7th]

S01.2 Open wound of nose
[5th]

7th characters for category S01
A—initial encounter
D—subsequent encounter
S—sequela

S01.21X Laceration without FB of nose
[7th]

S01.22X Laceration with FB of nose
[7th]

S01.23X Puncture wound without FB of nose
[7th]

S01.24X Puncture wound with FB of nose
[7th]

S01.25X Open bite of nose
[7th]
Bite of nose NOS
Excludes1: superficial bite of nose (S00.36, S00.37)

S01.3 Open wound of ear
[5th]

S01.31 Laceration without FB of ear
[6th]
> **S01.311 Laceration without FB of right ear**
> [7th]

 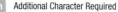

[4th] [5th] [6th] [7th] Additional Character Required   ✓ 3-character code   Unspecified laterality codes were excluded here.   •=New Code   ▲=Revised Code   *Excludes1*—Not coded here, do not use together   *Excludes2*—Not included here

S01.312 Laceration without FB of left ear
`7th`

S01.32 Laceration with FB of ear
`6th`
   S01.321 Laceration with FB of right ear
`7th`

> 7th characters for category S01
> A—initial encounter
> D—subsequent encounter
> S—sequela

   S01.322 Laceration with FB of left ear
`7th`

S01.33 Puncture wound without FB of ear
`6th`
   S01.331 Puncture wound without FB of right ear
`7th`

   S01.332 Puncture wound without FB of left ear
`7th`

S01.34 Puncture wound with FB of ear
`6th`
   S01.341 Puncture wound with FB of right ear
`7th`

   S01.342 Puncture wound with FB of left ear
`7th`

S01.35 Open bite of ear
`6th`
Bite of ear NOS
Excludes1: superficial bite of ear (S00.46, S00.47)
   S01.351 Open bite of right ear
`7th`

   S01.352 Open bite of left ear
`7th`

S01.4 Open wound of cheek and temporomandibular area
`5th`
S01.41 Laceration without FB of cheek and temporomandibular area
`6th`
   S01.411 Laceration without FB of right cheek and temporomandibular area
`7th`

   S01.412 Laceration without FB of left cheek and temporomandibular area
`7th`

S01.42 Laceration with FB of cheek and temporomandibular area
`6th`
   S01.421 Laceration with FB of right cheek and temporomandibular area
`7th`

   S01.422 Laceration with FB of left cheek and temporomandibular area
`7th`

S01.43 Puncture wound without FB of cheek and temporomandibular area
`6th`
   S01.431 Puncture wound without FB of right cheek and temporomandibular area
`7th`

   S01.432 Puncture wound without FB of left cheek and temporomandibular area
`7th`

S01.44 Puncture wound with FB of cheek and temporomandibular area
`6th`
   S01.441 Puncture wound with FB of right cheek and temporomandibular area
`7th`

   S01.442 Puncture wound with FB of left cheek and temporomandibular area
`7th`

S01.45 Open bite of cheek and temporomandibular area
`6th`
Bite of cheek and temporomandibular area NOS
Excludes2: superficial bite of cheek and temporomandibular area (S00.86, S00.87)
   S01.451 Open bite of right cheek and temporomandibular area
`7th`

   S01.452 Open bite of left cheek and temporomandibular area
`7th`

S01.5 Open wound of lip and oral cavity
`5th`
Excludes2: tooth dislocation (S03.2)
tooth fracture (S02.5)
S01.51 Laceration of lip and oral cavity without FB
`6th`
   S01.511 Laceration without FB of lip
`7th`

   S01.512 Laceration without FB of oral cavity
`7th`

S01.52 Laceration of lip and oral cavity with FB
`6th`
   S01.521 Laceration with FB of lip
`7th`

   S01.522 Laceration with FB of oral cavity
`7th`

S01.53 Puncture wound of lip and oral cavity without FB
`6th`
   S01.531 Puncture wound without FB of lip
`7th`

   S01.532 Puncture wound without FB of oral cavity
`7th`

S01.54 Puncture wound of lip and oral cavity with FB
`6th`
   S01.541 Puncture wound with FB of lip
`7th`

   S01.542 Puncture wound with FB of oral cavity
`7th`

S01.55 Open bite of lip and oral cavity
`6th`
   S01.551 Open bite of lip
`7th`
   Bite of lip NOS
   Excludes1: superficial bite of lip (S00.571)
   S01.552 Open bite of oral cavity
`7th`
   Bite of oral cavity NOS
   Excludes1: superficial bite of oral cavity (S00.572)

S01.8 Open wound of other parts of head
`5th`
S01.81X Laceration without FB of other part of head
`7th`

S01.82X Laceration with FB of other part of head
`7th`

S01.83X Puncture wound without FB of other part of head
`7th`

S01.84X Puncture wound with FB of other part of head
`7th`

S01.85X Open bite of other part of head
`7th`
Bite of other part of head NOS
Excludes1: superficial bite of other part of head (S00.85)

S01.9 Open wound of unspecified part of head
`5th`
S01.90X Unspecified open wound of unspecified part of head
`7th`

S01.91X Laceration without FB of unspecified part of head
`7th`

S01.92X Laceration with FB of unspecified part of head
`7th`

S01.93X Puncture wound without FB of unspecified part of head
`7th`

CHAPTER 19. INJURY, POISONING AND CERTAIN OTHER CONSEQUENCES OF EXTERNAL CAUSES (S01.312–S01.93X)

  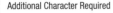 `6th` `7th` Additional Character Required   3-character code

Unspecified laterality codes were excluded here.
•=New Code
▲=Revised Code
Excludes1—Not coded here, do not use together
Excludes2—Not included here

CHAPTER 19. INJURY, POISONING AND CERTAIN OTHER CONSEQUENCES OF EXTERNAL CAUSES   (S01.94X–S02.632)

S01.94X **Puncture wound with FB of unspecified part of head**
[7th]

S01.95X **Open bite of unspecified part of head**
[7th]
Bite of head NOS
Excludes1: superficial bite of head NOS (S00.97)

S02 **FRACTURE OF SKULL AND FACIAL BONES**
[4th]
Note: A fracture not indicated as open or closed should be coded to closed
Code also any associated intracranial injury (S06.-)

S02.0 **Fracture of vault of skull**
Fracture of frontal bone
Fracture of parietal bone

▲S02.1 **Fracture of base of skull**
[5th]
Excludes1: orbit NOS (S02.8)
Excludes2: orbital floor (S02.3-)

> 7th characters for category S02
> A—initial encounter for closed fracture
> B—initial encounter for open fracture
> D—subsequent encounter for fracture with routine healing
> G—subsequent encounter for fracture with delayed healing
> K—subsequent encounter for fracture with nonunion
> S—sequela

     •**S02.101** **Fracture of base of skull, right side**
[7th]

     •**S02.102** **Fracture or base of skull, left side**
[7th]

     •**S02.109** **Fracture of base of skull, unspecified side**
[7th]

   S02.11 **Fracture of occiput**
[6th]

     •**S02.11A** **Type I occipital condyle fracture, right side**
[7th]

     •**S02.11B** **Type I occipital condyle fracture, left side**
[7th]

     ▲**S02.110** **Type I occipital condyle fracture, unspecified side**
[7th]

     •**S02.11C** **Type II occipital condyle fracture, right side**
[7th]

     •**S02.11D** **Type II occipital condyle fracture, left side**
[7th]

     ▲**S02.111** **Type II occipital condyle fracture, unspecified side**
[7th]

     •**S02.11E** **Type III occipital condyle fracture, right side**
[7th]

     •**S02.11F** **Type III occipital condyle fracture, left side**
[7th]

     ▲**S02.112** **Type III occipital condyle fracture, unspecified side**
[7th]

     S02.113 **Unspecified occipital condyle fracture**
[7th]

     •**S02.11G** **Other fracture of occiput, right side**
[7th]

     •**S02.11H** **Other fracture of occiput, left side**
[7th]

     ▲**S02.118** **Other fracture of occiput, unspecified side**
[7th]

     S02.119 **Unspecified fracture of occiput**
[7th]

> 7th characters for category S02
> A—initial encounter for closed fracture
> B—initial encounter for open fracture
> D—subsequent encounter for fracture with routine healing
> G—subsequent encounter for fracture with delayed healing
> K—subsequent encounter for fracture with nonunion
> S—sequela

S02.19X **Other fracture of base of skull**
[7th]
Fracture of anterior fossa of base of skull
Fracture of ethmoid or frontal sinus
Fracture of middle fossa of base of skull
Fracture of orbital roof
Fracture of posterior fossa of base of skull
Fracture of sphenoid
Fracture of temporal bone

S02.2XX **Fracture of nasal bones**
[7th]

S02.3 **Fracture of orbital floor**
[5th]
   •**S02.30X** **Fracture of orbital floor, unspecified side**
[7th]
Excludes1: orbit NOS (S02.8)
Excludes2: orbital roof (S02.1-)

   •**S02.31X** **Fracture of orbital floor, right side**
[7th]
Excludes1: orbit NOS (S02.8)
Excludes2: orbital roof (S02.1-)

   •**S02.32X** **Fracture of orbital floor, left side**
[7th]
Excludes1: orbit NOS (S02.8)
Excludes2: orbital roof (S02.1-)

S02.5XX **Fracture of tooth (traumatic)**
[7th]
Broken tooth
Excludes1: cracked tooth (nontraumatic) (K03.81)

S02.6 **Fracture of mandible**
[5th]
Fracture of lower jaw (bone)

   S02.60 **Fracture of mandible, unspecified**
[6th]
     ▲**S02.600** **Fracture of unspecified part of body of mandible, unspecified side**
[7th]

     •**S02.601** **Fracture of unspecified part of body of right mandible**
[7th]

     •**S02.602** **Fracture of unspecified part of body of left mandible**
[7th]

     S02.609 **Fracture of mandible, unspecified**
[7th]

> 7th characters for category S02
> A—initial encounter for closed fracture
> B—initial encounter for open fracture
> D—subsequent encounter for fracture with routine healing
> G—subsequent encounter for fracture with delayed healing
> K—subsequent encounter for fracture with nonunion
> S—sequela

   S02.61 **Fracture of condylar process of mandible**
[6th]
     •**S02.610** **Fracture of condylar process of mandible, unspecified side**
[7th]

     •**S02.611** **Fracture of condylar process of right mandible**
[7th]

     •**S02.612** **Fracture of condylar process of left mandible**
[7th]

   ▲**S02.62** **Fracture of subcondylar process of mandible**
[6th]
     •**S02.620** **Fracture of subcondylar process of mandible, unspecified side**
[7th]

     •**S02.621** **Fracture of subcondylar process of right mandible**
[7th]

     •**S02.622** **Fracture of subcondylar process of left mandible**
[7th]

   ▲**S02.63** **Fracture of coronoid process of mandible**
[6th]
     •**S02.630** **Fracture of process of mandible, unspecified side**
[7th]

     •**S02.631** **Fracture of subcondylar process of right mandible**
[7th]

     •**S02.632** **Fracture of subcondylar process of left mandible**
[7th]

  [4th] [5th] [6th] [7th] Additional Character Required   3-character code   Unspecified laterality codes were excluded here.   •=New Code ▲=Revised Code   *Excludes1*—Not coded here, do not use together   *Excludes2*—Not included here

▵**S02.64** **Fracture of ramus of mandible**

6th •**S02.640** **Fracture of ramus of mandible, unspecified side**
7th

•**S02.641** **Fracture of ramus of right mandible**
7th

•**S02.642** **Fracture of ramus of left mandible**
7th

▵**S02.65** **Fracture of angle of mandible**

6th •**S02.650** **Fracture of angle of mandible, unspecified side**
7th

•**S02.651** **Fracture of angle of right mandible**
7th

•**S02.652** **Fracture of angle of left mandible**
7th

S02.66X **Fracture of symphysis of mandible**
7th

▵**S02.67** **Fracture of alveolus of mandible**

6th •**S02.670** **Fracture of alveolus of mandible, unspecified side**
7th

7th characters for category S02
A—initial encounter for closed fracture
B—initial encounter for open fracture
D—subsequent encounter for fracture with routine healing
G—subsequent encounter for fracture with delayed healing
K—subsequent encounter for fracture with nonunion
S—sequela

•**S02.671** **Fracture of alveolus of right mandible**
7th

•**S02.672** **Fracture of alveolus of left mandible**
7th

S02.69X **Fracture of mandible of other specified site**
7th

▵**S02.8** **Fractures of other specified skull and facial bones**

5th •**S02.80X** **Fractures of other specified skull and facial bones, unspecified side**
7th   Fracture of orbit NOS
    Fracture of palate
    Excludes1: fracture of orbital floor (S02.3-)
      fracture of orbital roof (S02.1-)

•**S02.81X** **Fractures of other specified skull and facial bones, right side**
7th   Fracture of orbit NOS
    Fracture of palate
    Excludes1: fracture of orbital floor (S02.3-)
      fracture of orbital roof (S02.1-)

•**S02.82X** **Fractures of other specified skull and facial bones, left side**
7th   Fracture of orbit NOS
    Fracture of palate
    Excludes1: fracture of orbital floor (S02.3-)
      fracture of orbital roof (S02.1-)

S02.9 **Fracture of unspecified skull and facial bones**

5th **S02.91X** **Unspecified fracture of skull**
7th

S02.92X **Unspecified fracture of facial bones**
7th

S03 **DISLOCATION AND SPRAIN OF JOINTS AND LIGAMENTS OF HEAD**

4th *Includes:* avulsion of joint (capsule) or ligament of head
    laceration of cartilage, joint (capsule) or ligament of head
    sprain of cartilage, joint (capsule) or ligament of head
    traumatic hemarthrosis of joint or ligament of head
    traumatic rupture of joint or ligament of head
    traumatic subluxation of joint or ligament of head
    traumatic tear of joint or ligament of head

7th characters for category S03
A—initial encounter
D—subsequent encounter
S—sequela

Code also any associated open wound
Excludes2: Strain of muscle or tendon of head (S09.1)

▵**S03.0** **Dislocation of jaw**
5th   Dislocation of jaw (cartilage) (meniscus)
    Dislocation of mandible or of temporomandibular (joint)

•**S03.00X** **Dislocation of jaw, unspecified side**
7th

•**S03.01X** **Dislocation of jaw, right side**
7th

•**S03.02X** **Dislocation of jaw, left side**
7th

•**S03.03X** **Dislocation of jaw, bilateral**
7th

S03.1XX **Dislocation of septal cartilage of nose**
7th

S03.2XX **Dislocation of tooth**
7th

▵**S03.4** **Sprain of jaw**
5th   Sprain of temporomandibular (joint) (ligament)

•**S03.40X** **Sprain of jaw, unspecified side**
7th

•**S03.41X** **Sprain of jaw, right side**
7th

•**S03.42X** **Sprain of jaw, left side**
7th

•**S03.43X** **Sprain of jaw, bilateral**
7th

S05 **INJURY OF EYE AND ORBIT**

4th *Includes:* open wound of eye and orbit
Excludes2: 2nd cranial [optic] nerve injury (S04.0-)
    3rd cranial [oculomotor] nerve injury (S04.1-)

7th characters for categories S05 & S06
A—initial encounter
D—subsequent encounter
S—sequela

    open wound of eyelid and periocular area (S01.1-)
    orbital bone fracture (S02.1-, S02.3-, S02.8-)
    superficial injury of eyelid (S00.1–S00.2)

S05.0 **Injury of conjunctiva and corneal abrasion without FB**
5th *Excludes1:* FB in conjunctival sac (T15.1)
    FB in cornea (T15.0)

S05.01X **Injury of conjunctiva and corneal abrasion without FB, right eye**
7th

S05.02X **Injury of conjunctiva and corneal abrasion without FB, left eye**
7th

  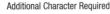 Additional Character Required   ✓ 3-character code   Unspecified laterality codes were excluded here.   •=New Code   ▵=Revised Code   *Excludes1*—Not coded here, do not use together   *Excludes2*—Not included here

S06 **INTRACRANIAL INJURY**
4th
Includes: traumatic brain injury
Code also any associated:
    open wound of head (S01.-)
    skull fracture (S02.-)
Excludes1: head injury NOS (S09.90)

7th characters for categories S05 & S06
A—initial encounter
D—subsequent encounter
S—sequela

S06.0 **Concussion**
5th
    Commotio cerebri
    Excludes1: concussion with other intracranial injuries classified in subcategories S06.1- to S06.6-, S06.81- and S06.82- code to specified intracranial injury

    S06.0X **Concussion**
    6th
        S06.0X0 **Concussion without LOC**
        7th

        S06.0X1 **Concussion with LOC of; 30 min or less**
        7th

        S06.0X9 **unspecified duration**
        7th   Concussion NOS

S06.3 **Focal traumatic brain injury**
5th
    Excludes1: any condition classifiable to S06.4–S06.6 focal cerebral edema (S06.1)

    S06.30 **Unspecified focal traumatic brain injury**
    6th
        S06.300 **Unspecified focal traumatic brain injury without LOC**
        7th

        S06.301 **Unspecified focal traumatic brain injury with LOC of; 30 min or less**
        7th

        S06.302 **31 min to 59 min**
        7th

        S06.303 **1 hour to 5 h 59 min**
        7th

        S06.304 **6 h to 24 h**
        7th

        S06.305 **greater than 24 h with return to pre-existing conscious level**
        7th

        S06.306 **greater than 24 h without return to pre-existing conscious level with patient surviving**
        7th

        S06.307 **any duration with death due to brain injury prior to regaining consciousness**
        7th

        S06.308 **any duration with death due to other cause prior to regaining consciousness**
        7th

        S06.309 **unspecified duration**
        7th   Unspecified focal traumatic brain injury NOS

    S06.31 **Contusion and laceration of right cerebrum**
    6th
        S06.310 **Contusion and laceration of right cerebrum without loss of consciousness**
        7th

        S06.311 **Contusion and laceration of right cerebrum with LOC of; 30 min or less**
        7th

        S06.312 **31 min to 59 min**
        7th

        S06.313 **1 hour to 5 h 59 min**
        7th

        S06.314 **6 h to 24 h**
        7th

        S06.315 **greater than 24 h with return to pre-existing conscious level**
        7th

        S06.316 **greater than 24 h without return to pre-existing conscious level with patient surviving**
        7th

        S06.317 **any duration with death due to brain injury prior to regaining consciousness**
        7th

        S06.318 **any duration with death due to other cause prior to regaining consciousness**
        7th

        S06.319 **unspecified duration**
        7th   Contusion and laceration of right cerebrum NOS

    S06.32 **Contusion and laceration of left cerebrum**
    6th
        S06.320 **Contusion and laceration of left cerebrum without loss of consciousness**
        7th

        S06.321 **Contusion and laceration of left cerebrum with LOC of; 30 min or less**
        7th

        S06.322 **31 min to 59 min**
        7th

        S06.323 **1 hour to 5 h 59 min**
        7th

        S06.324 **6 h to 24 h**
        7th

        S06.325 **greater than 24 h with return to - pre-existing conscious level**
        7th

        S06.326 **greater than 24 h without return to pre-existing conscious level with patient surviving**
        7th

        S06.327 **any duration with death due to brain injury prior to regaining consciousness**
        7th

        S06.328 **any duration with death due to other cause prior to regaining consciousness**
        7th

        S06.329 **unspecified duration**
        7th   Contusion and laceration of left cerebrum NOS

    S06.34 **Traumatic hemorrhage of right cerebrum**
    6th
        Traumatic intracerebral hemorrhage and hematoma of right cerebrum
        S06.340 **Traumatic hemorrhage of right cerebrum without LOC**
        7th

        S06.341 **Traumatic hemorrhage of right cerebrum with LOC of; 30 min or less**
        7th

        S06.342 **31 min to 59 min**
        7th

        S06.343 **1 h to 5 h 59 min**
        7th

7th characters for category S06
A—initial encounter
D—subsequent encounter
S—sequela

        S06.344 **6 h to 24 h**
        7th

        S06.345 **greater than 24 h with return to pre-existing conscious level**
        7th

        S06.346 **greater than 24 h without return to pre-existing conscious level with patient surviving**
        7th

        S06.347 **any duration with death due to brain injury prior to regaining consciousness**
        7th

CHAPTER 19. INJURY, POISONING AND CERTAIN OTHER CONSEQUENCES OF EXTERNAL CAUSES (S06–S06.347)

  Additional Character Required   3-character code   Unspecified laterality codes were excluded here.   •=New Code   ▲=Revised Code   *Excludes1*—Not coded here, do not use together   *Excludes2*—Not included here

S06.348 **7th** **any duration with death due to other cause prior to regaining consciousness**

S06.349 **7th** **unspecified duration**
Traumatic hemorrhage of right cerebrum NOS

S06.35 **6th** **Traumatic hemorrhage of left cerebrum**
Traumatic intracerebral hemorrhage and hematoma of left cerebrum

S06.350 **7th** **Traumatic hemorrhage of left cerebrum without LOC**

S06.351 **7th** **Traumatic hemorrhage of left cerebrum with LOC of; 30 min or less**

S06.352 **7th** **31 min to 59 min**

S06.353 **7th** **1 h to 5 h 59 min**

S06.354 **7th** **6 h to 24 h**

S06.355 **7th** **greater than 24 h with return to pre-existing conscious level**

S06.356 **7th** **greater than 24 h without return to pre-existing conscious level with patient surviving**

S06.357 **7th** **any duration with death due to brain injury prior to regaining consciousness**

S06.358 **7th** **any duration with death due to other cause prior to regaining consciousness**

S06.359 **7th** **unspecified duration**
Traumatic hemorrhage of left cerebrum NOS

S06.37 **6th** **Contusion, laceration, and hemorrhage of cerebellum**

S06.370 **7th** **Contusion, laceration, and hemorrhage of cerebellum without LOC**

S06.371 **7th** **Contusion, laceration, and hemorrhage of cerebellum with LOC of; 30 min or less**

S06.372 **7th** **31 min to 59 min**

S06.373 **7th** **1 hour to 5 h 59 min**

S06.374 **7th** **6 h to 24 h**

S06.375 **7th** **greater than 24 h with return to pre-existing conscious level**

S06.376 **7th** **greater than 24 h without return to pre-existing conscious level with patient surviving**

S06.377 **7th** **any duration with death due to brain injury prior to regaining consciousness**

S06.378 **7th** **any duration with death due to other cause prior to regaining consciousness**

S06.379 **7th** **unspecified duration**
Contusion, laceration, and hemorrhage of cerebellum NOS

S06.38 **6th** **Contusion, laceration, and hemorrhage of brainstem**

S06.380 **7th** **Contusion, laceration, and hemorrhage of brainstem without LOC**

S06.381 **7th** **Contusion, laceration, and hemorrhage of brainstem with LOC of; 30 min or less**

S06.382 **7th** **31 min to 59 min**

S06.383 **7th** **1 hour to 5 h 59 min**

S06.384 **7th** **6 h to 24 h**

S06.385 **7th** **greater than 24 h with return to pre-existing conscious level**

S06.386 **7th** **greater than 24 h without return to pre-existing conscious level with patient surviving**

S06.387 **7th** **any duration with death due to brain injury prior to regaining consciousness**

S06.388 **7th** **any duration with death due to other cause prior to regaining consciousness**

S06.389 **7th** **unspecified duration**
Contusion, laceration, and hemorrhage of brainstem NOS

S06.4 **5th** **Epidural hemorrhage**
Extradural hemorrhage NOS
Extradural hemorrhage (traumatic)

> **7th characters for category S06**
> A—initial encounter
> D—subsequent encounter
> S—sequela

S06.4X **6th** **Epidural hemorrhage**

S06.4X0 **7th** **Epidural hemorrhage without loss of consciousness**

S06.4X1 **7th** **Epidural hemorrhage with loss of consciousness of 30 minutes or less**

S06.4X2 **7th** **Epidural hemorrhage with loss of consciousness of 31 minutes to 59 minutes**

S06.4X3 **7th** **Epidural hemorrhage with loss of consciousness of 1 hour to 5 hours 59 minutes**

S06.4X4 **7th** **Epidural hemorrhage with loss of consciousness of 6 hours to 24 hours**

S06.4X5 **7th** **Epidural hemorrhage with loss of consciousness greater than 24 hours with return to pre-existing conscious level**

S06.4X6 **7th** **Epidural hemorrhage with loss of consciousness greater than 24 hours without return to pre-existing conscious level with patient surviving**

S06.4X7 **7th** **Epidural hemorrhage with loss of consciousness of any duration with death due to brain injury prior to regaining consciousness**

S06.4X8 **7th** **Epidural hemorrhage with loss of consciousness of any duration with death due to other causes prior to regaining consciousness**

S06.4X9 **7th** **Epidural hemorrhage with loss of consciousness of unspecified duration**
Epidural hemorrhage NOS

S06.5 **Traumatic subdural hemorrhage**

S06.5X **5th** **Traumatic subdural hemorrhage**

S06.5X0 **6th** **7th** **Traumatic subdural hemorrhage without LOC**

  Additional Character Required   ✓   3-character code   Unspecified laterality codes were excluded here.   •=New Code   ▲=Revised Code   *Excludes1*—Not coded here, do not use together   *Excludes2*—Not included here

CHAPTER 19. INJURY, POISONING AND CERTAIN OTHER CONSEQUENCES OF EXTERNAL CAUSES   (S06.5X1–S09.10X)

S06.5X1 Traumatic subdural hemorrhage with LOC of; 30 min or less
7th

S06.5X2 31 min to 59 min
7th

S06.5X3 1 hour to 5 h 59 min
7th

> 7th characters for category S06
> A—initial encounter
> D—subsequent encounter
> S—sequela

S06.5X4 6 h to 24 h
7th

S06.5X5 greater than 24 h with return to pre-existing conscious level
7th

S06.5X6 greater than 24 h without return to pre-existing conscious level with patient surviving
7th

S06.5X7 any duration with death due to brain injury before regaining consciousness
7th

S06.5X8 any duration with death due to other cause before regaining consciousness
7th

S06.5X9 unspecified duration
Traumatic subdural hemorrhage NOS
7th

S06.6 5th **Traumatic subarachnoid hemorrhage**
    S06.6X 6th **Traumatic subarachnoid hemorrhage**

S06.6X0 Traumatic subarachnoid hemorrhage without LOC
7th

S06.6X1 Traumatic subarachnoid hemorrhage with LOC of; 30 min or less
7th

S06.6X2 31 min to 59 min
7th

S06.6X3 1 hour to 5 h 59 min
7th

S06.6X4 6 h to 24 h
7th

S06.6X5 greater than 24 h with return to pre-existing conscious level
7th

S06.6X6 greater than 24 h without return to pre-existing conscious level with patient surviving
7th

S06.6X7 any duration with death due to brain injury prior to regaining consciousness
7th

S06.6X8 any duration with death due to other cause prior to regaining consciousness
7th

S06.6X9 unspecified duration
Traumatic subarachnoid hemorrhage NOS
7th

S06.8 5th **Other specified intracranial injuries**
    S06.89 6th **Other specified intracranial injury**
      Excludes1: concussion (S06.0X-)

S06.890 Other specified intracranial injury without LOC
7th

S06.891 Other specified intracranial injury with LOC of 30 min or less
7th

S06.892 Other specified intracranial injury with LOC of; 31 min to 59 min
7th

S06.893 1 hour to 5 h 59 min
7th

S06.894 6 h to 24 h
7th

S06.895 greater than 24 h with return to pre-existing conscious level
7th

S06.896 greater than 24 h without return to pre-existing conscious level with patient surviving
7th

S06.897 any duration with death due to brain injury prior to regaining consciousness
7th

S06.898 any duration with death due to other cause prior to regaining consciousness
7th

S06.899 unspecified duration
7th

S06.9 5th **Unspecified intracranial injury**
Brain injury NOS
Head injury NOS with LOC
Traumatic brain injury NOS
Excludes1: conditions classifiable to S06.0- to S06.8- code to specified intracranial injury
head injury NOS (S09.90)

    S06.9X 6th **Unspecified intracranial injury**

S06.9X0 Unspecified intracranial injury without LOC
7th

S06.9X1 Unspecified intracranial injury with LOC of; 30 min or less
7th

S06.9X2 31 min to 59 min
7th

S06.9X3 1 hour to 5 h 59 min
7th

S06.9X4 6 h to 24 h
7th

S06.9X5 greater than 24 h with return to pre-existing conscious level
7th

S06.9X6 greater than 24 h without return to pre-existing conscious level with patient surviving
7th

S06.9X7 any duration with death due to brain injury prior to regaining consciousness
7th

S06.9X8 any duration with death due to other cause prior to regaining consciousness
7th

S06.9X9 unspecified duration
7th

S09 **OTHER AND UNSPECIFIED INJURIES OF HEAD**

S09.0 4th **Injury of blood vessels of head, not elsewhere classified**
Excludes1: injury of cerebral blood vessels (S06.-)
injury of precerebral blood vessels (S15.-)

> 7th characters for category S09
> A—initial encounter
> D—subsequent encounter
> S—sequela

S09.1 5th **Injury of muscle and tendon of head**
Code also any associated open wound (S01.-)
Excludes2: sprain to joints and ligament of head (S03.9)

    S09.10X **Unspecified injury of muscle and tendon of head**
Injury of muscle and tendon of head NOS
7th

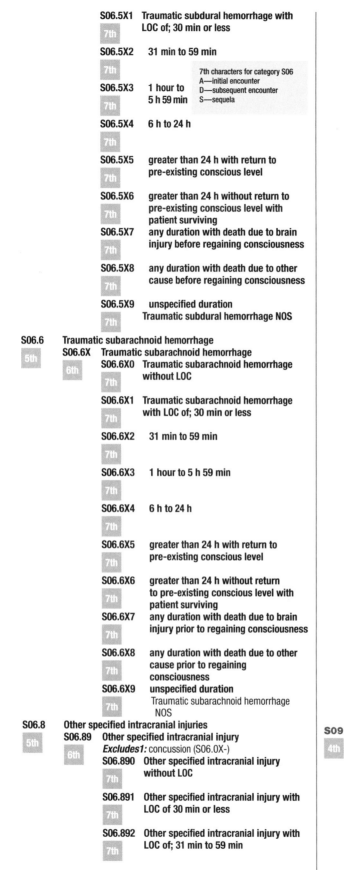

  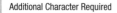 Additional Character Required   3-character code   Unspecified laterality codes were excluded here.   ●=New Code   ▲=Revised Code   *Excludes1*—Not coded here, do not use together   *Excludes2*—Not included here

280   PEDIATRIC ICD-10-CM 2017: A MANUAL FOR PROVIDER-BASED CODING

S09.11X   **Strain of muscle and tendon of head**
`7th`

S09.12X   **Laceration of muscle and tendon of head**
`7th`

S09.19X   **Other specified injury of muscle and tendon of head**
`7th`

S09.2   **Traumatic rupture of ear drum**
`5th`
Excludes1: traumatic rupture of ear drum due to blast injury (S09.31-)

7th characters for category S09
A—initial encounter
D—subsequent encounter
S—sequela

S09.21X   **Traumatic rupture of right ear drum**
`7th`

S09.22X   **Traumatic rupture of left ear drum**
`7th`

S09.8   **Other specified injuries of head**
`5th`

S09.9   **Unspecified injury of face and head**
`5th`
S09.90X   **Unspecified injury of head**
`7th`
    Head injury NOS
    Excludes1: brain injury NOS (S06.9-)
      head injury NOS with LOC (S06.9-)
      intracranial injury NOS (S06.9-)

S09.91X   **Unspecified injury of ear**
`7th`
    Injury of ear NOS

S09.92X   **Unspecified injury of nose**
`7th`
    Injury of nose NOS

S09.93X   **Unspecified injury of face**
`7th`
    Injury of face NOS
    Injuries to the neck (S10–S19)
    Includes: injuries of nape
    injuries of supraclavicular region
    injuries of throat
    Excludes2: burns and corrosions (T20–T32)
      effects of FB in esophagus (T18.1)
      effects of FB in larynx (T17.3)
      effects of FB in pharynx (T17.2)
      effects of FB in trachea (T17.4)
      frostbite (T33–T34)
      insect bite or sting, venomous (T63.4)

(S10–S19) INJURIES TO THE NECK

Includes: injuries of nape
  injuries of supraclavicular region
  injuries of throat
Excludes2: burns and corrosions (T20–T32)
  effects of FB in esophagus (T18.1)
  effects of FB in larynx (T17.3)
  effects of FB in pharynx (T17.2)
  effects of FB in trachea (T17.4)
  frostbite (T33–T34)
  insect bite or sting, venomous (T63.4)

7th characters for category S10 & S11
A—initial encounter
D—subsequent encounter
S—sequela

S10   **SUPERFICIAL INJURY OF NECK**
`4th`
S10.0XX   **Contusion of throat**
`7th`
    Contusion of cervical esophagus
    Contusion of larynx
    Contusion of pharynx
    Contusion of trachea

S10.1   **Other and unspecified superficial injuries of throat**
`5th`
S10.10X   **Unspecified superficial injuries of throat**
`7th`

S10.11X   **Abrasion of throat**
`7th`

S10.12X   **Blister (nonthermal) of throat**
`7th`

S10.14X   **External constriction of part of throat**
`7th`

S10.15X   **Superficial FB of throat**
`7th`
    Splinter in the throat

S10.16X   **Insect bite (nonvenomous) of throat**
`7th`

S10.17X   **Other superficial bite of throat**
`7th`
    Excludes1: open bite of throat (S11.85)

S10.8   **Superficial injury of other specified parts of neck**
`5th`
S10.80X   **Unspecified superficial injury of other specified part of neck**
`7th`

S10.81X   **Abrasion of other specified part of neck**
`7th`

S10.82X   **Blister (nonthermal) of other specified part of neck**
`7th`

S10.83X   **Contusion of other specified part of neck**
`7th`

S10.84X   **External constriction of other specified part of neck**
`7th`

S10.85X   **Superficial FB of other specified part of neck**
`7th`
    Splinter in other specified part of neck

S10.86X   **Insect bite of other specified part of neck**
`7th`

S10.87X   **Other superficial bite of other specified part of neck**
`7th`
    Excludes1: open bite of other specified parts of neck (S11.85)

S10.9   **Superficial injury of unspecified part of neck**
`5th`
S10.90X   **Unspecified superficial injury of unspecified part of neck**
`7th`

S10.91X   **Abrasion of unspecified part of neck**
`7th`

S10.92X   **Blister (nonthermal) of unspecified part of neck**
`7th`

S10.93X   **Contusion of unspecified part of neck**
`7th`

S10.94X   **External constriction of unspecified part of neck**
`7th`

S10.95X   **Superficial FB of unspecified part of neck**
`7th`

S10.96X   **Insect bite of unspecified part of neck**
`7th`

S10.97X   **Other superficial bite of unspecified part of neck**
`7th`

   Additional Character Required   3-character code   Unspecified laterality codes were excluded here.   •=New Code   ▲=Revised Code   *Excludes1*—Not coded here, do not use together   *Excludes2*—Not included here

CHAPTER 19. INJURY, POISONING AND CERTAIN OTHER CONSEQUENCES OF EXTERNAL CAUSES (S11–S14.101)

S11 **OPEN WOUND OF NECK**
`4th`

Code also any associated:
    spinal cord injury (S14.0, S14.1-)
    wound infection
Excludes2: open fracture of vertebra (S12.- with 7th character B)

S11.9 **Open wound of unspecified part of neck**
`5th`

    S11.91X **Laceration without FB of unspecified part of neck**
    `7th`

    S11.92X **Laceration with FB of unspecified part of neck**
    `7th`

    S11.93X **Puncture wound without FB of unspecified part of neck**
    `7th`

    S11.94X **Puncture wound with FB of unspecified part of neck**
    `7th`

    S11.95X **Open bite of unspecified part of neck**
    `7th`   Bite of neck NOS
        Excludes1: superficial bite of neck (S10.97)

S12 **FRACTURE OF CERVICAL VERTEBRA AND OTHER PARTS OF NECK**
`4th`

Note: A fracture not indicated as displaced or nondisplaced should be coded to displaced
A fracture not indicated as open or closed should be coded to closed
Includes: fracture of cervical neural arch
    fracture of cervical spine
    fracture of cervical spinous process
    fracture of cervical transverse process
    fracture of cervical vertebral arch
    fracture of neck
Code first any associated cervical spinal cord injury (S14.0, S14.1-)

7th characters for category S12.0–12.6
A—initial encounter for closed fracture
B—initial encounter for open fracture
D—subsequent encounter for fracture with routine healing
G—subsequent encounter for fracture with delayed healing
K—subsequent encounter for fracture with nonunion
S—sequela

S12.0 **Fracture of first cervical vertebra**
`5th` Atlas

    S12.00 **Unspecified fracture of first cervical vertebra**
    `6th`

        S12.000 **Unspecified displaced fracture of first cervical vertebra**
        `7th`

        S12.001 **Unspecified nondisplaced fracture of first cervical vertebra**
        `7th`

    S12.03 **Posterior arch fracture of first cervical vertebra**
    `6th`

        S12.030 **Displaced posterior arch fracture of first cervical vertebra**
        `7th`

        S12.031 **Nondisplaced posterior arch fracture of first cervical vertebra**
        `7th`

S12.1 **Fracture of second cervical vertebra**
`5th` Axis

    S12.10 **Unspecified fracture of second cervical vertebra**
    `6th`

        S12.100 **Unspecified displaced fracture of second cervical vertebra**
        `7th`

        S12.101 **Unspecified nondisplaced fracture of second cervical vertebra**
        `7th`

S12.2 **Fracture of third cervical vertebra**
`5th`

    S12.20 **Unspecified fracture of third cervical vertebra**
    `6th`

        S12.200 **Unspecified displaced fracture of third cervical vertebra**
        `7th`

        S12.201 **Unspecified nondisplaced fracture of third cervical vertebra**
        `7th`

S12.3 **Fracture of fourth cervical vertebra**
`5th`

    S12.30 **Unspecified fracture of fourth cervical vertebra**
    `6th`

        S12.300 **Unspecified displaced fracture of fourth cervical vertebra**
        `7th`

        S12.301 **Unspecified nondisplaced fracture of fourth cervical vertebra**
        `7th`

S12.4 **Fracture of fifth cervical vertebra**
`5th`

    S12.40 **Unspecified fracture of fifth cervical vertebra**
    `6th`

        S12.400 **Unspecified displaced fracture of fifth cervical vertebra**
        `7th`

        S12.401 **Unspecified nondisplaced fracture of fifth cervical vertebra**
        `7th`

S12.5 **Fracture of sixth cervical vertebra**
`5th`

    S12.50 **Unspecified fracture of sixth cervical vertebra**
    `6th`

        S12.500 **Unspecified displaced fracture of sixth cervical vertebra**
        `7th`

        S12.501 **Unspecified nondisplaced fracture of sixth cervical vertebra**
        `7th`

S12.6 **Fracture of seventh cervical vertebra**
`5th`

    S12.60 **Unspecified fracture of seventh cervical vertebra**
    `6th`

        S12.600 **Unspecified displaced fracture of seventh cervical vertebra**
        `7th`

        S12.601 **Unspecified nondisplaced fracture of seventh cervical vertebra**
        `7th`

S12.8XX **Fracture of other parts of neck**
`7th` Hyoid bone
    Larynx
    Thyroid cartilage
    Trachea

S12.9XX **Fracture of neck, unspecified**
`7th` Fracture of neck NOS
    Fracture of cervical spine NOS
    Fracture of cervical vertebra NOS

7th characters for category S12.8 & S12.9
A—initial encounter
D—subsequent encounter
S—sequela

S13 **DISLOCATION AND SPRAIN OF JOINTS AND LIGAMENTS AT NECK LEVEL**
`4th`

Includes: avulsion of joint or ligament at neck level
    laceration of cartilage, joint or ligament at neck level
    sprain of cartilage, joint or ligament at neck level
    traumatic hemarthrosis of joint or ligament at neck level
    traumatic rupture of joint or ligament at neck level
    traumatic subluxation of joint or ligament at neck level
    traumatic tear of joint or ligament at neck level
Code also any associated open wound
Excludes2: strain of muscle or tendon at neck level (S16.1)

7th characters for category S13
A—initial encounter
D—subsequent encounter
S—sequela

S13.4XX **Sprain of ligaments of cervical spine**
`7th` Sprain of anterior longitudinal (ligament), cervical
    Sprain of atlanto-axial (joints)
    Sprain of atlanto-occipital (joints)
    Whiplash injury of cervical spine

S14 **INJURY OF NERVES AND SPINAL CORD AT NECK LEVEL**
`4th`

Note: Code to highest level of cervical cord injury
Code also any associated:
    fracture of cervical vertebra (S12.0–S12.6.-)
    open wound of neck (S11.-)
    transient paralysis (R29.5)

7th characters for category S14
A—initial encounter
D—subsequent encounter
S—sequela

S14.0XX **Concussion and edema of cervical spinal cord**
`7th`

S14.1 **Other and unspecified injuries of cervical spinal cord**
`5th`

    S14.10 **Unspecified injury of cervical spinal cord**
    `6th`

        S14.101 **Unspecified injury at; C1 level of cervical spinal cord**
        `7th`

`4th` `5th` `6th` `7th` Additional Character Required   3-character code   Unspecified laterality codes were excluded here.   =New Code =Revised Code   ***Excludes1***—Not coded here, do not use together ***Excludes2***—Not included here

       PEDIATRIC ICD-10-CM 2017: A MANUAL FOR PROVIDER-BASED CODING

S14.102   C2 level of cervical spinal cord
7th

S14.103   C3 level of cervical spinal cord
7th

S14.104   C4 level of cervical spinal cord
7th

S14.105   C5 level of cervical spinal cord
7th

S14.106   C6 level of cervical spinal cord
7th

> 7th characters for category S14
> A—initial encounter
> D—subsequent encounter
> S—sequela

S14.107   C7 level of cervical spinal cord
7th

S14.108   C8 level of cervical spinal cord
7th

S14.109   unspecified level of cervical spinal cord
7th
     Injury of cervical spinal cord NOS

S14.2XX   Injury of nerve root of cervical spine
7th

S14.3XX   Injury of brachial plexus
7th

S14.4XX   Injury of peripheral nerves of neck
7th

S14.5XX   Injury of cervical sympathetic nerves
7th

S14.8XX   Injury of other specified nerves of neck
7th

> 7th characters for category S14, S15, & S16
> A—initial encounter
> D—subsequent encounter
> S—sequela

S14.9XX   Injury of unspecified nerves of neck
7th

S15   **INJURY OF BLOOD VESSELS AT NECK LEVEL**
4th
Code also any associated open wound (S11.-)

S15.8XX   Injury of other specified blood vessels at neck level
7th

S15.9XX   Injury of unspecified blood vessel at neck level
7th

S16   **INJURY OF MUSCLE, FASCIA AND TENDON AT NECK LEVEL**
4th
Code also any associated open wound (S11.-)
Excludes2: sprain of joint or ligament at neck level (S13.9)

S16.1XX   Strain of muscle, fascia and tendon at neck level
7th

S16.2XX   Laceration of muscle, fascia and tendon at neck level
7th

S16.8XX   Other specified injury of muscle, fascia and tendon at neck level
7th

S16.9XX   Unspecified injury of muscle, fascia and tendon at neck level
7th
Injuries to the thorax (S20–S29)
Includes: injuries of breast
   injuries of chest (wall)
   injuries of interscapular area
Excludes2: burns and corrosions (T20–T32)
   effects of FB in bronchus (T17.5)
   effects of FB in esophagus (T18.1)
   effects of FB in lung (T17.8)
   effects of FB in trachea (T17.4)
   frostbite (T33–T34)
   injuries of axilla
   injuries of clavicle
   injuries of scapular region
   injuries of shoulder
   insect bite or sting, venomous (T63.4)

(S20–S29) INJURIES TO THE THORAX

Includes: injuries of breast
   injuries of chest (wall)
   injuries of interscapular area
Excludes2: burns and corrosions (T20–T32)
   effects of FB in bronchus (T17.5)
   effects of FB in esophagus (T18.1)
   effects of FB in lung (T17.8)
   effects of FB in trachea (T17.4)
   frostbite (T33–T34)
   injuries of axilla
   injuries of clavicle
   injuries of scapular region
   injuries of shoulder
   insect bite or sting, venomous (T63.4)

> 7th characters for category S20
> A—initial encounter
> D—subsequent encounter
> S—sequela

S20   **SUPERFICIAL INJURY OF THORAX**
4th
   S20.0   **Contusion of breast**
5th
     S20.00X   Contusion of breast, unspecified breast
     7th

     S20.01X   Contusion of right breast
     7th

     S20.02X   Contusion of left breast
     7th

   S20.1   **Other and unspecified superficial injuries of breast**
5th
     S20.11   **Abrasion of breast**
     6th
       S20.111   Abrasion of breast, right breast
       7th

       S20.112   Abrasion of breast, left breast
       7th

       S20.119   Abrasion of breast, unspecified breast
       7th

     S20.12   **Blister (nonthermal) of breast**
     6th
       S20.121   Blister (nonthermal) of breast, right breast
       7th

       S20.122   Blister (nonthermal) of breast, left breast
       7th

       S20.129   Blister (nonthermal) of breast, unspecified breast
       7th

     S20.14   **External constriction of part of breast**
       S20.141   External constriction of part of breast, right breast
       7th

       S20.142   External constriction of part of breast, left breast
       7th

  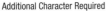

CHAPTER 19. INJURY, POISONING AND CERTAIN OTHER CONSEQUENCES OF EXTERNAL CAUSES (S20.15–S20.91X)

S20.15 **Superficial FB of breast**
6th
Splinter in the breast
S20.151 **Superficial FB of breast, right breast**
7th

S20.152 **Superficial FB of breast, left breast**
7th

S20.16 **Insect bite (nonvenomous) of breast**
6th
S20.161 **Insect bite (nonvenomous) of breast, right breast**
7th

S20.162 **Insect bite (nonvenomous) of breast, left breast**
7th

S20.17 **Other superficial bite of breast**
6th
Excludes1: open bite of breast (S21.05-)
S20.171 **Other superficial bite of breast, right breast**
7th

S20.172 **Other superficial bite of breast, left breast**
7th

7th characters for category S20
A—initial encounter
D—subsequent encounter
S—sequela

S20.2 **Contusion of thorax**
5th
S20.20X **Contusion of thorax, unspecified**
7th

S20.21 **Contusion of front wall of thorax**
6th
S20.211 **Contusion of right front wall of thorax**
7th

S20.212 **Contusion of left front wall of thorax**
7th

S20.219 **Contusion of unspecified front wall of thorax**
7th

S20.22 **Contusion of back wall of thorax**
6th
S20.221 **Contusion of right back wall of thorax**
7th

S20.222 **Contusion of left back wall of thorax**
7th

S20.229 **Contusion of unspecified back wall of thorax**
7th
Interscapular contusion

S20.3 **Other and unspecified superficial injuries of front wall of thorax**
5th
S20.30 **Unspecified superficial injuries of front wall of thorax**
6th
S20.301 **Unspecified superficial injuries of right front wall of thorax**
7th

S20.302 **Unspecified superficial injuries of left front wall of thorax**
7th

S20.309 **Unspecified superficial injuries of unspecified front wall of thorax**
7th

S20.31 **Abrasion of front wall of thorax**
6th
S20.311 **Abrasion of right front wall of thorax**
7th

S20.312 **Abrasion of left front wall of thorax**
7th

S20.319 **Abrasion of unspecified front wall of thorax**
7th

S20.36 **Insect bite (nonvenomous) of front wall of thorax**
6th
S20.361 **Insect bite (nonvenomous) of right front wall of thorax**
7th

S20.362 **Insect bite (nonvenomous) of left front wall of thorax**
7th

S20.369 **Insect bite (nonvenomous) of unspecified front wall of thorax**
7th

S20.37 **Other superficial bite of front wall of thorax**
6th
Excludes1: open bite of front wall of thorax (S21.14)
S20.371 **Other superficial bite of right front wall of thorax**
7th

S20.372 **Other superficial bite of left front wall of thorax**
7th

S20.379 **Other superficial bite of unspecified front wall of thorax**
7th

S20.4 **Other and unspecified superficial injuries of back wall of thorax**
5th
S20.40 **Unspecified superficial injuries of back wall of thorax**
6th
S20.401 **Unspecified superficial injuries of right back wall of thorax**
7th

S20.402 **Unspecified superficial injuries of left back wall of thorax**
7th

S20.409 **Unspecified superficial injuries of unspecified back wall of thorax**
7th

S20.41 **Abrasion of back wall of thorax**
6th
S20.411 **Abrasion of right back wall of thorax**
7th

S20.412 **Abrasion of left back wall of thorax**
7th

S20.419 **Abrasion of unspecified back wall of thorax**
7th

S20.46 **Insect bite (nonvenomous) of back wall of thorax**
6th
S20.461 **Insect bite (nonvenomous) of right back wall of thorax**
7th

S20.462 **Insect bite (nonvenomous) of left back wall of thorax**
7th

S20.469 **Insect bite (nonvenomous) of unspecified back wall of thorax**
7th

S20.47 **Other superficial bite of back wall of thorax**
6th
Excludes1: open bite of back wall of thorax (S21.24)
S20.471 **Other superficial bite of right back wall of thorax**
7th

S20.472 **Other superficial bite of left back wall of thorax**
7th

S20.479 **Other superficial bite of unspecified back wall of thorax**
7th

S20.9 **Superficial injury of unspecified parts of thorax**
5th
Excludes1: contusion of thorax NOS (S20.20)
S20.90X **Unspecified superficial injury of unspecified parts of thorax**
7th
Superficial injury of thoracic wall NOS
S20.91X **Abrasion of unspecified parts of thorax**
7th

  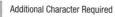 Additional Character Required   ✔ 3-character code   Unspecified laterality codes were excluded here.   •=New Code   ▲=Revised Code   *Excludes1*—Not coded here, do not use together   *Excludes2*—Not included here

S20.92X Blister (nonthermal) of unspecified parts of thorax

`7th`

S20.94X External constriction of unspecified parts of thorax

`7th`

S20.95X Superficial FB of unspecified parts of thorax

`7th`   Splinter in thorax NOS

S20.96X Insect bite (nonvenomous) of unspecified parts of thorax

`7th`

S20.97X Other superficial bite of unspecified parts of thorax

`7th`   *Excludes1:* open bite of thorax NOS (S21.95)

S21   **OPEN WOUND OF THORAX**

`4th`   **Code also** any associated injury, such as: rib fracture (S22.3-, S22.4-) wound infection

Excludes1: traumatic amputation (partial) of thorax (S28.1)

> 7th characters for category S21
> A—initial encounter
> D—subsequent encounter
> S—sequela

S21.1XX Open wound of front wall of thorax without penetration into thoracic cavity

`7th`

   S21.11 Laceration without FB of front wall of thorax without penetration into thoracic cavity

   `6th`

     S21.111 Laceration without FB of; right front wall of thorax without penetration into thoracic cavity

     `7th`

     S21.112 of left front wall of thorax without penetration into thoracic cavity

     `7th`

     S21.119 unspecified front wall of thorax without penetration into thoracic cavity

     `7th`

   S21.12 Laceration with FB of; front wall of thorax without penetration into thoracic cavity

   `6th`

     S21.121 right front wall of thorax without penetration into thoracic cavity

     `7th`

     S21.122 left front wall of thorax without penetration into thoracic cavity

     `7th`

     S21.129 unspecified front wall of thorax without penetration into thoracic cavity

     `7th`

   S21.13 Puncture wound without FB of; front wall of thorax without penetration into thoracic cavity

   `6th`

     S21.131 right front wall of thorax without penetration into thoracic cavity

     `7th`

     S21.132 left front wall of thorax without penetration into thoracic cavity

     `7th`

     S21.139 unspecified front wall of thorax without penetration into thoracic cavity

     `7th`

   S21.14 Puncture wound with FB of; front wall of thorax without penetration into thoracic cavity

   `6th`

     S21.141 right front wall of thorax without penetration into thoracic cavity

     `7th`

     S21.142 left front wall of thorax without penetration into thoracic cavity

     `7th`

     S21.149 unspecified front wall of thorax without penetration into thoracic cavity

     `7th`

S21.2 Open wound of back wall of thorax without penetration into thoracic cavity

`5th`

   S21.21 Laceration without FB of; back wall of thorax without penetration into thoracic cavity

   `6th`

     S21.211 right back wall of thorax without penetration into thoracic cavity

     `7th`

     S21.212 left back wall of thorax without penetration into thoracic cavity

     `7th`

     S21.219 unspecified back wall of thorax without penetration into thoracic cavity

     `7th`

   S21.22 Laceration with FB of; back wall of thorax without penetration into thoracic cavity

   `6th`

     S21.221 right back wall of thorax without penetration into thoracic cavity

     `7th`

     S21.222 left back wall of thorax without penetration into thoracic cavity

     `7th`

     S21.229 unspecified back wall of thorax without penetration into thoracic cavity

     `7th`

   S21.23 Puncture wound without FB of; back wall of thorax without penetration into thoracic cavity

   `6th`

     S21.231 right back wall of thorax without penetration into thoracic cavity

     `7th`

     S21.232 left back wall of thorax without penetration into thoracic cavity

     `7th`

     S21.239 unspecified back wall of thorax without penetration into thoracic cavity

     `7th`

   S21.24 Puncture wound with FB of; back wall of thorax without penetration into thoracic cavity

   `6th`

     S21.241 right back wall of thorax without penetration into thoracic cavity

     `7th`

     S21.242 left back wall of thorax without penetration into thoracic cavity

     `7th`

     S21.249 unspecified back wall of thorax without penetration into thoracic cavity

     `7th`

S21.9 Open wound of unspecified part of thorax

`5th`   Open wound of thoracic wall NOS

S21.91X Laceration without FB of unspecified part of thorax

`7th`

S21.92X Laceration with FB of unspecified part of thorax

`7th`

S21.93X Puncture wound without FB of unspecified part of thorax

`7th`

S21.94X Puncture wound with FB of unspecified part of thorax

`7th`

S21.95X Open bite of unspecified part of thorax

`7th`   *Excludes1:* superficial bite of thorax (S20.97)

CHAPTER 19. INJURY, POISONING AND CERTAIN OTHER CONSEQUENCES OF EXTERNAL CAUSES   (S20.92X–S21.95X)

    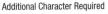 Additional Character Required   3-character code   Unspecified laterality codes were excluded here.   •=New Code   *Excludes1*—Not coded here, do not use together
    ▲=Revised Code   *Excludes2*—Not included here

PEDIATRIC ICD-10-CM 2017: A MANUAL FOR PROVIDER-BASED CODING   285

CHAPTER 19. INJURY, POISONING AND CERTAIN OTHER CONSEQUENCES OF EXTERNAL CAUSES (S22–S30.21X)

S22   FRACTURE OF RIB(S), STERNUM AND THORACIC SPINE

4th

Note: A fracture not indicated as displaced or nondisplaced should be coded to displaced

A fracture not indicated as open or closed should be coded to closed

Includes: fracture of thoracic neural arch
fracture of thoracic spinous process
fracture of thoracic transverse process
fracture of thoracic vertebra or of thoracic vertebral arch

Code first any associated:
injury of intrathoracic organ (S27.-)
spinal cord injury (S24.0-, S24.1-)

Excludes1: transection of thorax (S28.1)

Excludes2: fracture of clavicle (S42.0-)
fracture of scapula (S42.1-)

> 7th characters for category S22
> A—initial encounter for closed fracture
> B—initial encounter for open fracture
> D—subsequent encounter for fracture with routine healing
> G—subsequent encounter for fracture with delayed healing
> K—subsequent encounter for fracture with nonunion
> S—sequela

S22.3   **Fracture of one rib**

5th

S22.31X   **Fracture of one rib, right side**
7th

S22.32X   **Fracture of one rib, left side**
7th

S22.39X   **Fracture of one rib, unspecified side**
7th

S22.4   **Multiple fractures of ribs**

5th

Fractures of two or more ribs

Excludes1: flail chest (S22.5-)

S22.41X   **Multiple fractures of ribs, right side**
7th

S22.42X   **Multiple fractures of ribs, left side**
7th

S22.43X   **Multiple fractures of ribs, bilateral**
7th

S22.49X   **Multiple fractures of ribs, unspecified side**
7th

S22.5XX   **Flail chest**
7th

S22.9XX   **Fracture of bony thorax, part unspecified**
7th

S24   INJURY OF NERVES AND SPINAL CORD AT THORAX LEVEL

4th

Note: Code to highest level of thoracic spinal cord injury
Injuries to the spinal cord (S24.0 and S24.1) refer to the cord level and not bone level injury, and can affect nerve roots at and below the level given.

Code also any associated:
fracture of thoracic vertebra (S22.0-)
open wound of thorax (S21.-)
transient paralysis (R29.5)

> 7th characters for category S24
> A—initial encounter
> D—subsequent encounter
> S—sequela

Excludes2: injury of brachial plexus (S14.3)

S24.0XX   **Concussion and edema of thoracic spinal cord**
7th

S24.1   **Other and unspecified injuries of thoracic spinal cord**

5th

S24.10   **Unspecified injury of thoracic spinal cord**

6th

S24.101   **Unspecified injury at; T1 level of thoracic spinal cord**
7th

S24.102   T2–T6 level of thoracic spinal cord
7th

S24.103   T7–T10 level of thoracic spinal cord
7th

S24.104   T11–T12 level of thoracic spinal cord
7th

S24.109   **unspecified level of thoracic spinal cord**
7th
Injury of thoracic spinal cord NOS

S27   INJURY OF OTHER AND UNSPECIFIED INTRATHORACIC ORGANS

4th

Code also any associated open wound of thorax (S21.-)

Excludes2: injury of cervical esophagus (S10–S19)
injury of trachea (cervical) (S10–S19)

> 7th characters for category S27
> A—initial encounter
> D—subsequent encounter
> S—sequela

S27.0XX   **Traumatic pneumothorax**
7th
Excludes1: spontaneous pneumothorax (J93.-)

S27.3   **Other and unspecified injuries of lung**

5th

S27.30   **Unspecified injury of lung**

6th

S27.301   **Unspecified injury of lung, unilateral**
7th

S27.302   **Unspecified injury of lung, bilateral**
7th

S27.32   **Contusion of lung**

6th

S27.321   **Contusion of lung, unilateral**
7th

S27.322   **Contusion of lung, bilateral**
7th

S27.329   **Contusion of lung, unspecified**
7th

(S30–S39) INJURIES TO THE ABDOMEN, LOWER BACK, LUMBAR SPINE, PELVIS AND EXTERNAL GENITALS

Includes: injuries to the abdominal wall
injuries to the anus
injuries to the buttock
injuries to the external genitalia
injuries to the flank
injuries to the groin

Excludes2: burns and corrosions (T20–T32)
effects of FB in anus and rectum (T18.5)
effects of FB in genitourinary tract (T19.-)
effects of FB in stomach, small intestine and colon (T18.2–T18.4)
frostbite (T33–T34)
insect bite or sting, venomous (T63.4)

S30   SUPERFICIAL INJURY OF ABDOMEN, LOWER BACK, PELVIS AND EXTERNAL GENITALS

4th

Excludes2: superficial injury of hip (S70.-)

S30.0XX   **Contusion of lower back and pelvis**
7th
Contusion of buttock

> 7th characters for category S30
> A—initial encounter
> D—subsequent encounter
> S—sequela

S30.1XX   **Contusion of abdominal wall**
7th
Contusion of flank
Contusion of groin

S30.2   **Contusion of external genital organs**

5th

S30.20   **Contusion of unspecified external genital organ**

6th

S30.201   **Contusion of unspecified external genital organ, male**
7th

S30.202   **Contusion of unspecified external genital organ, female**
7th

S30.21X   **Contusion of penis**
7th

  Additional Character Required   3-character code   Unspecified laterality codes were excluded here.   •=New Code   ▲=Revised Code   **Excludes1**—Not coded here, do not use together   **Excludes2**—Not included here

S30.22X   Contusion of scrotum and testes

> `7th`

S30.23X   Contusion of vagina and vulva

> `7th`

S30.3XX   Contusion of anus

> `7th`

S30.8   Other superficial injuries of abdomen, lower back, pelvis and external genitals

> `5th`

    S30.81   Abrasion of abdomen, lower back, pelvis and external genitals

> `6th`

       S30.810   Abrasion of lower back and pelvis

> `7th`

       S30.811   Abrasion of abdominal wall

> `7th`

       S30.812   Abrasion of penis

> `7th`

       S30.813   Abrasion of scrotum and testes

> `7th`

       S30.814   Abrasion of vagina and vulva

> `7th`

       S30.815   Abrasion of unspecified external genital organs, male

> `7th`

       S30.816   Abrasion of unspecified external genital organs, female

> `7th`

7th characters for category S30
A—initial encounter
D—subsequent encounter
S—sequela

       S30.817   Abrasion of anus

> `7th`

    S30.82   Blister (nonthermal) of abdomen, lower back, pelvis and external genitals

> `6th`

       S30.820   Blister (non-thermal) of lower back and pelvis

> `7th`

       S30.821   Blister (nonthermal) of abdominal wall

> `7th`

       S30.822   Blister (nonthermal) of penis

> `7th`

       S30.823   Blister (nonthermal) of scrotum and testes

> `7th`

       S30.824   Blister (nonthermal) of vagina and vulva

> `7th`

       S30.825   Blister (nonthermal) of unspecified external genital organs, male

> `7th`

       S30.826   Blister (nonthermal) of unspecified external genital organs, female

> `7th`

       S30.827   Blister (nonthermal) of anus

> `7th`

    S30.84   External constriction of abdomen, lower back, pelvis and external genitals

> `6th`

       S30.840   External constriction of lower back and pelvis

> `7th`

       S30.841   External constriction of abdominal wall

> `7th`

S30.842   External constriction of penis

> `7th`

       Hair tourniquet syndrome of penis

       Use additional cause code to identify the constricting item (W49.0-)

S30.843   External constriction of scrotum and testes

> `7th`

S30.844   External constriction of vagina and vulva

> `7th`

S30.845   External constriction of unspecified external genital organs, male

> `7th`

S30.846   External constriction of unspecified external genital organs, female

> `7th`

S30.85   Superficial FB of abdomen, lower back, pelvis and external genitals

> `6th`

    Splinter in the abdomen, lower back, pelvis and external genitals

    S30.850   Superficial FB of; lower back and pelvis

> `7th`

    S30.851   abdominal wall

> `7th`

    S30.852   penis

> `7th`

    S30.853   scrotum and testes

> `7th`

    S30.854   vagina and vulva

> `7th`

    S30.855   unspecified external genital organs, male

> `7th`

    S30.856   unspecified external genital organs, female

> `7th`

    S30.857   anus

> `7th`

S30.86   Insect bite (nonvenomous) of abdomen, lower back, pelvis and external genitals

> `6th`

    S30.860   Insect bite (nonvenomous) of; lower back and pelvis

> `7th`

    S30.861   abdominal wall

> `7th`

    S30.862   penis

> `7th`

    S30.863   scrotum and testes

> `7th`

    S30.864   vagina and vulva

> `7th`

    S30.865   unspecified external genital organs, male

> `7th`

    S30.866   unspecified external genital organs, female

> `7th`

    S30.867   anus

> `7th`

  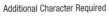 Additional Character Required   ✓   3-character code   Unspecified laterality codes were excluded here.   •=New Code   ▲=Revised Code   **Excludes1**—Not coded here, do not use together   **Excludes2**—Not included here

CHAPTER 19. INJURY, POISONING AND CERTAIN OTHER CONSEQUENCES OF EXTERNAL CAUSES   (S30.87–S31.123)

S30.87 **Other superficial bite of abdomen, lower back, pelvis and external genitals**
6th
Excludes1: open bite of abdomen, lower back, pelvis and external genitals (S31.05, S31.15, S31.25, S31.35, S31.45, S31.55)

S30.870 **Other superficial bite of; lower back and pelvis**
7th

S30.871 **abdominal wall**
7th

S30.872 **penis**
7th

S30.873 **scrotum and testes**
7th

S30.874 **vagina and vulva**
7th

S30.875 **unspecified external genital organs, male**
7th

S30.876 **unspecified external genital organs, female**
7th

S30.877 **anus**
7th

S30.9 **Unspecified superficial injury of abdomen, lower back, pelvis and external genitals**
5th

S30.91X **Unspecified superficial injury of; lower back and pelvis**
7th

S30.92X **abdominal wall**
7th

S30.93X **penis**
7th

S30.94X **scrotum and testes**
7th

S30.95X **vagina and vulva**
7th

S30.96X **unspecified external genital organs, male**
7th

S30.97X **unspecified external genital organs, female**
7th

S30.98X **anus**
7th

> 7th characters for categories S30 & S31
> A—initial encounter
> D—subsequent encounter
> S—sequela

S31 **OPEN WOUND OF ABDOMEN, LOWER BACK, PELVIS AND EXTERNAL GENITALS**
4th
Code also any associated:
    spinal cord injury (S24.0, S24.1-, S34.0-, S34.1-)
    wound infection

> For subcategory S31.0, use 6th character of 1 for penetration into the retroperitoneum, along with the appropriate 7th character.

Excludes1: traumatic amputation of part of abdomen, lower back and pelvis (S38.2-, S38.3)
Excludes2: open wound of hip (S71.00–S71.02)
    open fracture of pelvis (S32.1–S32.9 with 7th character B)

S31.0 **Open wound of lower back and pelvis**
5th

S31.01 **Laceration without FB of lower back and pelvis;**
6th
S31.010 **without penetration into retroperitoneum**
7th
    Laceration without FB of lower back and pelvis NOS

S31.02 **Laceration with FB of lower back and pelvis;**
6th
S31.020 **without penetration into retroperitoneum**
7th
    Laceration with FB of lower back and pelvis NOS

S31.03 **Puncture wound without FB of lower back and pelvis**
6th
S31.030 **Puncture wound without FB of lower back and pelvis without penetration into retroperitoneum**
7th
    Puncture wound without FB of lower back and pelvis NOS

S31.04 **Puncture wound with FB of lower back and pelvis**
6th
S31.040 **Puncture wound with FB of lower back and pelvis; without penetration into retroperitoneum**
7th
    Puncture wound with FB of lower back and pelvis NOS

S31.05 **Open bite of lower back and pelvis**
6th
    Bite of lower back and pelvis NOS
Excludes1: superficial bite of lower back and pelvis (S30.860, S30.870)
S31.050 **Open bite of lower back and pelvis without penetration into retroperitoneum**
7th
    Open bite of lower back and pelvis NOS

S31.1 **Open wound of abdominal wall without penetration into peritoneal cavity**
5th
    Open wound of abdominal wall NOS
Excludes2: open wound of abdominal wall with penetration into peritoneal cavity (S31.6-)

S31.11 **Laceration without FB of abdominal wall without penetration into peritoneal cavity**
6th
S31.110 **Laceration without FB of abdominal wall; RUQ without penetration into peritoneal cavity**
7th

> 7th characters for category S31
> A—initial encounter
> D—subsequent encounter
> S—sequela

S31.111 **LUQ without penetration into peritoneal cavity**
7th

S31.112 **epigastric region without penetration into peritoneal cavity**
7th

S31.113 **RLQ without penetration into peritoneal cavity**
7th

S31.114 **LLQ without penetration into peritoneal cavity**
7th

S31.115 **periumbilic region without penetration into peritoneal cavity**
7th

S31.119 **unspecified quadrant without penetration into peritoneal cavity**
7th

S31.12 **Laceration with FB of abdominal wall without penetration into peritoneal cavity**
6th
S31.120 **Laceration of abdominal wall with FB; RUQ without penetration into peritoneal cavity**
7th

S31.121 **LUQ without penetration into peritoneal cavity**
7th

S31.122 **epigastric region without penetration into peritoneal cavity**
7th

S31.123 **RLQ without penetration into peritoneal cavity**
7th

4th *5th* *6th* *7th*   Additional Character Required   ✔ 3-character code   Unspecified laterality codes were excluded here.   •=New Code   ▲=Revised Code   *Excludes1*—Not coded here, do not use together   *Excludes2*—Not included here

288   **PEDIATRIC ICD-10-CM 2017: A MANUAL FOR PROVIDER-BASED CODING**

S31.124 `7th` LLQ without penetration into peritoneal cavity

S31.125 `7th` periumbilic region without penetration into peritoneal cavity

S31.129 `7th` unspecified quadrant without penetration into peritoneal cavity

S31.13 `6th` **Puncture wound of abdominal wall without FB without penetration into peritoneal cavity**

S31.130 `7th` Puncture wound of abdominal wall without FB; RUQ without penetration into peritoneal cavity

S31.131 `7th` LUQ without penetration into peritoneal cavity

S31.132 `7th` epigastric region without penetration into peritoneal cavity

S31.133 `7th` RLQ without penetration into peritoneal cavity

S31.134 `7th` LLQ without penetration into peritoneal cavity

S31.135 `7th` periumbilic region without penetration into peritoneal cavity

S31.139 `7th` unspecified quadrant without penetration into peritoneal cavity

S31.14 `6th` **Puncture wound of abdominal wall with FB without penetration into peritoneal cavity**

S31.140 `7th` Puncture wound of abdominal wall with FB; RUQ without penetration into peritoneal cavity

7th characters for category S31
A—initial encounter
D—subsequent encounter
S—sequela

S31.141 `7th` LUQ without penetration into peritoneal cavity

S31.142 `7th` epigastric region without penetration into peritoneal cavity

S31.143 `7th` RLQ without penetration into peritoneal cavity

S31.144 `7th` LLQ without penetration into peritoneal cavity

S31.145 `7th` periumbilic region without penetration into peritoneal cavity

S31.149 `7th` unspecified quadrant without penetration into peritoneal cavity

S31.15 `6th` **Open bite of abdominal wall without penetration into peritoneal cavity**
Bite of abdominal wall NOS
Excludes1: superficial bite of abdominal wall (S30.871)

S31.150 `7th` Open bite of abdominal wall; RUQ without penetration into peritoneal cavity

S31.151 `7th` LUQ without penetration into peritoneal cavity

S31.152 `7th` epigastric region without penetration into peritoneal cavity

S31.153 `7th` RLQ without penetration into peritoneal cavity

S31.154 `7th` LLQ without penetration into peritoneal cavity

S31.155 `7th` periumbilic region without penetration into peritoneal cavity

S31.159 `7th` unspecified quadrant without penetration into peritoneal cavity

S31.2 **Open wound of penis**
S31.21X `5th` `7th` Laceration without FB of penis

S31.3 **Open wound of scrotum and testes**
S31.31X `5th` `7th` Laceration without FB of scrotum and testes

S31.4 **Open wound of vagina and vulva**
`5th` *Excludes1:* injury to vagina and vulva during delivery (O70.-, O71.4)

S31.41X `7th` Laceration without FB of vagina and vulva

S31.42X `7th` Laceration with FB of vagina and vulva

S31.43X `7th` Puncture wound without FB of vagina and vulva

S31.44X `7th` Puncture wound with FB of vagina and vulva

S31.45X `7th` Open bite of vagina and vulva
Bite of vagina and vulva NOS
Excludes1: superficial bite of vagina and vulva (S30.864, S30.874)

S31.8 **Open wound of other parts of abdomen, lower back and pelvis**
`5th`

S31.81 `6th` **Open wound of right buttock**

S31.811 `7th` Laceration without FB of right buttock

S31.812 `7th` Laceration with FB of right buttock

S31.813 `7th` Puncture wound without FB of right buttock

S31.814 `7th` Puncture wound with FB of right buttock

S31.815 `7th` Open bite of right buttock
Bite of right buttock NOS
Excludes1: superficial bite of buttock (S30.870)

S31.82 `6th` **Open wound of left buttock**

S31.821 `7th` Laceration without FB of left buttock

S31.822 `7th` Laceration with FB of left buttock

S31.823 `7th` Puncture wound without FB of left buttock

S31.824 `7th` Puncture wound with FB of left buttock

  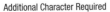 `4th` `5th` `6th` `7th` Additional Character Required   3-character code   Unspecified laterality codes were excluded here.   •=New Code   ▲=Revised Code   *Excludes1*—Not coded here, do not use together   *Excludes2*—Not included here

CHAPTER 19. INJURY, POISONING AND CERTAIN OTHER CONSEQUENCES OF EXTERNAL CAUSES   (S31.825–S32.399)

S31.825   **Open bite of left buttock**
`7th`
Bite of left buttock NOS
Excludes1: superficial bite of buttock (S30.870)

S31.83   **Open wound of anus**
`6th`

   S31.831   **Laceration without FB of anus**
`7th`

   S31.832   **Laceration with FB of anus**
`7th`

   S31.833   **Puncture wound without FB of anus**
`7th`

   S31.834   **Puncture wound with FB of anus**
`7th`

   S31.835   **Open bite of anus**
`7th`
Bite of anus NOS
Excludes1: superficial bite of anus (S30.877)

S32   FRACTURE OF LUMBAR SPINE AND PELVIS
`4th`

Note: A fracture not indicated as displaced or nondisplaced should be coded to displaced
A fracture not indicated as opened or closed should be coded to closed
Includes: fracture of lumbosacral neural arch
fracture of lumbosacral spinous process
fracture of lumbosacral transverse process
fracture of lumbosacral vertebra or of lumbosacral vertebral arch
Code first any associated spinal cord and spinal nerve injury (S34.-)
Excludes1: transection of abdomen (S38.3)
Excludes2: fracture of hip NOS (S72.0-)

> 7th characters for category S32
> A—initial encounter for closed fracture
> B—initial encounter for open fracture
> D—subsequent encounter for fracture with routine healing
> G—subsequent encounter for fracture with delayed healing
> K—subsequent encounter for fracture with nonunion
> S—sequela

S32.1   **Fracture of sacrum**
`5th`
For vertical fractures, code to most medial fracture extension
Use two codes if both a vertical and transverse fracture are present
Code also any associated fracture of pelvic ring (S32.8-)

   S32.10X   **Unspecified fracture of sacrum**
`7th`

   S32.11   **Zone I fracture of sacrum**
`6th`
Vertical sacral ala fracture of sacrum

     S32.110   **Nondisplaced Zone I fracture of sacrum**
`7th`

     S32.111   **Minimally displaced Zone I fracture of sacrum**
`7th`

     S32.112   **Severely displaced Zone I fracture of sacrum**
`7th`

     S32.119   **Unspecified Zone I fracture of sacrum**
`7th`

   S32.12   **Zone II fracture of sacrum**
`6th`
Vertical foraminal region fracture of sacrum

     S32.120   **Nondisplaced Zone II fracture of sacrum**
`7th`

     S32.121   **Minimally displaced Zone II fracture of sacrum**
`7th`

     S32.122   **Severely displaced Zone II fracture of sacrum**
`7th`

     S32.129   **Unspecified Zone II fracture of sacrum**
`7th`

S32.13   **Zone III fracture of sacrum**
`6th`
Vertical fracture into spinal canal region of sacrum

     S32.130   **Nondisplaced Zone III fracture of sacrum**
`7th`

     S32.131   **Minimally displaced Zone III fracture of sacrum**
`7th`

     S32.132   **Severely displaced Zone III fracture of sacrum**
`7th`

     S32.139   **Unspecified Zone III fracture of sacrum**
`7th`

   S32.14X   **Type 1 fracture of sacrum**
`7th`
Transverse flexion fracture of sacrum without displacement

   S32.15X   **Type 2 fracture of sacrum**
`7th`
Transverse flexion fracture of sacrum with posterior displacement

   S32.16X   **Type 3 fracture of sacrum**
`7th`
Transverse extension fracture of sacrum with anterior displacement

   S32.17X   **Type 4 fracture of sacrum**
`7th`
Transverse segmental comminution of upper sacrum

   S32.19X   **Other fracture of sacrum**
`7th`

S32.2XX   **Fracture of coccyx**
`7th`

S32.3   **Fracture of ilium**
`5th`
Excludes1: fracture of ilium with associated disruption of pelvic ring (S32.8-)

   S32.30   **Unspecified fracture of ilium**
`6th`

     S32.301   **Unspecified fracture of right ilium**
`7th`

     S32.302   **Unspecified fracture of left ilium**
`7th`

     S32.309   **Unspecified fracture of unspecified ilium**
`7th`

   S32.31   **Avulsion fracture of ilium**
`6th`

     S32.311   **Displaced avulsion fracture of right ilium**
`7th`

     S32.312   **Displaced avulsion fracture of left ilium**
`7th`

     S32.313   **Displaced avulsion fracture of unspecified ilium**
`7th`

     S32.314   **Nondisplaced avulsion fracture of right ilium**
`7th`

     S32.315   **Nondisplaced avulsion fracture of left ilium**
`7th`

     S32.316   **Nondisplaced avulsion fracture of unspecified ilium**
`7th`

   S32.39   **Other fracture of ilium**
`6th`

     S32.391   **Other fracture of right ilium**
`7th`

     S32.392   **Other fracture of left ilium**
`7th`

     S32.399   **Other fracture of unspecified ilium**
`7th`

  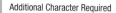 Additional Character Required   3-character code   Unspecified laterality codes were excluded here.   ■=New Code   ▲=Revised Code   *Excludes1*—Not coded here, do not use together   *Excludes2*—Not included here

S32.4   **Fracture of acetabulum**
[5th]   *Code also* any associated fracture of pelvic ring (S32.8-)

S32.40   **Unspecified fracture of acetabulum**
[6th]   **S32.401**   **Unspecified fracture of right acetabulum**
[7th]

     S32.402   **Unspecified fracture of left acetabulum**
[7th]

S32.41   **Fracture of anterior wall of acetabulum**
[6th]   **S32.411**   **Displaced fracture of anterior wall of right acetabulum**
[7th]

     S32.412   **Displaced fracture of anterior wall of left acetabulum**
[7th]

     S32.414   **Nondisplaced fracture of anterior wall of right acetabulum**
[7th]

     S32.415   **Nondisplaced fracture of anterior wall of left acetabulum**
[7th]

S32.42   **Fracture of posterior wall of acetabulum**
[6th]   **S32.421**   **Displaced fracture of posterior wall of right acetabulum**
[7th]

     S32.422   **Displaced fracture of posterior wall of left acetabulum**
[7th]

     S32.424   **Nondisplaced fracture of posterior wall of right acetabulum**
[7th]

     S32.425   **Nondisplaced fracture of posterior wall of left acetabulum**
[7th]

S32.43   **Fracture of anterior column [iliopubic] of acetabulum**
[6th]   **S32.431**   **Displaced fracture of anterior column [iliopubic] of right acetabulum**
[7th]

     S32.432   **Displaced fracture of anterior column [iliopubic] of left acetabulum**
[7th]

     S32.434   **Nondisplaced fracture of anterior column [iliopubic] of right acetabulum**
[7th]

> 7th characters for category S32
> A—initial encounter for closed fracture
> B—initial encounter for open fracture
> D—subsequent encounter for fracture with routine healing
> G—subsequent encounter for fracture with delayed healing
> K—subsequent encounter for fracture with nonunion
> S—sequela

     S32.435   **Nondisplaced fracture of anterior column [iliopubic] of left acetabulum**
[7th]

S32.44   **Fracture of posterior column [ilioischial] of acetabulum**
[6th]   **S32.441**   **Displaced fracture of posterior column [ilioischial] of right acetabulum**
[7th]

     S32.442   **Displaced fracture of posterior column [ilioischial] of left acetabulum**
[7th]

     S32.444   **Nondisplaced fracture of posterior column [ilioischial] of right acetabulum**
[7th]

     S32.445   **Nondisplaced fracture of posterior column [ilioischial] of left acetabulum**
[7th]

S32.45   **Transverse fracture of acetabulum**
[6th]   **S32.451**   **Displaced transverse fracture of right acetabulum**
[7th]

     S32.452   **Displaced transverse fracture of left acetabulum**
[7th]

     S32.454   **Nondisplaced transverse fracture of right acetabulum**
[7th]

     S32.455   **Nondisplaced transverse fracture of left acetabulum**
[7th]

     S32.456   **Nondisplaced transverse fracture of unspecified acetabulum**
[7th]

S32.46   **Associated transverse-posterior fracture of acetabulum**
[6th]   **S32.461**   **Displaced associated transverse-posterior fracture of right acetabulum**
[7th]

     S32.462   **Displaced associated transverse-posterior fracture of left acetabulum**
[7th]

     S32.464   **Nondisplaced associated transverse-posterior fracture of right acetabulum**
[7th]

     S32.465   **Nondisplaced associated transverse-posterior fracture of left acetabulum**
[7th]

S32.47   **Fracture of medial wall of acetabulum**
[6th]   **S32.471**   **Displaced fracture of medial wall of right acetabulum**
[7th]

     S32.472   **Displaced fracture of medial wall of left acetabulum**
[7th]

     S32.474   **Nondisplaced fracture of medial wall of right acetabulum**
[7th]

     S32.475   **Nondisplaced fracture of medial wall of left acetabulum**
[7th]

S32.48   **Dome fracture of acetabulum**
[6th]   **S32.481**   **Displaced dome fracture of right acetabulum**
[7th]

     S32.482   **Displaced dome fracture of left acetabulum**
[7th]

     S32.484   **Nondisplaced dome fracture of right acetabulum**
[7th]

     S32.485   **Nondisplaced dome fracture of left acetabulum**
[7th]

S32.49   **Other specified fracture of acetabulum**
[6th]   **S32.491**   **Other specified fracture of right acetabulum**
[7th]

     S32.492   **Other specified fracture of left acetabulum**
[7th]

S32.5   **Fracture of pubis**
[5th]   *Excludes1:* fracture of pubis with associated disruption of pelvic ring (S32.8-)

S32.50   **Unspecified fracture of pubis**
[6th]   **S32.501**   **Unspecified fracture of right pubis**
[7th]

     S32.502   **Unspecified fracture of left pubis**
[7th]

S32.51   **Fracture of superior rim of pubis**
[6th]   **S32.511**   **Fracture of superior rim of right pubis**
[7th]

  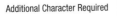 Additional Character Required   ✓ 3-character code   Unspecified laterality codes were excluded here.   •=New Code   ▲=Revised Code   *Excludes1*—Not coded here, do not use together   *Excludes2*—Not included here

S32.512   Fracture of superior rim of left pubis
7th

S32.59   Other specified fracture of pubis
6th
     S32.591   Other specified fracture of right pubis
     7th

     S32.592   Other specified fracture of left pubis
     7th

S32.6   Fracture of ischium
5th
Excludes1: fracture of ischium with associated disruption of pelvic ring (S32.8-)

S32.60   Unspecified fracture of ischium
6th
     S32.601   Unspecified fracture of right ischium
     7th

     S32.602   Unspecified fracture of left ischium
     7th

S32.61   Avulsion fracture of ischium
6th
     S32.611   Displaced avulsion fracture of right ischium
     7th

     S32.612   Displaced avulsion fracture of left ischium
     7th

     S32.614   Nondisplaced avulsion fracture of right ischium
     7th

     S32.615   Nondisplaced avulsion fracture of left ischium
     7th

S32.69   Other specified fracture of ischium
6th
     S32.691   Other specified fracture of right ischium
     7th

     S32.692   Other specified fracture of left ischium
     7th

S32.8   Fracture of other parts of pelvis
5th
Code also any associated:
     fracture of acetabulum (S32.4-)
     sacral fracture (S32.1-)

7th characters for category S32
A—initial encounter for closed fracture
B—initial encounter for open fracture
D—subsequent encounter for fracture with routine healing
G—subsequent encounter for fracture with delayed healing
K—subsequent encounter for fracture with nonunion
S—sequela

S32.81   Multiple fractures of pelvis with disruption of pelvic ring
6th
     Multiple pelvic fractures with disruption of pelvic circle

     S32.810   Multiple fractures of pelvis with stable disruption of pelvic ring
     7th

     S32.811   Multiple fractures of pelvis with unstable disruption of pelvic ring
     7th

S32.82X   Multiple fractures of pelvis without disruption of pelvic ring
7th
     Multiple pelvic fractures without disruption of pelvic circle

S32.89X   Fracture of other parts of pelvis
7th

S32.9XX   Fracture of unspecified parts of lumbosacral spine and pelvis
7th
     Fracture of lumbosacral spine NOS
     Fracture of pelvis NOS

S33   **DISLOCATION AND SPRAIN OF JOINTS AND LIGAMENTS OF LUMBAR SPINE AND PELVIS**
4th
Includes: avulsion of joint or ligament of lumbar spine and pelvis
     laceration of cartilage, joint or ligament of lumbar spine and pelvis
     sprain of cartilage, joint or ligament of lumbar spine and pelvis
     traumatic hemarthrosis of joint or ligament of lumbar spine and pelvis
     traumatic rupture of joint or ligament of lumbar spine and pelvis
     traumatic subluxation of joint or ligament of lumbar spine and pelvis
     traumatic tear of joint or ligament of lumbar spine and pelvis
Code also any associated open wound
Excludes1: nontraumatic rupture or displacement of lumbar intervertebral disc NOS (M51.-)
     obstetric damage to pelvic joints and ligaments (O71.6)
Excludes2: dislocation and sprain of joints and ligaments of hip (S73.-)
     strain of muscle of lower back and pelvis (S39.01-)

S33.5XX   Sprain of ligaments of lumbar spine
7th

S33.6XX   Sprain of sacroiliac joint
7th

7th characters for category S33
A—initial encounter
D—subsequent encounter
S—sequela

S33.8XX   Sprain of other parts of lumbar spine and pelvis
7th

S33.9XX   Sprain of unspecified parts of lumbar spine and pelvis
7th

S34   **INJURY OF LUMBAR AND SACRAL SPINAL CORD AND NERVES AT ABDOMEN, LOWER BACK AND PELVIS LEVEL**
4th
Note: Code to highest level of lumbar cord injury
     Injuries to the spinal cord (S34.0 and S34.1) refer to the cord level and not bone level injury, and can affect nerve roots at and below the level given.
Code also any associated: fracture of vertebra (S22.0-, S32.0-)
     open wound of abdomen, lower back and pelvis (S31.-)
     transient paralysis (R29.5)

S34.0   Concussion and edema of lumbar and sacral spinal cord
5th

7th characters for category S34
A—initial encounter
D—subsequent encounter
S—sequela

     S34.01   Concussion and edema of lumbar spinal cord
     6th

     S34.02X   Concussion and edema of sacral spinal cord
     7th
     Concussion and edema of conus medullaris

S34.1   Other and unspecified injury of lumbar and sacral spinal cord
5th
     S34.10   Unspecified injury to lumbar spinal cord (level)
     6th
         S34.101   Unspecified injury to; L1 level of lumbar spinal cord
         7th

         S34.102   L2 level of lumbar spinal cord
         7th

         S34.103   L3 level of lumbar spinal cord
         7th

         S34.104   L4 level of lumbar spinal cord
         7th

         S34.105   L5 level of lumbar spinal cord
         7th

         S34.109   unspecified level of lumbar spinal cord
         7th

     S34.12   Incomplete lesion of lumbar spinal cord (level)
     6th
         S34.121   Incomplete lesion of; L1 level of lumbar spinal cord
         7th

         S34.123   L3 level of lumbar spinal cord
         7th

   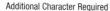   Additional Character Required   ✓   3-character code   Unspecified laterality codes were excluded here.   •=New Code   ▲=Revised Code   *Excludes1*—Not coded here, do not use together   *Excludes2*—Not included here

S34.124 **L4 level of lumbar spinal cord**
`7th`

S34.125 **L5 level of lumbar spinal cord**
`7th`

S34.129 **unspecified level of lumbar spinal cord**
`7th`

S34.13 **Other and unspecified injury to sacral spinal cord**
`6th`
Other injury to conus medullaris

S34.131 **Complete lesion of sacral spinal cord**
`7th`
Complete lesion of conus medullaris

S34.132 **Incomplete lesion of sacral spinal cord**
`7th`
Incomplete lesion of conus medullaris

S34.139 **Unspecified injury to sacral spinal cord**
`7th`
Unspecified injury of conus medullaris

S34.2 **Injury of nerve root of lumbar and sacral spine**
S34.21X **Injury of nerve root of lumbar spine**
`5th` `7th`

S34.22X **Injury of nerve root of sacral spine**
`7th`

S34.3XX **Injury of cauda equina**
`7th`

S34.4XX **Injury of lumbosacral plexus**
`7th`

S34.5XX **Injury of lumbar, sacral and pelvic sympathetic nerves**
`7th`
Injury of celiac ganglion or plexus
Injury of hypogastric plexus
Injury of mesenteric plexus (inferior) (superior)
Injury of splanchnic nerve

S34.6XX **Injury of peripheral nerve(s) at abdomen, lower back and pelvis level**
`7th`

S34.8XX **Injury of other nerves at abdomen, lower back and pelvis level**
`7th`

S34.9XX **Injury of unspecified nerves at abdomen, lower back and pelvis level**
`7th`

S36 **INJURY OF INTRA-ABDOMINAL ORGANS**
`4th`
Code also any associated open wound (S31.-)
S36.0 **Injury of spleen**
`5th`
   S36.03 **Laceration of spleen**
`6th`
      S36.030 **Superficial (capsular) laceration of spleen**
`7th`

7th characters for category S36
A—initial encounter
D—subsequent encounter
S—sequela

Laceration of spleen less than 1 cm
Minor laceration of spleen

S36.6 **Injury of rectum**
S36.60X **Unspecified injury of rectum**
`5th` `7th`

S36.62X **Contusion of rectum**
`7th`

S36.63X **Laceration of rectum**
`7th`

S36.9 **Injury of unspecified intra-abdominal organ**
`5th`
S36.90X **Unspecified injury of unspecified intra-abdominal organ**
`7th`

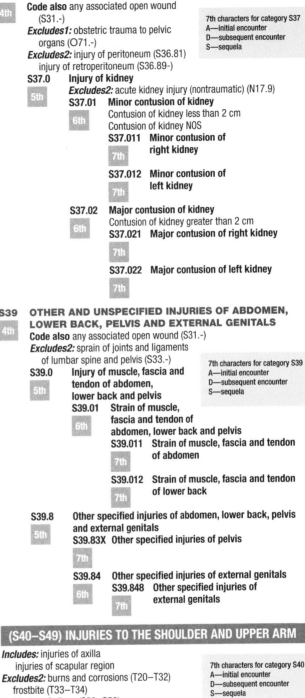

S37 **INJURY OF URINARY AND PELVIC ORGANS**
`4th`
Code also any associated open wound (S31.-)
Excludes1: obstetric trauma to pelvic organs (O71.-)
Excludes2: injury of peritoneum (S36.81) injury of retroperitoneum (S36.89-)

7th characters for category S37
A—initial encounter
D—subsequent encounter
S—sequela

S37.0 **Injury of kidney**
`5th`
Excludes2: acute kidney injury (nontraumatic) (N17.9)
   S37.01 **Minor contusion of kidney**
`6th`
Contusion of kidney less than 2 cm
Contusion of kidney NOS
      S37.011 **Minor contusion of right kidney**
`7th`

      S37.012 **Minor contusion of left kidney**
`7th`

   S37.02 **Major contusion of kidney**
`6th`
Contusion of kidney greater than 2 cm
      S37.021 **Major contusion of right kidney**
`7th`

      S37.022 **Major contusion of left kidney**
`7th`

S39 **OTHER AND UNSPECIFIED INJURIES OF ABDOMEN, LOWER BACK, PELVIS AND EXTERNAL GENITALS**
`4th`
Code also any associated open wound (S31.-)
Excludes2: sprain of joints and ligaments of lumbar spine and pelvis (S33.-)

7th characters for category S39
A—initial encounter
D—subsequent encounter
S—sequela

S39.0 **Injury of muscle, fascia and tendon of abdomen, lower back and pelvis**
`5th`
   S39.01 **Strain of muscle, fascia and tendon of abdomen, lower back and pelvis**
`6th`
      S39.011 **Strain of muscle, fascia and tendon of abdomen**
`7th`

      S39.012 **Strain of muscle, fascia and tendon of lower back**
`7th`

S39.8 **Other specified injuries of abdomen, lower back, pelvis and external genitals**
`5th`
   S39.83X **Other specified injuries of pelvis**
`7th`

   S39.84 **Other specified injuries of external genitals**
`6th`
      S39.848 **Other specified injuries of external genitals**
`7th`

(S40–S49) INJURIES TO THE SHOULDER AND UPPER ARM

Includes: injuries of axilla injuries of scapular region
Excludes2: burns and corrosions (T20–T32) frostbite (T33–T34) injuries of elbow (S50–S59) insect bite or sting, venomous (T63.4)

7th characters for category S40
A—initial encounter
D—subsequent encounter
S—sequela

S40 **SUPERFICIAL INJURY OF SHOULDER AND UPPER ARM**
`4th`
S40.0 **Contusion of shoulder and upper arm**
`4th`
   S40.01 **Contusion of shoulder**
`5th`
      S40.011 **Contusion of right shoulder**
`6th` `7th`

      S40.012 **Contusion of left shoulder**
`7th`

   S40.02 **Contusion of upper arm**
`6th`
      S40.021 **Contusion of right upper arm**
`7th`

`4th` `5th` `6th` `7th` Additional Character Required   ✓ 3-character code

Unspecified laterality codes were excluded here.

• =New Code
▲ =Revised Code

Excludes1—Not coded here, do not use together
Excludes2—Not included here

          S40.022   Contusion of left upper arm
          7th

S40.2   **Other superficial injuries of shoulder**
5th
    S40.21   **Abrasion of shoulder**
    6th   **S40.211**   Abrasion of right shoulder
          7th

          S40.212   Abrasion of left shoulder
          7th

    S40.22   **Blister (nonthermal) of shoulder**
    6th   **S40.221**   Blister (nonthermal) of right shoulder
          7th

          S40.222   Blister (nonthermal) of left shoulder
          7th

    S40.24   **External constriction of shoulder**
    6th   **S40.241**   External constriction of right shoulder
          7th

          S40.242   External constriction of left shoulder
          7th

    S40.25   **Superficial FB of shoulder**
    6th   Splinter in the shoulder
      S40.251   Superficial FB of right shoulder
          7th

      S40.252   Superficial FB of left shoulder
          7th

    S40.26   **Insect bite (nonvenomous) of shoulder**
    6th   **S40.261**   Insect bite (nonvenomous) of right shoulder
          7th

          S40.262   Insect bite (nonvenomous) of left shoulder
          7th

    S40.27   **Other superficial bite of shoulder**
    6th   *Excludes1:* open bite of shoulder (S41.05)
      S40.271   Other superficial bite of right shoulder
          7th

      S40.272   Other superficial bite of left shoulder
          7th

S40.8   **Other superficial injuries of upper arm**
5th
    S40.81   **Abrasion of upper arm**
    6th   **S40.811**   Abrasion of right upper arm
          7th

7th characters for category S40
A—initial encounter
D—subsequent encounter
S—sequela

      S40.812   Abrasion of left upper arm
          7th

    S40.82   **Blister (nonthermal) of upper arm**
    6th   **S40.821**   Blister (nonthermal) of right upper arm
          7th

      S40.822   Blister (nonthermal) of left upper arm
          7th

    S40.84   **External constriction of upper arm**
    6th   **S40.841**   External constriction of right upper arm
          7th

      S40.842   External constriction of left upper arm
          7th

    S40.85   **Superficial FB of upper arm**
    6th   Splinter in the upper arm

          S40.851   Superficial FB of right upper arm
          7th

          S40.852   Superficial FB of left upper arm
          7th

    S40.86   **Insect bite (nonvenomous) of upper arm**
    6th   **S40.861**   Insect bite (nonvenomous) of right upper arm
          7th

      S40.862   Insect bite (nonvenomous) of left upper arm
          7th

    S40.87   **Other superficial bite of upper arm**
    6th   *Excludes1:* open bite of upper arm (S41.14)
        Excludes2: other superficial bite of shoulder (S40.27-)
      S40.871   Other superficial bite of right upper arm
          7th

      S40.872   Other superficial bite of left upper arm
          7th

S40.9   **Unspecified superficial injury of shoulder and upper arm**
5th
    S40.91   **Unspecified superficial injury of shoulder**
    6th   **S40.911**   Unspecified superficial injury of right shoulder
          7th

      S40.912   Unspecified superficial injury of left shoulder
          7th

    S40.92   **Unspecified superficial injury of upper arm**
    6th   **S40.921**   Unspecified superficial injury of right upper arm
          7th

      S40.922   Unspecified superficial injury of left upper arm
          7th

7th characters for categories S40 & S41
A—initial encounter
D—subsequent encounter
S—sequela

S41   **OPEN WOUND OF SHOULDER AND UPPER ARM**
4th   **Code also** any associated wound infection
    Excludes1: traumatic amputation of shoulder and upper arm (S48.-)
    Excludes2: open fracture of shoulder and upper arm (S42.- with 7th character B or C)

    S41.0   **Open wound of shoulder**
    5th   **S41.01**   **Laceration without FB of shoulder**
        6th   **S41.011**   Laceration without FB of right shoulder
            7th

            S41.012   Laceration without FB of left shoulder
            7th

        S41.02   **Laceration with FB of shoulder**
        6th   **S41.021**   Laceration with FB of right shoulder
            7th

            S41.022   Laceration with FB of left shoulder
            7th

        S41.03   **Puncture wound without FB of shoulder**
        6th   **S41.031**   Puncture wound without FB of right shoulder
            7th

            S41.032   Puncture wound without FB of left shoulder
            7th

        S41.04   **Puncture wound with FB of shoulder**
        6th   **S41.041**   Puncture wound with FB of right shoulder
            7th

4th *5th* *6th* *7th*   Additional Character Required   ✓   3-character code   Unspecified laterality codes were excluded here.   •=New Code   ▲=Revised Code   *Excludes1*—Not coded here, do not use together   *Excludes2*—Not included here

294   **PEDIATRIC ICD-10-CM 2017: A MANUAL FOR PROVIDER-BASED CODING**

S41.042   Puncture wound with FB of left shoulder

S41.05   **Open bite of shoulder**
Bite of shoulder NOS
Excludes1: superficial bite of shoulder (S40.27)

S41.051   Open bite of right shoulder

S41.052   Open bite of left shoulder

S41.1   **Open wound of upper arm**

S41.11   **Laceration without FB of upper arm**

S41.111   Laceration without FB of right upper arm

S41.112   Laceration without FB of left upper arm

S41.12   **Laceration with FB of upper arm**

S41.121   Laceration with FB of right upper arm

S41.122   Laceration with FB of left upper arm

S41.13   **Puncture wound without FB of upper arm**

S41.131   Puncture wound without FB of right upper arm

S41.132   Puncture wound without FB of left upper arm

S41.14   **Puncture wound with FB of upper arm**

S41.141   Puncture wound with FB of right upper arm

S41.142   Puncture wound with FB of left upper arm

S41.15   **Open bite of upper arm**
Bite of upper arm NOS
Excludes1: superficial bite of upper arm (S40.87)

S41.151   Open bite of right upper arm

S41.152   Open bite of left upper arm

S42   FRACTURE OF SHOULDER AND UPPER ARM

Note: A fracture not indicated as displaced or nondisplaced should be coded to displaced
A fracture not indicated as open or closed should be coded to closed
Excludes1: traumatic amputation of shoulder and upper arm (S48.-)

S42.0   **Fracture of clavicle**

S42.00   **Fracture of unspecified part of clavicle**

S42.001   Fracture of unspecified part of right clavicle

S42.002   Fracture of unspecified part of left clavicle

S42.01   **Fracture of sternal end of clavicle**

> **7th characters for category S42**
> A—initial encounter for closed fracture
> B—initial encounter for open fracture
> D—subsequent encounter for fracture with routine healing
> G—subsequent encounter for fracture with delayed healing
> K—subsequent encounter for fracture with nonunion
> P—subsequent encounter for fracture with malunion
> S—sequela

S42.011   Anterior displaced fracture of sternal end of right clavicle

S42.012   Anterior displaced fracture of sternal end of left clavicle

S42.014   Posterior displaced fracture of sternal end of right clavicle

S42.015   Posterior displaced fracture of sternal end of left clavicle

S42.017   Nondisplaced fracture of sternal end of right clavicle

S42.018   Nondisplaced fracture of sternal end of left clavicle

S42.02   **Fracture of shaft of clavicle**

S42.021   Displaced fracture of shaft of right clavicle

S42.022   Displaced fracture of shaft of left clavicle

S42.024   Nondisplaced fracture of shaft of right clavicle

S42.025   Nondisplaced fracture of shaft of left clavicle

S42.03   **Fracture of lateral end of clavicle**
Fracture of acromial end of clavicle

S42.031   Displaced fracture of lateral end of right clavicle

S42.032   Displaced fracture of lateral end of left clavicle

S42.034   Nondisplaced fracture of lateral end of right clavicle

S42.035   Nondisplaced fracture of lateral end of left clavicle

S42.2   **Fracture of upper end of humerus**
Fracture of proximal end of humerus
Excludes2: fracture of shaft of humerus (S42.3-)
physeal fracture of upper end of humerus (S49.0-)

S42.20   **Unspecified fracture of upper end of; humerus**

S42.201   right humerus

S42.202   left humerus

S42.21   **Unspecified fracture of surgical neck of humerus**
Fracture of neck of humerus NOS

S42.211   Unspecified displaced fracture of surgical neck of right humerus

S42.212   Unspecified displaced fracture of surgical neck of left humerus

S42.214   Unspecified nondisplaced fracture of surgical neck of right humerus

S42.215   Unspecified nondisplaced fracture of surgical neck of left humerus

S42.22   **2-part fracture of surgical neck of humerus**

S42.221   2-part displaced fracture of surgical neck of right humerus

---

  Additional Character Required   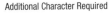 3-character code   Unspecified laterality codes were excluded here.   ■=New Code   ▲=Revised Code   *Excludes1* Not coded here, do not use together   *Excludes2*—Not included here

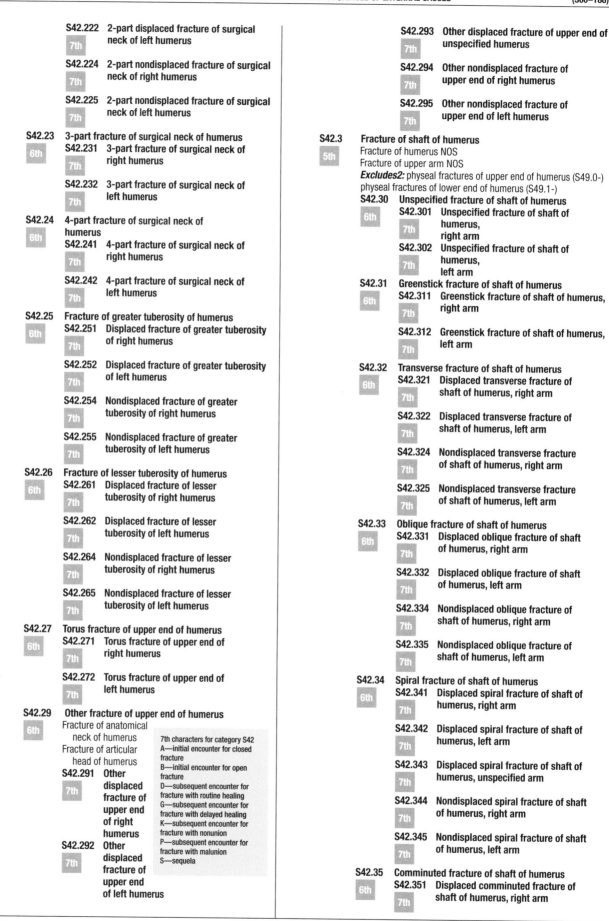

S42.222 2-part displaced fracture of surgical neck of left humerus
[7th]

S42.224 2-part nondisplaced fracture of surgical neck of right humerus
[7th]

S42.225 2-part nondisplaced fracture of surgical neck of left humerus
[7th]

S42.23 3-part fracture of surgical neck of humerus
[6th]
　S42.231 3-part fracture of surgical neck of right humerus
　[7th]

　S42.232 3-part fracture of surgical neck of left humerus
　[7th]

S42.24 4-part fracture of surgical neck of humerus
[6th]
　S42.241 4-part fracture of surgical neck of right humerus
　[7th]

　S42.242 4-part fracture of surgical neck of left humerus
　[7th]

S42.25 Fracture of greater tuberosity of humerus
[6th]
　S42.251 Displaced fracture of greater tuberosity of right humerus
　[7th]

　S42.252 Displaced fracture of greater tuberosity of left humerus
　[7th]

　S42.254 Nondisplaced fracture of greater tuberosity of right humerus
　[7th]

　S42.255 Nondisplaced fracture of greater tuberosity of left humerus
　[7th]

S42.26 Fracture of lesser tuberosity of humerus
[6th]
　S42.261 Displaced fracture of lesser tuberosity of right humerus
　[7th]

　S42.262 Displaced fracture of lesser tuberosity of left humerus
　[7th]

　S42.264 Nondisplaced fracture of lesser tuberosity of right humerus
　[7th]

　S42.265 Nondisplaced fracture of lesser tuberosity of left humerus
　[7th]

S42.27 Torus fracture of upper end of humerus
[6th]
　S42.271 Torus fracture of upper end of right humerus
　[7th]

　S42.272 Torus fracture of upper end of left humerus
　[7th]

S42.29 Other fracture of upper end of humerus
[6th]
Fracture of anatomical neck of humerus
Fracture of articular head of humerus
S42.291 Other displaced fracture of upper end of right humerus
[7th]
S42.292 Other displaced fracture of upper end of left humerus
[7th]

> 7th characters for category S42
> A—initial encounter for closed fracture
> B—initial encounter for open fracture
> D—subsequent encounter for fracture with routine healing
> G—subsequent encounter for fracture with delayed healing
> K—subsequent encounter for fracture with nonunion
> P—subsequent encounter for fracture with malunion
> S—sequela

S42.293 Other displaced fracture of upper end of unspecified humerus
[7th]

S42.294 Other nondisplaced fracture of upper end of right humerus
[7th]

S42.295 Other nondisplaced fracture of upper end of left humerus
[7th]

S42.3 Fracture of shaft of humerus
[5th]
Fracture of humerus NOS
Fracture of upper arm NOS
Excludes2: physeal fractures of upper end of humerus (S49.0-)
physeal fractures of lower end of humerus (S49.1-)

S42.30 Unspecified fracture of shaft of humerus
[6th]
　S42.301 Unspecified fracture of shaft of humerus, right arm
　[7th]
　S42.302 Unspecified fracture of shaft of humerus, left arm
　[7th]

S42.31 Greenstick fracture of shaft of humerus
[6th]
　S42.311 Greenstick fracture of shaft of humerus, right arm
　[7th]

　S42.312 Greenstick fracture of shaft of humerus, left arm
　[7th]

S42.32 Transverse fracture of shaft of humerus
[6th]
　S42.321 Displaced transverse fracture of shaft of humerus, right arm
　[7th]

　S42.322 Displaced transverse fracture of shaft of humerus, left arm
　[7th]

　S42.324 Nondisplaced transverse fracture of shaft of humerus, right arm
　[7th]

　S42.325 Nondisplaced transverse fracture of shaft of humerus, left arm
　[7th]

S42.33 Oblique fracture of shaft of humerus
[6th]
　S42.331 Displaced oblique fracture of shaft of humerus, right arm
　[7th]

　S42.332 Displaced oblique fracture of shaft of humerus, left arm
　[7th]

　S42.334 Nondisplaced oblique fracture of shaft of humerus, right arm
　[7th]

　S42.335 Nondisplaced oblique fracture of shaft of humerus, left arm
　[7th]

S42.34 Spiral fracture of shaft of humerus
[6th]
　S42.341 Displaced spiral fracture of shaft of humerus, right arm
　[7th]

　S42.342 Displaced spiral fracture of shaft of humerus, left arm
　[7th]

　S42.343 Displaced spiral fracture of shaft of humerus, unspecified arm
　[7th]

　S42.344 Nondisplaced spiral fracture of shaft of humerus, right arm
　[7th]

　S42.345 Nondisplaced spiral fracture of shaft of humerus, left arm
　[7th]

S42.35 Comminuted fracture of shaft of humerus
[6th]
　S42.351 Displaced comminuted fracture of shaft of humerus, right arm
　[7th]

  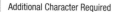 　Additional Character Required　　✔ 3-character code　　Unspecified laterality codes were excluded here.　　▪=New Code　　▲=Revised Code　　***Excludes1***—Not coded here, do not use together　***Excludes2***—Not included here

S42.352   Displaced comminuted fracture of shaft of humerus, left arm
`7th`

S42.354   Nondisplaced comminuted fracture of shaft of humerus, right arm
`7th`

S42.355   Nondisplaced comminuted fracture of shaft of humerus, left arm
`7th`

S42.36   Segmental fracture of shaft of humerus
`6th`

    S42.361   Displaced segmental fracture of shaft of humerus, right arm
`7th`

    S42.362   Displaced segmental fracture of shaft of humerus, left arm
`7th`

    S42.364   Nondisplaced segmental fracture of shaft of humerus, right arm
`7th`

    S42.365   Nondisplaced segmental fracture of shaft of humerus, left arm
`7th`

S42.39   Other fracture of shaft of humerus
`6th`

    S42.391   Other fracture of shaft of right humerus
`7th`

    S42.392   Other fracture of shaft of left humerus
`7th`

S42.4   Fracture of lower end of humerus
`5th`
    Fracture of distal end of humerus
    Excludes2: fracture of shaft of humerus (S42.3-)
      physeal fracture of lower end of humerus (S49.1-)

S42.40   Unspecified fracture of lower end of humerus
`6th`
    Fracture of elbow NOS

    S42.401   Unspecified fracture of lower end of right humerus
`7th`

    S42.402   Unspecified fracture of lower end of left humerus
`7th`

S42.41   Simple supracondylar fracture without intercondylar fracture of humerus
`6th`

    S42.411   Displaced simple supracondylar fracture without intercondylar fracture of right humerus
`7th`

    S42.412   Displaced simple supracondylar fracture without intercondylar fracture of left humerus
`7th`

    S42.414   Nondisplaced simple supracondylar fracture without intercondylar fracture of right humerus
`7th`

    S42.415   Nondisplaced simple supracondylar fracture without intercondylar fracture of left humerus
`7th`

S42.42   Comminuted supracondylar fracture without intercondylar fracture of humerus
`6th`

    S42.421   Displaced comminuted supracondylar fracture without intercondylar fracture of right humerus
`7th`

    S42.422   Displaced comminuted supracondylar fracture without intercondylar fracture of left humerus
`7th`

> **7th characters for category S42**
> A—initial encounter for closed fracture
> B—initial encounter for open fracture
> D—subsequent encounter for fracture with routine healing
> G—subsequent encounter for fracture with delayed healing
> K—subsequent encounter for fracture with nonunion
> P—subsequent encounter for fracture with malunion
> S—sequela

S42.424   Nondisplaced comminuted supracondylar fracture without intercondylar fracture of right humerus
`7th`

S42.425   Nondisplaced comminuted supracondylar fracture without intercondylar fracture of left humerus
`7th`

S42.43   Fracture (avulsion) of lateral epicondyle of humerus
`6th`

    S42.431   Displaced fracture (avulsion) of lateral epicondyle of right humerus
`7th`

    S42.432   Displaced fracture (avulsion) of lateral epicondyle of left humerus
`7th`

    S42.434   Nondisplaced fracture (avulsion) of lateral epicondyle of right humerus
`7th`

    S42.435   Nondisplaced fracture (avulsion) of lateral epicondyle of left humerus
`7th`

S42.44   Fracture (avulsion) of medial epicondyle of humerus
`6th`

    S42.441   Displaced fracture (avulsion) of medial epicondyle of right humerus
`7th`

    S42.442   Displaced fracture (avulsion) of medial epicondyle of left humerus
`7th`

    S42.444   Nondisplaced fracture (avulsion) of medial epicondyle of right humerus
`7th`

    S42.445   Nondisplaced fracture (avulsion) of medial epicondyle of left humerus
`7th`

    S42.447   Incarcerated fracture (avulsion) of medial epicondyle of right humerus
`7th`

    S42.448   Incarcerated fracture (avulsion) of medial epicondyle of left humerus
`7th`

S42.45   Fracture of lateral condyle of humerus
`6th`
    Fracture of capitellum of humerus

    S42.451   Displaced fracture of lateral condyle of right humerus
`7th`

    S42.452   Displaced fracture of lateral condyle of left humerus
`7th`

    S42.454   Nondisplaced fracture of lateral condyle of right humerus
`7th`

    S42.455   Nondisplaced fracture of lateral condyle of left humerus
`7th`

S42.46   Fracture of medial condyle of humerus
`6th`
    Trochlea fracture of humerus

    S42.461   Displaced fracture of medial condyle of right humerus
`7th`

    S42.462   Displaced fracture of medial condyle of left humerus
`7th`

    S42.464   Nondisplaced fracture of medial condyle of right humerus
`7th`

    S42.465   Nondisplaced fracture of medial condyle of left humerus
`7th`

S42.47   Transcondylar fracture of humerus
`6th`

    S42.471   Displaced transcondylar fracture of right humerus
`7th`

 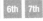   Additional Character Required   ✓   3-character code   Unspecified laterality codes were excluded here.   ✱=New Code   ▲=Revised Code   *Excludes1*—Not coded here, do not use together   *Excludes2*—Not included here

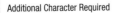

PEDIATRIC ICD-10-CM 2017: A MANUAL FOR PROVIDER-BASED CODING   297

S42.472 Displaced transcondylar fracture of left humerus
`7th`

S42.474 Nondisplaced transcondylar fracture of right humerus
`7th`

S42.475 Nondisplaced transcondylar fracture of left humerus
`7th`

S42.48 Torus fracture of lower end of humerus
`6th`
    S42.481 Torus fracture of lower end of right humerus
`7th`

    S42.482 Torus fracture of lower end of left humerus
`7th`

S42.49 Other fracture of lower end of humerus
`6th`
    S42.491 Other displaced fracture of lower end of right humerus
`7th`

    S42.492 Other displaced fracture of lower end of left humerus
`7th`

    S42.494 Other nondisplaced fracture of lower end of right humerus
`7th`

    S42.495 Other nondisplaced fracture of lower end of left humerus
`7th`

S42.9 Fracture of shoulder girdle, part unspecified
`5th`
Fracture of shoulder NOS

S42.91X Fracture of right shoulder girdle, part unspecified
`7th`

S42.92X Fracture of left shoulder girdle, part unspecified
`7th`

S43 DISLOCATION AND SPRAIN OF JOINTS AND LIGAMENTS OF SHOULDER GIRDLE
`4th`

Includes: avulsion of joint or ligament of shoulder girdle
    laceration of cartilage, joint or ligament of shoulder girdle
    sprain of cartilage, joint or ligament of shoulder girdle
    traumatic hemarthrosis of joint or ligament of shoulder girdle
    traumatic rupture of joint or ligament of shoulder girdle
    traumatic subluxation of joint or ligament of shoulder girdle
    traumatic tear of joint or ligament of shoulder girdle

Code also any associated open wound

Excludes2: strain of muscle, fascia and tendon of shoulder and upper arm (S46.-)

> 7th characters for category S43
> A—initial encounter
> D—subsequent encounter
> S—sequela

S43.0 Subluxation and dislocation of shoulder joint
`5th`
Dislocation of glenohumeral joint
Subluxation of glenohumeral joint

S43.00 Unspecified subluxation and dislocation of shoulder joint
`6th`
Dislocation of humerus NOS
Subluxation of humerus NOS

    S43.001 Unspecified subluxation of right shoulder joint
`7th`

    S43.002 Unspecified subluxation of left shoulder joint
`7th`

    S43.004 Unspecified dislocation of right shoulder joint
`7th`

    S43.005 Unspecified dislocation of left shoulder joint
`7th`

S43.01 Anterior subluxation and dislocation of humerus
`6th`

    S43.011 Anterior subluxation of right humerus
`7th`

    S43.012 Anterior subluxation of left humerus
`7th`

    S43.014 Anterior dislocation of right humerus
`7th`

    S43.015 Anterior dislocation of left humerus
`7th`

S43.02 Posterior subluxation and dislocation of humerus
`6th`
    S43.021 Posterior subluxation of right humerus
`7th`

    S43.022 Posterior subluxation of left humerus
`7th`

    S43.024 Posterior dislocation of right humerus
`7th`

    S43.025 Posterior dislocation of left humerus
`7th`

S43.03 Inferior subluxation and dislocation of humerus
`6th`
    S43.031 Inferior subluxation of right humerus
`7th`

    S43.032 Inferior subluxation of left humerus
`7th`

    S43.034 Inferior dislocation of right humerus
`7th`

    S43.035 Inferior dislocation of left humerus
`7th`

S43.08 Other subluxation and dislocation of shoulder joint
`6th`
    S43.081 Other subluxation of right shoulder joint
`7th`

    S43.082 Other subluxation of left shoulder joint
`7th`

    S43.084 Other dislocation of right shoulder joint
`7th`

    S43.085 Other dislocation of left shoulder joint
`7th`

S43.1 Subluxation and dislocation of acromioclavicular joint
`5th`
S43.10 Unspecified dislocation of acromioclavicular joint
`6th`
    S43.101 Unspecified dislocation of right acromioclavicular joint
`7th`

    S43.102 Unspecified dislocation of left acromioclavicular joint
`7th`

S43.11 Subluxation of acromioclavicular joint
    S43.111 Subluxation of right acromioclavicular joint
`7th`

    S43.112 Subluxation of left acromioclavicular joint
`7th`

S43.12 Dislocation of acromioclavicular joint, 100%–200% displacement
`6th`
    S43.121 Dislocation of right acromioclavicular joint, 100%–200% displacement
`7th`

    S43.122 Dislocation of left acromioclavicular joint, 100%–200% displacement
`7th`

`4th` `5th` `6th` `7th` Additional Character Required   ✓ 3-character code   Unspecified laterality codes were excluded here.   •=New Code   ▲=Revised Code   **Excludes1**—Not coded here, do not use together   **Excludes2**—Not included here

S43.13 Dislocation of acromioclavicular joint, greater than 200% displacement
6th
    S43.131 Dislocation of right acromioclavicular joint, greater than 200% displacement
       7th
    S43.132 Dislocation of left acromioclavicular joint, greater than 200% displacement
       7th

S43.14 Inferior dislocation of acromioclavicular joint
6th
    S43.141 Inferior dislocation of right acromioclavicular joint
       7th
    S43.142 Inferior dislocation of left acromioclavicular joint
       7th

S43.15 Posterior dislocation of acromioclavicular joint
6th
    S43.151 Posterior dislocation of right acromioclavicular joint
       7th
    S43.152 Posterior dislocation of left acromioclavicular joint
       7th

S43.2 Subluxation and dislocation of sternoclavicular joint
5th
    S43.20 Unspecified subluxation and dislocation of sternoclavicular joint
       6th
       S43.201 Unspecified subluxation of right sternoclavicular joint
          7th
       S43.202 Unspecified subluxation of left sternoclavicular joint
          7th
       S43.204 Unspecified dislocation of right sternoclavicular joint
          7th
       S43.205 Unspecified dislocation of left sternoclavicular joint
          7th

    S43.21 Anterior subluxation and dislocation of sternoclavicular joint
       6th

> 7th characters for category S43
> A—initial encounter
> D—subsequent encounter
> S—sequela

       S43.211 Anterior subluxation of right sternoclavicular joint
          7th
       S43.212 Anterior subluxation of left sternoclavicular joint
          7th
       S43.214 Anterior dislocation of right sternoclavicular joint
          7th
       S43.215 Anterior dislocation of left sternoclavicular joint
          7th

    S43.22 Posterior subluxation and dislocation of sternoclavicular joint
       6th
       S43.221 Posterior subluxation of right sternoclavicular joint
          7th
       S43.222 Posterior subluxation of left sternoclavicular joint
          7th
       S43.224 Posterior dislocation of right sternoclavicular joint
          7th
       S43.225 Posterior dislocation of left sternoclavicular joint
          7th

S43.3 Subluxation and dislocation of other and unspecified parts of shoulder girdle
5th
    S43.30 Subluxation and dislocation of unspecified parts of shoulder girdle
       6th
       Dislocation/subluxation of shoulder girdle NOS
       S43.301 Subluxation of unspecified parts of right shoulder girdle
          7th

       S43.302 Subluxation of unspecified parts of left shoulder girdle
          7th
       S43.304 Dislocation of unspecified parts of right shoulder girdle
          7th
       S43.305 Dislocation of unspecified parts of left shoulder girdle
          7th

    S43.31 Subluxation and dislocation of scapula
       6th
       S43.311 Subluxation of right scapula
          7th
       S43.312 Subluxation of left scapula
          7th
       S43.314 Dislocation of right scapula
          7th
       S43.315 Dislocation of left scapula
          7th

    S43.39 Subluxation and dislocation of other parts of shoulder girdle
       6th
       S43.391 Subluxation of other parts of right shoulder girdle
          7th
       S43.392 Subluxation of other parts of left shoulder girdle
          7th
       S43.394 Dislocation of other parts of right shoulder girdle
          7th
       S43.395 Dislocation of other parts of left shoulder girdle
          7th

S43.4 Sprain of shoulder joint
5th
    S43.40 Unspecified sprain of shoulder joint
       6th
       S43.401 Unspecified sprain of right shoulder joint
          7th
       S43.402 Unspecified sprain of left shoulder joint
          7th

    S43.41 Sprain of coracohumeral (ligament)
       6th
       S43.411 Sprain of right coracohumeral (ligament)
          7th
       S43.412 Sprain of left coracohumeral (ligament)
          7th

    S43.42 Sprain of rotator cuff capsule
       6th
       Excludes1: rotator cuff syndrome (complete) (incomplete), not specified as traumatic (M75.1-)
       Excludes2: injury of tendon of rotator cuff (S46.0-)
       S43.421 Sprain of right rotator cuff capsule
          7th
       S43.422 Sprain of left rotator cuff capsule
          7th

    S43.43 Superior glenoid labrum lesion
       6th
       SLAP lesion
       S43.431 Superior glenoid labrum lesion of right shoulder
          7th
       S43.432 Superior glenoid labrum lesion of left shoulder
          7th

    S43.49 Other sprain of shoulder joint
       6th
       S43.491 Other sprain of right shoulder joint
          7th

  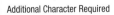 Additional Character Required   ✓ 3-character code   Unspecified laterality codes were excluded here.   •=New Code   ▲=Revised Code   *Excludes1*—Not coded here, do not use together   *Excludes2*—Not included here

S43.492   Other sprain of left shoulder joint
`7th`

S43.5   **Sprain of acromioclavicular joint**
`5th`
Sprain of acromioclavicular ligament
S43.51X   Sprain of right acromioclavicular joint
`7th`

S43.52X   Sprain of left acromioclavicular joint
`7th`

S43.6   **Sprain of sternoclavicular joint**
`5th`
S43.61X   Sprain of right sternoclavicular joint
`7th`

S43.62X   Sprain of left sternoclavicular joint
`7th`

> 7th characters for categories S43 & S46
> A—initial encounter
> D—subsequent encounter
> S—sequela

S43.8   **Sprain of other specified parts of shoulder girdle**
`5th`
S43.81X   Sprain of other specified parts of right shoulder girdle
`7th`

S43.82X   Sprain of other specified parts of left shoulder girdle
`7th`

S46   **INJURY OF MUSCLE, FASCIA AND TENDON AT SHOULDER AND UPPER ARM LEVEL**
`4th`
Code also any associated open wound (S41.-)
Excludes2: injury of muscle, fascia and tendon at elbow (S56.-)
sprain of joints and ligaments of shoulder girdle (S43.9)

S46.0   **Injury of muscle(s) and tendon(s) of the rotator cuff of shoulder**
`5th`
S46.00   Unspecified injury of muscle(s) and tendon(s) of the rotator cuff of shoulder
`6th`
    S46.001   Unspecified injury of muscle(s) and tendon(s) of the rotator cuff of right shoulder
    `7th`
    S46.002   Unspecified injury of muscle(s) and tendon(s) of the rotator cuff of left shoulder
    `7th`

S46.01   Strain of muscle(s) and tendon(s) of the rotator cuff of shoulder
`6th`
    S46.011   Strain of muscle(s) and tendon(s) of the rotator cuff of right shoulder
    `7th`
    S46.012   Strain of muscle(s) and tendon(s) of the rotator cuff of left shoulder
    `7th`

S46.02   Laceration of muscle(s) and tendon(s) of the rotator cuff of shoulder
`6th`
    S46.021   Laceration of muscle(s) and tendon(s) of the rotator cuff of right shoulder
    `7th`
    S46.022   Laceration of muscle(s) and tendon(s) of the rotator cuff of left shoulder
    `7th`

S46.09   Other injury of muscle(s) and tendon(s) of the rotator cuff of shoulder
`6th`
    S46.091   Other injury of muscle(s) and tendon(s) of the rotator cuff of right shoulder
    `7th`
    S46.092   Other injury of muscle(s) and tendon(s) of the rotator cuff of left shoulder
    `7th`

S46.91   Strain of unspecified muscle, fascia and tendon at shoulder and upper arm level
`6th`
    S46.911   Strain of unspecified muscle, fascia and tendon at shoulder and upper arm level, right arm
    `7th`
    S46.912   Strain of unspecified muscle, fascia and tendon at shoulder and upper arm level, left arm
    `7th`

S46.92   Laceration of unspecified muscle, fascia and tendon at shoulder and upper arm level
`6th`
    S46.921   Laceration of unspecified muscle, fascia and tendon at shoulder and upper arm level, right arm
    `7th`
    S46.922   Laceration of unspecified muscle, fascia and tendon at shoulder and upper arm level, left arm
    `7th`

S46.99   Other injury of unspecified muscle, fascia and tendon at shoulder and upper arm level
`6th`
    S46.991   Other injury of unspecified muscle, fascia and tendon at shoulder and upper arm level, right arm
    `7th`
    S46.992   Other injury of unspecified muscle, fascia and tendon at shoulder and upper arm level, left arm
    `7th`

S49   **OTHER AND UNSPECIFIED INJURIES OF SHOULDER AND UPPER ARM**
`4th`

S49.0   **Physeal fracture of upper end of humerus**
`5th`
S49.00   Unspecified physeal fracture of upper end of humerus
`6th`
    S49.001   Unspecified physeal fracture of upper end of humerus, right arm
    `7th`

> 7th characters for category S49
> A—initial encounter for closed fracture
> D—subsequent encounter for fracture with routine healing
> G—subsequent encounter for fracture with delayed healing
> K—subsequent encounter for fracture with nonunion
> P—subsequent encounter for fracture with malunion
> S—sequela

    S49.002   Unspecified physeal fracture of upper end of humerus, left arm
    `7th`

S49.01   Salter-Harris Type I physeal fracture of upper end of humerus
`6th`
    S49.011   Salter-Harris Type I physeal fracture of upper end of humerus, right arm
    `7th`
    S49.012   Salter-Harris Type I physeal fracture of upper end of humerus, left arm
    `7th`

S49.02   Salter-Harris Type II physeal fracture of upper end of humerus
`6th`
    S49.021   Salter-Harris Type II physeal fracture of upper end of humerus, right arm
    `7th`
    S49.022   Salter-Harris Type II physeal fracture of upper end of humerus, left arm
    `7th`

S49.03   Salter-Harris Type III physeal fracture of upper end of humerus
`6th`
    S49.031   Salter-Harris Type III physeal fracture of upper end of humerus, right arm
    `7th`
    S49.032   Salter-Harris Type III physeal fracture of upper end of humerus, left arm
    `7th`

S49.04   Salter-Harris Type IV physeal fracture of upper end of humerus
`6th`
    S49.041   Salter-Harris Type IV physeal fracture of upper end of humerus, right arm
    `7th`
    S49.042   Salter-Harris Type IV physeal fracture of upper end of humerus, left arm
    `7th`

S49.09   Other physeal fracture of upper end of humerus
`6th`
    S49.091   Other physeal fracture of upper end of humerus, right arm
    `7th`
    S49.092   Other physeal fracture of upper end of humerus, left arm
    `7th`

  Additional Character Required   3-character code   Unspecified laterality codes were excluded here.   •=New Code   ▲=Revised Code   ***Excludes1***—Not coded here, do not use together   ***Excludes2***—Not included here

S49.1   **Physeal fracture of lower end of humerus**

S49.10 | 5th   **Unspecified physeal fracture of lower end of humerus**

     S49.101 | 7th   Unspecified physeal fracture of lower end of humerus, right arm

     S49.102 | 7th   Unspecified physeal fracture of lower end of humerus, left arm

S49.11 | 6th   **Salter-Harris Type I physeal fracture of lower end of humerus**

     S49.111 | 7th   Salter-Harris Type I physeal fracture of lower end of humerus, right arm

     S49.112 | 7th   Salter-Harris Type I physeal fracture of lower end of humerus, left arm

S49.12 | 6th   **Salter-Harris Type II physeal fracture of lower end of humerus**

     S49.121 | 7th   Salter-Harris Type II physeal fracture of lower end of humerus, right arm

     S49.122 | 7th   Salter-Harris Type II physeal fracture of lower end of humerus, left arm

S49.13 | 6th   **Salter-Harris Type III physeal fracture of lower end of humerus**

     S49.131 | 7th   Salter-Harris Type III physeal fracture of lower end of humerus, right arm

     S49.132 | 7th   Salter-Harris Type III physeal fracture of lower end of humerus, left arm

S49.14 | 6th   **Salter-Harris Type IV physeal fracture of lower end of humerus**

     S49.141 | 7th   Salter-Harris Type IV physeal fracture of lower end of humerus, right arm

     S49.142 | 7th   Salter-Harris Type IV physeal fracture of lower end of humerus, left arm

S49.19 | 6th   **Other physeal fracture of lower end of humerus**

     S49.191 | 7th   Other physeal fracture of lower end of humerus, right arm

     S49.192 | 7th   Other physeal fracture of lower end of humerus, left arm

---

(S50–S59) INJURIES TO THE ELBOW AND FOREARM

Excludes2: burns and corrosions (T20–T32)
frostbite (T33–T34)
injuries of wrist and hand (S60–S69)
insect bite or sting, venomous (T63.4)

> 7th characters for category S50
> A—initial encounter
> D—subsequent encounter
> S—sequela

S50 | 4th   **SUPERFICIAL INJURY OF ELBOW AND FOREARM**

Excludes2: superficial injury of wrist and hand (S60.-)

S50.0 | 5th   **Contusion of elbow**

   S50.01X | 7th   Contusion of right elbow

   S50.02X | 7th   Contusion of left elbow

S50.1 | 5th   **Contusion of forearm**

   S50.11X | 7th   Contusion of right forearm

   S50.12X | 7th   Contusion of left forearm

S50.3 | 5th   **Other superficial injuries of elbow**

S50.31 | 6th   **Abrasion of elbow**

     S50.311 | 7th   Abrasion of right elbow

     S50.312 | 7th   Abrasion of left elbow

S50.32 | 6th   **Blister (nonthermal) of elbow**

     S50.321 | 7th   Blister (nonthermal) of right elbow

     S50.322 | 7th   Blister (nonthermal) of left elbow

S50.34 | 6th   **External constriction of elbow**

     S50.341 | 7th   External constriction of right elbow

     S50.342 | 7th   External constriction of left elbow

S50.35 | 6th   **Superficial FB of elbow**
Splinter in the elbow

     S50.351 | 7th   Superficial FB of right elbow

     S50.352 | 7th   Superficial FB of left elbow

S50.36 | 6th   **Insect bite (nonvenomous) of elbow**

     S50.361 | 7th   Insect bite (nonvenomous) of right elbow

     S50.362 | 7th   Insect bite (nonvenomous) of left elbow

S50.37 | 6th   **Other superficial bite of elbow**
Excludes1: open bite of elbow (S51.04)

     S50.371 | 7th   Other superficial bite of right elbow

     S50.372 | 7th   Other superficial bite of left elbow

S50.8 | 5th   **Other superficial injuries of forearm**

S50.81 | 6th   **Abrasion of forearm**

     S50.811 | 7th   Abrasion of right forearm

     S50.812 | 7th   Abrasion of left forearm

S50.82 | 6th   **Blister (nonthermal) of forearm**

     S50.821 | 7th   Blister (nonthermal) of right forearm

     S50.822 | 7th   Blister (nonthermal) of left forearm

S50.84 | 6th   **External constriction of forearm**

     S50.841 | 7th   External constriction of right forearm

     S50.842 | 7th   External constriction of left forearm

S50.85 | 6th   **Superficial FB of forearm**
Splinter in the forearm

     S50.851 | 7th   Superficial FB of right forearm

   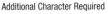   Additional Character Required   ✓ 3-character code

Unspecified laterality codes were excluded here.

●=New Code
▲=Revised Code

Excludes1 — Not coded here, do not use together
Excludes2 — Not included here

CHAPTER 19. INJURY, POISONING AND CERTAIN OTHER CONSEQUENCES OF EXTERNAL CAUSES (S50.852–S52.021)

S50.852 Superficial FB of left forearm
`7th`

S50.86 Insect bite (nonvenomous) of forearm
`6th`
  S50.861 Insect bite (nonvenomous) of right forearm
  `7th`

  S50.862 Insect bite (nonvenomous) of left forearm
  `7th`

S50.87 Other superficial bite of forearm
`6th`
Excludes1: open bite of forearm (S51.84)
  S50.871 Other superficial bite of right forearm
  `7th`

  S50.872 Other superficial bite of left forearm
  `7th`

S51 OPEN WOUND OF ELBOW AND FOREARM
`4th`
Code also any associated wound infection
Excludes1: open fracture of elbow and forearm (S52.- with open fracture 7th character)
    traumatic amputation of elbow and forearm (S58.-)
Excludes2: open wound of wrist and hand (S61.-)

> 7th characters for category S51
> A—initial encounter
> D—subsequent encounter
> S—sequela

S51.0 Open wound of elbow
`5th`
  S51.01 Laceration without FB of elbow
  `6th`
    S51.011 Laceration without FB of right elbow
    `7th`

    S51.012 Laceration without FB of left elbow
    `7th`

  S51.02 Laceration with FB of elbow
  `6th`
    S51.021 Laceration with FB of right elbow
    `7th`

    S51.022 Laceration with FB of left elbow
    `7th`

  S51.03 Puncture wound without FB of elbow
  `6th`
    S51.031 Puncture wound without FB of right elbow
    `7th`

    S51.032 Puncture wound without FB of left elbow
    `7th`

  S51.04 Puncture wound with FB of elbow
  `6th`
    S51.041 Puncture wound with FB of right elbow
    `7th`

    S51.042 Puncture wound with FB of left elbow
    `7th`

  S51.05 Open bite of elbow
  `6th`
  Bite of elbow NOS
  Excludes1: superficial bite of elbow (S50.36, S50.37)
    S51.051 Open bite, right elbow
    `7th`

    S51.052 Open bite, left elbow
    `7th`

S51.8 Open wound of forearm
`5th`
Excludes2: open wound of elbow (S51.0-)
  S51.81 Laceration without FB of forearm
  `6th`
    S51.811 Laceration without FB of right forearm
    `7th`

S51.812 Laceration without FB of left forearm
`7th`

S51.82 Laceration with FB of forearm
`6th`
  S51.821 Laceration with FB of right forearm
  `7th`

  S51.822 Laceration with FB of left forearm
  `7th`

S51.83 Puncture wound without FB of forearm
`6th`
  S51.831 Puncture wound without FB of right forearm
  `7th`

  S51.832 Puncture wound without FB of left forearm
  `7th`

S51.84 Puncture wound with FB of forearm
`6th`
  S51.841 Puncture wound with FB of right forearm
  `7th`

  S51.842 Puncture wound with FB of left forearm
  `7th`

S51.85 Open bite of forearm
`6th`
Bite of forearm NOS
Excludes1: superficial bite of forearm (S50.86, S50.87)
  S51.851 Open bite of right forearm
  `7th`

  S51.852 Open bite of left forearm
  `7th`

S52 FRACTURE OF FOREARM
`4th`
Note: A fracture not indicated as displaced or nondisplaced should be coded to displaced
A fracture not indicated as open or closed should be coded to closed
The open fracture designations are based on the Gustilo open fracture classification
Excludes1: traumatic amputation of forearm (S58.-)
Excludes2: fracture at wrist and hand level (S62.-)

> 7th characters for category S52
> A—initial encounter for closed fracture
> B—initial encounter for open fracture type I or II
> C—initial encounter for open fracture NOS
> D—subsequent encounter for closed fracture with routine healing
> G—subsequent encounter for closed fracture with delayed healing
> K—subsequent encounter for closed fracture with nonunion
> P—subsequent encounter for closed fracture with malunion
> S—sequela

S52.0 Fracture of upper end of ulna
`5th`
Fracture of proximal end of ulna
Excludes2: fracture of elbow NOS (S42.40-)
  fractures of shaft of ulna (S52.2-)
  S52.00 Unspecified fracture of upper end of ulna
  `6th`
    S52.001 Unspecified fracture of upper end of right ulna
    `7th`

    S52.002 Unspecified fracture of upper end of left ulna
    `7th`

  S52.01 Torus fracture of upper end of ulna
  `6th`
    S52.011 Torus fracture of upper end of right ulna
    `7th`

    S52.012 Torus fracture of upper end of left ulna
    `7th`

  S52.02 Fracture of olecranon process without intraarticular extension of ulna
  `6th`
    S52.021 Displaced fracture of olecranon process without intraarticular extension of right ulna
    `7th`

   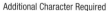 Additional Character Required   3-character code Unspecified laterality codes were excluded here. •=New Code ▲=Revised Code *Excludes1*—Not coded here, do not use together *Excludes2*—Not included here

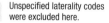

S52.022   Displaced fracture of olecranon process without intraarticular extension of left ulna
[7th]

S52.024   Nondisplaced fracture of olecranon process without intraarticular extension of right ulna
[7th]

S52.025   Nondisplaced fracture of olecranon process without intraarticular extension of left ulna
[7th]

S52.03 [6th]   Fracture of olecranon process with intraarticular extension of ulna

S52.031   Displaced fracture of olecranon process with intraarticular extension of right ulna
[7th]

S52.032   Displaced fracture of olecranon process with intraarticular extension of left ulna
[7th]

S52.034   Nondisplaced fracture of olecranon process with intraarticular extension of right ulna
[7th]

S52.035   Nondisplaced fracture of olecranon process with intraarticular extension of left ulna
[7th]

S52.04 [6th]   Fracture of coronoid process of ulna

S52.041   Displaced fracture of coronoid process of right ulna
[7th]

S52.042   Displaced fracture of coronoid process of left ulna
[7th]

S52.044   Nondisplaced fracture of coronoid process of right ulna
[7th]

S52.045   Nondisplaced fracture of coronoid process of left ulna
[7th]

S52.09 [6th]   Other fracture of upper end of ulna

S52.091   Other fracture of upper end of right ulna
[7th]

S52.092   Other fracture of upper end of left ulna
[7th]

S52.1 [5th]   **Fracture of upper end of radius**
Fracture of proximal end of radius
Excludes2: physeal fractures of upper end of radius (S59.2-)
    fracture of shaft of radius (S52.3-)

S52.10 [6th]   Unspecified fracture of upper end of radius

S52.101   Unspecified fracture of upper end of right radius
[7th]

S52.102   Unspecified fracture of upper end of left radius
[7th]

S52.11 [6th]   Torus fracture of upper end of radius

S52.111   Torus fracture of upper end of right radius
[7th]

S52.112   Torus fracture of upper end of left radius
[7th]

S52.12 [6th]   Fracture of head of radius

S52.121   Displaced fracture of head of right radius
[7th]

S52.122   Displaced fracture of head of left radius
[7th]

S52.124   Nondisplaced fracture of head of right radius
[7th]

S52.125   Nondisplaced fracture of head of left radius
[7th]

S52.13 [6th]   **Fracture of neck of radius**

S52.131   Displaced fracture of neck of right radius
[7th]

S52.132   Displaced fracture of neck of eft radius
[7th]

S52.134   Nondisplaced fracture of neck of right radius
[7th]

S52.135   Nondisplaced fracture of neck of left radius
[7th]

7th characters for category S52
A—initial encounter for closed fracture
B—initial encounter for open fracture type I or II
C—initial encounter for open fracture NOS
D—subsequent encounter for closed fracture with routine healing
G—subsequent encounter for closed fracture with delayed healing
K—subsequent encounter for closed fracture with nonunion
P—subsequent encounter for closed fracture with malunion
S—sequela

S52.18 [6th]   Other fracture of upper end of radius

S52.181   Other fracture of upper end of right radius
[7th]

S52.182   Other fracture of upper end of left radius
[7th]

S52.2 [5th]   **Fracture of shaft of ulna**

S52.20 [6th]   Unspecified fracture of shaft of ulna
Fracture of ulna NOS

S52.201   Unspecified fracture of shaft of right ulna
[7th]

S52.202   Unspecified fracture of shaft of left ulna
[7th]

S52.21 [6th]   Greenstick fracture of shaft of ulna

S52.211   Greenstick fracture of shaft of right ulna
[7th]

S52.212   Greenstick fracture of shaft of left ulna
[7th]

S52.22 [6th]   Transverse fracture of shaft of ulna

S52.221   Displaced transverse fracture of shaft of right ulna
[7th]

S52.222   Displaced transverse fracture of shaft of left ulna
[7th]

S52.224   Nondisplaced transverse fracture of shaft of right ulna
[7th]

S52.225   Nondisplaced transverse fracture of shaft of left ulna
[7th]

S52.23 [6th]   Oblique fracture of shaft of ulna

S52.231   Displaced oblique fracture of shaft of right ulna
[7th]

S52.232   Displaced oblique fracture of shaft of left ulna
[7th]

S52.234   Nondisplaced oblique fracture of shaft of right ulna
[7th]

S52.235   Nondisplaced oblique fracture of shaft of left ulna
[7th]

S52.24 [6th]   Spiral fracture of shaft of ulna

S52.241   Displaced spiral fracture of shaft of ulna, right arm
[7th]

4th 5th 6th 7th   Additional Character Required   ✔   3-character code   Unspecified laterality codes were excluded here.   •=New Code   ▲=Revised Code   *Excludes1*—Not coded here, do not use together   *Excludes2*—Not included here

PEDIATRIC ICD-10-CM 2017: A MANUAL FOR PROVIDER-BASED CODING   303

S52.242 **7th** Displaced spiral fracture of shaft of ulna, left arm

S52.244 **7th** Nondisplaced spiral fracture of shaft of ulna, right arm

S52.245 **7th** Nondisplaced spiral fracture of shaft of ulna, left arm

S52.25 6th Comminuted fracture of shaft of ulna

S52.251 **7th** Displaced comminuted fracture of shaft of ulna, right arm

S52.252 **7th** Displaced comminuted fracture of shaft of ulna, left arm

S52.254 **7th** Nondisplaced comminuted fracture of shaft of ulna, right arm

S52.255 **7th** Nondisplaced comminuted fracture of shaft of ulna, left arm

S52.26 6th Segmental fracture of shaft of ulna

S52.261 **7th** Displaced segmental fracture of shaft of ulna, right arm

S52.262 **7th** Displaced segmental fracture of shaft of ulna, left arm

S52.264 **7th** Nondisplaced segmental fracture of shaft of ulna, right arm

S52.265 **7th** Nondisplaced segmental fracture of shaft of ulna, left arm

S52.27 6th Monteggia's fracture of ulna
Fracture of upper shaft of ulna with dislocation of radial head

S52.271 **7th** Monteggia's fracture of right ulna

S52.272 **7th** Monteggia's fracture of left ulna

S52.28 6th Bent bone of ulna

S52.281 **7th** Bent bone of right ulna

S52.282 **7th** Bent bone of left ulna

S52.29 6th Other fracture of shaft of ulna

S52.291 **7th** Other fracture of shaft of right ulna

S52.292 **7th** Other fracture of shaft of left ulna

S52.3 5th Fracture of shaft of radius

S52.30 6th Unspecified fracture of shaft of radius

S52.301 **7th** Unspecified fracture of shaft of right radius

S52.302 **7th** Unspecified fracture of shaft of left radius

S52.31 6th Greenstick fracture of shaft of radius

S52.311 **7th** Greenstick fracture of shaft of radius, right arm

S52.312 **7th** Greenstick fracture of shaft of radius, left arm

S52.32 6th Transverse fracture of shaft of radius

S52.321 **7th** Displaced transverse fracture of shaft of right radius

S52.322 **7th** Displaced transverse fracture of shaft of left radius

S52.324 **7th** Nondisplaced transverse fracture of shaft of right radius

S52.325 **7th** Nondisplaced transverse fracture of shaft of left radius

S52.33 6th Oblique fracture of shaft of radius

S52.331 **7th** Displaced oblique fracture of shaft of right radius

S52.332 **7th** Displaced oblique fracture of shaft of left radius

S52.334 **7th** Nondisplaced oblique fracture of shaft of right radius

S52.335 **7th** Nondisplaced oblique fracture of shaft of left radius

S52.34 6th Spiral fracture of shaft of radius

S52.341 **7th** Displaced spiral fracture of shaft of radius, right arm

S52.342 **7th** Displaced spiral fracture of shaft of radius, left arm

S52.344 **7th** Nondisplaced spiral fracture of shaft of radius, right arm

S52.345 **7th** Nondisplaced spiral fracture of shaft of radius, left arm

S52.35 6th Comminuted fracture of shaft of radius

S52.351 **7th** Displaced comminuted fracture of shaft of radius, right arm

S52.352 **7th** Displaced comminuted fracture of shaft of radius, left arm

S52.354 **7th** Nondisplaced comminuted fracture of shaft of radius, right arm

S52.355 **7th** Nondisplaced comminuted fracture of shaft of radius, left arm

S52.36 6th Segmental fracture of shaft of radius

S52.361 **7th** Displaced segmental fracture of shaft of radius, right arm

S52.362 **7th** Displaced segmental fracture of shaft of radius, left arm

S52.364 **7th** Nondisplaced segmental fracture of shaft of radius, right arm

S52.365 **7th** Nondisplaced segmental fracture of shaft of radius, left arm

> 7th characters for category S52
> A—initial encounter for closed fracture
> B—initial encounter for open fracture type I or II
> C—initial encounter for open fracture NOS
> D—subsequent encounter for closed fracture with routine healing
> G—subsequent encounter for closed fracture with delayed healing
> K—subsequent encounter for closed fracture with nonunion
> P—subsequent encounter for closed fracture with malunion
> S—sequela

4th **5th** **6th** **7th** Additional Character Required ✓ 3-character code   Unspecified laterality codes were excluded here. •=New Code ▲=Revised Code *Excludes1*—Not coded here, do not use together *Excludes2*—Not included here

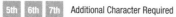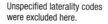

304   **PEDIATRIC ICD-10-CM 2017: A MANUAL FOR PROVIDER-BASED CODING**

S52.37   **Galeazzi's fracture**
6th   Fracture of lower shaft of radius with radioulnar joint dislocation

    S52.371   **Galeazzi's fracture of right radius**
7th

    S52.372   **Galeazzi's fracture of left radius**
7th

S52.38   **Bent bone of radius**
6th   **S52.381**   **Bent bone of right radius**
7th

    S52.382   **Bent bone of left radius**
7th

S52.39   **Other fracture of shaft of radius**
6th   **S52.391**   **Other fracture of shaft of radius, right arm**
7th

    S52.392   **Other fracture of shaft of radius, left arm**
7th

S52.5   **Fracture of lower end of radius**
5th   Fracture of distal end of radius
Excludes: physeal fractures of lower end of radius (S59.2-)

S52.50   **Unspecified fracture of the lower end of radius**
6th   **S52.501**   **Unspecified fracture of the lower end of right radius**
7th

    S52.502   **Unspecified fracture of the lower end of left radius**
7th

S52.51   **Fracture of radial styloid process**
6th   **S52.511**   **Displaced fracture of right radial styloid process**
7th

    S52.512   **Displaced fracture of left radial styloid process**
7th

    S52.514   **Nondisplaced fracture of right radial styloid process**
7th

    S52.515   **Nondisplaced fracture of left radial styloid process**
7th

S52.52   **Torus fracture of lower end of radius**
6th   **S52.521**   **Torus fracture of lower end of right radius**
7th

    S52.522   **Torus fracture of lower end of left radius**
7th

S52.53   **Colles' fracture**
6th   **S52.531**   **Colles' fracture of right radius**
7th

    S52.532   **Colles' fracture of left radius**
7th

S52.54   **Smith's fracture**
6th   **S52.541**   **Smith's fracture of right radius**
7th

    S52.542   **Smith's fracture of left radius**
7th

S52.55   **Other extraarticular fracture of lower end of radius**
6th   **S52.551**   **Other extraarticular fracture of lower end of right radius**
7th

S52.552   **Other extraarticular fracture of lower end of left radius**
7th

S52.56   **Barton's fracture**
6th   **S52.561**   **Barton's fracture of right radius**
7th

    S52.562   **Barton's fracture of left radius**
7th

S52.57   **Other intraarticular fracture of lower end of radius**
6th   **S52.571**   **Other intraarticular fracture of lower end of right radius**
7th

    S52.572   **Other intraarticular fracture of lower end of left radius**
7th

> 7th characters for category S52
> A—initial encounter for closed fracture
> B—initial encounter for open fracture type I or II
> C—initial encounter for open fracture NOS
> D—subsequent encounter for closed fracture with routine healing
> G—subsequent encounter for closed fracture with delayed healing
> K—subsequent encounter for closed fracture with nonunion
> P—subsequent encounter for closed fracture with malunion
> S—sequela

S52.59   **Other fractures of lower end of radius**
6th   **S52.591**   **Other fractures of lower end of right radius**
7th

    S52.592   **Other fractures of lower end of left radius**
7th

S52.6   **Fracture of lower end of ulna**
5th   **S52.60**   **Unspecified fracture of lower end of ulna**
6th   **S52.601**   **Unspecified fracture of lower end of right ulna**
7th

    S52.602   **Unspecified fracture of lower end of left ulna**
7th

S52.61   **Fracture of ulna styloid process**
6th   **S52.611**   **Displaced fracture of right ulna styloid process**
7th

    S52.612   **Displaced fracture of left ulna styloid process**
7th

    S52.614   **Nondisplaced fracture of right ulna styloid process**
7th

    S52.615   **Nondisplaced fracture of left ulna styloid process**
7th

S52.62   **Torus fracture of lower end of ulna**
6th   **S52.621**   **Torus fracture of lower end of right ulna**
7th

    S52.622   **Torus fracture of lower end of left ulna**
7th

S52.69   **Other fracture of lower end of ulna**
6th   **S52.691**   **Other fracture of lower end of right ulna**
7th

    S52.692   **Other fracture of lower end of left ulna**
7th

S52.9   **Unspecified fracture of forearm**
5th   **S52.91X**   **Unspecified fracture of right forearm**
7th

    S52.92X   **Unspecified fracture of left forearm**
7th

  Additional Character Required   ✓   3-character code   Unspecified laterality codes were excluded here.   •=New Code   ▲=Revised Code   *Excludes1*—Not coded here, do not use together   *Excludes2*—Not included here

S53 DISLOCATION AND SPRAIN OF JOINTS AND LIGAMENTS OF ELBOW

4th

Includes: avulsion of joint or ligament of elbow

laceration of cartilage, joint or ligament of elbow

sprain of cartilage, joint or ligament of elbow

traumatic hemarthrosis of joint or ligament of elbow

traumatic rupture of joint or ligament of elbow

traumatic subluxation of joint or ligament of elbow

traumatic tear of joint or ligament of elbow

Code also any associated open wound

Excludes2: strain of muscle, fascia and tendon at forearm level (S56.-)

> 7th characters for category S53
> A—initial encounter
> D—subsequent encounter
> S—sequela

S53.0 **Subluxation and dislocation of radial head**

5th

Dislocation of radiohumeral joint

Subluxation of radiohumeral joint

Excludes1: Monteggia's fracture-dislocation (S52.27-)

S53.00 **Unspecified subluxation and dislocation of radial head**

6th

S53.001 **Unspecified subluxation of right radial head**

7th

S53.002 **Unspecified subluxation of left radial head**

7th

S53.004 **Unspecified dislocation of right radial head**

7th

S53.005 **Unspecified dislocation of left radial head**

7th

S53.02 **Posterior subluxation and dislocation of radial head**

6th

Posteriolateral subluxation and dislocation of radial head

S53.021 **Posterior subluxation of right radial head**

7th

S53.022 **Posterior subluxation of left radial head**

7th

S53.024 **Posterior dislocation of right radial head**

7th

S53.025 **Posterior dislocation of left radial head**

7th

S53.03 **Nursemaid's elbow**

6th

S53.031 **Nursemaid's elbow, right elbow**

7th

S53.032 **Nursemaid's elbow, left elbow**

7th

S53.09 **Other subluxation and dislocation of radial head**

6th

S53.091 **Other subluxation of right radial head**

7th

S53.092 **Other subluxation of left radial head**

7th

S53.094 **Other dislocation of right radial head**

7th

S53.095 **Other dislocation of left radial head**

7th

S53.4 **Sprain of elbow**

5th

Excludes2: traumatic rupture of radial collateral ligament (S53.2-)

traumatic rupture of ulnar collateral ligament (S53.3-)

S53.40 **Unspecified sprain of elbow**

6th

S53.401 **Unspeci-fied sprain of right elbow**

7th

> 7th characters for category S53
> A—initial encounter
> D—subsequent encounter
> S—sequela

S53.402 **Unspeci-fied sprain of left elbow**

7th

S53.41 **Radiohumeral (joint) sprain**

6th

S53.411 **Radiohumeral (joint) sprain of right elbow**

7th

S53.412 **Radiohumeral (joint) sprain of left elbow**

7th

S53.42 **Ulnohumeral (joint) sprain**

6th

S53.421 **Ulnohumeral (joint) sprain of right elbow**

7th

S53.422 **Ulnohumeral (joint) sprain of left elbow**

7th

S53.43 **Radial collateral ligament sprain**

6th

S53.431 **Radial collateral ligament sprain of right elbow**

7th

S53.432 **Radial collateral ligament sprain of left elbow**

7th

S53.44 **Ulnar collateral ligament sprain**

6th

S53.441 **Ulnar collateral ligament sprain of right elbow**

7th

S53.442 **Ulnar collateral ligament sprain of left elbow**

7th

S53.49 **Other sprain of elbow**

6th

S53.491 **Other sprain of right elbow**

7th

S53.492 **Other sprain of left elbow**

7th

S56 INJURY OF MUSCLE, FASCIA AND TENDON AT FOREARM LEVEL

4th

Code also any associated open wound (S51.-)

Excludes2: injury of muscle, fascia and tendon at or below wrist (S66.-)

sprain of joints and ligaments of elbow (S53.4-)

S56.0 **Injury of flexor muscle, fascia and tendon of thumb at forearm level**

5th

S56.01 **Strain of flexor muscle, fascia and tendon of thumb at forearm level**

6th

> 7th characters for category S56
> A—initial encounter
> D—subsequent encounter
> S—sequela

S56.011 **Strain of flexor muscle, fascia and tendon of right thumb at forearm level**

7th

S56.012 **Strain of flexor muscle, fascia and tendon of left thumb at forearm level**

7th

S56.02 **Laceration of flexor muscle, fascia and tendon of thumb at forearm level**

6th

S56.021 **Laceration of flexor muscle, fascia and tendon of right thumb at forearm level**

7th

S56.022 **Laceration of flexor muscle, fascia and tendon of left thumb at forearm level**

7th

S56.1 **Injury of flexor muscle, fascia and tendon of other and unspecified finger at forearm level**

5th

 4th **5th** **6th** **7th** Additional Character Required

 ✓ 3-character code

Unspecified laterality codes were excluded here.

•=New Code
▲=Revised Code

Excludes1—Not coded here, do not use together

Excludes2—Not included here

S56.11 Strain of flexor muscle, fascia and tendon of other and unspecified finger at forearm level
6th
    S56.111 Strain of flexor muscle, fascia and tendon of right index finger at forearm level
    7th
    S56.112 Strain of flexor muscle, fascia and tendon of left index finger at forearm level
    7th
    S56.113 Strain of flexor muscle, fascia and tendon of right middle finger at forearm level
    7th
    S56.114 Strain of flexor muscle, fascia and tendon of left middle finger at forearm level
    7th
    S56.115 Strain of flexor muscle, fascia and tendon of right ring finger at forearm level
    7th
    S56.116 Strain of flexor muscle, fascia and tendon of left ring finger at forearm level
    7th
    S56.117 Strain of flexor muscle, fascia and tendon of right little finger at forearm level
    7th
    S56.118 Strain of flexor muscle, fascia and tendon of left little finger at forearm level
    7th

S56.12 Laceration of flexor muscle, fascia and tendon of other and unspecified finger at forearm level
6th
    S56.121 Laceration of flexor muscle, fascia and tendon of right index finger at forearm level
    7th
    S56.122 Laceration of flexor muscle, fascia and tendon of left index finger at forearm level
    7th
    S56.123 Laceration of flexor muscle, fascia and tendon of right middle finger at forearm level
    7th
    S56.124 Laceration of flexor muscle, fascia and tendon of left middle finger at forearm level
    7th
    S56.125 Laceration of flexor muscle, fascia and tendon of right ring finger at forearm level
    7th
    S56.126 Laceration of flexor muscle, fascia and tendon of left ring finger at forearm level
    7th
    S56.127 Laceration of flexor muscle, fascia and tendon of right little finger at forearm level
    7th
    S56.128 Laceration of flexor muscle, fascia and tendon of left little finger at forearm level
    7th

S56.2 Injury of other flexor muscle, fascia and tendon at forearm level
5th
  S56.21 Strain of other flexor muscle, fascia and tendon at forearm level
  6th
    S56.211 Strain of other flexor muscle, fascia and tendon at forearm level, right arm
    7th
    S56.212 Strain of other flexor muscle, fascia and tendon at forearm level, left arm
    7th

  S56.22 Laceration of other flexor muscle, fascia and tendon at forearm level
  6th
    S56.221 Laceration of other flexor muscle, fascia and tendon at forearm level, right arm
    7th
    S56.222 Laceration of other flexor muscle, fascia and tendon at forearm level, left arm
    7th

S56.3 Injury of extensor or abductor muscles, fascia and tendons of thumb at forearm level
5th

S56.31 Strain of extensor or abductor muscles, fascia and tendons of thumb at forearm level
6th
    S56.311 Strain of extensor or abductor muscles, fascia and tendons of right thumb at forearm level
    7th
    S56.312 Strain of extensor or abductor muscles, fascia and tendons of left thumb at forearm level
    7th

S56.32 Laceration of extensor or abductor muscles, fascia and tendons of thumb at forearm level
6th
    S56.321 Laceration of extensor or abductor muscles, fascia and tendons of right thumb at forearm level
    7th

> 7th characters for category S56
> A—initial encounter
> D—subsequent encounter
> S—sequela

    S56.322 Laceration of extensor or abductor muscles, fascia and tendons of left thumb at forearm level
    7th

S56.41 Strain of extensor muscle, fascia and tendon of other and unspecified finger at forearm level
6th
    S56.411 Strain of extensor muscle, fascia and tendon of right index finger at forearm level
    7th
    S56.412 Strain of extensor muscle, fascia and tendon of left index finger at forearm level
    7th
    S56.413 Strain of extensor muscle, fascia and tendon of right middle finger at forearm level
    7th
    S56.414 Strain of extensor muscle, fascia and tendon of left middle finger at forearm level
    7th
    S56.415 Strain of extensor muscle, fascia and tendon of right ring finger at forearm level
    7th
    S56.416 Strain of extensor muscle, fascia and tendon of left ring finger at forearm level
    7th
    S56.417 Strain of extensor muscle, fascia and tendon of right little finger at forearm level
    7th
    S56.418 Strain of extensor muscle, fascia and tendon of left little finger at forearm level
    7th

S56.42 Laceration of extensor muscle, fascia and tendon of other and unspecified finger at forearm level
6th
    S56.421 Laceration of extensor muscle, fascia and tendon of right index finger at forearm level
    7th
    S56.422 Laceration of extensor muscle, fascia and tendon of left index finger at forearm level
    7th
    S56.423 Laceration of extensor muscle, fascia and tendon of right middle finger at forearm level
    7th
    S56.424 Laceration of extensor muscle, fascia and tendon of left middle finger at forearm level
    7th
    S56.425 Laceration of extensor muscle, fascia and tendon of right ring finger at forearm level
    7th
    S56.426 Laceration of extensor muscle, fascia and tendon of left ring finger at forearm level
    7th
    S56.427 Laceration of extensor muscle, fascia and tendon of right little finger at forearm level
    7th

  4th 5th 6th 7th Additional Character Required ✓ 3-character code

Unspecified laterality codes were excluded here.

●=New Code
▲=Revised Code

Excludes1—Not coded here, do not use together
Excludes2—Not included here

CHAPTER 19. INJURY, POISONING AND CERTAIN OTHER CONSEQUENCES OF EXTERNAL CAUSES   (S56.428–S59.112)

S56.428 Laceration of extensor muscle, fascia and tendon of left little finger at forearm level
`7th`

S56.5 `5th` Injury of other extensor muscle, fascia and tendon at forearm level

    S56.51 `6th` Strain of other extensor muscle, fascia and tendon at forearm level

       S56.511 Strain of other extensor muscle, fascia and tendon at forearm level, right arm `7th`

       S56.512 Strain of other extensor muscle, fascia and tendon at forearm level, left arm `7th`

    S56.52 `6th` Laceration of other extensor muscle, fascia and tendon at forearm level

       S56.521 Laceration of other extensor muscle, fascia and tendon at forearm level, right arm `7th`

       S56.522 Laceration of other extensor muscle, fascia and tendon at forearm level, left arm `7th`

S56.8 `5th` Injury of other muscles, fascia and tendons at forearm level

    S56.81 `6th` Strain of other muscles, fascia and tendons at forearm level

       S56.811 Strain of other muscles, fascia and tendons at forearm level, right arm `7th`

       S56.812 Strain of other muscles, fascia and tendons at forearm level, left arm `7th`

    S56.82 `6th` Laceration of other muscles, fascia and tendons at forearm level

       S56.821 Laceration of other muscles, fascia and tendons at forearm level, right arm `7th`

       S56.822 Laceration of other muscles, fascia and tendons at forearm level, left arm `7th`

S56.9 `5th` Injury of unspecified muscles, fascia and tendons at forearm level

    S56.90 `6th` Unspecified injury of unspecified muscles, fascia and tendons at forearm level

       S56.901 Unspecified injury of unspecified muscles, fascia and tendons at forearm level, right arm `7th`

       S56.902 Unspecified injury of unspecified muscles, fascia and tendons at forearm level, left arm `7th`

    S56.91 `6th` Strain of unspecified muscles, fascia and tendons at forearm level

       S56.911 Strain of unspecified muscles, fascia and tendons at forearm level, right arm `7th`

       S56.912 Strain of unspecified muscles, fascia and tendons at forearm level, left arm `7th`

    S56.92 `6th` Laceration of unspecified muscles, fascia and tendons at forearm level

       S56.921 Laceration of unspecified muscles, fascia and tendons at forearm level, right arm `7th`

       S56.922 Laceration of unspecified muscles, fascia and tendons at forearm level, left arm `7th`

S59 `4th` OTHER AND UNSPECIFIED INJURIES OF ELBOW AND FOREARM

Excludes2: other and unspecified injuries of wrist and hand (S69.-)

> 7th characters for category S59
> A—initial encounter for closed fracture
> D—subsequent encounter for fracture with routine healing
> G—subsequent encounter for fracture with delayed healing
> K—subsequent encounter for fracture with nonunion
> P—subsequent encounter for fracture with malunion
> S—sequela

S59.0 `5th` Physeal fracture of lower end of ulna

    S59.00 `6th` Unspecified physeal fracture of lower end of ulna

       S59.001 Unspecified physeal fracture of lower end of ulna, right arm `7th`

       S59.002 Unspecified physeal fracture of lower end of ulna, left arm `7th`

    S59.01 `6th` Salter-Harris Type I physeal fracture of lower end of ulna

       S59.011 Salter-Harris Type I physeal fracture of lower end of ulna, right arm `7th`

       S59.012 Salter-Harris Type I physeal fracture of lower end of ulna, left arm `7th`

    S59.02 `6th` Salter-Harris Type II physeal fracture of lower end of ulna

       S59.021 Salter-Harris Type II physeal fracture of lower end of ulna, right arm `7th`

       S59.022 Salter-Harris Type II physeal fracture of lower end of ulna, left arm `7th`

    S59.03 `6th` Salter-Harris Type III physeal fracture of lower end of ulna

       S59.031 Salter-Harris Type III physeal fracture of lower end of ulna, right arm `7th`

       S59.032 Salter-Harris Type III physeal fracture of lower end of ulna, left arm `7th`

    S59.04 `6th` Salter-Harris Type IV physeal fracture of lower end of ulna

       S59.041 Salter-Harris Type IV physeal fracture of lower end of ulna, right arm `7th`

       S59.042 Salter-Harris Type IV physeal fracture of lower end of ulna, left arm `7th`

    S59.09 `6th` Other physeal fracture of lower end of ulna

       S59.091 Other physeal fracture of lower end of ulna, right arm `7th`

       S59.092 Other physeal fracture of lower end of ulna, left arm `7th`

S59.1 `5th` Physeal fracture of upper end of radius

    S59.10 `6th` Unspecified physeal fracture of upper end of radius

       S59.101 Unspecified physeal fracture of upper end of radius, right arm `7th`

       S59.102 Unspecified physeal fracture of upper end of radius, left arm `7th`

    S59.11 `6th` Salter-Harris Type I physeal fracture of upper end of radius

       S59.111 Salter-Harris Type I physeal fracture of upper end of radius, right arm `7th`

       S59.112 Salter-Harris Type I physeal fracture of upper end of radius, left arm `7th`

`4th` `5th` `6th` `7th` Additional Character Required   3-character code   Unspecified laterality codes were excluded here.   •=New Code   ▲=Revised Code   ***Excludes1***—Not coded here, do not use together   ***Excludes2***—Not included here

308   PEDIATRIC ICD-10-CM 2017: A MANUAL FOR PROVIDER-BASED CODING

S59.12 **6th** Salter-Harris Type II physeal fracture of upper end of radius

     S59.121 **7th** Salter-Harris Type II physeal fracture of upper end of radius, right arm

     S59.122 **7th** Salter-Harris Type II physeal fracture of upper end of radius, left arm

S59.13 **6th** Salter-Harris Type III physeal fracture of upper end of radius

     S59.131 **7th** Salter-Harris Type III physeal fracture of upper end of radius, right arm

     S59.132 **7th** Salter-Harris Type III physeal fracture of upper end of radius, left arm

S59.14 **6th** Salter-Harris Type IV physeal fracture of upper end of radius

     S59.141 **7th** Salter-Harris Type IV physeal fracture of upper end of radius, right arm

     S59.142 **7th** Salter-Harris Type IV physeal fracture of upper end of radius, left arm

S59.19 **6th** Other physeal fracture of upper end of radius

     S59.191 **7th** Other physeal fracture of upper end of radius, right arm

     S59.192 **7th** Other physeal fracture of upper end of radius, left arm

S59.2 **5th** Physeal fracture of lower end of radius

S59.20 **6th** Unspecified physeal fracture of lower end of radius

     S59.201 **7th** Unspecified physeal fracture of lower end of radius, right arm

     S59.202 **7th** Unspecified physeal fracture of lower end of radius, left arm

S59.21 **6th** Salter-Harris Type I physeal fracture of lower end of radius

     S59.211 **7th** Salter-Harris Type I physeal fracture of lower end of radius, right arm

     S59.212 **7th** Salter-Harris Type I physeal fracture of lower end of radius, left arm

S59.22 **6th** Salter-Harris Type II physeal fracture of lower end of radius

     S59.221 **7th** Salter-Harris Type II physeal fracture of lower end of radius, right arm

     S59.222 **7th** Salter-Harris Type II physeal fracture of lower end of radius, left arm

S59.23 **6th** Salter-Harris Type III physeal fracture of lower end of radius

     S59.231 **7th** Salter-Harris Type III physeal fracture of lower end of radius, right arm

     S59.232 **7th** Salter-Harris Type III physeal fracture of lower end of radius, left arm

S59.24 **6th** Salter-Harris Type IV physeal fracture of lower end of radius

     S59.241 **7th** Salter-Harris Type IV physeal fracture of lower end of radius, right arm

     S59.242 **7th** Salter-Harris Type IV physeal fracture of lower end of radius, left arm

S59.29 **6th** Other physeal fracture of lower end of radius

     S59.291 **7th** Other physeal fracture of lower end of radius, right arm

     S59.292 **7th** Other physeal fracture of lower end of radius, left arm

S59.8 Other specified injuries of elbow and forearm

S59.80 **5th** Other specified injuries of elbow

     S59.801 **7th** Other specified injuries of right elbow

> 7th characters for subcategory S59.8
> A—initial encounter
> D—subsequent encounter
> S—sequela

     S59.802 **7th** Other specified injuries of left elbow

S59.81 **6th** Other specified injuries of forearm

     S59.811 **7th** Other specified injuries right forearm

     S59.812 **7th** Other specified injuries left forearm

(S60–S69) INJURIES TO THE WRIST, HAND AND FINGERS

Excludes2: burns and corrosions (T20–T32)
     frostbite (T33–T34)
     insect bite or sting, venomous (T63.4)

S60 SUPERFICIAL INJURY OF WRIST, HAND AND FINGERS

S60.0 **4th** Contusion of finger without damage to nail

Excludes1: contusion involving nail (matrix) (S60.1)

S60.00X **5th** **7th** Contusion of unspecified finger without damage to nail

Contusion of finger(s) NOS

> 7th characters for category S60
> A—initial encounter
> D—subsequent encounter
> S—sequela

S60.01 Contusion of thumb without damage to nail

     S60.011 **6th** **7th** Contusion of right thumb without damage to nail

S60.02 **6th** Contusion of index finger without damage to nail

     S60.021 **7th** Contusion of right index finger without damage to nail

     S60.022 **7th** Contusion of left index finger without damage to nail

S60.03 **6th** Contusion of middle finger without damage to nail

     S60.031 **7th** Contusion of right middle finger without damage to nail

     S60.032 **7th** Contusion of left middle finger without damage to nail

S60.04 **6th** Contusion of ring finger without damage to nail

     S60.041 **7th** Contusion of right ring finger without damage to nail

     S60.042 **7th** Contusion of left ring finger without damage to nail

S60.05 **6th** Contusion of little finger without damage to nail

     S60.051 **7th** Contusion of right little finger without damage to nail

     S60.052 **7th** Contusion of left little finger without damage to nail

---

   Additional Character Required   ✓ 3-character code

Unspecified laterality codes were excluded here.

•=New Code
▲=Revised Code

Excludes1—Not coded here, do not use together
Excludes2—Not included here

CHAPTER 19. INJURY, POISONING AND CERTAIN OTHER CONSEQUENCES OF EXTERNAL CAUSES   (S60.1–S60.423)

S60.1 **5th** Contusion of finger with damage to nail

S60.11 **6th** Contusion of thumb with damage to nail

S60.111 **7th** Contusion of right thumb with damage to nail

S60.112 **7th** Contusion of left thumb with damage to nail

S60.12 **6th** Contusion of index finger with damage to nail

S60.121 **7th** Contusion of right index finger with damage to nail

S60.122 **7th** Contusion of left index finger with damage to nail

S60.13 **6th** Contusion of middle finger with damage to nail

S60.131 **7th** Contusion of right middle finger with damage to nail

S60.132 **7th** Contusion of left middle finger with damage to nail

S60.14 **6th** Contusion of ring finger with damage to nail

S60.141 **7th** Contusion of right ring finger with damage to nail

S60.142 **7th** Contusion of left ring finger with damage to nail

S60.15 **6th** Contusion of little finger with damage to nail

S60.151 **7th** Contusion of right little finger with damage to nail

S60.152 **7th** Contusion of left little finger with damage to nail

S60.2 **5th** Contusion of wrist and hand

Excludes2: contusion of fingers (S60.0-, S60.1-)

S60.21 **6th** Contusion of wrist

S60.211 **7th** Contusion of right wrist

S60.212 **7th** Contusion of left wrist

S60.22 **6th** Contusion of hand

S60.221 **7th** Contusion of right hand

S60.222 **7th** Contusion of left hand

S60.3 **5th** Other superficial injuries of thumb

S60.31 **6th** Abrasion of thumb

S60.311 **7th** Abrasion of right thumb

S60.312 **7th** Abrasion of left thumb

S60.32 **6th** Blister (nonthermal) of thumb

S60.321 **7th** Blister (nonthermal) of right thumb

S60.322 **7th** Blister (nonthermal) of left thumb

S60.34 **6th** External constriction of thumb

Hair tourniquet syndrome of thumb

Use additional cause code to identify the constricting item (W49.0-)

S60.341 **7th** External constriction of right thumb

S60.342 **7th** External constriction of left thumb

S60.35 **6th** Superficial FB of thumb

Splinter in the thumb

S60.351 **7th** Superficial FB of right thumb

S60.352 **7th** Superficial FB of left thumb

S60.36 **6th** Insect bite (nonvenomous) of thumb

S60.361 **7th** Insect bite (nonvenomous) of right thumb

S60.362 **7th** Insect bite (nonvenomous) of left thumb

S60.37 **6th** Other superficial bite of thumb

Excludes1: open bite of thumb (S61.05-, S61.15-)

S60.371 **7th** Other superficial bite of right thumb

S60.372 **7th** Other superficial bite of left thumb

> 7th characters for category S60
> A—initial encounter
> D—subsequent encounter
> S—sequela

S60.4 **5th** Other superficial injuries of other fingers

S60.41 **6th** Abrasion of fingers

S60.410 **7th** Abrasion of right index finger

S60.411 **7th** Abrasion of left index finger

S60.412 **7th** Abrasion of right middle finger

S60.413 **7th** Abrasion of left middle finger

S60.414 **7th** Abrasion of right ring finger

S60.415 **7th** Abrasion of left ring finger

S60.416 **7th** Abrasion of right little finger

S60.417 **7th** Abrasion of left little finger

S60.42 **6th** Blister (nonthermal) of fingers

S60.420 **7th** Blister (nonthermal) of right index finger

S60.421 **7th** Blister (nonthermal) of left index finger

S60.422 **7th** Blister (nonthermal) of right middle finger

S60.423 **7th** Blister (nonthermal) of left middle finger

4th **5th** **6th** **7th** Additional Character Required   ✓ 3-character code   Unspecified laterality codes were excluded here.   •=New Code ▲=Revised Code   ***Excludes1***—Not coded here, do not use together   ***Excludes2***—Not included here

310   **PEDIATRIC ICD-10-CM 2017: A MANUAL FOR PROVIDER-BASED CODING**

S60.424 Blister (nonthermal) of right ring finger
`7th`

S60.425 Blister (nonthermal) of left ring finger
`7th`

S60.426 Blister (nonthermal) of right little finger
`7th`

S60.427 Blister (nonthermal) of left little finger
`7th`

S60.44 External constriction of fingers
`6th`
Hair tourniquet syndrome of finger
Use additional cause code to identify the constricting item (W49.0-)

S60.440 External constriction of right index finger
`7th`

S60.441 External constriction of left index finger
`7th`

S60.442 External constriction of right middle finger
`7th`

S60.443 External constriction of left middle finger
`7th`

S60.444 External constriction of right ring finger
`7th`

S60.445 External constriction of left ring finger
`7th`

S60.446 External constriction of right little finger
`7th`

S60.447 External constriction of left little finger
`7th`

S60.45 Superficial FB of fingers
`6th`
Splinter in the finger(s)

S60.450 Superficial FB of right index finger
`7th`

S60.451 Superficial FB of left index finger
`7th`

S60.452 Superficial FB of right middle finger
`7th`

S60.453 Superficial FB of left middle finger
`7th`

S60.454 Superficial FB of right ring finger
`7th`

S60.455 Superficial FB of left ring finger
`7th`

S60.456 Superficial FB of right little finger
`7th`

S60.457 Superficial FB of left little finger
`7th`

S60.46 Insect bite (nonvenomous) of fingers
`6th`

S60.460 Insect bite (nonvenomous) of right index finger
`7th`

S60.461 Insect bite (nonvenomous) of left index finger
`7th`

S60.462 Insect bite (nonvenomous) of right middle finger
`7th`

S60.463 Insect bite (nonvenomous) of left middle finger
`7th`

S60.464 Insect bite (nonvenomous) of right ring finger
`7th`

S60.465 Insect bite (nonvenomous) of left ring finger
`7th`

S60.466 Insect bite (nonvenomous) of right little finger
`7th`

S60.467 Insect bite (nonvenomous) of left little finger
`7th`

S60.47 Other superficial bite of fingers
`6th`
Excludes1: open bite of fingers (S61.25-, S61.35-)

S60.470 Other superficial bite of right index finger
`7th`

7th characters for category S60
A—initial encounter
D—subsequent encounter
S—sequela

S60.471 Other superficial bite of left index finger
`7th`

S60.472 Other superficial bite of right middle finger
`7th`

S60.473 Other superficial bite of left middle finger
`7th`

S60.474 Other superficial bite of right ring finger
`7th`

S60.475 Other superficial bite of left ring finger
`7th`

S60.476 Other superficial bite of right little finger
`7th`

S60.477 Other superficial bite of left little finger
`7th`

S60.5 Other superficial injuries of hand
`5th`
Excludes2: superficial injuries of fingers (S60.3-, S60.4-)

S60.51 Abrasion of hand
`6th`
S60.511 Abrasion of right hand
`7th`

S60.512 Abrasion of left hand
`7th`

S60.52 Blister (nonthermal) of hand
`6th`
S60.521 Blister (nonthermal) of right hand
`7th`

S60.522 Blister (nonthermal) of left hand
`7th`

S60.54 External constriction of hand
`6th`
S60.541 External constriction of right hand
S60.542 External constriction of left hand

S60.55 Superficial FB of hand
`6th`
Splinter in the hand
S60.551 Superficial FB of right hand
`7th`

S60.552 Superficial FB of left hand
`7th`

  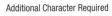 Additional Character Required   ✓ 3-character code   Unspecified laterality codes were excluded here.   •=New Code   ▲=Revised Code   *Excludes1*—Not coded here, do not use together   *Excludes2*—Not included here

S60.56 Insect bite (nonvenomous) of hand

   S60.561 **6th** Insect bite (nonvenomous) of right hand **7th**

   S60.562 Insect bite (nonvenomous) of left hand **7th**

S60.57 **6th** Other superficial bite of hand
Excludes1: open bite of hand (S61.45-)

   S60.571 Other superficial bite of hand of right hand **7th**

   S60.572 Other superficial bite of hand of left hand **7th**

S60.8 **5th** Other superficial injuries of wrist

S60.81 **6th** Abrasion of wrist

   S60.811 Abrasion of right wrist **7th**

   S60.812 Abrasion of left wrist **7th**

S60.82 **6th** Blister (nonthermal) of wrist

   S60.821 Blister (nonthermal) of right wrist **7th**

   S60.822 Blister (nonthermal) of left wrist **7th**

S60.84 **6th** External constriction of wrist

   S60.841 External constriction of right wrist **7th**

   S60.842 External constriction of left wrist **7th**

S60.85 **6th** Superficial FB of wrist
Splinter in the wrist

   S60.851 Superficial FB of right wrist **7th**

   S60.852 Superficial FB of left wrist **7th**

S60.86 **6th** Insect bite (nonvenomous) of wrist

   S60.861 Insect bite (nonvenomous) of right wrist **7th**

   S60.862 **7th** Insect bite (nonvenomous) of left wrist

> 7th characters for categories S60 & S61
> A—initial encounter
> D—subsequent encounter
> S—sequela

S60.87 **6th** Other superficial bite of wrist
Excludes1: open bite of wrist (S61.55)

   S60.871 Other superficial bite of right wrist **7th**

   S60.872 Other superficial bite of left wrist **7th**

S61 **4th** **OPEN WOUND OF WRIST, HAND AND FINGERS**
Code also any associated wound infection
Excludes1: open fracture of wrist, hand and finger (S62.- with 7th character B)
   traumatic amputation of wrist and hand (S68.-)

S61.0 **5th** Open wound of thumb without damage to nail
Excludes1: open wound of thumb with damage to nail (S61.1-)

   S61.01 **6th** Laceration without FB of thumb without damage to nail

---

   S61.011 Laceration without FB of right thumb without damage to nail **7th**

   S61.012 Laceration without FB of left thumb without damage to nail **7th**

S61.02 **6th** Laceration with FB of thumb without damage to nail

   S61.021 Laceration with FB of right thumb without damage to nail **7th**

   S61.022 Laceration with FB of left thumb without damage to nail **7th**

S61.03 **6th** Puncture wound without FB of thumb without damage to nail

   S61.031 **7th** Puncture wound without FB of right thumb without damage to nail

> 7th characters for category S61
> A—initial encounter
> D—subsequent encounter
> S—sequela

   S61.032 **7th** Puncture wound without FB of left thumb without damage to nail

S61.04 **6th** Puncture wound with FB of thumb without damage to nail

   S61.041 Puncture wound with FB of right thumb without damage to nail **7th**

   S61.042 Puncture wound with FB of left thumb without damage to nail **7th**

S61.05 **6th** Open bite of thumb without damage to nail
Bite of thumb NOS
Excludes1: superficial bite of thumb (S60.36-, S60.37-)

   S61.051 Open bite of right thumb without damage to nail **7th**

   S61.052 Open bite of left thumb without damage to nail **7th**

S61.1 **5th** Open wound of thumb with damage to nail

   S61.11 **6th** Laceration without FB of thumb with damage to nail

   S61.111 Laceration without FB of right thumb with damage to nail **7th**

   S61.112 Laceration without FB of left thumb with damage to nail **7th**

S61.12 **6th** Laceration with FB of thumb with damage to nail

   S61.121 Laceration with FB of right thumb with damage to nail **7th**

   S61.122 Laceration with FB of left thumb with damage to nail **7th**

S61.13 **6th** Puncture wound without FB of thumb with damage to nail

   S61.131 Puncture wound without FB of right thumb with damage to nail **7th**

   S61.132 Puncture wound without FB of left thumb with damage to nail **7th**

S61.14 **6th** Puncture wound with FB of thumb with damage to nail

   S61.141 Puncture wound with FB of right thumb with damage to nail **7th**

  4th **5th** **6th** **7th** Additional Character Required   3-character code   Unspecified laterality codes were excluded here.   •=New Code   *Excludes1*—Not coded here, do not use together
                                                                 ▲=Revised Code   *Excludes2*—Not included here

S61.142 **7th** Puncture wound with FB of left thumb with damage to nail

S61.15 **6th** Open bite of thumb with damage to nail
Bite of thumb with damage to nail NOS
Excludes1: superficial bite of thumb (S60.36-, S60.37-)

    S61.151 **7th** Open bite of right thumb with damage to nail

    S61.152 **7th** Open bite of left thumb with damage to nail

S61.2 **5th** Open wound of other finger without damage to nail
Excludes1: open wound of finger involving nail (matrix) (S61.3-)
Excludes2: open wound of thumb without damage to nail (S61.0-)

    S61.21 **6th** Laceration without FB of finger without damage to nail

       S61.210 **7th** Laceration without FB of right index finger without damage to nail

       S61.211 **7th** Laceration without FB of left index finger without damage to nail

       S61.212 **7th** Laceration without FB of right middle finger without damage to nail

       S61.213 **7th** Laceration without FB of left middle finger without damage to nail

       S61.214 **7th** Laceration without FB of right ring finger without damage to nail

       S61.215 **7th** Laceration without FB of left ring finger without damage to nail

       S61.216 **7th** Laceration without FB of right little finger without damage to nail

       S61.217 **7th** Laceration without FB of left little finger without damage to nail

    S61.22 **6th** Laceration with FB of finger without damage to nail

       S61.220 **7th** Laceration with FB of right index finger without damage to nail

       S61.221 **7th** Laceration with FB of left index finger without damage to nail

       S61.222 **7th** Laceration with FB of right middle finger without damage to nail

       S61.223 **7th** Laceration with FB of left middle finger without damage to nail

       S61.224 **7th** Laceration with FB of right ring finger without damage to nail

       S61.225 **7th** Laceration with FB of left ring finger without damage to nail

       S61.226 **7th** Laceration with FB of right little finger without damage to nail

       S61.227 **7th** Laceration with FB of left little finger without damage to nail

    S61.23 **6th** Puncture wound without FB of finger without damage to nail

       S61.230 **7th** Puncture wound without FB of right index finger without damage to nail

       S61.231 **7th** Puncture wound without FB of left index finger without damage to nail

       S61.232 **7th** Puncture wound without FB of right middle finger without damage to nail

       S61.233 **7th** Puncture wound without FB of left middle finger without damage to nail

       S61.234 **7th** Puncture wound without FB of right ring finger without damage to nail

       S61.235 **7th** Puncture wound without FB of left ring finger without damage to nail

       S61.236 **7th** Puncture wound without FB of right little finger without damage to nail

       S61.237 **7th** Puncture wound without FB of left little finger without damage to nail

    S61.24 **6th** Puncture wound with FB of finger without damage to nail

       S61.240 **7th** Puncture wound with FB of right index finger without damage to nail

> 7th characters for category S61
> A—initial encounter
> D—subsequent encounter
> S—sequela

       S61.241 **7th** Puncture wound with FB of left index finger without damage to nail

       S61.242 **7th** Puncture wound with FB of right middle finger without damage to nail

       S61.243 **7th** Puncture wound with FB of left middle finger without damage to nail

       S61.244 **7th** Puncture wound with FB of right ring finger without damage to nail

       S61.245 **7th** Puncture wound with FB of left ring finger without damage to nail

       S61.246 **7th** Puncture wound with FB of right little finger without damage to nail

       S61.247 **7th** Puncture wound with FB of left little finger without damage to nail

    S61.25 **6th** Open bite of finger without damage to nail
Bite of finger without damage to nail NOS
Excludes1: superficial bite of finger (S60.46-, S60.47-)

       S61.250 **7th** Open bite of right index finger without damage to nail

       S61.251 **7th** Open bite of left index finger without damage to nail

       S61.252 **7th** Open bite of right middle finger without damage to nail

       S61.253 **7th** Open bite of left middle finger without damage to nail

       S61.254 **7th** Open bite of right ring finger without damage to nail

       S61.255 **7th** Open bite of left ring finger without damage to nail

---

  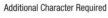 Additional Character Required   ✓   3-character code   Unspecified laterality codes were excluded here.   •=New Code   ▲=Revised Code   *Excludes1*—Not coded here, do not use together   *Excludes2*—Not included here

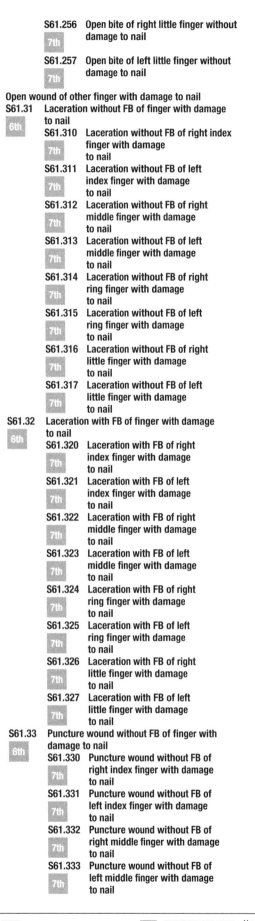

CHAPTER 19. INJURY, POISONING AND CERTAIN OTHER CONSEQUENCES OF EXTERNAL CAUSES (S61.256–S61.442)

S61.256 Open bite of right little finger without damage to nail [7th]

S61.257 Open bite of left little finger without damage to nail [7th]

S61.3 Open wound of other finger with damage to nail [5th]

S61.31 Laceration without FB of finger with damage to nail [6th]

S61.310 Laceration without FB of right index finger with damage to nail [7th]

S61.311 Laceration without FB of left index finger with damage to nail [7th]

S61.312 Laceration without FB of right middle finger with damage to nail [7th]

S61.313 Laceration without FB of left middle finger with damage to nail [7th]

S61.314 Laceration without FB of right ring finger with damage to nail [7th]

S61.315 Laceration without FB of left ring finger with damage to nail [7th]

S61.316 Laceration without FB of right little finger with damage to nail [7th]

S61.317 Laceration without FB of left little finger with damage to nail [7th]

S61.32 Laceration with FB of finger with damage to nail [6th]

S61.320 Laceration with FB of right index finger with damage to nail [7th]

S61.321 Laceration with FB of left index finger with damage to nail [7th]

S61.322 Laceration with FB of right middle finger with damage to nail [7th]

S61.323 Laceration with FB of left middle finger with damage to nail [7th]

S61.324 Laceration with FB of right ring finger with damage to nail [7th]

S61.325 Laceration with FB of left ring finger with damage to nail [7th]

S61.326 Laceration with FB of right little finger with damage to nail [7th]

S61.327 Laceration with FB of left little finger with damage to nail [7th]

S61.33 Puncture wound without FB of finger with damage to nail [6th]

S61.330 Puncture wound without FB of right index finger with damage to nail [7th]

S61.331 Puncture wound without FB of left index finger with damage to nail [7th]

S61.332 Puncture wound without FB of right middle finger with damage to nail [7th]

S61.333 Puncture wound without FB of left middle finger with damage to nail [7th]

S61.334 Puncture wound without FB of right ring finger with damage to nail [7th]

S61.335 Puncture wound without FB of left ring finger with damage to nail [7th]

S61.336 Puncture wound without FB of right little finger with damage to nail [7th]

S61.337 Puncture wound without FB of left little finger with damage to nail [7th]

S61.34 Puncture wound with FB of finger with damage to nail [6th]

S61.340 Puncture wound with FB of right index finger with damage to nail [7th]

S61.341 Puncture wound with FB of left index finger with damage to nail [7th]

S61.342 Puncture wound with FB of right middle finger with damage to nail [7th]

S61.343 Puncture wound with FB of left middle finger with damage to nail [7th]

> 7th characters for category S61
> A—initial encounter
> D—subsequent encounter
> S—sequela

S61.344 Puncture wound with FB of right ring finger with damage to nail [7th]

S61.345 Puncture wound with FB of left ring finger with damage to nail [7th]

S61.346 Puncture wound with FB of right little finger with damage to nail [7th]

S61.347 Puncture wound with FB of left little finger with damage to nail [7th]

S61.4 Open wound of hand [5th]

S61.41 Laceration without FB of hand [6th]

S61.411 Laceration without FB of right hand [7th]

S61.412 Laceration without FB of left hand [7th]

S61.42 Laceration with FB of hand [6th]

S61.421 Laceration with FB of right hand [7th]

S61.422 Laceration with FB of left hand [7th]

S61.43 Puncture wound without FB of hand [6th]

S61.431 Puncture wound without FB of right hand [7th]

S61.432 Puncture wound without FB of left hand [7th]

S61.44 Puncture wound with FB of hand [6th]

S61.441 Puncture wound with FB of right hand [7th]

S61.442 Puncture wound with FB of left hand [7th]

   Additional Character Required   ✓ 3-character code   Unspecified laterality codes were excluded here.   •=New Code   ▲=Revised Code   *Excludes1*—Not coded here, do not use together   *Excludes2*—Not included here

314   PEDIATRIC ICD-10-CM 2017: A MANUAL FOR PROVIDER-BASED CODING

S61.45 Open bite of hand
^{6th}
    Bite of hand NOS
    Excludes1: superficial bite of hand (S60.56-, S60.57-)
    S61.451 Open bite of right hand ^{7th}

    S61.452 Open bite of left hand ^{7th}

S61.5 Open wound of wrist
^{5th}
  S61.51 Laceration without FB of wrist
  ^{6th}
    S61.511 Laceration without FB of right wrist ^{7th}

    S61.512 Laceration without FB of left wrist ^{7th}

  S61.52 Laceration with FB of wrist
  ^{6th}
    S61.521 Laceration with FB of right wrist ^{7th}

    S61.522 Laceration with FB of left wrist ^{7th}

  S61.53 Puncture wound without FB of wrist
  ^{6th}
    S61.531 Puncture wound without FB of right wrist ^{7th}

    S61.532 Puncture wound without FB of left wrist ^{7th}

  S61.54 Puncture wound with FB of wrist
  ^{6th}
    S61.541 Puncture wound with FB of right wrist ^{7th}

    S61.542 Puncture wound with FB of left wrist ^{7th}

  S61.55 Open bite of wrist
  ^{6th}
    Bite of wrist NOS
    Excludes1: superficial bite of wrist (S60.86-, S60.87-)
    S61.551 Open bite of right wrist ^{7th}

    S61.552 Open bite of left wrist ^{7th}

S62 FRACTURE AT WRIST AND HAND LEVEL
^{4th}
Note: A fracture not indicated as displaced or nondisplaced should be coded to displaced
A fracture not indicated as open or closed should be coded to closed
Excludes1: traumatic amputation of wrist and hand (S68.-)
Excludes2: fracture of distal parts of ulna and radius (S52.-)

S62.0 Fracture of navicular [scaphoid] bone of wrist
^{5th}
  S62.00 Unspecified fracture of navicular [scaphoid] bone of wrist
  ^{6th}
    S62.001 Unspecified fracture of navicular [scaphoid] bone of right wrist ^{7th}
    S62.002 Unspecified fracture of navicular [scaphoid] bone of left wrist ^{7th}

> 7th characters for category S62
> A—initial encounter for closed fracture
> B—initial encounter for open fracture
> D—subsequent encounter for fracture with routine healing
> G—subsequent encounter for fracture with delayed healing
> K—subsequent encounter for fracture with nonunion
> P—subsequent encounter for fracture with malunion
> S—sequela

S62.01 Fracture of distal pole of navicular [scaphoid] bone of wrist
^{6th}
  Fracture of volar tuberosity of navicular [scaphoid] bone of wrist
  S62.011 Displaced fracture of distal pole of navicular [scaphoid] bone of right wrist ^{7th}
  S62.012 Displaced fracture of distal pole of navicular [scaphoid] bone of left wrist ^{7th}
  S62.014 Nondisplaced fracture of distal pole of navicular [scaphoid] bone of right wrist ^{7th}
  S62.015 Nondisplaced fracture of distal pole of navicular [scaphoid] bone of left wrist ^{7th}

S62.02 Fracture of middle third of navicular [scaphoid] bone of wrist
^{6th}
  S62.021 Displaced fracture of middle third of navicular [scaphoid] bone of right wrist ^{7th}
  S62.022 Displaced fracture of middle third of navicular [scaphoid] bone of left wrist ^{7th}
  S62.024 Nondisplaced fracture of middle third of navicular [scaphoid] bone of right wrist ^{7th}
  S62.025 Nondisplaced fracture of middle third of navicular [scaphoid] bone of left wrist ^{7th}

S62.03 Fracture of proximal third of navicular [scaphoid] bone of wrist
^{6th}
  S62.031 Displaced fracture of proximal third of navicular [scaphoid] bone of right wrist ^{7th}
  S62.032 Displaced fracture of proximal third of navicular [scaphoid] bone of left wrist ^{7th}
  S62.034 Nondisplaced fracture of proximal third of navicular [scaphoid] bone of right wrist ^{7th}
  S62.035 Nondisplaced fracture of proximal third of navicular [scaphoid] bone of left wrist ^{7th}

S62.1 Fracture of other and unspecified carpal bone(s)
^{5th}
Excludes2: fracture of scaphoid of wrist (S62.0-)
  S62.10 Fracture of unspecified carpal bone
  ^{6th}
    Fracture of wrist NOS
    S62.101 Fracture of unspecified carpal bone, right wrist ^{7th}

    S62.102 Fracture of unspecified carpal bone, left wrist ^{7th}

  S62.11 Fracture of triquetrum [cuneiform] bone of wrist
  ^{6th}
    S62.111 Displaced fracture of triquetrum [cuneiform] bone, right wrist ^{7th}

    S62.112 Displaced fracture of triquetrum [cuneiform] bone, left wrist ^{7th}

    S62.114 Nondisplaced fracture of triquetrum [cuneiform] bone, right wrist ^{7th}

    S62.115 Nondisplaced fracture of triquetrum [cuneiform] bone, left wrist ^{7th}

  S62.12 Fracture of lunate [semilunar]
  ^{6th}
    S62.121 Displaced fracture of lunate [semilunar], right wrist ^{7th}

  Additional Character Required   3-character code   Unspecified laterality codes were excluded here.   •=New Code   ▲=Revised Code   *Excludes1*—Not coded here, do not use together   *Excludes2*—Not included here

PEDIATRIC ICD-10-CM 2017: A MANUAL FOR PROVIDER-BASED CODING   315

CHAPTER 19. INJURY, POISONING AND CERTAIN OTHER CONSEQUENCES OF EXTERNAL CAUSES (S62.122–S62.244)

S62.122 Displaced fracture of lunate [semilunar], left wrist
7th

S62.124 Nondisplaced fracture of lunate [semilunar], right wrist
7th

S62.125 Nondisplaced fracture of lunate [semilunar], left wrist
7th

S62.13 Fracture of capitate [os magnum] bone
6th

S62.131 Displaced fracture of capitate [os magnum] bone, right wrist
7th

S62.132 Displaced fracture of capitate [os magnum] bone, left wrist
7th

S62.134 Nondisplaced fracture of capitate [os magnum] bone, right wrist
7th

S62.135 Nondisplaced fracture of capitate [os magnum] bone, left wrist
7th

S62.14 Fracture of body of hamate [unciform] bone
6th
Fracture of hamate [unciform] bone NOS

S62.141 Displaced fracture of body of hamate [unciform] bone, right wrist
7th

S62.142 Displaced fracture of body of hamate [unciform] bone, left wrist
7th

S62.144 Nondisplaced fracture of body of hamate [unciform] bone, right wrist
7th

S62.145 Nondisplaced fracture of body of hamate [unciform] bone, left wrist
7th

S62.15 Fracture of hook process of hamate [unciform] bone
6th
Fracture of unciform process of hamate [unciform] bone

S62.151 Displaced fracture of hook process of hamate [unciform] bone, right wrist
7th

S62.152 Displaced fracture of hook process of hamate [unciform] bone, left wrist
7th

S62.154 Nondisplaced fracture of hook process of hamate [unciform] bone, right wrist
7th

S62.155 Nondisplaced fracture of hook process of hamate [unciform] bone, left wrist
7th

S62.16 Fracture of pisiform
6th

S62.161 Displaced fracture of pisiform, right wrist
7th

S62.162 Displaced fracture of pisiform, left wrist
7th

S62.164 Nondisplaced fracture of pisiform, right wrist
7th

S62.165 Nondisplaced fracture of pisiform, left wrist
7th

S62.17 Fracture of trapezium [larger multangular]
6th

S62.171 Displaced fracture of trapezium [larger multangular], right wrist
7th

S62.172 Displaced fracture of trapezium [larger multangular], left wrist
7th

S62.174 Nondisplaced fracture of trapezium [larger multangular], right wrist
7th

S62.175 Nondisplaced fracture of trapezium [larger multangular], left wrist
7th

S62.18 Fracture of trapezoid [smaller multangular]
6th

S62.181 Displaced fracture of trapezoid [smaller multangular], right wrist
7th

S62.182 Displaced fracture of trapezoid [smaller multangular], left wrist
7th

S62.184 Nondisplaced fracture of trapezoid [smaller multangular], right wrist
7th

S62.185 Nondisplaced fracture of trapezoid [smaller multangular], left wrist
7th

S62.2 Fracture of first metacarpal bone
5th

S62.20 Unspecified fracture of first metacarpal bone
6th

S62.201 Unspecified fracture of first metacarpal bone, right hand
7th

S62.202 Unspecified fracture of first metacarpal bone, left hand
7th

S62.21 Bennett's fracture
6th

S62.211 Bennett's fracture, right hand
7th

S62.212 Bennett's fracture, left hand
7th

S62.22 Rolando's fracture
6th

S62.221 Displaced Rolando's fracture, right hand
7th

S62.222 Displaced Rolando's fracture, left hand
7th

S62.224 Nondisplaced Rolando's fracture, right hand
7th

S62.225 Nondisplaced Rolando's fracture, left hand
7th

> 7th characters for category S62
> A—initial encounter for closed fracture
> B—initial encounter for open fracture
> D—subsequent encounter for fracture with routine healing
> G—subsequent encounter for fracture with delayed healing
> K—subsequent encounter for fracture with nonunion
> P—subsequent encounter for fracture with malunion
> S—sequela

S62.23 Other fracture of base of first metacarpal bone
6th

S62.231 Other displaced fracture of base of first metacarpal bone, right hand
7th

S62.232 Other displaced fracture of base of first metacarpal bone, left hand
7th

S62.234 Other nondisplaced fracture of base of first metacarpal bone, right hand
7th

S62.235 Other nondisplaced fracture of base of first metacarpal bone, left hand
7th

S62.24 Fracture of shaft of first metacarpal bone
6th

S62.241 Displaced fracture of shaft of first metacarpal bone, right hand
7th

S62.242 Displaced fracture of shaft of first metacarpal bone, left hand
7th

S62.244 Nondisplaced fracture of shaft of first metacarpal bone, right hand
7th

  4th 5th 6th 7th Additional Character Required 3-character code | Unspecified laterality codes were excluded here. | •=New Code ▲=Revised Code | *Excludes1*—Not coded here, do not use together *Excludes2*—Not included here

S62.245 **7th** Nondisplaced fracture of shaft of first metacarpal bone, left hand

S62.25 **6th** Fracture of neck of first metacarpal bone
     S62.251 **7th** Displaced fracture of neck of first metacarpal bone, right hand
     S62.252 **7th** Displaced fracture of neck of first metacarpal bone, left hand
     S62.254 **7th** Nondisplaced fracture of neck of first metacarpal bone, right hand
     S62.255 **7th** Nondisplaced fracture of neck of first metacarpal bone, left hand

S62.29 **6th** Other fracture of first metacarpal bone
     S62.291 **7th** Other fracture of first metacarpal bone, right hand
     S62.292 **7th** Other fracture of first metacarpal bone, left hand

S62.3 **5th** Fracture of other and unspecified metacarpal bone
Excludes2: fracture of first metacarpal bone (S62.2-)
     S62.30 **6th** Unspecified fracture of other metacarpal bone
         S62.300 **7th** Unspecified fracture of second metacarpal bone, right hand
         S62.301 **7th** Unspecified fracture of second metacarpal bone, left hand
         S62.302 **7th** Unspecified fracture of third metacarpal bone, right hand
         S62.303 **7th** Unspecified fracture of third metacarpal bone, left hand
         S62.304 **7th** Unspecified fracture of fourth metacarpal bone, right hand
         S62.305 **7th** Unspecified fracture of fourth metacarpal bone, left hand
         S62.306 **7th** Unspecified fracture of fifth metacarpal bone, right hand
         S62.307 **7th** Unspecified fracture of fifth metacarpal bone, left hand

     S62.31 **6th** Displaced fracture of base of other metacarpal bone
         S62.310 **7th** Displaced fracture of base of second metacarpal bone, right hand
         S62.311 **7th** Displaced fracture of base of second metacarpal bone, left hand
         S62.312 **7th** Displaced fracture of base of third metacarpal bone, right hand
         S62.313 **7th** Displaced fracture of base of third metacarpal bone, left hand
         S62.314 **7th** Displaced fracture of base of fourth metacarpal bone, right hand
         S62.315 **7th** Displaced fracture of base of fourth metacarpal bone, left hand
         S62.316 **7th** Displaced fracture of base of fifth metacarpal bone, right hand

S62.317 **7th** Displaced fracture of base of fifth metacarpal bone, left hand

S62.32 **6th** Displaced fracture of shaft of other metacarpal bone
     S62.320 **7th** Displaced fracture of shaft of second metacarpal bone, right hand
     S62.321 **7th** Displaced fracture of shaft of second metacarpal bone, left hand
     S62.322 **7th** Displaced fracture of shaft of third metacarpal bone, right hand
     S62.323 **7th** Displaced fracture of shaft of third metacarpal bone, left hand
     S62.324 **7th** Displaced fracture of shaft of fourth metacarpal bone, right hand
     S62.325 **7th** Displaced fracture of shaft of fourth metacarpal bone, left hand
     S62.326 **7th** Displaced fracture of shaft of fifth metacarpal bone, right hand
     S62.327 **7th** Displaced fracture of shaft of fifth metacarpal bone, left hand

S62.33 **6th** Displaced fracture of neck of other metacarpal bone
     S62.330 **7th** Displaced fracture of neck of second metacarpal bone, right hand
     S62.331 **7th** Displaced fracture of neck of second metacarpal bone, left hand

> 7th characters for category S62
> A—initial encounter for closed fracture
> B—initial encounter for open fracture
> D—subsequent encounter for fracture with routine healing
> G—subsequent encounter for fracture with delayed healing
> K—subsequent encounter for fracture with nonunion
> P—subsequent encounter for fracture with malunion
> S—sequela

     S62.332 **7th** Displaced fracture of neck of third metacarpal bone, right hand
     S62.333 **7th** Displaced fracture of neck of third metacarpal bone, left hand
     S62.334 **7th** Displaced fracture of neck of fourth metacarpal bone, right hand
     S62.335 **7th** Displaced fracture of neck of fourth metacarpal bone, left hand
     S62.336 **7th** Displaced fracture of neck of fifth metacarpal bone, right hand
     S62.337 **7th** Displaced fracture of neck of fifth metacarpal bone, left hand

S62.34 **6th** Nondisplaced fracture of base of other metacarpal bone
     S62.340 **7th** Nondisplaced fracture of base of second metacarpal bone, right hand
     S62.341 **7th** Nondisplaced fracture of base of second metacarpal bone left hand
     S62.342 **7th** Nondisplaced fracture of base of third metacarpal bone, right hand

---

  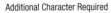 **Additional Character Required**   ✓ **3-character code**   Unspecified laterality codes were excluded here.   •=New Code   ▲=Revised Code   *Excludes1*—Not coded here, do not use together   *Excludes2*—Not included here

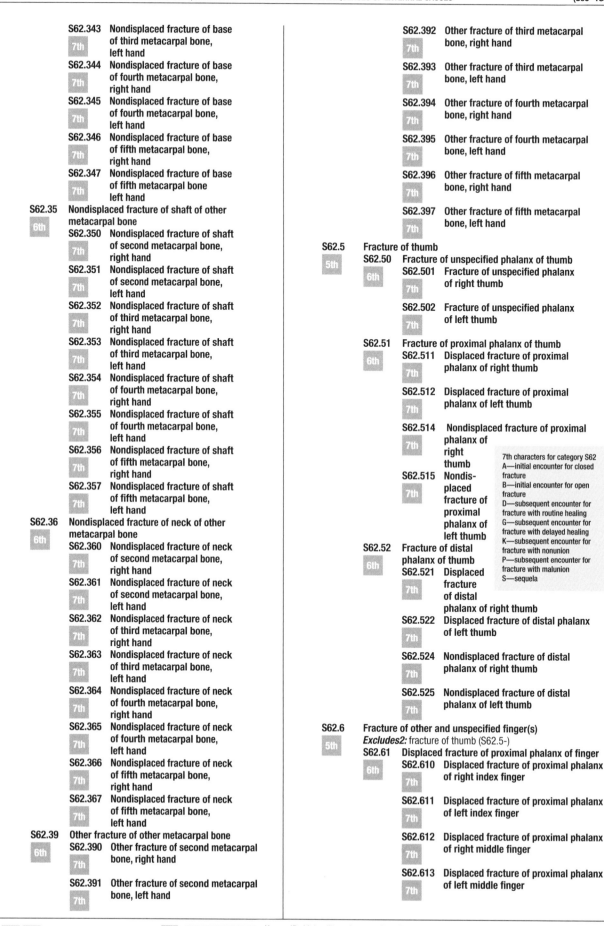

CHAPTER 19. INJURY, POISONING AND CERTAIN OTHER CONSEQUENCES OF EXTERNAL CAUSES   (S62.343–S62.613)

S62.343 7th Nondisplaced fracture of base of third metacarpal bone, left hand

S62.344 7th Nondisplaced fracture of base of fourth metacarpal bone, right hand

S62.345 7th Nondisplaced fracture of base of fourth metacarpal bone, left hand

S62.346 7th Nondisplaced fracture of base of fifth metacarpal bone, right hand

S62.347 7th Nondisplaced fracture of base of fifth metacarpal bone left hand

S62.35 6th **Nondisplaced fracture of shaft of other metacarpal bone**

S62.350 7th Nondisplaced fracture of shaft of second metacarpal bone, right hand

S62.351 7th Nondisplaced fracture of shaft of second metacarpal bone, left hand

S62.352 7th Nondisplaced fracture of shaft of third metacarpal bone, right hand

S62.353 7th Nondisplaced fracture of shaft of third metacarpal bone, left hand

S62.354 7th Nondisplaced fracture of shaft of fourth metacarpal bone, right hand

S62.355 7th Nondisplaced fracture of shaft of fourth metacarpal bone, left hand

S62.356 7th Nondisplaced fracture of shaft of fifth metacarpal bone, right hand

S62.357 7th Nondisplaced fracture of shaft of fifth metacarpal bone, left hand

S62.36 6th **Nondisplaced fracture of neck of other metacarpal bone**

S62.360 7th Nondisplaced fracture of neck of second metacarpal bone, right hand

S62.361 7th Nondisplaced fracture of neck of second metacarpal bone, left hand

S62.362 7th Nondisplaced fracture of neck of third metacarpal bone, right hand

S62.363 7th Nondisplaced fracture of neck of third metacarpal bone, left hand

S62.364 7th Nondisplaced fracture of neck of fourth metacarpal bone, right hand

S62.365 7th Nondisplaced fracture of neck of fourth metacarpal bone, left hand

S62.366 7th Nondisplaced fracture of neck of fifth metacarpal bone, right hand

S62.367 7th Nondisplaced fracture of neck of fifth metacarpal bone, left hand

S62.39 6th **Other fracture of other metacarpal bone**

S62.390 7th Other fracture of second metacarpal bone, right hand

S62.391 7th Other fracture of second metacarpal bone, left hand

S62.392 7th Other fracture of third metacarpal bone, right hand

S62.393 7th Other fracture of third metacarpal bone, left hand

S62.394 7th Other fracture of fourth metacarpal bone, right hand

S62.395 7th Other fracture of fourth metacarpal bone, left hand

S62.396 7th Other fracture of fifth metacarpal bone, right hand

S62.397 7th Other fracture of fifth metacarpal bone, left hand

S62.5 5th **Fracture of thumb**

S62.50 6th **Fracture of unspecified phalanx of thumb**

S62.501 7th Fracture of unspecified phalanx of right thumb

S62.502 7th Fracture of unspecified phalanx of left thumb

S62.51 6th **Fracture of proximal phalanx of thumb**

S62.511 7th Displaced fracture of proximal phalanx of right thumb

S62.512 7th Displaced fracture of proximal phalanx of left thumb

S62.514 7th Nondisplaced fracture of proximal phalanx of right thumb

S62.515 7th Nondisplaced fracture of proximal phalanx of left thumb

S62.52 6th **Fracture of distal phalanx of thumb**

S62.521 7th Displaced fracture of distal phalanx of right thumb

S62.522 7th Displaced fracture of distal phalanx of left thumb

S62.524 7th Nondisplaced fracture of distal phalanx of right thumb

S62.525 7th Nondisplaced fracture of distal phalanx of left thumb

> 7th characters for category S62
> A—initial encounter for closed fracture
> B—initial encounter for open fracture
> D—subsequent encounter for fracture with routine healing
> G—subsequent encounter for fracture with delayed healing
> K—subsequent encounter for fracture with nonunion
> P—subsequent encounter for fracture with malunion
> S—sequela

S62.6 5th **Fracture of other and unspecified finger(s)**
Excludes2: fracture of thumb (S62.5-)

S62.61 6th **Displaced fracture of proximal phalanx of finger**

S62.610 7th Displaced fracture of proximal phalanx of right index finger

S62.611 7th Displaced fracture of proximal phalanx of left index finger

S62.612 7th Displaced fracture of proximal phalanx of right middle finger

S62.613 7th Displaced fracture of proximal phalanx of left middle finger

---

 4th 5th 6th 7th   Additional Character Required   3-character code   Unspecified laterality codes were excluded here.   •=New Code   ▲=Revised Code   *Excludes1*—Not coded here, do not use together   *Excludes2*—Not included here

S62.614 7th Displaced fracture of proximal phalanx of right ring finger

S62.615 7th Displaced fracture of proximal phalanx of left ring finger

S62.616 7th Displaced fracture of proximal phalanx of right little finger

S62.617 7th Displaced fracture of proximal phalanx of left little finger

S62.62 6th Displaced fracture of medial phalanx of finger

S62.620 7th Displaced fracture of medial phalanx of right index finger

S62.621 7th Displaced fracture of medial phalanx of left index finger

S62.622 7th Displaced fracture of medial phalanx of right middle finger

S62.623 7th Displaced fracture of medial phalanx of left middle finger

S62.624 7th Displaced fracture of medial phalanx of right ring finger

S62.625 7th Displaced fracture of medial phalanx of left ring finger

S62.626 7th Displaced fracture of medial phalanx of right little finger

S62.627 7th Displaced fracture of medial phalanx of left little finger

S62.63 6th Displaced fracture of distal phalanx of finger

S62.630 7th Displaced fracture of distal phalanx of right index finger

S62.631 7th Displaced fracture of distal phalanx of left index finger

S62.632 7th Displaced fracture of distal phalanx of right middle finger

S62.633 7th Displaced fracture of distal phalanx of left middle finger

S62.634 7th Displaced fracture of distal phalanx of right ring finger

S62.635 7th Displaced fracture of distal phalanx of left ring finger

S62.636 7th Displaced fracture of distal phalanx of right little finger

S62.637 7th Displaced fracture of distal phalanx of left little finger

S62.64 6th Nondisplaced fracture of proximal phalanx of finger

S62.640 7th Nondisplaced fracture of proximal phalanx of right index finger

S62.641 7th Nondisplaced fracture of proximal phalanx of left index finger

S62.642 7th Nondisplaced fracture of proximal phalanx of right middle finger

S62.643 7th Nondisplaced fracture of proximal phalanx of left middle finger

S62.644 7th Nondisplaced fracture of proximal phalanx of right ring finger

S62.645 7th Nondisplaced fracture of proximal phalanx of left ring finger

S62.646 7th Nondisplaced fracture of proximal phalanx of right little finger

S62.647 7th Nondisplaced fracture of proximal phalanx of left little finger

S62.65 6th Nondisplaced fracture of medial phalanx of finger

S62.650 7th Nondisplaced fracture of medial phalanx of right index finger

S62.651 7th Nondisplaced fracture of medial phalanx of left index finger

S62.652 7th Nondisplaced fracture of medial phalanx of right middle finger

S62.653 7th Nondisplaced fracture of medial phalanx of left middle finger

S62.654 7th Nondisplaced fracture of medial phalanx of right ring finger

S62.655 7th Nondisplaced fracture of medial phalanx of left ring finger

S62.656 7th Nondisplaced fracture of medial phalanx of right little finger

S62.657 7th Nondisplaced fracture of medial phalanx of left little finger

> 7th characters for category S62
> A—initial encounter for closed fracture
> B—initial encounter for open fracture
> D—subsequent encounter for fracture with routine healing
> G—subsequent encounter for fracture with delayed healing
> K—subsequent encounter for fracture with nonunion
> P—subsequent encounter for fracture with malunion
> S—sequela

S62.66 6th Nondisplaced fracture of distal phalanx of finger

S62.660 7th Nondisplaced fracture of distal phalanx of right index finger

S62.661 7th Nondisplaced fracture of distal phalanx of left index finger

S62.662 7th Nondisplaced fracture of distal phalanx of right middle finger

S62.663 7th Nondisplaced fracture of distal phalanx of left middle finger

S62.664 7th Nondisplaced fracture of distal phalanx of right ring finger

S62.665 7th Nondisplaced fracture of distal phalanx of left ring finger

S62.666 7th Nondisplaced fracture of distal phalanx of right little finger

S62.667 7th Nondisplaced fracture of distal phalanx of left little finger

---

   Additional Character Required   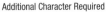 3-character code   Unspecified laterality codes were excluded here.   •=New Code   ▲=Revised Code   ***Excludes1***—Not coded here, do not use together   ***Excludes2***—Not included here

S63 **DISLOCATION AND SPRAIN OF JOINTS AND LIGAMENTS AT WRIST AND HAND LEVEL**
`4th`

Includes: avulsion of joint or ligament at wrist and hand level
    laceration of cartilage, joint or ligament at wrist and hand level
    sprain of cartilage, joint or ligament at wrist and hand level
    traumatic hemarthrosis of joint or ligament at wrist and hand level
    traumatic rupture of joint or ligament at wrist and hand level
    traumatic subluxation of joint or ligament at wrist and hand level
    traumatic tear of joint or ligament at wrist and hand level

> 7th characters for category S63
> A—initial encounter
> D—subsequent encounter
> S—sequela

Code also any associated open wound
Excludes2: strain of muscle, fascia and tendon of wrist and hand (S66.-)

S63.1 **Subluxation and dislocation of thumb**
`5th`

    S63.10 **Unspecified subluxation and dislocation of thumb**
    `6th`

        S63.101 **Unspecified subluxation of right thumb**
        `7th`

        S63.102 **Unspecified subluxation of left thumb**
        `7th`

        S63.104 **Unspecified dislocation of right thumb**
        `7th`

        S63.105 **Unspecified dislocation of left thumb**
        `7th`

    S63.11 **Subluxation and dislocation of metacarpophalangeal joint of thumb**
    `6th`

        S63.111 **Subluxation of metacarpophalangeal joint of right thumb**
        `7th`

        S63.112 **Subluxation of metacarpophalangeal joint of left thumb**
        `7th`

        S63.114 **Dislocation of metacarpophalangeal joint of right thumb**
        `7th`

        S63.115 **Dislocation of metacarpophalangeal joint of left thumb**
        `7th`

    S63.13 **Subluxation and dislocation of proximal interphalangeal joint of thumb**
    `6th`

        S63.131 **Subluxation of proximal interphalangeal joint of right thumb**
        `7th`

        S63.132 **Subluxation of proximal interphalangeal joint of left thumb**
        `7th`

        S63.134 **Dislocation of proximal interphalangeal joint of right thumb**
        `7th`

        S63.135 **Dislocation of proximal interphalangeal joint of left thumb**
        `7th`

    S63.14 **Subluxation and dislocation of distal interphalangeal joint of thumb**
    `6th`

        S63.141 **Subluxation of distal interphalangeal joint of right thumb**
        `7th`

        S63.142 **Subluxation of distal interphalangeal joint of left thumb**
        `7th`

        S63.144 **Dislocation of distal interphalangeal joint of right thumb**
        `7th`

        S63.145 **Dislocation of distal interphalangeal joint of left thumb**
        `7th`

S63.2 **Subluxation and dislocation of other finger(s)**
`5th`
Excludes2: subluxation and dislocation of thumb (S63.1-)

    S63.20 **Unspecified subluxation of other finger**
    `6th`

        S63.200 **Unspecified subluxation of right index finger**
        `7th`

        S63.201 **Unspecified subluxation of left index finger**
        `7th`

        S63.202 **Unspecified subluxation of right middle finger**
        `7th`

        S63.203 **Unspecified subluxation of left middle finger**
        `7th`

        S63.204 **Unspecified subluxation of right ring finger**
        `7th`

        S63.205 **Unspecified subluxation of left ring finger**
        `7th`

        S63.206 **Unspecified subluxation of right little finger**
        `7th`

        S63.207 **Unspecified subluxation of left little finger**
        `7th`

    S63.21 **Subluxation of metacarpophalangeal joint of finger**
    `6th`

        S63.210 **Subluxation of metacarpophalangeal joint of right index finger**
        `7th`

        S63.211 **Subluxation of metacarpophalangeal joint of left index finger**
        `7th`

        S63.212 **Subluxation of metacarpophalangeal joint of right middle finger**
        `7th`

        S63.213 **Subluxation of metacarpophalangeal joint of left middle finger**
        `7th`

        S63.214 **Subluxation of metacarpophalangeal joint of right ring finger**
        `7th`

> 7th characters for category S63
> A—initial encounter
> D—subsequent encounter
> S—sequela

        S63.215 **Subluxation of metacarpophalangeal joint of left ring finger**
        `7th`

        S63.216 **Subluxation of metacarpophalangeal joint of right little finger**
        `7th`

        S63.217 **Subluxation of metacarpophalangeal joint of left little finger**
        `7th`

    S63.23 **Subluxation of proximal interphalangeal joint of finger**
    `6th`

        S63.230 **Subluxation of proximal interphalangeal joint of right index finger**
        `7th`

        S63.231 **Subluxation of proximal interphalangeal joint of left index finger**
        `7th`

        S63.232 **Subluxation of proximal interphalangeal joint of right middle finger**
        `7th`

        S63.233 **Subluxation of proximal interphalangeal joint of left middle finger**
        `7th`

        S63.234 **Subluxation of proximal interphalangeal joint of right ring finger**
        `7th`

   Additional Character Required   3-character code   Unspecified laterality codes were excluded here.   •=New Code   ▲=Revised Code   *Excludes1*—Not coded here, do not use together   *Excludes2*—Not included here

320   PEDIATRIC ICD-10-CM 2017: A MANUAL FOR PROVIDER-BASED CODING

S63.235 `7th` Subluxation of proximal interphalangeal joint of left ring finger

S63.236 `7th` Subluxation of proximal interphalangeal joint of right little finger

S63.237 `7th` Subluxation of proximal interphalangeal joint of left little finger

S63.24 `6th` Subluxation of distal interphalangeal joint of finger

S63.240 `7th` Subluxation of distal interphalangeal joint of right index finger

S63.241 `7th` Subluxation of distal interphalangeal joint of left index finger

S63.242 `7th` Subluxation of distal interphalangeal joint of right middle finger

S63.243 `7th` Subluxation of distal interphalangeal joint of left middle finger

S63.244 `7th` Subluxation of distal interphalangeal joint of right ring finger

S63.245 `7th` Subluxation of distal interphalangeal joint of left ring finger

S63.246 `7th` Subluxation of distal interphalangeal joint of right little finger

S63.247 `7th` Subluxation of distal interphalangeal joint of left little finger

S63.26 `6th` Dislocation of metacarpophalangeal joint of finger

S63.260 `7th` Dislocation of metacarpophalangeal joint of right index finger

S63.261 `7th` Dislocation of metacarpophalangeal joint of left index finger

S63.262 `7th` Dislocation of metacarpophalangeal joint of right middle finger

S63.263 `7th` Dislocation of metacarpophalangeal joint of left middle finger

S63.264 `7th` Dislocation of metacarpophalangeal joint of right ring finger

S63.265 `7th` Dislocation of metacarpophalangeal joint of left ring finger

S63.266 `7th` Dislocation of metacarpophalangeal joint of right little finger

S63.267 `7th` Dislocation of metacarpophalangeal joint of left little finger

S63.28 `6th` Dislocation of proximal interphalangeal joint of finger

S63.280 `7th` Dislocation of proximal interphalangeal joint of right index finger

S63.281 `7th` Dislocation of proximal interphalangeal joint of left index finger

S63.282 `7th` Dislocation of proximal interphalangeal joint of right middle finger

S63.283 `7th` Dislocation of proximal interphalangeal joint of left middle finger

S63.284 `7th` Dislocation of proximal interphalangeal joint of right ring finger

S63.285 `7th` Dislocation of proximal interphalangeal joint of left ring finger

S63.286 `7th` Dislocation of proximal interphalangeal joint of right little finger

S63.287 `7th` Dislocation of proximal interphalangeal joint of left little finger

S63.29 `6th` Dislocation of distal interphalangeal joint of finger

S63.290 `7th` Dislocation of distal interphalangeal joint of right index finger

S63.291 `7th` Dislocation of distal interphalangeal joint of left index finger

S63.292 `7th` Dislocation of distal interphalangeal joint of right middle finger

S63.293 `7th` Dislocation of distal interphalangeal joint of left middle finger

S63.294 `7th` Dislocation of distal interphalangeal joint of right ring finger

S63.295 `7th` Dislocation of distal interphalangeal joint of left ring finger

S63.296 `7th` Dislocation of distal interphalangeal joint of right little finger

S63.297 `7th` Dislocation of distal interphalangeal joint of left little finger

S63.5 `5th` Other and unspecified sprain of wrist

S63.50 `6th` Unspecified sprain of wrist

S63.501 `7th` Unspecified sprain of right wrist

S63.502 `7th` Unspecified sprain of left wrist

S63.51 `6th` Sprain of carpal (joint)

S63.511 `7th` Sprain of carpal joint of right wrist

> 7th characters for category S63
> A—initial encounter
> D—subsequent encounter
> S—sequela

S63.512 `7th` Sprain of carpal joint of left wrist

S63.52 `6th` Sprain of radiocarpal joint
Excludes1: traumatic rupture of radiocarpal ligament (S63.32-)

S63.521 `7th` Sprain of radiocarpal joint of right wrist

S63.522 `7th` Sprain of radiocarpal joint of left wrist

S63.59 `6th` Other specified sprain of wrist

S63.591 `7th` Other specified sprain of right wrist

S63.592 `7th` Other specified sprain of left wrist

S63.6 `5th` Other and unspecified sprain of finger(s)
Excludes1: traumatic rupture of ligament of finger at metacarpophalangeal and interphalangeal joint(s) (S63.4-)

CHAPTER 19. INJURY, POISONING AND CERTAIN OTHER CONSEQUENCES OF EXTERNAL CAUSES (S63.235–S63.6)

 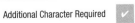 Additional Character Required `4th` `5th` `6th` `7th` ✓ 3-character code Unspecified laterality codes were excluded here. 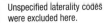 •=New Code ▲=Revised Code *Excludes1* Not coded here, do not use together *Excludes2*—Not included here

CHAPTER 19. INJURY, POISONING AND CERTAIN OTHER CONSEQUENCES OF EXTERNAL CAUSES   (S63.60–S65.212)

S63.60 **6th**   Unspecified sprain of thumb
- **S63.601** **7th**   Unspecified sprain of right thumb
- **S63.602** **7th**   Unspecified sprain of left thumb

S63.61 **6th**   Unspecified sprain of other and unspecified finger(s)
- **S63.610** **7th**   Unspecified sprain of right index finger
- **S63.611** **7th**   Unspecified sprain of left index finger
- **S63.612** **7th**   Unspecified sprain of right middle finger
- **S63.613** **7th**   Unspecified sprain of left middle finger
- **S63.614** **7th**   Unspecified sprain of right ring finger
- **S63.615** **7th**   Unspecified sprain of left ring finger
- **S63.616** **7th**   Unspecified sprain of right little finger
- **S63.617** **7th**   Unspecified sprain of left little finger

S63.62 **6th**   Sprain of interphalangeal joint of thumb
- **S63.621** **7th**   Sprain of interphalangeal joint of right thumb
- **S63.622** **7th**   Sprain of interphalangeal joint of left thumb

S63.63 **6th**   Sprain of interphalangeal joint of other and unspecified finger(s)
- **S63.630** **7th**   Sprain of interphalangeal joint of right index finger
- **S63.631** **7th**   Sprain of interphalangeal joint of left index finger
- **S63.632** **7th**   Sprain of interphalangeal joint of right middle finger
- **S63.633** **7th**   Sprain of interphalangeal joint of left middle finger
- **S63.634** **7th**   Sprain of interphalangeal joint of right ring finger
- **S63.635** **7th**   Sprain of interphalangeal joint of left ring finger
- **S63.636** **7th**   Sprain of interphalangeal joint of right little finger
- **S63.637** **7th**   Sprain of interphalangeal joint of left little finger

S63.64 **6th**   Sprain of metacarpophalangeal joint of thumb
- **S63.641** **7th**   Sprain of metacarpophalangeal joint of right thumb
- **S63.642** **7th**   Sprain of metacarpophalangeal joint of left thumb

S63.65 **6th**   Sprain of metacarpophalangeal joint of other and unspecified finger(s)
- **S63.650** **7th**   Sprain of metacarpophalangeal joint of right index finger
- **S63.651** **7th**   Sprain of metacarpophalangeal joint of left index finger
- **S63.652** **7th**   Sprain of metacarpophalangeal joint of right middle finger
- **S63.653** **7th**   Sprain of metacarpophalangeal joint of left middle finger
- **S63.654** **7th**   Sprain of metacarpophalangeal joint of right ring finger
- **S63.655** **7th**   Sprain of metacarpophalangeal joint of left ring finger
- **S63.656** **7th**   Sprain of metacarpophalangeal joint of right little finger
- **S63.657** **7th**   Sprain of metacarpophalangeal joint of left little finger

S63.68 **6th**   Other sprain of thumb
- **S63.681** **7th**   Other sprain of right thumb
- **S63.682** **7th**   Other sprain of left thumb

S63.69 **6th**   Other sprain of other and unspecified finger(s)
- **S63.690** **7th**   Other sprain of right index finger
- **S63.691** **7th**   Other sprain of left index finger
- **S63.692** **7th**   Other sprain of right middle finger
- **S63.693** **7th**   Other sprain of left middle finger
- **S63.694** **7th**   Other sprain of right ring finger
- **S63.695** **7th**   Other sprain of left ring finger
- **S63.696** **7th**   Other sprain of right little finger
- **S63.697** **7th**   Other sprain of left little finger

> 7th characters for category S63
> A—initial encounter
> D—subsequent encounter
> S—sequela

S65 **4th**   **INJURY OF BLOOD VESSELS AT WRIST AND HAND LEVEL**
   Code also any associated open wound (S61.-)

S65.2 **5th**   Injury of superficial palmar arch
- **S65.21** **6th**   Laceration of superficial palmar arch
  - **S65.211** **7th**   Laceration of superficial palmar arch of right hand
  - **S65.212** **7th**   Laceration of superficial palmar arch of left hand

> 7th characters for category S65
> A—initial encounter
> D—subsequent encounter
> S—sequela

  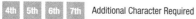 Additional Character Required   ✔ 3-character code   Unspecified laterality codes were excluded here.   •=New Code   ▲=Revised Code   *Excludes1*—Not coded here, do not use together   *Excludes2*—Not included here

322   PEDIATRIC ICD-10-CM 2017: A MANUAL FOR PROVIDER-BASED CODING

S65.29   Other specified injury of superficial palmar arch

6th   S65.291   Other specified injury of superficial palmar arch of right hand   **7th**

S65.292   Other specified injury of superficial palmar arch of left hand   **7th**

S65.3   Injury of deep palmar arch

5th   S65.30   Unspecified injury of deep palmar arch

6th   S65.301   Unspecified injury of deep palmar arch of right hand   **7th**

S65.302   Unspecified injury of deep palmar arch of left hand   **7th**

S65.31   Laceration of deep palmar arch

6th   S65.311   Laceration of deep palmar arch of right hand   **7th**

S65.312   Laceration of deep palmar arch of left hand   **7th**

S65.39   Other specified injury of deep palmar arch

6th   S65.391   Other specified injury of deep palmar arch of right hand   **7th**

S65.392   Other specified injury of deep palmar arch of left hand   **7th**

S65.9   Injury of unspecified blood vessel at wrist and hand level

5th   S65.91   Laceration of unspecified blood vessel at wrist and hand level

6th   S65.911   Laceration of unspecified blood vessel at wrist and hand level of right arm   **7th**

S65.912   Laceration of unspecified blood vessel at wrist and hand level of left arm   **7th**

S65.99   Other specified injury of unspecified blood vessel at wrist and hand level

6th   S65.991   Other specified injury of unspecified blood vessel at wrist and hand of right arm   **7th**

S65.992   Other specified injury of unspecified blood vessel at wrist and hand of left arm   **7th**

S66   **INJURY OF MUSCLE, FASCIA AND TENDON AT WRIST AND HAND LEVEL**

4th

Code also any associated open wound (S61.-)

Excludes2: sprain of joints and ligaments of wrist and hand (S63.-)

S66.01   Strain of long flexor muscle, fascia and tendon of thumb at wrist and hand level

6th   S66.011   Strain of long flexor muscle, fascia and tendon of right thumb at wrist and hand level   **7th**

> 7th characters for categories S65 & S66
> A—initial encounter
> D—subsequent encounter
> S—sequela

S66.012   Strain of long flexor muscle, fascia and tendon of left thumb at wrist and hand level   **7th**

S66.02   Laceration of long flexor muscle, fascia and tendon of thumb at wrist and hand level

6th   S66.021   Laceration of long flexor muscle, fascia and tendon of right thumb at wrist and hand level   **7th**

S66.022   Laceration of long flexor muscle, fascia and tendon of left thumb at wrist and hand level   **7th**

S66.11   Strain of flexor muscle, fascia and tendon of other and unspecified finger at wrist and hand level

6th

S66.110   Strain of flexor muscle, fascia and tendon of right index finger at wrist and hand level   **7th**

S66.111   Strain of flexor muscle, fascia and tendon of left index finger at wrist and hand level   **7th**

S66.112   Strain of flexor muscle, fascia and tendon of right middle finger at wrist and hand level   **7th**

S66.113   Strain of flexor muscle, fascia and tendon of left middle finger at wrist and hand level   **7th**

S66.114   Strain of flexor muscle, fascia and tendon of right ring finger at wrist and hand level   **7th**

S66.115   Strain of flexor muscle, fascia and tendon of left ring finger at wrist and hand level   **7th**

S66.116   Strain of flexor muscle, fascia and tendon of right little finger at wrist and hand level   **7th**

S66.117   Strain of flexor muscle, fascia and tendon of left little finger at wrist and hand level   **7th**

S66.21   Strain of extensor muscle, fascia and tendon of thumb at wrist and hand level

6th   S66.211   Strain of extensor muscle, fascia and tendon of right thumb at wrist and hand level   **7th**

S66.212   Strain of extensor muscle, fascia and tendon of left thumb at wrist and hand level   **7th**

S66.31   Strain of extensor muscle, fascia and tendon of other and unspecified finger at wrist and hand level

6th

S66.310   Strain of extensor muscle, fascia and tendon of right index finger at wrist and hand level   **7th**

S66.311   Strain of extensor muscle, fascia and tendon of left index finger at wrist and hand level   **7th**

S66.312   Strain of extensor muscle, fascia and tendon of right middle finger at wrist and hand level   **7th**

S66.313   Strain of extensor muscle, fascia and tendon of left middle finger at wrist and hand level   **7th**

S66.314   Strain of extensor muscle, fascia and tendon of right ring finger at wrist and hand level   **7th**

> 7th characters for category S66
> A—initial encounter
> D—subsequent encounter
> S—sequela

S66.315   Strain of extensor muscle, fascia and tendon of left ring finger at wrist and hand level   **7th**

S66.316   Strain of extensor muscle, fascia and tendon of right little finger at wrist and hand level   **7th**

S66.317   Strain of extensor muscle, fascia and tendon of left little finger at wrist and hand level   **7th**

S66.41   Strain of intrinsic muscle, fascia and tendon of thumb at wrist and hand level

6th   S66.411   Strain of intrinsic muscle, fascia and tendon of right thumb at wrist and hand level   **7th**

S66.412   Strain of intrinsic muscle, fascia and tendon of left thumb at wrist and hand level   **7th**

S66.51   Strain of intrinsic muscle, fascia and tendon of other and unspecified finger at wrist and hand level

6th

  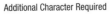   Additional Character Required   ✔   3-character code   Unspecified laterality codes were excluded here.   ●=New Code   ▲=Revised Code   *Excludes1*   Not coded here, do not use together   *Excludes2*—Not included here

S66.510 [7th] Strain of intrinsic muscle, fascia and tendon of right index finger at wrist and hand level

S66.511 [7th] Strain of intrinsic muscle, fascia and tendon of left index finger at wrist and hand level

S66.512 [7th] Strain of intrinsic muscle, fascia and tendon of right middle finger at wrist and hand level

S66.513 [7th] Strain of intrinsic muscle, fascia and tendon of left middle finger at wrist and hand level

S66.514 [7th] Strain of intrinsic muscle, fascia and tendon of right ring finger at wrist and hand level

S66.515 [7th] Strain of intrinsic muscle, fascia and tendon of left ring finger at wrist and hand level

S66.516 [7th] Strain of intrinsic muscle, fascia and tendon of right little finger at wrist and hand level

S66.517 [7th] Strain of intrinsic muscle, fascia and tendon of left little finger at wrist and hand level

S66.91 [6th] Strain of unspecified muscle, fascia and tendon at wrist and hand level

S66.911 [7th] Strain of unspecified muscle, fascia and tendon at wrist and hand level, right hand

S66.912 [7th] Strain of unspecified muscle, fascia and tendon at wrist and hand level, left hand

S67 [4th] **CRUSHING INJURY OF WRIST, HAND AND FINGERS**

Use additional code for all associated injuries, such as: fracture of wrist and hand (S62.-)
open wound of wrist and hand (S61.-)

S67.0 [5th] **Crushing injury of thumb**

S67.01X [7th] Crushing injury of right thumb

S67.02X [7th] Crushing injury of left thumb

S67.1 [5th] **Crushing injury of other and unspecified finger(s)**
Excludes2: crushing injury of thumb (S67.0-)

S67.19 [6th] Crushing injury of other finger(s)

S67.190 [7th] Crushing injury of right index finger

S67.191 [7th] Crushing injury of left index finger

S67.192 [7th] Crushing injury of right middle finger

S67.193 [7th] Crushing injury of left middle finger

S67.194 [7th] Crushing injury of right ring finger

S67.195 [7th] Crushing injury of left ring finger

S67.196 [7th] Crushing injury of right little finger

S67.197 [7th] Crushing injury of left little finger, initial encounter

S67.198 [7th] Crushing injury of other finger
Crushing injury of specified finger with unspecified laterality

S67.2 [5th] **Crushing injury of hand**
Excludes2: crushing injury of fingers (S67.1-)
crushing injury of thumb (S67.0-)

S67.21X [7th] Crushing injury of right hand

S67.22X [7th] Crushing injury of left hand

S67.3 [5th] **Crushing injury of wrist**

S67.31X [7th] Crushing injury of right wrist

S67.32X [7th] Crushing injury of left wrist

S67.4 [5th] **Crushing injury of wrist and hand**
Excludes1: crushing injury of hand alone (S67.2-)
crushing injury of wrist alone (S67.3-)
Excludes2: crushing injury of fingers (S67.1-)
crushing injury of thumb (S67.0-)

S67.41X [7th] Crushing injury of right wrist and hand

S67.42X [7th] Crushing injury of left wrist and hand

7th characters for category S67
A—initial encounter
D—subsequent encounter
S—sequela

(S70–S79) INJURIES TO THE HIP AND THIGH

Excludes2: burns and corrosions (T20–T32)
frostbite (T33–T34)
snake bite (T63.0-)
venomous insect bite or sting (T63.4-)

7th characters for category S70
A—initial encounter
D—subsequent encounter
S—sequela

S70 [4th] **SUPERFICIAL INJURY OF HIP AND THIGH**

S70.0 [5th] **Contusion of hip**

S70.01X [7th] Contusion of right hip

S70.02X [7th] Contusion of left hip

S70.1 [5th] **Contusion of thigh**

S70.11X [7th] Contusion of right thigh

S70.12X [7th] Contusion of left thigh

S70.2 [5th] **Other superficial injuries of hip**

S70.21 [6th] Abrasion of hip

S70.211 [7th] Abrasion, right hip

S70.212 [7th] Abrasion, left hip

S70.22 [6th] Blister (nonthermal) of hip

S70.221 [7th] Blister (nonthermal), right hip

S70.222 [7th] Blister (nonthermal), left hip

S70.24 [6th] External constriction of hip

S70.241 [7th] External constriction, right hip

S70.242 [7th] External constriction, left hip

[4th] [5th] [6th] [7th] Additional Character Required   3-character code   Unspecified laterality codes were excluded here.   •=New Code   ▲=Revised Code   *Excludes1*—Not coded here, do not use together   *Excludes2*—Not included here

S70.25 **Superficial FB of hip**
6th
Splinter in the hip
   S70.251 **Superficial FB, right hip**
   7th

   S70.252 **Superficial FB, left hip**
   7th

S70.26 **Insect bite (nonvenomous) of hip**
6th
   S70.261 **Insect bite (nonvenomous), right hip**
   7th

   S70.262 **Insect bite (nonvenomous), left hip**
   7th

S70.27 **Other superficial bite of hip**
6th
Excludes1: open bite of hip (S71.05-)
   S70.271 **Other superficial bite of hip, right hip**
   7th

   S70.272 **Other superficial bite of hip, left hip**
   7th

S70.3 **Other superficial injuries of thigh**
5th
S70.31 **Abrasion of thigh**
6th
   S70.311 **Abrasion, right thigh**
   7th

   S70.312 **Abrasion, left thigh**
   7th

S70.32 **Blister (nonthermal) of thigh**
6th
   S70.321 **Blister (nonthermal), right thigh**
   7th

   S70.322 **Blister (nonthermal), left thigh**
   7th

S70.34 **External constriction of thigh**
6th
   S70.341 **External constriction, right thigh**
   7th

   S70.342 **External constriction, left thigh**
   7th

S70.35 **Superficial FB of thigh**
6th
Splinter in the thigh
   S70.351 **Superficial FB, right thigh**
   7th

   S70.352 **Superficial FB, left thigh**
   7th

S70.36 **Insect bite (nonvenomous) of thigh**
6th
   S70.361 **Insect bite (nonvenomous), right thigh**
   7th

   S70.362 **Insect bite (nonvenomous), left thigh**
   7th

S70.37 **Other superficial bite of thigh**
6th
Excludes1: open bite of thigh (S71.15)
   S70.371 **Other superficial bite of right thigh**
   7th

   S70.372 **Other superficial bite of left thigh**
   7th

S71 **OPEN WOUND OF HIP AND THIGH**
4th
Code also any associated wound infection
Excludes1: open fracture of hip and thigh (S72.-)
traumatic amputation of hip and thigh (S78.-)
Excludes2: bite of venomous animal (T63.-)
open wound of ankle, foot and toes (S91.-)
open wound of knee and lower leg (S81.-)

7th characters for categories
S70 & S71
A—initial encounter
D—subsequent encounter
S—sequela

S71.0 **Open wound of hip**
5th
S71.01 **Laceration without FB of hip**
6th
   S71.011 **Laceration without FB, right hip**
   7th

   S71.012 **Laceration without FB, left hip**
   7th

S71.02 **Laceration with FB of hip**
6th
   S71.021 **Laceration with FB, right hip**
   7th

   S71.022 **Laceration with FB, left hip**
   7th

S71.03 **Puncture wound without FB of hip**
6th
   S71.031 **Puncture wound without FB, right hip**
   7th

   S71.032 **Puncture wound without FB, left hip**
   7th

S71.04 **Puncture wound with FB of hip**
6th
   S71.041 **Puncture wound with FB, right hip**
   7th

   S71.042 **Puncture wound with FB, left hip**
   7th

S71.05 **Open bite of hip**
6th
Bite of hip NOS
Excludes1: superficial bite of hip (S70.26, S70.27)
   S71.051 **Open bite, right hip**
   7th

   S71.052 **Open bite, left hip**
   7th

S71.1 **Open wound of thigh**
5th
S71.11 **Laceration without FB of thigh**
6th
   S71.111 **Laceration without FB, right thigh**
   7th
   S71.112 **Laceration without FB, left thigh**
   7th

7th characters for category S71
A—initial encounter
D—subsequent encounter
S—sequela

S71.12 **Laceration with FB of thigh**
6th
   S71.121 **Laceration with FB, right thigh**
   7th

   S71.122 **Laceration with FB, left thigh**
   7th

S71.13 **Puncture wound without FB of thigh**
6th
   S71.131 **Puncture wound without FB, right thigh**
   7th

   S71.132 **Puncture wound without FB, left thigh**
   7th

S71.14 **Puncture wound with FB of thigh**
6th

  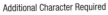 Additional Character Required   ✓   3-character code   Unspecified laterality codes were excluded here.   ●=New Code   ▲=Revised Code   *Excludes1*—Not coded here, do not use together   *Excludes2*—Not included here

S71.141 [7th] **Puncture wound with FB, right thigh**

S71.142 [7th] **Puncture wound with FB, left thigh**

S71.15 [6th] **Open bite of thigh**
Bite of thigh NOS
Excludes1: superficial bite of thigh (S70.37-)

S71.151 [7th] **Open bite, right thigh**

S71.152 [7th] **Open bite, left thigh**

S72 [4th] **FRACTURE OF FEMUR**
Please see full *ICD-10-CM* manual for seventh characters applicable to open fracture types IIIA, IIIB, or IIIC.
Note: A fracture not indicated as displaced or nondisplaced should be coded to displaced
A fracture not indicated as open or closed should be coded to closed
The open fracture designations are based on the Gustilo open fracture classification
Excludes1: traumatic amputation of hip and thigh (S78.-)
Excludes2: fracture of lower leg and ankle (S82.-)
  fracture of foot (S92.-)
  periprosthetic fracture of prosthetic implant of hip (T84.040, T84.041)

> 7th characters for category S72 except S72.47-
> A—initial encounter for closed fracture
> B—initial encounter for open fracture type I or II initial encounter for open fracture NOS
> D—subsequent encounter for closed fracture with routine healing
> E—subsequent encounter for open fracture type I or II with routine healing
> G—subsequent encounter for closed fracture with delayed healing
> H—subsequent encounter for open fracture type I or II with delayed healing
> K—subsequent encounter for closed fracture with nonunion
> M—subsequent encounter for open fracture type I or II with nonunion
> P—subsequent encounter for closed fracture with malunion
> Q—subsequent encounter for open fracture type I or II with malunion
> S—sequela

S72.0 [5th] **Fracture of head and neck of femur**
Excludes2: physeal fracture of upper end of femur (S79.0-)

S72.00 [6th] **Fracture of unspecified part of neck of femur**
Fracture of hip NOS
Fracture of neck of femur NOS

S72.001 [7th] **Fracture of unspecified part of neck of right femur**

S72.002 [7th] **Fracture of unspecified part of neck of left femur**

S72.03 [6th] **Midcervical fracture of femur**
Transcervical fracture of femur NOS

S72.031 [7th] **Displaced midcervical fracture of right femur**

S72.032 [7th] **Displaced midcervical fracture of left femur**

S72.034 [7th] **Nondisplaced midcervical fracture of right femur**

S72.035 [7th] **Nondisplaced midcervical fracture of left femur**

S72.04 [6th] **Fracture of base of neck of femur**
Cervicotrochanteric fracture of femur

S72.041 [7th] **Displaced fracture of base of neck of right femur**

S72.042 [7th] **Displaced fracture of base of neck of left femur**

S72.044 [7th] **Nondisplaced fracture of base of neck of right femur**

S72.045 [7th] **Nondisplaced fracture of base of neck of left femur**

S72.3 [5th] **Fracture of shaft of femur**

S72.30 [6th] **Unspecified fracture of shaft of femur**

S72.301 [7th] **Unspecified fracture of shaft of right femur**

S72.302 [7th] **Unspecified fracture of shaft of left femur**

S72.32 [6th] **Transverse fracture of shaft of femur**

S72.321 [7th] **Displaced transverse fracture of shaft of right femur**

S72.322 [7th] **Displaced transverse fracture of shaft of left femur**

S72.324 [7th] **Nondisplaced transverse fracture of shaft of right femur**

S72.325 [7th] **Nondisplaced transverse fracture of shaft of left femur**

S72.33 [6th] **Oblique fracture of shaft of femur**

S72.331 [7th] **Displaced oblique fracture of shaft of right femur**

S72.332 [7th] **Displaced oblique fracture of shaft of left femur**

S72.334 [7th] **Nondisplaced oblique fracture of shaft of right femur**

S72.335 [7th] **Nondisplaced oblique fracture of shaft of left femur**

S72.34 [6th] **Spiral fracture of shaft of femur**

S72.341 [7th] **Displaced spiral fracture of shaft of right femur**

S72.342 [7th] **Displaced spiral fracture of shaft of left femur**

S72.344 [7th] **Nondisplaced spiral fracture of shaft of right femur**

S72.345 [7th] **Nondisplaced spiral fracture of shaft of left femur**

> 7th characters for category S72 except S72.47-
> A—initial encounter for closed fracture
> B—initial encounter for open fracture type I or II initial encounter for open fracture NOS
> D—subsequent encounter for closed fracture with routine healing
> E—subsequent encounter for open fracture type I or II with routine healing
> G—subsequent encounter for closed fracture with delayed healing
> H—subsequent encounter for open fracture type I or II with delayed healing
> K—subsequent encounter for closed fracture with nonunion
> M—subsequent encounter for open fracture type I or II with nonunion
> P—subsequent encounter for closed fracture with malunion
> Q—subsequent encounter for open fracture type I or II with malunion
> S—sequela

S72.35 [6th] **Comminuted fracture of shaft of femur**

S72.351 [7th] **Displaced comminuted fracture of shaft of right femur**

S72.352 [7th] **Displaced comminuted fracture of shaft of left femur**

S72.354 [7th] **Nondisplaced comminuted fracture of shaft of right femur**

[4th] [5th] [6th] [7th] Additional Character Required   ✓ 3-character code   Unspecified laterality codes were excluded here.   •=New Code   ▲=Revised Code   *Excludes1*—Not coded here, do not use together   *Excludes2*—Not included here

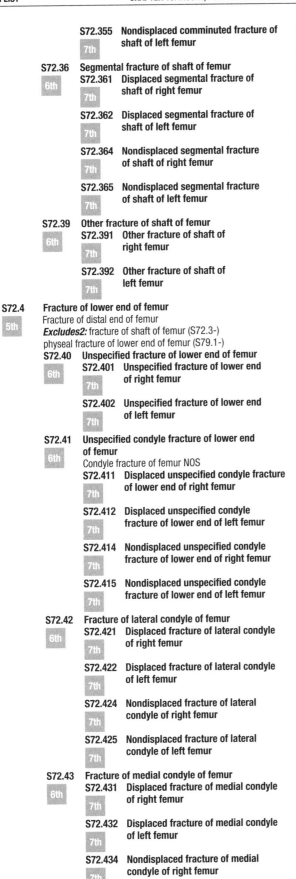

S72.355 **7th** Nondisplaced comminuted fracture of shaft of left femur

S72.36 **6th** Segmental fracture of shaft of femur

S72.361 **7th** Displaced segmental fracture of shaft of right femur

S72.362 **7th** Displaced segmental fracture of shaft of left femur

S72.364 **7th** Nondisplaced segmental fracture of shaft of right femur

S72.365 **7th** Nondisplaced segmental fracture of shaft of left femur

S72.39 **6th** Other fracture of shaft of femur

S72.391 **7th** Other fracture of shaft of right femur

S72.392 **7th** Other fracture of shaft of left femur

S72.4 **5th** Fracture of lower end of femur
Fracture of distal end of femur
Excludes2: fracture of shaft of femur (S72.3-)
physeal fracture of lower end of femur (S79.1-)

S72.40 **6th** Unspecified fracture of lower end of femur

S72.401 **7th** Unspecified fracture of lower end of right femur

S72.402 **7th** Unspecified fracture of lower end of left femur

S72.41 **6th** Unspecified condyle fracture of lower end of femur
Condyle fracture of femur NOS

S72.411 **7th** Displaced unspecified condyle fracture of lower end of right femur

S72.412 **7th** Displaced unspecified condyle fracture of lower end of left femur

S72.414 **7th** Nondisplaced unspecified condyle fracture of lower end of right femur

S72.415 **7th** Nondisplaced unspecified condyle fracture of lower end of left femur

S72.42 **6th** Fracture of lateral condyle of femur

S72.421 **7th** Displaced fracture of lateral condyle of right femur

S72.422 **7th** Displaced fracture of lateral condyle of left femur

S72.424 **7th** Nondisplaced fracture of lateral condyle of right femur

S72.425 **7th** Nondisplaced fracture of lateral condyle of left femur

S72.43 **6th** Fracture of medial condyle of femur

S72.431 **7th** Displaced fracture of medial condyle of right femur

S72.432 **7th** Displaced fracture of medial condyle of left femur

S72.434 **7th** Nondisplaced fracture of medial condyle of right femur

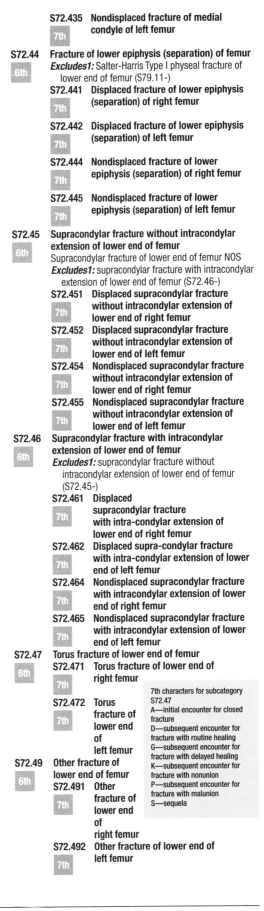

S72.435 **7th** Nondisplaced fracture of medial condyle of left femur

S72.44 **6th** Fracture of lower epiphysis (separation) of femur
Excludes1: Salter-Harris Type I physeal fracture of lower end of femur (S79.11-)

S72.441 **7th** Displaced fracture of lower epiphysis (separation) of right femur

S72.442 **7th** Displaced fracture of lower epiphysis (separation) of left femur

S72.444 **7th** Nondisplaced fracture of lower epiphysis (separation) of right femur

S72.445 **7th** Nondisplaced fracture of lower epiphysis (separation) of left femur

S72.45 **6th** Supracondylar fracture without intracondylar extension of lower end of femur
Supracondylar fracture of lower end of femur NOS
Excludes1: supracondylar fracture with intracondylar extension of lower end of femur (S72.46-)

S72.451 **7th** Displaced supracondylar fracture without intracondylar extension of lower end of right femur

S72.452 **7th** Displaced supracondylar fracture without intracondylar extension of lower end of left femur

S72.454 **7th** Nondisplaced supracondylar fracture without intracondylar extension of lower end of right femur

S72.455 **7th** Nondisplaced supracondylar fracture without intracondylar extension of lower end of left femur

S72.46 **6th** Supracondylar fracture with intracondylar extension of lower end of femur
Excludes1: supracondylar fracture without intracondylar extension of lower end of femur (S72.45-)

S72.461 **7th** Displaced supracondylar fracture with intra-condylar extension of lower end of right femur

S72.462 **7th** Displaced supra-condylar fracture with intra-condylar extension of lower end of left femur

S72.464 **7th** Nondisplaced supracondylar fracture with intracondylar extension of lower end of right femur

S72.465 **7th** Nondisplaced supracondylar fracture with intracondylar extension of lower end of left femur

S72.47 **6th** Torus fracture of lower end of femur

S72.471 **7th** Torus fracture of lower end of right femur

S72.472 **7th** Torus fracture of lower end of left femur

> 7th characters for subcategory S72.47
> A—initial encounter for closed fracture
> D—subsequent encounter for fracture with routine healing
> G—subsequent encounter for fracture with delayed healing
> K—subsequent encounter for fracture with nonunion
> P—subsequent encounter for fracture with malunion
> S—sequela

S72.49 **6th** Other fracture of lower end of femur

S72.491 **7th** Other fracture of lower end of right femur

S72.492 **7th** Other fracture of lower end of left femur

  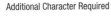 **4th 5th 6th 7th** Additional Character Required ✓ 3-character code | Unspecified laterality codes were excluded here. | 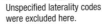•=New Code ▲=Revised Code | 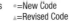*Excludes1*—Not coded here, do not use together *Excludes2*—Not included here

CHAPTER 19. INJURY, POISONING AND CERTAIN OTHER CONSEQUENCES OF EXTERNAL CAUSES   (S72.8–S76.211)

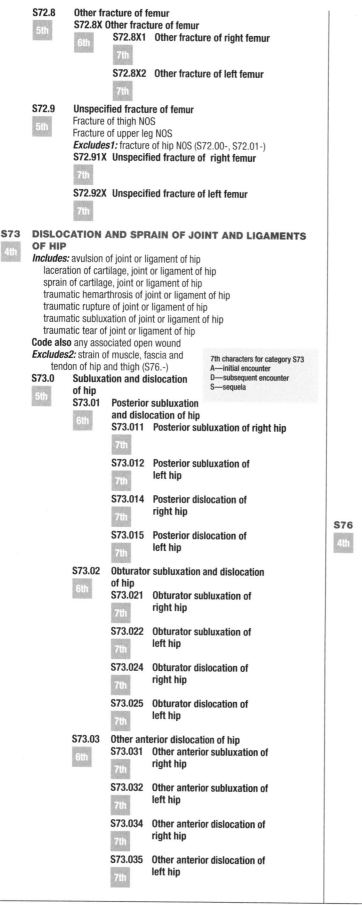

S72.8 **Other fracture of femur**
5th
    S72.8X Other fracture of femur
    6th
        S72.8X1   Other fracture of right femur
        7th

        S72.8X2   Other fracture of left femur
        7th

S72.9 **Unspecified fracture of femur**
5th
  Fracture of thigh NOS
  Fracture of upper leg NOS
  Excludes1: fracture of hip NOS (S72.00-, S72.01-)
  S72.91X Unspecified fracture of right femur
  7th

  S72.92X Unspecified fracture of left femur
  7th

S73 **DISLOCATION AND SPRAIN OF JOINT AND LIGAMENTS**
4th **OF HIP**
  Includes: avulsion of joint or ligament of hip
    laceration of cartilage, joint or ligament of hip
    sprain of cartilage, joint or ligament of hip
    traumatic hemarthrosis of joint or ligament of hip
    traumatic rupture of joint or ligament of hip
    traumatic subluxation of joint or ligament of hip
    traumatic tear of joint or ligament of hip
  Code also any associated open wound
  Excludes2: strain of muscle, fascia and
    tendon of hip and thigh (S76.-)

7th characters for category S73
A—initial encounter
D—subsequent encounter
S—sequela

S73.0 **Subluxation and dislocation**
5th **of hip**
  S73.01   **Posterior subluxation**
  6th   **and dislocation of hip**
    S73.011   Posterior subluxation of right hip
    7th

    S73.012   Posterior subluxation of left hip
    7th

    S73.014   Posterior dislocation of right hip
    7th

    S73.015   Posterior dislocation of left hip
    7th

  S73.02   **Obturator subluxation and dislocation**
  6th   **of hip**
    S73.021   Obturator subluxation of right hip
    7th

    S73.022   Obturator subluxation of left hip
    7th

    S73.024   Obturator dislocation of right hip
    7th

    S73.025   Obturator dislocation of left hip
    7th

  S73.03   **Other anterior dislocation of hip**
  6th   **S73.031**   Other anterior subluxation of right hip
    7th

    S73.032   Other anterior subluxation of left hip
    7th

    S73.034   Other anterior dislocation of right hip
    7th

    S73.035   Other anterior dislocation of left hip
    7th

S73.04 **Central dislocation of hip**
6th   **S73.041**   **Central subluxation of right hip**
    7th

    S73.042   **Central subluxation of left hip**
    7th

    S73.044   **Central dislocation of right hip**
    7th

    S73.045   **Central dislocation of left hip**
    7th

S73.1 **Sprain of hip**
5th
  S73.10   **Unspecified sprain of hip**
  6th   **S73.101**   **Unspecified sprain of right hip**
    7th

    S73.102   **Unspecified sprain of left hip**
    7th

  S73.11   **Iliofemoral ligament sprain of hip**
  6th   **S73.111**   **Iliofemoral ligament sprain of right hip**
    7th

    S73.112   **Iliofemoral ligament sprain of left hip**
    7th

  S73.12   **Ischiocapsular (ligament) sprain of hip**
  6th   **S73.121**   **Ischiocapsular ligament sprain of right hip**
    7th

    S73.122   **Ischiocapsular ligament sprain of left hip**
    7th

  S73.19   **Other sprain of hip**
  6th   **S73.191**   **Other sprain of right hip**
    7th

    S73.192   **Other sprain of left hip**
    7th

S76 **INJURY OF MUSCLE, FASCIA AND TENDON AT HIP**
4th **AND THIGH LEVEL**
  Code also any associated open wound
    (S71.-)
  Excludes2: injury of muscle, fascia and
    tendon at lower leg level (S86)
    sprain of joint and ligament of hip
    (S73.1)

7th characters for categories S73 & S76
A—initial encounter
D—subsequent encounter
S—sequela

S76.0 **Injury of muscle, fascia and**
5th **tendon of hip**
  S76.01   **Strain of muscle, fascia and tendon of hip**
  6th   **S76.011**   **Strain of muscle, fascia and tendon of right hip**
    7th

    S76.012   **Strain of muscle, fascia and tendon of left hip**
    7th

  S76.11   **Strain of quadriceps muscle, fascia and tendon**
  6th   **S76.111**   **Strain of right quadriceps muscle, fascia and tendon**
    7th

    S76.112   **Strain of left quadriceps muscle, fascia and tendon**
    7th

  S76.21   **Strain of adductor muscle, fascia and tendon of thigh**
  6th   **S76.211**   **Strain of adductor muscle, fascia and tendon of right thigh**
    7th

  6th 7th   Additional Character Required   ✓   3-character code   Unspecified laterality codes were excluded here.   •=New Code   ▲=Revised Code   ***Excludes1***—Not coded here, do not use together   ***Excludes2***—Not included here

S76.212 Strain of adductor muscle, fascia and tendon of left thigh
`7th`

S76.31 Strain of muscle, fascia and tendon of the posterior muscle group at thigh level
`6th`

S76.311 Strain of muscle, fascia and tendon of the posterior muscle group at thigh level, right thigh
`7th`

S76.312 Strain of muscle, fascia and tendon of the posterior muscle group at thigh level, left thigh
`7th`

S76.91 Strain of unspecified muscles, fascia and tendons at thigh level
`6th`

S76.911 Strain of unspecified muscles, fascia and tendons at thigh level, right thigh
`7th`

S76.912 Strain of unspecified muscles, fascia and tendons at thigh level, left thigh
`7th`

S79 OTHER AND UNSPECIFIED INJURIES OF HIP AND THIGH
`4th`
Note: A fracture not indicated as open or closed should be coded to closed

S79.0 Physeal fracture of upper end of femur
`5th`
Excludes1: apophyseal fracture of upper end of femur (S72.13-)
nontraumatic slipped upper femoral epiphysis (M93.0-)

S79.00 Unspecified physeal fracture of upper end of femur
`6th`

S79.001 Unspecified physeal fracture of upper end of right femur
`7th`

S79.002 Unspecified physeal fracture of upper end of left femur
`7th`

S79.01 Salter-Harris Type I physeal fracture of upper end of femur
`6th`
Acute on chronic slipped capital femoral epiphysis (traumatic)
Acute slipped capital femoral epiphysis (traumatic)
Capital femoral epiphyseal fracture
Excludes1: chronic slipped upper femoral epiphysis (nontraumatic) (M93.02-)

> 7th characters for subcategories S79.0–S79.1
> A—initial encounter for closed fracture
> D—subsequent encounter for fracture with routine healing
> G—subsequent encounter for fracture with delayed healing
> K—subsequent encounter for fracture with nonunion
> P—subsequent encounter for fracture with malunion
> S—sequela

S79.011 Salter-Harris Type I physeal fracture of upper end of right femur,
`7th`

S79.012 Salter-Harris Type I physeal fracture of upper end of left femur
`7th`

S79.09 Other physeal fracture of upper end of femur
`6th`

S79.091 Other physeal fracture of upper end of right femur
`7th`

S79.092 Other physeal fracture of upper end of left femur
`7th`

S79.1 Physeal fracture of lower end of femur
`5th`

S79.10 Unspecified physeal fracture of lower end of femur
`6th`

S79.101 Unspecified physeal fracture of lower end of right femur
`7th`

S79.102 Unspecified physeal fracture of lower end of left femur
`7th`

S79.11 Salter-Harris Type I physeal fracture of lower end of femur
`6th`

S79.111 Salter-Harris Type I physeal fracture of lower end of right femur
`7th`

S79.112 Salter-Harris Type I physeal fracture of lower end of left femur
`7th`

S79.12 Salter-Harris Type II physeal fracture of lower end of femur
`6th`

S79.121 Salter-Harris Type II physeal fracture of lower end of right femur
`7th`

S79.122 Salter-Harris Type II physeal fracture of lower end of left femur
`7th`

S79.13 Salter-Harris Type III physeal fracture of lower end of femur
`6th`

S79.131 Salter-Harris Type III physeal fracture of lower end of right femur
`7th`

S79.132 Salter-Harris Type III physeal fracture of lower end of left femur
`7th`

S79.14 Salter-Harris Type IV physeal fracture of lower end of femur
`6th`

S79.141 Salter-Harris Type IV physeal fracture of lower end of right femur
`7th`

S79.142 Salter-Harris Type IV physeal fracture of lower end of left femur
`7th`

S79.19 Other physeal fracture of lower end of femur
`6th`

S79.191 Other physeal fracture of lower end of right femur
`7th`

S79.192 Other physeal fracture of lower end of left femur
`7th`

S79.8 Other specified injuries of hip and thigh
`5th`

S79.81 Other specified injuries of hip
`6th`

S79.811 Other specified injuries of right hip
`7th`

S79.812 Other specified injuries of left hip
`7th`

> 7th characters for subcategory S79.8
> A—initial encounter
> D—subsequent encounter
> S—sequela

S79.82 Other specified injuries of thigh
`6th`

S79.821 Other specified injuries of right thigh
`7th`

S79.822 Other specified injuries of left thigh
`7th`

(S80–S89) INJURIES TO THE KNEE AND LOWER LEG

Excludes2: burns and corrosions (T20–T32)
frostbite (T33–T34)
injuries of ankle and foot, except fracture of ankle and malleolus (S90–S99)
insect bite or sting, venomous (T63.4)

S80 SUPERFICIAL INJURY OF KNEE AND LOWER LEG
`4th`
Excludes2: superficial injury of ankle and foot (S90.-)

S80.0 Contusion of knee

S80.01X Contusion of right knee
`5th`

S80.02X Contusion of left knee
`7th`

S80.1 Contusion of lower leg

S80.11X Contusion of right lower leg
`5th`

> 7th characters for category S80
> A—initial encounter
> D—subsequent encounter
> S—sequela

`7th`

`4th` `5th` `6th` `7th` Additional Character Required   ✔ 3-character code   Unspecified laterality codes were excluded here.   •=New Code ▲=Revised Code   *Excludes1*—Not coded here, do not use together   *Excludes2*—Not included here

CHAPTER 19. INJURY, POISONING AND CERTAIN OTHER CONSEQUENCES OF EXTERNAL CAUSES   (S80.12X–S81.812)

S80.12X   Contusion of left lower leg
`7th`

S80.2   Other superficial injuries of knee
`5th`

  S80.21   Abrasion of knee `6th`

    S80.211   Abrasion, right knee `7th`

    S80.212   Abrasion, left knee `7th`

  S80.22   Blister (nonthermal) of knee `6th`

    S80.221   Blister (nonthermal), right knee `7th`

    S80.222   Blister (nonthermal), left knee `7th`

  S80.24   External constriction of knee `6th`

    S80.241   External constriction, right knee `7th`

    S80.242   External constriction, left knee `7th`

  S80.25   Superficial FB of knee `6th`
Splinter in the knee

    S80.251   Superficial FB, right knee `7th`

    S80.252   Superficial FB, left knee `7th`

  S80.26   Insect bite (nonvenomous) of knee `6th`

    S80.261   Insect bite (nonvenomous), right knee `7th`

    S80.262   Insect bite (nonvenomous), left knee `7th`

  S80.27   Other superficial bite of knee `6th`
Excludes1: open bite of knee (S81.05-)

    S80.271   Other superficial bite of right knee `7th`

    S80.272   Other superficial bite of left knee `7th`

S80.8   Other superficial injuries of lower leg
`5th`

  S80.81   Abrasion of lower leg `6th`

    S80.811   Abrasion, right lower leg `7th`

    S80.812   Abrasion, left lower leg `7th`

  S80.82   Blister (nonthermal) of lower leg `6th`

    S80.821   Blister (nonthermal), right lower leg `7th`

    S80.822   Blister (nonthermal), left lower leg `7th`

  S80.84   External constriction of lower leg `6th`

    S80.841   External constriction, right lower leg `7th`

    S80.842   External constriction, left lower leg `7th`

  S80.85   Superficial FB of lower leg `6th`
Splinter in the lower leg

    S80.851   Superficial FB, right lower leg `7th`

    S80.852   Superficial FB, left lower leg `7th`

  S80.86   Insect bite (nonvenomous) of lower leg `6th`

    S80.861   Insect bite (nonvenomous), right lower leg `7th`

    S80.862   Insect bite (nonvenomous), left lower leg `7th`

  S80.87   Other superficial bite of lower leg `6th`
Excludes1: open bite of lower leg (S81.85-)

    S80.871   Other superficial bite, right lower leg `7th`

    S80.872   Other superficial bite, left lower leg `7th`

S81   **OPEN WOUND OF KNEE AND LOWER LEG** `4th`
Code also any associated wound infection
Excludes1: open fracture of knee and lower leg (S82.-)
traumatic amputation of lower leg (S88.-)
Excludes2: open wound of ankle and foot (S91.-)

S81.0   Open wound of knee `5th`

  S81.01   Laceration without FB of knee `6th`

> 7th characters for categories
> S80 & S81
> A—initial encounter
> D—subsequent encounter
> S—sequela

    S81.011   Laceration without FB, right knee `7th`

    S81.012   Laceration without FB, left knee

  S81.02   Laceration with FB of knee `6th`

    S81.021   Laceration with FB, right knee `7th`

    S81.022   Laceration with FB, left knee `7th`

  S81.03   Puncture wound without FB of knee `6th`

    S81.031   Puncture wound without FB, right knee `7th`

    S81.032   Puncture wound without FB, left knee `7th`

  S81.04   Puncture wound with FB of knee `6th`

    S81.041   Puncture wound with FB, right knee `7th`

    S81.042   Puncture wound with FB, left knee `7th`

  S81.05   Open bite of knee `6th`
Bite of knee NOS
Excludes1: superficial bite of knee (S80.27-)

    S81.051   Open bite, right knee `7th`

    S81.052   Open bite, left knee `7th`

S81.8   Open wound of lower leg `5th`

  S81.81   Laceration without FB of lower leg `6th`

    S81.811   Laceration without FB, right lower leg `7th`

    S81.812   Laceration without FB, left lower leg `7th`

    Additional Character Required   3-character code   Unspecified laterality codes were excluded here.   •=New Code   ▲=Revised Code   *Excludes1*—Not coded here, do not use together   *Excludes2*—Not included here

S81.82 **Laceration with FB of lower leg**

   [6th]   **S81.821** **Laceration with FB, right lower leg**

        [7th]

        S81.822 **Laceration with FB, left lower leg**

        [7th]

S81.83 **Puncture wound without FB of lower leg**

   [6th]   **S81.831** **Puncture wound without FB, right lower leg**

        [7th]

        S81.832 **Puncture wound without FB, left lower leg**

        [7th]

S81.84 **Puncture wound with FB of lower leg**

   [6th]   **S81.841** **Puncture wound with FB, right lower leg**

        [7th]

        S81.842 **Puncture wound with FB, left lower leg**

        [7th]

S81.85 **Open bite of lower leg**

   [6th]   Bite of lower leg NOS

       Excludes1: superficial bite of lower leg (S80.86-, S80.87-)

        S81.851 **Open bite, right lower leg**

        [7th]

        S81.852 **Open bite, left lower leg**

        [7th]

S82 **FRACTURE OF LOWER LEG, INCLUDING ANKLE**

 [4th]

Please see full *ICD-10-CM* manual for seventh characters applicable to open fracture types IIIA, IIIB, or IIIC.

Note: A fracture not indicated as displaced or nondisplaced should be coded to displaced

A fracture not indicated as open or closed should be coded to closed

The open fracture designations are based on the Gustilo open fracture classification

Includes: fracture of malleolus

Excludes1: traumatic amputation of lower leg (S88.-)

Excludes2: fracture of foot, except ankle (S92.-)

periprosthetic fracture of prosthetic implant of knee (T84.042, T84.043)

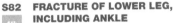

7th characters for category S82 except S82.16-, S82.31-, S82.81, & S81.82

A—initial encounter for closed fracture
B—initial encounter for open fracture type I or II
C—initial encounter for open fracture NOS
D—subsequent encounter for closed fracture with routine healing
E—subsequent encounter for open fracture type I or II with routine healing
G—subsequent encounter for closed fracture with delayed healing
H—subsequent encounter for open fracture type I or II with delayed healing
K—subsequent encounter for closed fracture with nonunion
M—subsequent encounter for open fracture type I or II with nonunion
P—subsequent encounter for closed fracture with malunion
Q—subsequent encounter for open fracture type I or II with malunion
S—sequela

S82.0 **Fracture of patella**

   [5th]   Knee cap

        S82.00 **Unspecified fracture of patella**

       [6th]   **S82.001** **Unspecified fracture of right patella**

           [7th]

           S82.002 **Unspecified fracture of left patella**

           [7th]

S82.1 **Fracture of upper end of tibia**

   [5th]   Fracture of proximal end of tibia

       Excludes2: fracture of shaft of tibia (S82.2-)

       physeal fracture of upper end of tibia (S89.0-)

        S82.10 **Unspecified fracture of upper end of tibia**

       [6th]   **S82.101** **Unspecified fracture of upper end of right tibia**

           [7th]

           S82.102 **Unspecified fracture of upper end of left tibia**

           [7th]

S82.16 **Torus fracture of upper end of tibia**

   [6th]   **S82.161** **Torus fracture of upper end of right tibia**

        [7th]

        S82.162 **Torus fracture of upper end of left tibia**

        [7th]

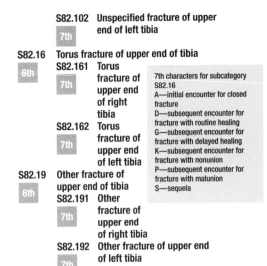

7th characters for subcategory S82.16
A—initial encounter for closed fracture
D—subsequent encounter for fracture with routine healing
G—subsequent encounter for fracture with delayed healing
K—subsequent encounter for fracture with nonunion
P—subsequent encounter for fracture with malunion
S—sequela

S82.19 **Other fracture of upper end of tibia**

   [6th]   **S82.191** **Other fracture of upper end of right tibia**

        [7th]

        S82.192 **Other fracture of upper end of left tibia**

        [7th]

S82.2 **Fracture of shaft of tibia**

   [5th]   **S82.20** **Unspecified fracture of shaft of tibia**

       [6th]   Fracture of tibia NOS

           S82.201 **Unspecified fracture of shaft of right tibia**

           [7th]

           S82.202 **Unspecified fracture of shaft of left tibia**

           [7th]

S82.24 **Spiral fracture of shaft of tibia**

   [6th]   Toddler fracture

        S82.241 **Displaced spiral fracture of shaft of right tibia**

        [7th]

        S82.242 **Displaced spiral fracture of shaft of left tibia**

        [7th]

        S82.244 **Nondisplaced spiral fracture of shaft of right tibia**

        [7th]

        S82.245 **Nondisplaced spiral fracture of shaft of left tibia**

        [7th]

S82.3 **Fracture of lower end of tibia**

   [5th]   *Excludes1:* bimalleolar fracture of lower leg (S82.84-)

       fracture of medial malleolus alone (S82.5-)

       Maisonneuve's fracture (S82.86-)

       pilon fracture of distal tibia (S82.87-)

       trimalleolar fractures of lower leg (S82.85-)

        S82.30 **Unspecified fracture of lower end of tibia**

       [6th]   **S82.301** **Unspecified fracture of lower end of right tibia**

           [7th]

           S82.302 **Unspecified fracture of lower end of left tibia**

           [7th]

S82.31 **Torus fracture of lower end of tibia**

   [6th]   **S82.311** **Torus fracture of lower end of right tibia**

        [7th]

        S82.312 **Torus fracture of lower end of left tibia**

        [7th]

7th characters for subcategory S82.31
A—initial encounter for closed fracture
D—subsequent encounter for fracture with routine healing
G—subsequent encounter for fracture with delayed healing
K—subsequent encounter for fracture with nonunion
P—subsequent encounter for fracture with malunion
S—sequela

S82.39 **Other fracture of lower end of tibia**

   [6th]   **S82.391** **Other fracture of lower end of right tibia**

        [7th]

 [4th] **[5th]** **[6th]** **[7th]**   Additional Character Required   ✓   3-character code

Unspecified laterality codes were excluded here.

●=New Code
▲=Revised Code

Excludes1—Not coded here, do not use together
Excludes2—Not included here

CHAPTER 19. INJURY, POISONING AND CERTAIN OTHER CONSEQUENCES OF EXTERNAL CAUSES   (S82.392–S82.892)

S82.392 Other fracture of lower end of left tibia
7th

S82.4 Fracture of shaft of fibula
5th
Excludes2: fracture of lateral malleolus alone (S82.6-)

  S82.40 Unspecified fracture of shaft of fibula
  6th
    S82.401 Unspecified fracture of shaft of right fibula
    7th

    S82.402 Unspecified fracture of shaft of left fibula
    7th

S82.5 Fracture of medial malleolus
5th
Excludes1: pilon fracture of distal tibia (S82.87-)
Salter-Harris type III of lower end of tibia (S89.13-)
Salter-Harris type IV of lower end of tibia (S89.14-)

  S82.51X Displaced fracture of medial malleolus of right tibia
  7th

  S82.52X Displaced fracture of medial malleolus of left tibia
  7th

  S82.54X Nondisplaced fracture of medial malleolus of right tibia
  7th

  S82.55X Nondisplaced fracture of medial malleolus of left tibia
  7th

S82.6 Fracture of lateral malleolus
5th
Excludes1: pilon fracture of distal tibia (S82.87-)

  S82.61X Displaced fracture of lateral malleolus of right fibula
  7th

  S82.62X Displaced fracture of lateral malleolus of left fibula
  7th

  S82.64X Nondisplaced fracture of lateral malleolus of right fibula
  7th

  S82.65X Nondisplaced fracture of lateral malleolus of left fibula
  7th

S82.8 Other fractures of lower leg
5th

  S82.81 Torus fracture of upper end of fibula
  6th
    S82.811 Torus fracture of upper end of right fibula
    7th

    S82.812 Torus fracture of upper end of left fibula
    7th

> 7th character for subcategories S82.81- & S82.82-
> A—initial encounter for closed fracture
> D—subsequent encounter for fracture with routine healing
> G—subsequent encounter for fracture with delayed healing
> K—subsequent encounter for fracture with nonunion
> P—subsequent encounter for fracture with malunion
> S—sequela

  S82.82 Torus fracture of lower end of fibula
  6th
    S82.821 Torus fracture of lower end of right fibula
    7th

    S82.822 Torus fracture of lower end of left fibula
    7th

  S82.83 Other fracture of upper and lower end of fibula
  6th
    S82.831 Other fracture of upper and lower end of right fibula
    7th

    S82.832 Other fracture of upper and lower end of left fibula
    7th

S82.84 Bimalleolar fracture of lower leg
6th
  S82.841 Displaced bimalleolar fracture of right lower leg
  7th

  S82.842 Displaced bimalleolar fracture of left lower leg
  7th

  S82.844 Nondisplaced bimalleolar fracture of right lower leg
  7th

  S82.845 Nondisplaced bimalleolar fracture of left lower leg
  7th

S82.85 Trimalleolar fracture of lower leg
6th
  S82.851 Displaced trimalleolar fracture of right lower leg
  7th

  S82.852 Displaced trimalleolar fracture of left lower leg
  7th

  S82.854 Nondisplaced trimalleolar fracture of right lower leg
  7th

  S82.855 Nondisplaced trimalleolar fracture of left lower leg
  7th

S82.86 Maisonneuve's fracture
6th
  S82.861 Displaced Maisonneuve's fracture of right leg
  7th

  S82.862 Displaced Maisonneuve's fracture of left leg
  7th

  S82.864 Nondisplaced Maisonneuve's fracture of right leg
  7th

  S82.865 Nondisplaced Maisonneuve's fracture of left leg
  7th

> 7th characters for category S82 except S82.16-, S82.31-, S82.81, & S81.82
> A—initial encounter for closed fracture
> B—initial encounter for open fracture type I or II
> C—initial encounter for open fracture NOS
> D—subsequent encounter for closed fracture with routine healing
> E—subsequent encounter for open fracture type I or II with routine healing
> G—subsequent encounter for closed fracture with delayed healing
> H—subsequent encounter for open fracture type I or II with delayed healing
> K—subsequent encounter for closed fracture with nonunion
> M—subsequent encounter for open fracture type I or II with nonunion
> P—subsequent encounter for closed fracture with malunion
> Q—subsequent encounter for open fracture type I or II with malunion
> S—sequela

S82.87 Pilon fracture of tibia
6th
  S82.871 Displaced pilon fracture of right tibia
  7th

  S82.872 Displaced pilon fracture of left tibia
  7th

  S82.874 Nondisplaced pilon fracture of right tibia
  7th

  S82.875 Nondisplaced pilon fracture of left tibia
  7th

S82.89 Other fractures of lower leg
6th
Fracture of ankle NOS
  S82.891 Other fracture of right lower leg
  7th

  S82.892 Other fracture of left lower leg
  7th

  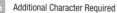

4th 5th 6th 7th Additional Character Required   ✓ 3-character code   Unspecified laterality codes were excluded here.   •=New Code ▲=Revised Code   *Excludes1*—Not coded here, do not use together *Excludes2*—Not included here

S83 DISLOCATION AND SPRAIN OF JOINTS AND LIGAMENTS OF KNEE
4th

Includes: avulsion of joint or ligament of knee
laceration of cartilage, joint or ligament of knee
sprain of cartilage, joint or ligament of knee
traumatic hemarthrosis of joint or ligament of knee
traumatic rupture of joint or ligament of knee
traumatic subluxation of joint or ligament of knee
traumatic tear of joint or ligament of knee

Code also any associated open wound

Excludes1: derangement of patella (M22.0–M22.3)
injury of patellar ligament (tendon) (S76.1-)
internal derangement of knee (M23.-)
old dislocation of knee (M24.36)
pathological dislocation of knee (M24.36)
recurrent dislocation of knee (M22.0)

Excludes2: strain of muscle, fascia and tendon of lower leg (S86.-)

S83.0 **Subluxation and dislocation of patella**
5th

  S83.00 **Unspecified subluxation and dislocation of patella**
  6th

7th characters for category S83
A—initial encounter
D—subsequent encounter
S—sequela

    S83.001 Unspecified subluxation of right patella
    7th

    S83.002 Unspecified subluxation of left patella
    7th

    S83.004 Unspecified dislocation of right patella
    7th

    S83.005 Unspecified dislocation of left patella
    7th

  S83.01 **Lateral subluxation and dislocation of patella**
  6th

    S83.011 Lateral subluxation of right patella
    7th

    S83.012 Lateral subluxation of left patella
    7th

    S83.014 Lateral dislocation of right patella
    7th

    S83.015 Lateral dislocation of left patella
    7th

  S83.09 **Other subluxation and dislocation of patella**
  6th

    S83.091 Other subluxation of right patella
    7th

    S83.092 Other subluxation of left patella
    7th

    S83.094 Other dislocation of right patella
    7th

    S83.095 Other dislocation of left patella
    7th

S83.1 **Subluxation and dislocation of knee**
5th

  Excludes2: instability of knee prosthesis (T84.022, T84.023)

  S83.10 **Unspecified subluxation and dislocation of knee**
  6th

    S83.101 Unspecified subluxation of right knee
    7th

    S83.102 Unspecified subluxation of left knee
    7th

    S83.104 Unspecified dislocation of right knee
    7th

    S83.105 Unspecified dislocation of left knee
    7th

S83.11 **Anterior subluxation and dislocation of proximal end of tibia**
6th

Posterior subluxation and dislocation of distal end of femur

    S83.111 Anterior subluxation of proximal end of tibia, right knee
    7th

    S83.112 Anterior subluxation of proximal end of tibia, left knee
    7th

    S83.114 Anterior dislocation of proximal end of tibia, right knee
    7th

    S83.115 Anterior dislocation of proximal end of tibia, left knee
    7th

S83.12 **Posterior subluxation and dislocation of proximal end of tibia**
6th

Anterior dislocation of distal end of femur

    S83.121 Posterior subluxation of proximal end of tibia, right knee
    7th

    S83.122 Posterior subluxation of proximal end of tibia, left knee
    7th

    S83.124 Posterior dislocation of proximal end of tibia, right knee
    7th

    S83.125 Posterior dislocation of proximal end of tibia, left knee
    7th

S83.13 **Medial subluxation and dislocation of proximal end of tibia**
6th

    S83.131 Medial subluxation of proximal end of tibia, right knee
    7th

    S83.132 Medial subluxation of proximal end of tibia, left knee
    7th

    S83.134 Medial dislocation of proximal end of tibia, right knee
    7th

    S83.135 Medial dislocation of proximal end of tibia, left knee
    7th

S83.14 **Lateral subluxation and dislocation of proximal end of tibia**
6th

    S83.141 Lateral subluxation of proximal end of tibia, right knee
    7th

    S83.142 Lateral subluxation of proximal end of tibia, left knee
    7th

    S83.144 Lateral dislocation of proximal end of tibia, right knee
    7th

    S83.145 Lateral dislocation of proximal end of tibia, left knee
    7th

S83.19 **Other subluxation and dislocation of knee**
6th

    S83.191 Other subluxation of right knee
    7th

    S83.192 Other subluxation of left knee
    7th

    S83.194 Other dislocation of right knee
    7th

   Additional Character Required 3-character code

Unspecified laterality codes were excluded here.

• =New Code
▲ =Revised Code

Excludes1—Not coded here, do not use together
Excludes2—Not included here

CHAPTER 19. INJURY, POISONING AND CERTAIN OTHER CONSEQUENCES OF EXTERNAL CAUSES (S83.195–S86.311)

S83.195 Other dislocation of left knee
7th

S83.4 **5th** **Sprain of collateral ligament of knee**

S83.40 **6th** Sprain of unspecified collateral ligament of knee

S83.401 **7th** Sprain of unspecified collateral ligament of right knee

S83.402 **7th** Sprain of unspecified collateral ligament of left knee

7th characters for category S83
A—initial encounter
D—subsequent encounter
S—sequela

S83.41 **6th** Sprain of medial collateral ligament of knee
Sprain of tibial collateral ligament

S83.411 **7th** Sprain of medial collateral ligament of right knee

S83.412 **7th** Sprain of medial collateral ligament of left knee

S83.42 **6th** Sprain of lateral collateral ligament of knee
Sprain of fibular collateral ligament

S83.421 **7th** Sprain of lateral collateral ligament of right knee

S83.422 **7th** Sprain of lateral collateral ligament of left knee

S83.5 **5th** Sprain of cruciate ligament of knee

S83.50 **6th** Sprain of unspecified cruciate ligament of knee

S83.501 **7th** Sprain of unspecified cruciate ligament of right knee

S83.502 **7th** Sprain of unspecified cruciate ligament of left knee

S83.51 **6th** Sprain of anterior cruciate ligament of knee

S83.511 **7th** Sprain of anterior cruciate ligament of right knee

S83.512 **7th** Sprain of anterior cruciate ligament of left knee

S83.52 **6th** Sprain of posterior cruciate ligament of knee

S83.521 **7th** Sprain of posterior cruciate ligament of right knee

S83.522 **7th** Sprain of posterior cruciate ligament of left knee

S83.6 **5th** Sprain of the superior tibiofibular joint and ligament

S83.60X **7th** Sprain of the superior tibiofibular joint and ligament, unspecified knee

S83.61X **7th** Sprain of the superior tibiofibular joint and ligament, right knee

S8362.X **7th** Sprain of the superior tibiofibular joint and ligament, left knee

S83.8 **5th** Sprain of other specified parts of knee

S83.8X **6th** Sprain of other specified parts of knee

S83.8X1 **7th** Sprain of other specified parts of right knee

S83.8X2 **7th** Sprain of other specified parts of left knee

S83.9 **5th** Sprain of unspecified site of knee

S83.91X **7th** Sprain of unspecified site of right knee

S83.92X **7th** Sprain of unspecified site of left knee

7th characters for categories
S83 & S86
A—initial encounter
D—subsequent encounter
S—sequela

S86 **4th** **INJURY OF MUSCLE, FASCIA AND TENDON AT LOWER LEG LEVEL**
Code also any associated open wound (S81.-)
Excludes2: injury of muscle, fascia and tendon at ankle (S96.-)
injury of patellar ligament (tendon) (S76.1-)
sprain of joints and ligaments of knee (S83.-)

S86.0 Injury of Achilles tendon

S86.00 **5th** Unspecified injury of Achilles tendon

S86.001 **6th** **7th** Unspecified injury of right Achilles tendon

S86.002 **7th** Unspecified injury of left Achilles tendon

S86.01 **6th** Strain of Achilles tendon

S86.011 **7th** Strain of right Achilles tendon

S86.012 **7th** Strain of left Achilles tendon

S86.02 **6th** Laceration of Achilles tendon

S86.021 **7th** Laceration of right Achilles tendon

S86.022 **7th** Laceration of left Achilles tendon

S86.09 **6th** Other specified injury of Achilles tendon

S86.091 **7th** Other specified injury of right Achilles tendon

S86.092 **7th** Other specified injury of left Achilles tendon

S86.1 **5th** Injury of other muscle(s) and tendon(s) of posterior muscle group at lower leg level

S86.11 **6th** Strain of other muscle(s) and tendon(s) of posterior muscle group at lower leg level

S86.111 **7th** Strain of other muscle(s) and tendon(s) of posterior muscle group at lower leg level, right leg

S86.112 **7th** Strain of other muscle(s) and tendon(s) of posterior muscle group at lower leg level, left leg

S86.2 **5th** Injury of muscle(s) and tendon(s) of anterior muscle group at lower leg level

S86.21 **6th** Strain of muscle(s) and tendon(s) of anterior muscle group at lower leg level

S86.211 **7th** Strain of muscle(s) and tendon(s) of anterior muscle group at lower leg level, right leg

S86.212 **7th** Strain of muscle(s) and tendon(s) of anterior muscle group at lower leg level, left leg

S86.3 **5th** Injury of muscle(s) and tendon(s) of peroneal muscle group at lower leg level

S86.31 **6th** Strain of muscle(s) and tendon(s) of peroneal muscle group at lower leg level

S86.311 **7th** Strain of muscle(s) and tendon(s) of peroneal muscle group at lower leg level, right leg

---

4th **5th** **6th** **7th** Additional Character Required ✓ 3-character code

Unspecified laterality codes were excluded here.

•=New Code
▲=Revised Code

Excludes1—Not coded here, do not use together
Excludes2—Not included here

334 PEDIATRIC ICD-10-CM 2017: A MANUAL FOR PROVIDER-BASED CODING

S86.312 **Strain of muscle(s) and tendon(s) of peroneal muscle group at lower leg level, left leg**
`7th`

S86.32 **Laceration of muscle(s) and tendon(s) of peroneal muscle group at lower leg level**
`6th`

S86.321 **Laceration of muscle(s) and tendon(s) of peroneal muscle group at lower leg level, right leg**
`7th`

> 7th characters for category S86
> A—initial encounter
> D—subsequent encounter
> S—sequela

S86.322 **Laceration of muscle(s) and tendon(s) of peroneal muscle group at lower leg level, left leg**
`7th`

S86.39 **Other injury of muscle(s) and tendon(s) of peroneal muscle group at lower leg level**
`6th`

S86.391 **Other injury of muscle(s) and tendon(s) of peroneal muscle group at lower leg level, right leg**
`7th`

S86.392 **Other injury of muscle(s) and tendon(s) of peroneal muscle group at lower leg level, left leg**
`7th`

S86.8 **Injury of other muscles and tendons at lower leg level**
`5th`

S86.81 **Strain of other muscles and tendons at lower leg level**
`6th`

S86.811 **Strain of other muscle(s) and tendon(s) at lower leg level, right leg**
`7th`

S86.812 **Strain of other muscle(s) and tendon(s) at lower leg level, left leg**
`7th`

S86.82 **Laceration of other muscles and tendons at lower leg level**
`6th`

S86.821 **Laceration of other muscle(s) and tendon(s) at lower leg level, right leg**
`7th`

S86.822 **Laceration of other muscle(s) and tendon(s) at lower leg level, left leg**
`7th`

S86.89 **Other injury of other muscles and tendons at lower leg level**
`6th`

S86.891 **Other injury of other muscle(s) and tendon(s) at lower leg level, right leg**
`7th`

S86.892 **Other injury of other muscle(s) and tendon(s) at lower leg level, left leg**
`7th`

S86.9 **Injury of unspecified muscle and tendon at lower leg level**
`5th`

S86.91 **Strain of unspecified muscle and tendon at lower leg level**
`6th`

S86.911 **Strain of unspecified muscle(s) and tendon(s) at lower leg level, right leg**
`7th`

S86.912 **Strain of unspecified muscle(s) and tendon(s) at lower leg level, left leg**
`7th`

S89 OTHER AND UNSPECIFIED INJURIES OF LOWER LEG
`4th`

Note: A fracture not indicated as open or closed should be coded to closed
Excludes2: other and unspecified injuries of ankle and foot (S99.-)

S89.0 **Physeal fracture of upper end of tibia**
`5th`

S89.00 **Unspecified physeal fracture of upper end of tibia**
`6th`

S89.001 **Unspecified physeal fracture of upper end of right tibia**
`7th`

> 7th characters for subcategories
> S89.0, S89.1, S89.2, and S89.3
> A—initial encounter for closed fracture
> D—subsequent encounter for fracture with routine healing
> G—subsequent encounter for fracture with delayed healing
> K—subsequent encounter for fracture with nonunion
> P—subsequent encounter for fracture with malunion
> S—sequela

S89.002 **Unspecified physeal fracture of upper end of left tibia**
`7th`

S89.01 **Salter-Harris Type I physeal fracture of upper end of tibia**
`6th`

S89.011 **Salter-Harris Type I physeal fracture of upper end of right tibia**
`7th`

S89.012 **Salter-Harris Type I physeal fracture of upper end of left tibia**
`7th`

S89.02 **Salter-Harris Type II physeal fracture of upper end of tibia**
`6th`

S89.021 **Salter-Harris Type II physeal fracture of upper end of right tibia**
`7th`

S89.022 **Salter-Harris Type II physeal fracture of upper end of left tibia**
`7th`

S89.03 **Salter-Harris Type III physeal fracture of upper end of tibia**
`6th`

S89.031 **Salter-Harris Type III physeal fracture of upper end of right tibia**
`7th`

S89.032 **Salter-Harris Type III physeal fracture of upper end of left tibia**
`7th`

S89.04 **Salter-Harris Type IV physeal fracture of upper end of tibia**
`6th`

S89.041 **Salter-Harris Type IV physeal fracture of upper end of right tibia**
`7th`

S89.042 **Salter-Harris Type IV physeal fracture of upper end of left tibia**
`7th`

S89.09 **Other physeal fracture of upper end of tibia**
`6th`

S89.091 **Other physeal fracture of upper end of right tibia**
`7th`

S89.092 **Other physeal fracture of upper end of left tibia**
`7th`

S89.1 **Physeal fracture of lower end of tibia**

S89.10 **Unspecified physeal fracture of lower end of tibia**
`5th`

S89.101 **Unspecified physeal fracture of lower end of right tibia**
`6th` `7th`

S89.102 **Unspecified physeal fracture of lower end of left tibia**
`7th`

S89.11 **Salter-Harris Type I physeal fracture of lower end of tibia**
`6th`

S89.111 **Salter-Harris Type I physeal fracture of lower end of right tibia**
`7th`

S89.112 **Salter-Harris Type I physeal fracture of lower end of left tibia**
`7th`

S89.12 **Salter-Harris Type II physeal fracture of lower end of tibia**
`6th`

S89.121 **Salter-Harris Type II physeal fracture of lower end of right tibia**
`7th`

S89.122 **Salter-Harris Type II physeal fracture of lower end of left tibia**
`7th`

S89.13 **Salter-Harris Type III physeal fracture of lower end of tibia**
`6th`

Excludes1: fracture of medial malleolus (adult) (S82.5-)

S89.131 **Salter-Harris Type III physeal fracture of lower end of right tibia**
`7th`

  Additional Character Required   ✓ 3-character code   Unspecified laterality codes were excluded here.   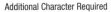 •=New Code   ▲=Revised Code   ***Excludes1***—Not coded here, do not use together   ***Excludes2***—Not included here

CHAPTER 19. INJURY, POISONING AND CERTAIN OTHER CONSEQUENCES OF EXTERNAL CAUSES (S89.132–S90.31X)

S89.132 Salter-Harris Type III physeal fracture of lower end of left tibia
`7th`

S89.14 `6th` **Salter-Harris Type IV physeal fracture of lower end of tibia**

Excludes1: fracture of medial malleolus (adult) (S82.5-)

> 7th characters for subcategories S89.0, S89.1, S89.2, and S89.3
> A—initial encounter for closed fracture
> D—subsequent encounter for fracture with routine healing
> G—subsequent encounter for fracture with delayed healing
> K—subsequent encounter for fracture with nonunion
> P—subsequent encounter for fracture with malunion
> S—sequela

S89.141 `7th` Salter-Harris Type IV physeal fracture of lower end of right tibia

S89.142 `7th` Salter-Harris Type IV physeal fracture of lower end of left tibia

S89.19 Other physeal fracture of lower end of tibia
S89.191 `7th` Other physeal fracture of lower end of right tibia

S89.192 `7th` Other physeal fracture of lower end of left tibia

S89.2 `5th` **Physeal fracture of upper end of fibula**
S89.20 `6th` Unspecified physeal fracture of upper end of fibula
S89.201 `7th` Unspecified physeal fracture of upper end of right fibula

S89.202 `7th` Unspecified physeal fracture of upper end of left fibula

S89.21 `6th` Salter-Harris Type I physeal fracture of upper end of fibula
S89.211 `7th` Salter-Harris Type I physeal fracture of upper end of right fibula

S89.212 `7th` Salter-Harris Type I physeal fracture of upper end of left fibula

S89.22 `6th` Salter-Harris Type II physeal fracture of upper end of fibula
S89.221 `7th` Salter-Harris Type II physeal fracture of upper end of right fibula

S89.222 `7th` Salter-Harris Type II physeal fracture of upper end of left fibula

S89.29 Other physeal fracture of upper end of fibula
S89.291 `7th` Other physeal fracture of upper end of right fibula

S89.292 `7th` Other physeal fracture of upper end of left fibula

S89.3 `5th` **Physeal fracture of lower end of fibula**
S89.30 `6th` Unspecified physeal fracture of lower end of fibula
S89.301 `7th` Unspecified physeal fracture of lower end of right fibula

S89.302 `7th` Unspecified physeal fracture of lower end of left fibula

S89.31 `6th` Salter-Harris Type I physeal fracture of lower end of fibula
S89.311 `7th` Salter-Harris Type I physeal fracture of lower end of right fibula

S89.312 `7th` Salter-Harris Type I physeal fracture of lower end of left fibula

S89.32 `6th` Salter-Harris Type II physeal fracture of lower end of fibula
S89.321 `7th` Salter-Harris Type II physeal fracture of lower end of right fibula

S89.322 `7th` Salter-Harris Type II physeal fracture of lower end of left fibula

S89.39 `6th` Other physeal fracture of lower end of fibula
S89.391 Other physeal fracture of lower end of right fibula

S89.392 `7th` Other physeal fracture of lower end of left fibula

S89.8 `5th` **Other specified injuries of lower leg**
S89.81X `7th` Other specified injuries of right lower leg

> 7th characters for subcategory S89.8
> A—initial encounter
> D—subsequent encounter
> S—sequela

S89.82X `7th` Other specified injuries of left lower leg

(S90–S99) INJURIES TO THE ANKLE AND FOOT

Excludes2: burns and corrosions (T20–T32)
fracture of ankle and malleolus (S82.-)
frostbite (T33–T34)
insect bite or sting, venomous (T63.4)

> 7th characters for category S90
> A—initial encounter
> D—subsequent encounter
> S—sequela

S90 `4th` **SUPERFICIAL INJURY OF ANKLE, FOOT AND TOES**
S90.0 `5th` **Contusion of ankle**
S90.01X `7th` Contusion of right ankle

S90.02X `7th` Contusion of left ankle

S90.1 `5th` **Contusion of toe without damage to nail**
S90.11 `6th` Contusion of great toe without damage to nail
S90.111 `7th` Contusion of right great toe without damage to nail

S90.112 `7th` Contusion of left great toe without damage to nail

S90.12 `6th` Contusion of lesser toe without damage to nail
S90.121 `7th` Contusion of right lesser toe(s) without damage to nail

S90.122 `7th` Contusion of left lesser toe(s) without damage to nail

S90.2 `5th` **Contusion of toe with damage to nail**
S90.21 `6th` Contusion of great toe with damage to nail
S90.211 `7th` Contusion of right great toe with damage to nail

S90.212 `7th` Contusion of left great toe with damage to nail

S90.22 `6th` Contusion of lesser toe with damage to nail
S90.221 `7th` Contusion of right lesser toe(s) with damage to nail

S90.222 `7th` Contusion of left lesser toe(s) with damage to nail

S90.3 `5th` **Contusion of foot**
Excludes2: contusion of toes (S90.1-, S90.2-)
S90.31X `7th` Contusion of right foot

`4th` `5th` `6th` `7th` Additional Character Required   3-character code

Unspecified laterality codes were excluded here.

•=New Code
▲=Revised Code

Excludes1—Not coded here, do not use together
Excludes2—Not included here

S90.32X   Contusion of left foot
`7th`

S90.4   Other superficial injuries of toe
`5th`
   S90.41   Abrasion of toe
`6th`
     S90.411   Abrasion, right great toe
`7th`

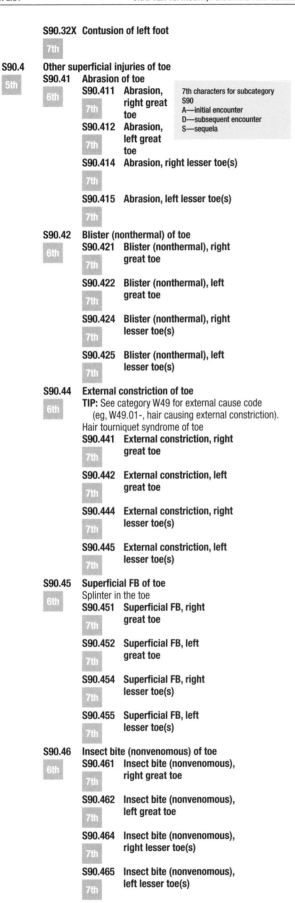

7th characters for subcategory S90
A—initial encounter
D—subsequent encounter
S—sequela

     S90.412   Abrasion, left great toe
`7th`

     S90.414   Abrasion, right lesser toe(s)
`7th`

     S90.415   Abrasion, left lesser toe(s)
`7th`

   S90.42   Blister (nonthermal) of toe
`6th`
     S90.421   Blister (nonthermal), right great toe
`7th`

     S90.422   Blister (nonthermal), left great toe
`7th`

     S90.424   Blister (nonthermal), right lesser toe(s)
`7th`

     S90.425   Blister (nonthermal), left lesser toe(s)
`7th`

   S90.44   External constriction of toe
`6th`
     TIP: See category W49 for external cause code (eg, W49.01-, hair causing external constriction).
     Hair tourniquet syndrome of toe
     S90.441   External constriction, right great toe
`7th`

     S90.442   External constriction, left great toe
`7th`

     S90.444   External constriction, right lesser toe(s)
`7th`

     S90.445   External constriction, left lesser toe(s)
`7th`

   S90.45   Superficial FB of toe
`6th`
     Splinter in the toe
     S90.451   Superficial FB, right great toe
`7th`

     S90.452   Superficial FB, left great toe
`7th`

     S90.454   Superficial FB, right lesser toe(s)
`7th`

     S90.455   Superficial FB, left lesser toe(s)
`7th`

   S90.46   Insect bite (nonvenomous) of toe
`6th`
     S90.461   Insect bite (nonvenomous), right great toe
`7th`

     S90.462   Insect bite (nonvenomous), left great toe
`7th`

     S90.464   Insect bite (nonvenomous), right lesser toe(s)
`7th`

     S90.465   Insect bite (nonvenomous), left lesser toe(s)
`7th`

   S90.47   Other superficial bite of toe
`6th`
     Excludes1: open bite of toe (S91.15-, S91.25-)
     S90.471   Other superficial bite of right great toe
`7th`

     S90.472   Other superficial bite of left great toe
`7th`

     S90.474   Other superficial bite of right lesser toe(s)
`7th`

     S90.475   Other superficial bite of left lesser toe(s)
`7th`

S90.5   Other superficial injuries of ankle
`5th`
   S90.51   Abrasion of ankle
`6th`
     S90.511   Abrasion, right ankle
`7th`

     S90.512   Abrasion, left ankle
`7th`

   S90.52   Blister (nonthermal) of ankle
`6th`
     S90.521   Blister (nonthermal), right ankle
`7th`

     S90.522   Blister (nonthermal), left ankle
`7th`

   S90.54   External constriction of ankle
`6th`
     S90.541   External constriction, right ankle
`7th`

     S90.542   External constriction, left ankle
`7th`

   S90.55   Superficial FB of ankle
`6th`
     Splinter in the ankle
     S90.551   Superficial FB, right ankle
`7th`

     S90.552   Superficial FB, left ankle
`7th`

   S90.56   Insect bite (nonvenomous) of ankle
`6th`
     S90.561   Insect bite (nonvenomous), right ankle
`7th`

     S90.562   Insect bite (nonvenomous), left ankle
`7th`

   S90.57   Other superficial bite of ankle
`6th`
     Excludes1: open bite of ankle (S91.05-)
     S90.571   Other superficial bite of ankle, right ankle
`7th`

     S90.572   Other superficial bite of ankle, left ankle
`7th`

S90.8   Other superficial injuries of foot
`5th`
   S90.81   Abrasion of foot
`6th`
     S90.811   Abrasion, right foot
`7th`

     S90.812   Abrasion, left foot

   S90.82   Blister (nonthermal) of foot
`6th`
     S90.821   Blister (nonthermal), right foot
`7th`

     S90.822   Blister (nonthermal), left foot
`7th`

CHAPTER 19. INJURY, POISONING AND CERTAIN OTHER CONSEQUENCES OF EXTERNAL CAUSES   (S90.32X–S90.822)

`4th` `5th` `6th` `7th`   Additional Character Required   ✓   3-character code   Unspecified laterality codes were excluded here.   •=New Code   ▲=Revised Code   *Excludes1*—Not coded here, do not use together   *Excludes2*—Not included here

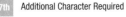

CHAPTER 19. INJURY, POISONING AND CERTAIN OTHER CONSEQUENCES OF EXTERNAL CAUSES   (S90.84–S91.154)

S90.84 **External constriction of foot**
6th

S90.841 **External constric-tion, right foot**
7th

S90.842 **External constric-tion, left foot**
7th

> 7th characters for subcategory S90
> A—initial encounter
> D—subsequent encounter
> S—sequela

S90.85 **Superficial FB of foot**
6th
Splinter in the foot

S90.851 **Superficial FB, right foot**
7th

S90.852 **Superficial FB, left foot**
7th

S90.86 **Insect bite (nonvenomous) of foot**
6th

S90.861 **Insect bite (nonvenomous), right foot**
7th

S90.862 **Insect bite (nonvenomous), left foot**
7th

S90.87 **Other superficial bite of foot**
6th
Excludes1: open bite of foot (S91.35-)

S90.871 **Other superficial bite of right foot**
7th

S90.872 **Other superficial bite of left foot**
7th

S91 **OPEN WOUND OF ANKLE, FOOT AND TOES**
4th
Code also any associated wound infection
Excludes1: open fracture of ankle, foot and toes (S92.-with 7th character B)
traumatic amputation of ankle and foot (S98.-)

> 7th characters for category S91
> A—initial encounter
> D—subsequent encounter
> S—sequela

S91.0 **Open wound of ankle**
5th

S91.01 **Laceration without FB of ankle**
6th

S91.011 **Laceration without FB, right ankle**
7th

S91.012 **Laceration without FB, left ankle**
7th

S91.02 **Laceration with FB of ankle**
6th

S91.021 **Laceration with FB, right ankle**
7th

S91.022 **Laceration with FB, left ankle**
7th

S91.03 **Puncture wound without FB of ankle**
6th

S91.031 **Puncture wound without FB, right ankle**
7th

S91.032 **Puncture wound without FB, left ankle**
7th

S91.04 **Puncture wound with FB of ankle**
6th

S91.041 **Puncture wound with FB, right ankle**
7th

S91.042 **Puncture wound with FB, left ankle**
7th

S91.05 **Open bite of ankle**
6th
Excludes1: superficial bite of ankle (S90.56-, S90.57-)

S91.051 **Open bite, right ankle**
7th

S91.052 **Open bite, left ankle**
7th

S91.1 **Open wound of toe without damage to nail**
5th

S91.11 **Laceration without FB of toe without damage to nail**
6th

S91.111 **Laceration without FB of right great toe without damage to nail**
7th

S91.112 **Laceration without FB of left great toe without damage to nail**
7th

S91.114 **Laceration without FB of right lesser toe(s) without damage to nail**
7th

S91.115 **Laceration without FB of left lesser toe(s) without damage to nail**
7th

S91.12 **Laceration with FB of toe without damage to nail**
6th

S91.121 **Laceration with FB of right great toe without damage to nail**
7th

S91.122 **Laceration with FB of left great toe without damage to nail**
7th

S91.124 **Laceration with FB of right lesser toe(s) without damage to nail**
7th

S91.125 **Laceration with FB of left lesser toe(s) without damage to nail**
7th

S91.13 **Puncture wound without FB of toe without damage to nail**
6th

S91.131 **Puncture wound without FB of right great toe without damage to nail**
7th

S91.132 **Puncture wound without FB of left great toe without damage to nail**
7th

S91.134 **Puncture wound without FB of right lesser toe(s) without damage to nail**
7th

S91.135 **Puncture wound without FB of left lesser toe(s) without damage to nail**
7th

S91.14 **Puncture wound with FB of toe without damage to nail**
6th

S91.141 **Puncture wound with FB of right great toe without damage to nail**
7th

S91.142 **Puncture wound with FB of left great toe without damage to nail**
7th

S91.144 **Puncture wound with FB of right lesser toe(s) without damage to nail**
7th

S91.145 **Puncture wound with FB of left lesser toe(s) without damage to nail**
7th

S91.15 **Open bite of toe without damage to nail**
6th
Bite of toe NOS
Excludes1: superficial bite of toe (S90.46-, S90.47-)

S91.151 **Open bite of right great toe without damage to nail**
7th

S91.152 **Open bite of left great toe without damage to nail**
7th

S91.154 **Open bite of right lesser toe(s) without damage to nail**
7th

   Additional Character Required   ✔ 3-character code   Unspecified laterality codes were excluded here.   •=New Code   ▲=Revised Code   *Excludes1*—Not coded here, do not use together   *Excludes2*—Not included here

S91.155 **7th** Open bite of left lesser toe(s) without damage to nail

S91.2 **5th** **Open wound of toe with damage to nail**
S91.21 **6th** Laceration without FB of toe with damage to nail
S91.211 **7th** Laceration without FB of right great toe with damage to nail

> 7th characters for category S91
> A—initial encounter
> D—subsequent encounter
> S—sequela

S91.212 **7th** Laceration without FB of left great toe with damage to nail
S91.214 **7th** Laceration without FB of right lesser toe(s) with damage to nail
S91.215 **7th** Laceration without FB of left lesser toe(s) with damage to nail

S91.22 **6th** Laceration with FB of toe with damage to nail
S91.221 **7th** Laceration with FB of right great toe with damage to nail
S91.222 **7th** Laceration with FB of left great toe with damage to nail
S91.224 **7th** Laceration with FB of right lesser toe(s) with damage to nail
S91.225 **7th** Laceration with FB of left lesser toe(s) with damage to nail

S91.23 **6th** Puncture wound without FB of toe with damage to nail
S91.231 **7th** Puncture wound without FB of right great toe with damage to nail
S91.232 **7th** Puncture wound without FB of left great toe with damage to nail
S91.234 **7th** Puncture wound without FB of right lesser toe(s) with damage to nail
S91.235 **7th** Puncture wound without FB of left lesser toe(s) with damage to nail

S91.24 **6th** Puncture wound with FB of toe with damage to nail
S91.241 **7th** Puncture wound with FB of right great toe with damage to nail
S91.242 **7th** Puncture wound with FB of left great toe with damage to nail
S91.244 **7th** Puncture wound with FB of right lesser toe(s) with damage to nail
S91.245 **7th** Puncture wound with FB of left lesser toe(s) with damage to nail

S91.25 **6th** Open bite of toe with damage to nail
Bite of toe with damage to nail NOS
Excludes1: superficial bite of toe (S90.46-, S90.47-)
S91.251 **7th** Open bite of right great toe with damage to nail
S91.252 **7th** Open bite of left great toe with damage to nail
S91.254 **7th** Open bite of right lesser toe(s) with damage to nail

S91.255 **7th** Open bite of left lesser toe(s) with damage to nail

S91.3 **5th** **Open wound of foot**
S91.31 **6th** Laceration without FB of foot
S91.311 **7th** Laceration without FB, right foot
S91.312 **7th** Laceration without FB, left foot

S91.32 **6th** Laceration with FB of foot
S91.321 **7th** Laceration with FB, right foot
S91.322 **7th** Laceration with FB, left foot

S91.33 **6th** Puncture wound without FB of foot
S91.331 **7th** Puncture wound without FB, right foot
S91.332 **7th** Puncture wound without FB, left foot

S91.34 **6th** Puncture wound with FB of foot
S91.341 **7th** Puncture wound with FB, right foot
S91.342 **7th** Puncture wound with FB, left foot

S91.35 **6th** Open bite of foot
Excludes1: superficial bite of foot (S90.86-, S90.87-)
S91.351 **7th** Open bite, right foot
S91.352 **7th** Open bite, left foot

S92 **4th** **FRACTURE OF FOOT AND TOE, EXCEPT ANKLE**
Note: A fracture not indicated as displaced or nondisplaced should be coded to displaced
A fracture not indicated as open or closed should be coded to closed
Excludes1: traumatic amputation of ankle and foot (S98.-)
Excludes2: fracture of ankle (S82.-)
fracture of malleolus (S82.-)

> 7th characters for category S92
> A—initial encounter for closed fracture
> B—initial encounter for open fracture
> D—subsequent encounter for fracture with routine healing
> G—subsequent encounter for fracture with delayed healing
> K—subsequent encounter for fracture with nonunion
> P—subsequent encounter for fracture with malunion
> S—sequela

S92.0 **5th** **Fracture of calcaneus**
Heel bone
Os calcis
Excludes2: physeal fracture of calcaneus (S99.0-)
S92.00 **6th** Unspecified fracture of calcaneus
S92.001 **7th** Unspecified fracture of right calcaneus
S92.002 **7th** Unspecified fracture of left calcaneus

S92.01 **6th** Fracture of body of calcaneus
S92.011 **7th** Displaced fracture of body of right calcaneus
S92.012 **7th** Displaced fracture of body of left calcaneus
S92.014 **7th** Nondisplaced fracture of body of right calcaneus

---

  Additional Character Required 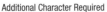 **3-character code** Unspecified laterality codes were excluded here. •=New Code ▲=Revised Code *Excludes1*—Not coded here, do not use together *Excludes2*—Not included here

CHAPTER 19. INJURY, POISONING AND CERTAIN OTHER CONSEQUENCES OF EXTERNAL CAUSES   (S92.015–S92.155)

S92.015   Nondisplaced fracture of body of left calcaneus
> **7th**

S92.02   Fracture of anterior process of calcaneus
> **6th**

    S92.021   Displaced fracture of anterior process of right calcaneus
> **7th**

    S92.022   Displaced fracture of anterior process of left calcaneus
> **7th**

    S92.024   Nondisplaced fracture of anterior process of right calcaneus
> **7th**

    S92.025   Nondisplaced fracture of anterior process of left calcaneus
> **7th**

S92.03   Avulsion fracture of tuberosity of calcaneus
> **6th**

    S92.031   Displaced avulsion fracture of tuberosity of right calcaneus
> **7th**

    S92.032   Displaced avulsion fracture of tuberosity of left calcaneus
> **7th**

    S92.034   Nondisplaced avulsion fracture of tuberosity of right calcaneus
> **7th**

    S92.035   Nondisplaced avulsion fracture of tuberosity of left calcaneus
> **7th**

S92.04   Other fracture of tuberosity of calcaneus
> **6th**

    S92.041   Displaced other fracture of tuberosity of right calcaneus
> **7th**

    S92.042   Displaced other fracture of tuberosity of left calcaneus
> **7th**

    S92.044   Nondisplaced other fracture of tuberosity of right calcaneus
> **7th**

    S92.045   Nondisplaced other fracture of tuberosity of left calcaneus
> **7th**

S92.05   Other extraarticular fracture of calcaneus
> **6th**

    S92.051   Displaced other extraarticular fracture of right calcaneus
> **7th**

    S92.052   Displaced other extraarticular fracture of left calcaneus
> **7th**

    S92.054   Nondisplaced other extraarticular fracture of right calcaneus
> **7th**

    S92.055   Nondisplaced other extraarticular fracture of left calcaneus
> **7th**

S92.06   Intraarticular fracture of calcaneus
> **6th**

    S92.061   Displaced intraarticular fracture of right calcaneus
> **7th**

    S92.062   Displaced intraarticular fracture of left calcaneus
> **7th**

    S92.064   Nondisplaced intraarticular fracture of right calcaneus
> **7th**

    S92.065   Nondisplaced intraarticular fracture of left calcaneus
> **7th**

S92.1   Fracture of talus
> **5th**

Astragalus

S92.10   Unspecified fracture of talus
> **6th**

    S92.101   Unspecified fracture of right talus
> **7th**

    S92.102   Unspecified fracture of left talus
> **7th**

S92.11   Fracture of neck of talus
> **6th**

    S92.111   Displaced fracture of neck of right talus
> **7th**

    S92.112   Displaced fracture of neck of left talus
> **7th**

    S92.114   Nondisplaced fracture of neck of right talus
> **7th**

    S92.115   Nondisplaced fracture of neck of left talus
> **7th**

S92.12   Fracture of body of talus
> **6th**

    S92.121   Displaced fracture of body of right talus
> **7th**

    S92.122   Displaced fracture of body of left talus
> **7th**

    S92.124   Nondisplaced fracture of body of right talus
> **7th**

    S92.125   Nondisplaced fracture of body of left talus
> **7th**

S92.13   Fracture of posterior process of talus
> **6th**

    S92.131   Displaced fracture of posterior process of right talus
> **7th**

    S92.132   Displaced fracture of posterior process of left talus
> **7th**

    S92.134   Nondisplaced fracture of posterior process of right talus
> **7th**

    S92.135   Nondisplaced fracture of posterior process of left talus
> **7th**

S92.14   Dome fracture of talus
> **6th**

Excludes1: osteochondritis dissecans (M93.2)

    S92.141   Displaced dome fracture of right talus
> **7th**

    S92.142   Displaced dome fracture of left talus
> **7th**

    S92.144   Nondisplaced dome fracture of right talus
> **7th**

    S92.145   Nondisplaced dome fracture of left talus
> **7th**

S92.15   Avulsion fracture (chip fracture) of talus
> **6th**

    S92.151   Displaced avulsion fracture (chip fracture) of right talus
> **7th**

    S92.152   Displaced avulsion fracture (chip fracture) of left talus
> **7th**

    S92.154   Nondisplaced avulsion fracture (chip fracture) of right talus
> **7th**

    S92.155   Nondisplaced avulsion fracture (chip fracture) of left talus
> **7th**

  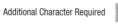   Additional Character Required   ✔ 3-character code   Unspecified laterality codes were excluded here.   •=New Code   ▲=Revised Code   ***Excludes1***—Not coded here, do not use together   ***Excludes2***—Not included here

S92.19   **Other fracture of talus**

S92.191   Other fracture of right talus
`7th`

S92.192   Other fracture of left talus
`7th`

> 7th characters for category S92
> A—initial encounter for closed fracture
> B—initial encounter for open fracture
> D—subsequent encounter for fracture with routine healing
> G—subsequent encounter for fracture with delayed healing
> K—subsequent encounter for fracture with nonunion
> P—subsequent encounter for fracture with malunion
> S—sequela

S92.2   **Fracture of other and unspecified tarsal bone(s)**
`5th`

S92.20   **Fracture of unspecified tarsal bone(s)**
`6th`

S92.201   Fracture of unspecified tarsal bone(s) of right foot
`7th`

S92.202   Fracture of unspecified tarsal bone(s) of left foot
`7th`

S92.21   **Fracture of cuboid bone**
`6th`

S92.211   Displaced fracture of cuboid bone of right foot
`7th`

S92.212   Displaced fracture of cuboid bone of left foot
`7th`

S92.214   Nondisplaced fracture of cuboid bone of right foot
`7th`

S92.215   Nondisplaced fracture of cuboid bone of left foot
`7th`

S92.22   **Fracture of lateral cuneiform**
`6th`

S92.221   Displaced fracture of lateral cuneiform of right foot
`7th`

S92.222   Displaced fracture of lateral cuneiform of left foot
`7th`

S92.224   Nondisplaced fracture of lateral cuneiform of right foot
`7th`

S92.225   Nondisplaced fracture of lateral cuneiform of left foot
`7th`

S92.23   **Fracture of intermediate cuneiform**
`6th`

S92.231   Displaced fracture of intermediate cuneiform of right foot
`7th`

S92.232   Displaced fracture of intermediate cuneiform of left foot
`7th`

S92.234   Nondisplaced fracture of intermediate cuneiform of right foot
`7th`

S92.235   Nondisplaced fracture of intermediate cuneiform of left foot
`7th`

S92.24   **Fracture of medial cuneiform**
`6th`

S92.241   Displaced fracture of medial cuneiform of right foot
`7th`

S92.242   Displaced fracture of medial cuneiform of left foot
`7th`

S92.244   Nondisplaced fracture of medial cuneiform of right foot
`7th`

S92.245   Nondisplaced fracture of medial cuneiform of left foot
`7th`

S92.25   **Fracture of navicular [scaphoid] of foot**
`6th`

S92.251   Displaced fracture of navicular [scaphoid] of right foot
`7th`

S92.252   Displaced fracture of navicular [scaphoid] of left foot
`7th`

S92.254   Nondisplaced fracture of navicular [scaphoid] of right foot
`7th`

S92.255   Nondisplaced fracture of navicular [scaphoid] of left foot
`7th`

S92.3   **Fracture of metatarsal bone(s)**
`5th`
Excludes2: physeal fracture of metatarsal (S99.1-)

S92.30   **Fracture of unspecified metatarsal bone(s)**
`6th`

S92.301   Fracture of unspecified metatarsal bone(s), right foot
`7th`

S92.302   Fracture of unspecified metatarsal bone(s), left foot
`7th`

S92.31   **Fracture of first metatarsal bone**
`6th`

S92.311   Displaced fracture of first metatarsal bone, right foot
`7th`

S92.312   Displaced fracture of first metatarsal bone, left foot
`7th`

S92.314   Nondisplaced fracture of first metatarsal bone, right foot
`7th`

S92.315   Nondisplaced fracture of first metatarsal bone, left foot
`7th`

S92.32   **Fracture of second metatarsal bone**
`6th`

S92.321   Displaced fracture of second metatarsal bone, right foot
`7th`

S92.322   Displaced fracture of second metatarsal bone, left foot
`7th`

S92.324   Nondisplaced fracture of second metatarsal bone, right foot
`7th`

S92.325   Nondisplaced fracture of second metatarsal bone, left foot
`7th`

S92.33   **Fracture of third metatarsal bone**
`6th`

S92.331   Displaced fracture of third metatarsal bone, right foot
`7th`

S92.332   Displaced fracture of third metatarsal bone, left foot
`7th`

S92.334   Nondisplaced fracture of third metatarsal bone, right foot
`7th`

S92.335   Nondisplaced fracture of third metatarsal bone, left foot
`7th`

S92.34   **Fracture of fourth metatarsal bone**
`6th`

S92.341   Displaced fracture of fourth metatarsal bone, right foot
`7th`

S92.342   Displaced fracture of fourth metatarsal bone, left foot
`7th`

S92.344   Nondisplaced fracture of fourth metatarsal bone, right foot
`7th`

S92.345   Nondisplaced fracture of fourth metatarsal bone, left foot
`7th`

  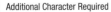   `4th` `5th` `6th` `7th` Additional Character Required   ✓ 3-character code   Unspecified laterality codes were excluded here.   •=New Code   ▲=Revised Code   *Excludes1*—Not coded here, do not use togethor   *Excludes2*—Not included here

CHAPTER 19. INJURY, POISONING AND CERTAIN OTHER CONSEQUENCES OF EXTERNAL CAUSES   (S92.35–S93.01X)

S92.35   **Fracture of fifth metatarsal bone**
`6th`

   S92.351   Displaced fracture of fifth metatarsal bone, right foot
`7th`

> 7th characters for category S92
> A—initial encounter for closed fracture
> B—initial encounter for open fracture
> D—subsequent encounter for fracture with routine healing
> G—subsequent encounter for fracture with delayed healing
> K—subsequent encounter for fracture with nonunion
> P—subsequent encounter for fracture with malunion
> S—sequela

   S92.352   Displaced fracture of fifth metatarsal bone, left foot
`7th`

   S92.354   Nondisplaced fracture of fifth metatarsal bone, right foot
`7th`

   S92.355   Nondisplaced fracture of fifth metatarsal bone, left foot
`7th`

S92.4   **Fracture of great toe**
`5th`
Excludes2: physeal fracture of phalanx of toe (S99.2-)

  S92.41   **Fracture of proximal phalanx of great toe**
`6th`

   S92.411   Displaced fracture of proximal phalanx of right great toe
`7th`

   S92.412   Displaced fracture of proximal phalanx of left great toe
`7th`

   S92.414   Nondisplaced fracture of proximal phalanx of right great toe
`7th`

   S92.415   Nondisplaced fracture of proximal phalanx of left great toe
`7th`

  S92.42   **Fracture of distal phalanx of great toe**
`6th`

   S92.421   Displaced fracture of distal phalanx of right great toe
`7th`

   S92.422   Displaced fracture of distal phalanx of left great toe
`7th`

   S92.424   Nondisplaced fracture of distal phalanx of right great toe
`7th`

   S92.425   Nondisplaced fracture of distal phalanx of left great toe
`7th`

  S92.49   **Other fracture of great toe**
`6th`

   S92.491   Other fracture of right great toe
`7th`

   S92.492   Other fracture of left great toe
`7th`

S92.5   **Fracture of lesser toe(s)**
`5th`
Excludes2: physeal fracture of toe (S99.2-)

  S92.51   **Fracture of proximal phalanx of lesser toe(s)**
`6th`

   S92.511   Displaced fracture of proximal phalanx of right lesser toe(s)
`7th`

   S92.512   Displaced fracture of proximal phalanx of left lesser toe(s)
`7th`

   S92.514   Nondisplaced fracture of proximal phalanx of right lesser toe(s)
`7th`

   S92.515   Nondisplaced fracture of proximal phalanx of left lesser toe(s)
`7th`

  S92.52   **Fracture of medial phalanx of lesser toe(s)**
`6th`

   S92.521   Displaced fracture of medial phalanx of right lesser toe(s)
`7th`

   S92.522   Displaced fracture of medial phalanx of left lesser toe(s)
`7th`

   S92.524   Nondisplaced fracture of medial phalanx of right lesser toe(s)
`7th`

   S92.525   Nondisplaced fracture of medial phalanx of left lesser toe(s)
`7th`

  S92.53   **Fracture of distal phalanx of lesser toe(s)**
`6th`

   S92.531   Displaced fracture of distal phalanx of right lesser toe(s)
`7th`

   S92.532   Displaced fracture of distal phalanx of left lesser toe(s)
`7th`

   S92.534   Nondisplaced fracture of distal phalanx of right lesser toe(s)
`7th`

   S92.535   Nondisplaced fracture of distal phalanx of left lesser toe(s)
`7th`

  S92.59   **Other fracture of lesser toe(s)**
`6th`

   S92.591   Other fracture of right lesser toe(s)
`7th`

   S92.592   Other fracture of left lesser toe(s)
`7th`

•S92.8   **Other fracture of foot**
`5th`

  •S92.81   **Other fracture of foot**
`6th`
   Sesamoid fracture of foot

   •S92.811   Other fracture of right foot
`7th`

   •S92.812   Other fracture of left foot
`7th`

S92.9   **Unspecified fracture of foot and toe**
`5th`

  S92.90   **Unspecified fracture of foot**
`6th`

   S92.901   Unspecified fracture of right foot
`7th`

   S92.902   Unspecified fracture of left foot
`7th`

  S92.91   **Unspecified fracture of toe**
`6th`

   S92.911   Unspecified fracture of right toe(s)
`7th`

   S92.912   Unspecified fracture of left toe(s)
`7th`

S93   DISLOCATION AND SPRAIN OF JOINTS AND LIGAMENTS AT ANKLE, FOOT AND TOE LEVEL
`4th`

Includes: avulsion of joint or ligament of ankle, foot and toe
   laceration of cartilage, joint or ligament of ankle, foot and toe
   sprain of cartilage, joint or ligament of ankle, foot and toe
   traumatic hemarthrosis of joint or ligament of ankle, foot and toe
   traumatic rupture of joint or ligament of ankle, foot and toe
   traumatic subluxation of joint or ligament of ankle, foot and toe
   traumatic tear of joint or ligament of ankle, foot and toe
Code also any associated open wound
Excludes2: strain of muscle and tendon of ankle and foot (S96.-)

S93.0   **Subluxation and dislocation of ankle joint**
`5th`
   Subluxation and dislocation of astragalus
   Subluxation and dislocation of fibula, lower end
   Subluxation and dislocation of talus or of tibia, lower end

  S93.01X   Subluxation of right ankle joint
`7th`

`4th` `5th` `6th` `7th`   Additional Character Required   ✓   3-character code   Unspecified laterality codes were excluded here.   •=New Code   ▲=Revised Code   *Excludes1*—Not coded here, do not use together   *Excludes2*—Not included here

S93.02X **7th** Subluxation of left ankle joint

7th characters for category S93
A—initial encounter
D—subsequent encounter
S—sequela

S93.04X **7th** Dislocation of right ankle joint

S93.05X **7th** Dislocation of left ankle joint

S93.1 **5th** Subluxation and dislocation of toe

S93.10 **6th** Unspecified subluxation and dislocation of toe
Dislocation/subluxation of toe NOS

    S93.101 **7th** Unspecified subluxation of right toe(s)

    S93.102 **7th** Unspecified subluxation of left toe(s)

    S93.104 **7th** Unspecified dislocation of right toe(s)

    S93.105 **7th** Unspecified dislocation of left toe(s)

S93.11 **6th** Dislocation of interphalangeal joint

    S93.111 **7th** Dislocation of interphalangeal joint of right great toe

    S93.112 **7th** Dislocation of interphalangeal joint of left great toe

    S93.114 **7th** Dislocation of interphalangeal joint of right lesser toe(s)

    S93.115 **7th** Dislocation of interphalangeal joint of left lesser toe(s)

S93.12 **6th** Dislocation of metatarsophalangeal joint

    S93.121 **7th** Dislocation of metatarsophalangeal joint of right great toe

    S93.122 **7th** Dislocation of metatarsophalangeal joint of left great toe

    S93.124 **7th** Dislocation of metatarsophalangeal joint of right lesser toe(s)

    S93.125 **7th** Dislocation of metatarsophalangeal joint of left lesser toe(s)

S93.13 **6th** Subluxation of interphalangeal joint

    S93.131 **7th** Subluxation of interphalangeal joint of right great toe

    S93.132 **7th** Subluxation of interphalangeal joint of left great toe

    S93.134 **7th** Subluxation of interphalangeal joint of right lesser toe(s)

    S93.135 **7th** Subluxation of interphalangeal joint of left lesser toe(s)

S93.14 **6th** Subluxation of metatarsophalangeal joint

    S93.141 **7th** Subluxation of metatarsophalangeal joint of right great toe

    S93.142 **7th** Subluxation of metatarsophalangeal joint of left great toe

    S93.144 **7th** Subluxation of metatarsophalangeal joint of right lesser toe(s)

    S93.145 **7th** Subluxation of metatarsophalangeal joint of left lesser toe(s)

S93.3 **5th** Subluxation and dislocation of foot
Excludes2: dislocation of toe (S93.1-)

S93.30 **6th** Unspecified subluxation and dislocation of foot
Dislocation of foot NOS
Subluxation of foot NOS

    S93.301 **7th** Unspecified subluxation of right foot

    S93.302 **7th** Unspecified subluxation of left foot

    S93.304 **7th** Unspecified dislocation of right foot

    S93.305 **7th** Unspecified dislocation of left foot

S93.31 **6th** Subluxation and dislocation of tarsal joint

    S93.311 **7th** Subluxation of tarsal joint of right foot

    S93.312 **7th** Subluxation of tarsal joint of left foot

    S93.314 **7th** Dislocation of tarsal joint of right foot

    S93.315 **7th** Dislocation of tarsal joint of left foot

S93.32 **6th** Subluxation and dislocation of tarsometatarsal joint

    S93.321 **7th** Subluxation of tarsometatarsal joint of right foot

    S93.322 **7th** Subluxation of tarsometatarsal joint of left foot

    S93.324 **7th** Dislocation of tarsometatarsal joint of right foot

    S93.325 **7th** Dislocation of tarsometatarsal joint of left foot

S93.33 **6th** Other subluxation and dislocation of foot

    S93.331 **7th** Other subluxation of right foot

    S93.332 **7th** Other subluxation of left foot

    S93.334 **7th** Other dislocation of right foot

    S93.335 **7th** Other dislocation of left foot

S93.4 **5th** Sprain of ankle
Excludes2: injury of Achilles tendon (S86.0-)

S93.40 **6th** Sprain of unspecified ligament of ankle
Sprain of ankle NOS
Sprained ankle NOS

    S93.401 **7th** Sprain of unspecified ligament of right ankle

    S93.402 **7th** Sprain of unspecified ligament of left ankle

S93.41 **6th** Sprain of calcaneofibular ligament

CHAPTER 19. INJURY, POISONING AND CERTAIN OTHER CONSEQUENCES OF EXTERNAL CAUSES (S93.02X–S93.41)

  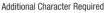 Additional Character Required 3-character code

Unspecified laterality codes were excluded here.

●=New Code
▲=Revised Code

Excludes1—Not coded here, do not use together
Excludes2—Not included here

CHAPTER 19. INJURY, POISONING AND CERTAIN OTHER CONSEQUENCES OF EXTERNAL CAUSES   (S93.411–S96.911)

S93.411   **[7th]**   Sprain of calcaneofibular ligament of right ankle

S93.412   **[7th]**   Sprain of calcaneofibular ligament of left ankle

S93.42 **[6th]**   Sprain of deltoid ligament

S93.421   **[7th]**   Sprain of deltoid ligament of right ankle

S93.422   **[7th]**   Sprain of deltoid ligament of left ankle

S93.43 **[6th]**   Sprain of tibiofibular ligament

S93.431   **[7th]**   Sprain of tibiofibular ligament of right ankle

S93.432   **[7th]**   Sprain of tibiofibular ligament of left ankle

S93.49 **[6th]**   Sprain of other ligament of ankle
Sprain of internal collateral ligament
Sprain of talofibular ligament

S93.491   **[7th]**   Sprain of other ligament of right ankle

S93.492   **[7th]**   Sprain of other ligament of left ankle

S93.5 **[5th]**   **Sprain of toe**

S93.50 **[6th]**   Unspecified sprain of toe

S93.501   **[7th]**   Unspecified sprain of right great toe

S93.502   **[7th]**   Unspecified sprain of left great toe

S93.504   **[7th]**   Unspecified sprain of right lesser toe(s)

S93.505   **[7th]**   Unspecified sprain of left lesser toe(s)

> 7th characters for category S93
> A—initial encounter
> D—subsequent encounter
> S—sequela

S93.51 **[6th]**   Sprain of interphalangeal joint of toe

S93.511   **[7th]**   Sprain of interphalangeal joint of right great toe

S93.512   **[7th]**   Sprain of interphalangeal joint of left great toe

S93.514   **[7th]**   Sprain of interphalangeal joint of right lesser toe(s)

S93.515   **[7th]**   Sprain of interphalangeal joint of left lesser toe(s)

S93.52 **[6th]**   Sprain of metatarsophalangeal joint of toe

S93.521   **[7th]**   Sprain of metatarsophalangeal joint of right great toe

S93.522   **[7th]**   Sprain of metatarsophalangeal joint of left great toe

S93.524   **[7th]**   Sprain of metatarsophalangeal joint of right lesser toe(s)

S93.525   **[7th]**   Sprain of metatarsophalangeal joint of left lesser toe(s)

S93.6 **[5th]**   **Sprain of foot**
Excludes2: sprain of metatarsophalangeal joint of toe (S93.52-)
sprain of toe (S93.5-)

S93.60 **[6th]**   Unspecified sprain of foot

S93.601   **[7th]**   Unspecified sprain of right foot

S93.602   **[7th]**   Unspecified sprain of left foot

S93.61 **[6th]**   Sprain of tarsal ligament of foot

S93.611   **[7th]**   Sprain of tarsal ligament of right foot

S93.612   **[7th]**   Sprain of tarsal ligament of left foot

S93.62 **[6th]**   Sprain of tarsometatarsal ligament of foot

S93.621   **[7th]**   Sprain of tarsometatarsal ligament of right foot

S93.622   **[7th]**   Sprain of tarsometatarsal ligament of left foot

S93.69 **[6th]**   Other sprain of foot

S93.691   **[7th]**   Other sprain of right foot

S93.692   **[7th]**   Other sprain of left foot

S96 **[4th]**   **INJURY OF MUSCLE AND TENDON AT ANKLE AND FOOT LEVEL**
Code also any associated open wound (S91.-)
Excludes2: injury of Achilles tendon (S86.0-)
sprain of joints and ligaments of ankle and foot (S93.-)

S96.01 **[6th]**   Strain of muscle and tendon of long flexor muscle of toe at ankle and foot level

S96.011   **[7th]**   Strain of muscle and tendon of long flexor muscle of toe at ankle and foot level, right foot

S96.012   **[7th]**   Strain of muscle and tendon of long flexor muscle of toe at ankle and foot level, left foot

S96.11 **[6th]**   Strain of muscle and tendon of long extensor muscle of toe at ankle and foot level

S96.111   **[7th]**   Strain of muscle and tendon of long extensor muscle of toe at ankle and foot level, right foot

S96.112   **[7th]**   Strain of muscle and tendon of long extensor muscle of toe at ankle and foot level, left foot

S96.21 **[6th]**   Strain of intrinsic muscle and tendon at ankle and foot level

S96.211   **[7th]**   Strain of intrinsic muscle and tendon at ankle and foot level, right foot

S96.212   **[7th]**   Strain of intrinsic muscle and tendon at ankle and foot level, left foot

S96.81 **[6th]**   Strain of other specified muscles and tendons at ankle and foot level

S96.811   **[7th]**   Strain of other specified muscles and tendons at ankle and foot level, right foot

S96.812   **[7th]**   Strain of other specified muscles and tendons at ankle and foot level, left foot

S96.91 **[6th]**   Strain of unspecified muscle and tendon at ankle and foot level

S96.911   **[7th]**   Strain of unspecified muscle and tendon at ankle and foot level, right foot

---

  Additional Character Required   **3-character code**   Unspecified laterality codes were excluded here.   •=New Code   ▲=Revised Code   *Excludes1*—Not coded here, do not use together   *Excludes2*—Not included here

S96.912   Strain of unspecified muscle and tendon at ankle and foot level, left foot
7th

S97   CRUSHING INJURY OF ANKLE AND FOOT
4th

Use additional code(s) for all associated injuries

S97.0   Crushing injury of ankle
5th

S97.01X   Crushing injury of right ankle
7th

> 7th characters for category S97
> A—initial encounter
> D—subsequent encounter
> S—sequela

S97.02X   Crushing injury of left ankle
7th

S97.1   Crushing injury of toe
5th

S97.10   Crushing injury of unspecified toe(s)
6th

S97.101   Crushing injury of unspecified right toe(s)
7th

S97.102   Crushing injury of unspecified left toe(s)
7th

S97.11   Crushing injury of great toe
6th

S97.111   Crushing injury of right great toe
7th

S97.112   Crushing injury of left great toe
7th

S97.12   Crushing injury of lesser toe(s)
6th

S97.121   Crushing injury of right lesser toe(s)
7th

S97.122   Crushing injury of left lesser toe(s)
7th

S97.8   Crushing injury of foot
5th

S97.81X   Crushing injury of right foot
7th

S97.82X   Crushing injury of left foot
7th

S99   OTHER AND UNSPECIFIED INJURIES OF ANKLE AND FOOT
4th

• **S99.0**   Physeal fracture of calcaneus
5th

• S99.00   Unspecified physeal fracture
6th

> 7th characters for subcategory S99.0-, S99.1-
> A—initial encounter for closed fracture
> B—initial encounter for open fracture
> D—subsequent encounter for fracture with routine healing
> G—subsequent encounter for fracture with delayed healing
> K—subsequent encounter for fracture with nonunion
> P—subsequent encounter for fracture with malunion
> S—sequela

• S99.001   Unspecified physeal fracture of right calcaneus
7th

• S99.002   Unspecified physeal fracture of left calcaneus
7th

• S99.01   Salter-Harris Type I physeal fracture
6th

• S99.011   Salter-Harris Type I physeal fracture of right calcaneus
7th

• S99.012   Salter-Harris Type I physeal fracture of left calcaneus
7th

• S99.02   Salter-Harris Type II physeal fracture
6th

• S99.021   Salter-Harris Type II physeal fracture of right calcaneus
7th

• S99.022   Salter-Harris Type II physeal fracture of left calcaneus
7th

• **S99.03**   Salter-Harris Type III physeal fracture
6th

• S99.031   Salter-Harris Type III physeal fracture of right calcaneus
7th

• S99.032   Salter-Harris Type III physeal fracture of left calcaneus
7th

• **S99.04**   Salter-Harris Type IV physeal fracture
6th

• S99.041   Salter-Harris Type IV physeal fracture of right calcaneus
7th

• S99.042   Salter-Harris Type IV physeal fracture of left calcaneus
7th

• **S99.09**   Other physeal fracture
6th

• S99.091   Other physeal fracture of right calcaneus
7th

• S99.092   Other physeal fracture of left calcaneus
7th

• **S99.1**   Physeal fracture of right metatarsal
5th

• S99.10   Unspecified physeal fracture
6th

• S99.101   Unspecified physeal fracture of right metatarsal
7th

• S99.102   Unspecified physeal fracture of left metatarsal
7th

• S99.11   Salter-Harris Type I physeal fracture of metatarsal
6th

• S99.111   Salter-Harris Type I physeal fracture of right metatarsal
7th

• S99.112   Salter-Harris Type I physeal fracture of left metatarsal
7th

• S99.12   Salter-Harris Type II physeal fracture of metatarsal
6th

• S99.121   Salter-Harris Type II physeal fracture of right metatarsal
7th

> 7th characters for subcategory S99.1-, S99.2-
> A—initial encounter for closed fracture
> B—initial encounter for open fracture
> D—subsequent encounter for fracture with routine healing
> G—subsequent encounter for fracture with delayed healing
> K—subsequent encounter for fracture with nonunion
> P—subsequent encounter for fracture with malunion
> S—sequela

• S99.122   Salter-Harris Type II physeal fracture of left metatarsal
7th

• S99.13   Salter-Harris Type III physeal fracture of metatarsal
6th

• S99.131   Salter-Harris Type III physeal fracture of right metatarsal
7th

• S99.132   Salter-Harris Type III physeal fracture of left metatarsal
7th

• S99.14   Salter-Harris Type IV physeal fracture of metatarsal
6th

• S99.141   Salter-Harris Type IV physeal fracture of right metatarsal
7th

• S99.142   Salter-Harris Type IV physeal fracture of left metatarsal
7th

• S99.19   Other physeal fracture of metatarsal
6th

• S99.191   Other physeal fracture of right metatarsal
7th

  Additional Character Required   3-character code   Unspecified laterality codes were excluded here.   •=New Code   ▲=Revised Code   *Excludes1*—Not coded here, do not use together   *Excludes2*—Not included here

CHAPTER 19. INJURY, POISONING AND CERTAIN OTHER CONSEQUENCES OF EXTERNAL CAUSES (S99.192–T16.2XX)

- S99.192   Other physeal fracture of left metatarsal
  - 7th

- S99.2   Physeal fracture of phalanx of toe
  - S99.20   Unspecified physeal fracture of phalanx of toe
  - 5th
    - S99.201   Unspecified physeal fracture of phalanx of right toe
      - 7th
    - S99.202   Unspecified physeal fracture of phalanx of left toe
      - 7th
  - S99.21   Salter-Harris Type I physeal fracture of phalanx of toe
  - 6th
    - S99.211   Salter-Harris Type I physeal fracture of phalanx of right toe
      - 7th
    - S99.212   Salter-Harris Type I physeal fracture of phalanx of left toe
      - 7th
  - S99.22   Salter-Harris Type II physeal fracture of phalanx of toe
  - 6th
    - S99.221   Salter-Harris Type II physeal fracture of phalanx of right toe
      - 7th
    - S99.222   Salter-Harris Type II physeal fracture of phalanx of left toe
      - 7th
  - S99.23   Salter-Harris Type III physeal fracture of phalanx of toe
  - 6th
    - S99.231   Salter-Harris Type III physeal fracture of phalanx of right toe
      - 7th
    - S99.232   Salter-Harris Type III physeal fracture of phalanx of left toe
      - 7th
  - S99.24   Salter-Harris Type IV physeal fracture of phalanx of toe
  - 6th
    - S99.241   Salter-Harris Type IV physeal fracture of phalanx of right toe
      - 7th
    - S99.242   Salter-Harris Type IV physeal fracture of phalanx of left toe
      - 7th
  - S99.29   Other physeal fracture of phalanx of toe
  - 6th
    - S99.291   Other physeal fracture of phalanx of right toe
      - 7th
    - S99.292   Other physeal fracture of phalanx of left toe
      - 7th

- S99.8   Other specified injuries of ankle and foot
  - 5th
  - S99.81   Other specified injuries of: ankle
  - 6th
    - S99.811   right ankle
      - 7th
    - S99.812   left ankle
      - 7th
  - S99.82   Other specified injuries of foot
  - 6th
    - S99.821   Other specified injuries of right foot
      - 7th
    - S99.822   Other specified injuries of left foot
      - 7th

- S99.9   Unspecified injury of ankle and foot
  - 5th
  - S99.91   Unspecified injury of ankle
  - 6th
    - S99.911   Unspecified injury of right ankle
      - 7th
    - S99.912   Unspecified injury of left ankle
      - 7th

(T07–T88) INJURY, POISONING AND CERTAIN OTHER CONSEQUENCES OF EXTERNAL CAUSES

(T07) INJURIES INVOLVING MULTIPLE BODY REGIONS

Excludes1: burns and corrosions (T20–T32)
frostbite (T33–T34)
insect bite or sting, venomous (T63.4)
sunburn (L55.-)

Note: No 7th characters are assigned to categories T07 and T14.

T07   UNSPECIFIED MULTIPLE INJURIES
✔
    Excludes1: injury NOS (T14)

(T14) INJURY OF UNSPECIFIED BODY REGION

T14   INJURY OF UNSPECIFIED BODY REGION
4th
    Excludes1: multiple unspecified injuries (T07)
    T14.8   Other injury of unspecified body region
        Abrasion NOS
        Contusion NOS
        Crush injury NOS
        Fracture NOS
        Skin injury NOS
        Vascular injury NOS
    T14.9   Unspecified injury
        T14.90   Injury, unspecified
        5th   Injury NOS
        T14.91   Suicide attempt
        Attempted suicide NOS

(T15–T19) EFFECTS OF FB ENTERING THROUGH NATURAL ORIFICE

Excludes2: FB accidentally left in operation wound (T81.5-)
FB in penetrating wound—See open wound by body region
residual FB in soft tissue (M79.5)
splinter, without open wound—See superficial injury by body region

T15   FB ON EXTERNAL EYE
4th
    Excludes2: FB in penetrating wound of orbit and eye ball (S05.4-, S05.5-)
        open wound of eyelid and periocular area (S01.1-)
        retained FB in eyelid (H02.8-)
        retained (old) FB in penetrating wound of orbit and eye ball (H05.5-, H44.6-, H44.7-)
        superficial FB of eyelid and periocular area (S00.25-)
    T15.0   FB in cornea
        T15.01X FB in cornea, right eye
        5th
            7th
        T15.02X FB in cornea, left eye
            7th
    T15.1   FB in conjunctival sac
        T15.11X FB in conjunctival sac, right eye
        5th
            7th
        T15.12X FB in conjunctival sac, left eye
            7th

7th characters for category S99.8- and S99.9-
A—initial encounter
D—subsequent encounter
S—sequela

T16   FB IN EAR
4th
    Includes: FB in auditory canal
    T16.1XX FB in right ear
        7th
    T16.2XX FB in left ear
        7th

  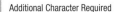 Additional Character Required   ✔ 3-character code   Unspecified laterality codes were excluded here.   •=New Code   ▲=Revised Code   ***Excludes1***—Not coded here, do not use together   ***Excludes2***—Not included here

T17   **FB IN RESPIRATORY TRACT**

`4th`

T17.0XX   **FB in nasal sinus**

`7th`

T17.1XX   **FB in nostril**
FB in nose NOS

`7th`

7th characters for category T17
A—initial encounter
D—subsequent encounter
S—sequela

T17.2   **FB in pharynx**
FB in nasopharynx
FB in throat NOS

`5th`

    T17.20   **Unspecified FB in pharynx**

`6th`

        T17.200   **Unspecified FB in pharynx causing asphyxiation**

`7th`

        T17.208   **Unspecified FB in pharynx causing other injury**

`7th`

    T17.22   **Food in pharynx**
Bones in pharynx
Seeds in pharynx

`6th`

        T17.220   **Food in pharynx causing asphyxiation**

`7th`

        T17.228   **Food in pharynx causing other injury**

`7th`

    T17.29   **Other foreign object in pharynx**

`6th`

        T17.290   **Other foreign object in pharynx causing asphyxiation**

`7th`

        T17.298   **Other foreign object in pharynx causing other injury**

`7th`

T17.3   **FB in larynx**

`5th`

    T17.30   **Unspecified FB in larynx**

`6th`

        T17.300   **Unspecified FB in larynx causing asphyxiation**

`7th`

        T17.308   **Unspecified FB in larynx causing other injury**

`7th`

    T17.31   **Gastric contents in larynx**
Aspiration of gastric contents into larynx
Vomitus in larynx

`6th`

        T17.310   **Gastric contents in larynx causing asphyxiation**

`7th`

        T17.318   **Gastric contents in larynx causing other injury**

`7th`

    T17.32   **Food in larynx**
Bones in larynx
Seeds in larynx

`6th`

        T17.320   **Food in larynx causing asphyxiation**

`7th`

        T17.328   **Food in larynx causing other injury**

`7th`

    T17.39   **Other foreign object in larynx**

`6th`

        T17.390   **Other foreign object in larynx causing asphyxiation**

`7th`

        T17.398   **Other foreign object in larynx causing other injury**

`7th`

T17.9   **FB in respiratory tract, part unspecified**

`5th`

    T17.90   **Unspecified FB in respiratory tract, part unspecified**

`6th`

        T17.900   **Unspecified FB in respiratory tract, part unspecified causing asphyxiation**

`7th`

        T17.908   **Unspecified FB in respiratory tract, part unspecified causing other injury**

`7th`

    T17.91   **Gastric contents in respiratory tract, part unspecified**
Aspiration of gastric contents into respiratory tract, part unspecified
Vomitus in trachea respiratory tract, part unspecified

`6th`

        T17.910   **Gastric contents in respiratory tract, part unspecified causing asphyxiation**

`7th`

        T17.918   **Gastric contents in respiratory tract, part unspecified causing other injury**

`7th`

    T17.92   **Food in respiratory tract, part unspecified**
Bones in respiratory tract, part unspecified
Seeds in respiratory tract, part unspecified

`6th`

        T17.920   **Food in respiratory tract, part unspecified causing asphyxiation**

`7th`

        T17.928   **Food in respiratory tract, part unspecified causing other injury**

`7th`

    T17.99   **Other foreign object in respiratory tract, part unspecified**

`6th`

        T17.990   **Other foreign object in respiratory tract, part unspecified in causing asphyxiation**

`7th`

        T17.998   **Other foreign object in respiratory tract, part unspecified causing other injury**

`7th`

T18   **FB IN ALIMENTARY TRACT**

`4th`

Excludes2: FB in pharynx (T17.2-)

T18.1   **FB in esophagus**

`5th`

Excludes2: FB in respiratory tract (T17.-)

7th characters for category T18
A—initial encounter
D—subsequent encounter
S—sequela

    T18.10   **Unspecified FB in esophagus**

`6th`

        T18.100   **Unspecified FB in esophagus causing compression of trachea**
Unspecified FB in esophagus causing obstruction of respiration

`7th`

        T18.108   **Unspecified FB in esophagus causing other injury**

`7th`

    T18.11   **Gastric contents in esophagus**
Vomitus in esophagus

`6th`

        T18.110   **Gastric contents in esophagus causing compression of trachea**
Gastric contents in esophagus causing obstruction of respiration

`7th`

        T18.118   **Gastric contents in esophagus causing other injury**

`7th`

    T18.12   **Food in esophagus**
Bones in esophagus
Seeds in esophagus

`6th`

        T18.120   **Food in esophagus causing compression of trachea**

`7th`

        T18.128   **Food in esophagus causing other injury**

`7th`

    T18.19   **Other foreign object in esophagus**

`6th`

        T18.190   **Other foreign object in esophagus causing compression of trachea**
Other FB in esophagus causing obstruction of respiration

`7th`

        T18.198   **Other foreign object in esophagus causing other injury**

`7th`

 `4th`   `5th`   `6th`   `7th`   Additional Character Required   ✓   3-character code

Unspecified laterality codes were excluded here.

•=New Code
▲=Revised Code

Excludes1—Not coded here, do not use together
Excludes2—Not included here

CHAPTER 19. INJURY, POISONING AND CERTAIN OTHER CONSEQUENCES OF EXTERNAL CAUSES   (T18.2XX–T20.012)

T18.2XX **FB in stomach**
`7th`

T18.3XX **FB in small intestine**
`7th`

T18.8 **FB in other parts of alimentary tract**
`7th`

T18.9XX **FB of alimentary tract, part unspecified**
`7th` FB in digestive system NOS
Swallowed FB NOS

T19 **FB IN XX GENITOURINARY TRACT**
`4th` ***Excludes2:*** complications due to implanted mesh (T83.7-)
mechanical complications of
contraceptive device (intrauterine)
(vaginal) (T83.3-)
presence of contraceptive device
(intrauterine) (vaginal) (Z97.5)

7th characters for category T19
A—initial encounter
D—subsequent encounter
S—sequela

T19.0XX **FB in urethra**
`7th`

T19.2XX **FB in vulva and vagina**
`7th`

T19.4XX **FB in penis**
`7th`

T19.8XX **FB in other parts of genitourinary tract**
`7th`

T19.9XX **FB in genitourinary tract, part unspecified**
`7th`

(T20–T32) BURNS AND CORROSIONS

GUIDELINES

The *ICD-10-CM* makes a distinction between burns and corrosions. The burn codes are for thermal burns, except sunburns, that come from a heat source, such as a fire or hot appliance. The burn codes are also for burns resulting from electricity and radiation. Corrosions are burns due to chemicals. The guidelines are the same for burns and corrosions.

Current burns (T20–T25) are classified by depth, extent and by agent (X code). Burns are classified by depth as first degree (erythema), second degree (blistering), and third degree (full-thickness involvement). Burns of the eye and internal organs (T26–T28) are classified by site, but not by degree.

Sequencing of burn and related condition codes

Sequence first the code that reflects the highest degree of burn when more than one burn is present.

When the reason for the admission or encounter is for treatment of external multiple burns, sequence first the code that reflects the burn of the highest degree.

When a patient has both internal and external burns, the circumstances of admission govern the selection of the principal diagnosis or first-listed diagnosis.

When a patient is admitted for burn injuries and other related conditions such as smoke inhalation and/or respiratory failure, the circumstances of admission govern the selection of the principal or first-listed diagnosis. Burns of the same local site

Classify burns

of the same local site (three-character category level, T20–T28) but of different degrees to the subcategory identifying the highest degree recorded in the diagnosis.

Non-healing burns

Non-healing burns are coded as acute burns.
Necrosis of burned skin should be coded as a non-healed burn.

Infected burn

For any documented infected burn site, use an additional code for the infection.

Assign separate codes for each burn site

When coding burns, assign separate codes for each burn site. Category T30, Burn and corrosion, body region unspecified is extremely vague and should rarely be used.

Burns and corrosions classified according to extent of body surface involved

Refer to category T31 for guidelines.

Encounters for treatment of sequela of burns

Encounters for the treatment of the late effects of burns or corrosions (i.e., scars or joint contractures) should be coded with a burn or corrosion code with the 7th character S for sequela.

Sequelae with a late effect code and current burn

When appropriate, both a code for a current burn or corrosion with 7th character A or D and a burn or corrosion code with 7th character S may be assigned on the same record (when both a current burn and sequelae of an old burn exist). Burns and corrosions do not heal at the same rate and a current healing wound may still exist with sequela of a healed burn or corrosion.

Use of an external cause code with burns and corrosions

An external cause code should be used with burns and corrosions to identify the source and intent of the burn, as well as the place where it occurred.

Includes: burns (thermal) from electrical heating appliances
burns (thermal) from electricity
burns (thermal) from flame
burns (thermal) from friction
burns (thermal) from hot air and hot gases
burns (thermal) from hot objects
burns (thermal) from lightning
burns (thermal) from radiation
chemical burn [corrosion] (external) (internal)
scalds
Excludes2: erythema [dermatitis] ab igne (L59.0)
radiation-related disorders of the skin and subcutaneous tissue (L55–L59)
sunburn (L55.-)

(T20–T25) BURNS AND CORROSIONS OF EXTERNAL BODY SURFACE, SPECIFIED BY SITE

Includes: burns and corrosions of first degree [erythema]
burns and corrosions of second degree [blisters]
[epidermal loss]
burns and corrosions of third degree [deep
necrosis of underlying tissue]
[full- thickness skin loss]

7th characters for categories T20–T25
A—initial encounter
D—subsequent encounter
S—sequela

Use additional code from category T31 or T32 to identify extent of body surface involved

T20 **BURN AND CORROSION OF HEAD, FACE, AND NECK**
`4th` ***Excludes2:*** burn and corrosion of ear drum (T28.41, T28.91)
burn and corrosion of eye and adnexa (T26.-)
burn and corrosion of mouth and pharynx (T28.0)

T20.0 **Burn of unspecified degree of head, face, and neck**
`5th` **Use additional external cause code** to identify the source, place and intent of the burn (X00–X19, X75–X77, X96–X98, Y92)

T20.00X **Burn of unspecified degree of head,**
`7th` **face, and neck, unspecified site**

T20.01 **Burn of unspecified degree of ear [any part,**
`6th` **except ear drum]**
Excludes2: burn of ear drum (T28.41-)

T20.011 **Burn of unspecified degree of right**
`7th` **ear [any part, except ear drum]**

T20.012 **Burn of unspecified degree of left ear**
`7th` **[any part, except ear drum]**

  Additional Character Required   3-character code

Unspecified laterality codes were excluded here.   •=New Code   ▲=Revised Code   ***Excludes1***—Not coded here, do not use together   ***Excludes2***—Not included here

348   PEDIATRIC ICD-10-CM 2017: A MANUAL FOR PROVIDER-BASED CODING

T20.02X [7th] Burn of unspecified degree of lip(s)

T20.03X [7th] Burn of unspecified degree of chin

T20.04X [7th] Burn of unspecified degree of nose (septum)

T20.05X [7th] Burn of unspecified degree of scalp [any part]

T20.06X [7th] Burn of unspecified degree of forehead and cheek

T20.07X [7th] Burn of unspecified degree of neck, initial encounter

T20.09X [7th] Burn of unspecified degree of multiple sites of head, face, and neck

T20.1 [5th] **Burn of first degree of head, face, and neck**
Use additional external cause code to identify the source, place and intent of the burn (X00–X19, X75–X77, X96–X98, Y92)

T20.10X [7th] Burn of first degree of head, face, and neck, unspecified site

T20.11 [6th] **Burn of first degree of ear [any part, except ear drum]**
Excludes2: burn of ear drum (T28.41-)

  T20.111 [7th] Burn of first degree of right ear [any part, except ear drum]

  T20.112 [7th] Burn of first degree of left ear [any part, except ear drum]

  T20.119 [7th] Burn of first degree of unspecified ear [any part, except ear drum]

T20.12X [7th] Burn of first degree of lip(s)

T20.13X [7th] Burn of first degree of chin

T20.14X [7th] Burn of first degree of nose (septum)

T20.15X [7th] Burn of first degree of scalp [any part]

T20.16X [7th] Burn of first degree of forehead and cheek

T20.17X [7th] Burn of first degree of neck

T20.19X [7th] Burn of first degree of multiple sites of head, face, and neck

T20.2 [5th] **Burn of second degree of head, face, and neck**
Use additional external cause code to identify the source, place and intent of the burn (X00–X19, X75–X77, X96–X98, Y92)

T20.20X [7th] Burn of second degree of head, face, and neck, unspecified site

T20.21 [6th] **Burn of second degree of ear [any part, except ear drum]**
Excludes2: burn of ear drum (T28.41-)

T20.211 [7th] Burn of second degree of right ear [any part, except ear drum]

T20.212 [7th] Burn of second degree of left ear [any part, except ear drum]

T20.219 [7th] Burn of second degree of unspecified ear [any part, except ear drum]

T20.22X [7th] Burn of second degree of lip(s)

T20.23X [7th] Burn of second degree of chin

T20.24X [7th] Burn of second degree of nose (septum)

T20.25X [7th] Burn of second degree of scalp [any part]

T20.26X [7th] Burn of second degree of forehead and cheek

T20.27X [7th] Burn of second degree of neck

T20.29X [7th] Burn of second degree of multiple sites of head, face, and neck

T20.3 [5th] **Burn of third degree of head, face, and neck**
Use additional external cause code to identify the source, place and intent of the burn (X00–X19, X75–X77, X96–X98, Y92)

T20.30X [7th] Burn of third degree of head, face, and neck, unspecified site

T20.31 [6th] **Burn of third degree of ear [any part, except ear drum]**
Excludes2: burn of ear drum (T28.41-)

  T20.311 [7th] Burn of third degree of right ear [any part, except ear drum]

  T20.312 [7th] Burn of third degree of left ear [any part, except ear drum]

  T20.319 [7th] Burn of third degree of unspecified ear [any part, except ear drum]

T20.32X [7th] Burn of third degree of lip(s)

T20.33X [7th] Burn of third degree of chin

T20.34X [7th] Burn of third degree of nose (septum)

T20.35X [7th] Burn of third degree of scalp [any part]

T20.36X [7th] Burn of third degree of forehead and cheek

T20.37X [7th] Burn of third degree of neck

T20.39X [7th] Burn of third degree of multiple sites of head, face, and neck

> 7th characters for categories
> T20–T25
> A—initial encounter
> D—subsequent encounter
> S—sequela

  4th 5th 6th 7th Additional Character Required

 3-character code

Unspecified laterality codes were excluded here.

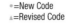 •=New Code
▲=Revised Code

Excludes1—Not coded here, do not use together
Excludes2—Not included here

(left margin, vertical text) CHAPTER 19. INJURY, POISONING AND CERTAIN OTHER CONSEQUENCES OF EXTERNAL CAUSES   (T21–T21.39X)

T21   BURN AND CORROSION OF TRUNK
4th

Includes: burns and corrosion of hip region
Excludes2: burns and corrosion of axilla (T22.- with fifth character 4)
burns and corrosion of scapular region (T22.- with fifth character 6)
burns and corrosion of shoulder (T22.- with fifth character 5)

T21.0   Burn of unspecified degree of trunk
5th
Use additional external cause code to identify the source, place and intent of the burn (X00–X19, X75–X77, X96–X98, Y92)

T21.00X   Burn of unspecified degree of trunk, unspecified site
7th

7th characters for categories
T20–T25
A—initial encounter
D—subsequent encounter
S—sequela

T21.01X   Burn of unspecified degree of chest wall
7th   Burn of unspecified degree of breast

T21.02X   Burn of unspecified degree of abdominal wall
7th   Burn of unspecified degree of flank or of groin

T21.03X   Burn of unspecified degree of upper back
7th   Burn of unspecified degree of interscapular region

T21.04X   Burn of unspecified degree of lower back
7th

T21.05X   Burn of unspecified degree of buttock
7th   Burn of unspecified degree of anus

T21.06X   Burn of unspecified degree of male genital region
7th   Burn of unspecified degree of penis or of scrotum or of testis

T21.07X   Burn of unspecified degree of female genital region
7th   Burn of unspecified degree of labium (majus) (minus) or of perineum
Burn of unspecified degree of vulva
Excludes2: burn of vagina (T28.3)

T21.09X   Burn of unspecified degree of other site of trunk
7th

T21.1   Burn of first degree of trunk
5th
Use additional external cause code to identify the source, place and intent of the burn (X00–X19, X75–X77, X96–X98, Y92)

T21.10X   Burn of first degree of trunk, unspecified site
7th

T21.11X   Burn of first degree of chest wall
7th   Burn of first degree of breast

T21.12X   Burn of first degree of abdominal wall
7th   Burn of first degree of flank OR OF GROIN

T21.13X   Burn of first degree of upper back
7th   Burn of first degree of interscapular region

T21.14X   Burn of first degree of lower back
7th

T21.15X   Burn of first degree of buttock
7th   Burn of first degree of anus

T21.16X   Burn of first degree of male genital region
7th   Burn of first degree of penis or of scrotum or of testis

7th characters for categories
T20–T25
A—initial encounter
D—subsequent encounter
S—sequela

T21.17X   Burn of first degree of female genital region
7th   Burn of first degree of labium (majus) (minus) or of perineum
Burn of first degree of vulva
Excludes2: burn of vagina (T28.3)

T21.19X   Burn of first degree of other site of trunk
7th

T21.2   Burn of second degree of trunk
5th
Use additional external cause code to identify the source, place and intent of the burn (X00–X19, X75–X77, X96–X98, Y92)

T21.20X   Burn of second degree of trunk, unspecified site
7th

T21.21X   Burn of second degree of chest wall
7th   Burn of second degree of breast

T21.22X   Burn of second degree of abdominal wall
7th   Burn of second degree of flank or of groin

T21.23X   Burn of second degree of upper back
7th   Burn of second degree of interscapular region

T21.24X   Burn of second degree of lower back
7th

T21.25X   Burn of second degree of buttock
7th   Burn of second degree of anus

T21.26X   Burn of second degree of male genital region
7th   Burn of second degree of penis or of scrotum or of testis

T21.27X   Burn of second degree of female genital region
7th   Burn of second degree of labium (majus) (minus) or of perineum
Burn of second degree of vulva
Excludes2: burn of vagina (T28.3)

T21.29X   Burn of second degree of other site of trunk
7th

T21.3   Burn of third degree of trunk
5th
Use additional external cause code to identify the source, place and intent of the burn (X00–X19, X75–X77, X96–X98, Y92)

T21.30X   Burn of third degree of trunk, unspecified site
7th

T21.31X   Burn of third degree of chest wall
7th   Burn of third degree of breast

T21.32X   Burn of third degree of abdominal wall
7th   Burn of third degree of flank OR GROIN

T21.33X   Burn of third degree of upper back
7th   Burn of third degree of interscapular region

T21.34X   Burn of third degree of lower back
7th

T21.35X   Burn of third degree of buttock
7th   Burn of third degree of anus

T21.36X   Burn of third degree of male genital region
7th   Burn of third degree of penis or of scrotum or of testis

T21.37X   Burn of third degree of female genital region
7th   Burn of third degree of labium (majus) (minus)
Burn of third degree of perineum
Burn of third degree of vulva
Excludes2: burn of vagina (T28.3)

T21.39X   Burn of third degree of other site of trunk
7th

  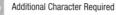 Additional Character Required   ✓ 3-character code

Unspecified laterality codes were excluded here.
•=New Code
▲=Revised Code
Excludes1—Not coded here, do not use together
Excludes2—Not included here

350   PEDIATRIC ICD-10-CM 2017: A MANUAL FOR PROVIDER-BASED CODING

T22 **BURN AND CORROSION OF SHOULDER AND UPPER LIMB, EXCEPT WRIST AND HAND**
`4th`

Excludes2: burn and corrosion of interscapular region (T21.-)
burn and corrosion of wrist and hand (T23.-)

T22.0 **Burn of unspecified degree of shoulder and upper limb, except wrist and hand**
`5th`

Use additional external cause code to identify the source, place and intent of the burn (X00–X19, X75–X77, X96–X98, Y92)

> 7th characters for categories
> T20–T25
> A—initial encounter
> D—subsequent encounter
> S—sequela

T22.00X **Burn of unspecified degree of shoulder and upper limb, except wrist and hand, unspecified site**
`7th`

T22.01 **Burn of unspecified degree of forearm**
`6th`

    T22.011 **Burn of unspecified degree of right forearm**
    `7th`

    T22.012 **Burn of unspecified degree of left forearm**
    `7th`

T22.02 **Burn of unspecified degree of elbow**
`6th`

    T22.021 **Burn of unspecified degree of right elbow**
    `7th`

    T22.022 **Burn of unspecified degree of left elbow**
    `7th`

T22.03 **Burn of unspecified degree of upper arm**
`6th`

    T22.031 **Burn of unspecified degree of right upper arm**
    `7th`

    T22.032 **Burn of unspecified degree of left upper arm**
    `7th`

T22.04 **Burn of unspecified degree of axilla**
`6th`

    T22.041 **Burn of unspecified degree of right axilla**
    `7th`

    T22.042 **Burn of unspecified degree of left axilla**
    `7th`

T22.05 **Burn of unspecified degree of shoulder**
`6th`

    T22.051 **Burn of unspecified degree of right shoulder**
    `7th`

    T22.052 **Burn of unspecified degree of left shoulder**
    `7th`

T22.06 **Burn of unspecified degree of scapular region**
`6th`

    T22.061 **Burn of unspecified degree of right scapular region**
    `7th`

    T22.062 **Burn of unspecified degree of left scapular region**
    `7th`

T22.09 **Burn of unspecified degree of multiple sites of shoulder and upper limb, except wrist and hand**
`6th`

    T22.091 **Burn of unspecified degree of multiple sites of right shoulder and upper limb, except wrist and hand**
    `7th`

    T22.092 **Burn of unspecified degree of multiple sites of left shoulder and upper limb, except wrist and hand**
    `7th`

T22.1 **Burn of first degree of shoulder and upper limb, except wrist and hand**
`5th`

Use additional external cause code to identify the source, place and intent of the burn (X00–X19, X75–X77, X96–X98, Y92)

T22.10X **Burn of first degree of shoulder and upper limb, except wrist and hand, unspecified site**
`7th`

T22.11 **Burn of first degree of forearm**
`6th`

    T22.111 **Burn of first degree of right forearm**
    `7th`

    T22.112 **Burn of first degree of left forearm**
    `7th`

T22.12 **Burn of first degree of elbow**
`6th`

    T22.121 **Burn of first degree of right elbow**
    `7th`

    T22.122 **Burn of first degree of left elbow**
    `7th`

T22.13 **Burn of first degree of upper arm**
`6th`

    T22.131 **Burn of first degree of right upper arm**
    `7th`

    T22.132 **Burn of first degree of left upper arm**
    `7th`

T22.14 **Burn of first degree of axilla**
`6th`

    T22.141 **Burn of first degree of right axilla**
    `7th`

    T22.142 **Burn of first degree of left axilla**
    `7th`

T22.15 **Burn of first degree of shoulder**
`6th`

    T22.151 **Burn of first degree of right shoulder**
    `7th`

    T22.152 **Burn of first degree of left shoulder**
    `7th`

T22.16 **Burn of first degree of scapular region**
`6th`

    T22.161 **Burn of first degree of right scapular region**
    `7th`

    T22.162 **Burn of first degree of left scapular region**
    `7th`

T22.19 **Burn of first degree of multiple sites of shoulder and upper limb, except wrist and hand**
`6th`

    T22.191 **Burn of first degree of multiple sites of right shoulder and upper limb, except wrist and hand**
    `7th`

    T22.192 **Burn of first degree of multiple sites of left shoulder and upper limb, except wrist and hand**
    `7th`

    T22.199 **Burn of first degree of multiple sites of unspecified shoulder and upper limb, except wrist and hand**
    `7th`

T22.2 **Burn of second degree of shoulder and upper limb, except wrist and hand**
`5th`

Use additional external cause code to identify the source, place and intent of the burn (X00–X19, X75–X77,X96–X98, Y92)

T22.20X **Burn of second degree of shoulder and upper limb, except wrist and hand, unspecified site**
`7th`

T22.21 **Burn of second degree of forearm**
`6th`

    T22.211 **Burn of second degree of right forearm**
    `7th`

    T22.212 **Burn of second degree of left forearm**
    `7th`

    T22.219 **Burn of second degree of unspecified forearm**
    `7th`

   Additional Character Required ✔ 3-character code   Unspecified laterality codes were excluded here.   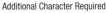=New Code =Revised Code   **Excludes1**—Not coded here, do not use together **Excludes2**—Not included here

CHAPTER 19. INJURY, POISONING AND CERTAIN OTHER CONSEQUENCES OF EXTERNAL CAUSES   (T22.22–T23.04)

T22.22 Burn of second degree of elbow
- **T22.221** [6th] Burn of second degree of right elbow [7th]
- **T22.222** Burn of second degree of left elbow [7th]

T22.23 Burn of second degree of upper arm
- **T22.231** [6th] Burn of second degree of right upper arm [7th]
- **T22.232** Burn of second degree of left upper arm [7th]

T22.24 Burn of second degree of axilla
- **T22.241** [6th] Burn of second degree of right axilla [7th]
- **T22.242** Burn of second degree of left axilla [7th]

T22.25 Burn of second degree of shoulder
- **T22.251** [6th] Burn of second degree of right shoulder [7th]
- **T22.252** Burn of second degree of left shoulder [7th]

T22.26 Burn of second degree of scapular region
- **T22.261** [6th] Burn of second degree of right scapular region [7th]
- **T22.262** Burn of second degree of left scapular region [7th]

T22.29 Burn of second degree of multiple sites of shoulder and upper limb, except wrist and hand
- **T22.291** [6th] Burn of second degree of multiple sites of right shoulder and upper limb, except wrist and hand [7th]
- **T22.292** Burn of second degree of multiple sites of left shoulder and upper limb, except wrist and hand [7th]

T22.3 [5th] Burn of third degree of shoulder and upper limb, except wrist and hand
Use additional external cause code to identify the source, place and intent of the burn (X00–X19, X75–X77, X96–X98, Y92)

T22.31 Burn of third degree of forearm
- **T22.311** [6th] Burn of third degree of right forearm [7th]
- **T22.312** Burn of third degree of left forearm [7th]
- **T22.319** Burn of third degree of unspecified forearm [7th]

T22.32 Burn of third degree of elbow
- **T22.321** [6th] Burn of third degree of right elbow [7th]
- **T22.322** Burn of third degree of left elbow [7th]

T22.33 Burn of third degree of upper arm
- **T22.331** [6th] Burn of third degree of right upper arm [7th]
- **T22.332** Burn of third degree of left upper arm [7th]

T22.34 Burn of third degree of axilla
- **T22.341** [6th] Burn of third degree of right axilla [7th]
- **T22.342** Burn of third degree of left axilla [7th]

T22.35 Burn of third degree of shoulder
- **T22.351** [6th] Burn of third degree of right shoulder [7th]
- **T22.352** Burn of third degree of left shoulder [7th]

T22.36 Burn of third degree of scapular region
- **T22.361** [6th] Burn of third degree of right scapular region [7th]
- **T22.362** Burn of third degree of left scapular region [7th]

T22.39 Burn of third degree of multiple sites of shoulder and upper limb, except wrist and hand
- **T22.391** [6th] Burn of third degree of multiple sites of right shoulder and upper limb, except wrist and hand [7th]
- **T22.392** Burn of third degree of multiple sites of left shoulder and upper limb, except wrist and hand [7th]

T23 [4th] BURN AND CORROSION OF WRIST AND HAND

T23.0 Burn of unspecified degree of wrist and hand
[5th] Use additional external cause code to identify the source, place and intent of the burn (X00–X19, X75–X77, X96–X98, Y92)

T23.00 [6th] Burn of unspecified degree of hand, unspecified site

	7th characters for categories T20–T25
	A—initial encounter
	D—subsequent encounter
	S—sequela

- **T23.001** Burn of unspecified degree of right hand, unspecified site [7th]
- **T23.002** Burn of unspecified degree of left hand, unspecified site [7th]
- **T23.009** Burn of unspecified degree of unspecified hand, unspecified site [7th]

T23.01 Burn of unspecified degree of thumb (nail)
- **T23.011** [6th] Burn of unspecified degree of right thumb (nail) [7th]
- **T23.012** Burn of unspecified degree of left thumb (nail) [7th]

T23.02 Burn of unspecified degree of single finger (nail) except thumb
- **T23.021** [6th] Burn of unspecified degree of single right finger (nail) except thumb [7th]
- **T23.022** Burn of unspecified degree of single left finger (nail) except thumb [7th]

T23.03 Burn of unspecified degree of multiple fingers (nail), not including thumb
- **T23.031** [6th] Burn of unspecified degree of multiple right fingers (nail), not including thumb [7th]
- **T23.032** Burn of unspecified degree of multiple left fingers (nail), not including thumb [7th]

T23.04 [6th] Burn of unspecified degree of multiple fingers (nail), including thumb

---

  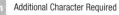 Additional Character Required   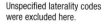 3-character code   Unspecified laterality codes were excluded here.   •=New Code   ▲=Revised Code   **Excludes1**—Not coded here, do not use together   **Excludes2**—Not included here

T23.041 Burn of unspecified degree of multiple right fingers (nail), including thumb `7th`

T23.042 Burn of unspecified degree of multiple left fingers (nail), including thumb `7th`

T23.05 `6th` Burn of unspecified degree of palm

T23.051 Burn of unspecified degree of right palm `7th`

T23.052 Burn of unspecified degree of left palm `7th`

T23.059 Burn of unspecified degree of unspecified palm `7th`

T23.06 `6th` Burn of unspecified degree of back of hand

T23.061 Burn of unspecified degree of back of right hand `7th`

T23.062 Burn of unspecified degree of back of left hand `7th`

T23.069 Burn of unspecified degree of back of unspecified hand `7th`

T23.07 `6th` Burn of unspecified degree of wrist

T23.071 Burn of unspecified degree of right wrist `7th`

T23.072 Burn of unspecified degree of left wrist `7th`

T23.09 `6th` Burn of unspecified degree of multiple sites of wrist and hand

T23.091 Burn of unspecified degree of multiple sites of right wrist and hand `7th`

T23.092 Burn of unspecified degree of multiple sites of left wrist and hand `7th`

T23.1 `5th` Burn of first degree of wrist and hand
Use additional external cause code to identify the source, place and intent of the burn (X00–X19, X75–X77, X96–X98, Y92)

T23.10 `6th` Burn of first degree of hand, unspecified site

T23.101 Burn of first degree of right hand, unspecified site `7th`

T23.102 Burn of first degree of left hand, unspecified site `7th`

T23.11 `6th` Burn of first degree of thumb (nail)

T23.111 Burn of first degree of right thumb (nail) `7th`

T23.112 Burn of first degree of left thumb (nail) `7th`

T23.12 `6th` Burn of first degree of single finger (nail) except thumb

T23.121 Burn of first degree of single right finger (nail) except thumb `7th`

T23.122 Burn of first degree of single left finger (nail) except thumb `7th`

7th characters for categories T20–T25
A—initial encounter
D—subsequent encounter
S—sequela

T23.13 `6th` Burn of first degree of multiple fingers (nail), not including thumb

T23.131 Burn of first degree of multiple right fingers (nail), not including thumb `7th`

T23.132 Burn of first degree of multiple left fingers (nail), not including thumb `7th`

T23.14 `6th` Burn of first degree of multiple fingers (nail), including thumb

T23.141 Burn of first degree of multiple right fingers (nail), including thumb `7th`

T23.142 Burn of first degree of multiple left fingers (nail), including thumb `7th`

T23.15 `6th` Burn of first degree of palm

T23.151 Burn of first degree of right palm `7th`

T23.152 Burn of first degree of left palm `7th`

T23.16 `6th` Burn of first degree of back of hand

T23.161 Burn of first degree of back of right hand `7th`

T23.162 Burn of first degree of back of left hand `7th`

T23.17 `6th` Burn of first degree of wrist

T23.171 Burn of first degree of right wrist `7th`

T23.172 Burn of first degree of left wrist `7th`

T23.19 `6th` Burn of first degree of multiple sites of wrist and hand

T23.191 Burn of first degree of multiple sites of right wrist and hand `7th`

T23.192 Burn of first degree of multiple sites of left wrist and hand `7th`

T23.2 `5th` Burn of second degree of wrist and hand
Use additional external cause code to identify the source, place and intent of the burn (X00–X19, X75–X77, X96–X98, Y92)

T23.20 `6th` Burn of second degree of hand, unspecified site

T23.201 Burn of second degree of right hand, unspecified site `7th`

T23.202 Burn of second degree of left hand, unspecified site `7th`

T23.21 `6th` Burn of second degree of thumb (nail)

T23.211 Burn of second degree of right thumb (nail) `7th`

T23.212 Burn of second degree of left thumb (nail) `7th`

T23.22 `6th` Burn of second degree of single finger (nail) except thumb

T23.221 Burn of second degree of single right finger (nail) except thumb `7th`

T23.222 Burn of second degree of single left finger (nail) except thumb `7th`

T23.23 `6th` Burn of second degree of multiple fingers (nail), not including thumb

---

  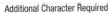 Additional Character Required ✓ 3-character code

Unspecified laterality codes were excluded here.

•=New Code
▲=Revised Code

Excludes1—Not coded here, do not use together
Excludes2—Not included here

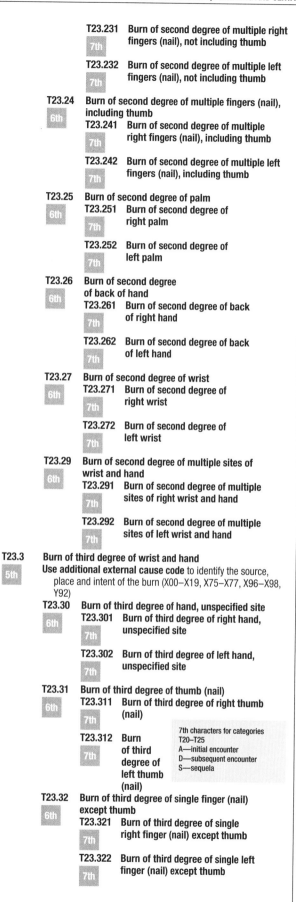

T23.231 Burn of second degree of multiple right fingers (nail), not including thumb [7th]

T23.232 Burn of second degree of multiple left fingers (nail), not including thumb [7th]

T23.24 [6th] Burn of second degree of multiple fingers (nail), including thumb

T23.241 Burn of second degree of multiple right fingers (nail), including thumb [7th]

T23.242 Burn of second degree of multiple left fingers (nail), including thumb [7th]

T23.25 [6th] Burn of second degree of palm

T23.251 Burn of second degree of right palm [7th]

T23.252 Burn of second degree of left palm [7th]

T23.26 [6th] Burn of second degree of back of hand

T23.261 Burn of second degree of back of right hand [7th]

T23.262 Burn of second degree of back of left hand [7th]

T23.27 [6th] Burn of second degree of wrist

T23.271 Burn of second degree of right wrist [7th]

T23.272 Burn of second degree of left wrist [7th]

T23.29 [6th] Burn of second degree of multiple sites of wrist and hand

T23.291 Burn of second degree of multiple sites of right wrist and hand [7th]

T23.292 Burn of second degree of multiple sites of left wrist and hand [7th]

T23.3 [5th] **Burn of third degree of wrist and hand**
Use additional external cause code to identify the source, place and intent of the burn (X00–X19, X75–X77, X96–X98, Y92)

T23.30 [6th] Burn of third degree of hand, unspecified site

T23.301 Burn of third degree of right hand, unspecified site [7th]

T23.302 Burn of third degree of left hand, unspecified site [7th]

T23.31 [6th] Burn of third degree of thumb (nail)

T23.311 Burn of third degree of right thumb (nail) [7th]

T23.312 [7th] Burn of third degree of left thumb (nail)

> 7th characters for categories
> T20–T25
> A—initial encounter
> D—subsequent encounter
> S—sequela

T23.32 [6th] Burn of third degree of single finger (nail) except thumb

T23.321 Burn of third degree of single right finger (nail) except thumb [7th]

T23.322 Burn of third degree of single left finger (nail) except thumb [7th]

T23.33 [6th] Burn of third degree of multiple fingers (nail), not including thumb

T23.331 Burn of third degree of multiple right fingers (nail), not including thumb [7th]

T23.332 Burn of third degree of multiple left fingers (nail), not including thumb [7th]

T23.34 [6th] Burn of third degree of multiple fingers (nail), including thumb

T23.341 Burn of third degree of multiple right fingers (nail), including thumb [7th]

T23.342 Burn of third degree of multiple left fingers (nail), including thumb [7th]

T23.35 [6th] Burn of third degree of palm

T23.351 Burn of third degree of right palm [7th]

T23.352 Burn of third degree of left palm [7th]

T23.36 [6th] Burn of third degree of back of hand

T23.361 Burn of third degree of back of right hand [7th]

T23.362 Burn of third degree of back of left hand [7th]

T23.37 [6th] Burn of third degree of wrist

T23.371 Burn of third degree of right wrist [7th]

T23.372 Burn of third degree of left wrist [7th]

T23.39 [6th] Burn of third degree of multiple sites of wrist and hand

T23.391 Burn of third degree of multiple sites of right wrist and hand [7th]

T23.392 Burn of third degree of multiple sites of left wrist and hand [7th]

T24 [4th] **BURN AND CORROSION OF LOWER LIMB, EXCEPT ANKLE AND FOOT**
Excludes2: burn and corrosion of ankle and foot (T25.-)
burn and corrosion of hip region (T21.-)

T24.0 [5th] **Burn of unspecified degree of lower limb, except ankle and foot**
Use additional external cause code to identify the source, place and intent of the burn (X00–X19, X75–X77, X96–X98, Y92)

> 7th characters for categories
> T20–T25
> A—initial encounter
> D—subsequent encounter
> S—sequela

T24.00 [6th] Burn of unspecified degree of unspecified site of lower limb, except ankle and foot

T24.001 Burn of unspecified degree of unspecified site of right lower limb, except ankle and foot [7th]

T24.002 Burn of unspecified degree of unspecified site of left lower limb, except ankle and foot [7th]

T24.01 [6th] Burn of unspecified degree of thigh

T24.011 Burn of unspecified degree of right thigh [7th]

T24.012 Burn of unspecified degree of left thigh [7th]

   Additional Character Required   3-character code   Unspecified laterality codes were excluded here.   •=New Code ▲=Revised Code   *Excludes1*—Not coded here, do not use together *Excludes2*—Not included here

354   **PEDIATRIC ICD-10-CM 2017: A MANUAL FOR PROVIDER-BASED CODING**

T24.02 Burn of unspecified degree of knee
 6th **T24.021** Burn of unspecified degree of right knee　**7th**

  T24.022 Burn of unspecified degree of left knee　**7th**

T24.03 Burn of unspecified degree of lower leg
 6th **T24.031** Burn of unspecified degree of right lower leg　**7th**

  T24.032 Burn of unspecified degree of left lower leg　**7th**

T24.09 Burn of unspecified degree of multiple sites of lower limb, except ankle and foot
 6th **T24.091** Burn of unspecified degree of multiple sites of right lower limb, except ankle and foot　**7th**

  T24.092 Burn of unspecified degree of multiple sites of left lower limb, except ankle and foot　**7th**

T24.1 Burn of first degree of lower limb, except ankle and foot
5th Use additional external cause code to identify the source, place and intent of the burn (X00–X19, X75–X77, X96–X98, Y92)

 T24.10 Burn of first degree of unspecified site of lower limb, except ankle and foot
 6th **T24.101** Burn of first degree of unspecified site of right lower limb, except ankle and foot　**7th**

  T24.102 Burn of first degree of unspecified site of left lower limb, except ankle and foot　**7th**

 T24.11 Burn of first degree of thigh
 6th **T24.111** Burn of first degree of right thigh　**7th**

  T24.112 Burn of first degree of left thigh　**7th**

 T24.12 Burn of first degree of knee
 6th **T24.121** Burn of first degree of right knee　**7th**

  T24.122 Burn of first degree of left knee　**7th**

 T24.13 Burn of first degree of lower leg
 6th **T24.131** Burn of first degree of right lower leg　**7th**

  T24.132 Burn of first degree of left lower leg　**7th**

 T24.19 Burn of first degree of multiple sites of lower limb, except ankle and foot
 6th **T24.191** Burn of first degree of multiple sites of right lower limb, except ankle and foot　**7th**

  T24.192 Burn of first degree of multiple sites of left lower limb, except ankle and foot　**7th**

T24.2 Burn of second degree of lower limb, except ankle and foot
5th Use additional external cause code to identify the source, place and intent of the burn (X00–X19, X75–X77, X96–X98, Y92)

 T24.20 Burn of second degree of unspecified site of lower limb, except ankle and foot
 6th **T24.201** Burn of second degree of unspecified site of right lower limb, except ankle and foot　**7th**

  T24.202 Burn of second degree of unspecified site of left lower limb, except ankle and foot　**7th**

T24.21 Burn of second degree of thigh
 6th **T24.211** Burn of second degree of right thigh　**7th**

  T24.212 Burn of second degree of left thigh　**7th**

> 7th characters for categories
> T20–T25
> A—initial encounter
> D—subsequent encounter
> S—sequela

T24.22 Burn of second degree of knee
 6th **T24.221** Burn of second degree of right knee　**7th**

  T24.222 Burn of second degree of left knee　**7th**

T24.23 Burn of second degree of lower leg
 6th **T24.231** Burn of second degree of right lower leg　**7th**

  T24.232 Burn of second degree of left lower leg　**7th**

T24.29 Burn of second degree of multiple sites of lower limb, except ankle and foot
 6th **T24.291** Burn of second degree of multiple sites of right lower limb, except ankle and foot　**7th**

  T24.292 Burn of second degree of multiple sites of left lower limb, except ankle and foot　**7th**

T24.3 Burn of third degree of lower limb, except ankle and foot
5th Use additional external cause code to identify the source, place and intent of the burn (X00–X19, X75–X77, X96–X98, Y92)

 T24.30 Burn of third degree of unspecified site of lower limb, except ankle and foot
 6th **T24.301** Burn of third degree of unspecified site of right lower limb, except ankle and foot　**7th**

  T24.302 Burn of third degree of unspecified site of left lower limb, except ankle and foot　**7th**

T24.31 Burn of third degree of thigh
 6th **T24.311** Burn of third degree of right thigh　**7th**

  T24.312 Burn of third degree of left thigh　**7th**

T24.32 Burn of third degree of knee
 6th **T24.321** Burn of third degree of right knee　**7th**

  T24.322 Burn of third degree of left knee　**7th**

T24.33 Burn of third degree of lower leg
 6th **T24.331** Burn of third degree of right lower leg　**7th**

  T24.332 Burn of third degree of left lower leg　**7th**

T24.39 Burn of third degree of multiple sites of lower limb, except ankle and foot
 6th **T24.391** Burn of third degree of multiple sites of right lower limb, except ankle and foot　**7th**

  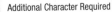 Additional Character Required　　✓ 3-character code　　Unspecified laterality codes were excluded here.　　◦=New Code　▲=Revised Code

Excludes1—Not coded here, do not use together
Excludes2—Not included here

CHAPTER 19. INJURY, POISONING AND CERTAIN OTHER CONSEQUENCES OF EXTERNAL CAUSES   (T24.392–T25.332)

T24.392   **7th**   Burn of third degree of multiple sites of left lower limb, except ankle and foot

T25   **4th**   **BURN AND CORROSION OF ANKLE AND FOOT**

T25.0   **5th**   Burn of unspecified degree of ankle and foot
Use additional external cause code to identify the source, place and intent of the burn (X00–X19, X75–X77, X96–X98, Y92)

> 7th characters for categories T20–T25
> A—initial encounter
> D—subsequent encounter
> S—sequela

T25.01   **6th**   Burn of unspecified degree of ankle

T25.011   **7th**   Burn of unspecified degree of right ankle

T25.012   **7th**   Burn of unspecified degree of left ankle

T25.02   **6th**   Burn of unspecified degree of foot
Excludes2: burn of unspecified degree of toe(s) (nail) (T25.03-)

T25.021   **7th**   Burn of unspecified degree of right foot

T25.022   **7th**   Burn of unspecified degree of left foot

T25.03   **6th**   Burn of unspecified degree of toe(s) (nail)

T25.031   **7th**   Burn of unspecified degree of right toe(s) (nail)

T25.032   **7th**   Burn of unspecified degree of left toe(s) (nail)

T25.09   **6th**   Burn of unspecified degree of multiple sites of ankle and foot

T25.091   **7th**   Burn of unspecified degree of multiple sites of right ankle and foot

T25.092   **7th**   Burn of unspecified degree of multiple sites of left ankle and foot

T25.1   **5th**   Burn of first degree of ankle and foot
Use additional external cause code to identify the source, place and intent of the burn (X00–X19, X75–X77, X96–X98, Y92)

T25.11   **6th**   Burn of first degree of ankle

T25.111   **7th**   Burn of first degree of right ankle

T25.112   **7th**   Burn of first degree of left ankle

T25.12   **6th**   Burn of first degree of foot
Excludes2: burn of first degree of toe(s) (nail) (T25.13-)

T25.121   **7th**   Burn of first degree of right foot

T25.122   **7th**   Burn of first degree of left foot

T25.13   **6th**   Burn of first degree of toe(s) (nail)

T25.131   **7th**   Burn of first degree of right toe(s) (nail)

T25.132   **7th**   Burn of first degree of left toe(s) (nail)

T25.19   **6th**   Burn of first degree of multiple sites of ankle and foot

T25.191   **7th**   Burn of first degree of multiple sites of right ankle and foot

T25.192   **7th**   Burn of first degree of multiple sites of left ankle and foot

T25.2   **5th**   Burn of second degree of ankle and foot
Use additional external cause code to identify the source, place and intent of the burn (X00–X19, X75–X77, X96–X98, Y92)

> 7th characters for category T25
> A—initial encounter
> D—subsequent encounter
> S—sequela

T25.21   **6th**   Burn of second degree of ankle

T25.211   **7th**   Burn of second degree of right ankle

T25.212   **7th**   Burn of second degree of left ankle

T25.22   **6th**   Burn of second degree of foot
Excludes2: burn of second degree of toe(s) (nail) (T25.23-)

T25.221   **7th**   Burn of second degree of right foot

T25.222   **7th**   Burn of second degree of left foot

T25.23   **6th**   Burn of second degree of toe(s) (nail)

T25.231   **7th**   Burn of second degree of right toe(s) (nail)

T25.232   **7th**   Burn of second degree of left toe(s) (nail)

T25.29   **6th**   Burn of second degree of multiple sites of ankle and foot

T25.291   **7th**   Burn of second degree of multiple sites of right ankle and foot

T25.292   **7th**   Burn of second degree of multiple sites of left ankle and foot

T25.3   **5th**   Burn of third degree of ankle and foot
Use additional external cause code to identify the source, place and intent of the burn (X00–X19, X75–X77, X96–X98, Y92)

T25.31   **6th**   Burn of third degree of ankle

T25.311   **7th**   Burn of third degree of right ankle

T25.312   **7th**   Burn of third degree of left ankle

T25.32   **6th**   Burn of third degree of foot
Excludes2: burn of third degree of toe(s) (nail) (T25.33–)

T25.321   **7th**   Burn of third degree of right foot

T25.322   **7th**   Burn of third degree of left foot

T25.33   **6th**   Burn of third degree of toe(s) (nail)

T25.331   **7th**   Burn of third degree of right toe(s) (nail)

T25.332   **7th**   Burn of third degree of left toe(s) (nail)

  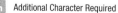

4th 5th 6th 7th Additional Character Required   ✓ 3-character code   Unspecified laterality codes were excluded here.   •=New Code   ▲=Revised Code   ***Excludes1***—Not coded here, do not use together   ***Excludes2***—Not included here

T25.39   Burn of third degree of multiple sites of ankle and foot

     T25.391   Burn of third degree of multiple sites of right ankle and foot

     T25.392   Burn of third degree of multiple sites of left ankle and foot

(T26–T28) BURNS AND CORROSIONS CONFINED TO EYE AND INTERNAL ORGANS

T26   **BURN AND CORROSION CONFINED TO EYE AND ADNEXA**

   T26.0   **Burn of eyelid and periocular area**

     Use additional external cause code to identify the source, place and intent of the burn (X00–X19, X75–X77, X96–X98, Y92)

> 7th characters for categories T26–T28
> A—initial encounter
> D—subsequent encounter
> S—sequela

     T26.01X   Burn of right eyelid and periocular area

     T26.02X   Burn of left eyelid and periocular area

T28   **BURN AND CORROSION OF OTHER INTERNAL ORGANS**

     Use additional external cause code to identify the source and intent of the burn (X00–X19, X75–X77, X96–X98) and external cause code to identify place (Y92)

     T28.0XX   Burn of mouth and pharynx

(T30–T32) BURNS AND CORROSIONS OF MULTIPLE AND UNSPECIFIED BODY REGIONS

T30   **BURN AND CORROSION, BODY REGION UNSPECIFIED**

   T30.0   **Burn of unspecified body region, unspecified degree**

     This code is not for inpatient use.

     Code to specified site and degree of burns

     Burn NOS

     Multiple burns NOS

> Note: No 7th characters are required for categories T30, T31, and T32.

   T30.4   **Corrosion of unspecified body region, unspecified degree**

     This code is not for inpatient use. Code to specified site and degree of corrosion

     Corrosion NOS

     Multiple corrosion NOS

T31   **BURNS CLASSIFIED ACCORDING TO EXTENT OF BODY SURFACE INVOLVED**

     Note: This category is to be used as the primary code only when the site of the burn is unspecified. It should be used as a supplementary code with categories T20–T25 when the site is specified.

     Please see full *ICD-10-CM* manual if reporting burns classified according to extent of body surface beyond 10% of body surface.

GUIDELINES

Assign codes from category T31, Burns classified according to extent of body surface involved, or T32, Corrosions classified according to extent of body surface involved, when the site of the burn is not specified or when there is a need for additional data. It is advisable to use category T31 as additional coding when needed to provide data for evaluating burn mortality, such as that needed by burn units. It is also advisable to use category T31 as an additional code for reporting purposes when there is mention of a third-degree burn involving 20 percent or more of the body surface.

Categories T31 and T32 are based on the classic "rule of nines" in estimating body surface involved: head and neck are assigned nine percent, each arm nine percent, each leg 18 percent, the anterior trunk 18 percent, posterior trunk 18 percent, and genitalia one percent.

Providers may change these percentage assignments where necessary to accommodate infants and children who have proportionately larger heads than adults, and patients who have large buttocks, thighs, or abdomen that involve burns.

     T31.0   Burns involving less than 10% of body surface

T32   **CORROSIONS CLASSIFIED ACCORDING TO EXTENT OF BODY SURFACE INVOLVED**

     Note: This category is to be used as the primary code only when the site of the corrosion is unspecified. It may be used as a supplementary code with categories T20–T25 when the site is specified.

     T32.0   Corrosions involving less than 10% of body surface

(T36–T50) POISONING BY, ADVERSE EFFECTS OF AND UNDERDOSING OF DRUGS, MEDICAMENTS AND BIOLOGICAL SUBSTANCES

GUIDELINES

Codes in categories T36–T65 are combination codes that include the substance that was taken as well as the intent. No additional external cause code is required for poisonings, toxic effects, adverse effects and underdosing codes.

Do not code directly from the Table of Drugs

Do not code directly from the Table of Drugs and Chemicals. Always refer back to the Tabular List. *Refer to the ICD-10-CM manual for the Table of Drugs.*

Use as many codes as necessary to describe

Use as many codes as necessary to describe completely all drugs, medicinal or biological substances.

If the same code would describe the causative agent

If the same code would describe the causative agent for more than one adverse reaction, poisoning, toxic effect or underdosing, assign the code only once.

If two or more drugs, medicinal or biological substances

If two or more drugs, medicinal or biological substances are reported, code each individually unless a combination code is listed in the Table of Drugs and Chemicals.

The occurrence of drug toxicity is classified in ICD-10-CM as follows:

ADVERSE EFFECT

When coding an adverse effect of a drug that has been correctly prescribed and properly administered, assign the appropriate code for the nature of the adverse effect followed by the appropriate code for the adverse effect of the drug (T36–T50). The code for the drug should have a 5th or 6th character "5" (for example T36.0X5-) Examples of the nature of an adverse effect are tachycardia, delirium, gastrointestinal hemorrhaging, vomiting, hypokalemia, hepatitis, renal failure, or respiratory failure.

POISONING

When coding a poisoning or reaction to the improper use of a medication (e.g., overdose, wrong substance given or taken in error, wrong route of administration), first assign the appropriate code from categories T36–T50. The poisoning codes have an associated intent as their 5th or 6th character (accidental, intentional self-harm, assault and undetermined. **Use additional code(s)** for all manifestations of poisonings.

If there is also a diagnosis of abuse or dependence of the substance, the abuse or dependence is assigned as an additional code.

Examples of poisoning include:

Error was made in drug prescription

Errors made in drug prescription or in the administration of the drug by provider, nurse, patient, or other person.

Overdose of a drug intentionally taken

If an overdose of a drug was intentionally taken or administered and resulted in drug toxicity, it would be coded as a poisoning.

  Additional Character Required   3-character code   Unspecified laterality codes were excluded here.   •=New Code   ▲=Revised Code   *Excludes1*—Not coded here, do not use together   *Excludes2*—Not included here

CHAPTER 19. INJURY, POISONING AND CERTAIN OTHER CONSEQUENCES OF EXTERNAL CAUSES (T36–T37.0X6)

Nonprescribed drug taken with correctly prescribed and properly administered drug

If a nonprescribed drug or medicinal agent was taken in combination with a correctly prescribed and properly administered drug, any drug toxicity or other reaction resulting from the interaction of the two drugs would be classified as a poisoning.

Interaction of drug(s) and alcohol

When a reaction results from the interaction of a drug(s) and alcohol, this would be classified as poisoning.

See Chapter 4 if poisoning is the result of insulin pump malfunctions.

UNDERDOSING

Underdosing refers to taking less of a medication than is prescribed by a provider or a manufacturer's instruction. For underdosing, assign the code from categories T36–T50 (fifth or sixth character "6").

Codes for underdosing should never be assigned as principal or first-listed codes. If a patient has a relapse or exacerbation of the medical condition for which the drug is prescribed because of the reduction in dose, then the medical condition itself should be coded.

Noncompliance (Z91.12-, Z91.13-) or complication of care (Y63.6–Y63.9) codes are to be used with an underdosing code to indicate intent, if known.

Toxic Effects

When a harmful substance is ingested or comes in contact with a person, this is classified as a toxic effect. The toxic effect codes are in categories T51–T65.

Toxic effect codes have an associated intent: accidental, intentional self-harm, assault and undetermined.

Includes: adverse effect of correct substance properly administered
  poisoning by overdose of substance
  poisoning by wrong substance given or taken in error
  underdosing by (inadvertently) (deliberately) taking less substance than
    prescribed or instructed
Code first, for adverse effects, the nature of the adverse effect, such as:
  adverse effect NOS (T88.7)
  aspirin gastritis (K29.-)
  blood disorders (D56–D76)
  contact dermatitis (L23–L25)
  dermatitis due to substances taken internally (L27.-)
  nephropathy (N14.0–N14.2)
Note: The drug giving rise to the adverse effect should be identified by use of codes from categories T36–T50 with fifth or sixth character 5.
Use additional code(s) to specify: manifestations of poisoning
  underdosing or failure in dosage during medical and surgical care (Y63.6, Y63.8–Y63.9)
  underdosing of medication regimen (Z91.12-, Z91.13-)
Excludes1: toxic reaction to local anesthesia in pregnancy (O29.3-)
Excludes2: abuse and dependence of psychoactive substances (F10–F19)
  abuse of non-dependence-producing substances (F55.-)
  drug reaction and poisoning affecting newborn (P00–P96)
  pathological drug intoxication (inebriation) (F10–F19)

T36 [4th] POISONING BY, ADVERSE EFFECT OF AND UNDERDOSING OF SYSTEMIC ANTIBIOTICS
  Excludes1: antineoplastic antibiotics (T45.1-)
    locally applied antibiotic NEC (T49.0)
    topically used antibiotic for ear, nose and throat (T49.6)
    topically used antibiotic for eye (T49.5)

  T36.0 [5th] Poisoning by, adverse effect of and underdosing of penicillins
    T36.0X [6th] Poisoning by, adverse effect of and underdosing of penicillins
      T36.0X1 [7th] Poisoning by penicillins, accidental (unintentional)
        Poisoning by penicillins NOS
      T36.0X5 [7th] Adverse effect of penicillins
      T36.0X6 [7th] Underdosing of penicillins

> 7th characters for categories T36–T50
> A—initial encounter
> D—subsequent encounter
> S—sequela

  T36.1 [5th] Poisoning by, adverse effect of and underdosing of cephalosporins and other beta-lactam antibiotics

  T36.1X [6th] Poisoning by, adverse effect of and underdosing of cephalosporins and other beta-lactam antibiotics
    T36.1X1 [7th] Poisoning by cephalosporins and other beta-lactam antibiotics, accidental (unintentional)
      Poisoning by cephalosporins and other beta-lactam antibiotics NOS
    T36.1X5 [7th] Adverse effect of cephalosporins and other beta-lactam antibiotics
    T36.1X6 [7th] Underdosing of cephalosporins and other beta-lactam antibiotics

  T36.3 [5th] Poisoning by, adverse effect of and underdosing of macrolides
    T36.3X [6th] Poisoning by, adverse effect of and underdosing of macrolides
      T36.3X1 [7th] Poisoning by macrolides, accidental (unintentional)
        Poisoning by macrolides NOS
      T36.3X5 [7th] Adverse effect of macrolides
      T36.3X6 [7th] Underdosing of macrolides

  T36.6 [5th] Poisoning by, adverse effect of and underdosing of rifampicins
    T36.6X [6th] Poisoning by, adverse effect of and underdosing of rifampicins
      T36.6X1 [7th] Poisoning by rifampicins, accidental (unintentional)
        Poisoning by rifampicins NOS
      T36.6X5 [7th] Adverse effect of rifampicins
      T36.6X6 [7th] Underdosing of rifampicins

  T36.8 [5th] Poisoning by, adverse effect of and underdosing of other systemic antibiotics
    T36.8X [6th] Poisoning by, adverse effect of and underdosing of other systemic antibiotics
      T36.8X1 [7th] Poisoning by other systemic antibiotics, accidental (unintentional)
        Poisoning by other systemic antibiotics NOS
      T36.8X5 [7th] Adverse effect of other systemic antibiotics
      T36.8X6 [7th] Underdosing of other systemic antibiotics

T37 [4th] POISONING BY, ADVERSE EFFECT OF AND UNDERDOSING OF OTHER SYSTEMIC ANTI-INFECTIVES AND ANTIPARASITICS
  Excludes1: anti-infectives topically used for ear, nose and throat (T49.6-)
    anti-infectives topically used for eye (T49.5-)
    locally applied anti-infectives NEC (T49.0-)

  T37.0 [5th] Poisoning by, adverse effect of and underdosing of sulfonamides
    T37.0X [6th] Poisoning by, adverse effect of and underdosing of sulfonamides
      T37.0X1 [7th] Poisoning by sulfonamides, accidental (unintentional)
        Poisoning by sulfonamides NOS
      T37.0X5 [7th] Adverse effect of sulfonamides
      T37.0X6 [7th] Underdosing of sulfonamides

  Additional Character Required   ✓ 3-character code   Unspecified laterality codes were excluded here.   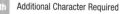 ●=New Code   ▲=Revised Code   *Excludes1*—Not coded here, do not use together   *Excludes2*—Not included here

T38 **POISONING BY, ADVERSE EFFECT OF AND UNDERDOSING OF HORMONES AND THEIR SYNTHETIC SUBSTITUTES AND ANTAGONISTS, NOT ELSEWHERE CLASSIFIED**

Excludes1: mineralocorticoids and their antagonists (T50.0-)
oxytocic hormones (T48.0-)
parathyroid hormones and derivatives (T50.9-)

T38.2 Poisoning by, adverse effect of and underdosing of antithyroid drugs

  T38.2X Poisoning by, adverse effect of and underdosing of antithyroid drugs

    T38.2X1 Poisoning by antithyroid drugs, accidental (unintentional)
      Poisoning by antithyroid drugs NOS

    T38.2X5 Adverse effect of antithyroid drugs

    T38.2X6 Underdosing of antithyroid drugs

T38.3 Poisoning by, adverse effect of and underdosing of insulin and oral hypoglycemic [antidiabetic] drugs

  T38.3X Poisoning by, adverse effect of and underdosing of insulin and oral hypoglycemic [antidiabetic] drugs

    T38.3X1 Poisoning by insulin and oral hypoglycemic [antidiabetic] drugs, accidental (unintentional)
      Poisoning by insulin and oral hypoglycemic [antidiabetic] drugs NOS

    T38.3X5 Adverse effect of insulin and oral hypoglycemic [antidiabetic] drugs

    T38.3X6 Underdosing of insulin and oral hypoglycemic [antidiabetic] drugs

T39 **POISONING BY, ADVERSE EFFECT OF AND UNDERDOSING OF NONOPIOID ANALGESICS, ANTIPYRETICS AND ANTIRHEUMATICS**

> 7th characters for categories
> T36–T50
> A—initial encounter
> D—subsequent encounter
> S—sequela

T39.0 Poisoning by, adverse effect of and underdosing of salicylates

  T39.01 Poisoning by, adverse effect of and underdosing of aspirin
  Poisoning by, adverse effect of and underdosing of acetylsalicylic acid

    T39.011 Poisoning by aspirin, accidental (unintentional)

    T39.012 Poisoning by aspirin, intentional self-harm

    T39.015 Adverse effect of aspirin

  T39.09 Poisoning by, adverse effect of and underdosing of other salicylates

    T39.091 Poisoning by salicylates, accidental (unintentional)
      Poisoning by salicylates NOS

    T39.092 Poisoning by salicylates, intentional self-harm

    T39.095 Adverse effect of salicylates

T39.1 Poisoning by, adverse effect of and underdosing of 4-Aminophenol derivatives

  T39.1X Poisoning by, adverse effect of and underdosing of 4-Aminophenol derivatives

    T39.1X1 Poisoning by 4-Aminophenol derivatives, accidental (unintentional)
      Poisoning by 4-Aminophenol derivatives NOS

    T39.1X2 Poisoning by 4-Aminophenol derivatives, intentional self-harm

    T39.1X5 Adverse effect of 4-Aminophenol derivatives

T39.3 Poisoning by, adverse effect of and underdosing of other nonsteroidal anti-inflammatory drugs [NSAID]

  T39.31 Poisoning by, adverse effect of and underdosing of propionic acid derivatives
  Poisoning by, adverse effect of and underdosing of fenoprofen/flurbiprofen/ ibuprofen/ketoprofen/ naproxen/oxaprozin

    T39.311 Poisoning by propionic acid derivatives, accidental (unintentional)

    T39.312 Poisoning by propionic acid derivatives, intentional self-harm

    T39.315 Adverse effect of propionic acid derivatives

  T39.39 Poisoning by, adverse effect of and under-dosing of other nonsteroidal anti-inflammatory drugs [NSAID]

    T39.391 Poisoning by other nonsteroidal anti-inflammatory drugs [NSAID], accidental (unintentional)
      Poisoning by other nonsteroidal anti-inflammatory drugs NOS

    T39.392 Poisoning by other nonsteroidal anti-inflammatory drugs [NSAID], intentional self-harm

    T39.395 Adverse effect of other nonsteroidal anti-inflammatory drugs [NSAID]

T40 **POISONING BY, ADVERSE EFFECT OF AND UNDERDOSING OF NARCOTICS AND PSYCHODYSLEPTICS [HALLUCINOGENS]**

Excludes2: drug dependence and related mental and behavioral disorders due to psychoactive substance use (F10.–F19.-)

T40.2 Poisoning by, adverse effect of and underdosing of other opioids

  T40.2X Poisoning by, adverse effect of and underdosing of other opioids

    T40.2X1 Poisoning by other opioids, accidental (unintentional)
      Poisoning by other opioids NOS

    T40.2X2 Poisoning by other opioids, intentional self-harm

    T40.2X5 Adverse effect of other opioids

T40.4 Poisoning by, adverse effect of and underdosing of other synthetic narcotics

  T40.4X Poisoning by, adverse effect of and underdosing of other synthetic narcotics

    T40.4X1 Poisoning by other synthetic narcotics, accidental (unintentional)
      Poisoning by other synthetic narcotics NOS

    T40.4X2 Poisoning by other synthetic narcotics, intentional self-harm

    T40.4X5 Adverse effect of other synthetic narcotics

  Additional Character Required　　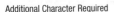 3-character code

Unspecified laterality codes were excluded here.　　•=New Code　▲=Revised Code

Excludes1—Not coded here, do not use together
Excludes2—Not included here

CHAPTER 19. INJURY, POISONING AND CERTAIN OTHER CONSEQUENCES OF EXTERNAL CAUSES   (T40.5–T43.3X6)

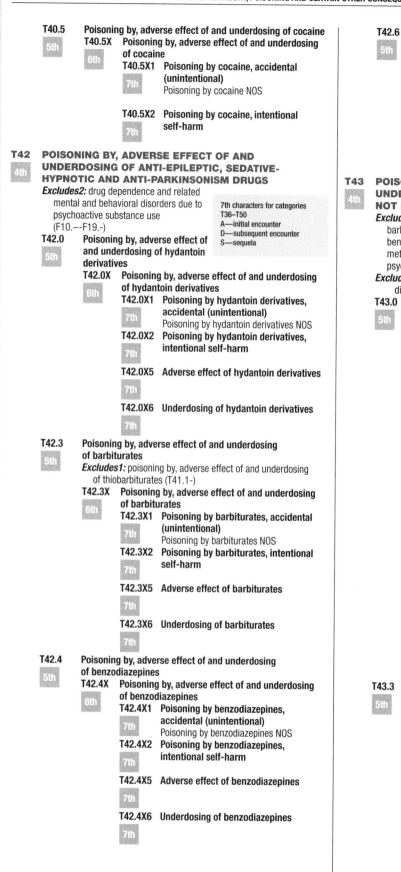

T40.5 **5th** Poisoning by, adverse effect of and underdosing of cocaine
   T40.5X **6th** Poisoning by, adverse effect of and underdosing of cocaine
      T40.5X1 **7th** Poisoning by cocaine, accidental (unintentional)
         Poisoning by cocaine NOS
      T40.5X2 **7th** Poisoning by cocaine, intentional self-harm

T42 **4th** **POISONING BY, ADVERSE EFFECT OF AND UNDERDOSING OF ANTI-EPILEPTIC, SEDATIVE-HYPNOTIC AND ANTI-PARKINSONISM DRUGS**
  Excludes2: drug dependence and related mental and behavioral disorders due to psychoactive substance use (F10.–-F19.-)

7th characters for categories T36–T50
A—initial encounter
D—subsequent encounter
S—sequela

T42.0 **5th** Poisoning by, adverse effect of and underdosing of hydantoin derivatives
   T42.0X **6th** Poisoning by, adverse effect of and underdosing of hydantoin derivatives
      T42.0X1 **7th** Poisoning by hydantoin derivatives, accidental (unintentional)
         Poisoning by hydantoin derivatives NOS
      T42.0X2 **7th** Poisoning by hydantoin derivatives, intentional self-harm
      T42.0X5 **7th** Adverse effect of hydantoin derivatives
      T42.0X6 **7th** Underdosing of hydantoin derivatives

T42.3 **5th** Poisoning by, adverse effect of and underdosing of barbiturates
  Excludes1: poisoning by, adverse effect of and underdosing of thiobarbiturates (T41.1-)
   T42.3X **6th** Poisoning by, adverse effect of and underdosing of barbiturates
      T42.3X1 **7th** Poisoning by barbiturates, accidental (unintentional)
         Poisoning by barbiturates NOS
      T42.3X2 **7th** Poisoning by barbiturates, intentional self-harm
      T42.3X5 **7th** Adverse effect of barbiturates
      T42.3X6 **7th** Underdosing of barbiturates

T42.4 **5th** Poisoning by, adverse effect of and underdosing of benzodiazepines
   T42.4X **6th** Poisoning by, adverse effect of and underdosing of benzodiazepines
      T42.4X1 **7th** Poisoning by benzodiazepines, accidental (unintentional)
         Poisoning by benzodiazepines NOS
      T42.4X2 **7th** Poisoning by benzodiazepines, intentional self-harm
      T42.4X5 **7th** Adverse effect of benzodiazepines
      T42.4X6 **7th** Underdosing of benzodiazepines

T42.6 **5th** Poisoning by, adverse effect of and underdosing of other antiepileptic and sedative-hypnotic drugs
  Poisoning by, adverse effect of and underdosing of methaqualone
  Poisoning by, adverse effect of and underdosing of valproic acid
  Excludes1: poisoning by, adverse effect of and underdosing of carbamazepine (T42.1-)
   T42.6X **6th** Poisoning by, adverse effect of and underdosing of other antiepileptic and sedative-hypnotic drugs
      T42.6X5 **7th** Adverse effect of other antiepileptic and sedative-hypnotic drugs

T43 **4th** **POISONING BY, ADVERSE EFFECT OF AND UNDERDOSING OF PSYCHOTROPIC DRUGS, NOT ELSEWHERE CLASSIFIED**
  Excludes1: appetite depressants (T50.5-)
    barbiturates (T42.3-)
    benzodiazepines (T42.4-)
    methaqualone (T42.6-)
    psychodysleptics [hallucinogens] (T40.7–T40.9-)
  Excludes2: drug dependence and related mental and behavioral disorders due to psychoactive substance use (F10.–-F19.-)

T43.0 **5th** Poisoning by, adverse effect of and underdosing of tricyclic and tetracyclic antidepressants
   T43.01 **6th** Poisoning by, adverse effect of and underdosing of tricyclic antidepressants
      T43.011 **7th** Poisoning by tricyclic antidepressants, accidental (unintentional)
         Poisoning by tricyclic antidepressants NOS
      T43.012 **7th** Poisoning by tricyclic antidepressants, intentional self-harm
      T43.015 **7th** Adverse effect of tricyclic antidepressants
      T43.016 **7th** Underdosing of tricyclic antidepressants
   T43.02 **6th** Poisoning by, adverse effect of and underdosing of tetracyclic antidepressants
      T43.021 **7th** Poisoning by tetracyclic antidepressants, accidental (unintentional)
         Poisoning by tetracyclic antidepressants NOS
      T43.022 **7th** Poisoning by tetracyclic antidepressants, intentional self-harm
      T43.025 **7th** Adverse effect of tetracyclic antidepressants
      T43.026 **7th** Underdosing of tetracyclic antidepressants

T43.3 **5th** Poisoning by, adverse effect of and underdosing of phenothiazine antipsychotics and neuroleptics
   T43.3X **6th** Poisoning by, adverse effect of and underdosing of phenothiazine antipsychotics and neuroleptics
      T43.3X1 **7th** Poisoning by phenothiazine antipsychotics and neuroleptics, accidental (unintentional)
         Poisoning by phenothiazine antipsychotics and neuroleptics NOS
      T43.3X2 **7th** Poisoning by phenothiazine antipsychotics and neuroleptics, intentional self-harm
      T43.3X5 **7th** Adverse effect of phenothiazine antipsychotics and neuroleptics
      T43.3X6 **7th** Underdosing of phenothiazine antipsychotics and neuroleptics

---

  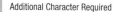 Additional Character Required   3-character code   Unspecified laterality codes were excluded here.   •=New Code   ▲=Revised Code   *Excludes1*—Not coded here, do not use together   *Excludes2*—Not included here

T43.6 Poisoning by, adverse effect of and underdosing of psychostimulants
`5th`

Excludes1: poisoning by, adverse effect of and underdosing of cocaine (T40.5-)

T43.62 Poisoning by, adverse effect of and underdosing of amphetamines
`6th`

Poisoning by, adverse effect of and underdosing of methamphetamines

T43.621 Poisoning by amphetamines, accidental (unintentional)
`7th`
Poisoning by amphetamines NOS

T43.622 Poisoning by amphetamines, intentional self-harm
`7th`

T43.625 Adverse effect of amphetamines
`7th`

T43.63 Poisoning by, adverse effect of and underdosing of methylphenidate
`6th`

T43.631 Poisoning by methylphenidate, accidental (unintentional)
`7th`
Poisoning by methylphenidate NOS

T43.632 Poisoning by methylphenidate, intentional self-harm
`7th`

T43.635 Adverse effect of methylphenidate
`7th`

T43.636 Underdosing of methylphenidate
`7th`

T43.9 Poisoning by, adverse effect of and underdosing of unspecified psychotropic drug
`5th`

T43.91X Poisoning by unspecified psychotropic drug, accidental (unintentional)
`7th`
Poisoning by psychotropic drug NOS

T43.92X Poisoning by unspecified psychotropic drug, intentional self-harm
`7th`

T43.95X Adverse effect of unspecified psychotropic drug
`7th`

T43.96X Underdosing of unspecified psychotropic drug
`7th`

T44 POISONING BY, ADVERSE EFFECT OF AND UNDERDOSING OF DRUGS PRIMARILY AFFECTING THE AUTONOMIC NERVOUS SYSTEM
`4th`

T44.5 Poisoning by, adverse effect of and underdosing of predominantly beta-adrenoreceptor agonists
`5th`

Excludes1: poisoning by, adverse effect of and underdosing of beta-adrenoreceptor agonists used in asthma therapy (T48.6-)

7th characters for categories T36–T50
A—initial encounter
D—subsequent encounter
S—sequela

T44.5X Poisoning by, adverse effect of and underdosing of predominantly beta-adrenoreceptor agonists
`6th`

T44.5X1 Poisoning by predominantly beta-adrenoreceptor agonists, accidental (unintentional)
`7th`
Poisoning by predominantly beta-adrenoreceptor agonists NOS

T44.5X2 Poisoning by predominantly beta-adrenoreceptor agonists, intentional self-harm
`7th`

T44.5X5 Adverse effect of predominantly beta-adrenoreceptor agonists
`7th`

T44.5X6 Underdosing of predominantly beta-adrenoreceptor agonists
`7th`

T45 POISONING BY, ADVERSE EFFECT OF AND UNDERDOSING OF PRIMARILY SYSTEMIC AND HEMATOLOGICAL AGENTS, NOT ELSEWHERE CLASSIFIED
`4th`

T45.0 Poisoning by, adverse effect of and underdosing of antiallergic and antiemetic drugs
`5th`

Excludes1: poisoning by, adverse effect of and underdosing of phenothiazine-based neuroleptics (T43.3)

T45.0X Poisoning by, adverse effect of and underdosing of antiallergic and antiemetic drugs
`6th`

T45.0X1 Poisoning by antiallergic and antiemetic drugs, accidental (unintentional)
`7th`
Poisoning by antiallergic and antiemetic drugs NOS

T45.0X5 Adverse effect of antiallergic and antiemetic drugs
`7th`

T45.4 Poisoning by, adverse effect of and underdosing of iron and its compounds
`5th`

T45.4X Poisoning by, adverse effect of and underdosing of iron and its compounds
`6th`

T45.4X1 Poisoning by iron and its compounds, accidental (unintentional)
`7th`
Poisoning by iron and its compounds NOS

T45.4X2 Poisoning by iron and its compounds, intentional self-harm
`7th`

T45.4X5 Adverse effect of iron and its compounds
`7th`

T46 POISONING BY, ADVERSE EFFECT OF AND UNDERDOSING OF AGENTS PRIMARILY AFFECTING THE CARDIOVASCULAR SYSTEM
`4th`

Excludes1: poisoning by, adverse effect of and underdosing of metaraminol (T44.4)

T46.0 Poisoning by, adverse effect of and underdosing of cardiac-stimulant glycosides and drugs of similar action
`5th`

T46.0X Poisoning by, adverse effect of and underdosing of cardiac-stimulant glycosides and drugs of similar action
`6th`

T46.0X1 Poisoning by cardiac-stimulant glycosides and drugs of similar action, accidental (unintentional)
`7th`
Poisoning by cardiac-stimulant glycosides and drugs of similar action NOS

T46.0X2 Poisoning by cardiac-stimulant glycosides and drugs of similar action, intentional self-harm
`7th`

T46.0X5 Adverse effect of cardiac-stimulant glycosides and drugs of similar action
`7th`

T47 POISONING BY, ADVERSE EFFECT OF AND UNDERDOSING OF AGENTS PRIMARILY AFFECTING THE GASTROINTESTINAL SYSTEM
`4th`

T47.8 Poisoning by, adverse effect of and underdosing of other agents primarily affecting gastrointestinal system
`5th`

T47.8X Poisoning by, adverse effect of and underdosing of other agents primarily affecting gastro-intestinal system
`6th`

T47.8X5 Adverse effect of other agents primarily affecting gastrointestinal system
`7th`

T48 POISONING BY, ADVERSE EFFECT OF AND UNDERDOSING OF AGENTS PRIMARILY ACTING ON SMOOTH AND SKELETAL MUSCLES AND THE RESPIRATORY SYSTEM
`4th`

T48.3 Poisoning by, adverse effect of and underdosing of antitussives
`5th`

T48.3X Poisoning by, adverse effect of and underdosing of antitussives
`6th`

7th characters for categories T48–T50
A—initial encounter
D—subsequent encounter
S—sequela

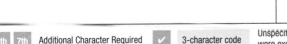

`4th` `5th` `6th` `7th` Additional Character Required	✔ 3-character code	Unspecified laterality codes were excluded here.	●—New Code ▲—Revised Code	*Excludes1*—Not coded here, do not use together *Excludes2*—Not included here

CHAPTER 19. INJURY, POISONING AND CERTAIN OTHER CONSEQUENCES OF EXTERNAL CAUSES   (T48.3X5–T52.8X2)

T48.3X5   Adverse effect of antitussives
`7th`

T48.5   Poisoning by, adverse effect of and underdosing of other anti-common-cold drugs
`5th`
Poisoning by, adverse effect of and underdosing of decongestants
Excludes2: poisoning by, adverse effect of and underdosing of antipyretics, NEC (T39.9-)
poisoning by, adverse effect of and underdosing of non-steroidal antiinflammatory drugs (T39.3-)
poisoning by, adverse effect of and underdosing of salicylates (T39.0-)

T48.5X   Poisoning by, adverse effect of and underdosing of other anti-common-cold drugs
`6th`
T48.5X5   Adverse effect of other anti-common-cold drugs
`7th`

T48.6   Poisoning by, adverse effect of and underdosing of antiasthmatics, not elsewhere classified
`5th`
Poisoning by, adverse effect of and underdosing of beta-adrenoreceptor agonists used in asthma therapy
Excludes1: poisoning by, adverse effect of and underdosing of beta-adrenoreceptor agonists not used in asthma therapy (T44.5)
poisoning by, adverse effect of and underdosing of anterior pituitary [adenohypophyseal] hormones (T38.8)

T48.6X   Poisoning by, adverse effect of and underdosing of antiasthmatics
`6th`
T48.6X1   Poisoning by antiasthmatics, accidental (unintentional)
`7th`
Poisoning by antiasthmatics NOS
T48.6X2   Poisoning by antiasthmatics, intentional self-harm
`7th`
T48.6X5   Adverse effect of anti-asthmatics
`7th`
T48.6X6   Underdosing of anti-asthmatics
`7th`

T50   **POISONING BY, ADVERSE EFFECT OF AND UNDERDOSING OF DIURETICS AND OTHER AND UNSPECIFIED DRUGS, MEDICAMENTS AND BIOLOGICAL SUBSTANCES**
`4th`
T50.0   Poisoning by, adverse effect of and underdosing of mineralocorticoids and their antagonists

T50.A   Poisoning by, adverse effect of and underdosing of bacterial vaccines
`5th`

7th characters for categories T36–T50
A—initial encounter
D—subsequent encounter
S—sequela

T50.A1   Poisoning by, adverse effect of and underdosing of pertussis vaccine, including combinations with a pertussis component
`6th`
T50.A15   Adverse effect of pertussis vaccine, including combinations with a pertussis component
`7th`
T50.A2   Poisoning by, adverse effect of and underdosing of mixed bacterial vaccines without a pertussis component
`6th`
T50.A25   Adverse effect of mixed bacterial vaccines without a pertussis component
`7th`
T50.A9   Poisoning by, adverse effect of and underdosing of other bacterial vaccines
`6th`
T50.A95   Adverse effect of other bacterial vaccines
`7th`
T50.A96   Underdosing of other bacterial vaccines
`7th`

T50.B9   Poisoning by, adverse effect of and underdosing of other viral vaccines
`6th`
T50.B95   Adverse effect of other viral vaccines
`7th`

T50.9   Poisoning by, adverse effect of and underdosing of other and unspecified drugs, medicaments and biological substances
`5th`
T50.90   Poisoning by, adverse effect of and underdosing of unspecified drugs, medicaments and biological substances
`6th`
T50.901   Poisoning by unspecified drugs, medicaments and biological substances, accidental (unintentional)
`7th`
T50.902   Poisoning by unspecified drugs, medicaments and biological substances, intentional self-harm
`7th`
T50.905   Adverse effect of unspecified drugs, medicaments and biological substances
`7th`
T50.99   Poisoning by, adverse effect of and underdosing of other drugs, medicaments and biological substances
`6th`
T50.995   Adverse effect of other drugs, medicaments and biological substances
`7th`

(T51–T65) TOXIC EFFECTS OF SUBSTANCES CHIEFLY NONMEDICINAL AS TO SOURCE

Note: When no intent is indicated code to accidental. Undetermined intent is only for use when there is specific documentation in the record that the intent of the toxic effect cannot be determined.
Use additional code(s): for all associated manifestations of toxic effect, such as:
respiratory conditions due to external agents (J60–J70)
personal history of FB fully removed (Z87.821)
to identify any retained FB, if applicable (Z18.-)
Excludes1: contact with and (suspected) exposure to toxic substances (Z77.-)

T52   **TOXIC EFFECT OF ORGANIC SOLVENTS**
`4th`
Excludes1: halogen derivatives of aliphatic and aromatic hydrocarbons (T53.-)

7th characters for categories T52–T65
A—initial encounter
D—subsequent encounter
S—sequela

T52.0   Toxic effects of petroleum products
`5th`
Toxic effects of gasoline [petrol]
Toxic effects of kerosene [paraffin oil]
Toxic effects of paraffin wax
Toxic effects of ether petroleum
Toxic effects of naphtha petroleum
Toxic effects of spirit petroleum

T52.0X   Toxic effects of petroleum products
T52.0X1   Toxic effect of petroleum products, accidental (unintentional)
`6th`
`7th`
Toxic effects of petroleum products NOS
T52.0X2   Toxic effects of petroleum products, intentional self-harm
`7th`

T52.8   Toxic effects of other organic solvents
`5th`
T52.8X   Toxic effects of other organic solvents
`6th`
T52.8X1   Toxic effects of other organic solvents, accidental (unintentional)
`7th`
Toxic effects of other organic solvents NOS
T52.8X2   Toxic effect of other organic solvents, intentional self-harm
`7th`

  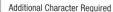   Additional Character Required   ✓   3-character code   Unspecified laterality codes were excluded here.   •=New Code   ▲=Revised Code   *Excludes1*—Not coded here, do not use together   *Excludes2*—Not included here

T54   **TOXIC EFFECT OF CORROSIVE SUBSTANCES**
`4th`

     T54.3   **Toxic effects of corrosive alkalis and alkali-like substances**
`5th`
       Toxic effects of potassium hydroxide
       Toxic effects of sodium hydroxide

       T54.3X   **Toxic effects of corrosive alkalis and alkali-like substances**
`6th`

         T54.3X1   **Toxic effect of corrosive alkalis and alkali-like substances, accidental (unintentional)**
`7th`
           Toxic effects of corrosive alkalis and alkali-like substances NOS

         T54.3X2   **Toxic effect of corrosive alkalis and alkali-like substances, intentional self-harm**
`7th`

T56   **TOXIC EFFECT OF METALS**
`4th`

    Includes: toxic effects of fumes and vapors of metals
       toxic effects of metals from all sources, except medicinal substances

    Use additional code to identify any retained metal FB, if applicable (Z18.0-, T18.1-)

    Excludes1: arsenic and its compounds (T57.0)
       manganese and its compounds (T57.2)

7th characters for categories T52–T65
A—initial encounter
D—subsequent encounter
S—sequela

     T56.0   **Toxic effects of lead and its compounds**
`5th`

       T56.0X   **Toxic effects of lead and its compounds**
`6th`

         T56.0X1   **Toxic effect of lead and its compounds, accidental (unintentional)**
`7th`
           Toxic effects of lead and its compounds NOS

T58   **TOXIC EFFECT OF CARBON MONOXIDE**
`4th`

    Includes: asphyxiation from carbon monoxide
       toxic effect of carbon monoxide from all sources

7th characters for categories T52–T65
A—initial encounter
D—subsequent encounter
S—sequela

     T58.0   **Toxic effect of carbon monoxide from motor vehicle exhaust**
`5th`
       Toxic effect of exhaust gas from gas engine
       Toxic effect of exhaust gas from motor pump

       T58.01X   **Toxic effect of carbon monoxide from motor vehicle exhaust, accidental (unintentional)**
`7th`

       T58.02X   **Toxic effect of carbon monoxide from motor vehicle exhaust, intentional self-harm**
`7th`

       T58.03X   **Toxic effect of carbon monoxide from motor vehicle exhaust, assault**
`7th`

       T58.04X   **Toxic effect of carbon monoxide from motor vehicle exhaust, undetermined**
`7th`

     T58.1   **Toxic effect of carbon monoxide from utility gas**
`5th`
       Toxic effect of acetylene
       Toxic effect of gas NOS used for lighting, heating, cooking
       Toxic effect of water gas

       T58.11X   **Toxic effect of carbon monoxide from utility gas, accidental (unintentional)**
`7th`

       T58.12X   **Toxic effect of carbon monoxide from utility gas, intentional self-harm**
`7th`

       T58.13X   **Toxic effect of carbon monoxide from utility gas, assault**
`7th`

       T58.14X   **Toxic effect of carbon monoxide from utility gas, undetermined**
`7th`

     T58.9   **Toxic effect of carbon monoxide from unspecified source**
`5th`
       T58.91X   **Toxic effect of carbon monoxide from unspecified source, accidental (unintentional)**
`7th`

       T58.92X   **Toxic effect of carbon monoxide from unspecified source, intentional self-harm**
`7th`

       T58.93X   **Toxic effect of carbon monoxide from unspecified source, assault**
`7th`

       T58.94X   **Toxic effect of carbon monoxide from unspecified source, undetermined**
`7th`

T59   **TOXIC EFFECT OF OTHER GASES, FUMES AND VAPORS**
`4th`

    Includes: aerosol propellants
    Excludes1: chlorofluorocarbons (T53.5)

7th characters for categories T52–T65
A—initial encounter
D—subsequent encounter
S—sequela

     T59.8   **Toxic effect of other specified gases, fumes and vapors**
`5th`

       T59.89   **Toxic effect of other specified gases, fumes and vapors**
`6th`

         T59.891   **Toxic effect of other specified gases, fumes and vapors, accidental (unintentional)**
`7th`

         T59.892   **Toxic effect of other specified gases, fumes and vapors, intentional self-harm**
`7th`

         T59.894   **Toxic effect of other specified gases, fumes and vapors, undetermined**
`7th`

T60   **TOXIC EFFECT OF PESTICIDES**
`4th`

    Includes: toxic effect of wood preservatives

     T60.0   **Toxic effect of organophosphate and carbamate insecticides**
`5th`

       T60.0X   **Toxic effect of organophosphate and carbamate insecticides**
`6th`

         T60.0X1   **Toxic effect of organophosphate and carbamate insecticides, accidental (unintentional)**
`7th`
           Toxic effect of organophosphate and carbamate insecticides NOS

         T60.0X2   **Toxic effect of organophosphate and carbamate insecticides, intentional self-harm**
`7th`

         T60.0X3   **Toxic effect of organophosphate and carbamate insecticides, assault**
`7th`

         T60.0X4   **Toxic effect of organophosphate and carbamate insecticides, undetermined**
`7th`

T62   **TOXIC EFFECT OF OTHER NOXIOUS SUBSTANCES EATEN AS FOOD**
`4th`

    Excludes1: allergic reaction to food, such as:
       anaphylactic shock (reaction) due to adverse food reaction (T78.0-)
       bacterial food borne intoxications (A05.-)
       dermatitis (L23.6, L25.4, L27.2)
       food protein-induced enterocolitis syndrome (K52.21)
       food protein-induced enteropathy (K52.22)
       gastroenteritis (noninfective) (K52.29)
       toxic effect of aflatoxin and other mycotoxins (T64)
       toxic effect of cyanides (T65.0-)
       toxic effect of hydrogen cyanide (T57.3-)
       toxic effect of mercury (T56.1-)

     T62.0   **Toxic effect of ingested mushrooms**
`5th`

       T62.0X   **Toxic effect of ingested mushrooms**
`6th`

         T62.0X1   **Toxic effect of ingested mushrooms, accidental (unintentional)**
`7th`
           Toxic effect of ingested mushrooms NOS

         T62.0X2   **Toxic effect of ingested mushrooms, intentional self-harm**
`7th`

Right margin: CHAPTER 19. INJURY, POISONING AND CERTAIN OTHER CONSEQUENCES OF EXTERNAL CAUSES   (T54–T62.0X2)

  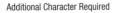   Additional Character Required   ✓   3-character code   Unspecified laterality codes were excluded here.   •=New Code   ▲=Revised Code   **Excludes1**   Not coded here, do not use together   **Excludes2**—Not included here

PEDIATRIC ICD-10-CM 2017: A MANUAL FOR PROVIDER-BASED CODING   363

CHAPTER 19. INJURY, POISONING AND CERTAIN OTHER CONSEQUENCES OF EXTERNAL CAUSES   (T63–T70.29X)

T63 **TOXIC EFFECT OF CONTACT WITH VENOMOUS ANIMALS AND PLANTS**
`4th`
Includes: bite or touch of venomous animal
    pricked or stuck by thorn or leaf
Excludes2: ingestion of toxic animal or plant (T61.-, T62.-)

T63.0   **Toxic effect of snake venom**
`5th`
    T63.00   **Toxic effect of unspecified snake venom**
`6th`
        T63.001   **Toxic effect of unspecified snake venom, accidental (unintentional)**
`7th`
            Toxic effect of unspecified snake venom NOS

T63.3   **Toxic effect of venom of spider**
`5th`
    T63.30   **Toxic effect of unspecified spider venom**
`6th`
        T63.301   **Toxic effect of unspecified spider venom, accidental (unintentional)**
`7th`

    T63.33   **Toxic effect of venom of brown recluse spider**
`6th`

T63.4   **Toxic effect of venom of other arthropods**
`5th`
    T63.42   **Toxic effect of venom of ants**
`6th`
        T63.421   **Toxic effect of venom of ants, accidental (unintentional)**
`7th`

    T63.44   **Toxic effect of venom of bees**
`6th`
        T63.441   **Toxic effect of venom of bees, accidental (unintentional)**
`7th`

    T63.45   **Toxic effect of venom of hornets**
`6th`
        T63.451   **Toxic effect of venom of hornets, accidental (unintentional)**
`7th`

    T63.46   **Toxic effect of venom of wasps**
`6th`
        Toxic effect of yellow jacket
        T63.461   **Toxic effect of venom of wasps, accidental (unintentional)**
`7th`

    T63.48   **Toxic effect of venom of other arthropod**
`6th`
        T63.481   **Toxic effect of venom of other arthropod, accidental (unintentional)**
`7th`

T63.6   **Toxic effect of contact with other venomous marine animals**
`5th`
    Excludes1: sea-snake venom (T63.09)
    Excludes2: poisoning by ingestion of shellfish (T61.78-)
    T63.62   **Toxic effect of contact with other jellyfish**
`6th`
        T63.621   **Toxic effect of contact with other jellyfish, accidental (unintentional)**
`7th`

T63.9   **Toxic effect of contact with unspecified venomous animal**
`5th`
    T63.91X   **Toxic effect of contact with unspecified venomous animal, accidental (unintentional)**
`7th`

T65 **TOXIC EFFECT OF OTHER AND UNSPECIFIED SUBSTANCES**
`4th`
T65.8   **Toxic effect of other specified substances**
`5th`
    T65.82   **Toxic effect of harmful algae and algae toxins**
`6th`
        Toxic effect of (harmful) algae bloom NOS
        Toxic effect of blue-green algae bloom
        Toxic effect of brown tide
        Toxic effect of cyanobacteria bloom
        Toxic effect of Florida red tide
        Toxic effect of pfiesteria piscicida
        Toxic effect of red tide
        T65.821   **Toxic effect of harmful algae and algae toxins, accidental (unintentional)**
`7th`
            Toxic effect of harmful algae and algae toxins NOS

> 7th characters for categories
> T52–T65
> A—initial encounter
> D—subsequent encounter
> S—sequela

T65.9   **Toxic effect of unspecified substance**
`5th`
    T65.91X   **Toxic effect of unspecified substance, accidental (unintentional)**
`7th`
        Poisoning NOS
    T65.92X   **Toxic effect of unspecified substance, intentional self-harm**
`7th`

(T66–T78) OTHER AND UNSPECIFIED EFFECTS OF EXTERNAL CAUSES

T67 **EFFECTS OF HEAT AND LIGHT**
`4th`
Excludes1: erythema [dermatitis] ab igne (L59.0)
    malignant hyperpyrexia due to anesthesia (T88.3)
    radiation-related disorders of the skin and subcutaneous tissue (L55–L59)
Excludes2: burns (T20–T31)
    sunburn (L55.-)
    sweat disorder due to heat (L74–L75)

> 7th characters for categories
> T67–T78
> A—initial encounter
> D—subsequent encounter
> S—sequela

T67.0XX   **Heatstroke and sun-stroke**
`7th`
    Heat apoplexy
    Heat pyrexia
    Siriasis
    Thermoplegia
    Use additional code(s) to identify any associated complications of heatstroke, such as:
        coma and stupor (R40.-)
        SIRS (R65.1-)

T67.1XX   **Heat syncope**
`7th`
    Heat collapse

T67.2XX   **Heat cramp**
`7th`

T67.3XX   **Heat exhaustion, anhydrotic**
`7th`
    Heat prostration due to water depletion
    Excludes1: heat exhaustion due to salt depletion (T67.4)

T67.4XX   **Heat exhaustion due to salt depletion**
`7th`
    Heat prostration due to salt (and water) depletion

T67.5XX   **Heat exhaustion, unspecified**
`7th`
    Heat prostration NOS

T68 **HYPOTHERMIA**
`7th`
Accidental hypothermia
Hypothermia NOS
Use additional code to identify source of exposure:
    Exposure to excessive cold of man-made origin (W93)
    Exposure to excessive cold of natural origin (X31)
Excludes1: hypothermia following anesthesia (T88.51)
    hypothermia not associated with low environmental temperature (R68.0)
    hypothermia of newborn (P80.-)
Excludes2: frostbite (T33–T34)

T70 **EFFECTS OF AIR PRESSURE AND WATER PRESSURE**
`4th`
T70.2   **Other and unspecified effects of high altitude**
`5th`
    Excludes2: polycythemia due to high altitude (D75.1)
    T70.20X   **Unspecified effects of high altitude**
`7th`

    T70.29X   **Other effects of high altitude**
`7th`
        Alpine sickness
        Anoxia due to high altitude
        Barotrauma NOS
        Hypobaropathy
        Mountain sickness

`4th` `5th` `6th` `7th`   Additional Character Required   ✓   3-character code   Unspecified laterality codes were excluded here.   •=New Code   ▲=Revised Code   *Excludes1*—Not coded here, do not use together   *Excludes2*—Not included here

T71 ASPHYXIATION
Mechanical suffocation
Traumatic suffocation
Excludes1: acute respiratory distress (syndrome) (J80)
  anoxia due to high altitude (T70.2)
  asphyxia NOS (R09.01)
  asphyxia from carbon monoxide (T58.-)
  asphyxia from inhalation of food or FB (T17.-)
  asphyxia from other gases, fumes and vapors (T59.-)
  respiratory distress (syndrome) in newborn (P22.-)

T71.1 **Asphyxiation due to mechanical threat to breathing** (5th)
Suffocation due to mechanical threat to breathing

T71.11 **Asphyxiation due to smothering under pillow** (6th)

T71.111 Asphyxiation due to smothering under pillow, accidental (7th)
Asphyxiation due to smothering under pillow NOS

T71.112 Asphyxiation due to smothering under pillow, intentional self-harm (7th)

T71.113 Asphyxiation due to smothering under pillow, assault (7th)

T71.114 Asphyxiation due to smothering under pillow, undetermined, initial encounter (7th)

T71.12 **Asphyxiation due to plastic bag** (6th)

T71.121 Asphyxiation due to plastic bag, accidental (7th)
Asphyxiation due to plastic bag NOS

T71.122 Asphyxiation due to plastic bag, intentional self-harm (7th)

T71.123 Asphyxiation due to plastic bag, assault (7th)

T71.124 Asphyxiation due to plastic bag, undetermined (7th)

T71.13 **Asphyxiation due to being trapped in bed linens** (6th)

T71.131 Asphyxiation due to being trapped in bed linens, accidental (7th)
Asphyxiation due to being trapped in bed linens NOS

T71.132 Asphyxiation due to being trapped in bed linens, intentional self-harm (7th)

T71.133 Asphyxiation due to being trapped in bed linens, assault (7th)

T71.134 Asphyxiation due to being trapped in bed linens, undetermined (7th)

T71.14 **Asphyxiation due to smothering under another person's body (in bed)** (6th)

T71.141 Asphyxiation due to smothering under another person's body (in bed), accidental (7th)
Asphyxiation due to smothering under another person's body (in bed) NOS

T71.143 Asphyxiation due to smothering under another person's body (in bed), assault (7th)

T71.144 Asphyxiation due to smothering under another person's body (in bed), undetermined (7th)

T71.15 **Asphyxiation due to smothering in furniture** (6th)

T71.151 Asphyxiation due to smothering in furniture, accidental (7th)

7th characters for categories T67–T78
A—initial encounter
D—subsequent encounter
S—sequela

Asphyxiation due to smothering in furniture NOS

T71.152 Asphyxiation due to smothering in furniture, intentional self-harm (7th)

T71.153 Asphyxiation due to smothering in furniture, assault (7th)

T71.154 Asphyxiation due to smothering in furniture, undetermined (7th)

T71.16 **Asphyxiation due to hanging** (6th)
Hanging by window shade cord
Use additional code for any associated injuries, such as:
  crushing injury of neck (S17.-)
  fracture of cervical vertebrae (S12.0–S12.2-)
  open wound of neck (S11.-)

T71.161 Asphyxiation due to hanging, accidental (7th)
Asphyxiation due to hanging NOS
Hanging NOS

T71.162 Asphyxiation due to hanging, intentional self-harm (7th)

T71.163 Asphyxiation due to hanging, assault (7th)

T71.164 Asphyxiation due to hanging, undetermined (7th)

T71.19 **Asphyxiation due to mechanical threat to breathing due to other causes** (6th)

T71.191 Asphyxiation due to mechanical threat to breathing due to other causes, accidental (7th)
Asphyxiation due to other causes NOS

T71.192 Asphyxiation due to mechanical threat to breathing due to other causes, intentional self-harm (7th)

T71.193 Asphyxiation due to mechanical threat to breathing due to other causes, assault (7th)

T71.194 Asphyxiation due to mechanical threat to breathing due to other causes, undetermined (7th)

T71.2 **Asphyxiation due to systemic oxygen deficiency due to low oxygen content in ambient air** (5th)
Suffocation due to systemic oxygen deficiency due to low oxygen content in ambient air

T71.21X Asphyxiation due to cave-in or falling earth (7th)
Use additional code for any associated cataclysm (X34–X38)

T71.22 **Asphyxiation due to being trapped in a car trunk** (6th)

T71.221 Asphyxiation due to being trapped in a car trunk, accidental (7th)

T71.222 Asphyxiation due to being trapped in a car trunk, intentional self-harm (7th)

T71.223 Asphyxiation due to being trapped in a car trunk, assault (7th)

T71.224 Asphyxiation due to being trapped in a car trunk, undetermined (7th)

  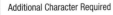 4th 5th 6th 7th Additional Character Required   ✔ 3-character code   Unspecified laterality codes were excluded here.   •=New Code   ▲=Revised Code   **Excludes1** Not coded here, do not use together   **Excludes2**—Not included here

CHAPTER 19. INJURY, POISONING AND CERTAIN OTHER CONSEQUENCES OF EXTERNAL CAUSES (T71.23–T78.01X)

T71.23 Asphyxiation due to being trapped in a (discarded) refrigerator
`6th`
> **T71.231** Asphyxiation due to being trapped in a (discarded) refrigerator, accidental `7th`
> **T71.232** Asphyxiation due to being trapped in a (discarded) refrigerator, intentional self-harm `7th`
> **T71.233** Asphyxiation due to being trapped in a (discarded) refrigerator, assault `7th`
> **T71.234** Asphyxiation due to being trapped in a (discarded) refrigerator, undetermined `7th`

T71.29X Asphyxiation due to being trapped in other low oxygen environment `7th`

T71.9XX Asphyxiation due to unspecified cause `7th`
Suffocation (by strangulation) due to unspecified cause
Suffocation NOS
Systemic oxygen deficiency due to low oxygen content in ambient air or due to due to mechanical threat to breathing due to unspecified cause
Traumatic asphyxia NOS

T74 ADULT AND CHILD ABUSE, NEGLECT AND OTHER MALTREATMENT, CONFIRMED `4th`
Sequence first the appropriate code from categories T74.- (Adult and child abuse, neglect and other maltreatment, confirmed) or T76.- (Adult and child abuse, neglect and other maltreatment, suspected) for abuse, neglect and other maltreatment, followed by any accompanying mental health or injury code(s).

If the documentation in the medical record states abuse or neglect it is coded as confirmed (T74.-). It is coded as suspected if it is documented as suspected (T76.-).

For cases of confirmed abuse or neglect an external cause code from the assault section (X92–Y08) should be added to identify the cause of any physical injuries. A perpetrator code (Y07) should be added when the perpetrator of the abuse is known. For suspected cases of abuse or neglect, do not report external cause or perpetrator code.

If a suspected case of abuse, neglect or mistreatment is ruled out during an encounter code Z04.71, Encounter for examination and observation following alleged physical adult abuse, ruled out, or code Z04.72, Encounter for examination and observation following alleged child physical abuse, ruled out, should be used, not a code from T76.

If a suspected case of alleged rape or sexual abuse is ruled out during an encounter code Z04.41, Encounter for examination and observation following alleged physical adult abuse, ruled out, or code Z04.42, Encounter for examination and observation following alleged rape or sexual abuse, ruled out, should be used, not a code from T76.
Use additional code, if applicable, to identify any associated current injury external cause code to identify perpetrator, if known (Y07.-)
Excludes1: abuse and maltreatment in pregnancy (O9A.3-, O9A.4-, O9A.5-)
adult and child maltreatment, suspected (T76.-)

T74.0 Neglect or abandonment, confirmed `5th`
> **T74.02X** Child neglect or abandonment, confirmed `7th`

T74.1 Physical abuse, confirmed `5th`
Excludes2: sexual abuse (T74.2-)
> **T74.12X** Child physical abuse, confirmed
> *Excludes2:* shaken infant syndrome (T74.4)

T74.2 Sexual abuse, confirmed `5th`
Rape, confirmed
Sexual assault, confirmed
> **T74.22X** Child sexual abuse, confirmed

> 7th characters for categories T67–T78
> A—initial encounter
> D—subsequent encounter
> S—sequela

T74.3 Psychological abuse, confirmed `5th`
> **T74.32X** Child psychological abuse, confirmed `7th`

T74.4XX Shaken infant syndrome `7th`

T74.9 Unspecified maltreatment, confirmed `5th`
> **T74.92X** Unspecified child maltreatment, confirmed `7th`

T75 OTHER AND UNSPECIFIED EFFECTS OF OTHER EXTERNAL CAUSES `4th`
Excludes1: adverse effects NEC (T78.-)
Excludes2: burns (electric) (T20–T31)
T75.1XX Unspecified effects of drowning and nonfatal submersion `7th`
Immersion
Excludes1: specified effects of drowning—*code to* effects
T75.3XX Motion sickness `7th`
Airsickness
Seasickness
Travel sickness
Use additional external cause code to identify vehicle or type of motion (Y92.81-, Y93.5-)
T75.4XX Electrocution `7th`
Shock from electric current
Shock from electroshock gun (taser)

T76 ADULT AND CHILD ABUSE, NEGLECT AND OTHER MALTREATMENT, SUSPECTED `4th`
Use additional code, if applicable, to identify any associated current injury
Excludes1: adult and child maltreatment, confirmed (T74.-)
suspected abuse and maltreatment in pregnancy (O9A.3-, O9A.4-, O9A.5-)
suspected adult physical abuse, ruled out (Z04.71)
suspected adult sexual abuse, ruled out (Z04.41)
suspected child physical abuse, ruled out (Z04.72)
suspected child sexual abuse, ruled out (Z04.42)
T76.0 Neglect or abandonment, suspected `5th`
> **T76.02X** Child neglect or abandonment, suspected `7th`

T76.1 Physical abuse, suspected `5th`
> **T76.12X** Child physical abuse, suspected `7th`

T76.2 Sexual abuse, suspected `5th`
Rape, suspected
Sexual abuse, suspected
Excludes1: alleged abuse, ruled out (Z04.7)
> **T76.22X** Child sexual abuse, suspected `7th`

T76.3 Psychological abuse, suspected `5th`
> **T76.32X** Child psychological abuse, suspected `7th`

T76.9 Unspecified maltreatment, suspected `5th`
> **T76.92X** Unspecified child maltreatment, suspected `7th`

T78 ADVERSE EFFECTS, NOT ELSEWHERE CLASSIFIED `4th`
Excludes2: complications of surgical and medical care NEC (T80–T88)
T78.0 Anaphylactic reaction due to food `5th`
Anaphylactic reaction due to adverse food reaction
Anaphylactic shock or reaction due to nonpoisonous foods
Anaphylactoid reaction due to food
> **T78.00X** Anaphylactic reaction due to unspecified food `7th`

> **T78.01X** Anaphylactic reaction due to peanuts `7th`

   Additional Character Required   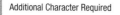 3-character code   Unspecified laterality codes were excluded here.   •=New Code   ▲=Revised Code   *Excludes1*—Not coded here, do not use together   *Excludes2*—Not included here

T78.02X   **Anaphylactic reaction due to shellfish (crustaceans)**
7th

T78.03X   **Anaphylactic reaction due to other fish**
7th

T78.04X   **Anaphylactic reaction due to fruits and vegetables**
7th

T78.05X   **Anaphylactic reaction due to tree nuts and seeds**
7th
    Excludes2: anaphylactic reaction due to peanuts (T78.01)

T78.06X   **Anaphylactic reaction due to food additives**
7th

T78.07X   **Anaphylactic reaction due to milk and dairy products**
7th

T78.08X   **Anaphylactic reaction due to eggs**
7th

T78.09X   **Anaphylactic reaction due to other food products**
7th

T78.2XX   **Anaphylactic shock, unspecified**
7th
    Allergic shock
    Anaphylactic reaction
    Anaphylaxis
    Excludes1: anaphylactic reaction or shock due to adverse effect of correct medicinal substance properly administered (T88.6)
      anaphylactic reaction or shock due to adverse food reaction (T78.0-)
      anaphylactic reaction or shock due to serum (T80.5-)

T78.3XX   **Angioneurotic edema**
7th
    Allergic angioedema
    Giant urticaria
    Quincke's edema
    Excludes1: serum urticaria (T80.6-)
      urticaria (L50.-)

T78.4   **Other and unspecified allergy**
5th
    Excludes1: specified types of allergic reaction such as:
      allergic diarrhea (K52.29)
      allergic gastroenteritis and colitis (K52.29)
      food protein-induced enterocolitis syndrome (K52.21)
      food protein-induced enteropathy (K52.22)
      dermatitis (L23–L25, L27.-)
      hay fever (J30.1)

    T78.40X   **Allergy, unspecified**
    7th
      Allergic reaction NOS
      Hypersensitivity NOS

(T79) CERTAIN EARLY COMPLICATIONS OF TRAUMA

T79   **CERTAIN EARLY COMPLICATIONS OF TRAUMA, NOT ELSEWHERE CLASSIFIED**
4th
    Excludes2: acute respiratory distress syndrome (J80)
      complications occurring during or following medical procedures (T80–T88)
      complications of surgical and medical care NEC (T80–T88)
      newborn respiratory distress syndrome (P22.0)

T79.4XX   **Traumatic shock**
7th
    Shock (immediate) (delayed) following injury
    Excludes1: anaphylactic shock due to adverse food reaction (T78.0-)
      anaphylactic shock due to correct medicinal substance properly administered (T88.6)
      anaphylactic shock due to serum (T80.5-)
      anaphylactic shock NOS (T78.2)
      anesthetic shock (T88.2)
      electric shock (T75.4)
      nontraumatic shock NEC (R57.-)

> 7th characters for category T79
> A—initial encounter
> D—subsequent encounter
> S—sequela

      obstetric shock (O75.1)
      postprocedural shock (T81.1-)
      septic shock (R65.21)
      shock complicating abortion or ectopic or molar pregnancy (O00–O07, O08.3)
      shock due to lightning (T75.01)
      shock NOS (R57.9)

T79.7XX   **Traumatic subcutaneous emphysema**
7th
    Excludes1: emphysema NOS (J43)
      emphysema (subcutaneous) resulting from a procedure (T81.82)

(T80–T88) COMPLICATIONS OF SURGICAL AND MEDICAL CARE, NOT ELSEWHERE CLASSIFIED

Use additional code for adverse effect, if applicable, to identify drug (T36–T50 with fifth or sixth character 5)

Use additional code(s) to identify the specified condition resulting from the complication

Use additional code to identify devices involved and details of circumstances (Y62–Y82)

Excludes2: any encounters with medical care for postprocedural conditions in which no complications are present, such as:
artificial opening status (Z93.-)
closure of external stoma (Z43.-)
fitting and adjustment of external prosthetic device (Z44.-)
burns and corrosions from local applications and irradiation (T20–T32)
complications of surgical procedures during pregnancy, childbirth and the puerperium (O00–O9A)
mechanical complication of respirator [ventilator] (J95.850)
poisoning and toxic effects of drugs and chemicals (T36–T65 with fifth or sixth character 1–4 or 6)
postprocedural fever (R50.82)
specified complications classified elsewhere, such as:
cerebrospinal fluid leak from spinal puncture (G97.0)
colostomy malfunction (K94.0-)
disorders of fluid and electrolyte imbalance (E86–E87)
functional disturbances following cardiac surgery (I97.0–I97.1)
intraoperative and postprocedural complications of specified body systems (D78.-, E36.-, E89.-, G97.3-, G97.4, H59.3-, H59.-, H95.2-, H95.3, I97.4-, I97.5, J95.6-, J95.7, K91.6-, L76.-, M96.-, N99.-)
ostomy complications (J95.0-, K94.-, N99.5-)
postgastric surgery syndromes (K91.1)
postlaminectomy syndrome NEC (M96.1)
postmastectomy lymphedema syndrome (I97.2)
postsurgical blind-loop syndrome (K91.2)
ventilator associated pneumonia (J95.851)

> 7th characters for category T80
> A—initial encounter
> D—subsequent encounter
> S—sequela

T80   **COMPLICATIONS FOLLOWING INFUSION, TRANSFUSION AND THERAPEUTIC INJECTION**
4th
    Includes: complications following perfusion
    Excludes2: bone marrow transplant rejection (T86.01)
      febrile nonhemolytic transfusion reaction (R50.84)
      fluid overload due to transfusion (E87.71)
      posttransfusion purpura (D69.51)
      transfusion associated circulatory overload (TACO) (E87.71)
      transfusion (red blood cell) associated hemochromatosis (E83.111)
      transfusion related acute lung injury (TRALI) (J95.84)

> 7th characters for category T80
> A—initial encounter
> D—subsequent encounter
> S—sequela

T80.0XX   **Air embolism following infusion, transfusion and therapeutic injection**
7th

T80.2   **Infections following infusion, transfusion and therapeutic injection**
5th
    Use additional code to identify the specific infection, such as: sepsis (A41.9)
    Use additional code (R65.2-) to identify severe sepsis, if applicable
    Excludes2: infections specified as due to prosthetic devices, implants and grafts (T82.6–T82.7, T83.5–T83.6, T84.5–T84.7, T85.7)
      postprocedural infections (T81.4-)

4th   5th   6th   7th   Additional Character Required   ✓   3-character code   Unspecified laterality codes were excluded here.   •=New Code   ▴=Revised Code   *Excludes1*—Not coded here, do not use together   *Excludes2*—Not included here

PEDIATRIC ICD-10-CM 2017: A MANUAL FOR PROVIDER-BASED CODING   367

T80.21 `6th` **Infection due to central venous catheter**
Infection due to pulmonary artery catheter (Swan-Ganz catheter)

T80.211 `7th` **Bloodstream infection due to central venous catheter**
Catheter-related bloodstream infection (CRBSI) NOS
Central line-associated bloodstream infection (CLABSI)
Bloodstream infection due to Hickman catheter/peripherally inserted central catheter (PICC)/portacath (port-a-cath)/pulmonary artery catheter/triple lumen catheter/umbilical venous catheter

T80.212 `7th` **Local infection due to central venous catheter**
Exit or insertion site infection
Local infection due to Hickman catheter/peripherally inserted central catheter (PICC)/portacath (port-a-cath)/pulmonary artery catheter/triple lumen catheter/umbilical venous catheter
Port or reservoir infection
Tunnel infection

T80.218 `7th` **Other infection due to central venous catheter**
Other central line-associated infection/Hickman catheter/peripherally inserted central catheter (PICC)/portacath (port-a-cath)/pulmonary artery catheter/triple lumen catheter/umbilical venous catheter

T80.219 `7th` **Unspecified infection due to central venous catheter**
Central line-associated infection NOS
Unspecified infection due to Hickman catheter/peripherally inserted central catheter (PICC)/portacath (port-a-cath)/pulmonary artery catheter/triple lumen catheter/umbilical venous catheter

T80.22X `7th` **Acute infection following transfusion, infusion, or injection of blood and blood products**

T80.29X `7th` **Infection following other infusion, transfusion and therapeutic injection**

T80.3 `5th` **ABO incompatibility reaction due to transfusion of blood or blood products**
Excludes1: minor blood group antigens reactions (Duffy) (E) (K(ell)) (Kidd) (Lewis) (M) (N) (P) (S) (T80.A)

T80.30X `7th` **ABO incompatibility reaction due to transfusion of blood or blood products, unspecified**
ABO incompatibility blood transfusion NOS
Reaction to ABO incompatibility from transfusion NOS

T80.5 `5th` **Anaphylactic reaction due to serum**
Allergic shock due to serum
Anaphylactic shock due to serum
Anaphylactoid reaction due to serum
Anaphylaxis due to serum
Excludes1: ABO incompatibility reaction due to transfusion of blood or blood products (T80.3-)
allergic reaction or shock NOS (T78.2)
anaphylactic reaction or shock NOS (T78.2)
anaphylactic reaction or shock due to adverse effect of correct medicinal substance properly administered (T88.6)
other serum reaction (T80.6-)

T80.51X `7th` **Anaphylactic reaction due to administration of blood and blood products**

T80.52X `7th` **Anaphylactic reaction due to vaccination**

T80.59X `7th` **Anaphylactic reaction due to other serum**

T80.6 `5th` **Other serum reactions**
Intoxication by serum
Protein sickness
Serum rash
Serum sickness
Serum urticaria
Excludes2: serum hepatitis (B16–B19)

T80.61X `7th` **Other serum reaction due to administration of blood and blood products**

T80.62X `7th` **Other serum reaction due to vaccination**

T80.69X `7th` **Other serum reaction due to other serum**

T80.8 `5th` **Other complications following infusion, transfusion and therapeutic injection**

T80.81 `6th` **Extravasation of vesicant agent**
Infiltration of vesicant agent

T80.810 `7th` **Extravasation of vesicant antineoplastic chemotherapy**
Infiltration of vesicant antineoplastic chemotherapy

T80.818 `7th` **Extravasation of other vesicant agent**
Infiltration of other vesicant agent

T80.89X `7th` **Other complications following infusion, transfusion and therapeutic injection**
Delayed serologic transfusion reaction (DSTR), unspecified incompatibility
Use additional code to identify graft-versus-host reaction, if applicable, (D89.81-)

T80.9 `5th` **Unspecified complication following infusion, transfusion and therapeutic injection**

T80.91 `6th` **Hemolytic transfusion reaction, unspecified incompatibility**
Excludes1: ABO incompatibility with hemolytic transfusion reaction (T80.31-)
Non-ABO incompatibility with hemolytic transfusion reaction (T80.A1-)
Rh incompatibility with hemolytic transfusion reaction (T80.41-)

T80.910 `7th` **Acute hemolytic transfusion reaction, unspecified incompatibility**

T80.911 `7th` **Delayed hemolytic transfusion reaction, unspecified incompatibility**

T80.919 `7th` **Hemolytic transfusion reaction, unspecified incompatibility, unspecified as acute or delayed**
Hemolytic transfusion reaction NOS

T80.92X `7th` **Unspecified transfusion reaction**
Transfusion reaction NOS

T81 `4th` **COMPLICATIONS OF PROCEDURES, NOT ELSEWHERE CLASSIFIED**
Use additional code for adverse effect, if applicable, to identify drug (T36–T50 with fifth or sixth character 5)
Excludes2: complications following immunization (T88.0–T88.1)
complications following infusion, transfusion and therapeutic injection (T80.-)
complications of transplanted organs and tissue (T86.-)
specified complications classified elsewhere, such as:
complication of prosthetic devices, implants and grafts (T82–T85)
dermatitis due to drugs and medicaments (L23.3, L24.4, L25.1, L27.0–L27.1)
endosseous dental implant failure (M27.6-)

  `4th` `5th` `6th` `7th` Additional Character Required   3-character code   Unspecified laterality codes were excluded here.   •=New Code   ▲=Revised Code   *Excludes1*—Not coded here, do not use together   *Excludes2*—Not included here

floppy iris syndrome (IFIS) (intraoperative) H21.81

intraoperative and postprocedural complications of specific body system (D78.-, E36.-, E89.-, G97.3-,G97.4, H59.3-, H59.-, H95.2-, H95.3, I97.4-, I97.5, J95, K91.-, L76.-, M96.-, N99.-)

ostomy complications (J95.0-, K94.-, N99.5-)

plateau iris syndrome (post-iridectomy) (postprocedural) H21.82

poisoning and toxic effects of drugs and chemicals (T36–T65 with fifth or sixth character 1–4 or 6)

T81.1 **Postprocedural shock**

Shock during or resulting from a procedure, not elsewhere classified

Excludes1: anaphylactic shock NOS (T78.2)

anaphylactic shock due to correct substance properly administered (T88.6)

anaphylactic shock due to serum (T80.5-)

anesthetic shock (T88.2)

electric shock (T75.4)

obstetric shock (O75.1)

septic shock (R65.21)

shock following abortion or ectopic or molar pregnancy (O00–O07, O08.3)

traumatic shock (T79.4)

7th characters for categories T81–T86
A—initial encounter
D—subsequent encounter
S—sequela

T81.10X **Postprocedural shock unspecified**

Collapse NOS during or resulting from a procedure, not elsewhere classified

Postprocedural failure of peripheral circulation

Postprocedural shock NOS

T81.11X **Postprocedural cardiogenic shock**

T81.12X **Postprocedural septic shock**

Postprocedural endotoxic shock resulting from a procedure, not elsewhere classified

Postprocedural gram-negative shock resulting from a procedure, not elsewhere classified

Code first underlying infection

Use additional code, to identify any associated acute organ dysfunction, if applicable

T81.19X **Other postprocedural shock**

Postprocedural hypovolemic shock

T81.3 **Disruption of wound, not elsewhere classified**

Disruption of any suture materials or other closure methods

Excludes1: breakdown (mechanical) of permanent sutures (T85.612)

displacement of permanent sutures (T85.622)

disruption of cesarean delivery wound (O90.0)

disruption of perineal obstetric wound (O90.1)

mechanical complication of permanent sutures NEC (T85.692)

7th characters for categories T81–T86
A—initial encounter
D—subsequent encounter
S—sequela

T81.30X **Disruption of wound, unspecified**

Disruption of wound NOS

T81.31X **Disruption of external operation (surgical) wound, not elsewhere classified**

Dehiscence of operation wound NOS

Disruption of operation wound NOS

Disruption or dehiscence of closure of cornea

Disruption or dehiscence of closure of mucosa

Disruption or dehiscence of closure of skin and subcutaneous tissue

Full-thickness skin disruption or dehiscence

Superficial disruption or dehiscence of operation wound

Excludes1: dehiscence of amputation stump (T87.81)

T81.33X **Disruption of traumatic injury wound repair**

Disruption or dehiscence of closure of traumatic laceration (external) (internal)

T81.8 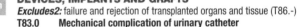 **Other complications of procedures, not elsewhere classified**

Excludes2: hypothermia following anesthesia (T88.51)

malignant hyperpyrexia due to anesthesia (T88.3)

T81.89X **Other complications of procedures, not elsewhere classified**

Use additional code to specify complication, such as: postprocedural delirium (F05)

T82 **COMPLICATIONS OF CARDIAC AND VASCULAR PROSTHETIC DEVICES, IMPLANTS AND GRAFTS**

Excludes2: failure and rejection of transplanted organs and tissue (T86.-)

T82.7XX **Infection and inflammatory reaction due to other cardiac and vascular devices, implants and grafts**

Use additional code to identify infection

T82.8 **Other specified complications of cardiac and vascular prosthetic devices, implants and grafts**

T82.84 **Pain due to cardiac and vascular prosthetic devices, implants and grafts**

T82.847 **Pain due to cardiac prosthetic devices, implants and grafts**

T82.848 **Pain due to vascular prosthetic devices, implants and grafts**

T82.89 **Other specified complication of cardiac and vascular prosthetic devices, implants and grafts**

T82.897 **Other specified complication of cardiac prosthetic devices, implants and grafts**

T82.898 **Other specified complication of vascular prosthetic devices, implants and grafts**

T83 **COMPLICATIONS OF GENITOURINARY PROSTHETIC DEVICES, IMPLANTS AND GRAFTS**

Excludes2: failure and rejection of transplanted organs and tissue (T86.-)

T83.0 **Mechanical complication of urinary catheter**

T83.09 **Other mechanical complication of urinary catheter**

Obstruction (mechanical) of urinary catheter

Perforation of urinary catheter

Protrusion of urinary catheter

T83.090 **Other mechanical complication of cystostomy catheter**

T83.098 **Other mechanical complication of other urinary catheter**

Other mechanical complication of Hopkins catheter

Other mechanical complication of ileostomy catheter

Other mechanical complication of urostomy catheter

T83.5 **Infection and inflammatory reaction due to prosthetic device, implant and graft in urinary system**

Use additional code to identify infection

▲**T83.51** **Infection and inflammatory reaction due to urinary catheter**

Excludes2: complications of stoma of urinary tract (N99.5-)

•**T83.510** **Infection and inflammatory reaction due to cystostomy catheter**

•**T83.511** **Infection and inflammatory reaction due to indwelling urethral catheter**

•**T83.518** **Infection and inflammatory reaction due to other urinary catheter**

Infection and inflammatory reaction due to Hopkins catheter or ileostomy catheter or urostomy catheter

▲**T83.59** **Infection and inflammatory reaction due to prosthetic device, implant and graft in urinary system**

| 4th 5th 6th 7th | Additional Character Required | | 3-character code | Unspecified laterality codes were excluded here. | •=New Code ▲=Revised Code | **Excludes1**—Not coded here, do not use together **Excludes2**—Not included here |

• **T83.591** **Infection and inflammatory reaction due to implanted urinary sphincter**
7th

• **T83.593** **Infection and inflammatory reaction due to other urinary stents**
7th
Infection and inflammatory reaction due to ileal conduit stents
Infection and inflammatory reaction due to nephroureteral stent

• **T83.598** **Infection and inflammatory reaction due to other prosthetic device, implant and graft in urinary system**
7th

T85 **COMPLICATIONS OF OTHER INTERNAL PROSTHETIC DEVICES, IMPLANTS AND GRAFTS**
4th
Excludes2: failure and rejection of transplanted organs and tissue (T86.-)

T85.0 **Mechanical complication of ventricular intracranial (communicating) shunt**
5th

T85.01X **Breakdown (mechanical) of ventricular intracranial (communicating) shunt**
7th

T85.02X **Displacement of ventricular intracranial (communicating) shunt**
7th
Malposition of ventricular intracranial (communicating) shunt

T85.03X **Leakage of ventricular intracranial (communicating) shunt**
7th

T85.09X **Other mechanical complication of ventricular intracranial (communicating) shunt**
7th
Obstruction (mechanical) of ventricular intracranial (communicating) shunt
Perforation of ventricular intracranial (communicating) shunt
Protrusion of ventricular intracranial (communicating) shunt

T86 **COMPLICATIONS OF TRANSPLANTED ORGANS AND TISSUE**
4th
Codes under category T86, Complications of transplanted organs and tissues, are for use for both complications and rejection of transplanted organs. A transplant complication code is only assigned if the complication affects the function of the transplanted organ.
Two codes are required to fully describe a transplant complication: the appropriate code from category T86 and a secondary code that identifies the complication.
Pre-existing conditions or conditions that develop after the transplant are not coded as complications unless they affect the function of the transplanted organs.
See I.C.21. for transplant organ removal status
See I.C.2. for malignant neoplasm associated with transplanted organ.
Use additional code to identify other transplant complications, such as:
graft-versus-host disease (D89.81-)
malignancy associated with organ transplant (C80.2)
post-transplant lymphoproliferative disorders (PTLD) (D47.Z1)

> 7th characters for categories T86–T88
> A—initial encounter
> D—subsequent encounter
> S—sequela

T86.0 **Complications of bone marrow transplant**
5th
T86.01X **Bone marrow transplant rejection**
7th

T86.02X **Bone marrow transplant failure**
7th

T86.1 **Complications of kidney transplant**
5th
Patients who have undergone kidney transplant may still have some form of CKD because the kidney transplant may not fully restore kidney function. Code T86.1- should be assigned for documented complications of a kidney transplant, such as transplant failure or rejection or other transplant complication. Code T86.1- should not be assigned for post kidney transplant patients who have CKD unless a transplant complication such as transplant failure or rejection is documented. If the documentation is unclear as to whether the patient has a complication of the transplant, query the provider.

Conditions that affect the function of the transplanted kidney, other than CKD, should be assigned a code from subcategory T86.1, Complications of transplanted organ, kidney, and a secondary code that identifies the complication.
For patients with CKD following a kidney transplant, but who do not have a complication such as failure or rejection, see section I.C.14. CKD and kidney transplant status.

T86.10X **Unspecified complication of kidney transplant**
7th

T86.11X **Kidney transplant rejection**
7th

T86.12X **Kidney transplant failure**
7th

T86.13X **Kidney transplant infection**
7th
Use additional code to specify infection

T86.19X **Other complication of kidney transplant**
7th

T86.2 **Complications of heart transplant**
5th
Excludes1: complication of:
artificial heart device (T82.5)
heart-lung transplant (T86.3)
T86.21X **Heart transplant rejection**
7th

T86.22X **Heart transplant failure**
7th

T86.4 **Complications of liver transplant**
5th
T86.41X **Liver transplant rejection**
7th

T86.42X **Liver transplant failure**
7th

T86.5XX **Complications of stem cell transplant**
7th
Complications from stem cells from peripheral blood
Complications from stem cells from umbilical cord

T86.8 **Complications of other transplanted organs and tissues**
5th
T86.81 **Complications of lung transplant**
6th
Excludes1: complication of heart-lung transplant (T86.3-)
T86.810 **Lung transplant rejection**
7th

T86.811 **Lung transplant failure**
7th

T86.9 **Complication of unspecified transplanted organ and tissue**
5th
T86.90X **Unspecified complication of unspecified transplanted organ and tissue**
7th

T88 **OTHER COMPLICATIONS OF SURGICAL AND MEDICAL CARE, NOT ELSEWHERE CLASSIFIED**
4th
Excludes2: complication following infusion, transfusion and therapeutic injection (T80.-)
complication following procedure NEC (T81.-)
complications of anesthesia in labor and delivery (O74.-)
complications of anesthesia in pregnancy (O29.-)
complications of anesthesia in puerperium (O89.-)
complications of devices, implants and grafts (T82–T85)
complications of obstetric surgery and procedure (O75.4)
dermatitis due to drugs and medicaments (L23.3, L24.4, L25.1, L27.0–L27.1)
poisoning and toxic effects of drugs and chemicals (T36–T65 with fifth or sixth character 1–4 or 6)
specified complications classified elsewhere

4th 5th 6th 7th Additional Character Required   3-character code

Unspecified laterality codes were excluded here.
•=New Code
▲=Revised Code
Excludes1—Not coded here, do not use together
Excludes2—Not included here

T88.1XX **Other complications following immunization, not elsewhere classified**

7th

Generalized vaccinia

Rash following immunization

Excludes1: vaccinia not from vaccine (B08.011)

Excludes2: anaphylactic shock due to serum (T80.5-)

other serum reactions (T80.6-)

postimmunization arthropathy (M02.2)

postimmunization encephalitis (G04.02)

postimmunization fever (R50.83)

T88.8XX **Other specified complications of surgical and medical care, NEC**

7th

Use additional code to identify the complication

T88.9XX **Complication of surgical and medical care, unspecified**

7th

4th 5th 6th 7th Additional Character Required ✓ 3-character code Unspecified laterality codes were excluded here. •=New Code ▲=Revised Code *Excludes1*—Not coded here, do not use together *Excludes2*—Not included here

PEDIATRIC ICD-10-CM 2017: A MANUAL FOR PROVIDER-BASED CODING 371

Chapter 20. External causes of morbidity (V00–Y99)

GUIDELINES

The external causes of morbidity codes should never be sequenced as the first-listed or principal diagnosis.

External cause codes are intended to provide data for injury research and evaluation of injury prevention strategies. These codes capture how the injury or health condition happened (cause), the intent (unintentional or accidental; or intentional, such as suicide or assault), the place where the event occurred the activity of the patient at the time of the event, and the person's status (e.g., civilian, military).

There is no national requirement for mandatory *ICD-10-CM* external cause code reporting. Unless a provider is subject to a state-based external cause code reporting mandate or these codes are required by a particular payer, reporting of *ICD-10-CM* codes in Chapter 20, External Causes of Morbidity, is not required. In the absence of a mandatory reporting requirement, providers are encouraged to voluntarily report external cause codes, as they provide valuable data for injury research and evaluation of injury prevention strategies.

General External Cause Coding Guidelines

USED WITH ANY CODE IN THE RANGE OF A00.0–T88.9, Z00–Z99

An external cause code may be used with any code in the range of A00.0–T88.9, Z00–Z99, classification that is a health condition due to an external cause. Though they are most applicable to injuries, they are also valid for use with such things as infections or diseases due to an external source, and other health conditions, such as a heart attack that occurs during strenuous physical activity.

EXTERNAL CAUSE CODE USED FOR LENGTH OF TREATMENT

Assign the external cause code, with the appropriate 7th character (initial encounter, subsequent encounter or sequela) for each encounter for which the injury or condition is being treated.

Most categories in chapter 20 have a 7th character requirement for each applicable code. Most categories in this chapter have three 7th character values: A, initial encounter, D, subsequent encounter and S, sequela. While the patient may be seen by a new or different provider over the course of treatment for an injury or condition, assignment of the 7th character for external cause should match the 7th character of the code assigned for the associated injury or condition for the encounter.

USE THE FULL RANGE OF EXTERNAL CAUSE CODES

Use the full range of external cause codes to completely describe the cause, the intent, the place of occurrence, and if applicable, the activity of the patient at the time of the event, and the patient's status, for all injuries, and other health conditions due to an external cause.

ASSIGN AS MANY EXTERNAL CAUSE CODES AS NECESSARY

Assign as many external cause codes as necessary to fully explain each cause. If only one external code can be recorded, assign the code most related to the principal diagnosis.

THE SELECTION OF THE APPROPRIATE EXTERNAL CAUSE CODE

The selection of the appropriate external cause code is guided by the Alphabetic Index of External Causes and by Inclusion and Exclusion notes in the Tabular List.

EXTERNAL CAUSE CODE CAN NEVER BE A PRINCIPAL DIAGNOSIS

An external cause code can never be a principal (first-listed) diagnosis.

COMBINATION EXTERNAL CAUSE CODES

Certain of the external cause codes are combination codes that identify sequential events that result in an injury, such as a fall which results in striking against an object. The injury may be due to either event or both. The combination external cause code used should correspond to the sequence of events regardless of which caused the most serious injury.

NO EXTERNAL CAUSE CODE NEEDED IN CERTAIN CIRCUMSTANCES

No external cause code from Chapter 20 is needed if the external cause and intent are included in a code from another chapter (e.g. T36.0X1- Poisoning by penicillins, accidental (unintentional)).

Place of Occurrence Guideline

Refer to category Y92.

Activity Code

Refer to category Y93.

Place of Occurrence, Activity, and Status Codes Used with other External Cause Code

When applicable, place of occurrence, activity, and external cause status codes are sequenced after the main external cause code(s). Regardless of the number of external cause codes assigned, there should be only one place of occurrence code, one activity code, and one external cause status code assigned to an encounter.

If the Reporting Format Limits the Number of External Cause Codes

If the reporting format limits the number of external cause codes that can be used in reporting clinical data, report the code for the cause/intent most related to the principal diagnosis. If the format permits capture of additional external cause codes, the cause/intent, including medical misadventures, of the additional events should be reported rather than the codes for place, activity, or external status.

Multiple External Cause Coding Guidelines

More than one external cause code is required to fully describe the external cause of an illness or injury. The assignment of external cause codes should be sequenced in the following priority:

If two or more events cause separate injuries, an external cause code should be assigned for each cause. The first-listed external cause code will be selected in the following order:

External codes for child and adult abuse take priority over all other external cause codes.

See Chapter 19, Child and Adult abuse guidelines.

External cause codes for terrorism events take priority over all other external cause codes except child and adult abuse.

External cause codes for cataclysmic events take priority over all other external cause codes except child and adult abuse and terrorism.

External cause codes for transport accidents take priority over all other external cause codes except cataclysmic events, child and adult abuse and terrorism.

Activity and external cause status codes are assigned following all causal (intent) external cause codes.

The first-listed external cause code should correspond to the cause of the most serious diagnosis due to an assault, accident, or self-harm, following the order of hierarchy listed above.

Child and Adult Abuse Guideline

Refer to category Y07.

Unknown or Undetermined Intent Guideline

If the intent (accident, self-harm, assault) of the cause of an injury or other condition is unknown or unspecified, code the intent as accidental intent. All transport accident categories assume accidental intent.

USE OF UNDETERMINED INTENT

External cause codes for events of undetermined intent are only for use if the documentation in the record specifies that the intent cannot be determined.

Sequelae (Late Effects) of External Cause Guidelines

SEQUELAE EXTERNAL CAUSE CODES

Sequelae are reported using the external cause code with the 7th character "S" for sequela. These codes should be used with any report of a late effect or sequela resulting from a previous injury.

SEQUELA EXTERNAL CAUSE CODE WITH A RELATED CURRENT INJURY

A sequela external cause code should never be used with a related current nature of injury code.

| 4th 5th 6th 7th | Additional Character Required | | 3-character code | •=New Code
▲=Revised Code | *Excludes1*—Not coded here, do not use together
Excludes2—Not included here |

CHAPTER 20. EXTERNAL CAUSES OF MORBIDITY   (V00–V00.148)

USE OF SEQUELA EXTERNAL CAUSE CODES FOR SUBSEQUENT VISITS

Use a late effect external cause code for subsequent visits when a late effect of the initial injury is being treated. Do not use a late effect external cause code for subsequent visits for follow-up care (e.g., to assess healing, to receive rehabilitative therapy) of the injury when no late effect of the injury has been documented.

Terrorism Guidelines See *ICD-10-CM* manual for full guidelines.

Cause of injury identified by the Federal Government (FBI) as terrorism
Cause of an injury is suspected to be the result of terrorism Code Y38.9, Terrorism, secondary effects

External cause status

Refer to category Y99.

Note: This chapter permits the classification of environmental events and circumstances as the cause of injury, and other adverse effects. Where a code from this section is applicable, it is intended that it shall be used secondary to a code from another chapter of the Classification indicating the nature of the condition. Most often, the condition will be classifiable to Chapter 19, Injury, poisoning and certain other consequences of external causes (S00–T88). Other conditions that may be stated to be due to external causes are classified in Chapters I to XVIII. For these conditions, codes from Chapter 20 should be used to provide additional information as to the cause of the condition.

ACCIDENTS (V00–X58)

(V00–V99) TRANSPORT ACCIDENTS

Note: This section is structured in 12 groups. Those relating to land transport accidents (V01–V89) reflect the victim's mode of transport and are subdivided to identify the victim's 'counterpart' or the type of event. The vehicle of which the injured person is an occupant is identified in the first two characters since it is seen as the most important factor to identify for prevention purposes. A transport accident is one in which the vehicle involved must be moving or running or in use for transport purposes at the time of the accident.

Use additional code to identify:
Airbag injury (W22.1)
Type of street or road (Y92.4-)
Use of cellular telephone and other electronic equipment at the time of the transport accident (Y93.C-)

Excludes1: agricultural vehicles in stationary use or maintenance (W31.-)
assault by crashing of motor vehicle (Y03.-)
automobile or motor cycle in stationary use or maintenance- code to type of accident
crashing of motor vehicle, undetermined intent (Y32)
intentional self-harm by crashing of motor vehicle (X82)

Excludes2: transport accidents due to cataclysm (X34–X38)
A traffic accident is any vehicle accident occurring on the public highway [i.e. originating on, terminating on, or involving a vehicle partially on the highway]. A vehicle accident is assumed to have occurred on the public highway unless another place is specified, except in the case of accidents involving only off-road motor vehicles, which are classified as nontraffic accidents unless the contrary is stated.
A nontraffic accident is any vehicle accident that occurs entirely in any place other than a public highway. Please see full *ICD-10-CM* manual for definitions of transport vehicles.

(V00–V09) PEDESTRIAN INJURED IN TRANSPORT ACCIDENT

Includes: person changing tire on transport vehicle
person examining engine of vehicle broken down in (on side of) road
Excludes1: fall due to non-transport collision with other person (W03)
pedestrian on foot falling (slipping) on ice and snow (W00.-)
struck or bumped by another person (W51)

7th characters for category V00
A—initial encounter
D—subsequent encounter
S—sequela

V00   PEDESTRIAN CONVEYANCE ACCIDENT

4th   **Use additional place of occurrence and activity external cause codes,** if known (Y92.-, Y93.-)

Excludes1: collision with another person without fall (W51)
fall due to person on foot colliding with another person on foot (W03)
fall from non-moving wheelchair, nonmotorized scooter and motorized mobility scooter without collision (W05.-)
pedestrian (conveyance) collision with other land transport vehicle (V01–V09)
pedestrian on foot falling (slipping) on ice and snow (W00.-)

V00.0   **Pedestrian on foot injured in collision with pedestrian conveyance**

5th

    V00.01X   **Pedestrian on foot injured in collision with roller-skater**

    7th

    V00.02X   **Pedestrian on foot injured in collision with skateboarder**

    7th

    V00.09X   **Pedestrian on foot injured in collision with other pedestrian conveyance**

    7th

V00.1   **Rolling-type pedestrian conveyance accident**

5th   **Excludes1:** accident with babystroller (V00.82-)
accident with wheelchair (powered) (V00.81-)
accident with motorized mobility scooter (V00.83-)

    V00.11   **In-line roller-skate accident**

    6th   **V00.111**   **Fall from in-line roller-skates**

        7th

        V00.112   **In-line roller-skater colliding with stationary object**

        7th

        V00.118   **Other in-line roller-skate accident**
        Excludes1: roller-skater collision with other land transport vehicle (V01–V09 with 5th character 1)

        7th

    V00.12   **Non-in- line roller-skate accident**

    6th   **V00.121**   **Fall from non-in-line roller-skates**

        7th

        V00.122   **Non-in-line roller-skater colliding with stationary object**

        7th

        V00.128   **Other non-in-line roller-skating accident**
        Excludes1: roller-skater collision with other land transport vehicle (V01–V09 with 5th character 1)

        7th

    V00.13   **Skateboard accident**

    6th   **V00.131**   **Fall from skateboard**

        7th

        V00.132   **Skateboarder colliding with stationary object**

        7th

        V00.138   **Other skateboard accident**
        Excludes1: skateboarder collision with other land transport vehicle (V01–V09 with 5th character 2)

        7th

    V00.14   **Scooter (nonmotorized) accident**

    6th   **Excludes1:** motorscooter accident (V20–V29)
    V00.141   **Fall from scooter (nonmotorized)**

        7th

        V00.142   **Scooter (nonmotorized) colliding with stationary object**

        7th

        V00.148   **Other scooter (nonmotorized) accident**
        Excludes1: scooter (nonmotorized) collision with other land transport vehicle (V01–V09 with fifth character 9)

        7th

     Additional Character Required   3-character code   •=New Code   ▲=Revised Code   **Excludes1**—Not coded here, do not use together   **Excludes2**—Not included here

374   **PEDIATRIC ICD-10-CM 2017: A MANUAL FOR PROVIDER-BASED CODING**

V00.15 **6th** **Heelies accident**
Rolling shoe
Wheeled shoe
Wheelies accident

> 7th characters for categories
> V00 and V01
> A—initial encounter
> D—subsequent encounter
> S—sequela

    V00.151 **7th** **Fall from heelies**

    V00.152 **7th** **Heelies colliding with stationary object**

    V00.158 **7th** **Other heelies accident**

V00.18 **6th** **Accident on other rolling-type pedestrian conveyance**
    V00.181 **7th** **Fall from other rolling-type pedestrian conveyance**

    V00.182 **7th** **Pedestrian on other rolling-type pedestrian conveyance colliding with stationary object**

    V00.188 **7th** **Other accident on other rolling-type pedestrian conveyance**

V00.2 **5th** **Gliding-type pedestrian conveyance accident**
  V00.21 **6th** **Ice-skates accident**
    V00.211 **7th** **Fall from ice-skates**

    V00.212 **7th** **Ice-skater colliding with stationary object**

    V00.218 **7th** **Other ice-skates accident**
      Excludes1: ice-skater collision with other land transport vehicle (V01–V09 with 5th character 9)

  V00.22 **6th** **Sled accident**
    V00.221 **7th** **Fall from sled**

    V00.222 **7th** **Sledder colliding with stationary object**

    V00.228 **7th** **Other sled accident**
      Excludes1: sled collision with other land transport vehicle (V01–V09 with 5th character 9)

V00.3 **5th** **Flat-bottomed pedestrian conveyance accident**
  V00.31 **6th** **Snowboard accident**
    V00.311 **7th** **Fall from snowboard**

    V00.312 **7th** **Snowboarder colliding with stationary object**

    V00.318 **7th** **Other snowboard accident**
      Excludes1: snowboarder collision with other land transport vehicle (V01–V09 with 5th character 9)

  V00.32 **6th** **Snow-ski accident**
    V00.321 **7th** **Fall from snow-skis**

    V00.322 **7th** **Snow-skier colliding with stationary object**

    V00.328 **7th** **Other snow-ski accident**
      Excludes1: snow-skier collision with other land transport vehicle (V01–V09 with 5th character 9)

  V00.38 **6th** **Other flat-bottomed pedestrian conveyance accident**

V00.381 **7th** **Fall from other flat-bottomed pedestrian conveyance**

V00.382 **7th** **Pedestrian on other flat-bottomed pedestrian conveyance colliding with stationary object**

V00.388 **7th** **Other accident on other flat-bottomed pedestrian conveyance**

V00.8 **5th** **Accident on other pedestrian conveyance**
  V00.81 **6th** **Accident with wheelchair (powered)**
    V00.811 **7th** **Fall from moving wheelchair (powered)**
      Excludes1: fall from non-moving wheelchair (W05.0)

    V00.812 **7th** **Wheelchair (powered) colliding with stationary object**

    V00.818 **7th** **Other accident with wheelchair (powered)**

  V00.82 **6th** **Accident with babystroller**
    V00.821 **7th** **Fall from babystroller**

    V00.822 **7th** **Babystroller colliding with stationary object**

    V00.828 **7th** **Other accident with babystroller**

V01 **4th** **PEDESTRIAN INJURED IN COLLISION WITH PEDAL CYCLE**
V01.0 **5th** **Pedestrian injured in collision with pedal cycle in nontraffic accident**
  V01.00X **7th** **Pedestrian on foot injured in collision with pedal cycle in nontraffic accident**
    Pedestrian NOS injured in collision with pedal cycle in nontraffic accident

  V01.01X **7th** **Pedestrian on roller-skates injured in collision with pedal cycle in nontraffic accident**

  V01.02X **7th** **Pedestrian on skateboard injured in collision with pedal cycle in nontraffic accident**

  V01.09X **7th** **Pedestrian with other conveyance injured in collision with pedal cycle in nontraffic accident**
    Pedestrian with babystroller injured in collision with pedal cycle in nontraffic accident
    Pedestrian on ice-skates or nonmotorized scooter or motorized mobility scooter or sled or snowboard or snow-skis or wheelchair (powered) injured in collision with pedal cycle in nontraffic accident

V01.1 **5th** **Pedestrian injured in collision with pedal cycle in traffic accident**
  V01.10X **7th** **Pedestrian on foot injured in collision with pedal cycle in traffic accident**
    Pedestrian NOS injured in collision with pedal cycle in traffic accident

  V01.11X **7th** **Pedestrian on roller-skates injured in collision with pedal cycle in traffic accident**

  V01.12X **7th** **Pedestrian on skateboard injured in collision with pedal cycle in traffic accident**

  V01.19X **7th** **Pedestrian with other conveyance injured in collision with pedal cycle in traffic accident**
    Pedestrian with babystroller injured in collision with pedal cycle in traffic accident
    Pedestrian on ice-skates or nonmotorized scooter or motorized mobility scooter or sled or snowboard or snow-skis or wheelchair (powered) injured in collision with pedal cycle in traffic accident

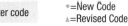
CHAPTER 20. EXTERNAL CAUSES OF MORBIDITY (V00.15–V01.19X)

  Additional Character Required   3-character code

•=New Code
▲=Revised Code

Excludes1—Not coded here, do not use together
Excludes2—Not included here

CHAPTER 20. EXTERNAL CAUSES OF MORBIDITY   (V01.9–V10.3XX)

V01.9   **5th**   Pedestrian injured in collision with pedal cycle, unspecified whether traffic or nontraffic accident

7th characters for categories
V01–V04
A—initial encounter
D—subsequent encounter
S—sequela

V01.90X   **7th**   Pedestrian on foot injured in collision with pedal cycle, unspecified whether traffic or nontraffic accident
Pedestrian NOS injured in collision with pedal cycle, unspecified whether traffic or nontraffic accident

V01.91X   **7th**   Pedestrian on roller-skates injured in collision with pedal cycle, unspecified whether traffic or nontraffic accident

V01.92X   **7th**   Pedestrian on skateboard injured in collision with pedal cycle, unspecified whether traffic or nontraffic accident

V01.99X   **7th**   Pedestrian with other conveyance injured in collision with pedal cycle, unspecified whether traffic or nontraffic accident
Pedestrian with babystroller injured in collision with pedal cycle, unspecified whether traffic or nontraffic accident
Pedestrian on ice-skates or nonmotorized scooter or motorized mobility scooter or sled or snowboard or snow-skis or wheelchair (powered) injured in collision with pedal cycle unspecified, whether traffic or nontraffic accident

V03   **4th**   **PEDESTRIAN INJURED IN COLLISION WITH CAR, PICK-UP TRUCK OR VAN**

V03.0   **5th**   Pedestrian injured in collision with car, pick-up truck or van in nontraffic accident

V03.00X   **7th**   Pedestrian on foot injured in collision with car, pick-up truck or van in nontraffic accident
Pedestrian NOS injured in collision with car, pick-up truck or van in nontraffic accident

V03.01X   **7th**   Pedestrian on roller-skates injured in collision with car, pick-up truck or van in nontraffic accident

V03.02X   **7th**   Pedestrian on skateboard injured in collision with car, pick-up truck or van in nontraffic accident

V03.09X   **7th**   Pedestrian with other conveyance injured in collision with car, pick-up truck or van in nontraffic accident
Pedestrian with babystroller injured in collision with car, pick-up truck or van in nontraffic accident
Pedestrian on ice-skates or nonmotorized scooter or motorized mobility scooter or sled or snowboard or snow-skis or wheelchair (powered) injured in collision with car, pick-up truck or van in nontraffic accident

V03.1   **5th**   Pedestrian injured in collision with car, pick-up truck or van in traffic accident

V03.10X   **7th**   Pedestrian on foot injured in collision with car, pick-up truck or van in traffic accident
Pedestrian NOS injured in collision with car, pick-up truck or van in traffic accident

V03.11X   **7th**   Pedestrian on roller-skates injured in collision with car, pick-up truck or van in traffic accident

V03.12X   **7th**   Pedestrian on skateboard injured in collision with car, pick-up truck or van in traffic accident

V03.19X   **7th**   Pedestrian with other conveyance injured in collision with car, pick-up truck or van in traffic accident
Pedestrian with babystroller injured in collision with car, pick-up truck or van in traffic accident
Pedestrian on ice-skates or nonmotorized scooter or motorized mobility scooter or sled or snowboard or snow-skis or wheelchair (powered) injured in collision with car, pick-up truck or van in traffic accident

V04   **4th**   **PEDESTRIAN INJURED IN COLLISION WITH HEAVY TRANSPORT VEHICLE OR BUS**
Excludes1: pedestrian injured in collision with military vehicle (V09.01, V09.21)

V04.0   **5th**   Pedestrian injured in collision with heavy transport vehicle or bus in nontraffic accident

V04.00X   **7th**   Pedestrian on foot injured in collision with heavy transport vehicle or bus in nontraffic accident
Pedestrian NOS injured in collision with heavy transport vehicle or bus in nontraffic accident

V04.01X   **7th**   Pedestrian on roller-skates injured in collision with heavy transport vehicle or bus in nontraffic accident

V04.02X   **7th**   Pedestrian on skateboard injured in collision with heavy transport vehicle or bus in nontraffic accident

V04.09X   **7th**   Pedestrian with other conveyance injured in collision with heavy transport vehicle or bus in nontraffic accident
Pedestrian with babystroller injured in collision with heavy transport vehicle or bus in nontraffic accident
Pedestrian on ice-skates or nonmotorized scooter or motorized mobility scooter or sled or snowboard or snow-skis or wheelchair (powered) injured in collision with heavy transport vehicle or bus in nontraffic accident

V04.1   **5th**   Pedestrian injured in collision with heavy transport vehicle or bus in traffic accident

V04.10X   **7th**   Pedestrian on foot injured in collision with heavy transport vehicle or bus in traffic accident
Pedestrian NOS injured in collision with heavy transport vehicle or bus in traffic accident

V04.11X   **7th**   Pedestrian on roller-skates injured in collision with heavy transport vehicle or bus in traffic accident

V04.12X   **7th**   Pedestrian on skateboard injured in collision with heavy transport vehicle or bus in traffic accident

V04.19X   **7th**   Pedestrian with other conveyance injured in collision with heavy transport vehicle or bus in traffic accident
Pedestrian with babystroller injured in collision with heavy transport vehicle or bus in traffic accident
Pedestrian on ice-skates or nonmotorized scooter or motorized mobility scooter or sled or snowboard or snow-skis or wheelchair (powered) injured in collision with heavy transport vehicle or bus in traffic accident

(V10–V19) PEDAL CYCLE RIDER INJURED IN TRANSPORT ACCIDENT

Includes: any non-motorized vehicle, excluding an animal-drawn vehicle, or a sidecar or trailer attached to the pedal cycle

Excludes2: rupture of pedal cycle tire (W37.0)

7th characters for categories
V10–V18
A—initial encounter
D—subsequent encounter
S—sequela

V10   **4th**   **PEDAL CYCLE RIDER INJURED IN COLLISION WITH PEDESTRIAN OR ANIMAL**
Excludes1: pedal cycle rider collision with animal-drawn vehicle or animal being ridden (V16.-)

V10.0XX   **7th**   Pedal cycle driver injured in collision with pedestrian or animal in nontraffic accident

V10.1XX   **7th**   Pedal cycle passenger injured in collision with pedestrian or animal in nontraffic accident

V10.2XX   **7th**   Unspecified pedal cyclist injured in collision with pedestrian or animal in nontraffic accident

V10.3XX   **7th**   Person boarding or alighting a pedal cycle injured in collision with pedestrian or animal

---

  Additional Character Required   3-character code

•=New Code
▲=Revised Code

Excludes1—Not coded here, do not use together
Excludes2—Not included here

V10.4XX Pedal cycle driver injured in collision with pedestrian or animal in traffic accident
> 7th

V10.5XX Pedal cycle passenger injured in collision with pedestrian or animal in traffic accident
> 7th

V10.9XX Unspecified pedal cyclist injured in collision with pedestrian or animal in traffic accident
> 7th

V11   **PEDAL CYCLE RIDER INJURED IN COLLISION WITH OTHER PEDAL CYCLE**
> 4th

V11.0XX Pedal cycle driver injured in collision with other pedal cycle in nontraffic accident
> 7th

V11.1XX Pedal cycle passenger injured in collision with other pedal cycle in nontraffic accident
> 7th

V11.2XX Unspecified pedal cyclist injured in collision with other pedal cycle in nontraffic accident
> 7th

V11.3XX Person boarding or alighting a pedal cycle injured in collision with other pedal cycle
> 7th

V11.4XX Pedal cycle driver injured in collision with other pedal cycle in traffic accident
> 7th

V11.5XX Pedal cycle passenger injured in collision with other pedal cycle in traffic accident
> 7th

V11.9XX Unspecified pedal cyclist injured in collision with other pedal cycle in traffic accident
> 7th

V13   **PEDAL CYCLE RIDER INJURED IN COLLISION WITH CAR, PICK-UP TRUCK OR VAN**
> 4th

V13.0XX Pedal cycle driver injured in collision with car, pick-up truck or van in nontraffic accident
> 7th

V13.1XX Pedal cycle passenger injured in collision with car, pick-up truck or van in nontraffic accident
> 7th

V13.2XX Unspecified pedal cyclist injured in collision with car, pick-up truck or van in nontraffic accident
> 7th

V13.3XX Person boarding or alighting a pedal cycle injured in collision with car, pick-up truck or van
> 7th

V13.4XX Pedal cycle driver injured in collision with car, pick-up truck or van in traffic accident
> 7th

V13.5XX Pedal cycle passenger injured in collision with car, pick-up truck or van in traffic accident
> 7th

V13.9XX Unspecified pedal cyclist injured in collision with car, pick-up truck or van in traffic accident
> 7th

V14   **PEDAL CYCLE RIDER INJURED IN COLLISION WITH HEAVY TRANSPORT VEHICLE OR BUS**
> 4th

Excludes1: pedal cycle rider injured in collision with military vehicle (V19.81)

V14.0XX Pedal cycle driver injured in collision with heavy transport vehicle or bus in nontraffic accident
> 7th

V14.1XX Pedal cycle passenger injured in collision with heavy transport vehicle or bus in nontraffic accident
> 7th

V14.2XX Unspecified pedal cyclist injured in collision with heavy transport vehicle or bus in nontraffic accident
> 7th

V14.3XX Person boarding or alighting a pedal cycle injured in collision with heavy transport vehicle or bus
> 7th

V14.4XX Pedal cycle driver injured in collision with heavy transport vehicle or bus in traffic accident
> 7th

V14.5XX Pedal cycle passenger injured in collision with heavy transport vehicle or bus in traffic accident
> 7th

V14.9XX Unspecified pedal cyclist injured in collision with heavy transport vehicle or bus in traffic accident
> 7th

V17   **PEDAL CYCLE RIDER INJURED IN COLLISION WITH FIXED OR STATIONARY OBJECT**
> 4th

V17.0XX Pedal cycle driver injured in collision with fixed or stationary object in nontraffic accident
> 7th

V17.1XX Pedal cycle passenger injured in collision with fixed or stationary object in nontraffic accident
> 7th

V17.2XX Unspecified pedal cyclist injured in collision with fixed or stationary object in nontraffic accident
> 7th

V17.3XX Person boarding or alighting a pedal cycle injured in collision with fixed or stationary object
> 7th

V17.4XX Pedal cycle driver injured in collision with fixed or stationary object in traffic accident
> 7th

V17.5XX Pedal cycle passenger injured in collision with fixed or stationary object in traffic accident
> 7th

V17.9XX Unspecified pedal cyclist injured in collision with fixed or stationary object in traffic accident
> 7th

V18   **PEDAL CYCLE RIDER INJURED IN NONCOLLISION TRANSPORT ACCIDENT**
> 4th

Includes: fall or thrown from pedal cycle (without antecedent collision)
> overturning pedal cycle NOS
> overturning pedal cycle without collision

V18.0XX Pedal cycle driver injured in noncollision transport accident in nontraffic accident
> 7th

V18.1XX Pedal cycle passenger injured in noncollision transport accident in nontraffic accident
> 7th

V18.2XX Unspecified pedal cyclist injured in noncollision transport accident in nontraffic accident
> 7th

V18.3XX Person boarding or alighting a pedal cycle injured in noncollision transport accident
> 7th

V18.4XX Pedal cycle driver injured in noncollision transport accident in traffic accident
> 7th

V18.5XX Pedal cycle passenger injured in noncollision transport accident in traffic accident
> 7th

V18.9XX Unspecified pedal cyclist injured in noncollision transport accident in traffic accident
> 7th

V19   **PEDAL CYCLE RIDER INJURED IN OTHER AND UNSPECIFIED TRANSPORT ACCIDENTS**
> 4th

V19.9XX Pedal cyclist (driver) (passenger) injured in unspecified traffic accident
> 7th
> Pedal cycle accident NOS

   Additional Character Required   3-character code

•=New Code
▲=Revised Code

Excludes1—Not coded here, do not use together
Excludes2—Not included here

CHAPTER 20. EXTERNAL CAUSES OF MORBIDITY (V20–V28.2XX)

(V20–V29) MOTORCYCLE RIDER INJURED IN TRANSPORT ACCIDENT

Includes: moped
   motorcycle with sidecar
   motorized bicycle
   motor scooter

Excludes1: three-wheeled motor vehicle (V30–V39)

> 7th characters for categories
> V20–V29
> A—initial encounter
> D—subsequent encounter
> S—sequela

V20 · 4th — **MOTORCYCLE RIDER INJURED IN COLLISION WITH PEDESTRIAN OR ANIMAL**
> **Excludes1:** motorcycle rider collision with animal-drawn vehicle or animal being ridden (V26.-)

V20.0XX · 7th — Motorcycle driver injured in collision with pedestrian or animal in nontraffic accident

V20.1XX · 7th — Motorcycle passenger injured in collision with pedestrian or animal in nontraffic accident

V20.2XX · 7th — Unspecified motorcycle rider injured in collision with pedestrian or animal in nontraffic accident

V20.3XX · 7th — Person boarding or alighting a motorcycle injured in collision with pedestrian or animal

V20.4XX · 7th — Motorcycle driver injured in collision with pedestrian or animal in traffic accident

V20.5XX · 7th — Motorcycle passenger injured in collision with pedestrian or animal in traffic accident

V20.9XX · 7th — Unspecified motorcycle rider injured in collision with pedestrian or animal in traffic accident

V21 · 4th — **MOTORCYCLE RIDER INJURED IN COLLISION WITH PEDAL CYCLE**
> **Excludes1:** motorcycle rider collision with animal-drawn vehicle or animal being ridden (V26.-)

V21.0XX · 7th — Motorcycle driver injured in collision or with pedal cycle in nontraffic accident

V21.1XX · 7th — Motorcycle passenger injured in collision with pedal cycle in nontraffic accident

V21.2XX · 7th — Unspecified motorcycle rider injured in collision with pedal cycle in nontraffic accident

V21.3XX · 7th — Person boarding or alighting a motorcycle injured in collision with pedal cycle

V21.4XX · 7th — Motorcycle driver injured in collision with pedal cycle in traffic accident

V21.5XX · 7th — Motorcycle passenger injured in collision with pedal cycle in traffic accident

V21.9XX · 7th — Unspecified motorcycle rider injured in collision with pedal cycle in traffic accident

V23 · 4th — **MOTORCYCLE RIDER INJURED IN COLLISION WITH CAR, PICK-UP TRUCK OR VAN**

V23.0XX · 7th — Motorcycle driver injured in collision with car, pick-up truck or van in nontraffic accident

V23.1XX · 7th — Motorcycle passenger injured in collision with car, pick-up truck or van in nontraffic accident

V23.2XX · 7th — Unspecified motorcycle rider injured in collision with car, pick-up truck or van in nontraffic accident

V23.3XX · 7th — Person boarding or alighting a motorcycle injured in collision with car, pick-up truck or van

V23.4XX · 7th — Motorcycle driver injured in collision with car, pick-up truck or van in traffic accident

V23.5XX · 7th — Motorcycle passenger injured in collision with car, pick-up truck or van in traffic accident

V23.9XX · 7th — Unspecified motorcycle rider injured in collision with car, pick-up truck or van in traffic accident

V24 · 4th — **MOTORCYCLE RIDER INJURED IN COLLISION WITH HEAVY TRANSPORT VEHICLE OR BUS**
> **Excludes1:** motorcycle rider injured in collision with military vehicle (V29.81)

V24.0XX · 7th — Motorcycle driver injured in collision with heavy transport vehicle or bus in nontraffic accident

V24.1XX · 7th — Motorcycle passenger injured in collision with heavy transport vehicle or bus in nontraffic accident

V24.2XX · 7th — Unspecified motorcycle rider injured in collision with heavy transport vehicle or bus in nontraffic accident

V24.3XX · 7th — Person boarding or alighting a motorcycle injured in collision with heavy transport vehicle or bus

V24.4XX · 7th — Motorcycle driver injured in collision with heavy transport vehicle or bus in traffic accident

V24.5XX · 7th — Motorcycle passenger injured in collision with heavy transport vehicle or bus in traffic accident

V24.9XX · 7th — Unspecified motorcycle rider injured in collision with heavy transport vehicle or bus in traffic accident

V27 · 4th — **MOTORCYCLE RIDER INJURED IN COLLISION WITH FIXED OR STATIONARY OBJECT**

V27.0XX · 7th — Motorcycle driver injured in collision with fixed or stationary object in nontraffic accident

V27.1XX · 7th — Motorcycle passenger injured in collision with fixed or stationary object in nontraffic accident

V27.2XX · 7th — Unspecified motorcycle rider injured in collision with fixed or stationary object in nontraffic accident

V27.3XX · 7th — Person boarding or alighting a motorcycle injured in collision with fixed or stationary object

V27.4XX · 7th — Motorcycle driver injured in collision with fixed or stationary object in traffic accident

V27.5XX · 7th — Motorcycle passenger injured in collision with fixed or stationary object in traffic accident

V27.9XX · 7th — Unspecified motorcycle rider injured in collision with fixed or stationary object in traffic accident

V28 · 4th — **MOTORCYCLE RIDER INJURED IN NONCOLLISION TRANSPORT ACCIDENT**
> **Includes:** fall or thrown from motorcycle (without antecedent collision)
> overturning motorcycle NOS
> overturning motorcycle without collision

V28.0XX · 7th — Motorcycle driver injured in noncollision transport accident in nontraffic accident

V28.1XX · 7th — Motorcycle passenger injured in noncollision transport accident in nontraffic accident

V28.2XX · 7th — Unspecified motorcycle rider injured in noncollision transport accident in nontraffic accident

---

   4th 5th 6th 7th   Additional Character Required   3-character code

•=New Code
▲=Revised Code

Excludes1—Not coded here, do not use together
Excludes2—Not included here

V28.3XX Person boarding or alighting a motorcycle injured in noncollision transport accident
`7th`

V28.4XX Motorcycle driver injured in noncollision transport accident in traffic accident
`7th`

V28.5XX Motorcycle passenger injured in noncollision transport accident in traffic accident
`7th`

V28.9XX Unspecified motorcycle rider injured in noncollision transport accident in traffic accident
`7th`

V29 `4th` MOTORCYCLE RIDER INJURED IN OTHER AND UNSPECIFIED TRANSPORT ACCIDENTS

7th characters for category V29
A—initial encounter
D—subsequent encounter
S—sequela

V29.0 `5th` Motorcycle driver injured in collision with other and unspecified motor vehicles in nontraffic accident

V29.00X Motorcycle driver injured in collision with unspecified motor vehicles in nontraffic accident
`7th`

V29.09X Motorcycle driver injured in collision with other motor vehicles in nontraffic accident
`7th`

V29.1 `5th` Motorcycle passenger injured in collision with other and unspecified motor vehicles in nontraffic accident

V29.10X Motorcycle passenger injured in collision with unspecified motor vehicles in nontraffic accident
`7th`

V29.19X Motorcycle passenger injured in collision with other motor vehicles in nontraffic accident
`7th`

V29.2 `5th` Unspecified motorcycle rider injured in collision with other and unspecified motor vehicles in nontraffic accident

V29.20X Unspecified motorcycle rider injured in collision with unspecified motor vehicles in nontraffic accident
`7th`
Motorcycle collision NOS, nontraffic

V29.29X Unspecified motorcycle rider injured in collision with other motor vehicles in nontraffic accident
`7th`

V29.3XX Motorcycle rider (driver) (passenger) injured in unspecified nontraffic accident
`7th`
Motorcycle accident NOS, nontraffic
Motorcycle rider injured in nontraffic accident NOS

V29.4 `5th` Motorcycle driver injured in collision with other and unspecified motor vehicles in traffic accident

V29.40X Motorcycle driver injured in collision with unspecified motor vehicles in traffic accident
`7th`

V29.49X Motorcycle driver injured in collision with other motor vehicles in traffic accident
`7th`

V29.5 `5th` Motorcycle passenger injured in collision with other and unspecified motor vehicles in traffic accident

V29.50X Motorcycle passenger injured in collision with unspecified motor vehicles in traffic accident
`7th`

V29.59X Motorcycle passenger injured in collision with other motor vehicles in traffic accident
`7th`

V29.6 `5th` Unspecified motorcycle rider injured in collision with other and unspecified motor vehicles in traffic accident

V29.60X Unspecified motorcycle rider injured in collision with unspecified motor vehicles in traffic accident
`7th`
Motorcycle collision NOS (traffic)

V29.69X Unspecified motorcycle rider injured in collision with other motor vehicles in traffic accident
`7th`

V29.8 `5th` Motorcycle rider (driver) (passenger) injured in other specified transport accidents

V29.81X Motorcycle rider (driver) (passenger) injured in transport accident with military vehicle
`7th`

V29.88X Motorcycle rider (driver) (passenger) injured in other specified transport accidents
`7th`

V29.9XX Motorcycle rider (driver) (passenger) injured in unspecified traffic accident
`7th`
Motorcycle accident NOS

(V30–V39) OCCUPANT OF THREE-WHEELED MOTOR VEHICLE INJURED IN TRANSPORT ACCIDENT

Includes: motorized tricycle
motorized rickshaw
three-wheeled motor car

Excludes1: all-terrain vehicles (V86.-)
motorcycle with sidecar (V20–V29)
vehicle designed primarily for off-road use (V86.-)

7th characters for categories V30–V39
A—initial encounter
D—subsequent encounter
S—sequela

V30 `4th` OCCUPANT OF THREE-WHEELED MOTOR VEHICLE INJURED IN COLLISION WITH PEDESTRIAN OR ANIMAL

Excludes1: three-wheeled motor vehicle collision with animal-drawn vehicle or animal being ridden (V36.-)

V30.0XX Driver of three-wheeled motor vehicle injured in collision with pedestrian or animal in nontraffic accident
`7th`

V30.1XX Passenger in three-wheeled motor vehicle injured in collision with pedestrian or animal in nontraffic accident
`7th`

V30.2XX Person on outside of three-wheeled motor vehicle injured in collision with pedestrian or animal in nontraffic accident
`7th`

V30.3XX Unspecified occupant of three-wheeled motor vehicle injured in collision with pedestrian or animal in nontraffic accident
`7th`

V30.4XX Person boarding or alighting a three-wheeled motor vehicle injured in collision with pedestrian or animal
`7th`

V30.5XX Driver of three-wheeled motor vehicle injured in collision with pedestrian or animal in traffic accident
`7th`

V30.6XX Passenger in three-wheeled motor vehicle injured in collision with pedestrian or animal in traffic accident
`7th`

V30.7XX Person on outside of three-wheeled motor vehicle injured in collision with pedestrian or animal in traffic accident
`7th`

V30.9XX Unspecified occupant of three-wheeled motor vehicle injured in collision with pedestrian or animal in traffic accident
`7th`

V32 `4th` OCCUPANT OF THREE-WHEELED MOTOR VEHICLE INJURED IN COLLISION WITH TWO- OR THREE-WHEELED MOTOR VEHICLE

V32.0XX Driver of three-wheeled motor vehicle injured in collision with two- or three-wheeled motor vehicle in nontraffic accident
`7th`

V32.1XX Passenger in three-wheeled motor vehicle injured in collision with two- or three-wheeled motor vehicle in nontraffic accident
`7th`

V32.2XX Person on outside of three-wheeled motor vehicle injured in collision with two- or three-wheeled motor vehicle in nontraffic accident
`7th`

V32.3XX Unspecified occupant of three-wheeled motor vehicle injured in collision with two- or three-wheeled motor vehicle in nontraffic accident
`7th`

V32.4XX Person boarding or alighting a three-wheeled motor vehicle injured in collision with two- or three-wheeled motor vehicle
`7th`

V32.5XX Driver of three-wheeled motor vehicle injured in collision with two- or three-wheeled motor vehicle in traffic accident
`7th`

   Additional Character Required
 3-character code
• =New Code
▲ =Revised Code
Excludes1 Not coded here, do not use together
Excludes2—Not included here

CHAPTER 20. EXTERNAL CAUSES OF MORBIDITY   (V32.6XX–V39.00X)

V32.6XX   Passenger in three-wheeled motor vehicle injured in collision with two- or three-wheeled motor vehicle in traffic accident
`7th`

V32.7XX   Person on outside of three-wheeled motor vehicle injured in collision with two- or three-wheeled motor vehicle in traffic accident
`7th`

V32.9XX   Unspecified occupant of three-wheeled motor vehicle injured in collision with two- or three-wheeled motor vehicle in traffic accident
`7th`

V33   **OCCUPANT OF THREE-WHEELED MOTOR VEHICLE INJURED IN COLLISION WITH CAR, PICK-UP TRUCK OR VAN**
`4th`

> 7th characters for categories
> V30–V39
> A—initial encounter
> D—subsequent encounter
> S—sequela

V33.0XX   Driver of three-wheeled motor vehicle injured in collision with car, pick-up truck or van in nontraffic accident
`7th`

V33.1XX   Passenger in three-wheeled motor vehicle injured in collision with car, pick-up truck or van in nontraffic accident
`7th`

V33.2XX   Person on outside of three-wheeled motor vehicle injured in collision with car, pick-up truck or van in nontraffic accident
`7th`

V33.3XX   Unspecified occupant of three-wheeled motor vehicle injured in collision with car, pick-up truck or van in nontraffic accident
`7th`

V33.4XX   Person boarding or alighting a three-wheeled motor vehicle injured in collision with car, pick-up truck or van
`7th`

V33.5XX   Driver of three-wheeled motor vehicle injured in collision with car, pick-up truck or van in traffic accident
`7th`

V33.6XX   Passenger in three-wheeled motor vehicle injured in collision with car, pick-up truck or van in traffic accident
`7th`

V33.7XX   Person on outside of three-wheeled motor vehicle injured in collision with car, pick-up truck or van in traffic accident
`7th`

V33.9XX   Unspecified occupant of three-wheeled motor vehicle injured in collision with car, pick-up truck or van in traffic accident
`7th`

V34   **OCCUPANT OF THREE-WHEELED MOTOR VEHICLE INJURED IN COLLISION WITH HEAVY TRANSPORT VEHICLE OR BUS**
`4th`

Excludes1: occupant of three-wheeled motor vehicle injured in collision with military vehicle (V39.81)

V34.0XX   Driver of three-wheeled motor vehicle injured in collision with heavy transport vehicle or bus in nontraffic accident
`7th`

V34.1XX   Passenger in three-wheeled motor vehicle injured in collision with heavy transport vehicle or bus in nontraffic accident
`7th`

V34.2XX   Person on outside of three-wheeled motor vehicle injured in collision with heavy transport vehicle or bus in nontraffic accident
`7th`

V34.3XX   Unspecified occupant of three-wheeled motor vehicle injured in collision with heavy transport vehicle or bus in nontraffic accident
`7th`

V34.4XX   Person boarding or alighting a three-wheeled motor vehicle injured in collision with heavy transport vehicle or bus
`7th`

V34.5XX   Driver of three-wheeled motor vehicle injured in collision with heavy transport vehicle or bus in traffic accident
`7th`

V34.6XX   Passenger in three-wheeled motor vehicle injured in collision with heavy transport vehicle or bus in traffic accident
`7th`

V34.7XX   Person on outside of three-wheeled motor vehicle injured in collision with heavy transport vehicle or bus in traffic accident
`7th`

V34.9XX   Unspecified occupant of three-wheeled motor vehicle injured in collision with heavy transport vehicle or bus in traffic accident
`7th`

V37   **OCCUPANT OF THREE-WHEELED MOTOR VEHICLE INJURED IN COLLISION WITH FIXED OR STATIONARY OBJECT**
`4th`

V37.0XX   Driver of three-wheeled motor vehicle injured in collision with fixed or stationary object in nontraffic accident
`7th`

V37.1XX   Passenger in three-wheeled motor vehicle injured in collision with fixed or stationary object in nontraffic accident
`7th`

V37.2XX   Person on outside of three-wheeled motor vehicle injured in collision with fixed or stationary object in nontraffic accident
`7th`

V37.3XX   Unspecified occupant of three-wheeled motor vehicle injured in collision with fixed or stationary object in nontraffic accident
`7th`

V37.4XX   Person boarding or alighting a three-wheeled motor vehicle injured in collision with fixed or stationary object
`7th`

V37.5XX   Driver of three-wheeled motor vehicle injured in collision with fixed or stationary object in traffic accident
`7th`

V37.6XX   Passenger in three-wheeled motor vehicle injured in collision with fixed or stationary object in traffic accident
`7th`

V37.7XX   Person on outside of three-wheeled motor vehicle injured in collision with fixed or stationary object in traffic accident
`7th`

V37.9XX   Unspecified occupant of three-wheeled motor vehicle injured in collision with fixed or stationary object in traffic accident
`7th`

V38   **OCCUPANT OF THREE-WHEELED MOTOR VEHICLE INJURED IN NONCOLLISION TRANSPORT ACCIDENT**
`4th`

Includes: fall or thrown from three-wheeled motor vehicle
> overturning of three-wheeled motor vehicle NOS
> overturning of three-wheeled motor vehicle without collision

V38.0XX   Driver of three-wheeled motor vehicle injured in noncollision transport accident in nontraffic accident
`7th`

V38.1XX   Passenger in three-wheeled motor vehicle injured in noncollision transport accident in nontraffic accident
`7th`

V38.2XX   Person on outside of three-wheeled motor vehicle injured in noncollision transport accident in nontraffic accident
`7th`

V38.3XX   Unspecified occupant of three-wheeled motor vehicle injured in noncollision transport accident in nontraffic accident
`7th`

V38.4XX   Person boarding or alighting a three-wheeled motor vehicle injured in noncollision transport accident
`7th`

V38.5XX   Driver of three-wheeled motor vehicle injured in noncollision transport accident in traffic accident
`7th`

V38.6XX   Passenger in three-wheeled motor vehicle injured in noncollision transport accident in traffic accident
`7th`

V38.7XX   Person on outside of three-wheeled motor vehicle injured in noncollision transport accident in traffic accident
`7th`

V38.9XX   Unspecified occupant of three-wheeled motor vehicle injured in noncollision transport accident in traffic accident
`7th`

V39   **OCCUPANT OF THREE-WHEELED MOTOR VEHICLE INJURED IN OTHER AND UNSPECIFIED TRANSPORT ACCIDENTS**
`4th`

V39.0   Driver of three-wheeled motor vehicle injured in collision with other and unspecified motor vehicles in nontraffic accident
`5th`

    V39.00X   Driver of three-wheeled motor vehicle injured in collision with unspecified motor vehicles in nontraffic accident
    `7th`

`4th` `5th` `6th` `7th`   Additional Character Required   3-character code

•=New Code
▲=Revised Code

Excludes1—Not coded here, do not use together
Excludes2—Not included here

V39.09X | 7th — Driver of three-wheeled motor vehicle injured in collision with other motor vehicles in nontraffic accident

V39.1 | 5th — Passenger in three-wheeled motor vehicle injured in collision with other and unspecified motor vehicles in nontraffic accident

> 7th characters for category V39
> A—initial encounter
> D—subsequent encounter
> S—sequela

V39.10X | 7th — Passenger in three-wheeled motor vehicle injured in collision with unspecified motor vehicles in nontraffic accident

V39.19X | 7th — Passenger in three-wheeled motor vehicle injured in collision with other motor vehicles in nontraffic accident

V39.2 | 5th — Unspecified occupant of three-wheeled motor vehicle injured in collision with other and unspecified motor vehicles in nontraffic accident

V39.20X | 7th — Unspecified occupant of three-wheeled motor vehicle injured in collision with unspecified motor vehicles in nontraffic accident
Collision NOS involving three-wheeled motor vehicle, nontraffic

V39.29X | 7th — Unspecified occupant of three-wheeled

V39.3XX | 7th — Occupant (driver) (passenger) of three-wheeled motor vehicle injured in unspecified nontraffic accident
Accident NOS involving three-wheeled motor vehicle, nontraffic
Occupant of three-wheeled motor vehicle injured in nontraffic accident NOS

V39.4 | 5th — Driver of three-wheeled motor vehicle injured in collision with other and unspecified motor vehicles in traffic accident

V39.40X | 7th — Driver of three-wheeled motor vehicle injured in collision with unspecified motor vehicles in traffic accident

V39.49X | 7th — Driver of three-wheeled motor vehicle injured in collision with other motor vehicles in traffic accident

V39.5 | 5th — Passenger in three-wheeled motor vehicle injured in collision with other and unspecified motor vehicles in traffic accident

V39.50X | 7th — Passenger in three-wheeled motor vehicle injured in collision with unspecified motor vehicles in traffic accident

V39.59X | 7th — Passenger in three-wheeled motor vehicle injured in collision with other motor vehicles in traffic accident

V39.6 | 5th — Unspecified occupant of three-wheeled motor vehicle injured in collision with other and unspecified motor vehicles in traffic accident

V39.60X | 7th — Unspecified occupant of three-wheeled motor vehicle injured in collision with unspecified motor vehicles in traffic accident
Collision NOS involving three-wheeled motor vehicle (traffic)

V39.69X | 7th — Unspecified occupant of three-wheeled motor vehicle injured in collision with other motor vehicles in traffic accident

V39.8 | 5th — Occupant (driver) (passenger) of three-wheeled motor vehicle injured in other specified transport accidents

V39.81X | 7th — Occupant (driver) (passenger) of three-wheeled motor vehicle injured in transport accident with military vehicle

V39.89X | 7th — Occupant (driver) (passenger) of three-wheeled motor vehicle injured in other specified transport accidents

V39.9XX | 7th — Occupant (driver) (passenger) of three-wheeled motor vehicle injured in unspecified traffic accident
Accident NOS involving three-wheeled motor vehicle

(V40–V49) CAR OCCUPANT INJURED IN TRANSPORT ACCIDENT

Includes: a four-wheeled motor vehicle designed primarily for carrying passengers
    automobile (pulling a trailer or camper)

Excludes1: bus (V50–V59)
    minibus (V50–V59)
    minivan (V50–V59)
    motorcoach (V70–V79)
    pick-up truck (V50–V59)
    sport utility vehicle (SUV) (V50–V59)

> 7th characters for categories
> V40–V49
> A—initial encounter
> D—subsequent encounter
> S—sequela

V40 | 4th — CAR OCCUPANT INJURED IN COLLISION WITH PEDESTRIAN OR ANIMAL
Excludes1: car collision with animal-drawn vehicle or animal being ridden (V46.-)

V40.0XX | 7th — Car driver injured in collision with pedestrian or animal in nontraffic accident

V40.1XX | 7th — Car passenger injured in collision with pedestrian or animal in nontraffic accident

V40.2XX | 7th — Person on outside of car injured in collision with pedestrian or animal in nontraffic accident

V40.3XX | 7th — Unspecified car occupant injured in collision with pedestrian or animal in nontraffic accident

V40.4XX | 7th — Person boarding or alighting a car injured in collision with pedestrian or animal

V40.5XX | 7th — Car driver injured in collision with pedestrian or animal in traffic accident

V40.6XX | 7th — Car passenger injured in collision with pedestrian or animal in traffic accident

V40.7XX | 7th — Person on outside of car injured in collision with pedestrian or animal in traffic accident

V40.9XX | 7th — Unspecified car occupant injured in collision with pedestrian or animal in traffic accident

V42 | 4th — CAR OCCUPANT INJURED IN COLLISION WITH TWO- OR THREE-WHEELED MOTOR VEHICLE

V42.0XX | 7th — Car driver injured in collision with two- or three-wheeled motor vehicle in nontraffic accident

V42.1XX | 7th — Car passenger injured in collision with two- or three-wheeled motor vehicle in nontraffic accident

V42.2XX | 7th — Person on outside of car injured in collision with two- or three-wheeled motor vehicle in nontraffic accident

V42.3XX | 7th — Unspecified car occupant injured in collision with two- or three-wheeled motor vehicle in nontraffic accident

V42.4XX | 7th — Person boarding or alighting a car injured in collision with two- or three-wheeled motor vehicle

V42.5XX | 7th — Car driver injured in collision with two- or three-wheeled motor vehicle in traffic accident

V42.6XX | 7th — Car passenger injured in collision with two- or three-wheeled motor vehicle in traffic accident

V42.7XX | 7th — Person on outside of car injured in collision with two- or three-wheeled motor vehicle in traffic accident

V42.9XX | 7th — Unspecified car occupant injured in collision with two- or three-wheeled motor vehicle in traffic accident

---

  Additional Character Required   ✓ 3-character code   •=New Code   ▲=Revised Code

Excludes1—Not coded here, do not use together
Excludes2—Not included here

CHAPTER 20. EXTERNAL CAUSES OF MORBIDITY   (V43–V44.3XX)

V43 **CAR OCCUPANT INJURED IN COLLISION WITH CAR, PICK-UP TRUCK OR VAN**
`4th`

V43.0 Car driver injured in collision with car, pick-up truck or van in nontraffic accident
`5th`

7th characters for categories
V40–V49
A—initial encounter
D—subsequent encounter
S—sequela

     V43.01X Car driver injured in collision with sport utility vehicle in nontraffic accident
`7th`

     V43.02X Car driver injured in collision with other type car in nontraffic accident
`7th`

     V43.03X Car driver injured in collision with pick-up truck in nontraffic accident
`7th`

     V43.04X Car driver injured in collision with van in nontraffic accident
`7th`

V43.1 Car passenger injured in collision with car, pick-up truck or van in nontraffic accident
`5th`

     V43.11X Car passenger injured in collision with sport utility vehicle in nontraffic accident
`7th`

     V43.12X Car passenger injured in collision with other type car in nontraffic accident
`7th`

     V43.13X Car passenger injured in collision with pick-up in nontraffic accident
`7th`

     V43.14X Car passenger injured in collision with van in nontraffic accident
`7th`

V43.2 Person on outside of car injured in collision with car, pick-up truck or van in nontraffic accident
`5th`

     V43.21X Person on outside of car injured in collision with sport utility vehicle in nontraffic accident
`7th`

     V43.22X Person on outside of car injured in collision with other type car in nontraffic accident
`7th`

     V43.23X Person on outside of car injured in collision with pick-up truck in nontraffic accident
`7th`

     V43.24X Person on outside of car injured in collision with van in nontraffic accident
`7th`

V43.3 Unspecified car occupant injured in collision with car, pick-up truck or van in nontraffic accident
`5th`

     V43.31X Unspecified car occupant injured in collision with sport utility vehicle in nontraffic accident
`7th`

     V43.32X Unspecified car occupant injured in collision with other type car in nontraffic accident
`7th`

     V43.33X Unspecified car occupant injured in collision with pick-up truck in nontraffic accident
`7th`

     V43.34X Unspecified car occupant injured in collision with van in nontraffic accident
`7th`

V43.4 Person boarding or alighting a car injured in collision with car, pick-up truck or van
`5th`

     V43.41X Person boarding or alighting a car injured in collision with sport utility vehicle, initial encounter
`7th`

     V43.42X Person boarding or alighting a car injured in collision with other type car
`7th`

     V43.43X Person boarding or alighting a car injured in collision with pick-up truck
`7th`

     V43.44X Person boarding or alighting a car injured in collision with van
`7th`

V43.5 Car driver injured in collision with car, pick-up truck or van in traffic accident
`5th`

     V43.51X Car driver injured in collision with sport utility vehicle in traffic accident
`7th`

     V43.52X Car driver injured in collision with other type car in traffic accident
`7th`

     V43.53X Car driver injured in collision with pick-up truck in traffic accident
`7th`

     V43.54X Car driver injured in collision with van in traffic accident
`7th`

V43.6 Car passenger injured in collision with car, pick-up truck or van in traffic accident
`5th`

     V43.61X Car passenger injured in collision with sport utility vehicle in traffic accident
`7th`

     V43.62X Car passenger injured in collision with other type car in traffic accident
`7th`

     V43.63X Car passenger injured in collision with pick-up truck in traffic accident
`7th`

     V43.64X Car passenger injured in collision with van in traffic accident
`7th`

V43.7 Person on outside of car injured in collision with car, pick-up truck or van in traffic accident
`5th`

     V43.71X Person on outside of car injured in collision with sport utility vehicle in traffic accident
`7th`

     V43.72X Person on outside of car injured in collision with other type car in traffic accident
`7th`

     V43.73X Person on outside of car injured in collision with pick-up truck in traffic accident
`7th`

     V43.74X Person on outside of car injured in collision with van in traffic accident
`7th`

V43.9 Unspecified car occupant injured in collision with car, pick-up truck or van in traffic accident
`5th`

     V43.91X Unspecified car occupant injured in collision with sport utility vehicle in traffic accident
`7th`

     V43.92X Unspecified car occupant injured in collision with other type car in traffic accident
`7th`

     V43.93X Unspecified car occupant injured in collision with pick-up truck in traffic accident
`7th`

     V43.94X Unspecified car occupant injured in collision with van in traffic accident
`7th`

V44 **CAR OCCUPANT INJURED IN COLLISION WITH HEAVY TRANSPORT VEHICLE OR BUS**
`4th`

Excludes1: car occupant injured in collision with military vehicle (V49.81)

V44.0XX Car driver injured in collision with heavy transport vehicle or bus in nontraffic accident
`7th`

V44.1XX Car passenger injured in collision with heavy transport vehicle or bus in nontraffic accident
`7th`

V44.2XX Person on outside of car injured in collision with heavy transport vehicle or bus in nontraffic accident
`7th`

V44.3XX Unspecified car occupant injured in collision with heavy transport vehicle or bus in nontraffic accident
`7th`

7th characters for categories
V40–V49
A—initial encounter
D—subsequent encounter
S—sequela

`4th` `5th` `6th` `7th`   Additional Character Required   ✓   3-character code

•=New Code
▲=Revised Code

Excludes1—Not coded here, do not use together
Excludes2—Not included here

V44.4XX Person boarding or alighting a car injured in collision with heavy transport vehicle or bus
`7th`

V44.5XX Car driver injured in collision with heavy transport vehicle or bus in traffic accident
`7th`

V44.6XX Car passenger injured in collision with heavy transport vehicle or bus in traffic accident
`7th`

V44.7XX Person on outside of car injured in collision with heavy transport vehicle or bus in traffic accident
`7th`

V44.9XX Unspecified car occupant injured in collision with heavy transport vehicle or bus in traffic accident
`7th`

V45 `4th` **CAR OCCUPANT INJURED IN COLLISION WITH RAILWAY TRAIN OR RAILWAY VEHICLE**

V45.0XX Car driver injured in collision with railway train or railway vehicle in nontraffic
`7th`

V45.1XX Car passenger injured in collision with railway train or railway vehicle in nontraffic accident
`7th`

V45.2XX Person on outside of car injured in collision with railway train or railway vehicle in nontraffic accident
`7th`

V45.3XX Unspecified car occupant injured in collision with railway train or railway vehicle in nontraffic accident
`7th`

V45.4XX Person boarding or alighting a car injured in collision with railway train or railway vehicle
`7th`

V45.5XX Car driver injured in collision with railway train or railway vehicle in traffic accident
`7th`

V45.6XX Car passenger injured in collision with railway train or railway vehicle in traffic accident
`7th`

V45.7XX Person on outside of car injured in collision with railway train or railway vehicle in traffic accident
`7th`

V45.9XX Unspecified car occupant injured in collision with railway train or railway vehicle in traffic accident
`7th`

V47 `4th` **CAR OCCUPANT INJURED IN COLLISION WITH FIXED OR STATIONARY OBJECT**

▲V47.0XX Car driver injured in collision with fixed or stationary object in nontraffic accident
`7th`

▲V47.1XX Car passenger injured in collision with fixed or stationary object in nontraffic accident
`7th`

▲V47.2XX Person on outside of car injured in collision with fixed or stationary object in nontraffic accident
`7th`

▲V47.3XX Unspecified car occupant injured in collision with fixed or stationary object in nontraffic accident
`7th`

▲V47.4XX Person boarding or alighting a car injured in collision with fixed or stationary object
`7th`

▲V47.5XX Car driver injured in collision with fixed or stationary object in traffic accident
`7th`

▲V47.6XX Car passenger injured in collision with fixed or stationary object in traffic accident
`7th`

▲V47.7XX Person on outside of car injured in collision with fixed or stationary object in traffic accident
`7th`

▲V47.9XX Unspecified car occupant injured in collision with fixed or stationary object in traffic accident
`7th`

V48 `4th` **CAR OCCUPANT INJURED IN NONCOLLISION TRANSPORT ACCIDENT**

Includes: overturning car NOS
overturning car without collision

V48.0XX Car driver injured in noncollision transport accident in nontraffic accident
`7th`

V48.1XX Car passenger injured in noncollision transport accident in nontraffic accident
`7th`

V48.2XX Person on outside of car injured in noncollision transport accident in nontraffic accident
`7th`

V48.3XX Unspecified car occupant injured in noncollision transport accident in nontraffic accident
`7th`

V48.4XX Person boarding or alighting a car injured in noncollision transport accident
`7th`

V48.5XX Car driver injured in noncollision transport accident in traffic accident
`7th`

V48.6XX Car passenger injured in noncollision transport accident in traffic accident
`7th`

V48.7XX Person on outside of car injured in noncollision transport accident in traffic accident
`7th`

V48.9XX Unspecified car occupant injured in noncollision transport accident in traffic accident
`7th`

V49 `4th` **CAR OCCUPANT INJURED IN OTHER AND UNSPECIFIED TRANSPORT ACCIDENTS**

V49.0 `5th` Driver injured in collision with other and unspecified motor vehicles in nontraffic accident

> 7th characters for categories V40–V49
> A—initial encounter
> D—subsequent encounter
> S—sequela

   V49.00X Driver injured in collision with unspecified motor vehicles in nontraffic accident
`7th`

   V49.09X Driver injured in collision with other motor vehicles in nontraffic accident
`7th`

V49.1 `5th` Passenger injured in collision with other and unspecified motor vehicles in nontraffic accident

   V49.10X Passenger injured in collision with unspecified motor vehicles in nontraffic accident
`7th`

   V49.19X Passenger injured in collision with other motor vehicles in nontraffic accident
`7th`

V49.2 `5th` Unspecified car occupant injured in collision with other and unspecified motor vehicles in nontraffic accident

   V49.20X Unspecified car occupant injured in collision with unspecified motor vehicles in nontraffic accident
`7th`
Car collision NOS, nontraffic

   V49.29X Unspecified car occupant injured in collision with other motor vehicles in nontraffic accident
`7th`

V49.3XX Car occupant (driver) (passenger) injured in unspecified nontraffic accident
`7th`
Car accident NOS, nontraffic
Car occupant injured in nontraffic accident NOS

V49.4 `5th` Driver injured in collision with other and unspecified motor vehicles in traffic accident

   V49.40X Driver injured in collision with unspecified motor vehicles in traffic accident
`7th`

   V49.49X Driver injured in collision with other motor vehicles in traffic accident
`7th`

`4th` `5th` `6th` `7th`   Additional Character Required   ✓   3-character code

*=New Code
▲=Revised Code

Excludes1   Not coded here, do not use together
Excludes2—Not included here

PEDIATRIC ICD-10-CM 2017: A MANUAL FOR PROVIDER-BASED CODING   383

V49.5 [5th] Passenger injured in collision with other and unspecified motor vehicles in traffic accident

V49.50X [7th] Passenger injured in collision with unspecified motor vehicles in traffic accident

V49.59X [7th] Passenger injured in collision with other motor vehicles in traffic accident

V49.6 [5th] Unspecified car occupant injured in collision with other and unspecified motor vehicles in traffic accident

V49.60X [7th] Unspecified car occupant injured in collision with other and unspecified motor vehicles in traffic accident
Car collision NOS (traffic)

V49.69X [7th] Unspecified car occupant injured in collision with other motor vehicles in traffic accident

V49.8 [5th] Car occupant (driver) (passenger) injured in other specified transport accidents

V49.81X [7th] Car occupant (driver) (passenger) injured in transport accident with military vehicle

V49.88X [7th] Car occupant (driver) (passenger) injured in other specified transport accidents

V49.9XX [7th] Car occupant (driver) (passenger) injured in unspecified traffic accident
Car accident NOS

(V50–V59) OCCUPANT OF PICK-UP TRUCK OR VAN OR SUV INJURED IN TRANSPORT ACCIDENT

Includes: a four or six wheel motor vehicle designed primarily for carrying passengers and property but weighing less than the local limit for classification as a heavy goods vehicle
Minibus, minivan, sport utility vehicle (SUV), truck, van

Excludes1: heavy transport vehicle (V60–V69)

7th characters for categories V50–V59
A—initial encounter
D—subsequent encounter
S—sequela

V50 [4th] OCCUPANT OF PICK-UP TRUCK OR VAN OR SUV INJURED IN COLLISION WITH PEDESTRIAN OR ANIMAL

Excludes1: pick-up truck or van collision with animal-drawn vehicle or animal being ridden (V56.-)

V50.0XX [7th] Driver of pick-up truck or van injured in collision with pedestrian or animal in nontraffic accident

V50.1XX [7th] Passenger in pick-up truck or van injured in collision with pedestrian or animal in nontraffic accident

V50.2XX [7th] Person on outside of pick-up truck or van injured in collision with pedestrian or animal in nontraffic accident

V50.3XX [7th] Unspecified occupant of pick-up truck or van injured in collision with pedestrian or animal in nontraffic accident

V50.4XX [7th] Person boarding or alighting a pick-up truck or van injured in collision with pedestrian or animal

V50.5XX [7th] Driver of pick-up truck or van injured in collision with pedestrian or animal in traffic accident

V50.6XX [7th] Passenger in pick-up truck or van injured in collision with pedestrian or animal in traffic accident

V50.7XX [7th] Person on outside of pick-up truck or van injured in collision with pedestrian or animal in traffic accident

V50.9XX [7th] Unspecified occupant of pick-up truck or van injured in collision with pedestrian or animal in traffic accident

V52 [4th] OCCUPANT OF PICK-UP TRUCK OR VAN OR SUV INJURED IN COLLISION WITH TWO- OR THREE-WHEELED MOTOR VEHICLE

V52.0XX [7th] Driver of pick-up truck or van injured in collision with two- or three-wheeled motor vehicle in nontraffic accident

V52.1XX [7th] Passenger in pick-up truck or van injured in collision with two- or three-wheeled motor vehicle in nontraffic accident

V52.2XX [7th] Person on outside of pick-up truck or van injured in collision with two- or three-wheeled motor vehicle in nontraffic accident

V52.3XX [7th] Unspecified occupant of pick-up truck or van injured in collision with two- or three-wheeled motor vehicle in nontraffic accident

V52.4XX [7th] Person boarding or alighting a pick-up truck or van injured in collision with two- or three-wheeled motor vehicle

V52.5XX [7th] Driver of pick-up truck or van injured in collision with two- or three-wheeled motor vehicle in traffic accident

V52.6XX [7th] Passenger in pick-up truck or van injured in collision with two- or three-wheeled motor vehicle in traffic accident

V52.7XX [7th] Person on outside of pick-up truck or van injured in collision with two- or three-wheeled motor vehicle in traffic accident

V52.9XX [7th] Unspecified occupant of pick-up truck or van injured in collision with two- or three-wheeled motor vehicle in traffic accident

V53 [4th] OCCUPANT OF PICK-UP TRUCK OR VAN OR SUV INJURED IN COLLISION WITH CAR, PICK-UP TRUCK OR VAN

7th characters for categories V50–V59
A—initial encounter
D—subsequent encounter
S—sequela

V53.0XX [7th] Driver of pick-up truck or van injured in collision with car, pick-up truck or van in nontraffic accident

V53.1XX [7th] Passenger in pick-up truck or van injured in collision with car, pick-up truck or van in nontraffic accident

V53.2XX [7th] Person on outside of pick-up truck or van injured in collision with car, pick-up truck or van in nontraffic accident

V53.3XX [7th] Unspecified occupant of pick-up truck or van injured in collision with car, pick-up truck or van in nontraffic accident

V53.4XX [7th] Person boarding or alighting a pick-up truck or van injured in collision with car, pick-up truck or van

V53.5XX [7th] Driver of pick-up truck or van injured in collision with car, pick-up truck or van in traffic accident

V53.6XX [7th] Passenger in pick-up truck or van injured in collision with car, pick-up truck or van in traffic accident

V53.7XX [7th] Person on outside of pick-up truck or van injured in collision with car, pick-up truck or van in traffic accident

V53.9XX [7th] Unspecified occupant of pick-up truck or van injured in collision with car, pick-up truck or van in traffic accident

V54 [4th] OCCUPANT OF PICK-UP TRUCK OR VAN OR SUV INJURED IN COLLISION WITH HEAVY TRANSPORT VEHICLE OR BUS

Excludes1: occupant of pick-up truck or van injured in collision with military vehicle (V59.81)

V54.0XX [7th] Driver of pick-up truck or van injured in collision with heavy transport vehicle or bus in nontraffic accident

V54.1XX [7th] Passenger in pick-up truck or van injured in collision with heavy transport vehicle or bus in nontraffic accident

[4th] [5th] [6th] [7th] Additional Character Required   ✔ 3-character code   •=New Code   ▲=Revised Code   **Excludes1**—Not coded here, do not use together   **Excludes2**—Not included here

384   PEDIATRIC ICD-10-CM 2017: A MANUAL FOR PROVIDER-BASED CODING

V54.2XX Person on outside of pick-up truck or van injured in collision with heavy transport vehicle or bus in nontraffic accident
7th

V54.3XX Unspecified occupant of pick-up truck or van injured in collision with heavy transport vehicle or bus in nontraffic accident
7th

V54.4XX Person boarding or alighting a pick-up truck or van injured in collision with heavy transport vehicle or bus
7th

V54.5XX Driver of pick-up truck or van injured in collision with heavy transport vehicle or bus in traffic accident
7th

V54.6XX Passenger in pick-up truck or van injured in collision with heavy transport vehicle or bus in traffic accident
7th

V54.7XX Person on outside of pick-up truck or van injured in collision with heavy transport vehicle or bus in traffic accident
7th

V54.9XX Unspecified occupant of pick-up truck or van injured in collision with heavy transport vehicle or bus in traffic accident
7th

V55 OCCUPANT OF PICK-UP TRUCK OR VAN OR SUV INJURED IN COLLISION WITH RAILWAY TRAIN OR RAILWAY VEHICLE
4th

V55.0XX Driver of pick-up truck or van injured in collision with railway train or railway vehicle in nontraffic accident
7th

V55.1XX Passenger in pick-up truck or van injured in collision with railway train or railway vehicle in nontraffic accident
7th

V55.2XX Person on outside of pick-up truck or van injured in collision with railway train or railway vehicle in nontraffic accident
7th

V55.3XX Unspecified occupant of pick-up truck or van injured in collision with railway train or railway vehicle in nontraffic accident
7th

V55.4XX Person boarding or alighting a pick-up truck or van injured in collision with railway train or railway vehicle
7th

V55.5XX Driver of pick-up truck or van injured in collision with railway train or railway vehicle in traffic accident
7th

V55.6XX Passenger in pick-up truck or van injured in collision with railway train or railway vehicle in traffic accident
7th

V55.7XX Person on outside of pick-up truck or van injured in collision with railway train or railway vehicle in traffic accident
7th

V55.9XX Unspecified occupant of pick-up truck or van injured in collision with railway train or railway vehicle in traffic accident
7th

V57 OCCUPANT OF PICK-UP TRUCK OR VAN OR SUV INJURED IN COLLISION WITH FIXED OR STATIONARY OBJECT
4th

V57.0XX Driver of pick-up truck or van injured in collision with fixed or stationary object in nontraffic accident
7th

V57.1XX Passenger in pick-up truck or van injured in collision with fixed or stationary object in nontraffic accident
7th

V57.2XX Person on outside of pick-up truck or van injured in collision with fixed or stationary object in nontraffic accident
7th

V57.3XX Unspecified occupant of pick-up truck or van injured in collision with fixed or stationary object in nontraffic accident
7th

V57.4XX Person boarding or alighting a pick-up truck or van injured in collision with fixed or stationary object
7th

V57.5XX Driver of pick-up truck or van injured in collision with fixed or stationary object in traffic accident
7th

V57.6XX Passenger in pick-up truck or van injured in collision with fixed or stationary object in traffic accident
7th

V57.7XX Person on outside of pick-up truck or van injured in collision with fixed or stationary object in traffic accident
7th

V57.9XX Unspecified occupant of pick-up truck or van injured in collision with fixed or stationary object in traffic accident
7th

V58 OCCUPANT OF PICK-UP TRUCK OR VAN OR SUV INJURED IN NONCOLLISION TRANSPORT ACCIDENT
4th
Includes: overturning pick-up truck or van NOS
overturning pick-up truck or van without collision

V58.0XX Driver of pick-up truck or van injured in noncollision transport accident in nontraffic accident
7th

V58.1XX Passenger in pick-up truck or van injured in noncollision transport accident in nontraffic accident
7th

V58.2XX Person on outside of pick-up truck or van injured in noncollision transport accident in nontraffic accident
7th

V58.3XX Unspecified occupant of pick-up truck or van injured in noncollision transport accident in nontraffic accident
7th

V58.4XX Person boarding or alighting a pick-up truck or van injured in noncollision transport accident
7th

V58.5XX Driver of pick-up truck or van injured in noncollision transport accident in traffic accident
7th

V58.6XX Passenger in pick-up truck or van injured in noncollision transport accident in traffic accident
7th

V58.7XX Person on outside of pick-up truck or van injured in noncollision transport accident in traffic accident
7th

> 7th characters for categories V50–V59
> A—initial encounter
> D—subsequent encounter
> S—sequela

V58.9XX Unspecified occupant of pick-up truck or van injured in noncollision transport accident in traffic accident
7th

V59 OCCUPANT OF PICK-UP TRUCK OR VAN OR SUV INJURED IN OTHER AND UNSPECIFIED TRANSPORT ACCIDENTS
4th

V59.0 Driver of pick-up truck or van injured in collision with other and unspecified motor vehicles in nontraffic accident
5th

    V59.00X Driver of pick-up truck or van injured in collision with unspecified motor vehicles in nontraffic accident
    7th

    V59.09X Driver of pick-up truck or van injured in collision with other motor vehicles in nontraffic accident
    7th

V59.1 Passenger in pick-up truck or van injured in collision with other and unspecified motor vehicles in nontraffic accident
5th

    V59.10X Passenger in pick-up truck or van injured in collision with unspecified motor vehicles in nontraffic accident
    7th

    V59.19X Passenger in pick-up truck or van injured in collision with other motor vehicles in nontraffic accident
    7th

V59.2 Unspecified occupant of pick-up truck or van injured in collision with other and unspecified motor vehicles in nontraffic accident
5th

    V59.20X Unspecified occupant of pick-up truck or van injured in collision with unspecified motor vehicles in nontraffic accident
    7th
    Collision NOS involving pick-up truck or van, nontraffic

    V59.29X Unspecified occupant of pick-up truck or van injured in collision with other motor vehicles in nontraffic accident
    7th

  Additional Character Required
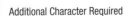 3-character code

⁕=New Code
▲=Revised Code

Excludes1—Not coded here, do not use together
Excludes2—Not included here

CHAPTER 20. EXTERNAL CAUSES OF MORBIDITY   (V59.3XX–V73.9XX)

V59.3XX Occupant (driver) (passenger) of pick-up truck or van injured in unspecified nontraffic accident
[7th]
Accident NOS involving pick-up truck or van, nontraffic
Occupant of pick-up truck or van injured in nontraffic accident NOS

V59.4 Driver of pick-up truck or van injured in collision with other and unspecified motor vehicles in traffic accident
[5th]
  V59.40X Driver of pick-up truck or van injured in collision with unspecified motor vehicles in traffic accident
[7th]

  V59.49X Driver of pick-up truck or van injured in collision with other motor vehicles in traffic accident
[7th]

V59.5 Passenger in pick-up truck or van injured in collision with other and unspecified motor vehicles in traffic accident
[5th]
  V59.50X Passenger in pick-up truck or van injured in collision with unspecified motor vehicles in traffic accident
[7th]

  V59.59X Passenger in pick-up truck or van injured in collision with other motor vehicles in traffic accident
[7th]

V59.6 Unspecified occupant of pick-up truck or van injured in collision with other and unspecified motor vehicles in traffic accident
[5th]
  V59.60X Unspecified occupant of pick-up truck or van injured in collision with unspecified motor vehicles in traffic accident
[7th]
  Collision NOS involving pick-up truck or van (traffic)

  V59.69X Unspecified occupant of pick-up truck or van injured in collision with other motor vehicles in traffic accident
[7th]

V59.8 Occupant (driver) (passenger) of pick-up truck or van injured in other specified transport accidents
[5th]
  V59.81X Occupant (driver) (passenger) of pick-up truck or van injured in transport accident with military vehicle
[7th]

  V59.88X Occupant (driver) (passenger) of pick-up truck or van injured in other specified transport accidents
[7th]

V59.9XX Occupant (driver) (passenger) of pick-up truck or van injured in unspecified traffic accident
[7th]
Accident NOS involving pick-up truck or van

(V70–V79) BUS OCCUPANT INJURED IN TRANSPORT ACCIDENT

Includes: motorcoach
Excludes1: minibus (V50–V59)

7th characters for categories V70–V79
A—initial encounter
D—subsequent encounter
S—sequela

V70 BUS OCCUPANT INJURED IN COLLISION WITH PEDESTRIAN OR ANIMAL
[4th]
Excludes1: bus collision with animal-drawn vehicle or animal being ridden (V76.-)

V70.0XX Driver of bus injured in collision with pedestrian or animal in nontraffic accident
[7th]

V70.1XX Passenger on bus injured in collision with pedestrian or animal in nontraffic accident
[7th]

V70.2XX Person on outside of bus injured in collision with pedestrian or animal in nontraffic accident
[7th]

V70.3XX Unspecified occupant of bus injured in collision with pedestrian or animal in nontraffic accident
[7th]

V70.4XX Person boarding or alighting from bus injured in collision with pedestrian or animal
[7th]

V70.5XX Driver of bus injured in collision with pedestrian or animal in traffic accident
[7th]

V70.6XX Passenger on bus injured in collision with pedestrian or animal in traffic accident
[7th]

V70.7XX Person on outside of bus injured in collision with pedestrian or animal in traffic accident
[7th]

V70.9XX Unspecified occupant of bus injured in collision with pedestrian or animal in traffic accident
[7th]

V72 BUS OCCUPANT INJURED IN COLLISION WITH TWO- OR THREE-WHEELED MOTOR VEHICLE
[4th]
V72.0XX Driver of bus injured in collision with two- or three-wheeled motor vehicle in nontraffic accident
[7th]

V72.1XX Passenger on bus injured in collision with two- or three-wheeled motor vehicle in nontraffic accident
[7th]

V72.2XX Person on outside of bus injured in collision with two- or three-wheeled motor vehicle in nontraffic accident
[7th]

V72.3XX Unspecified occupant of bus injured in collision with two- or three-wheeled motor vehicle in nontraffic accident
[7th]

V72.4XX Person boarding or alighting from bus injured in collision with two- or three-wheeled motor vehicle
[7th]

V72.5XX Driver of bus injured in collision with two- or three-wheeled motor vehicle in traffic accident, sequel
[7th]

V72.6XX Passenger on bus injured in collision with two- or three-wheeled motor vehicle in traffic accident
[7th]

7th characters for categories V70–V79
A—initial encounter
D—subsequent encounter
S—sequela

V72.7XX Person on outside of bus injured in collision with two- or three-wheeled motor vehicle in traffic accident
[7th]

V72.9XX Unspecified occupant of bus injured in collision with two- or three-wheeled motor vehicle in traffic accident
[7th]

V73 BUS OCCUPANT INJURED IN COLLISION WITH CAR, PICK-UP TRUCK OR VAN
[4th]
V73.0XX Driver of bus injured in collision with car, pick-up truck or van in nontraffic accident
[7th]

V73.1XX Passenger on bus injured in collision with car, pick-up truck or van in nontraffic accident
[7th]

V73.2XX Person on outside of bus injured in collision with car, pick-up truck or van in nontraffic accident
[7th]

V73.3XX Unspecified occupant of bus injured in collision with car, pick-up truck or van in nontraffic accident
[7th]

V73.4XX Person boarding or alighting from bus injured in collision with car, pick-up truck or van
[7th]

V73.5XX Driver of bus injured in collision with car, pick-up truck or van in traffic accident
[7th]

V73.6XX Passenger on bus injured in collision with car, pick-up truck or van in traffic accident
[7th]

V73.7XX Person on outside of bus injured in collision with car, pick-up truck or van in traffic accident
[7th]

V73.9XX Unspecified occupant of bus injured in collision with car, pick-up truck or van in traffic accident
[7th]

[4th] [5th] [6th] [7th]   Additional Character Required   ✔ 3-character code   •=New Code   ▲=Revised Code   *Excludes1*—Not coded here, do not use together   *Excludes2*—Not included here

V74   BUS OCCUPANT INJURED IN COLLISION WITH HEAVY TRANSPORT VEHICLE OR BUS

4th

Excludes1: bus occupant injured in collision with military vehicle (V79.81)

V74.0XX Driver of bus injured in collision with heavy transport vehicle or bus in nontraffic accident
   7th

V74.1XX Passenger on bus injured in collision with heavy transport vehicle or bus in nontraffic accident
   7th

V74.2XX Person on outside of bus injured in collision with heavy transport vehicle or bus in nontraffic accident
   7th

V74.3XX Unspecified occupant of bus injured in collision with heavy transport vehicle or bus in nontraffic accident
   7th

V74.4XX Person boarding or alighting from bus injured in collision with heavy transport vehicle or bus
   7th

V74.5XX Driver of bus injured in collision with heavy transport vehicle or bus in traffic accident
   7th

V74.6XX Passenger on bus injured in collision with heavy transport vehicle or bus in traffic accident
   7th

V74.7XX Person on outside of bus injured in collision with heavy transport vehicle or bus in traffic accident
   7th

V74.9XX Unspecified occupant of bus injured in collision with heavy transport vehicle or bus in traffic accident
   7th

V75   BUS OCCUPANT INJURED IN COLLISION WITH RAILWAY TRAIN OR RAILWAY VEHICLE

4th

V75.0XX Driver of bus injured in collision with railway train or railway vehicle in nontraffic accident
   7th

V75.1XX Passenger on bus injured in collision with railway train or railway vehicle in nontraffic accident
   7th

V75.2XX Person on outside of bus injured in collision with railway train or railway vehicle in nontraffic accident
   7th

V75.3XX Unspecified occupant of bus injured in collision with railway train or railway vehicle in nontraffic accident
   7th

V75.4XX Person boarding or alighting from bus injured in collision with railway train or railway vehicle
   7th

V75.5XX Driver of bus injured in collision with railway train or railway vehicle in traffic accident
   7th

V75.6XX Passenger on bus injured in collision with railway train or railway vehicle in traffic accident
   7th

V75.7XX Person on outside of bus injured in collision with railway train or railway vehicle in traffic accident
   7th

V75.9XX Unspecified occupant of bus injured in collision with railway train or railway vehicle in traffic accident
   7th

V77   BUS OCCUPANT INJURED IN COLLISION WITH FIXED OR STATIONARY OBJECT

4th

V77.0XX Driver of bus injured in collision with fixed or stationary object in nontraffic accident
   7th

V77.1XX Passenger on bus injured in collision with fixed or stationary object in nontraffic accident
   7th

V77.2XX Person on outside of bus injured in collision with fixed or stationary object in nontraffic accident
   7th

V77.3XX Unspecified occupant of bus injured in collision with fixed or stationary object in nontraffic accident
   7th

V77.4XX Person boarding or alighting from bus injured in collision with fixed or stationary object
   7th

V77.5XX Driver of bus injured in collision with fixed or stationary object in traffic accident
   7th

V77.6XX Passenger on bus injured in collision with fixed or stationary object in traffic accident
   7th

V77.7XX Person on outside of bus injured in collision with fixed or stationary object in traffic accident
   7th

V77.9XX Unspecified occupant of bus injured in collision with fixed or stationary object in traffic accident
   7th

V78   BUS OCCUPANT INJURED IN NONCOLLISION TRANSPORT ACCIDENT

4th

Includes: overturning bus NOS
overturning bus without collision

V78.0XX Driver of bus injured in noncollision transport accident in nontraffic accident
   7th

V78.1XX Passenger on bus injured in noncollision transport accident in nontraffic accident
   7th

V78.2XX Person on outside of bus injured in noncollision transport accident in nontraffic accident
   7th

V78.3XX Unspecified occupant of bus injured in noncollision transport accident in nontraffic accident
   7th

> 7th characters for categories
> V70–V79
> A—initial encounter
> D—subsequent encounter
> S—sequela

V78.4XX Person boarding or alighting from bus injured in noncollision transport accident
   7th

V78.5XX Driver of bus injured in noncollision transport accident in traffic accident
   7th

V78.6XX Passenger on bus injured in noncollision transport accident in traffic accident
   7th

V78.7XX Person on outside of bus injured in noncollision transport accident in traffic accident
   7th

V78.9XX Unspecified occupant of bus injured in noncollision transport accident in traffic accident
   7th

V79   BUS OCCUPANT INJURED IN OTHER AND UNSPECIFIED TRANSPORT ACCIDENTS

4th

V79.0 Driver of bus injured in collision with other and unspecified motor vehicles in nontraffic accident
   5th

    V79.00X Driver of bus injured in collision with unspecified motor vehicles in nontraffic accident
      7th

    V79.09X Driver of bus injured in collision with other motor vehicles in nontraffic accident
      7th

V79.1 Passenger on bus injured in collision with other and unspecified motor vehicles in nontraffic accident
   5th

    V79.10X Passenger on bus injured in collision with unspecified motor vehicles in nontraffic accident
      7th

    V79.19X Passenger on bus injured in collision with other motor vehicles in nontraffic accident
      7th

V79.2 Unspecified bus occupant injured in collision with other and unspecified motor vehicles in nontraffic accident
   5th

    V79.20X Unspecified bus occupant injured in collision with unspecified motor vehicles in nontraffic accident
      7th   Bus collision NOS, nontraffic

    V79.29X Unspecified bus occupant injured in collision with other motor vehicles in nontraffic accident
      7th

  Additional Character Required   3-character code

•=New Code
▲=Revised Code

Excludes1—Not coded here, do not use together
Excludes2—Not included here

CHAPTER 20. EXTERNAL CAUSES OF MORBIDITY (V79.3XX–V84.9XX)

V79.3XX Bus occupant (driver) (passenger) injured in unspecified nontraffic accident
7th
Bus accident NOS, nontraffic
Bus occupant injured in nontraffic accident NOS

V79.4 Driver of bus injured in collision with other and unspecified motor vehicles in traffic accident
5th

    V79.40X Driver of bus injured in collision with unspecified motor vehicles in traffic accident
    7th

    V79.49X Driver of bus injured in collision with other motor vehicles in traffic accident
    7th

V79.5 Passenger on bus injured in collision with other and unspecified motor vehicles in traffic accident
5th

    V79.50X Passenger on bus injured in collision with unspecified motor vehicles in traffic accident
    7th

    V79.59X Passenger on bus injured in collision with other motor vehicles in traffic accident
    7th

V79.6 Unspecified bus occupant injured in collision with other and unspecified motor vehicles in traffic accident
5th

    V79.60X Unspecified bus occupant injured in collision with unspecified motor vehicles in traffic accident
    7th
    Bus collision NOS (traffic)

    V79.69X Unspecified bus occupant injured in collision with other motor vehicles in traffic accident
    7th

V79.8 Bus occupant (driver) (passenger) injured in other specified transport accidents
5th

    V79.81X Bus occupant (driver) (passenger) injured in transport accidents with military vehicle
    7th

    V79.88X Bus occupant (driver) (passenger) injured in other specified transport accidents
    7th

V79.9XX Bus occupant (driver) (passenger) injured in unspecified traffic accident
7th
Bus accident NOS

(V80–V89) OTHER LAND TRANSPORT ACCIDENTS

V80 ANIMAL-RIDER OR OCCUPANT OF ANIMAL-DRAWN VEHICLE INJURED IN TRANSPORT ACCIDENT
4th

  V80.0 Animal-rider or occupant of animal-drawn vehicle injured by fall from or being thrown from animal or animal-drawn vehicle in noncollision accident
  5th

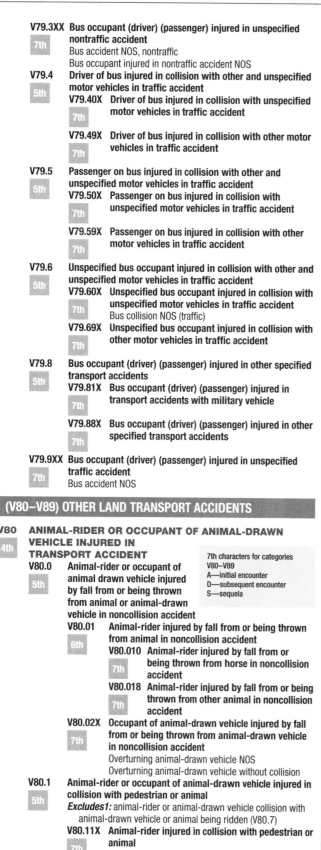

7th characters for categories
V80–V89
A—initial encounter
D—subsequent encounter
S—sequela

    V80.01 Animal-rider injured by fall from or being thrown from animal in noncollision accident
    6th

        V80.010 Animal-rider injured by fall from or being thrown from horse in noncollision accident
        7th

        V80.018 Animal-rider injured by fall from or being thrown from other animal in noncollision accident
        7th

    V80.02X Occupant of animal-drawn vehicle injured by fall from or being thrown from animal-drawn vehicle in noncollision accident
    7th
    Overturning animal-drawn vehicle NOS
    Overturning animal-drawn vehicle without collision

  V80.1 Animal-rider or occupant of animal-drawn vehicle injured in collision with pedestrian or animal
  5th
  Excludes1: animal-rider or animal-drawn vehicle collision with animal-drawn vehicle or animal being ridden (V80.7)

    V80.11X Animal-rider injured in collision with pedestrian or animal
    7th

    V80.12X Occupant of animal-drawn vehicle injured in collision with pedestrian or animal
    7th

  V80.4 Animal-rider or occupant of animal-drawn vehicle injured in collision with car, pick-up truck, van, heavy transport vehicle or bus
  5th
  Excludes1: animal-rider injured in collision with military vehicle (V80.910)
  occupant of animal-drawn vehicle injured in collision with military vehicle (V80.920)

    V80.41X Animal-rider injured in collision with car, pick-up truck, van, heavy transport vehicle or bus
    7th

    V80.42X Occupant of animal-drawn vehicle injured in collision with car, pick-up truck, van, heavy transport vehicle or bus
    7th

  V80.8 Animal-rider or occupant of animal-drawn vehicle injured in collision with fixed or stationary object
  5th

    V80.81X Animal-rider injured in collision with fixed or stationary object
    7th

    V80.82X Occupant of animal-drawn vehicle injured in collision with fixed or stationary object
    7th

  V80.9 Animal-rider or occupant of animal-drawn vehicle injured in other and unspecified transport accidents
  5th

7th characters for categories
V80–V89
A—initial encounter
D—subsequent encounter
S—sequela

    V80.91 Animal-rider injured in other and unspecified transport accidents
    6th

        V80.919 Animal-rider injured in unspecified transport accident
        7th
        Animal rider accident NOS

    V80.92 Occupant of animal-drawn vehicle injured in other and unspecified transport accidents
    6th

        V80.929 Occupant of animal-drawn vehicle injured in unspecified transport accident
        7th
        Animal-drawn vehicle accident NOS

V84 OCCUPANT OF SPECIAL VEHICLE MAINLY USED IN AGRICULTURE INJURED IN TRANSPORT ACCIDENT
4th
Includes: self-propelled farm machinery
    tractor (and trailer)
Excludes1: animal-powered farm machinery accident (W30.8-)
    contact with combine harvester (W30.0)
    special agricultural vehicle in stationary use or maintenance (W30.-)

V84.0XX Driver of special agricultural vehicle injured in traffic accident
7th

V84.1XX Passenger of special agricultural vehicle injured in traffic accident
7th

V84.2XX Person on outside of special agricultural vehicle injured in traffic accident
7th

V84.3XX Unspecified occupant of special agricultural vehicle injured in traffic accident
7th

V84.4XX Person injured while boarding or alighting from special agricultural vehicle
7th

V84.5XX Driver of special agricultural vehicle injured in nontraffic accident
7th

V84.6XX Passenger of special agricultural vehicle injured in nontraffic accident
7th

V84.7XX Person on outside of special agricultural vehicle injured in nontraffic accident
7th

V84.9XX Unspecified occupant of special agricultural vehicle injured in nontraffic accident
7th

   Additional Character Required   3-character code   •=New Code   *Excludes1*—Not coded here, do not use together
▲=Revised Code   *Excludes2*—Not included here

V86 **[4th]** **OCCUPANT OF SPECIAL ALL-TERRAIN OR OTHER OFF-ROAD MOTOR VEHICLE, INJURED IN TRANSPORT ACCIDENT**

Excludes1: special all-terrain vehicle in stationary use or maintenance (W31.-)
> sport-utility vehicle (V50–V59)
> three-wheeled motor vehicle designed for on-road use (V30–V39)

V86.0 **[5th]** **Driver of special all-terrain or other off-road motor vehicle injured in traffic accident**

  V86.02X **[7th]** **Driver of snowmobile injured in traffic accident**

  V86.03X **[7th]** **Driver of dune buggy injured in traffic accident**

  V86.09X **[7th]** **Driver of other special all-terrain or other off-road motor vehicle injured in traffic accident**
    Driver of dirt bike injured in traffic accident
    Driver of go cart injured in traffic accident
    Driver of golf cart injured in traffic accident

V86.1 **[5th]** **Passenger of special all-terrain or other off-road motor vehicle injured in traffic accident**

  V86.12X **[7th]** **Passenger of snowmobile injured in traffic accident**

  V86.13X **[7th]** **Passenger of dune buggy injured in traffic accident**

  V86.19X **[7th]** **Passenger of other special all-terrain or other off-road motor vehicle injured in traffic accident**
    Passenger of dirt bike injured in traffic accident
    Passenger of go cart injured in traffic accident
    Passenger of golf cart injured in traffic accident

V86.3 **[5th]** **Unspecified occupant of special all-terrain or other off-road motor vehicle injured in traffic accident**

  V86.32X **[7th]** **Unspecific occupant of snowmobile injured in traffic accident**

  V86.33X **[7th]** **Unspecified occupant of dune buggy injured in traffic accident**

  V86.39X **[7th]** **Unspecified occupant of other special all-terrain or other off-road motor vehicle injured in traffic accident**
    Passenger of dirt bike injured in traffic accident
    Passenger of go cart injured in traffic accident
    Passenger of golf cart injured in traffic accident

V86.5 **[5th]** **Driver of special all-terrain or other off-road motor vehicle injured in nontraffic accident**

  V86.52X **[7th]** **Driver of snowmobile injured in nontraffic accident**

  V86.53X **[7th]** **Driver of dune buggy injured in nontraffic accident**

  V86.59X **[7th]** **Driver of other special all-terrain or other off-road motor vehicle injured in nontraffic accident**
    Driver of dirt bike injured in nontraffic accident
    Driver of go cart injured in nontraffic accident
    Driver of golf cart injured in nontraffic accident

V86.6 **[5th]** **Passenger of special all-terrain or other off-road motor vehicle injured in nontraffic accident**

  V86.62X **[7th]** **Passenger of snowmobile injured in nontraffic accident**

  V86.63X **[7th]** **Passenger of dune buggy injured in nontraffic accident**

  V86.69X **[7th]** **Passenger of other special all-terrain or other off-road motor vehicle injured in nontraffic accident**
    Passenger of dirt bike injured in nontraffic accident
    Passenger of go cart injured in nontraffic accident
    Passenger of golf cart injured in nontraffic accident

V86.9 **[5th]** **Unspecified occupant of special all-terrain or other off-road motor vehicle injured in nontraffic accident**

  V86.92X **[7th]** **Unspecific occupant of snowmobile injured in nontraffic accident**

  V86.93X **[7th]** **Unspecified occupant of dune buggy injured in nontraffic accident**

  V86.99X **[7th]** **Unspecified occupant of other special all-terrain or other off-road motor vehicle injured in nontraffic accident**
    All-terrain motor-vehicle accident NOS
    Off-road motor-vehicle accident NOS
    Other motor-vehicle accident NOS
    Unspecified occupant of dirt bike injured in nontraffic accident
    Unspecified occupant of go cart injured in nontraffic accident
    Unspecified occupant of golf cart injured in nontraffic accident

V89 **[4th]** **MOTOR- OR NONMOTOR-VEHICLE ACCIDENT, TYPE OF VEHICLE UNSPECIFIED**

V89.0XX **[7th]** **Person injured in unspecified motor-vehicle accident, nontraffic**
  Motor-vehicle accident NOS, nontraffic

V89.1XX **[7th]** **Person injured in unspecified nonmotor-vehicle accident, nontraffic**
  Nonmotor-vehicle accident NOS (nontraffic)

V89.2XX **[7th]** **Person injured in unspecified motor-vehicle accident, traffic**
  Motor-vehicle accident [MVA] NOS
  Road (traffic) accident NOS

V89.3XX **[7th]** **Person injured in unspecified nonmotor-vehicle accident, traffic**
  Nonmotor-vehicle traffic accident NOS

V89.9XX **[7th]** **Person injured in unspecified vehicle accident**
  Collision NOS

> 7th characters for categories
> V80–V89
> A—initial encounter
> D—subsequent encounter
> S—sequela

(V90–V94) WATER TRANSPORT ACCIDENTS

V90 **[4th]** **DROWNING AND SUBMERSION DUE TO ACCIDENT TO WATERCRAFT**

Excludes1: fall into water not from watercraft (W16.-)
> water-transport-related drowning or submersion without accident to watercraft (V92.-)

> 7th characters for categories
> V90–V94
> A—initial encounter
> D—subsequent encounter
> S—sequela

V90.0 **[5th]** **Drowning and submersion due to watercraft overturning**

  V90.01X **[7th]** **Drowning and submersion due to passenger ship overturning**
    Drowning and submersion due to Ferry-boat overturning
    Drowning and submersion due to Liner overturning

  V90.02X **[7th]** **Drowning and submersion due to fishing boat overturning**

  V90.03X **[7th]** **Drowning and submersion due to other powered watercraft overturning**
    Drowning and submersion due to Hovercraft (on open water)/Jet ski overturning

  V90.04X **[7th]** **Drowning and submersion due to sailboat overturning**

  V90.05X **[7th]** **Drowning and submersion due to canoe or kayak overturning**

  V90.06X **[7th]** **Drowning and submersion due to (nonpowered) inflatable craft overturning**

  Additional Character Required   3-character code

•=New Code
▲=Revised Code

Excludes1—Not coded here, do not use together
Excludes2—Not included here

V90.08X **Drowning and submersion due to other unpowered watercraft overturning**
`7th`
Drowning and submersion due to windsurfer overturning

V90.09X **Drowning and submersion due to unspecified watercraft overturning**
`7th`
Drowning and submersion due to boat/ship/watercraft NOS overturning

V93.3 **Fall on board watercraft**
`5th`
Excludes1: fall due to collision of watercraft (V91.2-)

V93.32X **Fall on board fishing boat**
`7th`

V93.33X **Fall on board other powered watercraft**
`7th`
Fall on board Hovercraft/Jet ski (on open water)

V93.34X **Fall on board sailboat**
`7th`

V93.35X **Fall on board canoe or kayak**
`7th`

V93.36X **Fall on board (nonpowered) inflatable craft**
`7th`

V93.38X **Fall on board other unpowered watercraft**
`7th`

V93.39X **Fall on board unspecified watercraft**
`7th`
Fall on board boat/ship/watercraft NOS

V93.8 **Other injury due to other accident on board watercraft**
`5th`
Accidental poisoning by gases or fumes on watercraft

V93.82X **Other injury due to other accident on board fishing boat**
`7th`

V93.83X **Other injury due to other accident on board other powered watercraft**
`7th`
Other injury due to other accident on board Hovercraft
Other injury due to other accident on board Jet ski

V93.84X **Other injury due to other accident on board sailboat**
`7th`

V93.85X **Other injury due to other accident on board canoe or kayak**
`7th`

V93.86X **Other injury due to other accident on board (nonpowered) inflatable craft**
`7th`

V93.87X **Other injury due to other accident on board water-skis**
`7th`
Hit or struck by object while waterskiing

V93.88X **Other injury due to other accident on board other unpowered watercraft**
`7th`
Hit or struck by object while surfing
Hit or struck by object while on board windsurfer

V93.89X **Other injury due to other accident on board unspecified watercraft**
`7th`
Other injury due to other accident on board boat/ship/watercraft NOS

V94 **OTHER AND UNSPECIFIED WATER TRANSPORT ACCIDENTS**
`4th`
Excludes1: military watercraft accidents in military or war operations (Y36, Y37)

V94.3 **Injury to rider of (inflatable) watercraft being pulled behind other watercraft**
`5th`

V94.31X **Injury to rider of (inflatable) recreational watercraft being pulled behind other watercraft**
`7th`
Injury to rider of inner-tube pulled behind motor boat

V94.4XX **Injury to barefoot water-skier**
`7th`
Injury to person being pulled behind boat or ship

V94.9XX **Unspecified water transport accident**
`7th`
Water transport accident NOS
initial encounter accident
for definitions of transport

(W00–X58) OTHER EXTERNAL CAUSES OF ACCIDENTAL INJURY

(W00–W19) SLIPPING, TRIPPING, STUMBLING AND FALLS

Excludes1: assault involving a fall (Y01–Y02)
  fall from animal (V80.-)
  fall (in) (from) machinery (in operation) (W28–W31)
  fall (in) (from) transport vehicle (V01–V99)
  intentional self-harm involving a fall (X80–X81)

Excludes2: at risk for fall (history of fall) Z91.81 fall (in) (from) burning building (X00.-)
  fall into fire (X00–X04, X08–X09)

7th characters for categories W00–W19
A—initial encounter
D—subsequent encounter
S—sequela

W00 **FALL DUE TO ICE AND SNOW**
`4th`
Includes: pedestrian on foot falling (slipping) on ice and snow
Excludes1: fall on (from) ice and snow involving pedestrian conveyance (V00.-)
fall from stairs and steps not due to ice and snow (W10.-)

W00.0XX Fall on same level due to ice and snow
`7th`

W00.1XX Fall from stairs and steps due to ice and snow
`7th`

W00.2XX Other fall from one level to another due to ice and snow
`7th`

W00.9XX Unspecified fall due to ice and snow
`7th`

W01 **FALL ON SAME LEVEL FROM SLIPPING, TRIPPING AND STUMBLING**
`4th`
Includes: fall on moving sidewalk
Excludes1: fall due to bumping (striking) against object (W18.0-)
  fall in shower or bathtub (W18.2-)
  fall on same level NOS (W18.30)
  fall on same level from slipping, tripping and stumbling due to ice or snow (W00.0)
  fall off or from toilet (W18.1-)
  slipping, tripping and stumbling NOS (W18.40)
  slipping, tripping and stumbling without falling (W18.4-)

W01.0XX Fall on same level from slipping, tripping and stumbling without subsequent striking against object
`7th`
Falling over animal

W01.1 **Fall on same level from slipping, tripping and stumbling with subsequent striking against object**
`5th`

W01.11 **Fall on same level from slipping, tripping and stumbling with subsequent striking against sharp object**
`6th`

W01.110 Fall on same level from slipping, tripping and stumbling with subsequent striking against sharp glass
`7th`

W01.118 Fall on same level from slipping, tripping and stumbling with subsequent striking against other sharp object
`7th`

W01.119 Fall on same level from slipping, tripping and stumbling with subsequent striking against unspecified sharp object
`7th`

W01.19 **Fall on same level from slipping, tripping and stumbling with subsequent striking against other object**
`6th`

W01.190 Fall on same level from slipping, tripping and stumbling with subsequent striking against furniture
`7th`

  `4th` `5th` `6th` `7th`   Additional Character Required   ✓   3-character code

•=New Code
▲=Revised Code

Excludes1—Not coded here, do not use together
Excludes2—Not included here

W01.198 Fall on same level from slipping, tripping and stumbling with subsequent striking against other object
7th

W03 OTHER FALL ON SAME LEVEL DUE TO COLLISION WITH ANOTHER PERSON
7th
Fall due to non-transport collision with other person
Excludes1: collision with another person without fall (W51)
collision with another person without fall (W51)
crushed or pushed by a crowd or human stampede (W52)
fall involving pedestrian conveyance (V00-V09)
fall due to ice or snow (W00)
fall on same level NOS (W18.30)

W04 FALL WHILE BEING CARRIED OR SUPPORTED BY OTHER PERSONS
7th
Accidentally dropped while being carried

W05 FALL FROM NON-MOVING WHEELCHAIR, NONMOTORIZED SCOOTER AND MOTORIZED MOBILITY SCOOTER
7th
Excludes1: fall from moving wheelchair (powered) (V00.811)
fall from moving motorized mobility scooter (V00.831)
fall from nonmotorized scooter (V00.141)

W06 FALL FROM BED
7th

W07 FALL FROM CHAIR
7th

W08 FALL FROM OTHER FURNITURE
7th

W09 FALL ON AND FROM PLAYGROUND EQUIPMENT
4th
Excludes1: fall involving recreational machinery (W31)
W09.0XX Fall on or from playground slide
7th

W09.1XX Fall from playground swing
7th

W09.2XX Fall on or from jungle gym
7th

W09.8XX Fall on or from other playground equipment
7th

W10 FALL ON AND FROM STAIRS AND STEPS
4th
Excludes1: Fall from stairs and steps due to ice and snow (W00.1)
W10.0XX Fall (on) (from) escalator
7th

W10.1XX Fall (on) (from) sidewalk curb
7th

W10.2XX Fall (on) (from) incline
7th
Fall (on) (from) ramp

W10.8XX Fall (on) (from) other stairs and steps
7th

W10.9XX Fall (on) (from) unspecified stairs and steps
7th

W11 FALL ON AND FROM LADDER
7th

W13 FALL FROM, OUT OF OR THROUGH BUILDING OR STRUCTURE
4th
W13.0XX Fall from, out of or through balcony
7th
Fall from, out of or through railing

7th characters for categories W00-W19
A—initial encounter
D—subsequent encounter
S—sequela

W13.1XX Fall from, out of or through bridge
7th

W13.2XX Fall from, out of or through roof
7th

W13.3XX Fall through floor
7th

W13.4XX Fall from, out of or through window
7th
Excludes2: fall with subsequent striking against sharp glass (W01.110)

W14 FALL FROM TREE
7th

W15 FALL FROM CLIFF
7th

W16 FALL, JUMP OR DIVING INTO WATER
4th
Excludes1: accidental non-watercraft drowning and submersion not involving fall (W65–W74)
effects of air pressure from diving (W94.-)
fall into water from watercraft (V90–V94)
hitting an object or against bottom when falling from watercraft (V94.0)
Excludes2: striking or hitting diving board (W21.4)
W16.0 Fall into swimming pool
5th
Excludes1: fall into empty swimming pool (W17.3)
W16.01 Fall into swimming pool striking water surface
6th
W16.011 Fall into swimming pool striking water surface causing drowning and submersion
7th
Excludes1: drowning and submersion while in swimming pool without fall (W67)
W16.012 Fall into swimming pool striking water surface causing other injury
7th

W16.02 Fall into swimming pool striking bottom
6th
W16.021 Fall into swimming pool striking bottom causing drowning and submersion
7th
Excludes1: drowning and submersion while in swimming pool without fall (W67)
W16.022 Fall into swimming pool striking bottom causing other injury
7th

W16.03 Fall into swimming pool striking wall
6th
W16.031 Fall into swimming pool striking wall causing drowning and submersion
7th
Excludes1: drowning and submersion while in swimming pool without fall (W67)
W16.032 Fall into swimming pool striking wall causing other injury
7th

W16.1 Fall into natural body of water
5th
Fall into lake
Fall into open sea
Fall into river
Fall into stream
W16.11 Fall into natural body of water striking water surface
6th
W16.111 Fall into natural body of water striking water surface causing drowning and submersion
7th
Excludes1: drowning and submersion while in natural body of water without fall (W69)
W16.112 Fall into natural body of water striking water surface causing other injury
7th

W16.12 Fall into natural body of water striking bottom
6th

 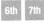 Additional Character Required   3-character code   •=New Code   *Excludes1—*Not coded here, do not use together
4th 5th 6th 7th   ▲=Revised Code   *Excludes2—*Not included here

W16.121 `7th` Fall into natural body of water striking bottom causing drowning and submersion

Excludes1: drowning and submersion while in natural body of water without fall (W69)

W16.122 `7th` Fall into natural body of water striking bottom causing other injury

W16.13 `6th` Fall into natural body of water striking side

W16.131 `7th` Fall into natural body of water striking side causing drowning and submersion

Excludes1: drowning and submersion while in natural body of water without fall (W69)

W16.132 `7th` Fall into natural body of water striking side causing other injury

W16.2 `5th` **Fall in (into) filled bathtub or bucket of water**

W16.21 `6th` **Fall in (into) filled bathtub**

Excludes1: fall into empty bathtub (W18.2)

W16.211 `7th` Fall in (into) filled bathtub causing drowning and submersion

Excludes1: drowning and submersion while in filled bathtub without fall (W65)

W16.212 `7th` Fall in (into) filled bathtub causing other injury

W16.22 `6th` **Fall in (into) bucket of water**

W16.221 `7th` Fall in (into) bucket of water causing drowning and submersion

W16.222 `7th` Fall in (into) bucket of water causing other injury

W16.5 `5th` **Jumping or diving into swimming pool**

W16.51 `6th` **Jumping or diving into swimming pool striking water surface**

W16.511 `7th` Jumping or diving into swimming pool striking water surface causing drowning and submersion

Excludes1: drowning and submersion while in swimming pool without jumping or diving (W67)

W16.512 `7th` Jumping or diving into swimming pool striking water surface causing other injury

W16.52 `6th` **Jumping or diving into swimming pool striking bottom**

W16.521 `7th` Jumping or diving into swimming pool striking bottom causing drowning and submersion

Excludes1: drowning and submersion while in swimming pool without jumping or diving (W67)

W16.522 `7th` Jumping or diving into swimming pool striking bottom causing other injury

W16.53 `6th` **Jumping or diving into swimming pool striking wall**

W16.531 `7th` Jumping or diving into swimming pool striking wall causing drowning and submersion

Excludes1: drowning and submersion while in swimming pool without jumping or diving (W67)

W16.532 `7th` Jumping or diving into swimming pool striking wall causing other injury

W16.6 `5th` **Jumping or diving into natural body of water**

Jumping or diving into lake
Jumping or diving into open sea
Jumping or diving into river
Jumping or diving into stream

> 7th characters for categories
> W00–W19
> A—initial encounter
> D—subsequent encounter
> S—sequela

W16.61 `6th` **Jumping or diving into natural body of water striking water surface**

W16.611 `7th` Jumping or diving into natural body of water striking water surface causing drowning and submersion

Excludes1: drowning and submersion while in natural body of water without jumping or diving (W69)

W16.612 Jumping or diving into natural body of water striking water surface causing other injury

W16.62 `6th` **Jumping or diving into natural body of water striking bottom**

W16.621 `7th` Jumping or diving into natural body of water striking bottom causing drowning and submersion

Excludes1: drowning and submersion while in natural body of water without jumping or diving (W69)

W16.622 `7th` Jumping or diving into natural body of water striking bottom causing other injury

W17 `4th` **OTHER FALL FROM ONE LEVEL TO ANOTHER**

W17.0XX `7th` **Fall into well**

W17.1XX `7th` **Fall into storm drain or manhole**

W17.2XX `7th` **Fall into hole**

Fall into pit

W17.3XX `7th` **Fall into empty swimming pool**

Excludes1: fall into filled swimming pool (W16.0-)

W17.4XX `7th` **Fall from dock**

W17.8 `5th` **Other fall from one level to another**

W17.81X `7th` **Fall down embankment (hill)***

W17.82X `7th` **Fall from (out of) grocery cart**

Fall due to grocery cart tipping over

W17.89X `7th` **Other fall from one level to another**

Fall from cherry picker/lifting device/ sky lift

W18 `4th` **OTHER SLIPPING, TRIPPING AND STUMBLING AND FALLS**

W18.0 `5th` **Fall due to bumping against object**

Striking against object with subsequent fall

Excludes1: fall on same level due to slipping, tripping, or stumbling with subsequent striking against object (W01.1-)

W18.00X `7th` **Striking against unspecified object with subsequent fall**

W18.01X `7th` **Striking against sports equipment with subsequent fall**

W18.02X `7th` **Striking against glass with subsequent fall**

W18.09X `7th` **Striking against other object with subsequent fall**

  `4th` `5th` `6th` `7th` Additional Character Required   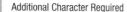 3-character code   •=New Code   ▲=Revised Code   *Excludes1*—Not coded here, do not use together   *Excludes2*—Not included here

W18.1 Fall from or off toilet
`5th`
   W18.11X Fall from or off toilet without subsequent striking against object
   `7th` Fall from (off) toilet NOS
   W18.12X Fall from or off toilet with subsequent striking against object
   `7th`

W18.2XX Fall in (into) shower or empty bathtub
   `7th` *Excludes1:* fall in full bathtub causing drowning or submersion (W16.21-)

W18.3 Other and unspecified fall on same level
`5th`
   W18.30X Fall on same level, unspecified
   `7th`

   W18.31X Fall on same level due to stepping on an object
   `7th` Fall on same level due to stepping on an animal
       Excludes1: slipping, tripping and stumbling without fall due to stepping on animal (W18.41)

   W18.39X Other fall on same level
   `7th`

W18.4 Slipping, tripping and stumbling without falling
`5th`
   Excludes1: collision with another person without fall (W51)
   W18.40X Slipping, tripping and stumbling without falling, unspecified
   `7th`

   W18.41X Slipping, tripping and stumbling without falling due to stepping on object
   `7th` Slipping, tripping and stumbling without falling due to stepping on animal
       Excludes1: slipping, tripping and stumbling with fall due to stepping on animal (W18.31)

   W18.42X Slipping, tripping and stumbling without falling due to stepping into hole or opening
   `7th`

   W18.43X Slipping, tripping and stumbling without falling due to stepping from one level to another
   `7th`

   W18.49X Other slipping, tripping and stumbling without falling
   `7th`

W19 UNSPECIFIED FALL
`7th` Accidental fall NOS

(W20–W49) EXPOSURE TO INANIMATE MECHANICAL FORCES

Excludes1: assault (X92–Y08)
   contact or collision with animals or persons (W50–W64)
   exposure to inanimate mechanical forces involving military or war operations (Y36.-, Y37.-)
   intentional self-harm (X71–X83)

7th characters for categories
W20–W49
A—initial encounter
D—subsequent encounter
S—sequela

W21 STRIKING AGAINST OR STRUCK BY SPORTS EQUIPMENT
`4th`
   Excludes1: assault with sports equipment (Y08.0-)
   striking against or struck by sports equipment with subsequent fall (W18.01)
   W21.0 Struck by hit or thrown ball
   `5th`
      W21.00X Struck by hit or thrown ball, unspecified type
      `7th`

      W21.01X Struck by football
      `7th`

      W21.02X Struck by soccer ball
      `7th`

      W21.03X Struck by baseball
      `7th`

W21.04X Struck by golf ball
`7th`

W21.05X Struck by basketball
`7th`

W21.06X Struck by volleyball
`7th`

W21.07X Struck by softball
`7th`

W21.09X Struck by other hit or thrown ball
`7th`

W21.1 Struck by bat, racquet or club
`5th`
   W21.11X Struck by baseball bat
   `7th`

   W21.12X Struck by tennis racquet
   `7th`

   W21.13X Struck by golf club
   `7th`

   W21.19X Struck by other bat, racquet or club
   `7th`

W21.2 Struck by hockey stick or puck
`5th`
   W21.21 Struck by hockey stick
   `6th`
      W21.210 Struck by ice hockey stick
      `7th`

      W21.211 Struck by field hockey stick
      `7th`

   W21.22 Struck by hockey puck
   `6th`
      W21.220 Struck by ice hockey puck
      `7th`

      W21.221 Struck by field hockey puck
      `7th`

W21.3 Struck by sports foot wear
`5th`
   W21.31X Struck by shoe cleats
   `7th` Stepped on by shoe cleats

   W21.32X Struck by skate blades
   `7th` Skated over by skate blades

   W21.39X Struck by other sports foot wear
   `7th`

W21.4XX Striking against diving board
`7th` **Use additional code** for subsequent falling into water, if applicable (W16.-)
W21.8 Striking against or struck by other sports equipment
`5th` **W21.81X Striking against or struck by football helmet**
   `7th`

   W21.89X Striking against or struck by other sports equipment
   `7th`

W21.9XX Striking against or struck by unspecified sports equipment
`7th`

W22 STRIKING AGAINST OR STRUCK BY OTHER OBJECTS
`4th`
   Excludes1: striking against or struck by object with subsequent fall (W18.09)
   W22.0 Striking against stationary object
   `5th` *Excludes1:* striking against stationary sports equipment (W21.8)

`4th` `5th` `6th` `7th` Additional Character Required	✓ 3-character code	•=New Code ▲=Revised Code	*Excludes1*—Not coded here, do not use together *Excludes2*—Not included here

CHAPTER 20. EXTERNAL CAUSES OF MORBIDITY (W22.01X–W49.9XX)

W22.01X Walked into wall
`7th`

W22.02X Walked into lamppost
`7th`

W22.03X Walked into furniture
`7th`

W22.04 Striking against wall of swimming pool
`6th`
  W22.041 Striking against wall of swimming pool causing drowning and submersion
  `7th`
    Excludes1: drowning and submersion while swimming without striking against wall (W67)
  W22.042 Striking against wall of swimming pool causing other injury
  `7th`

W22.09X Striking against other stationary object
`7th`

W22.1 Striking against or struck by automobile airbag
`5th`
  W22.10X Striking against or struck by unspecified automobile airbag
  `7th`

  W22.11X Striking against or struck by driver side automobile airbag
  `7th`

  W22.12X Striking against or struck by front passenger side automobile airbag
  `7th`

  W22.19X Striking against or struck by other automobile airbag
  `7th`

W22.8XX Striking against or struck by other objects
`7th`
  Striking against or struck by object NOS
  Excludes1: struck by thrown, projected or falling object (W20.-)

> 7th characters for categories W20–W49
> A—initial encounter
> D—subsequent encounter
> S—sequela

W23 CAUGHT, CRUSHED, JAMMED OR PINCHED IN OR BETWEEN OBJECTS
`4th`
Excludes1: injury caused by cutting or piercing instruments (W25–W27)
  injury caused by firearms malfunction (W32.1, W33.1-, W34.1-)
  injury caused by lifting and transmission devices (W24.-)
  injury caused by machinery (W28–W31)
  injury caused by nonpowered hand tools (W27.-)
  injury caused by transport vehicle being used as a means of transportation (V01–V99)
  injury caused by struck by thrown, projected or falling object (W20.-)
W23.0XX Caught, crushed, jammed, or pinched between moving objects
`7th`

W23.1XX Caught, crushed, jammed, or pinched between stationary objects
`7th`

W25 CONTACT WITH SHARP GLASS
`7th`
Code first any associated:
  injury due to flying glass from explosion or firearm discharge (W32–W40)
  transport accident (V00–V99)
Excludes1: fall on same level due to slipping, tripping and stumbling with subsequent striking against sharp glass (W01.10)
  striking against sharp glass with subsequent fall (W18.02)
Excludes 2: glass embedded in skin (W45)

W26 CONTACT WITH OTHER SHARP OBJECTS
`4th`
Excludes 2: glass embedded in skin (W45)
W26.0XX Contact with knife
`7th`

W26.1XX Contact with sword or dagger
`7th`
  Excludes1: contact with electric knife (W29.1)

•**W26.2XX** Contact with edge of stiff paper
`7th`
  Paper cut

•**W26.8XX** Contact with other sharp objects NEC
`7th`
  Contact with tin can lid

•**W25.9XX** Contact with unspecified sharp objects
`7th`

W28 CONTACT WITH POWERED LAWN MOWER
`7th`
Powered lawn mower (commercial) (residential)
Excludes1: contact with nonpowered lawn mower (W27.1)
Excludes2: exposure to electric current (W86.-)

W39 DISCHARGE OF FIREWORK
`7th`

W45 FB OR OBJECT ENTERING THROUGH SKIN
`4th`
Includes: foreign body or object embedded in skin
  nail embedded in skin
Excludes2: contact with hand tools (nonpowered) (powered) (W27–W29)
  contact with other sharp object(s) (W26.-)
  contact with sharp glass (W25.-)
  paper cut (W26.2-)
  struck by objects (W20–W22)
W45.0XX Nail entering through skin
`7th`

W45.8XX Other FB or object entering through skin
`7th`
  Splinter in skin NOS

W46 CONTACT WITH HYPODERMIC NEEDLE
`4th`
W46.0XX Contact with hypodermic needle
`7th`
  Hypodermic needle stick NOS

W46.1XX Contact with contaminated hypodermic needle
`7th`

W49 EXPOSURE TO OTHER INANIMATE MECHANICAL FORCES
`4th`
Includes: exposure to abnormal gravitational [G] forces
  exposure to inanimate mechanical forces NEC
Excludes1: exposure to inanimate mechanical forces involving military or war operations (Y36.-, Y37.-)
W49.0 Item causing external constriction
`5th`
  W49.01X Hair causing external constriction
  `7th`

  W49.02X String or thread causing external constriction
  `7th`

  W49.03X Rubber band causing external constriction
  `7th`

  W49.04X Ring or other jewelry causing external constriction
  `7th`

  W49.09X Other specified item causing external constriction
  `7th`

W49.9XX Exposure to other inanimate mechanical forces
`7th`

  Additional Character Required
 3-character code

•=New Code
▲=Revised Code

Excludes1—Not coded here, do not use together
Excludes2—Not included here

394 PEDIATRIC ICD-10-CM 2017: A MANUAL FOR PROVIDER-BASED CODING

(W50–W64) EXPOSURE TO ANIMATE MECHANICAL FORCES

Excludes1: Toxic effect of contact with venomous animals and plants (T63.-)

> **7th characters for categories W50–W64**
> A—initial encounter
> D—subsequent encounter
> S—sequela

W50 **ACCIDENTAL HIT, STRIKE, KICK, TWIST, BITE OR SCRATCH BY ANOTHER PERSON**
`4th`
Includes: hit, strike, kick, twist, bite, or scratch by another person NOS
Excludes1: assault by bodily force (Y04)
  struck by objects (W20–W22)

W50.0XX Accidental hit or strike by another person
`7th` Hit or strike by another person NOS

W50.1XX Accidental kick by another person
`7th` Kick by another person NOS

W50.2XX Accidental twist by another person
`7th` Twist by another person NOS

W50.3XX Accidental bite by another person
`7th` Human bite
  Bite by another person NOS

W50.4XX Accidental scratch by another person
`7th` Scratch by another person NOS

W51 **ACCIDENTAL STRIKING AGAINST OR BUMPED INTO BY ANOTHER PERSON**
`7th`
Excludes1: assault by striking against or bumping into by another person (Y04.2)
  fall due to collision with another person (W03)

W54 **CONTACT WITH DOG**
`4th`
Includes: contact with saliva, feces or urine of dog
W54.0XX Bitten by dog
`7th`

W54.1XX Struck by dog
`7th` Knocked over by dog

W54.8XX Other contact with dog
`7th`

W55 **CONTACT WITH OTHER MAMMALS**
`4th`
Includes: contact with saliva, feces or urine of mammal
Excludes1: animal being ridden—see transport accidents
  bitten or struck by dog (W54)
  bitten or struck by rodent (W53.-)
  contact with marine mammals (W56.-)
W55.0 **Contact with cat**
`5th`
  W55.01X **Bitten by cat**
  `7th`

  W55.03X **Scratched by cat**
  `7th`

  W55.09X **Other contact with cat**
  `7th`

(W65–W74) ACCIDENTAL NON-TRANSPORT DROWNING AND SUBMERSION

Excludes1: accidental drowning and submersion due to fall into water (W16.-)
  accidental drowning and submersion due to water transport accident (V90.-, V92.-)
Excludes2: accidental drowning and submersion due to cataclysm (X34–X39)

> **7th characters for categories W65–W74**
> A—initial encounter
> D—subsequent encounter
> S—sequela

W65 **ACCIDENTAL DROWNING AND SUBMERSION WHILE IN BATH-TUB**
`7th`
Excludes1: accidental drowning and submersion due to fall in (into) bathtub (W16.211)

W67 **ACCIDENTAL DROWNING AND SUBMERSION WHILE IN SWIMMING-POOL**
`7th`
Excludes1: accidental drowning and submersion due to fall into swimming pool (W16.011, W16.021, W16.031)
  accidental drowning and submersion due to striking into wall of swimming pool (W22.041)

W69 **ACCIDENTAL DROWNING AND SUBMERSION WHILE IN NATURAL WATER**
`7th`
Accidental drowning and submersion while in lake/open sea/river/stream
Excludes1: accidental drowning and submersion due to fall into natural body of water (W16.111, W16.121, W16.131)

(W85–W99) EXPOSURE TO ELECTRIC CURRENT, RADIATION AND EXTREME AMBIENT AIR TEMPERATURE AND PRESSURE

Excludes1: exposure to: failure in dosage of radiation or temperature during surgical and medical care (Y63.2–Y63.5)
  lightning (T75.0-)
  natural cold (X31)
  natural heat (X30)
  natural radiation NOS (X39)
  radiological procedure and radiotherapy (Y84.2)
  sunlight (X32)

> **7th characters for categories W85–W99**
> A—initial encounter
> D—subsequent encounter
> S—sequela

W86 **EXPOSURE TO OTHER SPECIFIED ELECTRIC CURRENT**
`7th`

W89 **EXPOSURE TO MAN-MADE VISIBLE AND ULTRAVIOLET LIGHT**
`4th`
Includes: exposure to welding light (arc)
Excludes1: exposure to sunlight (X32)
W89.1XX Exposure to tanning bed
`7th`

(X00–X08) EXPOSURE TO SMOKE, FIRE AND FLAMES

Excludes1: arson (X97)
Excludes2: explosions (W35–W40)
  lightning (T75.0-)
  transport accident (V01–V99)

> **7th characters for categories X00–X08**
> A—initial encounter
> D—subsequent encounter
> S—sequela

X00 **EXPOSURE TO UNCONTROLLED FIRE IN BUILDING OR STRUCTURE**
`4th`
X00.1XX **Exposure to smoke in uncontrolled fire in building or structure**
`7th`

X03 **EXPOSURE TO CONTROLLED FIRE, NOT IN BUILDING OR STRUCTURE**
`4th`
Includes: exposure to bon fire
  exposure to camp-fire
  exposure to trash fire
Includes: conflagration in building or structure
Code first any associated cataclysm
Excludes2: Exposure to ignition or melting of nightwear (X05)
  Exposure to ignition or melting of other clothing and apparel (X06.-)
  Exposure to other specified smoke, fire and flames (X08.-)
X03.1XX **Exposure to smoke in controlled fire, not in building or structure**
`7th`

  Additional Character Required   3-character code   •=New Code   ▲=Revised Code   ***Excludes1***—Not coded here, do not use together   ***Excludes2***—Not included here

PEDIATRIC ICD-10-CM 2017: A MANUAL FOR PROVIDER-BASED CODING   395

CHAPTER 20. EXTERNAL CAUSES OF MORBIDITY (X10–X78.2XX)

(X10–X19) CONTACT WITH HEAT AND HOT SUBSTANCES

Excludes1: exposure to excessive natural heat (X30)
exposure to fire and flames (X00–X09)

X10 **CONTACT WITH HOT DRINKS,**
4th **FOOD, FATS AND COOKING OILS**
X10.0XX **Contact with hot drinks**
7th

7th characters for categories
X10–X19
A—initial encounter
D—subsequent encounter
S—sequela

X10.1XX **Contact with hot food**
7th

X10.2XX **Contact with fats and cooking oils**
7th

X11 **CONTACT WITH HOT TAP-WATER**
4th *Includes:* contact with boiling tap-water
contact with boiling water NOS
Excludes1: contact with water heated on stove (X12)
X11.0XX **Contact with hot water in bath or tub**
7th *Excludes1:* contact with running hot water in bath or tub (X11.1)

X11.1XX **Contact with running hot water**
7th Contact with hot water running out of hose
Contact with hot water running out of tap
X11.8XX **Contact with other hot tap-water**
7th Contact with hot water in bucket
Contact with hot tap-water NOS

X12 **CONTACT WITH OTHER HOT FLUIDS**
7th Contact with water heated on stove
Excludes1: hot (liquid) metals (X18)

X13 **CONTACT WITH STEAM AND OTHER HOT VAPORS**
4th **X13.0XX** **Inhalation of steam and other hot vapors**
7th

X13.1XX **Other contact with steam and other hot vapors**
7th

X15 **CONTACT WITH HOT HOUSEHOLD APPLIANCES**
4th *Excludes1:* contact with heating appliances (X16)
contact with powered household appliances (W29.-)
exposure to controlled fire in building or structure due to household appliance (X02.8)
exposure to household appliances electrical current (W86.0)
X15.0XX **Contact with hot stove (kitchen)**
7th

X15.1XX **Contact with hot toaster**
7th

7th characters for categories
X10–X19
A—initial encounter
D—subsequent encounter
S—sequela

X15.2XX **Contact with hotplate**
7th

X15.3XX **Contact with hot saucepan or skillet**
7th

X15.8XX **Contact with other hot household appliances**
7th Contact with cooker/kettle/light bulbs

X16 **CONTACT WITH HOT HEATING APPLIANCES, RADIATORS**
7th **AND PIPES**
Excludes1: contact with powered appliances (W29.-)
exposure to controlled fire in building or structure due to appliance (X02.8)
exposure to industrial appliances electrical current (W86.1)

(X30–X39) EXPOSURE TO FORCES OF NATURE

X30 **EXPOSURE TO EXCESSIVE**
7th **NATURAL HEAT**
Exposure to excessive heat as the cause of sunstroke
Exposure to heat NOS
Excludes1: excessive heat of man-made origin (W92)
exposure to man-made radiation (W89)
exposure to sunlight (X32)
exposure to tanning bed (W89)

7th characters for categories
X30–X39
A—initial encounter
D—subsequent encounter
S—sequela

X31 **EXPOSURE TO EXCESSIVE NATURAL COLD**
7th Excessive cold as the cause of chilblains NOS
Excessive cold as the cause of immersion foot or hand
Exposure to cold NOS
Exposure to weather conditions

X32 **EXPOSURE TO SUNLIGHT**
7th *Excludes1:* man-made radiation (tanning bed) (W89)

(X50–X58) ACCIDENTAL EXPOSURE TO OTHER SPECIFIED FACTORS

•**X50** **OVEREXERTION FROM MOVEMENT**
4th •**X50.0XX** **Overexertion from strenuous**
7th **movement or load**
Lifting heavy objects
Lifting weights

7th characters for category X50
A—initial encounter
D—subsequent encounter
S—sequela

•**X50.1XX** **Overexertion from prolonged**
7th **static or awkward postures**
Prolonged or static bending
Prolonged or static kneeling
Prolonged or static reaching
Prolonged or static sitting
Prolonged or static standing
Prolonged or static twisting
•**X50.3XX** **Overexertion from repetitive movements**
7th Use of hand as hammer

•**X50.9XX** **Other and unspecified overexertion or strenuous movements**
7th **or postures**
Contact pressure
Contact stress

X58 **EXPOSURE TO OTHER SPECIFIED**
7th **FACTORS**
Accident NOS
Exposure NOS

7th characters for category X58
A—initial encounter
D—subsequent encounter
S—sequela

(X71–X83) INTENTIONAL SELF-HARM

Purposely self-inflicted injury
Suicide (attempted)

X72 **INTENTIONAL SELF-HARM BY**
7th **HANDGUN DISCHARGE**
Intentional self-harm by gun/pistol/revolver for single hand use
Excludes1: Very pistol (X74.8)

7th characters for category
X71–X83
A—initial encounter
D—subsequent encounter
S—sequela

X78 **INTENTIONAL SELF-HARM BY SHARP OBJECT**
4th **X78.0XX** **Intentional self-harm by sharp glass**
7th

X78.1XX **Intentional self-harm by knife**
7th

X78.2XX **Intentional self-harm by sword or dagger**
7th

   4th **5th** **6th** **7th** Additional Character Required 3-character code

•=New Code   *Excludes1*—Not coded here, do not use together
▲=Revised Code   *Excludes2*—Not included here

X78.8XX Intentional self-harm by other sharp object

`7th`

X78.9XX Intentional self-harm by unspecified sharp object

`7th`

(X92–Y09) ASSAULT

Adult and child abuse, neglect and maltreatment are classified as assault. Any of the assault codes may be used to indicate the external cause of any injury resulting from the confirmed abuse.

For confirmed cases of abuse, neglect and maltreatment, when the perpetrator is known, a code from Y07, Perpetrator of maltreatment and neglect, should accompany any other assault codes.

Includes: homicide

injuries inflicted by another person with intent
    to injure or kill, by any means

Excludes1: injuries due to legal intervention (Y35.-)
    injuries due to operations of war (Y36.-)
    injuries due to terrorism (Y38.-)

> 7th characters for categories
> X92–Y04
> A—initial encounter
> D—subsequent encounter
> S—sequela

X92 **ASSAULT BY DROWNING AND SUBMERSION**

`4th`

  X92.0XX Assault by drowning and submersion while in bathtub

`7th`

  X92.1XX Assault by drowning and submersion while in swimming pool

`7th`

  X92.2XX Assault by drowning and submersion after push into swimming pool

`7th`

  X92.3XX Assault by drowning and submersion in natural water

`7th`

  X92.8XX Other assault by drowning and submersion

`7th`

  X92.9XX Assault by drowning and submersion, unspecified

`7th`

X93 **ASSAULT BY HANDGUN DISCHARGE**

`7th`

Assault by discharge of gun for single hand use
Assault by discharge of pistol
Assault by discharge of revolver
Excludes1: Very pistol (X95.8)

X94 **ASSAULT BY RIFLE, SHOTGUN AND LARGER FIREARM DISCHARGE**

`4th`

Excludes1: airgun (X95.01)

  X94.1XX Assault by hunting rifle

`7th`

X95 **ASSAULT BY OTHER AND UNSPECIFIED FIREARM AND GUN DISCHARGE**

`4th`

  X95.0   Assault by gas, air or spring-operated guns

      X95.01X Assault by airgun discharge

`5th`

        Assault by BB gun discharge
        Assault by pellet gun discharge

      X95.02X Assault by paintball gun discharge

`7th`

      X95.09X Assault by other gas, air or spring-operated gun

`7th`

  X95.8XX Assault by other firearm discharge

`7th`

      Assault by very pistol [flare] discharge

  X95.9XX Assault by unspecified firearm discharge

`7th`

X97 **ASSAULT BY SMOKE, FIRE AND FLAMES**

`7th`

Assault by arson
Assault by cigarettes

X98 **ASSAULT BY STEAM, HOT VAPORS AND HOT OBJECTS**

`4th`

  X98.0XX Assault by steam or hot vapors

`7th`

  X98.1XX Assault by hot tap water

`7th`

  X98.2XX Assault by hot fluids

`7th`

  X98.3XX Assault by hot household appliances

`7th`

  X98.8XX Assault by other hot objects

`7th`

  X98.9XX Assault by unspecified hot objects

`7th`

X99 **ASSAULT BY SHARP OBJECT**

`4th`

Excludes1: assault by strike by sports equipment (Y08.0-)

  X99.0XX Assault by sharp glass

`7th`

  X99.1XX Assault by knife

`7th`

  X99.8XX Assault by other sharp object

`7th`

  X99.9XX Assault by unspecified sharp object

`7th`

      Assault by stabbing NOS

Y04 **ASSAULT BY BODILY FORCE**

`4th`

Excludes1: assault by:
    submersion (X92.-)
    use of weapon (X93–X95, X99, Y00)

  Y04.0XX Assault by unarmed brawl or fight

`7th`

  Y04.1XX Assault by human bite

`7th`

  Y04.2XX Assault by strike against or bumped into by another person

`7th`

  Y04.8XX Assault by other bodily force

`7th`

      Assault by bodily force NOS

Y07 **PERPETRATOR OF ASSAULT, MALTREATMENT AND NEGLECT**

`4th`

Adult and child abuse, neglect and maltreatment are classified as assault. Any of the assault codes may be used to indicate the external cause of any injury resulting from the confirmed abuse.

For confirmed cases of abuse, neglect and maltreatment, when the perpetrator is known, a code from Y07, Perpetrator of maltreatment and neglect, should accompany any other assault codes.

See Section I.C.19. Adult and child abuse, neglect and other maltreatment

Note: Codes from this category are for use only in cases of **confirmed abuse** (T74.-)

Selection of the correct perpetrator code is based on the relationship between the perpetrator and the victim

Includes: perpetrator of abandonment
    perpetrator of emotional neglect
    perpetrator of mental cruelty
    perpetrator of physical abuse
    perpetrator of physical neglect
    perpetrator of sexual abuse
    perpetrator of torture

`4th` `5th` `6th` `7th`   Additional Character Required   ✔   3-character code   •=New Code   ▲=Revised Code   *Excludes1*   Not coded here, do not use together   *Excludes2*—Not included here

Y07.0   **Spouse or partner, perpetrator of maltreatment and neglect**

5th

Spouse or partner, perpetrator of maltreatment and neglect against spouse or partner

Y07.01   Husband, perpetrator of maltreatment and neglect

Y07.02   Wife, perpetrator of maltreatment and neglect

Y07.03   Male partner, perpetrator of maltreatment and neglect

Y07.04   Female partner, perpetrator of maltreatment and neglect

Y07.1   **Parent (adoptive) (biological), perpetrator of maltreatment and neglect**

5th

Y07.11   Biological father, perpetrator of maltreatment and neglect

Y07.12   Biological mother, perpetrator of maltreatment and neglect

Y07.13   Adoptive father, perpetrator of maltreatment and neglect

Y07.14   Adoptive mother, perpetrator of maltreatment and neglect

Y07.4   **Other family member, perpetrator of maltreatment and neglect**

5th

Y07.41   Sibling, perpetrator of maltreatment and neglect

6th

Excludes1: stepsibling, perpetrator of maltreatment and neglect (Y07.435, Y07.436)

Y07.410   Brother, perpetrator of maltreatment and neglect

Y07.411   Sister, perpetrator of maltreatment and neglect

Y07.42   Foster parent, perpetrator of maltreatment and neglect

6th

Y07.420   Foster father, perpetrator of maltreatment and neglect

Y07.421   Foster mother, perpetrator of maltreatment and neglect

Y07.43   Stepparent or stepsibling, perpetrator of maltreatment and neglect

6th

Y07.430   Stepfather, perpetrator of maltreatment and neglect

Y07.432   Male friend of parent (co-residing in household), perpetrator of maltreatment and neglect

Y07.433   Stepmother, perpetrator of maltreatment and neglect

Y07.434   Female friend of parent (co-residing in household), perpetrator of maltreatment and neglect

Y07.435   Stepbrother, perpetrator or maltreatment and neglect

Y07.436   Stepsister, perpetrator of maltreatment and neglect

Y07.49   Other family member, perpetrator of maltreatment and neglect

6th

Y07.490   Male cousin, perpetrator of maltreatment and neglect

Y07.491   Female cousin, perpetrator of maltreatment and neglect

Y07.499   Other family member, perpetrator of maltreatment and neglect

Y07.5   **Non-family member, perpetrator of maltreatment and neglect**

5th

Y07.50   Unspecified non-family member, perpetrator of maltreatment and neglect

Y07.51   Daycare provider, perpetrator of maltreatment and neglect

6th

Y07.510   At-home childcare provider, perpetrator of maltreatment and neglect

Y07.511   Daycare center childcare provider, perpetrator of maltreatment and neglect

Y07.519   Unspecified daycare provider, perpetrator of maltreatment and neglect

Y07.53   Teacher or instructor, perpetrator of maltreatment and neglect

Coach, perpetrator of maltreatment and neglect

Y07.59   Other non-family member, perpetrator of maltreatment and neglect

Y07.9   **Unspecified perpetrator of maltreatment and neglect**

(Y21–Y33) EVENT OF UNDETERMINED INTENT

Undetermined intent is only for use when there is specific documentation in the record that the intent of the injury cannot be determined. If no such documentation is present, code to accidental (unintentional).

See full *ICD-10-CM* manual for codes in categories Y21–Y33.

(Y35–Y38) LEGAL INTERVENTION, OPERATIONS OF WAR, MILITARY OPERATIONS, AND TERRORISM

See full *ICD-10-CM* manual for codes in categories Y35–Y38.

(Y62–Y69) MISADVENTURES TO PATIENTS DURING SURGICAL AND MEDICAL CARE

Excludes2: breakdown or malfunctioning of medical device (during procedure) (after implantation) (ongoing use) (Y70–Y82)

Excludes 1: surgical and medical procedures as the cause of abnormal reaction of the patient, without mention of misadventure at the time of the procedure (Y83–Y84)

See full *ICD-10-CM* manual for codes in categories Y62–Y69.

(Y70–Y82) MEDICAL DEVICES ASSOCIATED WITH ADVERSE INCIDENTS IN DIAGNOSTIC AND THERAPEUTIC USE

Includes: breakdown or malfunction of medical devices (during use) (after implantation) (ongoing use)

Excludes2: misadventure to patients during surgical and medical care, classifiable to (Y62–Y69)

later complications following use of medical devices without breakdown or malfunctioning of device (Y83–Y84)

surgical and other medical procedures as the cause of abnormal reaction of the patient, or of later complication, without mention of misadventure at the time of the procedure (Y83–Y84)

See full *ICD-10-CM* manual for codes in categories Y70–Y82.

(Y83–Y84) SURGICAL AND OTHER MEDICAL PROCEDURES AS THE CAUSE OF ABNORMAL REACTION OF THE PATIENT, OR OF LATER COMPLICATION, WITHOUT MENTION OF MISADVENTURE AT THE TIME OF THE PROCEDURE

Excludes1: misadventures to patients during surgical and medical care, classifiable to (Y62–Y69)

Excludes2: breakdown or malfunctioning of medical device (after implantation) (during procedure) (ongoing use) (Y70–Y82)

See full *ICD-10-CM* manual for codes in categories Y83–Y84.

(Y90–Y99) SUPPLEMENTARY FACTORS RELATED TO CAUSES OF MORBIDITY CLASSIFIED ELSEWHERE

Note: These categories may be used to provide supplementary information concerning causes of morbidity. They are not to be used for single-condition coding.

Y90   **EVIDENCE OF ALCOHOL INVOLVEMENT DETERMINED BY BLOOD ALCOHOL LEVEL**

4th

Code first any associated alcohol related disorders (F10)

Y90.0   Blood alcohol level of less than 20 mg/100 ml

Y90.1   Blood alcohol level of 20–39 mg/100 ml

Y90.2   Blood alcohol level of 40–59 mg/100 ml

Y90.3   Blood alcohol level of 60–79 mg/100 ml

Y90.4   Blood alcohol level of 80–99 mg/100 ml

Y90.5   Blood alcohol level of 100–119 mg/100 ml

Y90.6   Blood alcohol level of 120–199 mg/100 ml

Y90.7   Blood alcohol level of 200–239 mg/100 ml

Y90.8   Blood alcohol level of 240 mg/100 ml or more

Y90.9   Presence of alcohol in blood, level not specified

  4th   5th   6th   7th   Additional Character Required   ✓   3-character code

•=New Code
▲=Revised Code

Excludes1—Not coded here, do not use together
Excludes2—Not included here

Y92 PLACE OF OCCURRENCE OF THE EXTERNAL CAUSE

4th

GUIDELINE

When applicable, place of occurrence, activity, and external cause status codes are sequenced after the main external cause code(s). Regardless of the number of external cause codes assigned, there should be only one place of occurrence code, one activity code, and one external cause status code assigned to an encounter.

Codes from category Y92, Place of occurrence of the external cause, are secondary codes for use after other external cause codes to identify the location of the patient at the time of injury or other condition.

Generally, a place of occurrence code is assigned only once, at the initial encounter for treatment. However, in the rare instance that a new injury occurs during hospitalization, an additional place of occurrence code may be assigned. No 7th characters are used for Y92.

Do not use place of occurrence code Y92.9 if the place is not stated or is not applicable.

The following category is for use, when relevant, to identify the place of occurrence of the external cause. Use in conjunction with an activity code. Place of occurrence should be recorded only at the **initial encounter** for treatment.

Y92.0 Non-institutional (private) residence as the place of occurrence of the external cause

5th

Excludes1: abandoned or derelict house (Y92.89)
home under construction but not yet occupied (Y92.6-)
institutional place of residence (Y92.1-)

Y92.00 Unspecified non-institutional (private) residence as the place of occurrence of the external cause

6th

- **Y92.000** Kitchen of unspecified non-institutional (private) residence as the place of occurrence of the external cause
- **Y92.001** Dining room of unspecified non-institutional (private) residence as the place of occurrence of the external cause
- **Y92.002** Bathroom of unspecified non-institutional (private) residence single-family (private) house as the place of occurrence of the external cause
- **Y92.003** Bedroom of unspecified non-institutional (private) residence as the place of occurrence of the external cause
- **Y92.007** Garden or yard of unspecified non-institutional (private) residence as the place of occurrence of the external cause
- **Y92.008** Other place in unspecified non-institutional (private) residence as the place of occurrence of the external cause
- **Y92.009** Unspecified place in unspecified non-institutional (private) residence as the place of occurrence of the external cause
  Home (NOS) as the place of occurrence of the external cause

Y92.1 Institutional (nonprivate) residence as the place of occurrence of the external cause

5th

Y92.10 Unspecified residential institution as the place of occurrence of the external cause

Y92.11 Children's home and orphanage as the place of occurrence of the external cause

6th

- **Y92.110** Kitchen in children's home and orphanage as the place of occurrence of the external cause
- **Y92.111** Bathroom in children's home and orphanage as the place of occurrence of the external cause
- **Y92.112** Bedroom in children's home and orphanage as the place of occurrence of the external cause
- **Y92.113** Driveway of children's home and orphanage as the place of occurrence of the external cause
- **Y92.114** Garage of children's home and orphanage as the place of occurrence of the external cause
- **Y92.115** Swimming-pool of children's home and orphanage as the place of occurrence of the external cause
- **Y92.116** Garden or yard of children's home and orphanage as the place of occurrence of the external cause
- **Y92.118** Other place in children's home and orphanage as the place of occurrence of the external cause
- **Y92.119** Unspecified place in children's home and orphanage as the place of occurrence of the external cause

Y92.15 Reform school as the place of occurrence of the external cause

6th

- **Y92.150** Kitchen in reform school as the place of occurrence of the external cause
- **Y92.151** Dining room in reform school as the place of occurrence of the external cause
- **Y92.152** Bathroom in reform school as the place of occurrence of the external cause
- **Y92.153** Bedroom in reform school as the place of occurrence of the external cause
- **Y92.154** Driveway of reform school as the place of occurrence of the external cause
- **Y92.155** Garage of reform school as the place of occurrence of the external cause
- **Y92.156** Swimming-pool of reform school as the place of occurrence of the external cause
- **Y92.157** Garden or yard of reform school as the place of occurrence of the external cause
- **Y92.158** Other place in reform school as the place of occurrence of the external cause
- **Y92.159** Unspecified place in reform school as the place of occurrence of the external cause

Y92.16 School dormitory as the place of occurrence of the external cause

6th

Excludes1: reform school as the place of occurrence of the external cause (Y92.15-)
school buildings and grounds as the place of occurrence of the external cause (Y92.2-)
school sports and athletic areas as the place of occurrence of the external cause (Y92.3-)

- **Y92.160** Kitchen in school dormitory as the place of occurrence of the external cause
- **Y92.161** Dining room in school dormitory as the place of occurrence of the external cause
- **Y92.162** Bathroom in school dormitory as the place of occurrence of the external cause
- **Y92.163** Bedroom in school dormitory as the place of occurrence of the external cause
- **Y92.168** Other place in school dormitory as the place of occurrence of the external cause
- **Y92.169** Unspecified place in school dormitory as the place of occurrence of the external cause

   Additional Character Required 3-character code

•=New Code
▲=Revised Code

Excludes1—Not coded here, do not use together
Excludes2—Not included here

Y92.2 **5th** **School, other institution and public administrative area as the place of occurrence of the external cause**
Building and adjacent grounds used by the general public or by a particular group of the public
Excludes1: building under construction as the place of occurrence of the external cause (Y92.6)
residential institution as the place of occurrence of the external cause (Y92.1)
school dormitory as the place of occurrence of the external cause (Y92.16-)
sports and athletics area of schools as the place of occurrence of the external cause (Y92.3-)

Y92.21 **6th** **School (private) (public) (state) as the place of occurrence of the external cause**

Y92.210 **Daycare center as the place of occurrence of the external cause**

Y92.211 **Elementary school as the place of occurrence of the external cause**
Kindergarten as the place of occurrence of the external cause

Y92.212 **Middle school as the place of occurrence of the external cause**

Y92.213 **High school as the place of occurrence of the external cause**

Y92.214 **College as the place of occurrence of the external cause**
University as the place of occurrence of the external cause

Y92.215 **Trade school as the place of occurrence of the external cause**

Y92.218 **Other school as the place of occurrence of the external cause**

Y92.219 **Unspecified school as the place of occurrence of the external cause**

Y92.22 **Religious institution as the place of occurrence of the external cause**
Church as the place of occurrence of the external cause
Mosque as the place of occurrence of the external cause
Synagogue as the place of occurrence of the external cause

Y92.25 **6th** **Cultural building as the place of occurrence of the external cause**

Y92.250 **Art Gallery as the place of occurrence of the external cause**

Y92.251 **Museum as the place of occurrence of the external cause**

Y92.252 **Music hall as the place of occurrence of the external cause**

Y92.253 **Opera house as the place of occurrence of the external cause**

Y92.254 **Theater (live) as the place of occurrence of the external cause**

Y92.258 **Other cultural public building as the place of occurrence of the external cause**

Y92.26 **Movie house or cinema as the place of occurrence of the external cause**

Y92.29 **Other specified public building as the place of occurrence of the external cause**
Assembly hall as the place of occurrence of the external cause
Clubhouse as the place of occurrence of the external cause

Y92.3 **5th** **Sports and athletics area as the place of occurrence of the external cause**

Y92.31 **6th** **Athletic court as the place of occurrence of the external cause**
Excludes1: tennis court in private home or garden (Y92.09)

Y92.310 **Basketball court as the place of occurrence of the external cause**

Y92.311 **Squash court as the place of occurrence of the external cause**

Y92.312 **Tennis court as the place of occurrence of the external cause**

Y92.318 **Other athletic court as the place of occurrence of the external cause**

Y92.32 **6th** **Athletic field as the place of occurrence of the external cause**

Y92.320 **Baseball field as the place of occurrence of the external cause**

Y92.321 **Football field as the place of occurrence of the external cause**

Y92.322 **Soccer field as the place of occurrence of the external cause**

Y92.328 **Other athletic field as the place of occurrence of the external cause**
Cricket field as the place of occurrence of the external cause
Hockey field as the place of occurrence of the external cause

Y92.33 **6th** **Skating rink as the place of occurrence of the external cause**

Y92.330 **Ice skating rink (indoor) (outdoor) as the place of occurrence of the external cause**

Y92.331 **Roller skating rink as the place of occurrence of the external cause**

Y92.34 **Swimming pool (public) as the place of occurrence of the external cause**
Excludes1: swimming pool in private home or garden (Y92.016)

Y92.39 **Other specified sports and athletic area as the place of occurrence of the external cause**
Golf-course/Gymnasium as the place of occurrence of the external cause

Y92.4 **5th** **Street, highway and other paved roadways as the place of occurrence of the external cause**
Excludes1: private driveway of residence (Y92.014, Y92.024, Y92.043, Y92.093, Y92.113, Y92.123, Y92.154, Y92.194)

Y92.41 **6th** **Street and highway as the place of occurrence of the external cause**

Y92.410 **Unspecified street and highway as the place of occurrence of the external cause**
Road NOS as the place of occurrence of the external cause

Y92.411 **Interstate highway as the place of occurrence of the external cause**
Freeway/Motorway as the place of occurrence of the external cause

Y92.412 **Parkway as the place of occurrence of the external cause**

Y92.413 **State road as the place of occurrence of the external cause**

Y92.414 **Local residential or business street as the place of occurrence of the external cause**

Y92.415 **Exit ramp or entrance ramp of street or highway as the place of occurrence of the external cause**

Y92.48 **6th** **Other paved roadways as the place of occurrence of the external cause**

Y92.480 **Sidewalk as the place of occurrence of the external cause**

Y92.481 **Parking lot as the place of occurrence of the external cause**

Y92.482 **Bike path as the place of occurrence of the external cause**

Y92.488 **Other paved roadways as the place of occurrence of the external cause**

Y92.7 **5th** **Farm as the place of occurrence of the external cause**
Ranch as the place of occurrence of the external cause
Excludes1: farmhouse and home premises of farm (Y92.01-)

•=New Code
▲=Revised Code

Excludes1—Not coded here, do not use together
Excludes2—Not included here

Y92.71 Barn as the place of occurrence of the external cause

Y92.72 Chicken coop as the place of occurrence of the external cause

Hen house as the place of occurrence of the external cause

Y92.73 Farm field as the place of occurrence of the external cause

Y92.74 Orchard as the place of occurrence of the external cause

Y92.79 Other farm location as the place of occurrence of the external cause

Y92.83 Recreation area as the place of occurrence of the external cause

 6th

     Y92.830 Public park as the place of occurrence of the external cause

     Y92.831 Amusement park as the place of occurrence of the external cause

     Y92.832 Beach/Seashore as the place of occurrence of the external cause

     Y92.833 Campsite as the place of occurrence of the external cause

     Y92.834 Zoological garden (Zoo) as the place of occurrence of the external cause

     Y92.838 Other recreation area as the place of occurrence of the external cause

Y93 ACTIVITY CODES

 4th

GUIDELINE

Note: Category Y93 is provided for use to indicate the activity of the person seeking healthcare for an injury or health condition, such as a heart attack while shoveling snow, which resulted from, or was contributed to, by the activity. These codes are appropriate for use for both acute injuries, such as those from chapter 19, and conditions that are due to the long-term, cumulative effects of an activity, such as those from chapter 13. They are also appropriate for use with external cause codes for cause and intent if identifying the activity provides additional information on the event. These codes should be used in conjunction with codes for external cause status (Y99) and place of occurrence (Y92).

Assign a code from category Y93, Activity code, to describe the activity of the patient at the time the injury or other health condition occurred.

An activity code is used only once, at the initial encounter for treatment. Only one code from Y93 should be recorded on a medical record.

The activity codes are not applicable to poisonings, adverse effects, misadventures or sequela.

Do not assign Y93.9, Unspecified activity, if the activity is not stated.

A code from category Y93 is appropriate for use with external cause and intent codes if identifying the activity provides additional information about the event.

Y93.0 Activities involving walking and running

 5th

Excludes1: activity, walking an animal (Y93.K1)
activity, walking or running on a treadmill (Y93.A1)

     Y93.01 Activity, walking, marching and hiking

Activity, walking, marching and hiking on level or elevated terrain

Excludes1: activity, mountain climbing (Y93.31)

     Y93.02 Activity, running

Y93.1 Activities involving water and water craft

5th

Excludes1: activities involving ice (Y93.2-)

     Y93.11 Activity, swimming

     Y93.12 Activity, springboard and platform diving

     Y93.13 Activity, water polo

     Y93.14 Activity, water aerobics and water exercise

     Y93.15 Activity, underwater diving and snorkeling

Activity, SCUBA diving

     Y93.16 Activity, rowing, canoeing, kayaking, rafting and tubing

     Y93.17 Activity, water skiing and wake boarding

     Y93.18 Activity, surfing, windsurfing and boogie boarding

Activity, water sliding

     Y93.19 Activity, other involving water and watercraft

Activity involving water NOS

Activity, parasailing

Activity, water survival training and testing

Y93.2 Activities involving ice and snow

5th

Excludes1: activity, shoveling ice and snow (Y93.H1)

     Y93.21 Activity, ice skating

Activity, figure skating (singles) (pairs)

Activity, ice dancing

Excludes1: activity, ice hockey (Y93.22)

     Y93.22 Activity, ice hockey

     Y93.23 Activity, snow (alpine) (downhill) skiing, snowboarding, sledding, tobogganing and snow tubing

Excludes1: activity, cross country skiing (Y93.24)

     Y93.24 Activity, cross country skiing

Activity, nordic skiing

     Y93.29 Activity, other involving ice and snow

Activity involving ice and snow NOS

Y93.3 Activities involving climbing, rappelling and jumping off

5th

Excludes1: activity, hiking on level or elevated terrain (Y93.01)
activity, jumping rope (Y93.56)
activity, trampoline jumping (Y93.44)

     Y93.31 Activity, mountain climbing, rock climbing and wall climbing

     Y93.32 Activity, rappelling

     Y93.33 Activity, BASE jumping

Activity, Building, Antenna, Span, Earth jumping

     Y93.34 Activity, bungee jumping

     Y93.35 Activity, hang gliding

     Y93.39 Activity, other involving climbing, rappelling and jumping off

Y93.4 Activities involving dancing and other rhythmic movement

5th

Excludes1: activity, martial arts (Y93.75)

     Y93.41 Activity, dancing

     Y93.42 Activity, yoga

     Y93.43 Activity, gymnastics

Activity, rhythmic gymnastics

Excludes1: activity, trampolining (Y93.44)

     Y93.44 Activity, trampolining

     Y93.45 Activity, cheerleading

     Y93.49 Activity, other involving dancing and other rhythmic movements

Y93.5 Activities involving other sports and athletics played individually

5th

Excludes1: activity, dancing (Y93.41)
     activity, gymnastic (Y93.43)
     activity, trampolining (Y93.44)
     activity, yoga (Y93.42)

     Y93.51 Activity, roller skating (inline) and skateboarding

     Y93.52 Activity, horseback riding

     Y93.53 Activity, golf

     Y93.54 Activity, bowling

     Y93.55 Activity, bike riding

     Y93.56 Activity, jumping rope

     Y93.57 Activity, non-running track and field events

Excludes1: activity, running (any form) (Y93.02)

     Y93.59 Activity, other involving other sports and athletics played individually

Excludes1: activities involving climbing, rappelling, and
         jumping (Y93.3-)
     activities involving ice and snow (Y93.2-)
     activities involving walking and running (Y93.0-)
     activities involving water and watercraft (Y93.1-)

Y93.6 Activities involving other sports and athletics played as a team or group

5th

Excludes1: activity, ice hockey (Y93.22)
activity, water polo (Y93.13)

     Y93.61 Activity, American tackle football

Activity, football NOS

     Y93.62 Activity, American flag or touch football

     Y93.63 Activity, rugby

     Y93.64 Activity, baseball

Activity, softball

     Y93.65 Activity, lacrosse and field hockey

     Y93.66 Activity, soccer

     Y93.67 Activity, basketball

 4th **5th** **6th** **7th** Additional Character Required   ✔ 3-character code

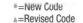
•=New Code   *Excludes1* Not coded here, do not use together
▲=Revised Code   *Excludes2*—Not included here

CHAPTER 20. EXTERNAL CAUSES OF MORBIDITY   (Y93.68–Y99.2)

Y93.68   **Activity, volleyball (beach) (court)**

Y93.6A   **Activity, physical games generally associated with school recess, summer camp and children**
    Including capture the flag/dodge ball/four square/kickball

Y93.69   **Activity, other involving other sports and athletics played as a team or group**
    Activity, cricket

Y93.7   **Activities involving other specified sports and athletics**

Y93.71   **Activity, boxing**

Y93.72   **Activity, wrestling**

Y93.73   **Activity, racquet and hand sports**
    Activity, handball/racquetball/squash/tennis

Y93.74   **Activity, Frisbee**

Y93.75   **Activity, martial arts**
    Activity, combatives

Y93.79   **Activity, other specified sports and athletics**
    Excludes1: sports and athletics activities specified in categories Y93.0–Y93.6

Y93.B   **Activities involving other muscle strengthening exercises**

Y93.B1   **Activity, exercise machines primarily for muscle strengthening**

Y93.B2   **Activity, push-ups, pull-ups, sit-ups**

Y93.B3   **Activity, free weights**
    Activity, barbells/dumbbells

Y93.B4   **Activity, pilates**

Y93.B9   **Activity, other involving muscle strengthening exercises**
    Excludes1: activities involving muscle strengthening specified in categories Y93.0–Y93.A

Y93.C   **Activities involving computer technology and electronic devices**
    Excludes1: activity, electronic musical keyboard or instruments (Y93.J-)

Y93.C1   **Activity, computer keyboarding**
    Activity, electronic game playing using keyboard or other stationary device

Y93.C2   **Activity, hand held interactive electronic device**
    Activity, cellular telephone and communication device
    Activity, electronic game playing using interactive device
    Excludes1: activity, electronic game playing using keyboard or other stationary device (Y93.C1)

Y93.C9   **Activity, other involving computer technology and electronic devices**

Y93.D   **Activities involving arts and handcrafts**
    Excludes1: activities involving playing musical instrument (Y93.J-)

Y93.D1   **Activity, knitting and crocheting**

Y93.D2   **Activity, sewing**

Y93.D3   **Activity, furniture building and finishing**
    Activity, furniture repair

Y93.D9   **Activity, other involving arts and handcrafts**

Y93.E   **Activities involving personal hygiene and interior property and clothing maintenance**
    Excludes1: activities involving cooking and grilling (Y93.G-)
    activities involving exterior property and land maintenance, building and construction (Y93.H-)
    activities involving caregiving (Y93.F-)
    activity, dishwashing (Y93.G1)
    activity, food preparation (Y93.G1)
    activity, gardening (Y93.H2)

Y93.E1   **Activity, personal bathing and showering**

Y93.E2   **Activity, laundry**

Y93.E3   **Activity, vacuuming**

Y93.E4   **Activity, ironing**

Y93.E5   **Activity, floor mopping and cleaning**

Y93.E6   **Activity, residential relocation**
    Activity, packing up and unpacking involved in moving to a new residence

Y93.E8   **Activity, other personal hygiene**

Y93.E9   **Activity, other interior property and clothing maintenance**

Y93.G   **Activities involving food preparation, cooking and grilling**

Y93.G1   **Activity, food preparation and clean up**
    Activity, dishwashing

Y93.G2   **Activity, grilling and smoking food**

Y93.G3   **Activity, cooking and baking**
    Activity, use of stove, oven and microwave oven

Y93.G9   **Activity, other involving cooking and grilling**

Y93.I   **Activities involving roller coasters and other types of external motion**

Y93.I1   **Activity, roller coaster riding**

Y93.I9   **Activity, other involving external motion**

Y93.J   **Activities involving playing musical instrument**
    Activity involving playing electric musical instrument

Y93.J1   **Activity, piano playing**
    Activity, musical keyboard (electronic) playing

Y93.J2   **Activity, drum and other percussion instrument playing**

Y93.J3   **Activity, string instrument playing**

Y93.J4   **Activity, winds and brass instrument playing**

Y93.K   **Activities involving animal care**
    Excludes1: activity, horseback riding (Y93.52)

Y93.K1   **Activity, walking an animal**

Y93.K2   **Activity, milking an animal**

Y93.K3   **Activity, grooming and shearing an animal**

Y93.K9   **Activity, other involving animal care**

Y93.8   **Activities, other specified**

Y93.81   **Activity, refereeing a sports activity**

Y93.82   **Activity, spectator at an event**

Y93.83   **Activity, rough housing and horseplay**

Y93.84   **Activity, sleeping**

•**Y93.85**   **Activity, choking game**
    Activity, blackout or fainting or pass out game

Y93.89   **Activity, other specified**

Y99   **EXTERNAL CAUSE STATUS**

GUIDELINE

A code from category Y99, External cause status, should be assigned whenever any other external cause code is assigned for an encounter, including an Activity code, except for the events noted below. Assign a code from category Y99, External cause status, to indicate the work status of the person at the time the event occurred. The status code indicates whether the event occurred during military activity, whether a non-military person was at work, whether an individual including a student or volunteer was involved in a non-work activity at the time of the causal event.

A code from Y99, External cause status, should be assigned, when applicable, with other external cause codes, such as transport accidents and falls. The external cause status codes are not applicable to poisonings, adverse effects, misadventures or late effects.

Do not assign a code from category Y99 if no other external cause codes (cause, activity) are applicable for the encounter.

An external cause status code is used only once, at the initial encounter for treatment. Only one code from Y99 should be recorded on a medical record.

Do not assign code Y99.9, Unspecified external cause status, if the status is not stated.

Note: A single code from category Y99 should be used in conjunction with the external cause code(s) assigned to a record to indicate the status of the person at the time the event occurred.

Y99.0   **Civilian activity done for income or pay**
    Civilian activity done for financial or other compensation
    Excludes1: military activity (Y99.1)
    volunteer activity (Y99.2)

Y99.2   **Volunteer activity**
    Excludes1: activity of child or other family member assisting in compensated work of other family member (Y99.8)

  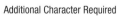   Additional Character Required   3-character code

•=New Code
▲=Revised Code

Excludes1—Not coded here, do not use together
Excludes2—Not included here

Y99.8 **Other external cause status**

Activity NEC

Activity of child or other family member assisting in compensated work of other family member

Hobby not done for income

Leisure activity

Off-duty activity of military personnel

Recreation or sport not for income or while a student

Student activity

Excludes1: civilian activity done for income or compensation (Y99.0)

military activity (Y99.1)

Y99.9 **Unspecified external cause status**

  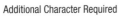 Additional Character Required 3-character code

•=New Code
▲=Revised Code

Excludes1 Not coded here, do not use together
Excludes2—Not included here

PEDIATRIC ICD-10-CM 2017: A MANUAL FOR PROVIDER-BASED CODING 403

Chapter 21. Factors influencing health status and contact with health services (Z00–Z99)

GUIDELINES

Note: The chapter specific guidelines provide additional information about the use of Z codes for specified encounters.

Use of Z codes in any healthcare setting

Z codes are for use in any healthcare setting. Z codes may be used as either a first-listed (principal diagnosis code in the inpatient setting) or secondary code, depending on the circumstances of the encounter. Certain Z codes may only be used as first-listed or principal diagnosis.

Z codes indicate a reason for an encounter

Z codes are not procedure codes. A corresponding procedure code must accompany a Z code to describe any procedure performed.

Categories of Z codes

CONTACT/EXPOSURE
Refer to categories Z20 and Z77.

INOCULATIONS AND VACCINATIONS
Refer to category Z23.

STATUS
Status codes indicate that a patient is either a carrier of a disease or has the sequelae or residual of a past disease or condition. This includes such things as the presence of prosthetic or mechanical devices resulting from past treatment. A status code is informative, because the status may affect the course of treatment and its outcome. A status code is distinct from a history code. The history code indicates that the patient no longer has the condition.

A status code should not be used with a diagnosis code from one of the body system chapters, if the diagnosis code includes the information provided by the status code. For example, code Z94.1, Heart transplant status, should not be used with a code from subcategory T86.2, Complications of heart transplant. The status code does not provide additional information. The complication code indicates that the patient is a heart transplant patient.

For encounters for weaning from a mechanical ventilator, assign a code from subcategory J96.1, Chronic respiratory failure, followed by code Z99.11, Dependence on respirator [ventilator] status.

The status Z codes/categories are:
Z14, Z15, Z16, Z17, Z18, Z21, Z22, Z28.3, Z33.1, Z66, Z67, Z68, Z74.01, Z76.82, Z78, Z79, Z88 (Except: Z88.9), Z89, Z90, Z91.0-, Z93, Z94, Z95, Z96,Z97, Z98, Z99

HISTORY (OF)
There are two types of history Z codes, personal and family. *Refer to categories or codes Z80, Z81, Z82, Z83, Z84, Z85, Z86, Z87, Z91.4-, Z91.5, Z91.8- (Except: Z91.83), Z92 (Except: Z92.0 and Z92.82)*

SCREENING
Refer to categories Z11, Z12 and Z13 (except: Z13.9).

OBSERVATION
Refer to categories Z03 and Z04 for further details.

AFTERCARE
Aftercare visit codes cover situations when the initial treatment of a disease has been performed and the patient requires continued care during the healing or recovery phase, or for the long-term consequences of the disease. The aftercare Z code should not be used if treatment is directed at a current, acute disease. The diagnosis code is to be used in these cases. Exceptions to this rule are codes Z51.0, Encounter for antineoplastic radiation therapy, and codes from subcategory Z51.1, Encounter for antineoplastic chemotherapy and immunotherapy. These codes are to be first-listed, followed by the diagnosis code when a patient's encounter is solely to receive radiation therapy, chemotherapy, or immunotherapy for the treatment of a neoplasm. If the reason for the encounter is more than one type of antineoplastic therapy, code Z51.0 and a code from subcategory Z51.1 may be assigned together, in which case one of these codes would be reported as a secondary diagnosis.

The aftercare Z codes should also not be used for aftercare for injuries. For aftercare of an injury, assign the acute injury code with the appropriate 7th character (for subsequent encounter).

The aftercare codes are generally first-listed to explain the specific reason for the encounter. An aftercare code may be used as an additional code when some type of aftercare is provided in addition to the reason for admission and no diagnosis code is applicable. An example of this would be the closure of a colostomy during an encounter for treatment of another condition.

Aftercare codes should be used in conjunction with other aftercare codes or diagnosis codes to provide better detail on the specifics of an aftercare encounter visit, unless otherwise directed by the classification. Should a patient receive multiple types of antineoplastic therapy during the same encounter, code Z51.0, Encounter for antineoplastic radiation therapy, and codes from subcategory Z51.1, Encounter for antineoplastic chemotherapy and immunotherapy, may be used together on a record. The sequencing of multiple aftercare codes depends on the circumstances of the encounter.

Certain aftercare Z code categories need a secondary diagnosis code to describe the resolving condition or sequelae. For others, the condition is included in the code title.

Additional Z code aftercare category terms include fitting and adjustment, and attention to artificial openings.

Status Z codes may be used with aftercare Z codes to indicate the nature of the aftercare. For example code Z95.1, Presence of aortocoronary bypass graft, may be used with code Z48.812, Encounter for surgical aftercare following surgery on the circulatory system, to indicate the surgery for which the aftercare is being performed. A status code should not be used when the aftercare code indicates the type of status, such as using Z43.0, Encounter for attention to tracheostomy, with Z93.0, Tracheostomy status.

The aftercare Z category/codes: Z42, Z43, Z44, Z45, Z46, Z47, Z48, Z49 and Z51

FOLLOW-UP
The follow-up codes are used to explain continuing surveillance following completed treatment of a disease, condition, or injury. *Refer to categories Z08 and Z09.*

DONOR
Refer to the *ICD-10-CM* manual.

COUNSELING
Counseling Z codes are used when a patient or family member receives assistance in the aftermath of an illness or injury, or when support is required in coping with family or social problems. They are not used in conjunction with a diagnosis code when the counseling component of care is considered integral to standard treatment.

The counseling Z codes/categories: Z30.0-, Z31.5, Z31.6-, Z32.2, Z32.3, Z69, Z70, Z71 and Z76.81

NEWBORNS AND INFANTS
Newborn Z codes/categories: Z05, Z76.1, Z00.1- and Z38

ROUTINE AND ADMINISTRATIVE EXAMINATIONS
Pre-operative examination and pre-procedural laboratory examination Z codes are for use only in those situations when a patient is being cleared for a procedure or surgery and no treatment is given.

Refer to the Z codes/categories for routine and administrative examinations: Z00, Z01, Z02 (except: Z02.9) and Z32.0-

MISCELLANEOUS Z CODES
The miscellaneous Z codes capture a number of other health care encounters that do not fall into one of the other categories. Certain of these codes identify the reason for the encounter; others are for use as additional codes that provide useful information on circumstances that may affect a patient's care and treatment.

PROPHYLACTIC ORGAN REMOVAL
For encounters specifically for prophylactic removal of an organ refer to the full *ICD-10-CM* manual guidelines.

MISCELLANEOUS Z CODES/CATEGORIES:
Z28, (except: Z28.3), Z40, Z41 (except: Z41.9), Z53, Z55, Z56, Z57,Z58, Z59, Z60, Z62, Z63, Z64, Z65, Z72, Z73, Z74 (except: Z74.01), Z75, Z76.0, Z76.3, Z76.4, Z76.5, Z91.1-, Z91.83 and Z91.89

  　Additional Character Required　　3-character code　　　*=New Code　　　***Excludes1***　Not coded here, do not use together
▲=Revised Code　　　***Excludes2***—Not included here

NONSPECIFIC Z CODES

Certain Z codes are so non-specific, or potentially redundant with other codes in the classification, that there can be little justification for their use in the inpatient setting. Their use in the outpatient setting should be limited to those instances when there is no further documentation to permit more precise coding. Otherwise, any sign or symptom or any other reason for visit that is captured in another code should be used.

NONSPECIFIC Z CODES:

Z02.9, Z04.9, Z13.9, Z41.9, Z52.9, Z86.59, Z88.9 and Z92.0

Z CODES THAT MAY ONLY BE PRINCIPAL/FIRST-LISTED DIAGNOSIS

The following Z codes/categories may only be reported as the principal/first-listed diagnosis, except when there are multiple encounters on the same day and the medical records for the encounters are combined: Z00, Z01, Z02, Z03, Z04, Z33.2, Z31.81, Z31.82, Z31.83, Z31.84, Z34, Z38, Z39, Z42, Z51.0, Z51.1-, Z52 (except: Z52.9), Z76.1, Z76.2 and Z99.12.

Note: Z codes represent reasons for encounters. A corresponding procedure code must accompany a Z code if a procedure is performed. Categories Z00–Z99 are provided for occasions when circumstances other than a disease, injury or external cause classifiable to categories A00–Y89 are recorded as 'diagnoses' or 'problems'. This can arise in two main ways:

a) When a person who may or may not be sick encounters the health services for some specific purpose, such as to receive limited care or service for a current condition, to donate an organ or tissue, to receive prophylactic vaccination (immunization), or to discuss a problem which is in itself not a disease or injury.

b) When some circumstance or problem is present which influences the person's health status but is not in itself a current illness or injury.

(Z00–Z13) PERSONS ENCOUNTERING HEALTH SERVICES FOR EXAMINATIONS

Note: Nonspecific abnormal findings disclosed at the time of these examinations are classified to categories R70–R94.

Excludes1: examinations related to pregnancy and reproduction (Z30–Z36, Z39.-) Codes in categories Z00–Z04 "may only be reported as the principal/first-listed diagnosis, except when there are multiple encounters on the same day and the medical records for the encounters are combined."

Z00 ENCOUNTER FOR GENERAL EXAMINATION WITHOUT COMPLAINT, SUSPECTED OR REPORTED DIAGNOSIS
`4th`

GUIDELINES

The codes are not to be used if the examination is for diagnosis of a suspected condition or for treatment purposes. In such cases the diagnosis code is used. During a routine exam, should a diagnosis or condition be discovered, it should be coded as an additional code. Pre-existing and chronic conditions and history codes may also be included as additional codes as long as the examination is for administrative purposes and not focused on any particular condition.

Some of the codes for routine health examinations distinguish between "with" and "without" abnormal findings. Code assignment depends on the information that is known at the time the encounter is being coded. For example, if no abnormal findings were found during the examination, but the encounter is being coded before test results are back, it is acceptable to assign the code for "without abnormal findings." When assigning a code for "with abnormal findings," additional code(s) should be assigned to identify the specific abnormal finding(s).

Excludes1: encounter for examination for administrative purposes (Z02.-)
Excludes2: encounter for pre-procedural examinations (Z01.81-) special screening examinations (Z11–Z13)

Z00.0 Encounter for general adult medical examination;
`5th` Encounter for adult periodic examination (annual) (physical) and any associated laboratory and radiologic examinations
   Excludes1: encounter for examination of sign or symptom— code to sign or symptom
   general health check-up of infant or child (Z00.12.-)
   Z00.00 without abnormal findings
      Encounter for adult health check-up NOS
   Z00.01 with abnormal findings
      Use additional code to identify abnormal findings

Z00.1 Encounter for newborn, infant and child health examinations
`5th`   **Z00.11 Newborn health examination.**
`6th`   *Refer to Chapter 16 for guidelines.*
    Health check for child under 29 days old
    Use additional code to identify any abnormal findings
    Excludes1: health check for child over 28 days old (Z00.12-)
    Z00.110 Health examination for newborn; under 8 days old
       Health check for newborn under 8 days old
    Z00.111 8 to 28 days old
       Health check for newborn 8 to 28 days old
       Newborn weight check

  Z00.12 Encounter for routine child health examination;
`6th`   Encounter for development testing of infant or child
       Health check (routine) for child over 28 days old
       Excludes1: health check for child under 29 days old (Z00.11-)
    health supervision of foundling or other healthy infant or child (Z76.1–Z76.2)
    newborn health examination (Z00.11-)

> *Tip: An abnormal finding can be defined as an acute illness/injury/finding, unstable chronic illness or abnormal screen*

    Z00.121 with abnormal findings
       Use additional code to identify abnormal findings
    Z00.129 without abnormal findings
       Encounter for routine child health examination NOS

Z00.2 Encounter for examination for period of rapid growth in childhood
Z00.3 Encounter for examination for adolescent development state
   Encounter for puberty development state

Z01 ENCOUNTER FOR OTHER SPECIAL EXAMINATION WITHOUT COMPLAINT, SUSPECTED OR REPORTED DIAGNOSIS
`4th`

GUIDELINES

The codes are not to be used if the examination is for diagnosis of a suspected condition or for treatment purposes. In such cases the diagnosis code is used. During a routine exam, should a diagnosis or condition be discovered, it should be coded as an additional code. Pre-existing and chronic conditions and history codes may also be included as additional codes as long as the examination is for administrative purposes and not focused on any particular condition.

Some of the codes for routine health examinations distinguish between "with" and "without" abnormal findings. Code assignment depends on the information that is known at the time the encounter is being coded. For example, if no abnormal findings were found during the examination, but the encounter is being coded before test results are back, it is acceptable to assign the code for "without abnormal findings." When assigning a code for "with abnormal findings," additional code(s) should be assigned to identify the specific abnormal finding(s).
Includes: routine examination of specific system
Note: Codes from category Z01 represent the reason for the encounter.
  A separate procedure code is required to identify any examinations or procedures performed
Excludes1: encounter for examination for administrative purposes (Z02.-)
  encounter for examination for suspected conditions, proven not to exist (Z03.-)
  encounter for laboratory and radiologic examinations as a component of general medical examinations (Z00.0-)
  encounter for laboratory, radiologic and imaging examinations for sign(s) and symptom(s)—**code to the sign(s) or symptom(s)**
Excludes2: screening examinations (Z11–Z13)
Z01.0 Encounter for examination of eyes and vision;
`5th` ***Excludes1:*** examination for driving license (Z02.4)
   Z01.00 without abnormal findings
      Encounter for examination of eyes and vision NOS
   Z01.01 with abnormal findings
      Use additional code to identify abnormal findings

  Additional Character Required   3-character code   •=New Code   ▲=Revised Code   ***Excludes1***—Not coded here, do not use together   ***Excludes2***—Not included here

Z01.1   **Encounter for examination of ears and hearing;**

> **Z01.10**   **Encounter for examination of ears and hearing without abnormal findings**
> Encounter for examination of ears and hearing NOS

> **Z01.11**   **Encounter for examination of ears and hearing with abnormal findings**
>> **Z01.110**   **Encounter for hearing examination following failed hearing screening**
>> **Z01.118**   **Encounter for examination of ears and hearing with other abnormal findings**
>> **Use additional code** to identify abnormal findings

> **Z01.12**   **Encounter for hearing conservation and treatment**

Z01.4   **Encounter for gynecological examination**

> *Excludes2:* pregnancy examination or test (Z32.0-)
> routine examination for contraceptive maintenance (Z30.4-)

> **Z01.41**   **Encounter for routine gynecological examination**
> Encounter for general gynecological examination with or without cervical smear
> Encounter for gynecological examination (general) (routine) NOS
> Encounter for pelvic examination (annual) (periodic)
> **Use additional code:** for screening for human papillomavirus, if applicable, (Z11.51)
> for screening vaginal pap smear, if applicable (Z12.72)
> to identify acquired absence of uterus, if applicable (Z90.71-)
> *Excludes1:* gynecologic examination status (Z08)
> screening cervical pap smear not a part of a routine gynecological examination (Z12.4)

>> **Z01.411**   **Encounter for gynecological examination (general) (routine); with abnormal findings**
>> **Use additional code** to identify abnormal findings
>> **Z01.419**   **without abnormal findings**

> **Z01.42**   **Encounter for cervical smear to confirm findings of recent normal smear following initial abnormal smear**

Z01.8   **Encounter for other specified special examinations**

> **Z01.81**   **Encounter for preprocedural examinations**
> Pre-operative examination and pre-procedural laboratory examination Z codes are for use only in those situations when a patient is being cleared for a procedure or surgery and no treatment is given.
> Encounter for preoperative examinations
> Encounter for radiological and imaging examinations as part of preprocedural examination

>> **Z01.810**   **Encounter for preprocedural; cardiovascular examination**
>> **Z01.811**   **respiratory examination**
>> **Z01.812**   **laboratory examination**
>> Blood and urine tests prior to treatment or procedure
>> **Z01.818**   **Encounter for other preprocedural examination**
>> Encounter for preprocedural examination NOS
>> Encounter for examinations prior to antineoplastic chemotherapy

> **Z01.82**   **Encounter for allergy testing**
> *Excludes1:* encounter for antibody response examination (Z01.84)

Z02   ENCOUNTER FOR ADMINISTRATIVE EXAMINATION

GUIDELINES

The codes are not to be used if the examination is for diagnosis of a suspected condition or for treatment purposes. In such cases the diagnosis code is used. During a routine exam, should a diagnosis or condition be discovered, it should be coded as an additional code. Pre-existing and chronic conditions and history codes may also be included as additional codes as long as the examination is for administrative purposes and not focused on any particular condition.

Some of the codes for routine health examinations distinguish between "with" and "without" abnormal findings. Code assignment depends on the information that is known at the time the encounter is being coded. For

example, if no abnormal findings were found during the examination, but the encounter is being coded before test results are back, it is acceptable to assign the code for "without abnormal findings." When assigning a code for "with abnormal findings," additional code(s) should be assigned to identify the specific abnormal finding(s).

Z02.0   **Encounter for examination for admission to educational institution**
Encounter for examination for admission to preschool (education)
Encounter for examination for re-admission to school following illness or medical treatment

Z02.5   **Encounter for examination for participation in sport**
Excludes1: blood-alcohol and blood-drug test (Z02.83)

Z02.7   **Encounter for issue of medical certificate**
Excludes1: encounter for general medical examination (Z00–Z01, Z02.0–Z02.6, Z02.8– Z02.9)

> **Z02.71**   **Encounter for disability determination**
> Encounter for issue of medical certificate of incapacity or invalidity
> **Z02.79**   **Encounter for issue of other medical certificate**

Z02.8   **Encounter for other administrative examinations**

> **Z02.82**   **Encounter for adoption services**
> **Z02.83**   **Encounter for blood-alcohol and blood-drug test**
> **Use additional code** for findings of alcohol or drugs in blood (R78.-)

> **Z02.89**   **Encounter for other administrative examinations**
> Encounter for examination for admission to prison
> Encounter for examination for admission to summer camp
> Encounter for immigration or naturalization examination
> Encounter for premarital examination
> *Excludes1:* health supervision of foundling or other healthy infant or child (Z76.1–Z76.2)

Z03   ENCOUNTER FOR MEDICAL OBSERVATION FOR SUSPECTED DISEASES AND CONDITIONS RULED OUT

GUIDELINES

This observation category is for use in very limited circumstances when a person is being observed for a suspected condition that is ruled out. The observation codes are not for use if an injury or illness or any signs or symptoms related to the suspected condition are present. In such cases the diagnosis/symptom code is used with the corresponding external cause code. The observation codes are to be used as principal diagnosis only. Additional codes may be used in addition to the observation code but only if they are unrelated to the suspected condition being observed.

This category is to be used when a person without a diagnosis is suspected of having an abnormal condition, without signs or symptoms, which requires study, but after examination and observation, is ruled out. This category is also for use for administrative and legal observation status.

Excludes1: contact with and (suspected) exposures hazardous to health (Z77.-)
newborn observation for suspected condition, ruled out (P00–P04)
person with feared complaint in whom no diagnosis is made (Z71.1)
signs or symptoms under study- code to signs or symptoms

Z03.6   **Encounter for observation for suspected toxic effect from ingested substance ruled out**
Encounter for observation for suspected adverse effect from drug
Encounter for observation for suspected poisoning

Z03.7   **Encounter for suspected maternal and fetal conditions ruled out**

GUIDELINES

Codes from subcategory Z03.7 may either be used as a first-listed or as an additional code assignment depending on the case. They are for use in very limited circumstances on a maternal record when an encounter is for a suspected maternal or fetal condition that is ruled out during that encounter (for example, a maternal or fetal condition may be suspected due to an abnormal test result). These codes should not be used when the condition is confirmed. In those cases, the confirmed condition should be coded. In addition, these codes are not for use if an illness or any signs or symptoms related to the suspected condition or problem are present. In such cases the diagnosis/symptom code is used.

Additional codes may be used in addition to the code from subcategory Z03.7, but only if they are unrelated to the suspected condition being evaluated. Codes from subcategory Z03.7 may

---

not be used for encounters for antenatal screening of mother. For encounters for suspected fetal condition that are inconclusive following testing and evaluation, assign the appropriate code from category O35, O36, O40 or O41.

Encounter for suspected maternal and fetal conditions not found

Excludes1: known or suspected fetal anomalies affecting management of mother, not ruled out (O26.-, O35.-, O36.-, O40.-, O41.-)

Z03.73   **Encounter for suspected; fetal anomaly ruled out**

Z03.74   **problem with fetal growth ruled out**

Z03.79   **maternal and fetal conditions ruled out**

Z03.8   **Encounter for observation for other suspected diseases and conditions ruled out**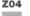

    Z03.81   **Encounter for observation for suspected exposure to; biological agents ruled out**

        Z03.810   **anthrax ruled out**

        Z03.818   **other biological agents ruled out**

    Z03.89   **Encounter for observation for other suspected diseases and conditions ruled out**

Z04   ENCOUNTER FOR EXAMINATION AND OBSERVATION FOR OTHER REASONS

GUIDELINES

This observation category (excludes Z04.9) is for use in very limited circumstances when a person is being observed for a suspected condition that is ruled out. The observation codes are not for use if an injury or illness or any signs or symptoms related to the suspected condition are present. In such cases the diagnosis/symptom code is used with the corresponding external cause code. The observation codes are to be used as principal diagnosis only. Additional codes may be used in addition to the observation code but only if they are unrelated to the suspected condition being observed.

Includes: encounter for examination for medicolegal reasons

This category is to be used when a person without a diagnosis is suspected of having an abnormal condition, without signs or symptoms, which requires study, but after examination and observation, is ruled out.

This category is also for use for administrative and legal observation status.

Z04.1   **Encounter for examination and observation following; transport accident**

Excludes1: encounter for examination and observation following work accident (Z04.2)

Z04.2   **work accident**

Z04.3   **other accident**

Z04.4   **Encounter for examination and observation following alleged rape**

Encounter for examination and observation of victim following alleged rape

Encounter for examination and observation of victim following alleged sexual abuse

    Z04.42   **Encounter for examination and observation following alleged child rape**

Suspected child rape, ruled out

Suspected child sexual abuse, ruled out

Z04.7   **Encounter for examination and observation following alleged; physical abuse**

    Z04.72   **child physical abuse**

Suspected child physical abuse, ruled out

Excludes1: confirmed case of child physical abuse (T74.-)

encounter for examination and observation following alleged child sexual abuse (Z04.42)

suspected case of child physical abuse, not ruled out (T76.-)

Z04.8   **Encounter for examination and observation for other specified reasons**

Encounter for examination and observation for request for expert evidence

Z04.9   **Encounter for examination and observation for unspecified reason**

Code is a nonspecific Z code, refer to Chapter 21 for guidelines.

Z05   ENCOUNTER FOR OBSERVATION AND EVALUATION OF NEWBORN FOR SUSPECTED DISEASES AND CONDITIONS RULED OUT

This category is to be used for newborns, within the neonatal period (the first 28 days of life), who are suspected of having an abnormal condition but without signs or symptoms, and which, after examination and observation, is ruled out.

Excludes2: newborn observation for suspected condition, related to exposure from the mother or birth process (P00–P04)

- **Z05.0**   **Observation and evaluation of newborn for suspected cardiac condition ruled out**

- **Z05.1**   **Observation and evaluation of newborn for suspected infectious condition ruled out**

- **Z05.2**   **Observation and evaluation of newborn for suspected neurological condition ruled out**

- **Z05.3**   **Observation and evaluation of newborn for suspected respiratory condition ruled out**

- **Z05.4**   **Observation and evaluation of newborn for suspected genetic, metabolic or immunologic condition ruled out**

    - **Z05.41**   **Observation and evaluation of newborn for suspected genetic condition ruled out**

    - **Z05.42**   **Observation and evaluation of newborn for suspected metabolic condition ruled out**

    - **Z05.43**   **Observation and evaluation of newborn for suspected immunologic condition ruled out**

- **Z05.5**   **Observation and evaluation of newborn for suspected gastrointestinal condition ruled out**

- **Z05.6**   **Observation and evaluation of newborn for suspected genitourinary condition ruled out**

- **Z05.7**   **Observation and evaluation of newborn for suspected skin and subcutaneous tissue or musculoskeletal condition ruled out**

    - **Z05.71**   **Observation and evaluation of newborn for suspected skin and subcutaneous tissue condition ruled out**

    - **Z05.72**   **Observation and evaluation of newborn for suspected musculoskeletal condition ruled out**

    - **Z05.73**   **Observation and evaluation of newborn for suspected connective tissue condition ruled out**

- **Z05.8**   **Observation and evaluation of newborn for other specified suspected condition ruled out**

- **Z05.9**   **Observation and evaluation of newborn for unspecified suspected condition ruled out**

Z08   ENCOUNTER FOR FOLLOW-UP EXAMINATION AFTER COMPLETED TREATMENT FOR MALIGNANT NEOPLASM

GUIDELINES

The follow-up codes are used to explain continuing surveillance following completed treatment of a disease, condition, or injury. They imply that the condition has been fully treated and no longer exists. They should not be confused with aftercare codes, or injury codes with a 7th character for subsequent encounter, that explain ongoing care of a healing condition or its sequelae. Follow-up codes may be used in conjunction with history codes to provide the full picture of the healed condition and its treatment. The follow-up code is sequenced first, followed by the history code.

A follow-up code may be used to explain multiple visits. Should a condition be found to have recurred on the follow-up visit, then the diagnosis code for the condition should be assigned in place of the follow-up code.

Medical surveillance following completed treatment

Use additional code to identify any acquired absence of organs (Z90.-)

Use additional code to identify the personal history of malignant neoplasm (Z85.-)

Excludes1: aftercare following medical care (Z43–Z49, Z51)

Z09   ENCOUNTER FOR FOLLOW-UP EXAMINATION AFTER COMPLETED TREATMENT FOR CONDITIONS OTHER THAN MALIGNANT NEOPLASM

GUIDELINES

The follow-up codes are used to explain continuing surveillance following completed treatment of a disease, condition, or injury. They imply that the condition has been fully treated and no longer exists. They should not be confused with aftercare codes, or injury codes with a 7th character for subsequent encounter, that explain ongoing care of a healing condition

---

or its sequelae. Follow-up codes may be used in conjunction with history codes to provide the full picture of the healed condition and its treatment. The follow-up code is sequenced first, followed by the history code.

A follow-up code may be used to explain multiple visits. Should a condition be found to have recurred on the follow-up visit, then the diagnosis code for the condition should be assigned in place of the follow-up code.

Medical surveillance following completed treatment

Use additional code to identify any applicable history of disease code (Z86.-. Z87.-)

Excludes1: aftercare following medical care (Z43–Z49, Z51)
    surveillance of contraception (Z30.4-)
    surveillance of prosthetic and other medical devices (Z44–Z46)

Z11 ENCOUNTER FOR SCREENING FOR INFECTIOUS AND PARASITIC DISEASES
4th

GUIDELINES

Screening is the testing for disease or disease precursors in seemingly well individuals so that early detection and treatment can be provided for those who test positive for the disease (e.g., screening mammogram).

The testing of a person to rule out or confirm a suspected diagnosis because the patient has some sign or symptom is a diagnostic examination, not a screening. In these cases, the sign or symptom is used to explain the reason for the test.

A screening code may be a first-listed code if the reason for the visit is specifically the screening exam. It may also be used as an additional code if the screening is done during an office visit for other health problems. A screening code is not necessary if the screening is inherent to a routine examination, such as a pap smear done during a routine pelvic examination. Should a condition be discovered during the screening then the code for the condition may be assigned as an additional diagnosis.

The Z code indicates that a screening exam is planned. A procedure code is required to confirm that the screening was performed.

Excludes1: encounter for diagnostic examination-code to sign or symptom

Z11.0 Encounter for screening for; intestinal infectious diseases
Z11.1 respiratory tuberculosis
Z11.2 other bacterial diseases
Z11.3 infections with a predominantly sexual mode of transmission
    Excludes2: encounter for screening for HIV (Z11.4)
    encounter for screening for human papillomavirus (Z11.51)
Z11.4 HIV
Z11.5 Encounter for screening for; other viral diseases
5th
    Excludes2: encounter for screening for viral intestinal disease (Z11.0)
    Z11.51 human papillomavirus (HPV)
    Z11.59 other viral diseases
Z11.6 Encounter for screening for other protozoal diseases and helminthiases
    Excludes2: encounter for screening for protozoal intestinal disease (Z11.0)
Z11.8 Encounter for screening for other infectious and parasitic diseases
    Encounter for screening for chlamydia or rickettsial or spirochetal or mycoses
Z11.9 Encounter for screening for infectious and parasitic diseases, unspecified

Z12 ENCOUNTER FOR SCREENING FOR MALIGNANT NEOPLASMS
4th

GUIDELINES

Screening is the testing for disease or disease precursors in seemingly well individuals so that early detection and treatment can be provided for those who test positive for the disease (e.g., screening mammogram).

The testing of a person to rule out or confirm a suspected diagnosis because the patient has some sign or symptom is a diagnostic examination. In these cases, the sign or symptom is used to explain the reason for the test.

A screening code may be a first-listed code if the reason for the visit is specifically the screening exam. It may also be used as an additional code if the screening is done during an office visit for other health problems. A screening code is not necessary if the screening is inherent to a routine examination, such as a pap smear done during a routine pelvic

examination. Should a condition be discovered during the screening then the code for the condition may be assigned as an additional diagnosis.

The Z code indicates that a screening exam is planned. A procedure code is required to confirm that the screening was performed.

Use additional code to identify any family history of malignant neoplasm (Z80.-)

Excludes1: encounter for diagnostic examination-code to sign or symptom
Z12.3 Encounter for screening for malignant neoplasm of breast
5th
    Z12.31 Encounter for screening mammogram for malignant neoplasm of breast
      Excludes1: inconclusive mammogram (R92.2)
    Z12.39 Encounter for other screening for malignant neoplasm of breast
Z12.8 Encounter for screening for malignant neoplasm of; other sites
5th
    Z12.82 nervous system
    Z12.89 other sites
Z12.9 Encounter for screening for malignant neoplasm, site unspecified

Z13 ENCOUNTER FOR SCREENING FOR OTHER DISEASES AND DISORDERS
4th

GUIDELINES

Screening is the testing for disease or disease precursors in seemingly well individuals so that early detection and treatment can be provided for those who test positive for the disease (e.g., screening mammogram).

The testing of a person to rule out or confirm a suspected diagnosis because the patient has some sign or symptom is a diagnostic examination, not a screening. In these cases, the sign or symptom is used to explain the reason for the test.

A screening code may be a first-listed code if the reason for the visit is specifically the screening exam. It may also be used as an additional code if the screening is done during an office visit for other health problems. A screening code is not necessary if the screening is inherent to a routine examination, such as a pap smear done during a routine pelvic examination. Should a condition be discovered during the screening then the code for the condition may be assigned as an additional diagnosis.

The Z code indicates that a screening exam is planned. A procedure code is required to confirm that the screening was performed. Excludes Z13.9.

Excludes1: encounter for diagnostic examination-code to sign or symptom
Z13.0 Encounter for screening for; diseases of the blood and blood-forming organs and certain disorders involving the immune mechanism
Z13.1 DM
Z13.2 nutritional, metabolic and other endocrine disorders
5th
    Z13.21 nutritional disorder
    Z13.22 metabolic disorder
6th
      Z13.220 lipoid disorders
       Encounter for screening for cholesterol level or hypercholesterolemia or hyperlipidemia
      Z13.228 other metabolic disorders
    Z13.29 other suspected endocrine disorder
      Excludes1: encounter for screening for DM (Z13.1)
Z13.4 certain developmental disorders in childhood
    Encounter for screening for developmental handicaps in early childhood
    Excludes1: routine development testing of infant or child (Z00.1-)
Z13.5 eye and ear disorders
    Excludes2: encounter for general hearing examination (Z01.1-)
    encounter for general vision examination (Z01.0-)
Z13.6 cardiovascular disorders
Z13.7 genetic and chromosomal anomalies
5th
    Excludes1: genetic testing for procreative management (Z31.4-)
    Z13.71 Encounter for nonprocreative screening for genetic disease carrier status
    Z13.79 Encounter for other screening for genetic and chromosomal anomalies
Z13.8 Encounter for screening for; other specified diseases and disorders
5th
    Excludes2: screening for malignant neoplasms (Z12.-)
    Z13.81 digestive system disorders
6th
      Z13.810 upper gastrointestinal disorder

  4th 5th 6th 7th Additional Character Required   3-character code

•=New Code
▲=Revised Code

Excludes1 Not coded here, do not use together
Excludes2—Not included here

CHAPTER 21. FACTORS INFLUENCING HEALTH STATUS AND CONTACT WITH HEALTH SERVICES   (Z13.811–Z20.6)

Z13.811   **lower gastrointestinal disorder**
     Excludes1: encounter for screening for intestinal infectious disease (Z11.0)

Z13.818   **other digestive system disorders**

Z13.82   **Encounter for screening for musculoskeletal disorder**

 Z13.828   **other musculoskeletal disorder**

Z13.83   **respiratory disorder NEC**
     Excludes1: encounter for screening for respiratory tuberculosis (Z11.1)

Z13.84   **dental disorders**

Z13.85   **Encounter for screening for nervous system disorders**

 Z13.850   **traumatic brain injury**

Z13.858   **other nervous system disorders**

Z13.88   **disorder due to exposure to contaminants**
     Excludes1: those exposed to contaminants without suspected disorders (Z57.-, Z77.-)

Z13.89   **other disorder**
     Encounter for screening for genitourinary disorders

Z13.9   **Encounter for screening, unspecified**
     Code is a nonspecific Z code, refer to Chapter 21 for guidelines.

(Z14–Z15) GENETIC CARRIER AND GENETIC SUSCEPTIBILITY TO DISEASE

Z14   **GENETIC CARRIER**

 Genetic carrier status indicates that a person carries a gene, associated with a particular disease, which may be passed to offspring who may develop that disease. The person does not have the disease and is not at risk of developing the disease. Refer to Chapter 21 for status guidelines.

Z14.0   **Hemophilia A carrier**

 Z14.01   **Asymptomatic hemophilia A carrier**

Z14.02   **Symptomatic hemophilia A carrier**

Z14.1   **Cystic fibrosis carrier**

Z14.8   **Genetic carrier of other disease**

(Z16) RESISTANCE TO ANTIMICROBIAL DRUGS

Z16   **RESISTANCE TO ANTIMICROBIAL DRUGS**

 This code indicates that a patient has a condition that is resistant to antimicrobial drug treatment. Sequence the infection code first. This is a status category, refer to Chapter 21 for status guidelines.
Note: The codes in this category are provided for use as additional codes to identify the resistance and non-responsiveness of a condition to antimicrobial drugs.
Code first the infection
Excludes1: MRSA infection (A49.02)
     MRSA infection in diseases classified elsewhere (B95.62)
     MRSA pneumonia (J15.212)
     Sepsis due to MRSA (A41.02)

Z16.1   **Resistance to beta lactam antibiotics**

 Z16.10   **Resistance to unspecified beta lactam antibiotics**

Z16.11   **Resistance to penicillins**
     Resistance to amoxicillin or ampicillin

Z16.12   **Extended spectrum beta lactamase (ESBL) resistance**

Z16.19   **other specified beta lactam antibiotics**
     Resistance to cephalosporins

Z16.2   **Resistance to; other antibiotics**

 Z16.20   **unspecified antibiotic**
     Resistance to antibiotics NOS

Z16.21   **vancomycin**

Z16.22   **vancomycin related antibiotics**

Z16.23   **quinolones and fluoroquinolones**

Z16.24   **multiple antibiotics**

Z16.29   **other single specified antibiotic**
     Resistance to aminoglycosides or macrolides or sulfonamides or tetracyclines

Z16.3   **Resistance to; other antimicrobial drugs**

 Excludes1: resistance to antibiotics (Z16.1-, Z16.2-)

Z16.30   **unspecified antimicrobial drugs**
     Drug resistance NOS

Z16.32   **antifungal drug(s)**

Z16.33   **antiviral drug(s)**

 Z16.341   **single antimycobacterial drug**
     Resistance to antimycobacterial drug NOS

Z16.342   **multiple antimycobacterial drugs**

Z16.39   **other specified antimicrobial drug**

(Z18) RETAINED FB FRAGMENTS

Z18   **RETAINED FB FRAGMENTS**

 This is a status category, refer to Chapter 21 for status guidelines.
Includes: embedded fragment (status)
     embedded splinter (status)
     retained FB status
Excludes1: artificial joint prosthesis status (Z96.6-)
     FB accidentally left during a procedure (T81.5-)
     FB entering through orifice (T15–T19)
     in situ cardiac device (Z95.-)
     organ or tissue replaced by means other than transplant (Z96.-, Z97.-)
     organ or tissue replaced by transplant (Z94.-)
     personal history of retained FB fully removed Z87.821
     superficial FB (non-embedded splinter)—code to superficial FB, by site

Z18.1   **Retained metal fragments;**

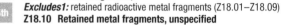 *Excludes1:* retained radioactive metal fragments (Z18.01–Z18.09)

Z18.10   **Retained metal fragments, unspecified**
     Retained metal fragment NOS

Z18.11   **Retained magnetic metal fragments**

Z18.12   **Retained nonmagnetic metal fragments**

Z18.2   **Retained plastic fragments**
     Acrylics fragments
     Diethylhexylphthalates fragments
     Isocyanate fragments

Z18.3   **Retained organic fragments**

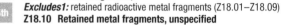 **Z18.31**   **Retained animal quills or spines**

Z18.32   **Retained tooth**

Z18.33   **Retained wood fragments**

Z18.39   **Other retained organic fragments**

Z18.8   **Other specified retained FB**

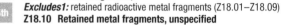 **Z18.81**   **Retained glass fragments**

Z18.83   **Retained stone or crystalline fragments**
     Retained concrete or cement fragments

Z18.89   **Other specified retained FB fragments**

Z18.9   **Retained FB fragments, unspecified material**

(Z20–Z29) PERSONS WITH POTENTIAL HEALTH HAZARDS RELATED TO COMMUNICABLE DISEASES

GUIDELINES

Category Z20 indicates contact with, and suspected exposure to, communicable diseases. These codes are for patients who do not show any sign or symptom of a disease but are suspected to have been exposed to it by close personal contact with an infected individual or are in an area where a disease is epidemic.

     Contact/exposure codes may be used as a first-listed code to explain an encounter for testing, or, more commonly, as a secondary code to identify a potential risk.

Z20   **CONTACT WITH AND (SUSPECTED) EXPOSURE TO COMMUNICABLE DISEASES**

 Excludes1: carrier of infectious disease (Z22.-)
     diagnosed current infectious or parasitic disease -see Alphabetic Index
Excludes2: personal history of infectious and parasitic diseases (Z86.1-)

Z20.0   **Contact with and (suspected) exposure to intestinal infectious diseases;**

 Z20.01   **due to E. coli**

Z20.09   **other intestinal infectious diseases**

Z20.1   **Contact with and (suspected) exposure to; tuberculosis**

Z20.2   **infections with a predominantly sexual mode of transmission**

Z20.3   **rabies**

Z20.4   **rubella**

Z20.5   **viral hepatitis**

Z20.6   **HIV**
     Excludes1: asymptomatic HIV
     HIV infection status (Z21)

   Additional Character Required   3-character code   •=New Code   *Excludes1*—Not coded here, do not use together
    ▲=Revised Code   *Excludes2*—Not included here

Z20.7   pediculosis, acariasis and other infestations
Z20.8   Contact with and (suspected) exposure to; other communicable diseases
    [5th]
Z20.81   other bacterial communicable diseases
    [6th]
Z20.810   anthrax
Z20.811   meningococcus
Z20.818   other bacterial communicable diseases
Z20.82   Contact with and (suspected) exposure to; other viral communicable diseases
    [6th]
Z20.820   varicella
Z20.828   other viral communicable diseases
Z20.89   other communicable diseases
Z20.9   unspecified communicable disease

Z21 ASYMPTOMATIC HIV INFECTION STATUS

This code indicates that a patient has tested positive for HIV but has manifested no signs or symptoms of the disease. This is a status code, refer to Chapter 21 for status guidelines.
HIV positive NOS
Code first HIV disease complicating pregnancy, childbirth and the puerperium, if applicable (O98.7-)
Excludes1: acquired immunodeficiency syndrome (B20)
    contact with HIV (Z20.6)
    exposure to HIV (Z20.6)
    HIV disease (B20)
    inconclusive laboratory evidence of HIV (R75)

Z22 CARRIER OF INFECTIOUS DISEASE

Carrier status indicates that a person harbors the specific organisms of a disease without manifest symptoms and is capable of transmitting the infection. This is a status category, refer to Chapter 21 for status guidelines.
Includes: colonization status
    suspected carrier
Excludes2: carrier of viral hepatitis (B18.-)
Z22.1   Carrier of other intestinal infectious diseases
Z22.2   Carrier of diphtheria
Z22.3   Carrier of other specified bacterial diseases
    [5th]
Z22.31   Carrier of bacterial disease due to; meningococci
Z22.32   Carrier of bacterial disease due to staphylococci
    [6th]
Z22.321   Carrier or suspected carrier of MSSA
      MSSA colonization
Z22.322   Carrier or suspected carrier of MRSA
      MRSA colonization
Z22.33   Carrier of bacterial disease due to streptococci
    [6th]
Z22.330   Carrier of Group B streptococcus
      Excludes1: carrier of streptococcus group B (GBS) complicating pregnancy, childbirth and the puerperium (O99.82-)
Z22.338   Carrier of other streptococcus
Z22.39   Carrier of other specified bacterial diseases
Z22.4   Carrier of infections with a predominantly sexual mode of transmission
▲Z22.5   Carrier of viral hepatitis
Z22.6   Carrier of human T-lymphotropic virus type-1 [HTLV-1] infection
Z22.8   Carrier of other infectious diseases
Z22.9   Carrier of infectious disease, unspecified

Z23 ENCOUNTER FOR IMMUNIZATION

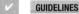

GUIDELINES

Code Z23 is for encounters for inoculations and vaccinations. It indicates that a patient is being seen to receive a prophylactic inoculation against a disease. Procedure
Tip: Z23 should be reported for every vaccine encounter
codes are required to identify the actual administration of the injection and the type(s) of immunizations given. Code Z23 may be used as a secondary code if the inoculation is given as a routine part of preventive health care, such as a well-baby visit.
Code first any routine childhood examination
Note: procedure codes are required to identify the types of immunizations given

Z28 IMMUNIZATION NOT CARRIED OUT AND UNDERIMMUNIZATION STATUS

Includes: vaccination not carried out
Z28.0   Immunization not carried out due to; contraindication
    [5th]
Z28.01   acute illness of patient
Z28.02   chronic illness or condition of patient
Z28.03   immune compromised state of patient
Z28.04   patient allergy to vaccine or component
Z28.09   other contraindication
Z28.1   Immunization not carried out due to patient decision for reasons of belief or group pressure
    Immunization not carried out because of religious belief
Z28.2   Immunization not carried out due to; patient decision for other and unspecified reason
    [5th]
Z28.20   patient decision for unspecified reason
Z28.21   patient refusal
Z28.29   patient decision for other reason
Z28.3   Underimmunization status
    This is a status code, refer to Chapter 21 for status guidelines.
    Delinquent immunization status
    Lapsed immunization schedule status
Z28.8   Immunization not carried out; for other reason
    [5th]
Z28.81   due to patient having had the disease
Z28.82   because of caregiver refusal
      Immunization not carried out because of parental or guardian refusal
      Excludes1: immunization not carried out because of caregiver refusal because of religious belief (Z28.1)
Z28.89   for other reason
Z28.9   Immunization not carried out for unspecified reason

Z29 ENCOUNTER FOR PROPHYLACTIC MEASURES

Excludes 1: desensitization to allergens (Z51.6)
    prophylactic surgery (Z40.-)
●Z29.1   Encounter for prophylactic therapy
    Encounter for administration of immunoglobulin
    [5th]
    ●Z29.11   Encounter for prophylactic immunotherapy for respiratory syncytial virus (RSV)
    ●Z29.12   Encounter for prophylactic antivenin
    ●Z29.13   Encounter for prophylactic Rho(D) immune globulin
    ●Z29.14   Encounter for prophylactic rabies immune globin
●Z29.3   Encounter for prophylactic fluoride administration
●Z29.8   Encounter for other specified prophylactic measures
●Z29.9   Encounter for prophylactic measures, unspecified

(Z30–Z39) PERSONS ENCOUNTERING HEALTH SERVICES IN CIRCUMSTANCES RELATED TO REPRODUCTION

Z30 ENCOUNTER FOR CONTRACEPTIVE MANAGEMENT

Z30.0   Encounter for general counseling and advice on contraception
    Refer to Chapter 21 for guidelines on counseling.
    [5th]
Z30.01   Encounter for initial prescription of; contraceptives
    [6th]
    Excludes1: encounter for surveillance of contraceptives (Z30.4-)
Z30.011   contraceptive pills
Z30.012   emergency contraception
    Encounter for postcoital contraception
Z30.013   injectable contraceptive
Z30.014   intrauterine contraceptive device
    Excludes1: encounter for insertion of intrauterine contraceptive device (Z30.430, Z30.432)
●Z30.015   vaginal ring hormonal contraceptive
●Z30.016   transdermal patch hormonal contraceptive device
●Z30.017   implantable subdermal contraceptive
Z30.018   other contraceptives
    Encounter for initial prescription of barrier contraception or diaphragm
Z30.019   contraceptives, unspecified
Z30.02   Counseling and instruction in natural family planning to avoid pregnancy

---

Z30.09 **Encounter for other general counseling and advice on contraception**
Encounter for family planning advice NOS

Z30.4 **Encounter for surveillance of contraceptives**

5th **Z30.40** **Encounter for surveillance of unspecified**

Z30.41 **Encounter for surveillance of contraceptive pills**
Encounter for repeat prescription for contraceptive pill

Z30.42 **Encounter for surveillance of injectable contraceptive**

Z30.43 **Encounter for surveillance of intrauterine**
6th contraceptive device

Z30.430 **Encounter for insertion of intrauterine contraceptive device**

Z30.431 **Encounter for routine checking of intrauterine contraceptive device**

Z30.432 **Encounter for removal of intrauterine contraceptive device**

Z30.433 **Encounter for removal and reinsertion of intrauterine contraceptive device**
replacement of intrauterine contraceptive device

•**Z30.44** **Encounter for surveillance of vaginal ring hormonal contraceptive device**

•**Z30.45** **Encounter for surveillance of transdermal patch hormonal contraceptive device**

•**Z30.46** **Encounter for surveillance of implantable subdermal contraceptive**
Encounter for checking, reinsertion or removal of implantable subdermal contraceptive

Z30.49 **Encounter for surveillance of other contraceptives**
Encounter for surveillance of barrier contraception
Encounter for surveillance of diaphragm

Z30.8 **Encounter for other contraceptive management**
Encounter for postvasectomy sperm count
Encounter for routine examination for contraceptive maintenance
Excludes1: sperm count following sterilization reversal (Z31.42)
　　　sperm count for fertility testing (Z31.41)

Z30.9 **Encounter for contraceptive management, unspecified**

Z31 **ENCOUNTER FOR PROCREATIVE MANAGEMENT**
4th ***Excludes1:*** complications associated with artificial fertilization (N98.-)
　　female infertility (N97.-)
　　male infertility (N46.-)

Z31.5 **Encounter for genetic counseling**
Refer to Chapter 21 for guidelines on counseling.

Z31.6 **Encounter for general counseling and advice on procreation**
5th *Refer to Chapter 21 for guidelines on counseling.*

Z31.69 **Encounter for other general counseling and advice on procreation**

Z32 **ENCOUNTER FOR PREGNANCY TEST AND CHILDBIRTH**
4th **AND CHILDCARE INSTRUCTION**

Z32.0 **Encounter for pregnancy test**

5th **GUIDELINES**

The codes are not to be used if the examination is for diagnosis of a suspected condition or for treatment purposes. In such cases the diagnosis code is used. During a routine exam, should a diagnosis or condition be discovered, it should be coded as an additional code. Pre-existing and chronic conditions and history codes may also be included as additional codes as long as the examination is for administrative purposes and not focused on any particular condition.

　Some of the codes for routine health examinations distinguish between "with" and "without" abnormal findings. Code assignment depends on the information that is known at the time the encounter is being coded. For example, if no abnormal findings were found during the examination, but the encounter is being coded before test results are back, it is acceptable to assign the code for "without abnormal findings." When assigning a code for "with abnormal findings," additional code(s) should be assigned to identify the specific abnormal finding(s).

Z32.00 **Encounter for pregnancy test, result unknown**
Encounter for pregnancy test NOS

Z32.01 **Encounter for pregnancy test, result positive**

Z32.02 **Encounter for pregnancy test, result negative**

Z33 **PREGNANT STATE**
4th **Z33.1** **Pregnant state, incidental**
This is a status code, refer to Chapter 21 for status guidelines.
Pregnant state NOS
Excludes1: complications of pregnancy (O00–O9A)

Z38 **LIVEBORN INFANTS ACCORDING TO PLACE OF BIRTH**
4th **AND TYPE OF DELIVERY**

GUIDELINES

When coding the birth episode in a newborn record, assign a code from category Z38, Liveborn infants according to place of birth and type of delivery, as the principal diagnosis. A code from category Z38 is assigned only once, to a newborn at the time of birth and throughout the initial stay at the birth hospital. If a newborn is transferred to another institution, a code from category Z38 should not be used at the receiving hospital.

　A code from category Z38 is used only on the newborn record, not on the mother's record. Codes in category Z38 "may only be reported as the principal/first-listed diagnosis, except when there are multiple encounters on the same day and the medical records for the encounters are combined." Refer to Chapter 16 for further guidelines.

Z38.0 **Single liveborn infant, born in hospital**
5th Single liveborn infant, born in birthing center or other health care facility

Z38.00 **Single liveborn infant, delivered vaginally**

Z38.01 **Single liveborn infant, delivered by cesarean**

Z38.1 **Single liveborn infant, born outside hospital**

Z38.2 **Single liveborn infant, unspecified as to place of birth**
Single liveborn infant NOS

Z38.3 **Twin liveborn infant, born in hospital**
5th **Z38.30** **Twin liveborn infant, delivered vaginally**

Z38.31 **Twin liveborn infant, delivered by cesarean**

Z38.4 **Twin liveborn infant, born outside hospital**

Z38.5 **Twin liveborn infant, unspecified as to place of birth**

Z38.6 **Other multiple liveborn infant, born in hospital**

5th **Z38.61** **Triplet liveborn infant, delivered vaginally**

Z38.62 **Triplet liveborn infant, delivered by cesarean**

Z38.63 **Quadruplet liveborn infant, delivered vaginally**

Z38.64 **Quadruplet liveborn infant, delivered by cesarean**

Z38.65 **Quintuplet liveborn infant, delivered vaginally**

Z38.66 **Quintuplet liveborn infant, delivered by cesarean**

Z38.68 **Other multiple liveborn infant, delivered vaginally**

Z38.69 **Other multiple liveborn infant, delivered by cesarean**

(Z40–Z53) ENCOUNTERS FOR OTHER SPECIFIC HEALTH CARE

Categories Z40–Z53 are intended for use to indicate a reason for care. They may be used for patients who have already been treated for a disease or injury, but who are receiving aftercare or prophylactic care, or care to consolidate the treatment, or to deal with a residual state.

Z41 **ENCOUNTER FOR PROCEDURES FOR PURPOSES OTHER**
4th **THAN REMEDYING HEALTH STATE**

Z41.2 **Encounter for routine and ritual male circumcision**

Z41.8 **Encounter for other procedures for purposes other than remedying health state**

Z43 **ENCOUNTER FOR ATTENTION TO ARTIFICIAL OPENINGS**

4th **GUIDELINES**

Aftercare visit codes cover situations when the initial treatment of a disease has been performed and the patient requires continued care during the healing or recovery phase, or for the long-term consequences of the disease. The aftercare Z code should not be used if treatment is directed at a current, acute disease. The diagnosis code is to be used in these cases.
Refer to Chapter 21 for aftercare guidelines.
Includes: closure of artificial openings
　　passage of sounds or bougies through artificial openings
　　reforming artificial openings
　　removal of catheter from artificial openings
　　toilet or cleansing of artificial openings
Excludes1: artificial opening status only, without need for care (Z93.-)
　　complications of external stoma (J95.0-, K94.-, N99.5-)
Excludes2: fitting and adjustment of prosthetic and other devices (Z44–Z46)

Z43.1 **Encounter for attention to gastrostomy**

4th **5th** **6th** **7th**　Additional Character Required　　✓　3-character code　　•=New Code　　***Excludes1***—Not coded here, do not use together
　▲=Revised Code　　***Excludes2***—Not included here

412　　　PEDIATRIC ICD-10-CM 2017: A MANUAL FOR PROVIDER-BASED CODING

Z48 ENCOUNTER FOR OTHER POSTPROCEDURAL AFTERCARE
4th

GUIDELINES

Aftercare visit codes cover situations when the initial treatment of a disease has been performed and the patient requires continued care during the healing or recovery phase, or for the long-term consequences of the disease. The aftercare Z code should not be used if treatment is directed at a current, acute disease. The diagnosis code is to be used in these cases.
Refer to Chapter 21 for aftercare guidelines
Excludes1: encounter for follow-up examination after completed treatment (Z08–Z09)
Excludes2: encounter for attention to artificial openings (Z43.-)
encounter for fitting and adjustment of prosthetic and other devices (Z44–Z46)

Z48.0 Encounter for; attention to dressings, sutures and drains
5th
    Excludes1: encounter for planned postprocedural wound closure (Z48.1)
    Z48.00 change or removal of nonsurgical wound dressing
         change or removal of wound dressing NOS
    Z48.01 change or removal of surgical wound dressing
    Z48.02 removal of sutures
         removal of staples
    Z48.03 change or removal of drains

Z48.1 planned postprocedural wound closure
    Excludes1: encounter for attention to dressings and sutures (Z48.0-)

Z48.2 Encounter for aftercare following; organ transplant
5th
    Z48.21 heart transplant
    Z48.22 kidney transplant
    Z48.23 liver transplant
    Z48.24 lung transplant
    Z48.28 multiple organ transplant
      6th   **Z48.280 heart-lung transplant**
         Z48.288 multiple organ transplant
    Z48.29 other organ transplant
      6th   **Z48.290 bone marrow transplant**
         Z48.298 other organ transplant

Z48.3 Aftercare following surgery for neoplasm
    Use additional code to identify the neoplasm

Z48.8 Encounter for other specified postprocedural aftercare

Z51 ENCOUNTER FOR OTHER AFTERCARE AND MEDICAL CARE
4th

GUIDELINES

Aftercare visit codes cover situations when the initial treatment of a disease has been performed and the patient requires continued care during the healing or recovery phase, or for the long-term consequences of the disease. The aftercare Z code should not be used if treatment is directed at a current, acute disease. The diagnosis code is to be used in these cases. Refer to Chapter 21 for aftercare guidelines.
Code also condition requiring care
Excludes1: follow-up examination after treatment (Z08–Z09)
Excludes2: follow-up examination for medical surveillance after treatment (Z08–Z09)

Z51.0 Encounter for antineoplastic; radiation therapy
    May only be reported as the principal/first-listed diagnosis, except when there are multiple encounters on the same day and the medical records for the encounters are combined."

Z51.1 chemotherapy and immunotherapy
5th
    Codes Z51.1- may only be reported as the principal/first-listed diagnosis, except when there are multiple encounters on the same day and the medical records for the encounters are combined."
    Excludes2: encounter for chemotherapy and immunotherapy for non-neoplastic condition—code to condition
    Z51.11 chemotherapy
    Z51.12 immunotherapy

Z51.5 Encounter for palliative care
Z51.6 Encounter for desensitization to allergens

Z51.8 Encounter for other specified aftercare
5th
    Excludes1: holiday relief care (Z75.5)
    Z51.81 Encounter for therapeutic drug level monitoring
         Code also any long-term (current) drug therapy (Z79.-)
         Excludes1: encounter for blood-drug test for administrative or medicolegal reasons (Z02.83)
    Z51.89 Encounter for other specified aftercare

Z53 PERSONS ENCOUNTERING HEALTH SERVICES FOR SPECIFIC PROCEDURES AND TREATMENT, NOT CARRIED OUT
4th

Z53.0 Procedure and treatment not carried out because of contraindication
5th
    Z53.01 Procedure and treatment not carried out due to patient smoking
    Z53.09 Procedure and treatment not carried out because of other contraindication

Z53.2 Procedure and treatment not carried out because of patient's decision for other and unspecified reasons
5th
    Z53.20 Procedure and treatment not carried out because of patient's decision for unspecified reasons
    Z53.21 Procedure and treatment not carried out due to patient leaving prior to being seen by healthcare provider
    Z53.29 Procedure and treatment not carried out because of patient's decision for other reasons

• Z53.3 Procedure converted to open procedure
5th
    • Z53.31 Laparoscopic surgical procedure converted to open procedure
    • Z53.32 Thoracoscopic surgical procedure converted to open procedure
    • Z53.33 Arthroscopic surgical procedure converted to open procedure
    • Z53.39 Other specified procedure converted to open procedure

Z53.8 Procedure and treatment not carried out for other reasons
Z53.9 Procedure and treatment not carried out, unspecified reason

(Z55–Z65) PERSONS WITH POTENTIAL HEALTH HAZARDS RELATED TO SOCIOECONOMIC AND PSYCHOSOCIAL CIRCUMSTANCES

Z55 PROBLEMS RELATED TO EDUCATION AND LITERACY
4th
Excludes1: disorders of psychological development (F80–F89)
Z55.0 Illiteracy and low-level literacy
Z55.1 Schooling unavailable and unattainable
Z55.2 Failed school examinations
Z55.3 Underachievement in school
Z55.4 Educational maladjustment and discord with teachers and classmates
Z55.8 Other problems related to education and literacy
    Problems related to inadequate teaching
Z55.9 Problems related to education and literacy, unspecified
    Academic problems NOS

Z59 PROBLEMS RELATED TO HOUSING AND ECONOMIC CIRCUMSTANCES
4th
Excludes2: problems related to upbringing (Z62.-)
Z59.0 Homelessness
Z59.1 Inadequate housing
    Lack of heating
    Restriction of space
    Technical defects in home preventing adequate care
    Unsatisfactory surroundings
    Excludes1: problems related to the natural and physical environment (Z77.1-)
Z59.5 Extreme poverty

Z60 PROBLEMS RELATED TO SOCIAL ENVIRONMENT
4th
Z60.3 Acculturation difficulty
    Problem with migration
    Problem with social transplantation

  Additional Character Required   **3-character code**

•=New Code
▲=Revised Code
Excludes1—Not coded here, do not use together
Excludes2—Not included here

CHAPTER 21. FACTORS INFLUENCING HEALTH STATUS AND CONTACT WITH HEALTH SERVICES   (Z60.4–Z69.010)

Z60.4   **Social exclusion and rejection**
Exclusion and rejection on the basis of personal characteristics, such as unusual physical appearance, illness or behavior
Excludes1: target of adverse discrimination such as for racial or religious reasons (Z60.5)

Z60.5   **Target of (perceived) adverse discrimination and persecution**
Excludes1: social exclusion and rejection (Z60.4)

Z60.8   **Other problems related to social environment**

Z60.9   **Problem related to social environment, unspecified**

Z62   **PROBLEMS RELATED TO UPBRINGING**
Includes: current and past negative life events in childhood
current and past problems of a child related to upbringing
Excludes2: maltreatment syndrome (T74.-)
problems related to housing and economic circumstances (Z59.-)

Z62.0   **Inadequate parental supervision and control**

Z62.1   **Parental overprotection**

Z62.2   **Upbringing away from parents**
Excludes1: problems with boarding school (Z59.3)

> **Z62.21**   **Child in welfare custody**
> Child in care of non-parental family member
> Child in foster care
> *Excludes2:* problem for parent due to child in welfare custody (Z63.5)
>
> **Z62.22**   **Institutional upbringing**
> Child living in orphanage or group home

Z62.8   **Other specified problems related to upbringing**

> **Z62.81**   **Personal history of abuse in childhood**
>
> > **Z62.810**   **Personal history of; physical and sexual abuse in childhood**
> > *Excludes1:* current child physical abuse (T74.12, T76.12)
> > current child sexual abuse (T74.22, T76.22)
> >
> > **Z62.811**   **psychological abuse in childhood**
> > *Excludes1:* current child psychological abuse (T74.32, T76.32)
> >
> > **Z62.812**   **neglect in childhood**
> > *Excludes1:* current child neglect (T74.02, T76.02)
> >
> > **Z62.819**   **unspecified abuse in childhood**
> > *Excludes1:* current child abuse NOS (T74.92, T76.92)
>
> **Z62.82**   **Parent-child conflict**
>
> > **Z62.820**   **Parent-biological child conflict**
> > Parent-child problem NOS
> >
> > **Z62.821**   **Parent-adopted child conflict**
> >
> > **Z62.822**   **Parent-foster child conflict**
>
> **Z62.89**   **Other specified problems related to upbringing**
>
> > **Z62.890**   **Parent-child estrangement NEC**
> >
> > **Z62.891**   **Sibling rivalry**

Z63   **OTHER PROBLEMS RELATED TO PRIMARY SUPPORT GROUP, INCLUDING FAMILY CIRCUMSTANCES**
Excludes2: maltreatment syndrome (T74.-, T76)
parent-child problems (Z62.-)
problems related to negative life events in childhood (Z62.-)
problems related to upbringing (Z62.-)

Z63.3   **Absence of family member**
Excludes1: absence of family member due to disappearance and death (Z63.4)
absence of family member due to separation and divorce (Z63.5)

> **Z63.31**   **Absence of family member due to military deployment**
> Individual or family affected by other family member being on military deployment
> *Excludes1:* family disruption due to return of family member from military deployment (Z63.71)
>
> **Z63.32**   **Other absence of family member**

Z63.4   **Disappearance and death of family member**
Assumed death of family member
Bereavement

Z63.5   **Disruption of family by separation and divorce**

Z63.7   **Other stressful life events affecting family and household**

Z63.71   **Stress on family due to return of family member from military deployment**
Individual or family affected by family member having returned from military deployment (current or past conflict)

Z63.72   **Alcoholism and drug addiction in family**

Z63.79   **Other stressful life events affecting family and household**
Anxiety (normal) about sick person in family
Health problems within family
Ill or disturbed family member
Isolated family

Z63.8   **Other specified problems related to primary support group**
Family discord NOS
Family estrangement NOS
High expressed emotional level within family
Inadequate family support NOS
Inadequate or distorted communication within family

Z63.9   **Problem related to primary support group, unspecified**
Relationship disorder NOS

Z65   **PROBLEMS RELATED TO OTHER PSYCHOSOCIAL CIRCUMSTANCES**

Z65.8   **Other specified problems related to psychosocial circumstances**

Z65.9   **Problem related to unspecified psychosocial circumstances**

(Z66) DO NOT RESUSCITATE STATUS

Z66   **DO NOT RESUSCITATE**
This code may be used when it is documented by the provider that a patient is on do not resuscitate status at any time during the stay. This is a status code, *refer to Chapter 21 for status guidelines.*
DNR status

(Z67) BLOOD TYPE

(Z68) BODY MASS INDEX [BMI]

Z68   **BODY MASS INDEX [BMI]**
This is a status category, refer to Chapter 21 for status guidelines. Kilograms per meters squared
Note: BMI adult codes are for use for persons 21 years of age or older.
BMI pediatric codes are for use for persons 2–20 years of age. These percentiles are based on the growth charts published by the Centers for Disease Control and Prevention (CDC)

Z68.5   **BMI pediatric**

> **Z68.51**   **BMI pediatric, less than 5th percentile for age**
>
> **Z68.52**   **BMI pediatric, 5th percentile to less than 85th percentile for age**
>
> **Z68.53**   **BMI pediatric, 85th percentile to less than 95th percentile for age**
>
> **Z68.54**   **BMI pediatric, greater than or equal to 95th percentile for age**

(Z69–Z76) PERSONS ENCOUNTERING HEALTH SERVICES IN OTHER CIRCUMSTANCES

Z69   **ENCOUNTER FOR MENTAL HEALTH SERVICES FOR VICTIM AND PERPETRATOR OF ABUSE**

GUIDELINES

Counseling Z codes are used when a patient or family member receives assistance in the aftermath of an illness or injury, or when support is required in coping with family or social problems. They are not used in conjunction with a diagnosis code when the counseling component of care is considered integral to standard treatment.
Includes: counseling for victims and perpetrators of abuse

Z69.0   **Encounter for mental health services for child abuse problems**

> **Z69.01**   **Encounter for mental health services for; parental child abuse**
>
> > **Z69.010**   **victim of parental child abuse**

     Additional Character Required   3-character code   •=New Code   *Excludes1*—Not coded here, do not use together
    ▲=Revised Code   *Excludes2*—Not included here

Z69.011   perpetrator of parental child abuse
> *Excludes1:* encounter for mental health services for non-parental child abuse (Z69.02-)

Z69.02   **Encounter for mental health services for; non-parental child abuse**
> Z69.020   victim of non-parental child abuse
> Z69.021   perpetrator of non-parental child abuse

Z69.1   **Encounter for mental health services for; spousal or partner abuse problems**
> Z69.11   victim of spousal or partner abuse
> Z69.12   perpetrator of spousal or partner abuse

Z69.8   **Encounter for mental health services for victim or perpetrator of other abuse**
> Z69.81   **Encounter for mental health services for victim of other abuse**
> Encounter for rape victim counseling
> Z69.82   **Encounter for mental health services for perpetrator of other abuse**

Z71   PERSONS ENCOUNTERING HEALTH SERVICES FOR OTHER COUNSELING AND MEDICAL ADVICE, NEC
Refer to category Z69 for guideline.
Excludes2: contraceptive or procreation counseling (Z30–Z31)
sex counseling (Z70.-)

Z71.0   **Person encountering health services to consult on behalf of another person**
> Person encountering health services to seek advice or treatment for non-attending third party
> *Excludes2:* anxiety (normal) about sick person in family (Z63.7)
> expectant (adoptive) parent(s) pre-birth pediatrician visit (Z76.81)

Z71.3   **Dietary counseling and surveillance**
> **Use additional code** for any associated underlying medical condition
> **Use additional code** to identify body mass index (BMI), if known (Z68.-)

Z71.4   **Alcohol abuse counseling and surveillance**
> **Use additional code** for alcohol abuse or dependence (F10.-)
> Z71.41   **Alcohol abuse counseling and surveillance of alcoholic**
> Z71.42   **Counseling for family member of alcoholic**
> Counseling for significant other, partner, or friend of alcoholic

Z71.6   **Tobacco abuse counseling**
> **Use additional code** for nicotine dependence (F17.-)

Z71.7   **HIV counseling**

Z71.8   **Other specified counseling**
> *Excludes2:* counseling for contraception (Z30.0-)
> counseling for genetics (Z31.5)
> counseling for procreative management (Z31.6-)
> Z71.81   **Spiritual or religious counseling**
> Z71.89   **Other specified counseling**

Z71.9   **Counseling, unspecified**
> Encounter for medical advice NOS

Z72   PROBLEMS RELATED TO LIFESTYLE
Excludes2: problems related to life-management difficulty (Z73.-)
problems related to socioeconomic and psychosocial circumstances (Z55–Z65)

Z72.0   **Tobacco use**
> Tobacco use NOS
> *Excludes1:* history of tobacco dependence (Z87.891)
> nicotine dependence (F17.2-)
> tobacco dependence (F17.2-)
> tobacco use during pregnancy (O99.33-)

Z72.3   **Lack of physical exercise**

Z72.4   **Inappropriate diet and eating habits**
> *Excludes1:* behavioral eating disorders of infancy or childhood (F98.2.–F98.3)
> eating disorders (F50.-)
> lack of adequate food (Z59.4)
> malnutrition and other nutritional deficiencies (E40–E64)

Z72.5   **High risk sexual behavior**
> Promiscuity
> *Excludes1:* paraphilias (F65)
> Z72.51   **High risk heterosexual behavior**
> Z72.52   **High risk homosexual behavior**
> Z72.53   **High risk bisexual behavior**

Z72.6   **Gambling and betting**
> *Excludes1:* compulsive or pathological gambling (F63.0)

Z73   PROBLEMS RELATED TO LIFE MANAGEMENT DIFFICULTY
Excludes2: problems related to socioeconomic and psychosocial circumstances (Z55– Z65)

Z73.8   **Other problems related to life management difficulty**
> Z73.81   **Behavioral insomnia of childhood**
> > Z73.810   **Behavioral insomnia of childhood, sleep-onset association type**
> > Z73.811   **Behavioral insomnia of childhood, limit setting type**
> > Z73.812   **Behavioral insomnia of childhood, combined type**
> > Z73.819   **Behavioral insomnia of childhood, unspecified type**
> Z73.82   **Dual sensory impairment**
> Z73.89   **Other problems related to life management difficulty**

Z73.9   **Problem related to life management difficulty, unspecified**

Z74   PROBLEMS RELATED TO CARE PROVIDER DEPENDENCY
Excludes2: dependence on enabling machines or devices NEC (Z99.-)

Z74.2   **Need for assistance at home and no other household member able to render care**

Z75   PROBLEMS RELATED TO MEDICAL FACILITIES AND OTHER HEALTH CARE
Z75.0   **Medical services not available in home**
> *Excludes1:* no other household member able to render care (Z74.2)

Z76   PERSONS ENCOUNTERING HEALTH SERVICES IN OTHER CIRCUMSTANCES
Z76.0   **Encounter for issue of repeat prescription**
> Encounter for issue of repeat prescription for appliance or medicaments or spectacles
> *Excludes2:* issue of medical certificate (Z02.7)
> repeat prescription for contraceptive (Z30.4-)
> Codes Z76.1 and Z76.2 may only be reported as the principal/first-listed diagnosis, except when there are multiple encounters on the same day and the medical records for the encounters are combined.

Z76.1   **Encounter for health supervision and care of foundling**
> *Refer to Chapter 16 for guidelines.*

Z76.2   **Encounter for health supervision and care of other healthy infant and child**
> Encounter for medical or nursing care or supervision of healthy infant under circumstances such as adverse socioeconomic conditions at home or such as awaiting foster or adoptive placement or such as maternal illness or such as number of children at home preventing or interfering with normal care

Z76.5   **Malingerer [conscious simulation]**
> Person feigning illness (with obvious motivation)
> *Excludes1:* factitious disorder (F68.1-)
> peregrinating patient (F68.1-)

Z76.8   **Persons encountering health services in other specified circumstances**
> Z76.81   **Expectant parent(s) prebirth pediatrician visit**
> > Refer to Chapter 21 for guidelines on counseling.
> > Pre-adoption pediatrician visit for adoptive parent(s)
> Z76.82   **Awaiting organ transplant status**
> > This is a status code, refer to Chapter 21 for status guidelines.
> > Patient waiting for organ availability
> Z76.89   **Persons encountering health services in other specified circumstances**
> > Persons encountering health services NOS

CHAPTER 21. FACTORS INFLUENCING HEALTH STATUS AND CONTACT WITH HEALTH SERVICES   (Z77–Z80.6)

(Z77–Z99) PERSONS WITH POTENTIAL HEALTH HAZARDS RELATED TO FAMILY AND PERSONAL HISTORY AND CERTAIN CONDITIONS INFLUENCING HEALTH STATUS

GUIDELINES

Contact/exposure codes may be used as a first-listed code to explain an encounter for testing, or, more commonly, as a secondary code to identify a potential risk.
Code also any follow-up examination (Z08–Z09)

Z77 [4th] **OTHER CONTACT WITH AND (SUSPECTED) EXPOSURES HAZARDOUS TO HEALTH**
> **Includes:** contact with and (suspected) exposures to potential hazards to health
> **Excludes2:** contact with and (suspected) exposure to communicable diseases (Z20.-)
> exposure to (parental) (environmental) tobacco smoke in the perinatal period (P96.81)
> newborn affected by noxious substances transmitted via placenta or breast milk (P04.-)
> occupational exposure to risk factors (Z57.-)
> retained FB (Z18.-)
> retained FB fully removed (Z87.821)
> toxic effects of substances chiefly nonmedicinal as to source (T51–T65)

Z77.0 [5th] **Contact with and (suspected) exposure to hazardous, chiefly nonmedicinal, chemicals**
  Z77.01 [6th] **Contact with and (suspected) exposure to; hazardous metals**
    Z77.010 arsenic
    Z77.011 lead
    Z77.012 uranium
      Excludes1: retained depleted uranium fragments (Z18.01)
    Z77.018 other hazardous metals
      Contact with and (suspected) exposure to chromium compounds or nickel dust
  Z77.02 [6th] **Contact with and (suspected) exposure to; hazardous aromatic compounds**
    Z77.020 aromatic amines
    Z77.021 benzene
    Z77.028 other hazardous aromatic compounds
      Aromatic dyes NOS
      Polycyclic aromatic hydrocarbons
  Z77.09 [6th] **Contact with and (suspected) exposure to; other hazardous, chiefly nonmedicinal, chemicals**
    Z77.090 asbestos
    Z77.098 other hazardous, chiefly nonmedicinal, chemicals
      Dyes NOS

Z77.1 [5th] **Contact with and (suspected) exposure to; environmental pollution and hazards in the physical environment**
  Z77.12 hazards in the physical environment
    Z77.120 [6th] **mold (toxic)**

Z77.2 [5th] **other hazardous substances**
  Z77.21 potentially hazardous body fluids
  Z77.22 environmental tobacco smoke (acute) (chronic)
    Exposure to second hand tobacco smoke (acute) (chronic)
    Passive smoking (acute) (chronic)
    Excludes1: nicotine dependence (F17.-)
      tobacco use (Z72.0)
    Excludes2: occupational exposure to environmental tobacco smoke (Z57.31)
  Z77.29 other hazardous substances

Z78 [4th] **OTHER SPECIFIED HEALTH STATUS**
This is a status category, refer to Chapter 21 for status guidelines.
> **Excludes2:** asymptomatic HIV infection status (Z21)
> postprocedural status (Z93–Z99)
> sex reassignment status (Z87.890)

Z78.1 Physical restraint status
May be used when it is documented by the provider that a patient has been put in restraints during the current encounter. Please note that this code should not be reported when it is documented by the provider that a patient is temporarily restrained during a procedure.

Z79 [4th] **LONG TERM (CURRENT) DRUG THERAPY**

GUIDELINES

Codes from this category indicate a patient's continuous use of a prescribed drug (including such things as aspirin therapy) for the long-term treatment of a condition or for prophylactic use. It is not for use for patients who have addictions to drugs. This subcategory is not for use of medications for detoxification or maintenance programs to prevent withdrawal symptoms in patients with drug dependence (e.g., methadone maintenance for opiate dependence). Assign the appropriate code for the drug dependence instead.

Assign a code from Z79 if the patient is receiving a medication for an extended period as a prophylactic measure (such as for the prevention of deep vein thrombosis) or as treatment of a chronic condition (such as arthritis) or a disease requiring a lengthy course of treatment (such as cancer). Do not assign a code from category Z79 for medication being administered for a brief period of time to treat an acute illness or injury (such as a course of antibiotics to treat acute bronchitis). This is a status category, refer to Chapter 21 for status guidelines.
Includes: long term (current) drug use for prophylactic purposes
Code also any therapeutic drug level monitoring (Z51.81)
Excludes2: drug abuse and dependence (F11–F19)
> drug use complicating pregnancy, childbirth, and the puerperium (O99.32-)

Z79.1 Long term (current) use of; non-steroidal anti-inflammatories (NSAID)
> **Excludes2:** long term (current) use of aspirin (Z79.82)
> long term (current) use of oral antidiabetic or oral hypoglycemic drugs (Z79.84)

Z79.2 antibiotics
Z79.4 insulin
Z79.5 steroids
  [5th] **Z79.51 inhaled steroids**
  Z79.52 systemic steroids
Z79.8 Other long term (current) drug therapy
  [5th] **Z79.82 Long term (current) use of aspirin**
  •**Z79.84 Long term (current) use of oral hypoglycemic drugs**
    Long term use of oral antidiabetic drugs
    Excludes2: long term (current) use of insulin (Z79.4)
  Z79.89 Other long term (current) drug therapy
    [6th] **Z79.899 Other long term (current) drug therapy**

Z80 [4th] **FAMILY HISTORY OF PRIMARY MALIGNANT NEOPLASM**

GUIDELINES

Family history codes are for use when a patient has a family member(s) who has had a particular disease that causes the patient to be at higher risk of also contracting the disease. family history codes may be used in conjunction with screening codes to explain the need for a test or procedure. History codes are also acceptable on any medical record regardless of the reason for visit. A history of an illness, even if no longer present, is important information that may alter the type of treatment ordered.

Z80.3 Family history of malignant neoplasm of breast
  Conditions classifiable to C50.-
Z80.4 Family history of malignant neoplasm of genital organs
  [5th] Conditions classifiable to C51-C63
  Z80.41 Family history of malignant neoplasm of ovary
  Z80.43 Family history of malignant neoplasm of testis
  Z80.49 Family history of malignant neoplasm of other genital organs
Z80.5 Family history of malignant neoplasm of urinary tract
  [5th] Conditions classifiable to C64–C68
  Z80.51 Family history of malignant neoplasm of kidney
  Z80.52 Family history of malignant neoplasm of bladder
Z80.6 Family history of leukemia
  Conditions classifiable to C91–C95

   Additional Character Required   3-character code   •=New Code   ▲=Revised Code   *Excludes1*—Not coded here, do not use together   *Excludes2*—Not included here

Z80.7 Family history of other malignant neoplasms of lymphoid, hematopoietic and related tissues
Conditions classifiable to C81–C90, C96.-

Z80.8 Family history of malignant neoplasm of other organs or systems
Conditions classifiable to C00–C14, C40–C49, C69–C79

Z80.9 Family history of malignant neoplasm, unspecified
Conditions classifiable to C80.1

Z81 FAMILY HISTORY OF MENTAL AND BEHAVIORAL DISORDERS
`4th`

GUIDELINES

Family history codes are for use when a patient has a family member(s) who has had a particular disease that causes the patient to be at higher risk of also contracting the disease. family history codes may be used in conjunction with screening codes to explain the need for a test or procedure. History codes are also acceptable on any medical record regardless of the reason for visit. A history of an illness, even if no longer present, is important information that may alter the type of treatment ordered.

Z81.0 Family history of intellectual disabilities
Conditions classifiable to F70–F79

Z81.8 Family history of other mental and behavioral disorders
Conditions classifiable elsewhere in F01–F99

Z82 FAMILY HISTORY OF CERTAIN DISABILITIES AND CHRONIC DISEASES (LEADING TO DISABLEMENT)
`4th`

GUIDELINES

Family history codes are for use when a patient has a family member(s) who has had a particular disease that causes the patient to be at higher risk of also contracting the disease. family history codes may be used in conjunction with screening codes to explain the need for a test or procedure. History codes are also acceptable on any medical record regardless of the reason for visit. A history of an illness, even if no longer present, is important information that may alter the type of treatment ordered.

Z82.0 Family history of; epilepsy and other diseases of the nervous system
Conditions classifiable to G00–G99

Z82.1 blindness and visual loss
Conditions classifiable to H54.-

Z82.2 deafness and hearing loss
Conditions classifiable to H90–H91

Z82.4 Family history of; ischemic heart disease and other diseases of the circulatory system
`5th`
Conditions classifiable to I00–I52, I65–I99

  Z82.41 sudden cardiac death

  Z82.49 ischemic heart disease and other diseases of the circulatory system

Z82.5 Family history of asthma and other chronic lower respiratory diseases
Conditions classifiable to J40–J47
Excludes2: family history of other diseases of the respiratory system (Z83.6)

Z82.6 Family history of; arthritis and other diseases of the musculoskeletal system and connective tissue
`5th`
Conditions classifiable to M00–M99

  Z82.61 arthritis

  Z82.62 osteoporosis

  Z82.69 other diseases of the musculoskeletal system and connective tissue

Z82.7 Family history of; congenital malformations, deformations and chromosomal abnormalities
`5th`
Conditions classifiable to Q00–Q99

  Z82.71 polycystic kidney

  Z82.79 other congenital malformations, deformations and chromosomal abnormalities

Z83 FAMILY HISTORY OF OTHER SPECIFIC DISORDERS
`4th`

GUIDELINES

Family history codes are for use when a patient has a family member(s) who has had a particular disease that causes the patient to be at higher risk of also contracting the disease. family history codes may be used in conjunction with screening codes to explain the need for a test or procedure. History codes are also acceptable on any medical record regardless of the reason for visit. A history of an illness, even if no longer present, is important information that may alter the type of treatment ordered.
Excludes2: contact with and (suspected) exposure to communicable disease in the family (Z20.-)

Z83.2 Family history of; diseases of the blood and blood-forming organs and certain disorders involving the immune mechanism
Conditions classifiable to D50–D89

Z83.3 DM
Conditions classifiable to E08–E13

Z83.4 other endocrine, nutritional and metabolic diseases
`5th`
Conditions classifiable to E00–E07, E15–E88

  Z83.41 multiple endocrine neoplasia syndrome

  •**Z83.42 familial hypercholesterolemia**

  Z83.49 other endocrine, nutritional and metabolic diseases

Z83.5 eye and ear disorders
`5th`

  Z83.51 eye disorders
`6th`
    Conditions classifiable to H00–H53, H55–H59
    Excludes2: family history of blindness and visual loss (Z82.1)

    Z83.511 glaucoma

    Z83.518 other specified eye disorder

Z83.6 other diseases of the respiratory system
Conditions classifiable to J00–J39, J60–J99
Excludes2: family history of asthma and other chronic lower respiratory diseases (Z82.5)

Z83.7 diseases of the digestive system
`5th`
Conditions classifiable to K00–K93

  Z83.71 colonic polyps
  Excludes1: family history of malignant neoplasm of digestive organs (Z80.0)

  Z83.79 other diseases of the digestive system

Z84 FAMILY HISTORY OF OTHER CONDITIONS
`4th`

GUIDELINES

Family history codes are for use when a patient has a family member(s) who has had a particular disease that causes the patient to be at higher risk of also contracting the disease. family history codes may be used in conjunction with screening codes to explain the need for a test or procedure. History codes are also acceptable on any medical record regardless of the reason for visit. A history of an illness, even if no longer present, is important information that may alter the type of treatment ordered.

Z84.1 Family history of disorders of kidney and ureter
Conditions classifiable to N00–N29

Z84.8 Family history of other specified conditions
`5th`
  Z84.81 Family history of carrier of genetic disease

  •**Z84.82 Family history of sudden Infant death syndrome**

  Z84.89 Family history of other specified conditions

Z85 PERSONAL HISTORY OF MALIGNANT NEOPLASM
`4th`

GUIDELINES

Personal history codes explain a patient's past medical condition that no longer exists and is not receiving any treatment, but that has the potential for recurrence, and therefore may require continued monitoring. These codes may be used in conjunction with follow-up codes to explain the need for a test or procedure. History codes are also acceptable on any medical record regardless of the reason for visit. A history of an illness, even if no longer present, is important information that may alter the type of treatment ordered.
Code first any follow-up examination after treatment of malignant neoplasm (Z08)
Use additional code to identify: alcohol use and dependence (F10.-)
  exposure to environmental tobacco smoke (Z77.22)
  history of tobacco dependence (Z87.891)
  occupational exposure to environmental tobacco smoke (Z57.31)
  tobacco dependence (F17.-)
  tobacco use (Z72.0)
Excludes2: personal history of benign neoplasm (Z86.01-)
  personal history of carcinoma-in-situ (Z86.00-)

`4th` `5th` `6th` `7th` Additional Character Required   3-character code

•=New Code
▲=Revised Code

Excludes1—Not coded here, do not use together
Excludes2—Not included here

Z85.5 Personal history of malignant neoplasm of urinary tract
5th
Conditions classifiable to C64–C68
Z85.50 Personal history of malignant neoplasm of; unspecified urinary tract organ
Z85.51 bladder
Z85.52 kidney
6th
Excludes1: personal history of malignant neoplasm of renal pelvis (Z85.53)
Z85.520 Personal history of; malignant carcinoid tumor of kidney
Conditions classifiable to C7A.093
Z85.528 other malignant neoplasm of kidney
Conditions classifiable to C64

Z85.6 Leukemia
Conditions classifiable to C91–C95
Excludes1: leukemia in remission C91.0–C95.9 with 5th character 1

Z85.7 Personal history of other malignant neoplasms of lymphoid, hematopoietic and related tissues
5th
Z85.71 Personal history of; Hodgkin lymphoma
Conditions classifiable to C81
Z85.72 non-Hodgkin lymphomas
Conditions classifiable to C82–C85
Z85.79 other malignant neoplasms of lymphoid, hematopoietic and related tissues
Conditions classifiable to C88–C90, C96
Excludes1: multiple myeloma in remission (C90.01)
plasma cell leukemia in remission (C90.11)
plasmacytoma in remission (C90.21)

Z85.8 Malignant neoplasms of other organs and systems
5th
Conditions classifiable to C00–C14, C40–C49, C69–C79, C7A.098
Z85.83 Personal history of malignant neoplasm of; bone and soft tissue
6th
Z85.830 bone
Z85.831 soft tissue
Excludes2: personal history of malignant neoplasm of skin (Z85.82-)
Z85.84 Personal history of; malignant neoplasm of eye and nervous tissue
6th
Z85.840 eye
Z85.841 brain
Z85.848 other parts of nervous tissue
Z85.85 Personal history of; malignant neoplasm of endocrine glands
6th
Z85.850 thyroid
Z85.858 other endocrine glands
Z85.89 other organs and systems

Z85.9 Personal history of malignant neoplasm, unspecified
Conditions classifiable to C7A.00, C80.1

Z86 PERSONAL HISTORY OF CERTAIN OTHER DISEASES
4th

GUIDELINES

Personal history codes explain a patient's past medical condition that no longer exists and is not receiving any treatment, but that has the potential for recurrence, and therefore may require continued monitoring. These codes may be used in conjunction with follow-up codes to explain the need for a test or procedure. History codes are also acceptable on any medical record regardless of the reason for visit. A history of an illness, even if no longer present, is important information that may alter the type of treatment ordered.
Code first any follow-up examination after treatment (Z09)

Z86.1 Personal history of infectious and parasitic diseases
5th
Conditions classifiable to A00–B89, B99
Excludes1: personal history of infectious diseases specific to a body system
sequelae of infectious and parasitic diseases (B90–B94)
Z86.11 Personal history of; tuberculosis
Z86.13 malaria
Z86.14 MRSA infection
Personal history of MRSA infection
Z86.19 other infectious and parasitic diseases

Z86.2 Personal history of diseases of the blood and blood-forming organs and certain disorders involving the immune mechanism
Conditions classifiable to D50–D89

Z86.3 Personal history of endocrine, nutritional and metabolic diseases
5th
Conditions classifiable to E00–E88
Z86.39 other endocrine, nutritional and metabolic disease

Z86.5 Personal history of; mental and behavioral disorders
5th
Conditions classifiable to F40–F59
Z86.59 other mental and behavioral disorders
Code is a nonspecific Z code, refer to Chapter 21 for guidelines.

Z86.6 Personal history of; diseases of the nervous system and sense organs
5th
Conditions classifiable to G00–G99, H00–H95
Z86.61 infections of the central nervous system
Personal history of encephalitis
Personal history of meningitis
Z86.69 other diseases of the nervous system and sense organs

Z86.7 Personal history of; diseases of the circulatory system
5th
Conditions classifiable to I00–I99
Z86.73 TIA and cerebral infarction without residual deficits
Personal history of prolonged reversible ischemic neurological deficit (PRIND)
Personal history of stroke NOS without residual deficits
Excludes1: personal history of traumatic brain injury (Z87.820)
sequelae of cerebrovascular disease (I69.-)
Z86.74 sudden cardiac arrest
Personal history of sudden cardiac death successfully resuscitated
Z86.79 other diseases of the circulatory system

Z87 PERSONAL HISTORY OF OTHER DISEASES AND CONDITIONS
4th

GUIDELINES

Personal history codes explain a patient's past medical condition that no longer exists and is not receiving any treatment, but that has the potential for recurrence, and therefore may require continued monitoring. These codes may be used in conjunction with follow-up codes to explain the need for a test or procedure. History codes are also acceptable on any medical record regardless of the reason for visit. A history of an illness, even if no longer present, is important information that may alter the type of treatment ordered.
Code first any follow-up examination after treatment (Z09)

Z87.0 Personal history of; diseases of the respiratory system
5th
Conditions classifiable to J00–J99
Z87.01 pneumonia (recurrent)
Z87.09 other diseases of the respiratory system

Z87.3 Personal history of diseases of the musculoskeletal system and connective tissue
5th
Conditions classifiable to M00–M99
Excludes2: personal history of (healed) traumatic fracture (Z87.81)
Z87.39 other diseases of the musculoskeletal system and connective tissue

Z87.4 Personal history of; diseases of genitourinary system
5th
Conditions classifiable to N00–N99
Z87.44 diseases of urinary system
6th
Excludes1: personal history of malignant neoplasm of cervix uteri (Z85.41)
Z87.440 urinary (tract) infections
Z87.441 nephrotic syndrome
Z87.442 urinary calculi
Personal history of kidney stones
Z87.448 other diseases of urinary system

 4th 5th 6th 7th Additional Character Required   3-character code

•=New Code
▲=Revised Code

Excludes1—Not coded here, do not use together
Excludes2—Not included here

Z87.7   **Personal history of (corrected) congenital malformations**

`5th` Conditions classifiable to Q00–Q89 that have been repaired or corrected

Excludes1: congenital malformations that have been partially corrected or repair but which still require medical treatment—**code to condition**

Excludes2: other postprocedural states (Z98.-)
personal history of medical treatment (Z92.-)
presence of cardiac and vascular implants and grafts (Z95.-)
presence of other devices (Z97.-)
presence of other functional implants (Z96.-)
transplanted organ and tissue status (Z94.-)

Z87.71   **Personal history of; (corrected) congenital malformations of genitourinary system**

`6th`   **Z87.710**   (corrected) hypospadias

    Z87.718   other specified (corrected) congenital malformations of genitourinary system

Z87.72   **Personal history of; (corrected) congenital malformations of nervous system and sense organs**

`6th`   **Z87.720**   (corrected) congenital malformations of eye

    Z87.721   (corrected) congenital malformations of ear

    Z87.728   other specified (corrected) congenital malformations of nervous system and sense organs

Z87.73   **Personal history of; (corrected) congenital malformations of digestive system**

`6th`   **Z87.730**   (corrected) cleft lip and palate

    Z87.738   other specified (corrected) congenital malformations of digestive system

Z87.74   **Personal history of; (corrected) congenital malformations of heart and circulatory system**

Z87.75   **(corrected) congenital malformations of respiratory system**

Z87.76   **(corrected) congenital malformations of integument, limbs and musculoskeletal system**

Z87.79   **other (corrected) congenital malformations**

`6th`   **Z87.790**   (corrected) congenital malformations of face and neck

    Z87.798   other (corrected) congenital malformations

Z87.8   **Personal history of; other specified conditions**

`5th`   **Z87.82**   **other (healed) physical injury and trauma**

`6th` Conditions classifiable to S00–T88, except traumatic fractures

    Z87.820   **traumatic brain injury**

      Excludes1: personal history of TIA, and cerebral infarction without residual deficits (Z86.73)

    Z87.821   **retained FB fully removed**

    Z87.828   **other (healed) physical injury and trauma**

   Z87.89   **Personal history of; other specified conditions**

`6th`   **Z87.891**   **nicotine dependence**

      Excludes1: current nicotine dependence (F17.2-)

    Z87.892   **anaphylaxis**

      Code also allergy status such as:
      allergy status to drugs, medicaments and biological substances (Z88.-)
      allergy status, other than to drugs and biological substances (Z91.0-)

    Z87.898   **other specified conditions**

Z88   **ALLERGY STATUS TO DRUGS, MEDICAMENTS AND BIOLOGICAL SUBSTANCES**

`4th` This is a status category (excluding Z88.9), refer to Chapter 21 for status guidelines.

Excludes2: Allergy status, other than to drugs and biological substances (Z91.0-)

Z88.0   **Allergy status to; penicillin**

Z88.1   **other antibiotic agents status**

Z88.2   **sulfonamides status**

Z88.3   **other anti-infective agents status**

Z88.4   **anesthetic agent status**

Z88.5   **narcotic agent status**

Z88.6   **analgesic agent status**

Z88.7   **serum and vaccine status**

Z88.8   **other drugs, medicaments and biological substances status**

Z88.9   **unspecified drugs, medicaments and biological substances status**

Code is a nonspecific Z code, refer to Chapter 21 for guidelines.

Z90   **ACQUIRED ABSENCE OF ORGANS, NEC**

`4th` This is a status category, refer to Chapter 21 for status guidelines.

Includes: postprocedural or post-traumatic loss of body part NEC

Excludes1: congenital absence—see Alphabetical Index

Excludes2: postprocedural absence of endocrine glands (E89.-)

Note: Use only if there are no complications or malfunctions of the organ or tissue replaced, the amputation site, or the equipment on which the patient is dependent.

Z90.4   **Acquired absence of; other specified parts of digestive tract**

`5th`   **Z90.49**   **other specified parts of digestive tract**

Z90.5   **Acquired absence of: kidney**

Z90.7   **genital organ(s)**

`5th` *Excludes1:* personal history of sex reassignment (Z87.890)

Excludes2: female genital mutilation status (N90.81-)

   Z90.79   **other genital organ(s)**

Z90.8   **Acquired absence of; other organs**

`5th`   **Z90.81**   **spleen**

   Z90.89   **other organs**

Z91   **PERSONAL RISK FACTORS, NEC**

Excludes2: contact with and (suspected) exposures hazardous to health (Z77.-)
exposure to pollution and other problems related to physical environment (Z77.1-)
personal history of physical injury and trauma (Z87.81, Z87.82-)
occupational exposure to risk factors (Z57.-)

Z91.0   **Allergy status, other than to drugs and biological substances**

`5th` *This is a status sub-category, refer to Chapter 21 for status guidelines.*

Excludes2: Allergy status to drugs, medicaments, and biological substances (Z88.-)

   Z91.01   **Food allergy status**

`6th` *Excludes2:* food additives allergy status (Z91.02)

    Z91.010   **Allergy to; peanuts**

    Z91.011   **milk products**

      Excludes1: lactose intolerance (E73.-)

    Z91.012   **eggs**

    Z91.013   **seafood**

      Allergy to shellfish or octopus or squid ink

    Z91.018   **other foods**

      nuts other than peanuts

   Z91.03   **Insect allergy status**

`6th`   **Z91.030**   **Bee allergy status**

    Z91.038   **Other insect allergy status**

   Z91.04   **Nonmedicinal substance allergy status**

`6th`   **Z91.040**   **Latex allergy status**

      Latex sensitivity status

    Z91.041   **Radiographic dye allergy status**

      Allergy status to contrast media used for diagnostic X-ray procedure

    Z91.048   **Other nonmedicinal substance allergy status**

Z91.1   **Patient's noncompliance with medical treatment and regimen**

`5th`   **Z91.12**   **Patient's intentional underdosing of medication regimen**

`6th` **Code first** underdosing of medication (T36–T50) with fifth or sixth character 6

Excludes1: adverse effect of prescribed drug taken as directed- code to adverse effect
poisoning (overdose) -code to poisoning

    Z91.120   **Patient's intentional underdosing of medication regimen due to financial hardship**

    Z91.128   **Patient's intentional underdosing of medication regimen for other reason**

   Z91.14   **Patient's other noncompliance with medication regimen**

      Patient's underdosing of medication NOS

   Z91.15   **Patient's noncompliance with renal dialysis**

`4th` `5th` `6th` `7th`   Additional Character Required   ✓   3-character code

•=New Code   *Excludes1*—Not coded here, do not use together
▲=Revised Code   *Excludes2*—Not included here

Z91.19 Patient's noncompliance with other medical treatment and regimen

Z91.4 Personal history of psychological trauma, NEC

 GUIDELINES

Personal history codes explain a patient's past medical condition that no longer exists and is not receiving any treatment, but that has the potential for recurrence, and therefore may require continued monitoring. These codes may be used in conjunction with follow-up codes to explain the need for a test or procedure. History codes are also acceptable on any medical record regardless of the reason for visit. A history of an illness, even if no longer present, is important information that may alter the type of treatment ordered.

Z91.49 Other personal history of psychological trauma, NEC

Z91.5 Personal history of self-harm

GUIDELINES

Personal history codes explain a patient's past medical condition that no longer exists and is not receiving any treatment, but that has the potential for recurrence, and therefore may require continued monitoring. These codes may be used in conjunction with follow-up codes to explain the need for a test or procedure. History codes are also acceptable on any medical record regardless of the reason for visit. A history of an illness, even if no longer present, is important information that may alter the type of treatment ordered.

Personal history of parasuicide

Personal history of self-poisoning

Personal history of suicide attempt

Z91.8 Other specified personal risk factors, NEC

 GUIDELINES

Personal history codes explain a patient's past medical condition that no longer exists and is not receiving any treatment, but that has the potential for recurrence, and therefore may require continued monitoring. These codes may be used in conjunction with follow-up codes to explain the need for a test or procedure. History codes are also acceptable on any medical record regardless of the reason for visit. A history of an illness, even if no longer present, is important information that may alter the type of treatment ordered. Excludes code Z91.83.

Z91.81 History of falling

At risk for falling

Z91.83 Wandering in diseases classified elsewhere

Code first underlying disorder such as:

Alzheimer's disease (G30.-)

autism or pervasive developmental disorder (F84.-)

intellectual disabilities (F70–F79)

unspecified dementia with behavioral disturbance (F03.9-)

Z91.89 Other specified personal risk factors, NEC

Z92 PERSONAL HISTORY OF MEDICAL TREATMENT

 GUIDELINES

Personal history codes explain a patient's past medical condition that no longer exists and is not receiving any treatment, but that has the potential for recurrence, and therefore may require continued monitoring. These codes may be used in conjunction with follow-up codes to explain the need for a test or procedure. History codes are also acceptable on any medical record regardless of the reason for visit. A history of an illness, even if no longer present, is important information that may alter the type of treatment ordered. Excludes codes Z92.0 and Z92.82.

Excludes2: postprocedural states (Z98.-)

Z92.2 Personal history of; drug therapy

Excludes2: long term (current) drug therapy (Z79.-)

Z92.21 antineoplastic chemotherapy

Z92.22 monoclonal drug therapy

Z92.24 steroid therapy

Z92.240 inhaled steroid therapy

Z92.241 systemic steroid therapy

steroid therapy NOS

Z92.25 immunosuppression therapy

Excludes2: personal history of steroid therapy (Z92.24)

Z92.29 other drug therapy

Z92.8 Personal history of; other medical treatment

Z92.81 extracorporeal membrane oxygenation (ECMO)

Z93 ARTIFICIAL OPENING STATUS

Note: Use only if there are no complications or malfunctions of the organ or tissue replaced, the amputation site, or the equipment on which the patient is dependent. This is a status category, refer to Chapter 21 for status guidelines.

Excludes1: artificial openings requiring attention or management (Z43.-)

complications of external stoma (J95.0-, K94.-, N99.5-)

Z93.0 Tracheostomy status

Z93.1 Gastrostomy status

Z93.2 Ileostomy status

Z93.3 Colostomy status

Z93.4 Other artificial openings of gastrointestinal tract status

Z93.5 Cystostomy status

Z93.50 Unspecified cystostomy status

Z93.51 Cutaneous-vesicostomy status

Z93.52 Appendico-vesicostomy status

Z93.59 Other cystostomy status

Z94 TRANSPLANTED ORGAN AND TISSUE STATUS

Note: Use only if there are no complications or malfunctions of the organ or tissue replaced, the amputation site, or the equipment on which the patient is dependent. This is a status category, refer to Chapter 21 for status guidelines.

Includes: organ or tissue replaced by heterogenous or homogenous transplant

Excludes1: complications of transplanted organ or tissue—see Alphabetical Index

Excludes2: presence of vascular grafts (Z95.-)

Z94.0 Kidney transplant status

Z94.1 Heart transplant status

Excludes1: artificial heart status (Z95.812)

heart-valve replacement status (Z95.2–Z95.4)

Z95 PRESENCE OF CARDIAC AND VASCULAR IMPLANTS AND GRAFTS

This is a status category, refer to Chapter 21 for status guidelines.

Excludes1: complications of cardiac and vascular devices, implants and grafts (T82.-)

Z95.0 Presence of cardiac pacemaker

Presence of cardiac resynchronization therapy (CRT-P) pacemaker

Excludes1: adjustment or management of cardiac pacemaker (Z45.0-)

presence of automatic (implantable) cardiac defibrillator with synchronous cardiac pacemaker (Z95.810)

Z95.2 Presence of prosthetic heart valve

Presence of heart valve NOS

Z95.3 Presence of xenogenic heart valve

Z95.4 Presence of other heart-valve replacement

Z97 PRESENCE OF OTHER DEVICES

Excludes1: complications of internal prosthetic devices, implants and grafts (T82–T85)

fitting and adjustment of prosthetic and other devices (Z44–Z46)

Z97.5 Presence of (intrauterine) contraceptive device

checking, reinsertion or removal of contraceptive device (Z30.43)

Excludes1: checking, reinsertion or removal of implantable subdermal contraceptive (Z30.46)

checking, reinsertion or removal of intrauterine contraceptive device (Z30.43-)

Z97.8 Presence of other specified devices

   Additional Character Required   3-character code   •=New Code   ▲=Revised Code   ***Excludes1***—Not coded here, do not use together   ***Excludes2***—Not included here

Z98   OTHER POSTPROCEDURAL STATES

[4th] This is a status category, refer to Chapter 21 for status guidelines.

Excludes2: aftercare (Z43–Z49, Z51)

     follow-up medical care (Z08–Z09)

     postprocedural complication—see Alphabetical Index

Z98.2   Presence of cerebrospinal fluid drainage device

     Presence of CSF shunt

Z98.8   Other specified postprocedural states

[5th]   **Z98.85   Transplanted organ removal status**

     Assign code Z98.85, Transplanted organ removal status, to indicate that a transplanted organ has been previously removed. This code should not be assigned for the encounter in which the transplanted organ is removed. The complication necessitating removal of the transplant organ should be assigned for that encounter.

     See Chapter 19 for information on the coding of organ transplant complications.

     Transplanted organ previously removed due to complication, failure, rejection or infection

     Excludes1: encounter for removal of transplanted organ—code to complication of transplanted organ (T86.-)

     Z98.87   Personal history of in utero procedure

[6th]   **Z98.871   Personal history of in utero procedure while a fetus**

   ▲**Z98.89   Other specified postprocedural states**

[6th]   •**Z98.890   Other specified postprocedural states**

     Personal history of surgery, NEC

Z99   DEPENDENCE ON ENABLING MACHINES AND DEVICES, NEC

[4th] This is a status category, refer to Chapter 21 for status guidelines.

Z99.1   Dependence on respirator

[5th]   Dependence on ventilator

     Z99.11   Dependence on respirator [ventilator] status

     For encounters for weaning from a mechanical ventilator, assign a code from subcategory J96.1, Chronic respiratory failure, followed by code Z99.11, Dependence on respirator [ventilator] status.

Z99.2   Dependence on renal dialysis

     Hemodialysis status

     Peritoneal dialysis status

     Presence of arteriovenous shunt for dialysis

     Renal dialysis status NOS

     Excludes1: encounter for fitting and adjustment of dialysis catheter (Z49.0-)

     Excludes2: noncompliance with renal dialysis (Z91.15)

[4th] [5th] [6th] [7th]   Additional Character Required   ✓   3-character code

•=New Code   ▲=Revised Code

Excludes1—Not coded here, do not use together

Excludes2—Not included here

ICD-10-CM EXTERNAL CAUSE
OF INJURIES TABLE

These tables are inserted for ease to locate an external cause code from a transport accident.
If not listed here, refer to the index.

ICD-10-CM EXTERNAL CAUSE OF INJURIES TABLE

Activity of the Person Injured	Pedestrian Conveyance	Collides with: Car/Pick-up Truck/Van	Bike	Bus/HTV	Fixed Object	Pedestrian or Animal	Other (NOS)	Unspecified	Train/Train car	2 or 3 Motor Wheeler	Non-Motor Vehicle[a]
Pedestrian on foot	V00.01 R / V00.02 S / V00.09 O	V03.00 N / V03.10 T / V03.90 U	V01.00 N / V01.10 T / V01.90 U	V04.00 N / V04.10 T / V04.90 U	Refer to W22		V09.09 N / V09.29 T	V09.00 N / V09.20 T	V05.00 N / V05.10 T / V05.90 U	V02.00 N / V02.10 T / V02.90 U	V06.00 N / V06.10 T / V06.90 U
In-line skater (I)/ Roller skater (R)		V03.01 N / V03.11 T / V03.91 U	V01.01 N / V01.11 T / V01.91 U	V04.01 N / V04.11 T / V04.91 U	V00.112 I / V00.122 R	V00.118 I / V00.128 R	V00.118 I / V00.128 R		V05.01 N / V05.11 T / V05.91 U	V02.01 N / V02.11 T / V02.91 U	V06.01 N / V06.11 T / V06.91 U
Skateboarder		V03.02 N / V03.12 T / V03.92 U	V01.02 N / V01.12 T / V01.92 U	V04.02 N / V04.12 T / V04.92 U	V00.132	V00.138	V00.138		V05.02 N / V05.12 T / V05.92 U	V02.02 N / V02.12 T / V02.92 U	V06.02 N / V06.12 T / V06.92 U
Other (NOS)		V03.09 N / V03.19 T / V03.99 U	V01.09 N / V01.19 T / V01.99 U	V04.09 N / V04.19 T / V04.99 U					V05.09 N / V05.19 T / V05.99 U	V02.09 N / V02.19 T / V02.99 U	V06.09 N / V06.19 T / V06.99 U
Scooter (Non-motorized)		V03.09 N / V03.19 T / V03.99 U	V01.09 N / V01.19 T / V01.99 U	V04.09 N / V04.19 T / V04.99 U	V00.142				V05.09 N / V05.19 T / V05.99 U	V02.09 N / V02.19 T / V02.99 U	V06.09 N / V06.19 T / V06.99 U
Heelies		V03.09 N / V03.19 T / V03.99 U	V01.09 N / V01.19 T / V01.99 U	V04.09 N / V04.19 T / V04.99 U	V00.152				V05.09 N / V05.19 T / V05.99 U	V02.09 N / V02.19 T / V02.99 U	V06.09 N / V06.19 T / V06.99 U
Ice-skater		V03.09 N / V03.19 T / V03.99 U	V01.09 N / V01.19 T / V01.99 U	V04.09 N / V04.19 T / V04.99 U	V00.212				V05.09 N / V05.19 T / V05.99 U	V02.09 N / V02.19 T / V02.99 U	V06.09 N / V06.19 T / V06.99 U
Sledder		V03.09 N / V03.19 T / V03.99 U	V01.09 N / V01.19 T / V01.99 U	V04.09 N / V04.19 T / V04.99 U	V00.222				V05.09 N / V05.19 T / V05.99 U	V02.09 N / V02.19 T / V02.99 U	V06.09 N / V06.19 T / V06.99 U
Snowboarder		V03.09 N / V03.19 T / V03.99 U	V01.09 N / V01.19 T / V01.99 U	V04.09 N / V04.19 T / V04.99 U	V00.312				V05.09 N / V05.19 T / V05.99 U	V02.09 N / V02.19 T / V02.99 U	V06.09 N / V06.19 T / V06.99 U
Snowskier		V03.09 N / V03.19 T / V03.99 U	V01.09 N / V01.19 T / V01.99 U	V04.09 N / V04.19 T / V04.99 U	V00.322				V05.09 N / V05.19 T / V05.99 U	V02.09 N / V02.19 T / V02.99 U	V06.09 N / V06.19 T / V06.99 U
Wheelchair		V03.09 N / V03.19 T / V03.99 U	V01.09 N / V01.19 T / V01.99 U	V04.09 N / V04.19 T / V04.99 U	V00.812				V05.09 N / V05.19 T / V05.99 U	V02.09 N / V02.19 T / V02.99 U	V06.09 N / V06.19 T / V06.99 U
Bike											
Driver		V13.0 N / V13.4 T	V11.0 N / V11.4 T	V14.0 N / V14.4 T	V17.0 N / V17.4 T	V10.0 N / V10.4 T	V19.09 N / V19.49 T	V19.00 N / V19.40 T	V15.0 N / V15.4 T	V12.0 N / V12.4 T	V16.0 N / V16.4 T
Passenger		V13.1 N / V13.5 T	V11.1 N / V11.5 T	V14.1 N / V14.5 T	V17.1 N / V17.5 T	V10.1 N / V10.5 T	V19.19 N / V19.59 T	V19.10 N / V19.50 T	V15.1 N / V15.5 T	V12.1 N / V12.5 T	V16.1 N / V16.5 T
Boarding		V13.3	V11.3	V14.3	V17.3	V10.3			V15.3	V12.3	V16.3
Unspecified		V13.2 N / V13.9 T	V11.2 N / V11.9 T	V14.2 N / V14.9 T	V17.2 N / V17.9 T	V10.2 N / V10.9 T	V19.29 N / V19.69 T	V19.20 N / V19.60 T	V15.2 N / V15.9 T	V12.2 N / V12.9 T	V16.2 N / V16.9 T

[a]Non-motor vehicle includes streetcar, animal drawn vehicle, animal being ridden

I = In-line skates; R = roller skates; N = nontraffic accident; T = traffic accident; U = unspecified whether traffic or not

*Refer to the index

Activity of the Person Injured	Collides with										
	Pedestrian Conveyance	Car/Pick-up Truck/Van	Bike	Bus/HTV	Fixed Object	Pedestrian or Animal	Other (NOS)	Unspecified	Train/Train car	2 or 3 Motor Wheeler	Non-Motor Vehicle[a]
Motorcycle/Motor Scooter/Moped											
Driver		V23.0 N V23.4 T	V21.0 N V21.4 T	V24.0 N V24.4 T	V27.0 N V27.4 T	V20.0 N V20.4 T	V29.09 N V29.49 T	V29.00 N V29.40 T	V25.0 N V25.4 T	V22.00 N V22.4 T	V26.0 N V26.4 T
Passenger		V23.1 N V23.5 T	V21.1 N V21.5 T	V24.1 N V24.5 T	V27.1 N V27.5 T	V20.1 N V20.5 T	V29.19 N V29.59 T	V29.10 N V29.50 T	V25.1 N V25.5 T	V22.1 N V22.5 T	V26.1 N V26.5 T
Boarding		V23.3	V21.3	V24.3	V27.3	V20.3			V25.3	V22.3	V26.3
Unspecified		V23.2 N V23.9 T	V21.2 N V21.9 T	V24.2 N V24.9 T	V27.2 N V27.9 T	V20.2 N V20.9 T	V29.29 N V29.69 T	V29.20 N V29.60 T	V25.2 N V25.9 T	V22.2 N V22.9 T	V26.2 N V26.9 T
3-wheel vehicle											
Driver		V33.0 N V33.5 T	V31.0 N V31.5 T	V34.0 N V34.5 T	V37.0 N V37.5 T	V30.0 N V30.5 T	V39.09 N V39.49 T	V39.00 N V39.40 T	V35.0 N V35.5 T	V32.0 N V32.5 T	V36.0 N V36.5 T
Passenger		V33.1 N V33.6 T	V31.1 N V31.6 T	V34.1 N V34.6 T	V37.1 N V37.6 T	V30.1 N V30.6 T	V39.19 N V39.59 T	V39.10 N V39.50	V35.1 N V35.6 T	V32.1 N V32.6 T	V36.1 N V36.6 T
Rider on outside		V33.2 N V33.7 T	V31.2 N V31.7 T	V34.2 N V34.7 T	V37.2 N V37.7 T	V30.2 N V30.7 T			V35.2 N V35.7 T	V32.2 N V32.7 T	V36.2 N V36.7 T
Boarding		V33.4	V31.4	V34.4	V37.4	V30.4			V35.4	V32.4	V36.4
Unspecified		V33.3 N V33.9 T	V31.3 N V31.9 T	V34.3 N V34.9 T	V37.3 N V37.9 T	V30.3 N V30.9 T	V39.29 N V39.69 T	V39.20 N V39.60 T	V35.3 N V35.9 T	V32.3 N V32.9 T	V36.3 N V36.9 T
Car											
Driver		V43.0- N V43.5- T	V41.0 N V41.5 T	V44.0 N V44.5 T	V47.0- N V47.5- T	V40.0 N V40.5 T	V49.09N V49.49 T	V49.00N V49.40 T	V45.0 N V45.5 T	V42.0 N V42.5 T	
Passenger		V43.1- N V43.6- T	V41.1 N V41.6 T	V44.1 N V44.6 T	V47.1- N V47.6- T	V40.1 N V40.6 T	V49.19N V49.59 T	V49.10 N V49.50 T	V45.1 N V45.6 T	V42.1 N V42.6 T	
Rider on outside		V43.2- N V43.7- T	V41.2 N V41.7 T	V44.2 N V44.7 T	V47.2- N V47.7- T	V40.2 N V40.7 T		V59.3 N V59.9 T	V45.2 N V45.7 T	V42.2 N V42.7 T	
Boarding		V43.4-	V41.4	V44.4	V47.4-	V40.4			V45.4	V42.4	
Unspecified		V43.3- N V43.9- T	V41.3 N V41.9 T	V44.3 N V44.9 T	V47.3- N V47.9- T	V40.3 N V40.9 T	V49.29N V49.69 T	V49.20 N V49.60 T	V45.3 N V45.9 T	V42.3 N V42.9 T	
Pick-Up Truck/ Van/SUV											
Driver		V53.0 N V53.5 T	V51.0 N V51.5 T	V54.0 N V54.5 T	V57.0 N V57.5 T	V50.0 N V50.5 T	V59.09 N V59.49 T	V59.00 N V59.40 T	V55.0 N V55.5 T	V52.0 N V52.5 T	
Passenger		V53.1 N V53.6 T	V51.1 N V51.6 T	V54.1 N V54.6 T	V57.1 N V57.6 T	V50.1 N V50.6 T	V59.19 N V59.59 T	V59.10 N V59.50 T	V55.1 N V55.6 T	V52.1 N V52.6 T	
Rider on outside		V53.2 N V53.7 T	V51.2 N V51.7 T	V54.2 N V54.7 T	V57.2 N V57.7 T	V50.2 N V50.7 T			V55.2 N V55.7 T	V52.2 N V52.7 T	
Boarding		V53.4	V51.4	V54.4	V57.4	V50.4			V55.4	V52.4	
Unspecified		V53.3 N V53.9 T	V51.3 N V51.9 T	V54.3 N V54.9 T	V57.3 N V57.9 T	V50.3 N V50.9 T	V59.29 N V59.69 T	V59.20 N V59.60 T	V55.3 N V55.9 T	V52.3 N V52.9 T	

[a]Non-motor vehicle includes streetcar, animal drawn vehicle, animal being ridden

I = In-line skates; R = roller skates; N = nontraffic accident; T = traffic accident; U = unspecified whether traffic or not

*Refer to the index

ICD-10-CM EXTERNAL CAUSE OF INJURIES TABLE

ICD-10-CM EXTERNAL CAUSE OF INJURIES TABLE

Activity of the Person Injured	Pedestrian Conveyance	Collides with									
		Car/Pick-up Truck/Van	Bike	Bus/HTV	Fixed Object	Pedestrian or Animal	Other (NOS)	Unspecified	Train/Train car	2 or 3 Motor Wheeler	Non-Motor Vehicle[a]
Bus											
Driver		V73.0 N / V73.5 T	V71.0 N / V71.5 T	V74.0 N / V74.5 T	V77.0 N / V77.5 T	V70.0 N / V70.5 T	V79.09N / V79.49 T	V79.00N / V79.40 T	V75.0 N / V75.5 T	V72.0 N / V72.5 T	V76.0 N / V76.5 T
Passenger		V73.1 N / V73.6 T	V71.1 N / V71.6 T	V74.1 N / V74.6 T	V77.1 N / V77.6 T	V70.1 N / V70.6 T	V79.19N / V79.59 T	V79.10 N / V79.50 T	V75.1 N / V75.6 T	V72.1 N / V72.6 T	V76.1 N / V76.6 T
Rider on outside		V73.2 N / V73.7 T	V71.2 N / V71.7 T	V74.2 N / V74.7 T	V77.2 N / V77.7 T	V70.2 N / V70.7 T		V79.3 N / V79.9 T	V75.2 N / V75.7 T	V72.2 N / V72.7 T	V76.2 N / V76.7 T
Boarding		V73.4	V71.4	V74.4	V77.4	V70.4			V75.4	V72.4	V76.4
Unspecified		V73.3 N / V73.9 T	V71.3 N / V71.9 T	V74.3 N / V74.9 T	V77.3 N / V77.9 T	V70.3 N / V70.9 T	V79.29N / V79.69 T	V79.20 N / V79.60 T	V75.3 N / V75.9 T	V72.3 N / V72.9 T	V76.3 N / V76.9 T
Animal Rider		V80.41	V80.21	V80.41	V80.81	*	V80.918	V80.919	V80.61	V80.31	V06.09
Animal-Drawn Vehicle		V80.42	V80.22	V80.42	V80.82	*	V80.928	V80.929	V80.62	V80.32	V06.09

Injured Person	Special Agriculture Vehicle	Vehicle		
		Snowmobile	Dune Buggy	Other ATV (eg, go-cart, golf cart, dirt bike)
Driver	V84.0 T / V84.5 N	V86.02 T / V86.52 N	V86.03 T / V86.53 N	V86.09 T / V86.59 N
Passenger	V84.1 T / V84.6 N	V86.12 T / V86.62 N	V86.13 T / V86.63 N	V86.19 T / V86.69 N
Outside rider	V84.2 T / V84.7 N	V86.22 T / V86.72 N	V86.23 T / V86.73 N	V86.29 T / V86.79 N
Unspecified	V84.3 T / V84.9 N	V86.32 T / V86.92 N	V86.33 T / V86.93 N	V86.39 T / V86.99 N
Boarding	V84.4	V86.42	V86.43	V86.49

[a]Non-motor vehicle includes streetcar, animal drawn vehicle, animal being ridden
I = In-line skates; R = roller skates; N = nontraffic accident; T = traffic accident; U = unspecified whether traffic or not
*Refer to the index

ICD-10-CM EXTERNAL CAUSE
OF INJURIES INDEX

A

Abandonment (causing exposure to weather conditions) (with intent to injure or kill) NEC X58

Abuse (adult) (child) (mental) (physical) (sexual) X58

Accident (to) X58

  aircraft (in transit) (powered) — *see also* Accident, transport, aircraft
    due to, caused by cataclysm — *see* Forces of nature, by type
  animal-rider — *see* Accident, transport, animal-rider
  animal-drawn vehicle — *see* Accident, transport, animal-drawn vehicle occupant
  automobile — *see* Accident, transport, car occupant
  bare foot water skiier V94.4
  boat, boating — *see also* Accident, watercraft
    striking swimmer
      powered V94.11
      unpowered V94.12
  bus — *see* Accident, transport, bus occupant
  cable car, not on rails V98.0
    on rails — *see* Accident, transport, streetcar occupant
  car — *see* Accident, transport, car occupant
  caused by, due to
    animal NEC W64
    chain hoist W24.0
    cold (excessive) — *see* Exposure, cold
    corrosive liquid, substance — *see* Table of Drugs and Chemicals
    cutting or piercing instrument — *see* Contact, with, by type of instrument
    drive belt W24.0
    electric
      current — *see* Exposure, electric current
      motor (see also Contact, with, by type of machine) W31.3
        current (of) W86.8
    environmental factor NEC X58
    explosive material — *see* Explosion
    fire, flames — *see* Exposure, fire
    firearm missile — *see* Discharge, firearm by type
    heat (excessive) — *see* Heat
    hot — *see* Contact, with, hot
    ignition — *see* Ignition
    lifting device W24.0
    lightning — *see* subcategory T75.0
      causing fire — *see* Exposure, fire
    machine, machinery — *see* Contact, with, by type of machine
    natural factor NEC X58
    pulley (block) W24.0
    radiation — *see* Radiation
    steam X13.1
      inhalation X13.0
      pipe X16
    thunderbolt — *see* subcategory T75.0
      causing fire — *see* Exposure, fire
    transmission device W24.1
  diving — *see also* Fall, into, water
    with
      drowning or submersion — *see* Drowning
  ice yacht V98.2
  in
    medical, surgical procedure
      as, or due to misadventure — *see* Misadventure
      causing an abnormal reaction or later complication without mention of misadventure
        (see also Complication of or following, by type of procedure) Y84.9
  land yacht V98.1
  late effect of — *see* W00-X58 with 7th character S
  logging car — *see* Accident, transport, industrial vehicle occupant
  machine, machinery — *see also* Contact, with, by type of machine
    on board watercraft V93.69
      explosion — *see* Explosion, in, watercraft
      fire — *see* Burn, on board watercraft
      powered craft V93.63
        ferry boat V93.61
        fishing boat V93.62
        jetskis V93.63
        liner V93.61
        merchant ship V93.60
        passenger ship V93.61
        sailboat V93.64
  mobility scooter (motorized) — *see* Accident, transport, pedestrian, conveyance, specified type NEC
  motor scooter — *see* Accident, transport, motorcyclist
  motor vehicle NOS (traffic) (see also Accident, transport) V89.2
    nontraffic V89.0
    three-wheeled NOS — *see* Accident, transport, three-wheeled motor vehicle occupant

Accident (to), *continued*

  motorcycle NOS — *see* Accident, transport, motorcyclist
  nonmotor vehicle NOS (nontraffic) (see also Accident, transport) V89.1
    traffic NOS V89.3
  nontraffic (victim's mode of transport NOS) V88.9
    collision (between) V88.7
      bus and truck V88.5
      car and:
        bus V88.3
        pickup V88.2
        three-wheeled motor vehicle V88.0
        train V88.6
        truck V88.4
        two-wheeled motor vehicle V88.0
        van V88.2
      specified vehicle NEC and:
        three-wheeled motor vehicle V88.1
        two-wheeled motor vehicle V88.1
    known mode of transport — *see* Accident, transport, by type of vehicle
    noncollision V88.8
  on board watercraft V93.8-
    inflatable V93.86
      in tow
        recreational V94.31
        specified NEC V94.32
  parachutist V97.29
    entangled in object V97.21
    injured on landing V97.22
  pedal cycle — *see* Accident, transport, pedal cyclist
  pedestrian (on foot)
    with
      another pedestrian W51
        with fall W03
          due to ice or snow W00.0
      transport vehicle — *see* Accident, transport
    on pedestrian conveyance — *see* Accident, transport, pedestrian, conveyance
  quarry truck — *see* Accident, transport, industrial vehicle occupant
  railway vehicle (any) (in motion) — *see* Accident, transport, railway vehicle occupant
    due to cataclysm — *see* Forces of nature, by type
  scooter (non-motorized) — *see* Accident, transport, pedestrian, conveyance, scooter
  skateboard — *see* Accident, transport, pedestrian, conveyance, skateboard
  ski (ing) — *see* Accident, transport, pedestrian, conveyance
    lift V98.3
  specified cause NEC X58
  streetcar — *see* Accident, transport, streetcar occupant
  traffic (victim's mode of transport NOS) V87.9
    collision (between) V87.7
      bus and truck V87.5
      car and:
        bus V87.3
        pickup V87.2
        three-wheeled motor vehicle V87.0
        train V87.6
        truck V87.4
        two-wheeled motor vehicle V87.0
        van V87.2
      specified vehicle NEC and:
        three-wheeled motor vehicle V87.1
        two-wheeled motor vehicle V87.1
    known mode of transport — *see* Accident, transport, by type of vehicle
    noncollision V87.8
  transport (involving injury to) V99
    agricultural vehicle occupant (nontraffic) V84.-
    aircraft V97.8-
      occupant injured (in)
        nonpowered craft accident V96.9
          balloon V96.0-
          glider V96.2-
          hang glider V96.1-
          specified craft NEC V96.8
        powered craft accident V95.9
          fixed wing NEC
            commercial V95.3-
            private V95.2-
          glider (powered) V95.1-
          helicopter V95.0-
          specified craft NEC V95.8
          ultralight V95.1-
        specified accident NEC V97.0
        while boarding or alighting V97.1

Accident (to), *continued*
- person (injured by)
  - falling from, in or on aircraft V97.0
  - machinery on aircraft V97.89
  - on ground with aircraft involvement V97.39
  - while boarding or alighting aircraft V97.1
- airport (battery-powered) passenger vehicle — *see* Accident, transport, industrial vehicle occupant
- all-terrain vehicle occupant (nontraffic) V86.99
  - driver V86.59
  - dune buggy — *see* Accident, transport, dune buggy occupant
  - hanger-on V86.79
  - passenger V86.69
- animal-drawn vehicle occupant (in) V80.929
  - collision (with)
    - animal V80.12
      - being ridden V80.711
    - animal-drawn vehicle V80.721
    - fixed or stationary object V80.82
    - military vehicle V80.920
    - nonmotor vehicle V80.791
    - pedestrian V80.12
    - specified motor vehicle NEC V80.52
    - streetcar V80.731
  - noncollision V80.02
  - specified circumstance NEC V80.928
- animal-rider V80.919
  - collision (with)
    - animal V80.11
      - being ridden V80.710
    - animal-drawn vehicle V80.720
    - fixed or stationary object V80.81
    - nonmotor vehicle V80.790
    - pedestrian V80.11
    - specified motor vehicle NEC V80.51
    - streetcar V80.730
  - noncollision V80.018
    - specified as horse rider V80.010
  - specified circumstance NEC V80.918
- bus occupant V79.9
  - collision (with)
  - driver
    - collision (with)
      - noncollision accident (traffic) V78.5
        - nontraffic V78.0
    - noncollision accident (traffic) V78.9
      - nontraffic V78.3
    - while boarding or alighting V78.4
    - noncollision accident (traffic) V78.7
      - nontraffic V78.2
  - passenger
    - collision (with)
      - noncollision accident (traffic) V78.6
        - nontraffic V78.1
  - specified type NEC V79.88
    - military vehicle V79.81
- cable car, not on rails V98.0
  - on rails — *see* Accident, transport, streetcar occupant
- car occupant V49.9
  - ambulance occupant — *see* Accident, transport, ambulance occupant
  - collision (with)
    - animal being ridden (traffic) V46.9
      - nontraffic V46.3
        - while boarding or alighting V46.4
    - animal-drawn vehicle (traffic) V46.9
      - nontraffic V46.3
      - while boarding or alighting V46.4
    - car (traffic) V43.92
      - nontraffic V43.32
      - while boarding or alighting V43.42
    - motor vehicle NOS (traffic) V49.60
      - nontraffic V49.20
      - specified type NEC (traffic) V49.69
        - nontraffic V49.29
    - pickup truck (traffic) V43.93
      - nontraffic V43.13
      - while boarding or alighting V43.43
    - specified vehicle NEC (traffic) V46.9
      - nontraffic V46.3
      - while boarding or alighting V46.4

Accident (to), *continued*
- sport utility vehicle (traffic) V43.91
  - nontraffic V43.31
  - while boarding or alighting V43.41
- stationary object (traffic) V47.92
  - while boarding or alighting V47.4
- streetcar (traffic) V46.9
  - nontraffic V46.3
  - while boarding or alighting V46.4
- van (traffic) V43.94
  - nontraffic V43.34
  - while boarding or alighting V43.44
- driver
  - collision (with)
    - animal being ridden (traffic) V46.5
      - nontraffic V46.0
    - animal-drawn vehicle (traffic) V46.5
      - nontraffic V46.0
    - car (traffic) V43.52
      - nontraffic V43.02
    - motor vehicle NOS (traffic) V49.40
      - nontraffic V49.00
      - specified type NEC (traffic) V49.49
        - nontraffic V49.09
    - pickup truck (traffic) V43.53
      - nontraffic V43.03
    - specified vehicle NEC (traffic) V46.5
      - nontraffic V46.0
    - sport utility vehicle (traffic) V43.51
      - nontraffic V43.01
    - streetcar (traffic) V46.5
      - nontraffic V46.0
    - van (traffic) V43.54
      - nontraffic V43.04
  - noncollision accident (traffic) V48.5
    - nontraffic V48.0
- noncollision accident (traffic) V48.9
  - nontraffic V48.3
  - while boarding or alighting V48.4
- nontraffic V49.3
- hanger-on
  - collision (with)
    - animal being ridden (traffic) V46.7
      - nontraffic V46.2
    - animal-drawn vehicle (traffic) V46.7
      - nontraffic V46.2
    - car (traffic) V43.72
      - nontraffic V43.22
    - pickup truck (traffic) V43.73
      - nontraffic V43.23
    - specified vehicle NEC (traffic) V46.7
      - nontraffic V46.2
    - sport utility vehicle (traffic) V43.71
      - nontraffic V43.21
    - stationary object (traffic) V47.7
      - nontraffic V47.2
    - streetcar (traffic) V46.7
      - nontraffic V46.2
    - van (traffic) V43.74
      - nontraffic V43.24
  - noncollision accident (traffic) V48.7
    - nontraffic V48.2
- passenger
  - collision (with)
    - animal being ridden (traffic) V46.6
      - nontraffic V46.1
    - animal-drawn vehicle (traffic) V46.6
      - nontraffic V46.1
    - car (traffic) V43.62
      - nontraffic V43.12
    - motor vehicle NOS (traffic) V49.50
      - nontraffic V49.10
      - specified type NEC (traffic) V49.59
        - nontraffic V49.19
    - pickup truck (traffic) V43.63
      - nontraffic V43.13
    - specified vehicle NEC (traffic) V46.6
      - nontraffic V46.1
    - sport utility vehicle (traffic) V43.61
      - nontraffic V43.11
    - streetcar (traffic) V46.6
      - nontraffic V46.1

Accident (to), *continued*
    van (traffic) V43.64
      nontraffic V43.14
    noncollision accident (traffic) V48.6
      nontraffic V48.1
    specified type NEC V49.88
  due to cataclysm — *see* Forces of nature, by type
  ice yacht V98.2
  industrial vehicle occupant (nontraffic) V83.-
  land yacht V98.1
  logging car — *see* Accident, transport, industrial vehicle occupant
  motorcoach — *see* Accident, transport, bus occupant
  motorcyclist V29.9
    collision (with)
      animal being ridden (traffic) V26.9
        nontraffic V26.2
        while boarding or alighting V26.3
      animal-drawn vehicle (traffic) V26.9
        nontraffic V26.2
        while boarding or alighting V26.3
      motor vehicle NOS (traffic) V29.60
        nontraffic V29.20
        specified type NEC (traffic) V29.69
          nontraffic V29.29
      specified vehicle NEC (traffic) V26.9
        nontraffic V26.2
        while boarding or alighting V26.3
      streetcar (traffic) V26.9
        nontraffic V26.2
        while boarding or alighting V26.3
    driver
      collision (with)
        animal being ridden (traffic) V26.4
          nontraffic V26.0
        animal-drawn vehicle (traffic) V26.4
          nontraffic V26.0
        specified vehicle NEC (traffic) V26.4
          nontraffic V26.0
        streetcar (traffic) V26.4
          nontraffic V26.0
      noncollision accident (traffic) V28.4
        nontraffic V28.0
    noncollision accident (traffic) V28.9
      nontraffic V28.2
      while boarding or alighting V28.3
    nontraffic V29.3
    passenger
      collision (with)
        animal being ridden (traffic) V26.5
          nontraffic V26.1
        animal-drawn vehicle (traffic) V26.5
          nontraffic V26.1
        specified vehicle NEC (traffic) V26.5
        streetcar (traffic) V26.5
          nontraffic V26.1
      noncollision accident (traffic) V28.5
        nontraffic V28.1
    specified type NEC V29.88
    military vehicle V29.81
  motor vehicle NEC occupant (traffic) V86.39
  occupant (of)
    aircraft (powered) V95.9
      nonpowered V96.9
      specified NEC V95.8
    airport battery-powered vehicle — *see* Accident, transport, industrial vehicle
        occupant
    all-terrain vehicle (ATV) — *see* Accident, transport, all-terrain vehicle occupant
    animal-drawn vehicle — *see* Accident, transport, animal-drawn vehicle occupant
    automobile — *see* Accident, transport, car occupant
    balloon V96.00
    battery-powered vehicle — *see* Accident, transport, industrial vehicle occupant
    bicycle — *see* Accident, transport, pedal cyclist
      motorized — *see* Accident, transport, motorcycle rider
    boat NEC — *see* Accident, watercraft
    bus — *see* Accident, transport, bus occupant
    cable car (on rails) — *see also* Accident, transport, streetcar occupant
      not on rails V98.0
    car — *see also* Accident, transport, car occupant
      cable (on rails) — *see also* Accident, transport, streetcar occupant
      not on rails V98.0
    coach — *see* Accident, transport, bus occupant
    farm machinery (self-propelled) — *see* Accident, transport, agricultural vehicle
        occupant

Accident (to), *continued*
  forklift — *see* Accident, transport, industrial vehicle occupant
  glider (unpowered) V96.20
    hang V96.10
    powered (microlight) (ultralight) — *see* Accident, transport, aircraft, occupant,
          powered, glider
  glider (unpowered)NEC V96.20
  hang-glider V96.10
  heavy (transport)vehicle — *see* Accident, transport, truck occupant
  ice-yacht V98.2
  kite (carrying person) V96.8
  land-yacht V98.1
  microlight — *see* Accident, transport, aircraft, occupant, powered, glider
  motor scooter — *see* Accident, transport, motorcycle
  motorcycle (with sidecar) — *see* Accident, transport, motorcycle
  pedal cycle — *see also* Accident, transport, pedal cyclist
  pick-up (truck) — *see* Accident, transport, pickup truck occupant
  railway (train) (vehicle) (subterranean) (elevated) — *see* Accident, transport, railway
        vehicle occupant
    motorized — *see* Accident, transport, three-wheeled motor vehicle
    pedal driven — *see* Accident, transport, pedal cyclist
  ship NOS V94.9
  ski-lift (chair) (gondola) V98.3
  sport utility vehicle — *see* Accident, transport, car occupant
  streetcar (interurban) (operating on public street or highway) — *see* Accident,
        transport, streetcar occupant
  three-wheeled vehicle (motorized) — *see also* Accident, transport, three-wheeled
        motor vehicle occupant
    nonmotorized — *see* Accident, transport, pedal cycle
  tractor (farm) (and trailer) — *see* Accident, transport, agricultural vehicle occupant
  train — *see* Accident, transport, railway vehicle occupant
  tram — *see* Accident, transport, streetcar occupant
  tricycle — *see* Accident, transport, pedal cycle
    motorized — *see* Accident, transport, three-wheeled motor vehicle
  trolley — *see* Accident, transport, streetcar occupant
  ultralight — *see* Accident, transport, aircraft, occupant, powered, glider
  van — *see* Accident, transport, van occupant
  vehicle NEC V89.9
    heavy transport — *see* Accident, transport, truck occupant
    motor (traffic)NEC V89.2
      nontraffic NEC V89.0
  watercraft NOS V94.9
    causing drowning — *see* Drowning, resulting from accident to boat
parachutist V97.29
  after accident to aircraft — *see* Accident, transport, aircraft
  entangled in object V97.21
  injured on landing V97.22
pedal cyclist V19.9
  noncollision accident (traffic) V18.4
    nontraffic V18.0
  noncollision accident (traffic) V18.9
    nontraffic V18.2
    while boarding or alighting V18.3
  nontraffic V19.3
  passenger
    noncollision accident (traffic) V18.5
      nontraffic V18.1
  specified type NEC V19.88
  military vehicle V19.81
pedestrian
  conveyance (occupant) V09.9
    babystroller V00.828
      collision (with) V09.9
        stationary object V00.822
        vehicle V09.9
          nontraffic V09.00
          traffic V09.20
      fall V00.821
      nontraffic V09.1
        involving motor vehicle NEC V09.00
      traffic V09.3
        involving motor vehicle NEC V09.20
    flat-bottomed NEC V00.388
      collision (with) V09.9
        stationary object V00.382
        vehicle V09.9
          nontraffic V09.00
          traffic V09.20
      fall V00.381
      nontraffic V09.1
        involving motor vehicle NEC V09.00

Accident (to), *continued*
 snow
  board — *see* Accident, transport, pedestrian, conveyance, snow board
  ski- — *see* Accident, transport, pedestrian, conveyance, skis (snow)
  traffic V09.3
   involving motor vehicle NEC V09.20
 gliding type NEC V00.288
  collision (with) V09.9
   stationary object V00.282
   vehicle V09.9
    nontraffic V09.00
     traffic V09.20
  fall V00.281
  heelies — *see* Accident, transport, pedestrian, conveyance, heelies
  ice skate — *see* Accident, transport, pedestrian, conveyance, ice skate
  nontraffic V09.1
   involving motor vehicle NEC V09.00
  sled — *see* Accident, transport, pedestrian, conveyance, sled
  traffic V09.3
   involving motor vehicle NEC V09.20
   wheelies — *see* Accident, transport, pedestrian, conveyance, heelies
 heelies V00.158
  fall V00.151
 ice skates V00.218
  collision (with) V09.9
   vehicle V09.9
    nontraffic V09.00
     traffic V09.20
  fall V00.211
  nontraffic V09.1
   involving motor vehicle NEC V09.00
  traffic V09.3
   involving motor vehicle NEC V09.20
 motorized mobility scooter V00.838
  collision with stationary object V00.832
  fall from V00.831
  nontraffic V09.1
   involving motor vehicle V09.00
    military V09.01
    specified type NEC V09.09
 roller skates (non in-line) V00.128
  collision (with) V09.9
   stationary object V00.122
   vehicle V09.9
    nontraffic V09.00
     traffic V09.20
  fall V00.121
  in-line V00.118
   collision- — *see also* Accident, transport, pedestrian, conveyance
     occupant, roller skates, collision
    with stationary object V00.112
   fall V00.111
   nontraffic V09.1
    involving motor vehicle NEC V09.00
   traffic V09.3
    involving motor vehicle NEC V09.20
 rolling shoes V00.158
  fall V00.151
 rolling type NEC V00.188
  collision (with) V09.9
   stationary object V00.182
   vehicle V09.9
    nontraffic V09.00
     traffic V09.20
  fall V00.181
  in-line roller skate — *see* Accident, transport, pedestrian, conveyance, roller
    skate, in-line
  nontraffic V09.1
   involving motor vehicle NEC V09.00
  roller skate — *see* Accident, transport, pedestrian, conveyance, roller skate
  scooter (non-motorized) — *see* Accident, transport, pedestrian, conveyance, scooter
  skateboard — *see* Accident, transport, pedestrian, conveyance, skateboard
  traffic V09.3
   involving motor vehicle NEC V09.20
 scooter (non-motorized) V00.148
  collision (with) V09.9
   vehicle V09.9
    nontraffic V09.00
     traffic V09.20
  fall V00.141

Accident (to), *continued*
  nontraffic V09.1
   involving motor vehicle NEC V09.00
  traffic V09.3
   involving motor vehicle NEC V09.20
 skate board V00.138
  collision (with) V09.9
   stationary object V00.132
   vehicle V09.9
    nontraffic V09.00
     traffic V09.20
  fall V00.131
  nontraffic V09.1
   involving motor vehicle NEC V09.00
  traffic V09.3
   involving motor vehicle NEC V09.20
 sled V00.228
  collision (with) V09.9
   vehicle V09.9
    nontraffic V09.00
     traffic V09.20
  fall V00.221
  nontraffic V09.1
   involving motor vehicle NEC V09.00
  traffic V09.3
   involving motor vehicle NEC V09.20
 skis (snow) V00.328
  collision (with) V09.9
   vehicle V09.9
    nontraffic V09.00
     traffic V09.20
  fall V00.321
  nontraffic V09.1
   involving motor vehicle NEC V09.00
  traffic V09.3
   involving motor vehicle NEC V09.20
 snow board V00.318
  collision (with) V09.9
   vehicle V09.9
    nontraffic V09.00
     traffic V09.20
  fall V00.311
  nontraffic V09.1
   involving motor vehicle NEC V09.00
  traffic V09.3
   involving motor vehicle NEC V09.20
 specified type NEC V00.898
  collision (with) V09.9
   stationary object V00.892
   vehicle V09.9
    nontraffic V09.00
     traffic V09.20
  fall V00.891
  nontraffic V09.1
   involving motor vehicle NEC V09.00
  traffic V09.3
   involving motor vehicle NEC V09.20
 traffic V09.3
  involving motor vehicle V09.20
   military V09.21
   specified type NEC V09.29
 wheelchair (powered) V00.818
  collision (with) V09.9
   stationary object V00.812
   vehicle V09.9
    nontraffic V09.00
     traffic V09.20
  fall V00.811
  nontraffic V09.1
   involving motor vehicle NEC V09.00
  traffic V09.3
   involving motor vehicle NEC V09.20
 wheeled shoe V00.158
  fall V00.151
 on foot — *see also* Accident, pedestrian
  collision (with)
   vehicle V09.9
    nontraffic V09.00
     traffic V09.20
  nontraffic V09.1
   involving motor vehicle V09.00
    military V09.01
    specified type NEC V09.09

Accident (to), *continued*
  traffic V09.3
    involving motor vehicle V09.20
      military V09.21
      specified type NEC V09.29
  person NEC (unknown way or transportation) V99
    collision (between)
      bus (with)
        heavy transport vehicle (traffic) V87.5
          nontraffic V88.5
      car (with)
        nontraffic V88.5
        bus (traffic) V87.3
          nontraffic V88.3
        heavy transport vehicle (traffic) V87.4
          nontraffic V88.4
        pick-up truck or van (traffic) V87.2
          nontraffic V88.2
        train or railway vehicle (traffic) V87.6
          nontraffic V88.6
        two-or three-wheeled motor vehicle (traffic) V87.0
          nontraffic V88.0
      motor vehicle (traffic)NEC V87.7
        nontraffic V88.7
      two-or three-wheeled vehicle (with) (traffic)
        motor vehicle NEC V87.1
          nontraffic V88.1
      nonmotor vehicle (collision) (noncollision) (traffic) V87.9
        nontraffic V88.9
  pickup truck occupant V59.9
    collision (with)
      animal (traffic) V50.9
        animal being ridden (traffic) V56.9
          nontraffic V56.3
            while boarding or alighting V56.4
        animal-drawn vehicle (traffic) V56.9
          nontraffic V56.3
            while boarding or alighting V56.4
        motor vehicle NOS (traffic) V59.60
          nontraffic V59.20
          specified type NEC (traffic) V59.69
            nontraffic V59.29
        specified vehicle NEC (traffic) V56.9
          nontraffic V56.3
            while boarding or alighting V56.4
        streetcar (traffic) V56.9
          nontraffic V56.3
            while boarding or alighting V56.4
      driver
        collision (with)
          animal being ridden (traffic) V56.5
            nontraffic V56.0
          animal-drawn vehicle (traffic) V56.5
            nontraffic V56.0
          motor vehicle NOS (traffic) V59.40
            nontraffic V59.00
            specified type NEC (traffic) V59.49
              nontraffic V59.09
          specified vehicle NEC (traffic) V56.5
            nontraffic V56.0
          streetcar (traffic) V56.5
            nontraffic V56.0
        noncollision accident (traffic) V58.5
          nontraffic V58.0
      noncollision accident (traffic) V58.9
        nontraffic V58.3
        while boarding or alighting V58.4
      nontraffic V59.3
      hanger-on
        collision (with)
          animal being ridden (traffic) V56.7
            nontraffic V56.2
          animal-drawn vehicle (traffic) V56.7
            nontraffic V56.2
          specified vehicle NEC (traffic) V56.7
            nontraffic V56.2
          streetcar (traffic) V56.7
            nontraffic V56.2
        noncollision accident (traffic) V58.7
          nontraffic V58.2
      passenger

Accident (to), *continued*
    collision (with)
        animal being ridden (traffic) V56.6
          nontraffic V56.1
        animal-drawn vehicle (traffic) V56.6
          nontraffic V56.1
        motor vehicle NOS (traffic) V59.50
          nontraffic V59.10
          specified type NEC (traffic) V59.59
            nontraffic V59.19
        specified vehicle NEC (traffic) V56.6
          nontraffic V56.1
        streetcar (traffic) V56.6
          nontraffic V56.1
      noncollision accident (traffic) V58.6
        nontraffic V58.1
  specified type NEC V59.88
  military vehicle V59.81
  railway vehicle occupant V81.9
    collision (with) V81.3
      motor vehicle (non-military) (traffic) V81.1
        military V81.83
        nontraffic V81.0
      rolling stock V81.2
      specified object NEC V81.3
    during derailment V81.7
    explosion V81.81
    fall (in railway vehicle) V81.5
      during derailment V81.7
      from railway vehicle V81.6
        during derailment V81.7
        while boarding or alighting V81.4
    fire V81.81
    object falling onto train V81.82
    specified type NEC V81.89
    while boarding or alighting V81.4
  ski lift V98.3
  specified NEC V98.8
  sport utility vehicle occupant
    collision (with)
  streetcar occupant V82.9
    collision (with) V82.3
      motor vehicle (traffic) V82.1
        nontraffic V82.0
      rolling stock V82.2
    during derailment V82.7
    fall (in streetcar) V82.5
      during derailment V82.7
      from streetcar V82.6
        during derailment V82.7
        while boarding or alighting V82.4
      while boarding or alighting V82.4
    specified type NEC V82.8
    while boarding or alighting V82.4
  three-wheeled motor vehicle occupant V39.9
    collision (with)
      motor vehicle NOS (traffic) V39.60
        nontraffic V39.20
        specified type NEC (traffic) V39.69
          nontraffic V39.29
    driver
      collision (with)
        motor vehicle NOS (traffic) V39.40
          nontraffic V39.00
          specified type NEC (traffic) V39.49
            nontraffic V39.09
      noncollision accident (traffic) V38.5
        nontraffic V38.0
    noncollision accident (traffic) V38.9
      nontraffic V38.3
      while boarding or alighting V38.4
    nontraffic V39.3
    hanger-on
      noncollision accident (traffic) V38.7
        nontraffic V38.2
    passenger
      collision (with)
        motor vehicle NOS (traffic) V39.50
          nontraffic V39.10
          specified type NEC (traffic) V39.59
            nontraffic V39.19
      noncollision accident (traffic) V38.6
        nontraffic V38.1

Accident (to), *continued*

    specified type NEC V39.89

      military vehicle V39.81

   tractor (farm) (and trailer) — *see* Accident, transport, agricultural vehicle occupant

   tram — *see* Accident, transport, streetcar

   trolley — *see* Accident, transport, streetcar

   truck (heavy)occupant V69.9

    collision (with)

     animal (traffic) V60.9

      being ridden (traffic) V66.9

       nontraffic V66.3

        while boarding or alighting V66.4

      nontraffic V60.3

      while boarding or alighting V60.4

     animal-drawn vehicle (traffic) V66.9

      nontraffic V66.3

      while boarding or alighting V66.4

     bus (traffic) V64.9

      nontraffic V64.3

      while boarding or alighting V64.4

     car (traffic) V63.9

      nontraffic V63.3

      while boarding or alighting V63.4

     motor vehicle NOS (traffic) V69.60

      nontraffic V69.20

      specified type NEC (traffic) V69.69

       nontraffic V69.29

     pedal cycle (traffic) V61.9

      nontraffic V61.3

      while boarding or alighting V61.4

     pickup truck (traffic) V63.9

      nontraffic V63.3

      while boarding or alighting V63.4

     railway vehicle (traffic) V65.9

      nontraffic V65.3

      while boarding or alighting V65.4

     specified vehicle NEC (traffic) V66.9

      nontraffic V66.3

      while boarding or alighting V66.4

     stationary object (traffic) V67.9

      nontraffic V67.3

      while boarding or alighting V67.4

     streetcar (traffic) V66.9

      nontraffic V66.3

      while boarding or alighting V66.4

     three wheeled motor vehicle (traffic) V62.9

      nontraffic V62.3

      while boarding or alighting V62.4

     truck (traffic) V64.9

      nontraffic V64.3

      while boarding or alighting V64.4

     two wheeled motor vehicle (traffic) V62.9

      nontraffic V62.3

      while boarding or alighting V62.4

     van (traffic) V63.9

      nontraffic V63.3

      while boarding or alighting V63.4

    driver

     collision (with)

      animal (traffic) V60.5

       being ridden (traffic) V66.5

        nontraffic V66.0

       nontraffic V60.0

      animal-drawn vehicle (traffic) V66.5

       nontraffic V66.0

      bus (traffic) V64.5

       nontraffic V64.0

      car (traffic) V63.5

       nontraffic V63.0

      motor vehicle NOS (traffic) V69.40

       nontraffic V69.00

       specified type NEC (traffic) V69.49

        nontraffic V69.09

      pedal cycle (traffic) V61.5

       nontraffic V61.0

      pickup truck (traffic) V63.5

       nontraffic V63.0

      railway vehicle (traffic) V65.5

       nontraffic V65.0

      specified vehicle NEC (traffic) V66.5

       nontraffic V66.0

      stationary object (traffic) V67.5

       nontraffic V67.0

Accident (to), *continued*

      streetcar (traffic) V66.5

       nontraffic V66.0

      three wheeled motor vehicle (traffic) V62.5

       nontraffic V62.0

      truck (traffic) V64.5

       nontraffic V64.0

      two wheeled motor vehicle (traffic) V62.5

       nontraffic V62.0

      van (traffic) V63.5

       nontraffic V63.0

     noncollision accident (traffic) V68.5

      nontraffic V68.0

   hanger-on

    collision (with)

     animal (traffic) V60.7

      being ridden (traffic) V66.7

       nontraffic V66.2

       nontraffic V60.2

     animal-drawn vehicle (traffic) V66.7

      nontraffic V66.2

     bus (traffic) V64.7

      nontraffic V64.2

     car (traffic) V63.7

      nontraffic V63.2

     pedal cycle (traffic) V61.7

      nontraffic V61.2

     pickup truck (traffic) V63.7

      nontraffic V63.2

     railway vehicle (traffic) V65.7

      nontraffic V65.2

     specified vehicle NEC (traffic) V66.7

      nontraffic V66.2

     stationary object (traffic) V67.7

      nontraffic V67.2

     streetcar (traffic) V66.7

      nontraffic V66.2

     three wheeled motor vehicle (traffic) V62.7

      nontraffic V62.2

     truck (traffic) V64.7

      nontraffic V64.2

     two wheeled motor vehicle (traffic) V62.7

      nontraffic V62.2

     van (traffic) V63.7

      nontraffic V63.2

    noncollision accident (traffic) V68.7

     nontraffic V68.2

   noncollision accident (traffic) V68.9

    nontraffic V68.3

    while boarding or alighting V68.4

   nontraffic V69.3

   passenger

    collision (with)

     animal (traffic) V60.6

      being ridden (traffic) V66.6

       nontraffic V66.1

       nontraffic V60.1

     animal-drawn vehicle (traffic) V66.6

      nontraffic V66.1

     bus (traffic) V64.6

      nontraffic V64.1

     car (traffic) V63.6

      nontraffic V63.1

     motor vehicle NOS (traffic) V69.50

      nontraffic V69.10

      specified type NEC (traffic) V69.59

       nontraffic V69.19

     pedal cycle (traffic) V61.6

      nontraffic V61.1

     pickup truck (traffic) V63.6

      nontraffic V63.1

     railway vehicle (traffic) V65.6

      nontraffic V65.1

     specified vehicle NEC (traffic) V66.6

      nontraffic V66.1

     stationary object (traffic) V67.6

      nontraffic V67.1

     streetcar (traffic) V66.6

      nontraffic V66.1

     three wheeled motor vehicle (traffic) V62.6

      nontraffic V62.1

     truck (traffic) V64.6

      nontraffic V64.1

Accident (to), *continued*
  two wheeled motor vehicle (traffic) V62.6
    nontraffic V62.1
  van (traffic) V63.6
    nontraffic V63.1
  noncollision accident (traffic) V68.6
    nontraffic V68.1
  pickup — *see* Accident, transport, pickup truck occupant
  specified type NEC V69.88
    military vehicle V69.81
van occupant V59.9
  collision (with)
    animal (traffic) V50.9
      being ridden (traffic) V56.9
        nontraffic V56.3
          while boarding or alighting V56.4
    animal-drawn vehicle (traffic) V56.9
      nontraffic V56.3
        while boarding or alighting V56.4
    motor vehicle NOS (traffic) V59.60
      nontraffic V59.20
        specified type NEC (traffic) V59.69
          nontraffic V59.29
    specified vehicle NEC (traffic) V56.9
      nontraffic V56.3
        while boarding or alighting V56.4
    streetcar (traffic) V56.9
      nontraffic V56.3
        while boarding or alighting V56.4
  driver
    collision (with)
      animal being ridden (traffic) V56.5
        nontraffic V56.0
      animal-drawn vehicle (traffic) V56.5
        nontraffic V56.0
      motor vehicle NOS (traffic) V59.40
        nontraffic V59.00
          specified type NEC (traffic) V59.49
            nontraffic V59.09
      specified vehicle NEC (traffic) V56.5
      streetcar (traffic) V56.5
        nontraffic V56.0
    noncollision accident (traffic) V58.5
      nontraffic V58.0
  noncollision accident (traffic) V58.9
    nontraffic V58.3
      while boarding or alighting V58.4
  nontraffic V59.3
  hanger-on
    collision (with)
      animal being ridden (traffic) V56.7
        nontraffic V56.2
      animal-drawn vehicle (traffic) V56.7
        nontraffic V56.2
      specified vehicle NEC (traffic) V56.7
        nontraffic V56.2
      streetcar (traffic) V56.7
        nontraffic V56.2
    noncollision accident (traffic) V58.7
      nontraffic V58.2
  passenger
    collision (with)
      animal being ridden (traffic) V56.6
        nontraffic V56.1
      animal-drawn vehicle (traffic) V56.6
      motor vehicle NOS (traffic) V59.50
        nontraffic V59.10
          specified type NEC (traffic) V59.59
            nontraffic V59.19
      specified vehicle NEC (traffic) V56.6
        nontraffic V56.1
      streetcar (traffic) V56.6
        nontraffic V56.1
    noncollision accident (traffic) V58.6
      nontraffic V58.1
  specified type NEC V59.88
    military vehicle V59.81
  watercraft occupant — *see* Accident, watercraft
vehicle NEC V89.9
  animal-drawn NEC — *see* Accident, transport, animal-drawn vehicle occupant
  special
    agricultural — *see* Accident, transport, agricultural vehicle occupant

Accident (to), *continued*
  three-wheeled NEC (motorized) — *see* Accident, transport, three-wheeled motor vehicle occupant
  watercraft V94.9
    causing
      drowning — *see* Drowning, due to, accident to, watercraft
      injury NEC V91.89
        crushed between craft and object V91.19
          powered craft V91.1-
          unpowered craft V91.1-
        fall on board V91.29
          powered craft V91.2-
          unpowered craft V91.2-
        fire on board causing burn V91.09
          powered craft V91.0-
          unpowered craft V91.0-
        hit by falling object V91.39
          powered craft V91.3-
          unpowered craft V91.3-
        specified type NEC V91.89
          powered craft V91.8-
          unpowered craft V91.8-
    nonpowered, struck by
      nonpowered vessel V94.22
      powered vessel V94.21
    specified type NEC V94.89
    striking swimmer
      powered V94.11
      unpowered V94.12
Acid throwing (assault) Y08.89
Activity (involving) (of victim at time of event) Y93.9
  aerobic and step exercise (class) Y93.A3
  alpine skiing Y93.23
  animal care NEC Y93.K9
  arts and handcrafts NEC Y93.D9
  athletics NEC Y93.79
  athletics played as a team or group NEC Y93.69
  athletics played individually NEC Y93.59
  baking Y93.G3
  ballet Y93.41
  barbells Y93.B3
  BASE (Building, Antenna, Span, Earth)jumping Y93.33
  baseball Y93.64
  basketball Y93.67
  bathing (personal) Y93.E1
  beach volleyball Y93.68
  bike riding Y93.55
  blackout game Y93.85
  boogie boarding Y93.18
  bowling Y93.54
  boxing Y93.71
  brass instrument playing Y93.J4
  building construction Y93.H3
  bungee jumping Y93.34
  calisthenics Y93.A2
  canoeing (in calm and turbulent water) Y93.16
  capture the flag Y93.6A
  cardiorespiratory exercise NEC Y93.A9
  caregiving (providing)NEC Y93.F9
    bathing Y93.F1
    lifting Y93.F2
  cellular
    communication device Y93.C2
    telephone Y93.C2
  challenge course Y93.A5
  cheerleading Y93.45
  choking game Y93.85
  circuit training Y93.A4
  cleaning
    floor Y93.E5
  climbing NEC Y93.39
    mountain Y93.31
    rock Y93.31
    wall Y93.31
  clothing care and maintenance NEC Y93.E9
  combatives Y93.75
  computer
    keyboarding Y93.C1
    technology NEC Y93.C9
  confidence course Y93.A5
  construction (building) Y93.H3
  cooking and baking Y93.G3

Activity (involving) (of victim at time of event), *continued*
   cool down exercises Y93.A2
   cricket Y93.69
   crocheting Y93.D1
   cross country skiing Y93.24
   dancing (all types) Y93.41
   digging
      dirt Y93.H1
   dirt digging Y93.H1
   dishwashing Y93.G1
   diving (platform) (springboard) Y93.12
      underwater Y93.15
   dodge ball Y93.6A
   downhill skiing Y93.23
   drum playing Y93.J2
   dumbbells Y93.B3
   electronic
      devices NEC Y93.C9
         hand held interactive Y93.C2
      game playing (using) (with)
         interactive device Y93.C2
         keyboard or other stationary device Y93.C1
   elliptical machine Y93.A1
   exercise (s)
      machines ((primarily) for)
         cardiorespiratory conditioning Y93.A1
         muscle strengthening Y93.B1
      muscle strengthening (non-machine)NEC Y93.B9
   external motion NEC Y93.I9
      rollercoaster Y93.I1
   fainting game Y93.85
   field hockey Y93.65
   figure skating (pairs) (singles) Y93.21
   flag football Y93.62
   floor mopping and cleaning Y93.E5
   food preparation and clean up Y93.G1
   football (American)NOS Y93.61
      flag Y93.62
      tackle Y93.61
      touch Y93.62
   four square Y93.6A
   free weights Y93.B3
   frisbee (ultimate) Y93.74
   furniture
      building Y93.D3
      finishing Y93.D3
      repair Y93.D3
   game playing (electronic)
      using keyboard or other stationary device Y93.C1
      using interactive device Y93.C2
   gardening Y93.H2
   golf Y93.53
   grass drills Y93.A6
   grilling and smoking food Y93.G2
   grooming and shearing an animal Y93.K3
   guerilla drills Y93.A6
   gymnastics (rhythmic) Y93.43
   handball Y93.73
   handcrafts NEC Y93.D9
   hand held interactive electronic device Y93.C2
   hang gliding Y93.35
   hiking (on level or elevated terrain) Y93.01
   hockey (ice) Y93.22
      field Y93.65
   horseback riding Y93.52
   household (interior)maintenance NEC Y93.E9
   ice NEC Y93.29
      dancing or skating Y93.21
      hockey Y93.22
   inline roller skating Y93.51
   ironing Y93.E4
   judo Y93.75
   jumping (off)NEC Y93.39
      BASE (Building, Antenna, Span, Earth) Y93.33
      bungee Y93.34
      jacks Y93.A2
      rope Y93.56
   jumping jacks Y93.A2
   jumping rope Y93.56
   karate Y93.75
   kayaking (in calm and turbulent water) Y93.16
   keyboarding (computer) Y93.C1

Activity (involving) (of victim at time of event), *continued*
   kickball Y93.6A
   knitting Y93.D1
   lacrosse Y93.65
   land maintenance NEC Y93.H9
   landscaping Y93.H2
   laundry Y93.E2
   machines (exercise)
      primarily for cardiorespiratory conditioning Y93.A1
      primarily for muscle strengthening Y93.B1
   maintenance
      exterior building NEC Y93.H9
      household (interior)NEC Y93.E9
      land Y93.H9
      property Y93.H9
   marching (on level or elevated terrain) Y93.01
   martial arts Y93.75
   microwave oven Y93.G3
   milking an animal Y93.K2
   mopping (floor) Y93.E5
   mountain climbing Y93.31
   muscle strengthening
      exercises (non-machine)NEC Y93.B9
      machines Y93.B1
   musical keyboard (electronic)playing Y93.J1
   nordic skiing Y93.24
   obstacle course Y93.A5
   oven (microwave) Y93.G3
   packing up and unpacking in moving to a new residence Y93.E6
   parasailing Y93.19
   percussion instrument playing NEC Y93.J2
   personal
      bathing and showering Y93.E1
      hygiene NEC Y93.E8
      showering Y93.E1
   physical games generally associated with school recess, summer camp and children
             Y93.6A
   physical training NEC Y93.A9
   piano playing Y93.J1
   pilates Y93.B4
   platform diving Y93.12
   playing musical instrument
      brass instrument Y93.J4
      drum Y93.J2
      musical keyboard (electronic) Y93.J1
      percussion instrument NEC Y93.J2
      piano Y93.J1
      string instrument Y93.J3
      winds instrument Y93.J4
   property maintenance
      exterior NEC Y93.H9
      interior NEC Y93.E9
   pruning (garden and lawn) Y93.H2
   pull-ups Y93.B2
   push-ups Y93.B2
   racquetball Y93.73
   rafting (in calm and turbulent water) Y93.16
   raking (leaves) Y93.H1
   rappelling Y93.32
   refereeing a sports activity Y93.81
   residential relocation Y93.E6
   rhythmic gymnastics Y93.43
   rhythmic movement NEC Y93.49
   riding
      horseback Y93.52
      rollercoaster Y93.I1
   rock climbing Y93.31
   rollercoaster riding Y93.I1
   roller skating (inline) Y93.51
   rough housing and horseplay Y93.83
   rowing (in calm and turbulent water) Y93.16
   rugby Y93.63
   running Y93.02
   SCUBA diving Y93.15
   sewing Y93.D2
   shoveling Y93.H1
      dirt Y93.H1
      snow Y93.H1
   showering (personal) Y93.E1
   sit-ups Y93.B2
   skateboarding Y93.51

Activity (involving) (of victim at time of event), *continued*
skating (ice) Y93.21
    roller Y93.51
skiing (alpine) (downhill) Y93.23
    cross country Y93.24
    nordic Y93.24
    water Y93.17
sledding (snow) Y93.23
sleeping (sleep) Y93.84
smoking and grilling food Y93.G2
snorkeling Y93.15
snow NEC Y93.29
    boarding Y93.23
    shoveling Y93.H1
    sledding Y93.23
    tubing Y93.23
soccer Y93.66
softball Y93.64
specified NEC Y93.89
spectator at an event Y93.82
sports NEC Y93.79
    sports played as a team or group NEC Y93.69
    sports played individually NEC Y93.59
springboard diving Y93.12
squash Y93.73
stationary bike Y93.A1
step (stepping) exercise (class) Y93.A3
stepper machine Y93.A1
stove Y93.G3
string instrument playing Y93.J3
surfing Y93.18
    wind Y93.18
swimming Y93.11
tap dancing Y93.41
tennis Y93.73
tobogganing Y93.23
touch football Y93.62
track and field events (non-running) Y93.57
    running Y93.02
trampoline Y93.44
treadmill Y93.A1
trimming shrubs Y93.H2
tubing (in calm and turbulent water) Y93.16
    snow Y93.23
ultimate frisbee Y93.74
underwater diving Y93.15
unpacking in moving to a new residence Y93.E6
use of stove, oven and microwave oven Y93.G3
vacuuming Y93.E3
volleyball (beach) (court) Y93.68
wake boarding Y93.17
walking an animal Y93.K1
walking (on level or elevated terrain) Y93.01
    an animal Y93.K1
wall climbing Y93.31
warm up and cool down exercises Y93.A2
water NEC Y93.19
    aerobics Y93.14
    craft NEC Y93.19
    exercise Y93.14
    polo Y93.13
    skiing Y93.17
    sliding Y93.18
    survival training and testing Y93.19
weeding (garden and lawn) Y93.H2
wind instrument playing Y93.J4
windsurfing Y93.18
wrestling Y93.72
yoga Y93.42
Adverse effect of drugs — *see* Table of Drugs and Chemicals
Air
pressure
    change, rapid
        during
            ascent W94.29
                while (in) (surfacing from)
                    aircraft W94.23
                    deep water diving W94.21
                    underground W94.22
            descent W94.39
                in
                    aircraft W94.31
                    water W94.32

Air, *continued*
high, prolonged W94.0
low, prolonged W94.12
    due to residence or long visit at high altitude W94.11
Alpine sickness W94.11
Altitude sickness W94.11
Anaphylactic shock, anaphylaxis — *see* Table of Drugs and Chemicals
Andes disease W94.11
Arachnidism, arachnoidism X58
Arson (with intent to injure or kill) X97
Asphyxia, asphyxiation
by
    food (bone) (*seed*) (*see* categories T17 and) T18
    gas — *see also* Table of Drugs and Chemicals
from
    fire — *see also* Exposure, fire
    ignition — *see* Ignition
    vomitus T17.81
Aspiration
food (any type) (into respiratory tract) (with asphyxia, obstruction respiratory tract, suffocation) (*see* categories T17 and) T18
foreign body — *see* Foreign body, aspiration
vomitus (with asphyxia, obstruction respiratory tract, suffocation) T17.81
Assassination (attempt) — *see* Assault
Assault (homicidal) (by) (in) Y09
bite (of human being) Y04.1
bodily force Y04.8
    bite Y04.1
    bumping into Y04.2
    sexual (*see* subcategories T74.0,) T76.0
    unarmed fight Y04.0
brawl (hand) (fists) (foot) (unarmed) Y04.0
burning, burns (by fire)NEC X97
    acid Y08.89
    caustic, corrosive substance Y08.89
    chemical from swallowing caustic, corrosive substance — *see* Table of Drugs and Chemicals
    cigarette (s) X97
    hot object X98.9
        fluid NEC X98.2
        household appliance X98.3
        specified NEC X98.8
        steam X98.0
        tap water X98.1
        vapors X98.0
    scalding X97
    steam X98.0
    vitriol Y08.89
caustic, corrosive substance (gas) Y08.89
crashing of
    aircraft Y08.81
    motor vehicle Y03.8
        pushed in front of Y02.0
        run over Y03.0
        specified NEC Y03.8
cutting or piercing instrument X99.9
    dagger X99.2
    glass X99.0
    knife X99.1
    specified NEC X99.8
    sword X99.2
dagger X99.2
drowning (in) X92.9
    bathtub X92.0
    natural water X92.3
    specified NEC X92.8
    swimming pool X92.1
        following fall X92.2
dynamite X96.8
explosive (s) (material) X96.9
fight (hand) (fists) (foot) (unarmed) Y04.0
    with weapon — *see* Assault, by type of weapon
fire X97
firearm X95.9
    airgun X95.01
    handgun X93
    hunting rifle X94.1
    larger X94.9
        specified NEC X94.8
    machine gun X94.2
    shotgun X94.0
    specified NEC X95.8

Assault (homicidal) (by) (in), *continued*
gunshot (wound)NEC — *see* Assault, firearm, by type
incendiary device X97
injury Y09
to child due to criminal abortion attempt NEC Y08.89
knife X99.1
late effect of — *see* X92-Y08 with 7th character S
placing before moving object NEC Y02.8
motor vehicle Y02.0
poisoning — *see* categories T36-T65 with 7th character S
puncture, any part of body — *see* Assault, cutting or piercing instrument
pushing
before moving object NEC Y02.8
motor vehicle Y02.0
subway train Y02.1
train Y02.1
from high place Y01
rape T74.2-
scalding —X97
sexual (by bodily force) T74.2-
shooting — *see* Assault, firearm
specified means NEC Y08.89
stab, any part of body — *see* Assault, cutting or piercing instrument
steam X98.0
striking against
other person Y04.2
sports equipment Y08.09
baseball bat Y08.02
hockey stick Y08.01
struck by
sports equipment Y08.09
baseball bat Y08.02
hockey stick Y08.01
submersion — *see* Assault, drowning
violence Y09
weapon Y09
blunt Y00
cutting or piercing — *see* Assault, cutting or piercing instrument
firearm — *see* Assault, firearm
wound Y09
cutting — *see* Assault, cutting or piercing instrument
gunshot — *see* Assault, firearm
knife X99.1
piercing — *see* Assault, cutting or piercing instrument
puncture — *see* Assault, cutting or piercing instrument
stab — *see* Assault, cutting or piercing instrument
Attack by mammals NEC W55.89
Avalanche — *see* Landslide

B

Barotitis, barodontalgia, barosinusitis, barotrauma (otitic) (sinus)- — *see* Air, pressure
Battered (baby) (child) (person) (syndrome) X58
Bean in nose (*see* categories T17 and) T18
Bed set on fire NEC — *see* Exposure, fire, uncontrolled, building, bed
Bending, injury in — *see* category Y93
Bends- — *see* Air, pressure, change
Bite, bitten by
alligator W58.01
arthropod (nonvenomous)NEC W57
bull W55.21
cat W55.01
cow W55.21
crocodile W58.11
dog W54.0
goat W55.31
hoof stock NEC W55.31
horse W55.11
human being (accidentally) W50.3
with intent to injure or kill Y04.1
as, or caused by, a crowd or human stampede (with fall) W52
assault Y04.1
in
fight Y04.1
insect (nonvenomous) W57
lizard (nonvenomous) W59.01
mammal NEC W55.81
marine W56.31
marine animal (nonvenomous) W56.81
millipede W57
moray eel W56.51
mouse W53.01

Bite, bitten by, *continued*
person (s) (accidentally) W50.3
with intent to injure or kill Y04.1
as, or caused by, a crowd or human stampede (with fall) W52
assault Y04.1
in
fight Y04.1
pig W55.41
raccoon W55.51
rat W53.11
reptile W59.81
lizard W59.01
snake W59.11
turtle W59.21
terrestrial W59.81
rodent W53.81
mouse W53.01
rat W53.11
specified NEC W53.81
squirrel W53.21
shark W56.41
sheep W55.31
snake (nonvenomous) W59.11
spider (nonvenomous) W57
squirrel W53.21
Blizzard X37.2
Blood alcohol level Y90.-
Blow X58
Blowing up — *see* Explosion
Brawl (hand) (fists) (foot) Y04.0
Breakage (accidental) (part of)
ladder (causing fall) W11
scaffolding (causing fall) W12
Broken
glass, contact with — *see* Contact, with, glass
Bumping against, into (accidentally)
object NEC W22.8
with fall — *see* Fall, due to, bumping against, object
caused by crowd or human stampede (with fall) W52
sports equipment W21.9
person (s) W51
with fall W03
due to ice or snow W00.0
assault Y04.2
caused by, a crowd or human stampede (with fall) W52
sports equipment W21.9
Burn, burned, burning (accidental) (by) (from) (on)
acid NEC — *see* Table of Drugs and Chemicals
bed linen — *see* Exposure, fire, uncontrolled, in building, bed
blowtorch X08.8
with ignition of clothing NEC X06.2
nightwear X05
bonfire, campfire (controlled) — *see* also Exposure, fire, controlled, not in building
uncontrolled — *see* Exposure, fire, uncontrolled, not in building
candle X08.8
with ignition of clothing NEC X06.2
nightwear X05
caustic liquid, substance (external) (internal)NEC — *see* Table of Drugs and Chemicals
chemical (external) (internal) — *see* also Table of Drugs and Chemicals
cigar (s) or cigarette(s) X08.8
with ignition of clothing NEC X06.2
nightwear X05
clothes, clothing NEC (from controlled fire) X06.2
with conflagration — *see* Exposure, fire, uncontrolled, building
not in building or structure — *see* Exposure, fire, uncontrolled, not in building
cooker (hot) X15.8
stated as undetermined whether accidental or intentional Y27.3
electric blanket X16
engine (hot) X17
fire, flames — *see* Exposure, fire
flare, Very pistol — *see* Discharge, firearm NEC
heat
from appliance (electrical) (household) (cooking object) X15.-
stated as undetermined whether accidental or intentional Y27.3
in local application or packing during medical or surgical procedure Y63.5
heating
appliance, radiator or pipe X16
hot
air X14.1
cooker X15.8
drink X10.0
engine X17

Burn, burned, burning (accidental) (by) (from) (on), *continued*
 fat X10.2
 fluid NEC X12
 food X10.1
 gases X14.1
 heating appliance X16
 household appliance NEC X15.8
 kettle X15.8
 liquid NEC X12
 machinery X17
 metal (molten) (liquid)NEC X18
 object (not producing fire or flames)NEC X19
 oil (cooking) X10.2
 pipe (s) X16
 radiator X16
 saucepan (glass) (metal) X15.3
 stove (kitchen) X15.0
 substance NEC X19
  caustic or corrosive NEC — *see* Table of Drugs and Chemicals
 toaster X15.1
 tool X17
 vapor X13.1
 water (tap) — *see* Contact, with, hot, tap water
hotplate X15.2
ignition — *see* Ignition
inflicted by other person X97
 by hot objects, hot vapor, and steam — *see* Assault, burning, hot object
internal, from swallowed caustic, corrosive liquid, substance — *see* Table of Drugs and
      Chemicals
iron (hot) X15.8
 stated as undetermined whether accidental or intentional Y27.3
kettle (hot) X15.8
 stated as undetermined whether accidental or intentional Y27.3
lamp (flame) X08.8
 with ignition of clothing NEC X06.2
  nightwear X05
lighter (cigar) (cigarette) X08.8
 with ignition of clothing NEC X06.2
  nightwear X05
lightning — *see* subcategory T75.0
 causing fire — *see* Exposure, fire
liquid (boiling) (hot)NEC X12
 stated as undetermined whether accidental or intentional Y27.2
on board watercraft
 due to
  accident to watercraft V91.09
   powered craft V91.0-
   unpowered craft V91.0-
  fire on board V93.0-
  specified heat source NEC on board V93.19
   ferry boat V93.11
   fishing boat V93.12
   jetskis V93.13
   liner V93.11
   merchant ship V93.10
   passenger ship V93.11
   powered craft NEC V93.13
   sailboat V93.14
machinery (hot) X17
matches X08.8
 with ignition of clothing NEC X06.2
  nightwear X05
mattress — *see* Exposure, fire, uncontrolled, building, bed
medicament, externally applied Y63.5
metal (hot) (liquid) (molten)NEC X18
nightwear (nightclothes, nightdress, gown, pajamas, robe) X05
object (hot)NEC X19
pipe (hot) X16
 smoking X08.8
  with ignition of clothing NEC X06.2
   nightwear X05
powder — *see* Powder burn
radiator (hot) X16
saucepan (hot) (glass) (metal) X15.3
 stated as undetermined whether accidental or intentional Y27.3
self-inflicted X76
 stated as undetermined whether accidental or intentional Y26
steam X13.1
 pipe X16
  stated as undetermined whether accidental or intentional Y27.8
 stated as undetermined whether accidental or intentional Y27.0

Burn, burned, burning (accidental) (by) (from) (on), *continued*
 stove (hot) (kitchen) X15.0
  stated as undetermined whether accidental or intentional Y27.3
 substance (hot)NEC X19
  boiling X12
   stated as undetermined whether accidental or intentional Y27.2
  molten (metal) X18
  hot
   household appliance X77.3
   object X77.9
 stated as undetermined whether accidental or intentional Y27.0
 therapeutic misadventure
  heat in local application or packing during medical or surgical procedure Y63.5
  overdose of radiation Y63.2
 toaster (hot) X15.1
  stated as undetermined whether accidental or intentional Y27.3
 tool (hot) X17
 torch, welding X08.8
  with ignition of clothing NEC X06.2
   nightwear X05
 trash fire (controlled) — *see* Exposure, fire, controlled, not in building
  uncontrolled — *see* Exposure, fire, uncontrolled, not in building
 vapor (hot) X13.1
  stated as undetermined whether accidental or intentional Y27.0
 Very pistol — *see* Discharge, firearm NEC
Butted by animal W55-

C

Caisson disease - — *see* Air, pressure, change
Campfire (exposure to) (controlled) — *see also* Exposure, fire, controlled, not in building
 uncontrolled — *see* Exposure, fire, uncontrolled, not in building Car sickness T75.3
Cat
 bite W55.01
 scratch W55.03
Cataclysm, cataclysmic (any injury)NEC — *see* Forces of nature
Catching fire — *see* Exposure, fire
Caught
 between
  folding object W23.0
  objects (moving) (stationary and moving) W23.0
   and machinery — *see* Contact, with, by type of machine
   stationary W23.1
  sliding door and door frame W23.0
 by, in
  machinery (moving parts of) — *see* Contact, with, by type of machine
  washing-machine wringer W23.0
 under packing crate (due to losing grip) W23.1
Cave-in caused by cataclysmic earth surface movement or eruption — *see* Landslide
Change (s)in air pressure - — *see* Air, pressure, change
Choked, choking (on) (any object except food or vomitus)
 food (bone) (*see*d) (*see* categories T17 and) T18
 vomitus T17.81-
Cloudburst (any injury) X37.8
Cold, exposure to (accidental) (excessive) (extreme) (natural) (place) NEC — *see*
      Exposure, cold
Collapse
 building W20.1
  burning (uncontrolled fire) X00.2
 dam or man-made structure (causing earth movement) X36.0
 machinery — *see* Contact, with, by type of machine
 structure W20.1
  burning (uncontrolled fire) X00.2
Collision (accidental) NEC (*see also* Accident, transport) V89.9
 pedestrian W51
  with fall W03
   due to ice or snow W00.0
   involving pedestrian conveyance — *see* Accident, transport, pedestrian, conveyance
  and
   crowd or human stampede (with fall) W52
   object W22.8
    with fall — *see* Fall, due to, bumping against, object
 person (s) — *see* Collision, pedestrian
 transport vehicle NEC V89.9
  and
   avalanche, fallen or not moving — *see* Accident, transport
    falling or moving — *see* Landslide
   landslide, fallen or not moving — *see* Accident, transport
    falling or moving — *see* Landslide
  due to cataclysm — *see* Forces of nature, by type
Combustion, spontaneous — *see* Ignition

Complication (delayed) of or following (medical or surgical procedure) Y84.9
  with misadventure — *see* Misadventure
  amputation of limb (s) Y83.5
  anastomosis (arteriovenous) (blood vessel) (gastrojejunal) (tendon) (natural or artificial
          material) Y83.2
  aspiration (of fluid) Y84.4
    tissue Y84.8
  biopsy Y84.8
  blood
    sampling Y84.7
    transfusion
        procedure Y84.8
  bypass Y83.2
  catheterization (urinary) Y84.6
    cardiac Y84.0
  colostomy Y83.3
  cystostomy Y83.3
  dialysis (kidney) Y84.1
  drug — *see* Table of Drugs and Chemicals
  due to misadventure — *see* Misadventure
  duodenostomy Y83.3
  electroshock therapy Y84.3
  external stoma, creation of Y83.3
  formation of external stoma Y83.3
  gastrostomy Y83.3
  graft Y83.2
  hypothermia (medically-induced) Y84.8
  implant, implantation (of)
    artificial
      internal device (cardiac pacemaker) (electrodes in brain) (heart valve prosthesis)
          (orthopedic) Y83.1
      material or tissue (for anastomosis or bypass) Y83.2
        with creation of external stoma Y83.3
      natural tissues (for anastomosis or bypass) Y83.2
        with creation of external stoma Y83.3
  infusion
    procedure Y84.8
  injection — *see* Table of Drugs and Chemicals
    procedure Y84.8
  insertion of gastric or duodenal sound Y84.5
  insulin-shock therapy Y84.3
  paracentesis (abdominal) (thoracic) (aspirative) Y84.4
  procedures other than surgical operation — *see* Complication of or following, by type of
          procedure
  radiological procedure or therapy Y84.2
  removal of organ (partial) (total)NEC Y83.6
  sampling
    blood Y84.7
    fluid NEC Y84.4
    tissue Y84.8
  shock therapy Y84.3
  surgical operation NEC (*see also* Complication of or following, by type of operation) Y83.9
    reconstructive NEC Y83.4
      with
        anastomosis, bypass or graft Y83.2
        formation of external stoma Y83.3
    specified NEC Y83.8
  transfusion — *see also* Table of Drugs and Chemicals
    procedure Y84.8
  transplant, transplantation (heart) (kidney) (liver) (whole organ, any) Y83.0
    partial organ Y83.4
  ureterostomy Y83.3
  vaccination — *see also* Table of Drugs and Chemicals
    procedure Y84.8
Compression
  divers' squeeze - — *see* Air, pressure, change
  trachea by
    food (lodged in esophagus) (*see* categories T17 and T18
    vomitus (lodged in esophagus) T17.81- Conflagration — *see* Exposure, fire, uncontrolled
          Constriction (external)
  hair W49.01
  jewelry W49.04
  ring W49.04
  rubber band W49.03
  specified item NEC W49.09
  string W49.02
  thread W49.02

Contact (accidental)
  with
    abrasive wheel (metalworking) W31.1
    alligator W58.0-
    amphibian W62.9
      frog W62.0
      toad W62.1
    animal (nonvenomous) NEC W64 (refer to specific animal by name in alphabetical order
          under "contact")
      marine W56.8-
    animate mechanical force NEC W64
    arrow W21.89
      not thrown, projected or falling W45.8
    arthropods (nonvenomous) W57
    axe W27.0
    band-saw (industrial) W31.2
    bayonet — *see* Bayonet wound
    bee (s) X58
    bench-saw (industrial) W31.2
    bird W61.9-
    blender W29.0
    boiling water X12
      stated as undetermined whether accidental or intentional Y27.2
    bore, earth-drilling or mining (land) (seabed) W31.0
    buffalo W55.39
    bull W55.2-
    bumper cars W31.81
    camel W55.39
    can
      lid W26.8
      opener W27.4
        powered W29.0
    cat W55.09
      bite W55.01
      scratch W55.03
    caterpillar (venomous) X58
    centipede (venomous) X58
    chain
      hoist W24.0
        agricultural operations W30.89
      saw W29.3
    chicken W61.3-
    chisel W27.0
    circular saw W31.2
    cobra X58
    combine (harvester) W30.0
    conveyer belt W24.1
    cooker (hot) X15.8
      stated as undetermined whether accidental or intentional Y27.3
    coral X58
    cotton gin W31.82
    cow W55.2-
    crocodile W58.1-
    dagger W26.1
      stated as undetermined whether accidental or intentional Y28.2
    dairy equipment W31.82
    dart W21.89
      not thrown, projected or falling W26.8
    deer W55.39
    derrick W24.0
      agricultural operations W30.89
        hay W30.2
    dog W54.-
    dolphin W56.0-
    donkey W55.39
    drill (powered) W29.8
      earth (land) (seabed) W31.0
      nonpowered W27.8
    drive belt W24.0
      agricultural operations W30.89
    dry ice — *see* Exposure, cold, man-made
    dryer (clothes) (powered) (spin) W29.2
    duck W61.69
    earth (-)
      drilling machine (industrial) W31.0
      scraping machine in stationary use W31.83
    edge of stiff paper W26.2
    electric
      beater W29.0
      blanket X16
      fan W29.2
        commercial W31.82

Contact (accidental), *continued*
    knife W29.1
    mixer W29.0
  elevator (building) W24.0
    agricultural operations W30.89
      grain W30.3
  engine (s), hot NEC X17
  excavating machine W31.0
  farm machine W30.9
  feces — *see* Contact, with, by type of animal
  fer de lance X58
  fish W56.5-
  flying horses W31.81
  forging (metalworking)machine W31.1
  fork W27.4
  forklift (truck) W24.0
    agricultural operations W30.89
  frog W62.0
  garden
    cultivator (powered) W29.3
      riding W30.89
    fork W27.1
  gas turbine W31.3
  Gila monster X58
  giraffe W55.39
  glass (sharp) (broken) W25
    with subsequent fall W18.02
    assault X99.0
    due to fall — *see* Fall, by type
    stated as undetermined whether accidental or intentional Y28.0
  goat W55.3-
  goose W61.5-
  hand
    saw W27.0
    tool (not powered)NEC W27.8
      powered W29.8
  harvester W30.0
  hay-derrick W30.2
  heat NEC X19
    from appliance (electrical) (household) — *see* Contact, with, hot, household appliance
    heating appliance X16
  heating
    appliance (hot) X16
    pad (electric) X16
  hedge-trimmer (powered) W29.3
  hoe W27.1
  hoist (chain) (shaft)NEC W24.0
    agricultural W30.89
  hoof stock NEC W55.3-
  hornet (s) X58
  horse W55.1-
  hot
    air X14.1
      inhalation X14.0
    cooker X15.8
    drinks X10.0
    engine X17
    fats X10.2
    fluids NEC X12
      assault X98.2
      undetermined whether accidental or intentional Y27.2
    food X10.1
    gases X14.1
      inhalation X14.0
    heating appliance X16
    household appliance X15.-
      assault X98.3
      object NEC X19
        assault X98.8
        stated as undetermined whether accidental or intentional Y27.9
      stated as undetermined whether accidental or intentional Y27.3
    kettle X15.8
    light bulb X15.8
    liquid NEC (*see also* Burn) X12
      drinks X10.0
      stated as undetermined whether accidental or intentional Y27.2
      tap water X11.8
        stated as undetermined whether accidental or intentional Y27.1
    machinery X17
    metal (molten) (liquid)NEC X18
    object (not producing fire or flames)NEC X19

Contact (accidental), *continued*
  oil (cooking) X10.2
  pipe X16
  plate X15.2
  radiator X16
  saucepan (glass) (metal) X15.3
  skillet X15.3
  stove (kitchen) X15.0
  substance NEC X19
  tap-water X11.8
    assault X98.1
    heated on stove X12
      stated as undetermined whether accidental or intentional Y27.2
    in bathtub X11.0
    running X11.1
    stated as undetermined whether accidental or intentional Y27.1
  toaster X15.1
  tool X17
  vapors X13.1
    inhalation X13.0
  water (tap) X11.8
    boiling X12
      stated as undetermined whether accidental or intentional Y27.2
    heated on stove X12
      stated as undetermined whether accidental or intentional Y27.2
    in bathtub X11.0
    running X11.1
    stated as undetermined whether accidental or intentional Y27.1
hotplate X15.2
ice-pick W27.4
insect (nonvenomous)NEC W57
kettle (hot) X15.8
knife W26.0
  assault X99.1
  electric W29.1
  stated as undetermined whether accidental or intentional Y28.1
  suicide (attempt) X78.1
lathe (metalworking) W31.1
  turnings W45.8
  woodworking W31.2
lawnmower (powered) (ridden) W28
  causing electrocution W86.8
  unpowered W27.1
lift, lifting (devices) W24.0
  agricultural operations W30.89
  shaft W24.0
liquefied gas — *see* Exposure, cold, man-made
liquid air, hydrogen, nitrogen — *see* Exposure, cold, man-made
lizard (nonvenomous) W59.09
  bite W59.01
  strike W59.02
llama W55.39
macaw W61.1-
machine, machinery W31.9
  abrasive wheel W31.1
  agricultural including animal-powered W30.-
  band or bench or circular saw W31.2
  commercial NEC W31.82
  drilling, metal (industrial) W31.1
  earth-drilling W31.0
  earthmoving or scraping W31.89
  excavating W31.89
  forging machine W31.1
  gas turbine W31.3
  hot X17
  internal combustion engine W31.3
  land drill W31.0
  lathe W31.1
  lifting (devices) W24.0
  metal drill W31.1
  metalworking (industrial) W31.1
  milling, metal W31.1
  mining W31.0
  molding W31.2
  overhead plane W31.2
  power press, metal W31.1
  prime mover W31.3
  printing W31.89
  radial saw W31.2
  recreational W31.81
  roller-coaster W31.81
  rolling mill, metal W31.1
  sander W31.2

Contact (accidental), *continued*
    seabed drill W31.0
    shaft
      hoist W31.0
      lift W31.0
    specified NEC W31.89
    spinning W31.89
    steam engine W31.3
    transmission W24.1
    undercutter W31.0
    water driven turbine W31.3
    weaving W31.89
    woodworking or forming (industrial) W31.2
  mammal (feces) (urine) W55.89
    marine W56.39 (refer to specific animal by name)
      specified NEC W56.3-
    specified NEC W55.8-
  marine
    animal W56.8- (refer to specific animal by name)
  meat
    grinder (domestic) W29.0
      industrial W31.82
      nonpowered W27.4
    slicer (domestic) W29.0
      industrial W31.82
  merry go round W31.81
  metal, hot (liquid) (molten)NEC X18
  millipede W57
  nail W45.0
    gun W29.4
  needle (sewing) W27.3
    hypodermic W46.0
      contaminated W46.1
  object (blunt)NEC
    hot NEC X19
    sharp NEC W26.8
      inflicted by other person NEC W26.8
      self-inflicted X78.9
  orca W56.2-
  overhead plane W31.2
  paper (as sharp object) W26.2
  paper-cutter W27.5
  parrot W61.0-
  pig W55.4-
  pipe, hot X16
  pitchfork W27.1
  plane (metal) (wood) W27.0
    overhead W31.2
  plant thorns, spines, sharp leaves or other mechanisms W60
  powered
    garden cultivator W29.3
    household appliance, implement, or machine W29.8
    saw (industrial) W31.2
      hand W29.8
  printing machine W31.89
  psittacine bird W61.2-
    strike W61.22
  pulley (block) (transmission) W24.0
    agricultural operations W30.89
  raccoon W55.5-
  radial-saw (industrial) W31.2
  radiator (hot) X16
  rake W27.1
  rattlesnake X58
  reaper W30.0
  reptile W59.8- (refer to specific reptile by name)
  rivet gun (powered) W29.4
  rodent (feces) (urine) W53.8-
    mouse W53.0-
    rat W53.1-
    specified NEC W53.8-
    squirrel W53.2-
  roller coaster W31.81
  rope NEC W24.0
    agricultural operations W30.89
  saliva — *see* Contact, with, by type of animal
  sander W29.8
    industrial W31.2
  saucepan (hot) (glass) (metal) X15.3

Contact (accidental), *continued*
  saw W27.0
    band (industrial) W31.2
    bench (industrial) W31.2
    chain W29.3
    hand W27.0
  sawing machine, metal W31.1
  scissors W27.2
  scorpion X58
  screwdriver W27.0
    powered W29.8
  sea
    anemone, cucumber or urchin (spine) X58
    lion W56.1-
  sewing-machine (electric) (powered) W29.2
    not powered W27.8
  shaft (hoist) (lift) (transmission)NEC W24.0
    agricultural W30.89
  shark W56.4-
  shears (hand) W27.2
    powered (industrial) W31.1
      domestic W29.2
  sheep W55.3-
  shovel W27.8
  snake (nonvenomous) W59.11
  spade W27.1
  spider (venomous) X58
  spin-drier W29.2
  spinning machine W31.89
  splinter W45.8
  sports equipment W21.9
  staple gun (powered) W29.8
  steam X13.1
    engine W31.3
    inhalation X13.0
    pipe X16
    shovel W31.89
  stove (hot) (kitchen) X15.0
  substance, hot NEC X19
    molten (metal) X18
  sword W26.1
    assault X99.2
    stated as undetermined whether accidental or intentional Y28.2
  tarantula X58
  thresher W30.0
  tin can lid W26.8
  toad W62.1
  toaster (hot) X15.1
  tool W27.8
    hand (not powered) W27.8
      auger W27.0
      axe W27.0
      can opener W27.4
      chisel W27.0
      fork W27.4
      garden W27.1
      handsaw W27.0
      hoe W27.1
      ice-pick W27.4
      kitchen utensil W27.4
      manual
        lawn mower W27.1
        sewing machine W27.8
      meat grinder W27.4
      needle (sewing) W27.3
        hypodermic W46.0
          contaminated W46.1
      paper cutter W27.5
      pitchfork W27.1
      rake W27.1
      scissors W27.2
      screwdriver W27.0
      specified NEC W27.8
      workbench W27.0
    hot X17
    powered W29.8
      blender W29.0
        commercial W31.82
      can opener W29.0
        commercial W31.82
      chainsaw W29.3

Contact (accidental), *continued*
    clothes dryer W29.2
      commercial W31.82
    dishwasher W29.2
      commercial W31.82
    edger W29.3
    electric fan W29.2
      commercial W31.82
    electric knife W29.1
    food processor W29.0
      commercial W31.82
    garbage disposal W29.0
      commercial W31.82
    garden tool W29.3
    hedge trimmer W29.3
    ice maker W29.0
      commercial W31.82
    kitchen appliance W29.0
      commercial W31.82
    lawn mower W28
    meat grinder W29.0
      commercial W31.82
    mixer W29.0
      commercial W31.82
    rototiller W29.3
    sewing machine W29.2
      commercial W31.82
    washing machine W29.2
      commercial W31.82
  transmission device (belt, cable, chain, gear, pinion, shaft) W24.1
    agricultural operations W30.89
  turbine (gas) (water-driven) W31.3
  turkey W61.4-
  turtle (nonvenomous) W59.2-
    terrestrial W59.8-
  under-cutter W31.0
  vehicle
    agricultural use (transport) — *see* Accident, transport, agricultural vehicle
      not on public highway W30.81
    industrial use (transport) — *see* Accident, transport, industrial vehicle
      not on public highway W31.83
    off-road use (transport) — *see* Accident, transport, all-terrain or off-road vehicle
      not on public highway W31.83
  venomous animal/plant X58
  viper X58
  washing-machine (powered) W29.2
  wasp X58
  weaving-machine W31.89
  winch W24.0
    agricultural operations W30.89
  wire NEC W24.0
    agricultural operations W30.89
  wood slivers W45.8
  yellow jacket X58
  zebra W55.39
Coup de soleil X32
Crash
  aircraft (in transit) (powered) V95.9
    balloon V96.01
    fixed wing NEC (private) V95.21
      commercial V95.31
    glider V96.21
      hang V96.11
      powered V95.11
    helicopter V95.01
    microlight V95.11
    nonpowered V96.9
      specified NEC V96.8
    powered NEC V95.8
    stated as
      homicide (attempt) Y08.81
      suicide (attempt) X83.0
    ultralight V95.11
  transport vehicle NEC (*see also* Accident, transport) V89.9
Crushed (accidentally) X58
  between objects (moving) (stationary and moving) W23.0
    stationary W23.1
  by
    alligator W58.03
    avalanche NEC — *see* Landslide
    cave-in W20.0
      caused by cataclysmic earth surface movement — *see* Landslide
    crocodile W58.13

Crushed (accidentally), *continued*
  crowd or human stampede W52
  falling
    aircraft V97.39
    earth, material W20.0
      caused by cataclysmic earth surface movement — *see* Landslide
    object NEC W20.8
  landslide NEC — *see* Landslide
  lizard (nonvenomous) W59.09
  machinery — *see* Contact, with, by type of machine
  reptile NEC W59.89
  snake (nonvenomous) W59.13
  in
    machinery — *see* Contact, with, by type of machine
Cut, cutting (any part of body) (accidental) — *see also* Contact, with, by object or machine
  during medical or surgical treatment as misadventure — *see* Index to Diseases and Injuries, Complications
  inflicted by other person — *see* Assault, cutting or piercing instrument
  machine NEC (*see also* Contact, with, by type of machine) W31.9
  self-inflicted — *see* Suicide, cutting or piercing instrument
  suicide (attempt) — *see* Suicide, cutting or piercing instrument
Cyclone (any injury) X37.1

D

Dehydration from lack of water X58
Deprivation X58
Derailment (accidental)
  railway (rolling stock) (train) (vehicle) (without antecedent collision) V81.7
    with antecedent collision — *see* Accident, transport, railway vehicle occupant
  streetcar (without antecedent collision) V82.7
    with antecedent collision — *see* Accident, transport, streetcar occupant
Descent
  parachute (voluntary) (without accident to aircraft) V97.29
    due to accident to aircraft — *see* Accident, transport, aircraft
Desertion X58
Destitution X58
Disability, late effect or sequela of injury — *see* Sequelae
Discharge (accidental)
  airgun W34.010
    assault X95.01
    stated as undetermined whether accidental or intentional Y24.0
  BB gun — *see* Discharge, airgun
  firearm (accidental) W34.00
    assault X95.9
    handgun (pistol) (revolver) W32.0
      assault X93
      stated as undetermined whether accidental or intentional Y22
    homicide (attempt) X95.9
    hunting rifle W33.02
      assault X94.1
      stated as undetermined whether accidental or intentional Y23.1
    larger W33.00
      assault X94.9
      hunting rifle — *see* Discharge, firearm, hunting rifle
      shotgun — *see* Discharge, firearm, shotgun
      specified NEC W33.09
        assault X94.8
        stated as undetermined whether accidental or intentional Y23.8
      stated as undetermined whether accidental or intentional Y23.9
      using rubber bullet
        injuring
          bystander Y35.042
          law enforcement personnel Y35.041
          suspect Y35.043
    machine gun W33.03
      assault X94.2
      stated as undetermined whether accidental or intentional Y23.3
    pellet gun — *see* Discharge, airgun
    shotgun W33.01
      assault X94.0
      stated as undetermined whether accidental or intentional Y23.0
    specified NEC W34.09
      assault X95.8
      stated as undetermined whether accidental or intentional Y24.8
    stated as undetermined whether accidental or intentional Y24.9
    Very pistol W34.09
      assault X95.8
      stated as undetermined whether accidental or intentional Y24.8
  firework (s) W39
    stated as undetermined whether accidental or intentional Y25
  gas-operated gun NEC W34.018

Discharge (accidental), *continued*
    airgun — *see* Discharge, airgun
    assault X95.09
    paintball gun — *see* Discharge, paintball gun
    stated as undetermined whether accidental or intentional Y24.8
    gun NEC — *see also* Discharge, firearm NEC
      air — *see* Discharge, airgun
      BB — *see* Discharge, airgun
      for single hand use — *see* Discharge, firearm, handgun
      hand — *see* Discharge, firearm, handgun
      machine — *see* Discharge, firearm, machine gun
      other specified — *see* Discharge, firearm NEC
      paintball — *see* Discharge, paintball gun
      pellet — *see* Discharge, airgun
    handgun — *see* Discharge, firearm, handgun
    machine gun — *see* Discharge, firearm, machine gun
    paintball gun W34.011
      assault X95.02
      stated as undetermined whether accidental or intentional Y24.8
    rifle (hunting) — *see* Discharge, firearm, hunting rifle
    shotgun — *see* Discharge, firearm, shotgun
    spring-operated gun NEC W34.018
      assault / homicide (attempt) X95.09
      stated as undetermined whether accidental or intentional Y24.8
Diver's disease, palsy, paralysis, squeeze - — *see* Air, pressure
Diving (into water) — *see* Accident, diving
Dog bite W54.0
Dragged by transport vehicle NEC (*see also* Accident, transport) V09.9
Drinking poison (accidental) — *see* Table of Drugs and Chemicals
Dropped (accidentally)while being carried or supported by other person W04
Drowning (accidental) W74
  assault X92.9
  due to
    accident (to)
      machinery — *see* Contact, with, by type of machine
      watercraft V90.89
        burning V90.29
          powered V90.2-
          unpowered V90.2-
        crushed V90.39
          powered V90.3-
          unpowered V90.3-
        overturning V90.09
          powered V90.0-
          unpowered V90.0-
        sinking V90.19
          powered V90.1-
          unpowered V90.1-
        specified type NEC V90.89
          powered V90.8-
          unpowered V90.8-
    avalanche — *see* Landslide
    cataclysmic
      earth surface movement NEC — *see* Forces of nature, earth movement
      storm — *see* Forces of nature, cataclysmic storm
    cloudburst X37.8
    cyclone X37.1
    fall overboard (from) V92.09
      powered craft V92.0-
      unpowered craft V92.0-
      resulting from
        accident to watercraft — *see* Drowning, due to, accident to, watercraft
        being washed overboard (from) V92.29
          powered craft V92.2-
          unpowered craft V92.2-
        motion of watercraft V92.19
          powered craft V92.1-
          unpowered craft V92.1-
    hurricane X37.0
    jumping into water from watercraft (involved in accident) — *see also* Drowning, due to, accident to, watercraft
      without accident to or on watercraft W16.711
    torrential rain X37.8
  following
    fall
      into
        bathtub W16.211
        bucket W16.221
        fountain — *see* Drowning, following, fall, into, water, specified NEC
        quarry — *see* Drowning, following, fall, into, water, specified NEC
        reservoir — *see* Drowning, following, fall, into, water, specified NEC
        swimming-pool W16.011

Drowning (accidental), *continued*
      striking
        bottom W16.021
        wall W16.031
      stated as undetermined whether accidental or intentional Y21.3
      water NOS W16.41
        natural (lake) (open sea) (river) (stream) (pond) W16.111
          striking
            bottom W16.121
            side W16.131
        specified NEC W16.311
          striking
            bottom W16.321
            wall W16.331
    overboard NEC — *see* Drowning, due to, fall overboard
    jump or dive
      from boat W16.711
        striking bottom W16.721
      into
        fountain — *see* Drowning, following, jump or dive, into, water, specified NEC
        quarry — *see* Drowning, following, jump or dive, into, water, specified NEC
        reservoir — *see* Drowning, following, jump or dive, into, water, specified NEC
        swimming-pool W16.511
          striking
            bottom W16.521
            wall W16.531
        water NOS W16.91
          natural (lake) (open sea) (river) (stream) (pond) W16.611
          specified NEC W16.811
            striking
             bottom W16.821
             wall W16.831
          striking bottom W16.621
  in
    bathtub (accidental) W65
      assault X92.0
      following fall W16.211
        stated as undetermined whether accidental or intentional Y21.1
      stated as undetermined whether accidental or intentional Y21.0
    lake — *see* Drowning, in, natural water
    natural water (lake) (open sea) (river) (stream) (pond) W69
      assault X92.3
      following
        dive or jump W16.611
          striking bottom W16.621
        fall W16.111
          striking
           bottom W16.121
           side W16.131
      stated as undetermined whether accidental or intentional Y21.4
    quarry — *see* Drowning, in, specified place NEC
    quenching tank — *see* Drowning, in, specified place NEC
    reservoir — *see* Drowning, in, specified place NEC
    river — *see* Drowning, in, natural water
    sea — *see* Drowning, in, natural water
    specified place NEC W73
      assault X92.8
      following
        dive or jump W16.811
          striking
           bottom W16.821
           wall W16.831
        fall W16.311
          striking
           bottom W16.321
           wall W16.331
      stated as undetermined whether accidental or intentional Y21.8
    stream — *see* Drowning, in, natural water
    swimming-pool W67
      assault X92.1
        following fall X92.2
      following
        dive or jump W16.511
          striking
           bottom W16.521
           wall W16.531
        fall W16.011
          striking
           bottom W16.021
           wall W16.031
      stated as undetermined whether accidental or intentional Y21.2
        following fall Y21.3
        following fall X71.2

Drowning (accidental), *continued*
    resulting from accident to watercraft *see* Drowning, due to, accident, watercraft
    self-inflicted X71.9
    stated as undetermined whether accidental or intentional Y21.9

E

Earth (surface)movement NEC — *see* Forces of nature, earth movement
Earth falling (on) W20.0
    caused by cataclysmic earth surface movement or eruption — *see* Landslide
Earthquake (any injury) X34
Effect (s) (adverse)of
    air pressure (any)- — *see* Air, pressure
    cold, excessive (exposure to) — *see* Exposure, cold
    heat (excessive) — *see* Heat
    hot place (weather) — *see* Heat
    insolation X30
    late — *see* Sequelae
    motion — *see* Motion
    radiation — *see* Radiation
    travel — *see* Travel
Electric shock (accidental) (by) (in) — *see* Exposure, electric current Electrocution
            (accidental) — *see* Exposure, electric current
            Endotracheal tube wrongly placed during anesthetic
            procedure Entanglement
    in
        bed linen, causing suffocation — *see* category T71
        wheel of pedal cycle V19.88
Entry of foreign body or material — *see* Foreign body
Environmental pollution related condition- *see* Z57
Exhaustion
    cold — *see* Exposure, cold
    due to excessive exertion — *see* category Y93
    heat — *see* Heat
Explosion (accidental) (of) (with secondary fire) W40.9
    acetylene W40.1
    aerosol can W36.1
    air tank (compressed) (in machinery) W36.2
    aircraft (in transit) (powered)NEC V95.9
        balloon V96.05
        fixed wing NEC (private) V95.25
            commercial V95.35
        glider V96.25
            hang V96.15
            powered V95.15
        helicopter V95.05
        microlight V95.15
        nonpowered V96.9
            specified NEC V96.8
        powered NEC V95.8
        ultralight V95.15
    anesthetic gas in operating room W40.1
    bicycle tire W37.0
    blasting (cap) (materials) W40.0
    boiler (machinery), not on transport vehicle W35
        on watercraft — *see* Explosion, in, watercraft
    butane W40.1
    caused by other person X96.9
    coal gas W40.1
    detonator W40.0
    dump (munitions) W40.8
    dynamite W40.0
        in
            assault X96.8
    explosive (material) W40.9
        gas W40.1
        specified NEC W40.8
            in
    factory (munitions) W40.8
    firearm (parts)NEC W34.19
        airgun W34.110
        BB gun W34.110
        gas, air or spring-operated gun NEC W34.118
        hangun W32.1
        hunting rifle W33.12
        larger firearm W33.10
            specified NEC W33.19
        machine gun W33.13
        paintball gun W34.111
        pellet gun W34.110
        shotgun W33.11
        Very pistol [flare] W34.19
    fire-damp W40.1

Explosion (accidental) (of) (with secondary fire), *continued*
    fireworks W39
    gas (coal) (explosive) W40.1
        cylinder W36.9
            aerosol can W36.1
            air tank W36.2
            pressurized W36.3
            specified NEC W36.8
    gasoline (fumes) (tank)not in moving motor vehicle W40.1
        in motor vehicle — *see* Accident, transport, by type of vehicle
    grain store W40.8
    handgun (parts) — *see* Explosion, firearm, hangun (parts)
    homicide (attempt) X96.9
        specified NEC X96.8
    hose, pressurized W37.8
    hot water heater, tank (in machinery) W35
        on watercraft — *see* Explosion, in, watercraft
    in, on
        dump W40.8
        factory W40.8
        watercraft V93.59
            powered craft V93.53
                ferry boat V93.51
                fishing boat V93.52
                jetskis V93.53
                liner V93.51
                merchant ship V93.50
                passenger ship V93.51
                sailboat V93.54
    machinery — *see also* Contact, with, by type of machine
        on board watercraft — *see* Explosion, in, watercraft
        pressure vessel — *see* Explosion, by type of vessel
    methane W40.1
    missile NEC W40.8
    munitions (dump) (factory) W40.8
    pipe, pressurized W37.8
    pressure, pressurized
        cooker W38
        gas tank (in machinery) W36.3
        hose W37.8
        pipe W37.8
        specified device NEC W38
        tire W37.8
            bicycle W37.0
        vessel (in machinery) W38
    propane W40.1
    self-inflicted X75
    steam or water lines (in machinery) W37.8
    stove W40.9
    stated as undetermined whether accidental or intentional Y25
    tire, pressurized W37.8
        bicycle W37.0
    undetermined whether accidental or intentional Y25
    vehicle tire NEC W37.8
        bicycle W37.0
Exposure (to) X58
    air pressure change — *see* Air, pressure
    cold (accidental) (excessive) (extreme) (natural) (place) X31
        assault Y08.89
        due to
            man-made conditions W93.8
                dry ice (contact) W93.01
                    inhalation W93.02
                liquid air (contact) (hydrogen) (nitrogen) W93.11
                    inhalation W93.12
                refrigeration unit (deep freeze) W93.2
            weather (conditions) X31
        self-inflicted X83.2
    due to abandonment or neglect X58
    electric current W86.8
        appliance (faulty) W86.8
            domestic W86.0
        caused by other person Y08.89
        conductor (faulty) W86.1
        control apparatus (faulty) W86.1
        electric power generating plant, distribution station W86.1
        electroshock gun — *see* Exposure, electric current, taser
        high-voltage cable W85
        lightning — *see* subcategory T75.0
        live rail W86.8
        misadventure in medical or surgical procedure in electroshock therapy Y63.4
        motor (electric) (faulty) W86.8
            domestic W86.0

Exposure (to), *continued*

self-inflicted X83.1
specified NEC W86.8
domestic W86.0
stun gun — *see* Exposure, electric current, taser
taser W86.8
assault Y08.89
self-harm (intentional) X83.8
undetermined intent Y33
third rail W86.8
transformer (faulty) W86.1
transmission lines W85
environmental tobacco smoke X58
excessive
cold — *see* Exposure, cold
heat (natural)NEC X30
man-made W92
factor (s)NOS X58
environmental NEC X58
man-made NEC W99
natural NEC — *see* Forces of nature
specified NEC X58
fire, flames (accidental) X08.8
assault X97
campfire — *see* Exposure, fire, controlled, not in building
controlled (in)
with ignition (of)clothing (*see also* Ignition, clothes) X06.2
nightwear X05
bonfire — *see* Exposure, fire, controlled, not in building
brazier (in building or structure) — *see also* Exposure, fire, controlled, building
not in building or structure — *see* Exposure, fire, controlled, not in building
building or structure X02.0
with
fall from building X02.3
injury due to building collapse X02.2
from building X02.5
smoke inhalation X02.1
hit by object from building X02.4
specified mode of injury NEC X02.8
fireplace, furnace or stove — *see* Exposure, fire, controlled, building
not in building or structure X03.0
with
fall X03.3
smoke inhalation X03.1
hit by object X03.4
specified mode of injury NEC X03.8
trash — *see* Exposure, fire, controlled, not in building
fireplace — *see* Exposure, fire, controlled, building
fittings or furniture (in building or structure) (uncontrolled) — *see* Exposure, fire, uncontrolled, building
forest (uncontrolled) — *see* Exposure, fire, uncontrolled, not in building
grass (uncontrolled) — *see* Exposure, fire, uncontrolled, not in building
hay (uncontrolled) — *see* Exposure, fire, uncontrolled, not in building
ignition of highly flammable material X04
in, of, on, starting in
machinery — *see* Contact, with, by type of machine
motor vehicle (in motion) (*see also* Accident, transport, occupant by type of vehicle) V87.8
with collision — *see* Collision
railway rolling stock, train, vehicle V81.81
with collision — *see* Accident, transport, railway vehicle occupant
street car (in motion) V82.8
with collision — *see* Accident, transport, streetcar occupant
transport vehicle NEC — *see also* Accident, transport
with collision — *see* Collision
watercraft (in transit) (not in transit) V91.09
localized — *see* Burn, on board watercraft, due to, fire on board
powered craft V91.03
ferry boat V91.01
fishing boat V91.02
jet skis V91.03
liner V91.01
merchant ship V91.00
passenger ship V91.01
unpowered craft V91.08
canoe V91.05
inflatable V91.06
kayak V91.05
sailboat V91.04
surf-board V91.08
waterskis V91.07
windsurfer V91.08

Exposure (to), *continued*

lumber (uncontrolled) — *see* Exposure, fire, uncontrolled, not in building
prairie (uncontrolled) — *see* Exposure, fire, uncontrolled, not in building
resulting from
explosion — *see* Explosion
lightning X08.8
self-inflicted X76
specified NEC X08.8
started by other person X97
stove — *see* Exposure, fire, controlled, building
stated as undetermined whether accidental or intentional Y26
tunnel (uncontrolled) — *see* Exposure, fire, uncontrolled, not in building
uncontrolled
in building or structure X00.0
with
fall from building X00.3
injury due to building collapse X00.2
jump from building X00.5
smoke inhalation X00.1
bed X08.00
due to
cigarette X08.01
specified material NEC X08.09
furniture NEC X08.20
due to
cigarette X08.21
specified material NEC X08.29
hit by object from building X00.4
sofa X08.10
due to
cigarette X08.11
specified material NEC X08.19
specified mode of injury NEC X00.8
not in building or structure (any) X01.0
with
fall X01.3
smoke inhalation X01.1
hit by object X01.4
specified mode of injury NEC X01.8
undetermined whether accidental or intentional Y26
forces of nature NEC — *see* Forces of nature
G-forces (abnormal) W49.9
gravitational forces (abnormal) W49.9
heat (natural)NEC — *see* Heat
high-pressure jet (hydraulic) (pneumatic) W49.9
hydraulic jet W49.9
inanimate mechanical force W49.9
jet, high-pressure (hydraulic) (pneumatic) W49.9
lightning — *see* subcategory T75.0
causing fire — *see* Exposure, fire
mechanical forces NEC W49.9
animate NEC W64
inanimate NEC W49.9
noise W42.9
supersonic W42.0
noxious substance — *see* Table of Drugs and Chemicals
pneumatic jet W49.9
prolonged in deep-freeze unit or refrigerator W93.2
radiation — *see* Radiation
smoke — *see also* Exposure, fire
tobacco, second hand Z77.22
specified factors NEC X58
sunlight X32
man-made (sun lamp) W89.8
tanning bed W89.1
supersonic waves W42.0
transmission line (s), electric W85
vibration W49.9
waves
infrasound W49.9
sound W42.9
supersonic W42.0
weather NEC — *see* Forces of nature
External cause status Y99.9
child assisting in compensated work for family Y99.8
civilian activity done for financial or other compensation Y99.0
civilian activity done for income or pay Y99.0
family member assisting in compensated work for other family member Y99.8
hobby not done for income Y99.8
leisure activity Y99.8
military activity Y99.1
off-duty activity of military personnel Y99.8

External cause status, *continued*
  recreation or sport not for income or while a student Y99.8
  specified NEC Y99.8
  student activity Y99.8
  volunteer activity Y99.2

F

Factors, supplemental
  alcohol
    blood level Y90.-
  environmental-pollution-related condition- *see* Z57
  nosocomial condition Y95
  work-related condition Y99.0
Failure
  in suture or ligature during surgical procedure Y65.2
  mechanical, of instrument or apparatus (any) (during any medical or surgical procedure) Y65.8
  sterile precautions (during medical and surgical care) — *see* Misadventure, failure, sterile precautions, by type of procedure
  to
    introduce tube or instrument Y65.4
      endotracheal tube during anesthesia Y65.3
    make curve (transport vehicle)NEC — *see* Accident, transport
    remove tube or instrument Y65.4
Fall, falling (accidental) W19
  building W20.1
    burning (uncontrolled fire) X00.3
  down
    embankment W17.81
    escalator W10.0
    hill W17.81
    ladder W11
    ramp W10.2
    stairs, steps W10.9
  due to
    bumping against
      object W18.00
        sharp glass W18.02
        specified NEC W18.09
        sports equipment W18.01
      person W03
        due to ice or snow W00.0
        on pedestrian conveyance — *see* Accident, transport, pedestrian, conveyance
    collision with another person W03
      due to ice or snow W00.0
      involving pedestrian conveyance — *see* Accident, transport, pedestrian, conveyance
    grocery cart tipping over W17.82
    ice or snow W00.9
      from one level to another W00.2
        on stairs or steps W00.1
      involving pedestrian conveyance — *see* Accident, transport, pedestrian, conveyance
      on same level W00.0
    slipping (on moving sidewalk) W01.0
      with subsequent striking against object W01.10
        furniture W01.190
        sharp object W01.119
          glass W01.110
          power tool or machine W01.111
          specified NEC W01.118
        specified NEC W01.198
    striking against
      object W18.00
        sharp glass W18.02
        specified NEC W18.09
        sports equipment W18.01
      person W03
        due to ice or snow W00.0
        on pedestrian conveyance — *see* Accident, transport, pedestrian, conveyance
  earth (with asphyxia or suffocation (by pressure)) — *see* Earth, falling
  from, off, out of
    aircraft NEC (with accident to aircraft NEC) V97.0
      while boarding or alighting V97.1
    balcony W13.0
    bed W06
    boat, ship, watercraft NEC (with drowning or submersion) — *see* Drowning, due to, fall overboard
      with hitting bottom or object V94.0
    bridge W13.1
    building W13.9
      burning (uncontrolled fire) X00.3
    cavity W17.2
    chair W07

Fall, falling (accidental), *continued*
  cherry picker W17.89
  cliff W15
  dock W17.4
  embankment W17.81
  escalator W10.0
  flagpole W13.8
  furniture NEC W08
  grocery cart W17.82
  haystack W17.89
  high place NEC W17.89
    stated as undetermined whether accidental or intentional Y30
  hole W17.2
  incline W10.2
  ladder W11
  lifting device W17.89
  machine, machinery — *see also* Contact, with, by type of machine
    not in operation W17.89
  manhole W17.1
  mobile elevated work platform [MEWP] W17.89
  motorized mobility scooter W05.2
  one level to another NEC W17.89
    intentional, purposeful, suicide (attempt) X80
    stated as undetermined whether accidental or intentional Y30
  pit W17.2
  playground equipment W09.8
    jungle gym W09.2
    slide W09.0
    swing W09.1
  quarry W17.89
  railing W13.9
  ramp W10.2
  roof W13.2
  scaffolding W12
  scooter (nonmotorized) W05.1
    motorized mobility W05.2
  sky lift W17.89
  stairs, steps W10.9
    curb W10.1
    due to ice or snow W00.1
    escalator W10.0
    incline W10.2
    ramp W10.2
    sidewalk curb W10.1
    specified NEC W10.8
  stepladder W11
  storm drain W17.1
  streetcar NEC V82.6
    with antecedent collision — *see* Accident, transport, streetcar occupant
    while boarding or alighting V82.4
  structure NEC W13.8
    burning (uncontrolled fire) X00.3
  table W08
  toilet W18.11
    with subsequent striking against object W18.12
  train NEC V81.6
    during derailment (without antecedent collision) V81.7
      with antecedent collision — *see* Accident, transport, railway vehicle occupant
    while boarding or alighting V81.4
  transport vehicle after collision — *see* Accident, transport, by type of vehicle, collision
  tree W14
  vehicle (in motion)NEC (*see also* Accident, transport) V89.9
    motor NEC (*see also* Accident, transport, occupant, by type of vehicle) V87.8
    stationary W17.89
      while boarding or alighting — *see* Accident, transport, by type of vehicle, while boarding or alighting
  viaduct W13.8
  wall W13.8
  watercraft — *see also* Drowning, due to, fall overboard
    with hitting bottom or object V94.0
  well W17.0
  wheelchair, non-moving W05.0
    powered — *see* Accident, transport, pedestrian, conveyance occupant, specified type NEC
  window W13.4
  in, on
    aircraft NEC V97.0
      with accident to aircraft V97.0
      while boarding or alighting V97.1
    bathtub (empty) W18.2
      filled W16.212
        causing drowning W16.211

Fall, falling (accidental), *continued*
  escalator W10.0
  incline W10.2
  ladder W11
  machine, machinery — *see* Contact, with, by type of machine
  object, edged, pointed or sharp (with cut) — *see* Fall, by type
  playground equipment W09.8
    jungle gym W09.2
    slide W09.0
    swing W09.1
  ramp W10.2
  scaffolding W12
  shower W18.2
    causing drowning W16.211
  staircase, stairs, steps W10.9
    curb W10.1
    due to ice or snow W00.1
    escalator W10.0
    incline W10.2
    specified NEC W10.8
  streetcar (without antecedent collision) V82.5
    with antecedent collision — *see* Accident, transport, streetcar occupant
    while boarding or alighting V82.4
  train (without antecedent collision) V81.5
    with antecedent collision — *see* Accident, transport, railway vehicle occupant
    during derailment (without antecedent collision) V81.7
      with antecedent collision — *see* Accident, transport, railway vehicle occupant
    while boarding or alighting V81.4
  transport vehicle after collision — *see* Accident, transport, by type of vehicle, collision
  watercraft V93.39
    due to
      accident to craft V91.29
        powered craft V91.2-
        unpowered craft V91.2-
      powered craft V93.3-
      unpowered craft V93.3-
  into
    cavity W17.2
    dock W17.4
    fire — *see* Exposure, fire, by type
    haystack W17.89
    hole W17.2
    lake — *see* Fall, into, water
    manhole W17.1
    moving part of machinery — *see* Contact, with, by type of machine
    ocean — *see* Fall, into, water
    opening in surface NEC W17.89
    pit W17.2
    pond — *see* Fall, into, water
    quarry W17.89
    river — *see* Fall, into, water
    shaft W17.89
    storm drain W17.1
    stream — *see* Fall, into, water
    swimming pool — *see also* Fall, into, water, in, swimming pool
      empty W17.3
    tank W17.89
    water W16.42
      causing drowning W16.41
      from watercraft — *see* Drowning, due to, fall overboard
      hitting diving board W21.4
      in
        bathtub W16.212
          causing drowning W16.211
        bucket W16.222
          causing drowning W16.221
        natural body of water W16.112
          causing drowning W16.111
          striking
            bottom W16.122
              causing drowning W16.121
            side W16.132
              causing drowning W16.131
        specified water NEC W16.312
          causing drowning W16.311
          striking
            bottom W16.322
              causing drowning W16.321
            wall W16.332
              causing drowning W16.331
        swimming pool W16.012
          causing drowning W16.011
          striking

Fall, falling (accidental), *continued*
            bottom W16.022
              causing drowning W16.021
            wall W16.032
              causing drowning W16.031
        utility bucket W16.222
          causing drowning W16.221
    well W17.0
  involving
    bed W06
    chair W07
    furniture NEC W08
    glass — *see* Fall, by type
    playground equipment W09.8
      jungle gym W09.2
      slide W09.0
      swing W09.1
    roller blades — *see* Accident, transport, pedestrian, conveyance
    skateboard (s) — *see* Accident, transport, pedestrian, conveyance
    skates (ice) (in line) (roller) — *see* Accident, transport, pedestrian, conveyance
    skis — *see* Accident, transport, pedestrian, conveyance
    table W08
    wheelchair, non-moving W05.0
      powered — *see* Accident, transport, pedestrian, conveyance, specified type NEC
  object — *see* Struck by, object, falling
  off
    toilet W18.11
      with subsequent striking against object W18.12
  on same level W18.30
    due to
      specified NEC W18.39
      stepping on an object W18.31
  out of
    bed W06
    building NEC W13.8
    chair W07
    furniture NEC W08
    wheelchair, non-moving W05.0
      powered — *see* Accident, transport, pedestrian, conveyance, specified type NEC
    window W13.4
  over
    animal W01.0
    cliff W15
    embankment W17.81
    small object W01.0
  rock W20.8
  same level W18.30
    from
      being crushed, pushed, or stepped on by a crowd or human stampede W52
      collision, pushing, shoving, by or with other person W03
      slipping, stumbling, tripping W01.0
    involving ice or snow W00.0
      involving skates (ice) (roller), skateboard, skis — *see* Accident, transport, pedestrian, conveyance
  snowslide (avalanche) — *see* Landslide
  stone W20.8
  structure W20.1
    burning (uncontrolled fire) X00.3
  through
    bridge W13.1
    floor W13.3
    roof W13.2
    wall W13.8
    window W13.4
  timber W20.8
  tree (caused by lightning) W20.8
  while being carried or supported by other person (s) W04

Fallen on by
  animal (not being ridden)NEC W55.89
Felo-de-se — *see* Suicide
Fight (hand) (fists) (foot) — *see* Assault, fight Fire (accidental) — *see* Exposure, fire Firearm discharge — *see* Discharge, firearm
Fireworks (explosion) W39
Flash burns from explosion — *see* Explosion
Flood (any injury) (caused by) X38
  collapse of man-made structure causing earth movement X36.0
  tidal wave — *see* Forces of nature, tidal wave
Food (any type) in
  air passages (with asphyxia, obstruction, or suffocation) (*see* categories T17 and) T18
  alimentary tract causing asphyxia (due to compression of trachea) (*see* categories T17 and) T18

Forces of nature X39.8
  avalanche X36.1
    causing transport accident — *see* Accident, transport, by type of vehicle
  blizzard X37.2
  cataclysmic storm X37.9
    with flood X38
    blizzard X37.2
    cloudburst X37.8
    cyclone X37.1
    dust storm X37.3
    hurricane X37.0
    specified storm NEC X37.8
    storm surge X37.0
    tornado X37.1
    twister X37.1
    typhoon X37.0
  cloudburst X37.8
  cold (natural) X31
  cyclone X37.1
  dam collapse causing earth movement X36.0
  dust storm X37.3
  earth movement X36.1
    earthquake X34
    caused by dam or structure collapse X36.0
  earthquake X34
  flood (caused by) X38
    dam collapse X36.0
    tidal wave — *see* Forces of nature, tidal wave
  heat (natural) X30
  hurricane X37.0
  landslide X36.1
    causing transport accident — *see* Accident, transport, by type of vehicle
  lightning — *see* subcategory T75.0
    causing fire — *see* Exposure, fire
  mudslide X36.1
    causing transport accident — *see* Accident, transport, by type of vehicle
  specified force NEC X39.8
  storm surge X37.0
  structure collapse causing earth movement X36.0
  sunlight X32
  tidal wave X37.41
    due to
      earthquake X37.41
      landslide X37.43
      storm X37.42
      volcanic eruption X37.41
  tornado X37.1
  tsunami X37.41
  twister X37.1
  typhoon X37.0
  volcanic eruption X35
Foreign body
  aspiration — *see* Index to Diseases and Injuries, Foreign body, respiratory tract
  entering through skin W45.8
    can lid W26.8
    nail W45.0
    paper W26.2
    specified NEC W45.8
    splinter W45.8
Forest fire (exposure to) — *see* Exposure, fire, uncontrolled, not in building
Found injured X58
  from exposure (to) — *see* Exposure
  on
    highway, road (way), street V89.9
    railway right of way V81.9
Fracture (circumstances unknown or unspecified) X58
  due to specified cause NEC X58
Frostbite X31
  due to man-made conditions — *see* Exposure, cold, man-made
Frozen — *see* Exposure, cold

G

Gunshot wound W34.00

H

Hailstones, injured by X39.8
Hanged herself or himself — *see* Hanging, self-inflicted
Hanging (accidental) (*see also* category) T71
Heat (effects of) (excessive) X30
  due to
    man-made conditions W92
      on board watercraft V93.29

Heat (effects of) (excessive), *continued*
        fishing boat V93.22
        merchant ship V93.20
        passenger ship V93.21
        sailboat V93.24
        specified powered craft NEC V93.23
    weather (conditions) X30
  from
    electric heating apparatus causing burning X16
  inappropriate in local application or packing in medical or surgical procedure Y63.5
Hemorrhage
  delayed following medical or surgical treatment without mention of misadventure — *see* Index to Diseases and Injuries, Complication(s)
  during medical or surgical treatment as misadventure — *see* Index to Diseases and Injuries, Complication(s)
High
  altitude (effects)- — *see* Air, pressure, low
  level of radioactivity, effects — *see* Radiation
  pressure (effects)- — *see* Air, pressure, high
  temperature, effects — *see* HeatHit, hitting (accidental)by — *see* Struck by Hitting against — *see* Striking against Hot
  place, effects — *see also* Heat
  weather, effects X30
House fire (uncontrolled) — *see* Exposure, fire, uncontrolled, building
Humidity, causing problem X39.8
Hunger X58
Hurricane (any injury) X37.0
Hypobarism, hypobaropathy - — *see* Air, pressure, low

I

Ictus
  caloris — *see also* Heat
  solaris X30
Ignition (accidental) (*see also* Exposure, fire) X08.8
  anesthetic gas in operating room W40.1
  apparel X06.2
    from highly flammable material X04
    nightwear X05
  bed linen (sheets) (spreads) (pillows) (mattress) — *see* Exposure, fire, uncontrolled, building, bed
  benzine X04
  clothes, clothing NEC (from controlled fire) X06.2
    from
      highly flammable material X04
  ether X04
    in operating room W40.1
  explosive material — *see* Explosion
  gasoline X04
  jewelry (plastic) (any) X06.0
  kerosene X04
  material
    explosive — *see* Explosion
    highly flammable with secondary explosion X04
  nightwear X05
  paraffin X04
  petrol X04
Immersion (accidental) — *see also* Drowning
  hand or foot due to cold (excessive) X31
Implantation of quills of porcupine W55.89
Inanition (from) (hunger) X58
  thirst X58
Inappropriate operation performed
  correct operation on wrong side or body part (wrong side) (wrong site) Y65.53
  operation intended for another patient done on wrong patient Y65.52
  wrong operation performed on correct patient Y65.51
Incident, adverse
  device
    anesthesiology Y70.-
    cardiovascular Y71.-
    gastroenterology Y73.-
    general
      hospital Y74.-
      surgical Y81.-
    gynecological Y76.-
    medical Y82.9
      specified type NEC Y82.8
    neurological Y75.-
    obstetrical Y76.-
    ophthalmic Y77.-
    orthopedic Y79.-
    otorhinolaryngological Y72.-
    personal use Y74.-

Incident, adverse, *continued*
    physical medicine Y80.-
    plastic surgical Y81.-
    radiological Y78.-
    urology Y73.-
Incineration (accidental) — *see* Exposure, fireInfanticide — *see* Assault
Infrasound waves (causing injury) W49.9
Ingestion
    foreign body (causing injury) (with obstruction) T17 or T18
    poisonous
        plant (s) X58
        substance NEC — *see* Table of Drugs and Chemicals
Inhalation
    excessively cold substance, man-made — *see* Exposure, cold, man-made
    food (any type) (into respiratory tract) (with asphyxia, obstruction respiratory tract, suffocation) (*see* categories T17 and) T18
    foreign body — *see* Foreign body, aspiration
    gastric contents (with asphyxia, obstruction respiratory passage, suffocation) T17.81-
    hot air or gases X14.0
    liquid air, hydrogen, nitrogen W93.12
    steam X13.0
        assault X98.0
        stated as undetermined whether accidental or intentional Y27.0
    toxic gas — *see* Table of Drugs and Chemicals
    vomitus (with asphyxia, obstruction respiratory passage, suffocation) T17.81-
Injury, injured (accidental(ly) NOS X58
    by, caused by, from
        assault — *see* Assault
    homicide (*see also* Assault) Y09
    inflicted (by)
        other person
            stated as
                accidental X58
                undetermined whether accidental or intentional Y33
        purposely (inflicted) by other person(s) — *see* Assault
        self-inflicted X83.8
            stated as accidental X58
        specified cause NEC X58
        undetermined whether accidental or intentional Y33
Insolation, effects X30
Insufficient nourishment X58
Interruption of respiration (by)
    food (lodged in esophagus) (*see* categories T17 and) T18
    vomitus (lodged in esophagus) T17.81- Intoxication
    drug — *see* Table of Drugs and Chemicals
    poison — *see* Table of Drugs and Chemicals

J

Jammed (accidentally)
    between objects (moving) (stationary and moving) W23.0
        stationary W23.1
Jumped, jumping
    before moving object NEC X81.8
        motor vehicle X81.0
        subway train X81.1
        train X81.1
        undetermined whether accidental or intentional Y31
    from
        boat (into water) voluntarily, without accident (to or on boat) W16.712
            with
                accident to or on boat — *see* Accident, watercraft
                drowning or submersion W16.711
            striking bottom W16.722
                causing drowning W16.721
        building (*see also* Jumped, from, high place) W13.9
            burning (uncontrolled fire) X00.5
        high place NEC W17.89
            suicide (attempt) X80
            undetermined whether accidental or intentional Y30
        structure (*see also* Jumped, from, high place) W13.9
            burning (uncontrolled fire) X00.5
    into water W16.92
        causing drowning W16.91
        from, off watercraft — *see* Jumped, from, boat
        in
            natural body W16.612
                causing drowning W16.611
                striking bottom W16.622
                  causing drowning W16.621

Jumped, jumping, *continued*
    specified place NEC W16.812
        causing drowning W16.811
        striking
            bottom W16.822
                causing drowning W16.821
            wall W16.832
                causing drowning W16.831
    swimming pool W16.512
        causing drowning W16.511
        striking
            bottom W16.522
                causing drowning W16.521
            wall W16.532
                causing drowning W16.531

K

Kicked by
    animal NEC W55.82
    person (s) (accidentally) W50.1
        with intent to injure or kill Y04.0
        as, or caused by, a crowd or human stampede (with fall) W52
        assault Y04.0
        in
            fight Y04.0
Kicking against
    object W22.8
        sports equipment W21.9
        stationary wW22.09
            sports equipment W21.89
    person — *see* Striking against, person
    sports equipment W21.9
Knocked down (accidentally) (by) NOS X58
    animal (not being ridden)NEC — *see also* Struck by, by type of animal
    crowd or human stampede W52
    person W51
        in brawl, fight Y04.0
    transport vehicle NEC (*see also* Accident, transport) V09.9

L

Laceration NEC — *see* Injury
Lack of
    care (helpless person) (infant) (newborn) X58
    food except as result of abandonment or neglect X58
        due to abandonment or neglect X58
    water except as result of transport accident X58
        due to transport accident — *see* Accident, transport, by type
        helpless person, infant, newborn X58
Landslide (falling on transport vehicle) X36.1
    caused by collapse of man-made structure X36.0
Late effect — *see* Sequelae
Lightning (shock) (stroke) (struck by) — *see* subcategory T75.0
    causing fire — *see* Exposure, fire
Loss of control (transport vehicle) NEC — *see* Accident, transport
Lying before train, vehicle or other moving object X81.8
    subway train X81.1
    train X81.1
    undetermined whether accidental or intentional Y31

M

Malfunction (mechanism or component) (of)
    firearm W34.10
        airgun W34.110
        BB gun W34.110
        gas, air or spring-operated gun NEC W34.118
        handgun W32.1
        hunting rifle W33.12
        larger firearm W33.10
            specified NEC W33.19
        machine gun W33.13
        paintball gun W34.111
        pellet gun W34.110
        shotgun W33.11
        specified NEC W34.19
        Very pistol [flare] W34.19
    handgun — *see* Malfunction, firearm, handgun
Maltreatment — *see* Perpetrator
Mangled (accidentally) NOS X58
Manhandling (in brawl, fight) Y04.0
Manslaughter (nonaccidental) — *see* Assault
Mauled by animal NEC W55.89

Medical procedure, complication of (delayed or as an abnormal reaction without mention of misadventure) — *see* Complication of or following, by specified type of procedure
  due to or as a result of misadventure — *see* Misadventure
Melting (due to fire) — *see also* Exposure, fire
  apparel NEC X06.3
  clothes, clothing NEC X06.3
    nightwear X05
  fittings or furniture (burning building) (uncontrolled fire) X00.8
  nightwear X05
  plastic jewelry X06.1
Mental cruelty X58
Military operations (injuries to military and civilians occuring during peacetime on military property and during routine military exercises and operations) (by) (from) (involving) — *Refer to ICD-10-CM Manual*
Misadventure (s) to patient(s)during surgical or medical care Y69
  contaminated medical or biological substance (blood, drug, fluid) Y64.9
    administered (by)NEC Y64.9
      immunization Y64.1
      infusion Y64.0
      injection Y64.1
      specified means NEC Y64.8
      transfusion Y64.0
      vaccination Y64.1
  excessive amount of blood or other fluid during transfusion or infusion Y63.0
  failure
    in dosage Y63.9
      electroshock therapy Y63.4
      inappropriate temperature (too hot or too cold)in local application and packing Y63.5
      infusion
        excessive amount of fluid Y63.0
        incorrect dilution of fluid Y63.1
      insulin-shock therapy Y63.4
      nonadministration of necessary drug or biological substance Y63.6
      overdose — *see* Table of Drugs and Chemicals
        radiation, in therapy Y63.2
      radiation
        overdose Y63.2
      specified procedure NEC Y63.8
      transfusion
        excessive amount of blood Y63.0
    mechanical, of instrument or apparatus (any) (during any procedure) Y65.8
    sterile precautions (during procedure) Y62.9
      aspiration of fluid or tissue (by puncture or catheterization, except heart) Y62.6
      biopsy (except needle aspiration) Y62.8
        needle (aspirating) Y62.6
      blood sampling Y62.6
      catheterization Y62.6
        heart Y62.5
      dialysis (kidney) Y62.2
      endoscopic examination Y62.4
      enema Y62.8
      immunization Y62.3
      infusion Y62.1
      injection Y62.3
      needle biopsy Y62.6
      paracentesis (abdominal) (thoracic) Y62.6
      perfusion Y62.2
      puncture (lumbar) Y62.6
      removal of catheter or packing Y62.8
      specified procedure NEC Y62.8
      surgical operation Y62.0
      transfusion Y62.1
      vaccination Y62.3
    suture or ligature during surgical procedure Y65.2
    to introduce or to remove tube or instrument — *see* Failure, to
  hemorrhage — *see* Index to Diseases and Injuries, Complication(s)
  inadvertent exposure of patient to radiation Y63.3
  inappropriate
    operation performed — *see* Inappropriate operation performed
    temperature (too hot or too cold) in local application or packing Y63.5
  infusion (*see also* Misadventure, by type, infusion) Y69
    excessive amount of fluid Y63.0
    incorrect dilution of fluid Y63.1
    wrong fluid Y65.1
  nonadministration of necessary drug or biological substance Y63.6
  overdose — *see* Table of Drugs and Chemicals
    radiation (in therapy) Y63.2
  perforation — *see* Index to Diseases and Injuries, Complication(s)
  performance of inappropriate operation — *see* Inappropriate operation performed
  puncture — *see* Index to Diseases and Injuries, Complication(s)
  specified type NEC Y65.8

Misadventure (s) to patient(s)during surgical or medical care, *continued*
  failure
    suture or ligature during surgical operation Y65.2
    to introduce or to remove tube or instrument — *see* Failure, to
  infusion of wrong fluid Y65.1
  performance of inappropriate operation — *see* Inappropriate operation performed
  transfusion of mismatched blood Y65.0
  wrong
    fluid in infusion Y65.1
    placement of endotracheal tube during anesthetic procedure Y65.3
  transfusion — *see* Misadventure, by type, transfusion
    excessive amount of blood Y63.0
    mismatched blood Y65.0
  wrong
    drug given in error — *see* Table of Drugs and Chemicals
    fluid in infusion Y65.1
    placement of endotracheal tube during anesthetic procedure Y65.3
Mismatched blood in transfusion Y65.0
Motion sickness T75.3
Mountain sickness W94.11
Mudslide (of cataclysmic nature) — *see* Landslide

N

Nail, contact with W45.0
  gun W29.4
Noise (causing injury) (pollution) W42.9
  supersonic W42.0
Nonadministration (of)
  drug or biological substance (necessary) Y63.6
  surgical and medical care Y66
Nosocomial condition Y95

O

Object
  falling
    from, in, on, hitting
      machinery — *see* Contact, with, by type of machine
  set in motion by
    accidental explosion or rupture of pressure vessel W38
    firearm — *see* Discharge, firearm, by type
    machine (ry) — *see* Contact, with, by type of machine
Overdose (drug) — *see* Table of Drugs and Chemicals
  radiation Y63.2
Overexertion
  due to
    other or unspecified movement X50.9
    prolonged static or awkward postures X50.1
    repetitive movements X50.3
    strenuous movement X50.0
Overexposure (accidental) (to)
  cold (*see also* Exposure, cold) X31
    due to man-made conditions — *see* Exposure, cold, man-made
  heat (*see also* Heat) X30
  radiation — *see* Radiation
  radioactivity W88.0
  sun (sunburn) X32
  weather NEC — *see* Forces of nature
  wind NEC — *see* Forces of nature Overheated — *see* Heat Overturning (accidental)
  machinery — *see* Contact, with, by type of machine
  transport vehicle NEC (*see also* Accident, transport) V89.9
  watercraft (causing drowning, submersion) — *see also* Drowning, due to, accident to, watercraft, overturning
    causing injury except drowning or submersion — *see* Accident, watercraft, causing, injury NEC

P

Parachute descent (voluntary) (without accident to aircraft) V97.29
  due to accident to aircraft — *see* Accident, transport, aircraft
Pecked by bird W61.99
Perforation during medical or surgical treatment as misadventure — *see* Index to Diseases and Injuries, Complication(s)
Perpetrator, perpetration, of assault, maltreatment and neglect (by) Y07.-
Piercing — *see* Contact, with, by type of object or machine
Pinched
  between objects (moving) (stationary and moving) W23.0
    stationary W23.1
Pinned under machine (ry) — *see* Contact, with, by type of machine
Place of occurrence Y92.9
  abandoned house Y92.89
  airplane Y92.813
  airport Y92.520

Place of occurrence, *continued*

  ambulatory health services establishment NEC Y92.538
  ambulatory surgery center Y92.530
  amusement park Y92.831
  apartment (co-op) Y92.039
    bathroom Y92.031
    bedroom Y92.032
    kitchen Y92.030
    specified NEC Y92.038
  assembly hall Y92.29
  bank Y92.510
  barn Y92.71
  baseball field Y92.320
  basketball court Y92.310
  beach Y92.832
  boat Y92.814
  bowling alley Y92.39
  bridge Y92.89
  building under construction Y92.61
  bus Y92.811
    station Y92.521
  cafe Y92.511
  campsite Y92.833
  campus — *see* Place of occurrence, school
  canal Y92.89
  car Y92.810
  casino Y92.59
  church Y92.22
  cinema Y92.26
  clubhouse Y92.29
  coal pit Y92.64
  college (community) Y92.214
  condominium — *see* apartment
  construction area — Y92.6-
  convalescent home — Y92.129-
  court-house Y92.240
  cricket ground Y92.328
  cultural building Y92.25-
  dancehall Y92.252
  day nursery Y92.210
  dentist office Y92.531
  derelict house Y92.89
  desert Y92.820
  dock NOS Y92.89
  dockyard Y92.62
  doctor's office Y92.531
  dormitory — *see* institutional, school dormitory
  dry dock Y92.62
  factory (building) (premises) Y92.63
  farm (land under cultivation) (outbuildings) Y92.7-
  football field Y92.321
  forest Y92.821
  freeway Y92.411
  gallery Y92.250
  garage (commercial) Y92.59 (refer to specific residence)
  gas station Y92.524
  gasworks Y92.69
  golf course Y92.39
  gravel pit Y92.64
  grocery Y92.512
  gymnasium Y92.39
  handball court Y92.318
  harbor Y92.89
  harness racing course Y92.39
  healthcare provider office Y92.531
  highway (interstate) Y92.411
  hill Y92.828
  hockey rink Y92.330
  home — *see* residence
  hospice — Y92.129-
  hospital Y92.23-
    patient room Y92.23-
  hotel Y92.59
  house — *see also* residence
    abandoned Y92.89
    under construction Y92.61
  industrial and construction area (yard) Y92.6-
  kindergarten Y92.211
  lacrosse field Y92.328
  lake Y92.828
  library Y92.241
  mall Y92.59

Place of occurrence, *continued*

  market Y92.512
  marsh Y92.828
  military base — Y92.13-
  mosque Y92.22
  motel Y92.59
  motorway (interstate) Y92.411
  mountain Y92.828
  movie-house Y92.26
  museum Y92.251
  music-hall Y92.252
  not applicable Y92.9
  nuclear power station Y92.69
  nursing home — Y92.129-
  office building Y92.59
  offshore installation Y92.65
  opera-house Y92.253
  orphanage — Y92.11-
  outpatient surgery center Y92.530
  park (public) Y92.830
    amusement Y92.831
  parking garage Y92.89
    lot Y92.481
  pavement Y92.480
  physician office Y92.531
  polo field Y92.328
  pond Y92.828
  post office Y92.242
  power station Y92.69
  prairie Y92.828
  prison — Y92.14-
  public
    administration building Y92.24-
    building NEC Y92.29
    hall Y92.29
    place NOS Y92.89
  race course Y92.39
  railway line (bridge) Y92.85
  ranch (outbuildings) Y92.7-
  recreation area Y92.838 (refer to specific sites)
  religious institution Y92.22
  reform school — *see* institutional, reform school
  residence (non-institutional) (private) Y92.009
    apartment Y92.039
      bathroom Y92.031
      bedroom Y92.032
      kitchen Y92.030
      specified NEC Y92.038
    boarding house Y92.04-
    home, unspecified Y92.009
      bathroom Y92.002
      bedroom Y92.003
      dining room Y92.001
      garden Y92.007
      kitchen Y92.000
    house, single family Y92.019
      bathroom Y92.012
      bedroom Y92.013
      dining room Y92.011
      driveway Y92.014
      garage Y92.015
      garden Y92.017
      kitchen Y92.010
      specified NEC Y92.018
      swimming pool Y92.016
      yard Y92.017
    institutional Y92.10
      hospice — Y92.12-
      military base Y92.13-
      nursing home Y92.12-
      orphanage Y92.119
        bathroom Y92.111
        bedroom Y92.112
        driveway Y92.113
        garage Y92.114
        garden Y92.116
        kitchen Y92.110
        specified NEC Y92.118
        swimming pool Y92.115
        yard Y92.116
      reform school Y92.15-
      school dormitory Y92.169

Place of occurrence, *continued*
    bathroom Y92.162
    bedroom Y92.163
    dining room Y92.161
    kitchen Y92.160
    specified NEC Y92.168
  specified NEC Y92.199
    bathroom Y92.192
    bedroom Y92.193
    dining room Y92.191
    driveway Y92.194
    garage Y92.195
    garden Y92.197
    kitchen Y92.190
    specified NEC Y92.198
    swimming pool Y92.196
    yard Y92.197
  mobile home Y92.029
    bathroom Y92.022
    bedroom Y92.023
    dining room Y92.021
    driveway Y92.024
    garage Y92.025
    garden Y92.027
    kitchen Y92.020
    specified NEC Y92.028
    swimming pool Y92.026
    yard Y92.027
  specified place in residence NEC Y92.008
  specified residence type NEC Y92.09-
restaurant Y92.511
riding school Y92.39
river Y92.828
road Y92.488
rodeo ring Y92.39
rugby field Y92.328
same day surgery center Y92.530
sand pit Y92.64
school (private) (public) (state) Y92.219
    college Y92.214
    daycare center Y92.210
    elementary school Y92.211
    high school Y92.213
    kindergarten Y92.211
    middle school Y92.212
    specified NEC Y92.218
    trace school Y92.215
    university Y92.214
    vocational school Y92.215
sea (shore) Y92.832
senior citizen center Y92.29
service area (refer to specific site)
shipyard Y92.62
shop (commercial) Y92.513
sidewalk Y92.480
skating rink (roller) Y92.331
    ice Y92.330
soccer field Y92.322
specified place NEC Y92.89
sports area Y92.39 (also refer to specific sites)
    athletic
        court Y92.31-
        field Y92.32-
    golf course Y92.39
    gymnasium Y92.39
    riding school Y92.39
    stadium Y92.39
    swimming pool Y92.34
squash court Y92.311
stadium Y92.39
steeple chasing course Y92.39
store Y92.512
stream Y92.828
street and highway Y92.410
    bike path Y92.482
    freeway Y92.411
    highway ramp Y92.415
    interstate highway Y92.411
    local residential or business street Y92.414
    motorway Y92.411

Place of occurrence, *continued*
        parkway Y92.412
        parking lot Y92.481
        sidewalk Y92.480
        specified NEC Y92.488
        state road Y92.413
    subway car Y92.816
    supermarket Y92.512
    swamp Y92.828
    swimming pool (public) Y92.34
        private (at) Y92.095 (refer to specific residence)
    synagogue Y92.22
    tennis court Y92.312
    theater Y92.254
    trade area Y92.59 (refer to specific site)
    trailer park, residential — *see* mobile home
    trailer site NOS Y92.89
    train Y92.815
        station Y92.522
    truck Y92.812
    tunnel under construction Y92.69
    urgent (health)care center Y92.532
    university Y92.214
    vehicle (transport) Y92.818
        airplane Y92.813
        boat Y92.814
        bus Y92.811
        car Y92.810
        specified NEC Y92.818
        subway car Y92.816
        train Y92.815
        truck Y92.812
    warehouse Y92.59
    water reservoir Y92.89
    wilderness area Y92.82-
    workshop Y92.69
    yard, private Y92.096 (refer to specific residence)
    youth center Y92.29
    zoo (zoological garden) Y92.834
Poisoning (accidental) (by) — *see also* Table of Drugs and Chemicals
    by plant, thorns, spines, sharp leaves or other mechanisms NEC X58
    carbon monoxide
        generated by
            motor vehicle — *see* Accident, transport
            watercraft (in transit) (not in transit) V93.8-
    caused by injection of poisons into skin by plant thorns, spines, sharp leaves X58
        marine or sea plants (venomous) X58
    exhaust gas
        generated by
            motor vehicle — *see* Accident, transport
            watercraft (in transit) (not in transit) V93.89
                ferry boat V93.81
                fishing boat V93.82
                jet skis V93.83
                liner V93.81
                merchant ship V93.80
                passenger ship V93.81
                powered craft NEC V93.83
    fumes or smoke due to
        explosion (*see also* Explosion) W40.9
        fire — *see* Exposure, fire
        ignition — *see* Ignition
Powder burn (by) (from)
    airgun W34.110
    BB gun W34.110
    firearm NEC W34.19
    gas, air or spring-operated gun NEC W34.118
    handgun W32.1
    hunting rifle W33.12
    larger firearm W33.10
        specified NEC W33.19
    machine gun W33.13
    paintball gun W34.111
    pellet gun W34.110
    shotgun W33.11
    Very pistol [flare] W34.19
Premature cessation (of)surgical and medical care Y66
Privation (food) (water) X58

Procedure (operation)
  correct, on wrong side or body part (wrong side) (wrong site) Y65.53
  intended for another patient done on wrong patient Y65.52
  performed on patient not scheduled for surgery Y65.52
  performed on wrong patient Y65.52
  wrong, performed on correct patient Y65.51
Prolonged
  sitting in transport vehicle — *see* Travel, by type of vehicle
  stay in
    high altitude as cause of anoxia, barodontalgia, barotitis or hypoxia W94.11
    weightless environment X52
Pulling, excessive — *see* category Y93
Puncture, puncturing — *see also* Contact, with, by type of object or machine
  by
    plant thorns, spines, sharp leaves or other mechanisms NEC W60
    during medical or surgical treatment as misadventure — *see* Index to Diseases and Injuries, Complication(s)
Pushed, pushing (accidental) (injury in) (overexertion) — *see* category Y93
  by other person (s) (accidental) W51
    with fall W03
      due to ice or snow W00.0
    as, or caused by, a crowd or human stampede (with fall) W52
    before moving object NEC Y02.8
      motor vehicle Y02.0
      subway train Y02.1
      train Y02.1
    from
      high place NEC
        in accidental circumstances W17.89
        stated as
          intentional, homicide (attempt) Y01
          undetermined whether accidental or intentional Y30
    transport vehicle NEC (*see also* Accident, transport) V89.9

R

Radiation (exposure to) (refer to *ICD-10-CM* manual for more)
  infrared (heaters and lamps) W90.1
    excessive heat from W92
  ionized, ionizing (particles, artificially accelerated)
    radioisotopes W88.1
    specified NEC W88.8
    x-rays W88.0
  light sources (man-made visible and ultraviolet) W89.9
    natural X32
    specified NEC W89.8
    tanning bed W89.1
    welding light W89.0
  man-made visible light W89.9
    specified NEC W89.8
    tanning bed W89.1
    welding light W89.0
  microwave W90.8
  misadventure in medical or surgical procedure Y63.2
  natural NEC X39.08
  overdose (in medical or surgical procedure) Y63.2
  sun X32
  ultraviolet (light) (man-made) W89.9
    natural X32
    specified NEC W89.8
    tanning bed W89.1
    welding light W89.0
  x-rays (hard) (soft) W88.0
Range disease W94.11
Rape (attempted) T74.2-
Rat bite W53.11
Reaction, abnormal to medical procedure (*see also* Complication of or following, by type of procedure) Y84.9
  with misadventure — *see* Misadventure
  biologicals or drugs or vaccine — *see* Table of Drugs and Chemicals
Recoil
  airgun W34.110
  BB gun W34.110
  firearm NEC W34.19
  gas, air or spring-operated gun NEC W34.118
  handgun W32.1
  hunting rifle W33.12
  larger firearm W33.10
    specified NEC W33.19
  machine gun W33.13
  paintball gun W34.111
  pellet W34.110

Recoil, *continued*
  shotgun W33.11
  Very pistol [flare] W34.19
Reduction in
  atmospheric pressure - — *see* Air, pressure, change
Rock falling on or hitting (accidentally) (person) W20.8
  in cave-in W20.0
Run over (accidentally) (by)
  animal (not being ridden)NEC W55.89
  machinery — *see* Contact, with, by specified type of machine
  transport vehicle NEC (*see also* Accident, transport) V09.9
    motor NEC V09.20
Running
  before moving object X81.8
    motor vehicle X81.0
Running off, away
  animal (being ridden) (*see also* Accident, transport) V80.918
    not being ridden W55.89
  animal-drawn vehicle NEC (*see also* Accident, transport) V80.928
  highway, road (way), street
  transport vehicle NEC (*see also* Accident, transport) V89.9
Rupture pressurized devices — *see* Explosion, by type of device

S

Saturnism — *see* Table of Drugs and Chemicals, lead
Scald, scalding (accidental) (by) (from) (in) X19
  air (hot) X14.1
  gases (hot) X14.1
  liquid (boiling) (hot)NEC X12
    stated as undetermined whether accidental or intentional Y27.2
  local application of externally applied substance in medical or surgical care Y63.5
  metal (molten) (liquid) (hot)NEC X18
  self-inflicted X77.9
  stated as undetermined whether accidental or intentional Y27.8
  steam X13.1
    assault X98.0
    stated as undetermined whether accidental or intentional Y27.0
  vapor (hot) X13.1
    assault X98.0
    stated as undetermined whether accidental or intentional Y27.0
Scratched by
  cat W55.03
  person (s) (accidentally) W50.4
    with intent to injure or kill Y04.0
    as, or caused by, a crowd or human stampede (with fall) W52
    assault Y04.0
    in
      fight Y04.0
Seasickness T75.3
Self-harm NEC — *see also* **External cause by type, undetermined whether accidental or intentional**
  intentional — *see* Suicide
  poisoning NEC — *see* Table of drugs and biologicals, accident
Self-inflicted (injury)NEC — *see also* External cause by type, undetermined whether accidental or intentional
  intentional — *see* Suicide
  poisoning NEC — *see* Table of drugs and biologicals, accident
Sequelae (of)
Use original code to define how the injury occurred with 7th character S
Shock
  electric — *see* Exposure, electric current
  from electric appliance (any) (faulty) W86.8
    domestic W86.0
Shooting, shot (accidental(ly)) — *see also* Discharge, firearm, by type
  herself or himself — *see* Discharge, firearm by type, self-inflicted
  inflicted by other person — *see* Discharge, firearm by type, homicide
    accidental — *see* Discharge, firearm, by type of firearm
  self-inflicted — *see* Discharge, firearm by type, suicide
    accidental — *see* Discharge, firearm, by type of firearm
  suicide (attempt) — *see* Discharge, firearm by type, suicide
Shoving (accidentally) by other person — *see* Pushed, by other person
Sickness
  alpine W94.11
  motion — *see* Motion
  mountain W94.11
Sinking (accidental)
  watercraft (causing drowning, submersion) — *see also* Drowning, due to, accident to, watercraft, sinking
    causing injury except drowning or submersion — *see* Accident, watercraft, causing, injury NEC
Siriasis X32

Slashed wrists — *see* Cut, self-inflicted
Slipping (accidental) (on same level) (with fall) W01.0
    on
        ice W00.0
            with skates — *see* Accident, transport, pedestrian, conveyance
        mud W01.0
        oil W01.0
        snow W00.0
            with skis — *see* Accident, transport, pedestrian, conveyance
        surface (slippery) (wet)NEC W01.0
    without fall W18.40
        due to
            specified NEC W18.49
            stepping from one level to another W18.43
            stepping into hole or opening W18.42
            stepping on object W18.41
Sliver, wood, contact with W45.8
Smoldering (due to fire) — *see* Exposure, fire
Sodomy (attempted)by force T74.2-
Sound waves (causing injury) W42.9
    supersonic W42.0
Splinter, contact with W45.8
Stab, stabbing — *see* Cut
Starvation X58
Status of external cause Y99.-
Stepped on
    by
        animal (not being ridden)NEC W55.89
        crowd or human stampede W52
        person W50.0
Stepping on
    object W22.8
        with fall W18.31
        sports equipment W21.9
        stationary W22.09
            sports equipment W21.89
    person W51
        by crowd or human stampede W52
    sports equipment W21.9
Sting
    arthropod, nonvenomous W57
    insect, nonvenomous W57
Storm (cataclysmic) — *see* Forces of nature, cataclysmic storm
Straining, excessive — *see* category Y93
Strangling — *see* Strangulation
Strangulation (accidental) — *see* category T71
Strenuous movements — *see* category Y93
Striking against
    airbag (automobile) W22.10
        driver side W22.11
        front passenger side W22.12
        specified NEC W22.19
    bottom when
        diving or jumping into water (in) W16.822
            causing drowning W16.821
            from boat W16.722
                causing drowning W16.721
            natural body W16.622
                causing drowning W16.821
            swimming pool W16.522
                causing drowning W16.521
        falling into water (in) W16.322
            causing drowning W16.321
            fountain — *see* Striking against, bottom when, falling into water, specified NEC
            natural body W16.122
                causing drowning W16.121
            reservoir — *see* Striking against, bottom when, falling into water, specified NEC
            specified NEC W16.322
                causing drowning W16.321
            swimming pool W16.022
                causing drowning W16.021
    diving board (swimming-pool) W21.4
    object W22.8
        with
            drowning or submersion — *see* Drowning
            fall — *see* Fall, due to, bumping against, object
        caused by crowd or human stampede (with fall) W52
        furniture W22.03
        lamppost W22.02
        sports equipment W21.9
        stationary W22.09
            sports equipment W21.89

Striking against, *continued*
    wall W22.01
    person (s) W51
        with fall W03
            due to ice or snow W00.0
        as, or caused by, a crowd or human stampede (with fall) W52
        assault Y04.2
    sports equipment W21.9
    wall (when) W22.01
        diving or jumping into water (in) W16.832
            causing drowning W16.831
            swimming pool W16.532
                causing drowning W16.531
        falling into water (in) W16.332
            causing drowning W16.331
            fountain — *see* Striking against, wall when, falling into water, specified NEC
            natural body W16.132
                causing drowning W16.131
            reservoir — *see* Striking against, wall when, falling into water, specified NEC
            specified NEC W16.332
                causing drowning W16.331
            swimming pool W16.032
                causing drowning W16.031
        swimming pool (when) W22.042
            causing drowning W22.041
            diving or jumping into water W16.532
                causing drowning W16.531
            falling into water W16.032
                causing drowning W16.031
Struck (accidentally) by
    airbag (automobile) W22.10
        driver side W22.11
        front passenger side W22.12
        specified NEC W22.19
    alligator W58.02
    animal (not being ridden)NEC W55.89
    avalanche — *see* Landslide
    ball (hit) (thrown) W21.00
        assault Y08.09
        baseball W21.03
        basketball W21.05
        golf ball W21.04
        football W21.01
        soccer W21.02
        softball W21.07
        specified NEC W21.09
        volleyball W21.06
    bat or racquet
        baseball bat W21.11
            assault Y08.02
        golf club W21.13
            assault Y08.09
        specified NEC W21.19
            assault Y08.09
        tennis racquet W21.12
            assault Y08.09
    bullet — *see also* Discharge, firearm by type
    crocodile W58.12
    dog W54.1
    flare, Very pistol — *see* Discharge, firearm NEC
    hailstones X39.8
    hockey (ice)
        field
            puck W21.221
            stick W21.211
        puck W21.220
        stick W21.210
            assault Y08.01
    landslide — *see* Landslide
    lightning — *see* subcategory T75.0
        causing fire — *see* Exposure, fire
    machine — *see* Contact, with, by type of machine
    mammal NEC W55.89
        marine W56.32
    marine animal W56.82
    object W22.8
        blunt W22.8
            assault Y00
            undetermined whether accidental or intentional Y29
        falling W20.8
            from, in, on
                building W20.1

Suicide, suicidal (attempted) (by) X83.8
  blunt object X79
  burning, burns X76
    hot object X77.9
      fluid NEC X77.2
      household appliance X77.3
      specified NEC X77.8
      steam X77.0
      tap water X77.1
      vapors X77.0
  caustic substance — *see* Table of Drugs and Chemicals
  cold, extreme X83.2
  collision of motor vehicle with
    motor vehicle X82.0
    specified NEC X82.8
    train X82.1
    tree X82.2
  cut (any part of body) X78.9
  cutting or piercing instrument X78.9
    dagger X78.2
    glass X78.0
    knife X78.1
    specified NEC X78.8
    sword X78.2
  drowning (in) X71.9
    bathtub X71.0
    natural water X71.3
    specified NEC X71.8
    swimming pool X71.1
      following fall X71.2
  electrocution X83.1
  explosive (s) (material) X75
  fire, flames X76
  firearm X74.9
    airgun X74.01
    handgun X72
    hunting rifle X73.1
    larger X73.9
      specified NEC X73.8
    machine gun X73.2
    -- paintball gun X74.02
    shotgun X73.0
    specified NEC X74.8
  hanging X83.8
  hot object — *see* Suicide, burning, hot object
  jumping
    before moving object X81.8
      motor vehicle X81.0
      subway train X81.1
      train X81.1
    from high place X80
  lying before moving object, train, vehicle X81.8
  poisoning — *see* Table of Drugs and Chemicals
  puncture (any part of body) — *see* Suicide, cutting or piercing instrument
  scald — *see* Suicide, burning, hot object
  sharp object (any) — *see* Suicide, cutting or piercing instrument
  shooting — *see* Suicide, firearm
  specified means NEC X83.8
  stab (any part of body) — *see* Suicide, cutting or piercing instrument
  steam, hot vapors X77.0
  strangulation X83.8
  submersion — *see* Suicide, drowning
  suffocation X83.8
  wound NEC X83.8
Sunstroke X32
Supersonic waves (causing injury) W42.0
Surgical procedure, complication of (delayed or as an abnormal reaction without mention of misadventure) — *see also* Complication of or following, by type of procedure
  due to or as a result of misadventure — *see* Misadventure
Swallowed, swallowing
  foreign body T18
  poison — *see* Table of Drugs and Chemicals
  substance
    caustic or corrosive — *see* Table of Drugs and Chemicals
    poisonous — *see* Table of Drugs and Chemicals

T

Tackle in sport W03
Terrorism (involving) Y38.8-
Thirst X58

Thrown (accidentally)
  against part (any) of or object in transport vehicle (in motion) NEC — *see also* Accident, transport
  from
    high place, homicide (attempt) Y01
    machinery — *see* Contact, with, by type of machine
    transport vehicle NEC (*see also* Accident, transport) V89.9
  off — *see* Thrown, from
Thunderbolt — *see* subcategory T75.0
  causing fire — *see* Exposure, fire
Tidal wave (any injury)NEC — *see* Forces of nature, tidal wave
Took
  overdose (drug) — *see* Table of Drugs and Chemicals
  poison — *see* Table of Drugs and Chemicals
Tornado (any injury) X37.1
Torrential rain (any injury) X37.8
Torture X58
Trampled by animal NEC W55.89
Trapped (accidentally)
  between objects (moving) (stationary and moving) — *see* Caught
  by part (any)of
    motorcycle V29.88
    pedal cycle V19.88
    transport vehicle NEC (*see also* Accident, transport) V89.9
Travel (effects) (sickness) T75.3
Tree falling on or hitting (accidentally) (person) W20.8
Tripping
  over
    animal W01.0
    carpet, rug or (small)object W22.8
      with fall W18.09
    person W51
      with fall W03
        due to ice or snow W00.0
  without fall W18.40
    due to
      specified NEC W18.49
      stepping from one level to another W18.43
      stepping into hole or opening W18.42
      stepping on object W18.41
Twisted by person (s) (accidentally) W50.2
  with intent to injure or kill Y04.0
  as, or caused by, a crowd or human stampede (with fall) W52
  assault Y04.0
  in fight Y04.0
Twisting, excessive — *see* category Y93

U

Underdosing of necessary drugs, medicaments or biological substances Y63.6

V

Vibration (causing injury) W49.9
Volcanic eruption (any injury) X35
Vomitus, gastric contents in air passages (with asphyxia, obstruction or suffocation) T17.81-

W

Walked into stationary object (any) W22.09
  furniture W22.03
  lamppost W22.02
  wall W22.01
War operations (injuries to military personnel and civilians during war, civil insurrection and peacekeeping missions) (by) (from) (involving) — *Refer to ICD-10-CM Manual*
Washed
  away by flood — *see* Flood
  off road by storm (transport vehicle) — *see* Forces of nature, cataclysmic storm
Weather exposure NEC — *see* Forces of nature
Weightlessness (causing injury) (effects of) (in spacecraft, real or simulated) X52
Work related condition Y99.0
Wound (accidental) NEC (*see also* Injury) X58
  battle (*see also* War operations) Y36.90
  gunshot — *see* Discharge, firearm by type
Wrong
  device implanted into correct surgical site Y65.51
  fluid in infusion Y65.1
  procedure (operation)on correct patient Y65.51
  patient, procedure performed on Y65.52

Table of Drugs and Chemicals

The following table is a quick reference for all poisonings (accidental/unintentional, intentional/self-harm, assault), adverse effects, and underdosing as a result of a specific drug or chemical. The drugs/chemicals are listed alphabetically with their respective subcategory code. Every code is listed with a dash (-) to indicate that the next character is missing and should be reported with the fifth or sixth character as follows:

1	Poisoning, accidental, unintentional
2	Poisoning, intentional, self-harm
3	Poisoning, assault
4	Poisoning, undetermined
5	Adverse effect
6	Underdosing

DO NOT CODE FROM THE TABLE—ALWAYS REFER TO THE TABULAR. If the code requires an "encounter type," please refer to the tabular for more details.

EXAMPLE

Accidental Poisoning From Lysol—Initial Encounter
Lysol is listed as T54.1X-.
Lysol accidental poisoning would be T54.1X1-.
Lysol accidental poisoning, initial encounter, would be T54.1X1A.

Underdosing of Barbiturate—Follow-up Encounter
Barbiturate is listed as T42.3X-.
Underdosing of barbiturate would be T42.3X6-.
Underdosing of barbiturate, subsequent encounter, would be T42.3X6D.

Drug/Chemical	Code
1-propanol	T51.3X-
2-propanol	T51.2X-
2,4-D (dichlorophen-oxyacetic acid)	T60.3X-
2,4-toluene diisocyanate	T65.0X-
2,4,5-T (trichloro-phenoxyacetic acid)	T60.1X-
14-hydroxydihydro-morphinone	T40.2X-
ABOB	T37.5X-
Abrine	T62.2X-
Abrus (seed)	T62.2X-
Absinthe (beverage)	T51.0X-
Acaricide	T60.8X-
Acebutolol	T44.7X-
Acecarbromal	T42.6X-
Aceclidine	T44.1X-
Acedapsone	T37.0X-
Acefylline piperazine	T48.6X-
Acemorphan	T40.2X-
Acenocoumarin / Acenocoumarol	T45.51-
Acepifylline	T48.6X-
Acepromazine	T43.3X-
Acesulfamethoxypyridazine	T37.0X-
Acetal	T52.8X-
Acetaldehyde (vapor)	T52.8X-
liquid	T65.89-
P-Acetamidophenol	T39.1X-
Acetaminophen	T39.1X-
Acetaminosalol	T39.1X-
Acetanilide	T39.1X-
Acetarsol	T37.3X-
Acetazolamide	T50.2X-
Acetiamine	T45.2X-

Drug/Chemical	Code
Acetic	
acid	T54.2X-
w/sodium acetate (ointment)	T49.3X-
ester (solvent) (vapor)	T52.8X-
irrigating solution	T50.3X-
medicinal (lotion)	T49.2X-
anhydride	T65.89-
ether (vapor)	T52.8X-
Acetohexamide	T38.3X-
Acetohydroxamic acid	T50.99-
Acetomenaphthone	T45.7X-
Acetomorphine	T40.1X-
Acetone (oils)	T52.4X-
Acetonitrile	T52.8X-
Acetophenazine	T43.3X-
Acetophenetedin	T39.1X-
Acetophenone	T52.4X-
Acetorphine	T40.2X-
Acetosulfone (sodium)	T37.1X-
Acetrizoate (sodium)	T50.8X-
Acetrizoic acid	T50.8X-
Acetyl (bromide) (chloride)	T53.6X-
Acetylcarbromal	T42.6X-
Acetylcholine (chloride)	T44.1X-
derivative	T44.1X-
Acetylcysteine	T48.4X-
Acetyldigitoxin	T46.0X-
Acetyldigoxin	T46.0X-
Acetyldihydrocodeine	T40.2X-
Acetyldihydrocodeinone	T40.2X-
Acetylene (gas)	T59.89-
dichloride	T53.6X-
incomplete combustion of	T58.1-
industrial	T59.89-
tetrachloride	T53.6X-
vapor	T53.6X-

1-PROPANOL–ACETYLENE (GAS)

Drug/Chemical	Code
Acetylpheneturide	T42.6X-
Acetylphenylhydrazine	T39.8X-
Acetylsalicylic acid (salts)	T39.01-
enteric coated	T39.01-
Acetylsulfamethoxypyridazine	T37.0X-
Achromycin	T36.4X-
ophthalmic preparation	T49.5X-
topical NEC	T49.0X-
Aciclovir	T37.5X-
Acid (corrosive)NEC	T54.2X-
Acidifying agent NEC	T50.90-
Acipimox	T46.6X-
Acitretin	T50.99-
Aclarubicin	T45.1X-
Aclatonium napadisilate	T48.1X-
Aconite (wild)	T46.99-
Aconitine	T46.99-
Aconitum ferox	T46.99-
Acridine	T65.6X-
vapor	T59.89-
Acriflavine	T37.9-
Acriflavinium chloride	T49.0X-
Acrinol	T49.0X-
Acrisorcin	T49.0X-
Acrivastine	T45.0X-
Acrolein (gas)	T59.89-
liquid	T54.1X-
Acrylamide	T65.89-
Acrylic resin	T49.3X-
Acrylonitrile	T65.89-
Actaea spicata	T62.2X-
berry	T62.1X-
Acterol	T37.3X-
ACTH	T38.81-
Actinomycin C	T45.1X-
Actinomycin D	T45.1X-
Activated charcoal—*see also Charcoal, medicinal*	T47.6X-
Acyclovir	T37.5X-
Adenine	T45.2X-
arabinoside	T37.5X-
Adenosine (phosphate)	T46.2X-
ADH	T38.89-
Adhesive NEC	T65.89-
Adicillin	T36.0X-
Adiphenine	T44.3X-
Adipiodone	T50.8X-

Drug/Chemical	Code
Adjunct, pharmaceutical	T50.90-
Adrenal (extract, cortex or medulla) (gluco or mineral corticoids) (hormones)	T38.0X-
ENT agent	T49.6X-
ophthalmic preparation	T49.5X-
topical NEC	T49.0X-
Adrenaline / Adrenalin	T44.5X-
Adrenergic NEC	T44.90-
blocking agent NEC	T44.8X-
beta, heart	T44.7X-
specified NEC	T44.99-
Adrenochrome	
(mono)semicarbazone	T46.99-
derivative	T46.99-
Adrenocorticotrophic hormone	T38.81-
Adrenocorticotrophin	T38.81-
Adriamycin	T45.1X-
Aerosol spray NEC	T65.9-
Aerosporin	T36.8X-
ENT agent	T49.6X-
ophthalmic preparation	T49.5X-
topical NEC	T49.0X-
Aethusa cynapium	T62.2X-
Afghanistan black	T40.7X-
Aflatoxin	T64.0-
Afloqualone	T42.8X-
African boxwood	T62.2X-
Agar	T47.4X-
Agonist (predominantly)	
- alpha-adrenoreceptor	T44.4X-
beta-adrenoreceptor	T44.5X-
Agricultural agent NEC	T65.9-
Agrypnal	T42.3X-
AHLG	T50.Z1-
Air contaminant (s) type NOS	T65.9-
Ajmaline	T46.2X-
Akee	T62.1X-
Akrinol	T49.0X-
Akritoin	T37.8X-
Alacepril	T46.4X-
Alantolactone	T37.4X-
Albamycin	T36.8X-
Albendazole	T37.4X-
Albumin	T45.8X-
Albuterol	T48.6X-
Albutoin	T42.0X-
Alclometasone	T49.0X-

Drug/Chemical	Code
Alcohol	T51.9-
allyl	T51.8X-
amyl / butyl/ propyl	T51.3X-
antifreeze / methyl	T51.1X-
beverage (grain, ethyl)	T51.0X-
dehydrated / denatured	T51.0X-
deterrent NEC	T50.6X-
diagnostic (gastric function)	T50.8X-
industrial	T51.0X-
isopropyl	T51.2X-
preparation for consumption	T51.0X-
radiator	T51.1X-
rubbing	T51.2X-
specified type NEC	T51.8X-
surgical	T51.0X-
vapor (any type of Alcohol)	T59.89-
wood	T51.1X-
Alcuronium (chloride)	T48.1X-
Aldactone	T50.0X-
Aldesulfone sodium	T37.1X-
Aldicarb	T60.0X-
Aldomet	T46.5X-
Aldosterone	T50.0X-
Aldrin (dust)	T60.1X-
Alexitol sodium	T47.1X-
Alfacalcidol	T45.2X-
Alfadolone	T41.1X-
Alfaxalone	T41.1X-
Alfentanil	T40.4X-
Alfuzosin (hydrochloride)	T44.8X-
Algae (harmful) (toxin)	T65.821
Algeldrate	T47.1X-
Algin	T47.8X-
Alglucerase	T45.3X-
Alidase	T45.3X-
Alimemazine	T43.3X-
Aliphatic thiocyanates	T65.0X-
Alizapride	T45.0X-
Alkali (caustic)	T54.3X-
Alkaline antiseptic solution (aromatic)	T49.6X-
Alkalinizing agents (medicinal)	T50.90-
Alkalizing agent NEC	T50.90-
Alka-seltzer	T39.01-
Alkavervir	T46.5X-
Alkonium (bromide)	T49.0X-
Alkylating drug NEC	T45.1X-
antimyeloproliferative or lymphatic	T45.1X-

Drug/Chemical	Code
Alkylisocyanate	T65.0X-
Allantoin	T49.4X-
Allegron	T43.01-
Allethrin	T49.0X-
Allobarbital	T42.3X-
Allopurinol	T50.4X-
Allyl	
Alcohol	T51.8X-
disulfide	T46.6X-
Allylestrenol	T38.5X-
Allylisopropylacetylurea	T42.6X-
Allylisopropylmalonylurea	T42.3X-
Allylthiourea	T49.3X-
Allyltribromide	T42.6X-
Allypropymal	T42.3X-
Almagate	T47.1X-
Almasilate	T47.1X-
Almitrine	T50.7X-
Aloes	T47.2X-
Aloglutamol	T47.1X-
Aloin	T47.2X-
Aloxidone	T42.2X-
Alpha	
acetyldigoxin	T46.0X-
adrenergic blocking drug	T44.6X-
amylase	T45.3X-
tocoferol (acetate) toco	T45.2X-
tocopherol	T45.2X-
Alphadolone	T41.1X-
Alphaprodine	T40.4X-
Alphaxalone	T41.1X-
Alprazolam	T42.4X-
Alprenolol	T44.7X-
Alprostadil	T46.7X-
Alsactide	T38.81-
Alseroxylon	T46.5X-
Alteplase	T45.61-
Altizide	T50.2X-
Altretamine	T45.1X-
Alum (medicinal)	T49.4X-
nonmedicinal (ammonium) (potassium)	T56.89-
Aluminium, aluminum	
acetate / chloride	T49.2X-
solution	T49.0X-
aspirin / bis (acetylsalicylate)	T39.01-
carbonate (gel, basic)	T47.1X-
chlorhydroxide-complex	T47.1X-

Drug/Chemical	Code
Aluminium, aluminum, continued	
clofibrate	T46.6X-
diacetate	T49.2X-
glycinate	T47.1X-
hydroxide (gel)	T47.1X-
hydroxide-magn. carb. gel	T47.1X-
magnesium silicate	T47.1X-
nicotinate	T46.7X-
ointment (surgical) (topical)	T49.3X-
phosphate / silicate (sodium)	T47.1X-
salicylate	T39.09-
subacetate	T49.2X-
sulfate	T49.0X-
tannate	T47.6X-
Alurate	T42.3X-
Alverine	T44.3X-
Alvodine	T40.2X-
Amanita phalloides	T62.0X-
Amanitine	T62.0X-
Amantadine	T42.8X-
Ambazone	T49.6X-
Ambenonium (chloride)	T44.0X-
Ambroxol	T48.4X-
Ambuphylline	T48.6X-
Ambutonium bromide	T44.3X-
Amcinonide	T49.0X-
Amdinocilline	T36.0X-
Ametazole	T50.8X-
Amethocaine (regional, spinal)	T41.3X-
Amethopterin	T45.1X-
Amezinium metilsulfate	T44.99-
Amfebutamone	T43.29-
Amfepramone	T50.5X-
Amfetamine	T43.62-
Amfetaminil	T43.62-
Amfomycin	T36.8X-
Amidefrine mesilate	T48.5X-
Amidone	T40.3X-
Amidopyrine	T39.2X-
Amidotrizoate	T50.8X-
Amiflamine	T43.1X-
Amikacin	T36.5X-
Amikhelline	T46.3X-
Amiloride	T50.2X-
Aminacrine	T49.0X-
Amineptine	T43.01-
Aminitrozole	T37.3X-

Drug/Chemical	Code
Amino acids	T50.3X-
Aminoacetic acid (derivatives)	T50.3X-
Aminoacridine	T49.0X-
Aminobenzoic acid (-p)	T49.3X-
4-Aminobutyric acid	T43.8X-
Aminocaproic acid	T45.62-
Aminoethylisothiourium	T45.8X-
Aminofenazone	T39.2X-
Aminoglutethimide	T45.1X-
Aminohippuric acid	T50.8X-
Aminomethylbenzoic acid	T45.69-
Aminometradine	T50.2X-
Aminopentamide	T44.3X-
Aminophenazone	T39.2X-
Aminophenol	T54.0X-
4-Aminophenol derivatives	T39.1X-
Aminophenylpyridone	T43.59-
Aminophylline	T48.6X-
Aminopterin sodium	T45.1X-
Aminopyrine	T39.2X-
8-Aminoquinoline drugs	T37.2X-
Aminorex	T50.5X-
Aminosalicylic acid	T37.1X-
Aminosalylum	T37.1X-
Amiodarone	T46.2X-
Amiphenazole	T50.7X-
Amiquinsin	T46.5X-
Amisometradine	T50.2X-
Amisulpride	T43.59-
Amitriptyline	T43.01-
Amitriptylinoxide	T43.01-
Amlexanox	T48.6X-
Ammonia (fumes/vapor) (gas)	T59.89-
aromatic spirit	T48.99-
liquid (household)	T54.3X-
Ammoniated mercury	T49.0X-
Ammonium	
acid tartrate	T49.5X-
bromide	T42.6X-
carbonate	T54.3X-
chloride	T50.99-
expectorant	T48.4X-
compounds (household)NEC	T54.3X-
fumes (any usage)	T59.89-
industrial	T54.3X-
ichthyosulronate	T49.4X-
mandelate	T37.9-

Drug/Chemical	Code
Ammonium, continued	
sulfamate	T60.3X-
sulfonate resin	T47.8X-
Amobarbital (sodium)	T42.3X-
Amodiaquine	T37.2X-
Amopyroquin (e)	T37.2X-
Amoxapine	T43.01-
Amoxicillin	T36.0X-
Amperozide	T43.59-
Amphenidone	T43.59-
Amphetamine NEC	T43.62-
Amphomycin	T36.8X-
Amphotalide	T37.4X-
Amphotericin B	T36.7X-
topical	T49.0X-
Ampicillin	T36.0X-
Amprotropine	T44.3X-
Amsacrine	T45.1X-
Amygdaline	T62.2X-
Amyl	
acetate	T52.8X-
vapor	T59.89-
alcohol	T51.3X-
chloride	T53.6X-
formate	T52.8X-
nitrite	T46.3X-
propionate	T65.89-
Amylase	T47.5X-
Amyleine, regional	T41.3X-
Amylene	
dichloride	T53.6X-
hydrate	T51.3X-
Amylmetacresol	T49.6X-
Amylobarbitone	T42.3X-
Amylocaine, regional (infiltration) (subcutaneous) (nerve block) (spinal) (topical)	T41.3X-
Amylopectin	T47.6X-
Amytal (sodium)	T42.3X-
Anabolic steroid	T38.7X-
Analeptic NEC	T50.7X-
Analgesic	T39.9-
anti-inflammatory NEC	T39.9-
propionic acid derivative	T39.31-
antirheumatic NEC	T39.4X-
aromatic NEC	T39.1X-
narcotic NEC	T40.60-
non-narcotic NEC	T39.9-

Drug/Chemical	Code
Analgesic, continued	
pyrazole	T39.2X-
specified NEC	T39.8X-
Analgin	T39.2X-
Anamirta cocculus	T62.1X-
Ancillin	T36.0X-
Ancrod	T45.69-
Androgen	T38.7X-
Androgen-estrogen mixture	T38.7X-
Androstalone	T38.7X-
Androstanolone	T38.7X-
Androsterone	T38.7X-
Anemone pulsatilla	T62.2X-
Anesthesia	
caudal	T41.3X-
endotracheal	T41.0X-
epidural	T41.3X-
inhalation	T41.0X-
local (nerve or plexus blocking)	T41.3X-
mucosal	T41.3X-
muscle relaxation	T48.1X-
potentiated	T41.20-
rectal (general)	T41.20-
local	T41.3X-
regional	T41.3X-
surface	T41.3X-
Anesthetic NEC	T41.41
with muscle relaxant	T41.20-
general	T41.20-
local	T41.3X-
gaseous NEC	T41.0X-
general NEC	T41.20-
halogenated hydrocarbon derivatives NEC	T41.0X-
infiltration NEC	T41.3X-
intravenous NEC	T41.1X-
local NEC	T41.3X-
rectal (general)	T41.20-
local	T41.3X-
regional NEC / spinal NEC	T41.3X-
thiobarbiturate	T41.1X-
topical	T41.3X-
Aneurine	T45.2X-
Angio-Conray	T50.8X-
Angiotensin	T44.5X-
Angiotensinamide	T44.99-
Anhydrohydroxy-progesterone	T38.5X-

Drug/Chemical	Code
Anhydron	T50.2X-
Anileridine	T40.4X-
Aniline (dye) (liquid)	T65.3X-
analgesic	T39.1X-
derivatives, therapeutic NEC	T39.1X-
vapor	T65.3X-
Aniscoropine	T44.3X-
Anise oil	T47.5X-
Anisidine	T65.3X-
Anisindione	T45.51-
Anisotropine methyl-bromide	T44.3X-
Anistreplase	T45.61-
Anorexiant (central)	T50.5X-
Anorexic agents	T50.5X-
Ansamycin	T36.6X-
Ant (bite) (sting)	T63.421
Antabuse	T50.6X-
Antacid NEC	T47.1X-
Antagonist	
Aldosterone	T50.0X-
alpha-adrenoreceptor	T44.6X-
anticoagulant	T45.7X-
beta-adrenoreceptor	T44.7X-
extrapyramidal NEC	T44.3X-
folic acid	T45.1X-
H2 receptor	T47.0X-
heavy metal	T45.8X-
narcotic analgesic	T50.7X-
opiate	T50.7X-
pyrimidine	T45.1X-
serotonin	T46.5X-
Antazolin (e)	T45.0X-
Anterior pituitary hormone NEC	T38.81-
Anthelmintic NEC	T37.4X-
Anthiolimine	T37.4X-
Anthralin	T49.4X-
Anthramycin	T45.1X-
Antiadrenergic NEC	T44.8X-
Antiallergic NEC	T45.0X-
Anti-anemic (drug) (preparation)	T45.8X-
Antiandrogen NEC	T38.6X-
Antianxiety drug NEC	T43.50-
Antiaris toxicaria	T65.89-
Antiarteriosclerotic drug	T46.6X-
Antiasthmatic drug NEC	T48.6X-

Drug/Chemical	Code
Antibiotic NEC	T36.9-
aminoglycoside	T36.5X-
anticancer	T45.1X-
antifungal	T36.7X-
antimycobacterial	T36.5X-
antineoplastic	T45.1X-
cephalosporin (group)	T36.1X-
chloramphenicol (group)	T36.2X-
ENT	T49.6X-
eye	T49.5X-
fungicidal (local)	T49.0X-
intestinal	T36.8X-
b-lactam NEC	T36.1X-
local	T49.0X-
macrolides	T36.3X-
polypeptide	T36.8X-
specified NEC	T36.8X-
tetracycline (group)	T36.4X-
throat	T49.6X-
Anticancer agents NEC	T45.1X-
Anticholesterolemic drug NEC	T46.6X-
Anticholinergic NEC	T44.3X-
Anticholinesterase	T44.0X-
organophosphorus	T44.0X-
insecticide	T60.0X-
nerve gas	T59.89-
reversible	T44.0X-
ophthalmological	T49.5X-
Anticoagulant NEC	T45.51-
Antagonist	T45.7X-
Anti-common-cold drug NEC	T48.5X-
Anticonvulsant	T42.71
barbiturate	T42.3X-
combination (with barbiturate)	T42.3X-
hydantoin	T42.0X-
hypnotic NEC	T42.6X-
oxazolidinedione	T42.2X-
pyrimidinedione	T42.6X-
specified NEC	T42.6X-
succinimide	T42.2X-
Anti-D immunoglobulin (human)	T50.Z1-
Antidepressant	T43.20-
monoamine oxidase inhibitor	T43.1X-
SSNRI	T43.21-
SSRI	T43.22-
specified NEC	T43.29-

Drug/Chemical	Code
Antidepressant, continued	
tetracyclic	T43.02-
triazolopyridine	T43.21-
tricyclic	T43.01-
Antidiabetic NEC	T38.3X-
biguanide	T38.3X-
and sulfonyl combined	T38.3X-
combined	T38.3X-
sulfonylurea	T38.3X-
Antidiarrheal drug NEC	T47.6X-
absorbent	T47.6X-
Antidiphtheria serum	T50.Z1-
Antidiuretic hormone	T38.89-
Antidote NEC	T50.6X-
heavy metal	T45.8X-
Antidysrhythmic NEC	T46.2X-
Antiemetic drug	T45.0X-
Antiepilepsy agent	T42.71
combination or mixed	T42.5X-
specified, NEC	T42.6X-
Antiestrogen NEC	T38.6X-
Antifertility pill	T38.4X-
Antifibrinolytic drug	T45.62-
Antifilarial drug	T37.4X-
Antiflatulent	T47.5X-
Antifreeze	T65.9-
alcohol	T51.1X-
ethylene glycol	T51.8X-
Antifungal	
antibiotic (systemic)	T36.7X-
anti-infective NEC	T37.9-
disinfectant, local	T49.0X-
nonmedicinal (spray)	T60.3X-
topical	T49.0X-
Anti-gastric-secretion drug NEC	T47.1X-
Antigonadotrophin NEC	T38.6X-
Antihallucinogen	T43.50-
Antihelmintics	T37.4X-
Antihemophilic	
factor	T45.8X-
fraction	T45.8X-
globulin concentrate	T45.7X-
human plasma	T45.8X-
plasma, dried	T45.7X-
Antihemorrhoidal preparation	T49.2X-
Antiheparin drug	T45.7X-

Drug/Chemical	Code
Antihistamine	T45.0X-
Antihookworm drug	T37.4X-
Anti-human lymphocytic globulin	T50.Z1-
Antihyperlipidemic drug	T46.6X-
Antihypertensive drug NEC	T46.5X-
Anti-infective NEC	T37.9-
anthelmintic	T37.4X-
antibiotics	T36.9-
specified NEC	T36.8X-
antimalarial	T37.2X-
antimycobacterial NEC	T37.1X-
antibiotics	T36.5X-
antiprotozoal NEC	T37.3X-
blood	T37.2X-
antiviral	T37.5X-
arsenical	T37.8X-
bismuth, local	T49.0X-
ENT	T49.6X-
eye NEC	T49.5X-
heavy metals NEC	T37.8X-
local NEC	T49.0X-
specified NEC	T49.0X-
mixed	T37.9-
ophthalmic preparation	T49.5X-
topical NEC	T49.0X-
Anti-inflammatory drug NEC	T39.39-
local	T49.0X-
nonsteroidal NEC	T39.39-
propionic acid derivative	T39.31-
specified NEC	T39.39-
Antikaluretic	T50.3X-
Antiknock (tetraethyl lead)	T56.0X-
Antilipemic drug NEC	T46.6X-
Antimalarial	T37.2X-
prophylactic NEC	T37.2X-
pyrimidine derivative	T37.2X-
Antimetabolite	T45.1X-
Antimitotic agent	T45.1X-
Antimony (compounds) (vapor) NEC	T56.89-
anti-infectives	T37.8X-
dimercaptosuccinate	T37.3X-
hydride	T56.89-
pesticide (vapor)	T60.8X-
potassium (sodium)tartrate	T37.8X-
sodium dimercaptosuccinate	T37.3X-
tartrated	T37.8X-

ANTIMUSCARINIC NEC–ARSPHENAMINE (SILVER)

Drug/Chemical	Code
Antimuscarinic NEC	T44.3X-
Antimycobacterial drug NEC	T37.1X-
antibiotics	T36.5X-
combination	T37.1X-
Antinausea drug	T45.0X-
Antinematode drug	T37.4X-
Antineoplastic NEC	T45.1X-
alkaloidal	T45.1X-
antibiotics	T45.1X-
combination	T45.1X-
estrogen	T38.5X-
steroid	T38.7X-
Antiparasitic drug (systemic)	T37.9-
local	T49.0X-
specified NEC	T37.8X-
Antiparkinsonism drug NEC	T42.8X-
Antiperspirant NEC	T49.2X-
Antiphlogistic NEC	T39.4X-
Antiplatyhelmintic drug	T37.4X-
Antiprotozoal drug NEC	T37.3X-
blood	T37.2X-
local	T49.0X-
Antipruritic drug NEC	T49.1X-
Antipsychotic drug	T43.50-
specified NEC	T43.59-
Antipyretic	T39.9-
specified NEC	T39.8X-
Antipyrine	T39.2X-
Antirabies hyperimmune serum	T50.Z1-
Antirheumatic NEC	T39.4X-
Antirigidity drug NEC	T42.8X-
Antischistosomal drug	T37.4X-
Antiscorpion sera	T50.Z1-
Antiseborrheics	T49.4X-
Antiseptics (external) (medicinal)	T49.0X-
Antistine	T45.0X-
Antitapeworm drug	T37.4X-
Antitetanus immunoglobulin	T50.Z1-
Antithyroid drug NEC	T38.2X-
Antitoxin	T50.Z1-
Antitrichomonal drug	T37.3X-
Antituberculars	T37.1X-
antibiotics	T36.5X-
Antitussive NEC	T48.3X-
codeine mixture	T40.2X-
opiate	T40.2X-
Antivaricose drug	T46.8X-

Drug/Chemical	Code
Antivenin, antivenom (sera)	T50.Z1-
crotaline	T50.Z1-
spider bite	T50.Z1-
Antivertigo drug	T45.0X-
Antiviral drug NEC	T37.5X-
eye	T49.5X-
Antiwhipworm drug	T37.4X-
Antrol—see also specific chemical	T60.9-
fungicide	T60.9-
ANTU (alpha naphthylthiourea)	T60.4X-
Apalcillin	T36.0X-
APC	T48.5X-
Aplonidine	T44.4X-
Apomorphine	T47.7X-
Appetite depressants, central	T50.5X-
Apraclonidine (hydrochloride)	T44.4X-
Apresoline	T46.5X-
Aprindine	T46.2X-
Aprobarbital	T42.3X-
Apronalide	T42.6X-
Aprotinin	T45.62-
Aptocaine	T41.3X-
Aqua fortis	T54.2X-
Ara-A	T37.5X-
Ara-C	T45.1X-
Arachis oil	T49.3X-
cathartic	T47.4X-
Aralen	T37.2X-
Arecoline	T44.1X-
Arginine	T50.99-
glutamate	T50.99-
Argyrol	T49.0X-
ENT agent	T49.6X-
ophthalmic preparation	T49.5X-
Aristocort	T38.0X-
ENT agent	T49.6X-
ophthalmic preparation	T49.5X-
topical NEC	T49.0X-
Aromatics, corrosive	T54.1X-
disinfectants	T54.1X-
Arsenate of lead	T57.0X-
herbicide	T57.0X-
Arsenic, arsenicals (compounds) (dust) (vapor)NEC	T57.0X-
anti-infectives	T37.8X-
pesticide (dust) (fumes)	T57.0X-
Arsine (gas)	T57.0X-
Arsphenamine (silver)	T37.8X-

Drug/Chemical	Code	Drug/Chemical	Code
Arsthinol	T37.3X-	Azapetine	T46.7X-
Artane	T44.3X-	Azapropazone	T39.2X-
Arthropod (venomous)NEC	T63.481	Azaribine	T45.1X-
Articaine	T41.3X-	Azaserine	T45.1X-
Asbestos	T57.8X-	Azatadine	T45.0X-
Ascaridole	T37.4X-	Azatepa	T45.1X-
Ascorbic acid	T45.2X-	Azathioprine	T45.1X-
Asiaticoside	T49.0X-	Azelaic acid	T49.0X-
Asparaginase	T45.1X-	Azelastine	T45.0X-
Aspidium (oleoresin)	T37.4X-	Azidocillin	T36.0X-
Aspirin (aluminum) (soluble)	T39.01-	Azidothymidine	T37.5X-
Aspoxicillin	T36.0X-	Azinphos (ethyl) (methyl)	T60.0X-
Astemizole	T45.0X-	Aziridine (chelating)	T54.1X-
Astringent (local)	T49.2X-	Azithromycin	T36.3X-
specified NEC	T49.2X-	Azlocillin	T36.0X-
Astromicin	T36.5X-	Azobenzene smoke	T65.3X-
Ataractic drug NEC	T43.50-	acaricide	T60.8X-
Atenolol	T44.7X-	Azosulfamide	T37.0X-
Atonia drug, intestinal	T47.4X-	AZT	T37.5X-
Atophan	T50.4X-	Aztreonam	T36.1X-
Atracurium besilate	T48.1X-	Azulfidine	T37.0X-
Atropine	T44.3X-	Azuresin	T50.8X-
derivative	T44.3X-	Bacampicillin	T36.0X-
methonitrate	T44.3X-	Bacillus	
Attapulgite	T47.6X-	lactobacillus	T47.8X-
Auramine	T65.89-	subtilis	T47.6X-
dye	T65.6X-	Bacimycin	T49.0X-
fungicide	T60.3X-	ophthalmic preparation	T49.5X-
Auranofin	T39.4X-	Bacitracin zinc	T49.0X-
Aurantiin	T46.99-	with neomycin	T49.0X-
Aureomycin	T36.4X-	ENT agent	T49.6X-
ophthalmic preparation	T49.5X-	ophthalmic preparation	T49.5X-
topical NEC	T49.0X-	topical NEC	T49.0X-
Aurothioglucose	T39.4X-	Baclofen	T42.8X-
Aurothioglycanide	T39.4X-	Baking soda	T50.99-
Aurothiomalate sodium	T39.4X-	BAL	T45.8X-
Aurotioprol	T39.4X-	Bambuterol	T48.6X-
Automobile fuel	T52.0X-	Bamethan (sulfate)	T46.7X-
Autonomic nervous system agent NEC	T44.90-	Bamifylline	T48.6X-
Avlosulfon	T37.1X-	Bamipine	T45.0X-
Avomine	T42.6X-	Baneberry—see Actaea spicata	
Axerophthol	T45.2X-	Banewort—see Belladonna	
Azacitidine	T45.1X-	Barbenyl	T42.3X-
Azacyclonol	T43.59-	Barbexaclone	T42.6X-
Azadirachta	T60.2X-	Barbital (sodium)	T42.3X-
Azanidazole	T37.3X-	Barbitone	T42.3X-

Drug/Chemical	Code
Barbiturate NEC	T42.3X-
with tranquilizer	T42.3X-
anesthetic (intravenous)	T41.1X-
Barium (carbonate) (chloride) (sulfite)	T57.8X-
diagnostic agent	T50.8X-
pesticide / rodenticide	T60.4X-
sulfate (medicinal)	T50.8X-
Barrier cream	T49.3X-
Basic fuchsin	T49.0X-
Battery acid or fluid	T54.2X-
Bay rum	T51.8X-
BCG (vaccine)	T50.A9-
BCNU	T45.1X-
Bearsfoot	T62.2X-
Beclamide	T42.6X-
Beclomethasone	T44.5X-
Bee (sting) (venom)	T63.441
Befunolol	T49.5X-
Bekanamycin	T36.5X-
Belladonna—see Nightshade	T44.3X-
Bemegride	T50.7X-
Benactyzine	T44.3X-
Benadryl	T45.0X-
Benaprizine	T44.3X-
Benazepril	T46.4X-
Bencyclane	T46.7X-
Bendazol	T46.3X-
Bendrofluazide	T50.2X-
Bendroflumethiazide	T50.2X-
Benemid	T50.4X-
Benethamine penicillin	T36.0X-
Benexate	T47.1X-
Benfluorex	T46.6X-
Benfotiamine	T45.2X-
Benisone	T49.0X-
Benomyl	T60.0X-
Benoquin	T49.8X-
Benoxinate	T41.3X-
Benperidol	T43.4X-
Benproperine	T48.3X-
Benserazide	T42.8X-
Bentazepam	T42.4X-
Bentiromide	T50.8X-
Bentonite	T49.3X-
Benzalbutyramide	T46.6X-

Drug/Chemical	Code
Benzalkonium (chloride)	T49.0X-
ophthalmic preparation	T49.5X-
Benzamidosalicylate (calcium)	T37.1X-
Benzamine	T41.3X-
lactate	T49.1X-
Benzamphetamine	T50.5X-
Benzapril hydrochloride	T46.5X-
Benzathine benzylpenicillin	T36.0X-
Benzathine penicillin	T36.0X-
Benzatropine	T42.8X-
Benzbromarone	T50.4X-
Benzcarbimine	T45.1X-
Benzedrex	T44.99-
Benzedrine (amphetamine)	T43.62-
Benzenamine	T65.3X-
Benzene	T52.1X-
homologues (acetyl) (dimethyl) (methyl) (solvent)	T52.2X-
Benzethonium (chloride)	T49.0X-
Benzfetamine	T50.5X-
Benzhexol	T44.3X-
Benzhydramine (chloride)	T45.0X-
Benzidine	T65.89-
Benzilonium bromide	T44.3X-
Benzimidazole	T60.3X-
Benziodarone	T46.3X-
Benznidazole	T37.3X-
Benzocaine	T41.3X-
Benzodiapin	T42.4X-
Benzodiazepine NEC	T42.4X-
Benzoic acid	T49.0X-
with salicylic acid	T49.0X-
Benzoin (tincture)	T48.5X-
Benzol (benzene)	T52.1X-
vapor	T52.0X-
Benzomorphan	T40.2X-
Benzonatate	T48.3X-
Benzophenones	T49.3X-
Benzopyrone	T46.99-
Benzothiadiazides	T50.2X-
Benzoxonium chloride	T49.0X-
Benzoyl peroxide	T49.0X-
Benzoylpas calcium	T37.1X-
Benzperidin	T43.59-
Benzperidol	T43.59-
Benzphetamine	T50.5X-
Benzpyrinium bromide	T44.1X-

BARBITURATE NEC–BENZPYRINIUM BROMIDE

Drug/Chemical	Code
Benzquinamide	T45.0X-
Benzthiazide	T50.2X-
Benztropine	
anticholinergic	T44.3X-
antiparkinson	T42.8X-
Benzydamine	T49.0X-
Benzyl	
acetate	T52.8X-
alcohol	T49.0X-
benzoate	T49.0X-
Benzoic acid	T49.0X-
morphine	T40.2X-
nicotinate	T46.6X-
penicillin	T36.0X-
Benzylhydrochlorthia-zide	T50.2X-
Benzylpenicillin	T36.0X-
Benzylthiouracil	T38.2X-
Bephenium hydroxy-naphthoate	T37.4X-
Bepridil	T46.1X-
Bergamot oil	T65.89-
Bergapten	T50.99-
Berries, poisonous	T62.1X-
Beryllium (compounds)	T56.7X-
b-acetyldigoxin	T46.0X-
beta adrenergic blocking agent, heart	T44.7X-
b-benzalbutyramide	T46.6X-
Betacarotene	T45.2X-
b-eucaine	T49.1X-
Beta-Chlor	T42.6X-
b-galactosidase	T47.5X-
Betahistine	T46.7X-
Betaine	T47.5X-
Betamethasone	T49.0X-
topical	T49.0X-
Betamicin	T36.8X-
Betanidine	T46.5X-
b-sitosterol (s)	T46.6X-
Betaxolol	T44.7X-
Betazole	T50.8X-
Bethanechol	T44.1X-
chloride	T44.1X-
Bethanidine	T46.5X-
Betoxycaine	T41.3X-
Betula oil	T49.3X-
Bevantolol	T44.7X-
Bevonium metilsulfate	T44.3X-
Bezafibrate	T46.6X-

Drug/Chemical	Code
Bezitramide	T40.4X-
BHA	T50.99-
Bhang	T40.7X-
BHC (medicinal)	T49.0X-
nonmedicinal (vapor)	T53.6X-
Bialamicol	T37.3X-
Bibenzonium bromide	T48.3X-
Bibrocathol	T49.5X-
Bichloride of mercury—*see Mercury, chloride*	
Bichromates (calcium) (potassium) (sodium) (crystals)	T57.8X-
fumes	T56.2X-
Biclotymol	T49.6X-
Bicucculine	T50.7X-
Bifemelane	T43.29-
Biguanide derivatives, oral	T38.3X-
Bile salts	T47.5X-
Biligrafin	T50.8X-
Bilopaque	T50.8X-
Binifibrate	T46.6X-
Binitrobenzol	T65.3X-
Bioflavonoid (s)	T46.99-
Biological substance NEC	T50.90-
Biotin	T45.2X-
Biperiden	T44.3X-
Bisacodyl	T47.2X-
Bisbentiamine	T45.2X-
Bisbutiamine	T45.2X-
Bisdequalinium (salts) (diacetate)	T49.6X-
Bishydroxycoumarin	T45.51-
Bismarsen	T37.8X-
Bismuth salts	T47.6X-
aluminate	T47.1X-
anti-infectives	T37.8X-
formic iodide	T49.0X-
glycolylarsenate	T49.0X-
nonmedicinal (compounds)NEC	T65.9-
subcarbonate	T47.6X-
subsalicylate	T37.8X-
sulfarsphenamine	T37.8X-
Bisoprolol	T44.7X-
Bisoxatin	T47.2X-
Bisulepin (hydrochloride)	T45.0X-
Bithionol	T37.8X-
anthelminthic	T37.4X-
Bitolterol	T48.6X-
Bitoscanate	T37.4X-
Bitter almond oil	T62.8X-

Drug/Chemical	Code
Bittersweet	T62.2X-
Black	
flag	T60.9-
henbane	T62.2X-
leaf (40)	T60.9-
widow spider (bite)	T63.31-
antivenin	T50.Z1-
Blast furnace gas (carbon monoxide)	T58.8X-
Bleach	T54.9-
Bleaching agent (medicinal)	T49.4X-
Bleomycin	T45.1X-
Blockain (infiltration) (topical) (subcutaneous) (nerve block)	T41.3X-
Blockers, calcium channel	T46.1X-
Blood (derivatives) (natural) (plasma) (whole) (substitute)	T45.8X-
dried	T45.8X-
drug affecting NEC	T45.9-
expander NEC	T45.8X-
fraction NEC	T45.8X-
Blue velvet	T40.2X-
Bone meal	T62.8X-
Bonine	T45.0X-
Bopindolol	T44.7X-
Boracic acid	T49.0X-
ENT agent	T49.6X-
ophthalmic preparation	T49.5X-
Borane complex	T57.8X-
Borate (s)	T57.8X-
buffer	T50.99-
cleanser	T54.9-
sodium	T57.8X-
Borax (cleanser)	T54.9-
Bordeaux mixture	T60.3X-
Boric acid	T49.0X-
ENT agent	T49.6X-
ophthalmic preparation	T49.5X-
Bornaprine	T44.3X-
Boron	T57.8X-
hydride NEC	T57.8X-
fumes or gas	T57.8X-
trifluoride	T59.89-
Botox	T48.29-
Botulinus anti-toxin (type A, B)	T50.Z1-
Brake fluid vapor	T59.89-
Brallobarbital	T42.3X-
Bran (wheat)	T47.4X-
Brass (fumes)	T56.89-

Drug/Chemical	Code
Brasso	T52.0X-
Bretylium tosilate	T46.2X-
Brevital (sodium)	T41.1X-
Brinase	T45.3X-
British antilewisite	T45.8X-
Brodifacoum	T60.4X-
Bromal (hydrate)	T42.6X-
Bromazepam	T42.4X-
Bromazine	T45.0X-
Brombenzylcyanide	T59.3X-
Bromelains	T45.3X-
Bromethalin	T60.4X-
Bromhexine	T48.4X-
Bromide salts	T42.6X-
Bromindione	T45.51-
Bromine	
compounds (medicinal)	T42.6X-
sedative	T42.6X-
vapor	T59.89-
Bromisoval	T42.6X-
Bromisovalum	T42.6X-
Bromobenzylcyanide	T59.3X-
Bromochlorosalicylani-lide	T49.0X-
Bromocriptine	T42.8X-
Bromodiphenhydramine	T45.0X-
Bromoform	T42.6X-
Bromophenol blue reagent	T50.99-
Bromopride	T47.8X-
Bromosalicylchloranitide	T49.0X-
Bromosalicylhydroxamic acid	T37.1X-
Bromo-seltzer	T39.1X-
Bromoxynil	T60.3X-
Bromperidol	T43.4X-
Brompheniramine	T45.0X-
Bromsulfophthalein	T50.8X-
Bromural	T42.6X-
Bromvaletone	T42.6X-
Bronchodilator NEC	T48.6X-
Brotizolam	T42.4X-
Brovincamine	T46.7X-
Brown recluse spider (bite) (venom)	T63.33-
Brown spider (bite) (venom)	T63.39-
Broxaterol	T48.6X-
Broxuridine	T45.1X-
Broxyquinoline	T37.8X-
Bruceine	T48.29-

Drug/Chemical	Code
Brucia	T62.2X-
Brucine	T65.1X-
Bryonia	T47.2X-
Buclizine	T45.0X-
Buclosamide	T49.0X-
Budesonide	T44.5X-
Budralazine	T46.5X-
Bufferin	T39.01-
Buflomedil	T46.7X-
Buformin	T38.3X-
Bufotenine	T40.99-
Bufrolin	T48.6X-
Bufylline	T48.6X-
Bulk filler	T50.5X-
cathartic	T47.4X-
Bumetanide	T50.1X-
Bunaftine	T46.2X-
Bunamiodyl	T50.8X-
Bunazosin	T44.6X-
Bunitrolol	T44.7X-
Buphenine	T46.7X-
Bupivacaine (infiltration) (Nerve block) (spinal)	T41.3X-
Bupranolol	T44.7X-
Buprenorphine	T40.4X-
Bupropion	T43.29-
Burimamide	T47.1X-
Buserelin	T38.89-
Buspirone	T43.59-
Busulfan, busulphan	T45.1X-
Butabarbital (sodium)	T42.3X-
Butabarbitone	T42.3X-
Butabarpal	T42.3X-
Butacaine	T41.3X-
Butalamine	T46.7X-
Butalbital	T42.3X-
Butallylonal	T42.3X-
Butamben	T41.3X-
Butamirate	T48.3X-
Butane (distributed in mobile container or through pipes)	T59.89-
incomplete combustion	T58.1-
Butanilicaine	T41.3X-
Butanol	T51.3X-
Butanone, 2-butanone	T52.4X-
Butantrone	T49.4X-
Butaperazine	T43.3X-
Butazolidin	T39.2X-

Drug/Chemical	Code
Butetamate	T48.6X-
Butethal	T42.3X-
Butethamate	T44.3X-
Buthalitone (sodium)	T41.1X-
Butisol (sodium)	T42.3X-
Butizide	T50.2X-
Butobarbital (sodium)	T42.3X-
Butobarbitone	T42.3X-
Butoconazole (nitrate)	T49.0X-
Butorphanol	T40.4X-
Butriptyline	T43.01-
Butropium bromide	T44.3X-
Buttercups	T62.2X-
Butyl	
acetate (secondary)	T52.8X-
alcohol	T51.3X-
aminobenzoate	T41.3X-
butyrate	T52.8X-
carbinol or carbitol	T51.3X-
cellosolve	T52.3X-
chloral (hydrate)	T42.6X-
formate or lactate or propionate	T52.8X-
scopolamine bromide	T44.3X-
thiobarbital sodium	T41.1X-
Butylated hydroxy-anisole	T50.99-
Butylchloral hydrate	T42.6X-
Butyltoluene	T52.2X-
Butyn	T41.3X-
Butyrophenone (-based tranquilizers)	T43.4X-
Cabergoline	T42.8X-
Cacodyl, cacodylic acid	T57.0X-
Cactinomycin	T45.1X-
Cade oil	T49.4X-
Cadexomer iodine	T49.0X-
Cadmium (chloride) (fumes) (oxide)	T56.3X-
sulfide (medicinal)NEC	T49.4X-
Cadralazine	T46.5X-
Caffeine	T43.61-
Calabar bean	T62.2X-
Caladium seguinum	T62.2X-
Calamine (lotion)	T49.3X-
Calcifediol	T45.2X-
Calciferol	T45.2X-
Calcitonin	T50.99-
Calcitriol	T45.2X-

Drug/Chemical	Code
Calcium	T50.3X-
actylsalicylate	T39.01-
benzamidosalicylate	T37.1X-
bromide or bromolactobionate	T42.6X-
carbaspirin	T39.01-
carbimide	T50.6X-
carbonate	T47.1X-
chloride (anhydrous)	T50.99-
cyanide	T57.8X-
dioctyl sulfosuccinate	T47.4X-
disodium edathamil	T45.8X-
disodium edetate	T45.8X-
dobesilate	T46.99-
EDTA	T45.8X-
ferrous citrate	T45.4X-
folinate	T45.8X-
glubionate	T50.3X-
gluconate or – gluconogalactogluconate	T50.3X-
hydrate, hydroxide	T54.3X-
hypochlorite	T54.3X-
iodide	T48.4X-
ipodate	T50.8X-
lactate	T50.3X-
leucovorin	T45.8X-
mandelate	T37.9-
oxide	T54.3X-
pantothenate	T45.2X-
phosphate	T50.3X-
salicylate	T39.09-
salts	T50.3X-
Calculus-dissolving drug	T50.99-
Calomel	T49.0X-
Caloric agent	T50.3X-
Calusterone	T38.7X-
Camazepam	T42.4X-
Camomile	T49.0X-
Camoquin	T37.2X-
Camphor	
insecticide	T60.2X-
medicinal	T49.8X-
Camylofin	T44.3X-
Cancer chemo drug regimen	T45.1X-
Candeptin	T49.0X-
Candicidin	T49.0X-
Cannabinol	T40.7X-
Cannabis (derivatives)	T40.7X-

Drug/Chemical	Code
Canned heat	T51.1X-
Canrenoic acid	T50.0X-
Canrenone	T50.0X-
Cantharides, cantharidin, cantharis	T49.8X-
Canthaxanthin	T50.99-
Capillary-active drug NEC	T46.90-
Capreomycin	T36.8X-
Capsicum	T49.4X-
Captafol	T60.3X-
Captan	T60.3X-
Captodiame, captodiamine	T43.59-
Captopril	T46.4X-
Caramiphen	T44.3X-
Carazolol	T44.7X-
Carbachol	T44.1X-
Carbacrylamine (resin)	T50.3X-
Carbamate (insecticide)	T60.0X-
Carbamate (sedative)	T42.6X-
herbicide or insecticide	T60.0X-
Carbamazepine	T42.1X-
Carbamide	T47.3X-
peroxide	T49.0X-
topical	T49.8X-
Carbamylcholine chloride	T44.1X-
Carbaril	T60.0X-
Carbarsone	T37.3X-
Carbaryl	T60.0X-
Carbaspirin	T39.01-
Carbazochrome (salicylate) (sodium sulfonate)	T49.4X-
Carbenicillin	T36.0X-
Carbenoxolone	T47.1X-
Carbetapentane	T48.3X-
Carbethyl salicylate	T39.09-
Carbidopa (with levodopa)	T42.8X-
Carbimazole	T38.2X-
Carbinol	T51.1X-
Carbinoxamine	T45.0X-
Carbiphene	T39.8X-
Carbitol	T52.3X-
Carbo medicinalis	T47.6X-
Carbocaine (infiltration) (topical) (subcutaneous) (nerve block)	T41.3X-
Carbocisteine	T48.4X-
Carbocromen	T46.3X-
Carbol fuchsin	T49.0X-
Carbolic acid—see also Phenol	T54.0X-
Carbolonium (bromide)	T48.1X-

Drug/Chemical	Code
Carbomycin	T36.8X-
Carbon	
bisulfide (liquid) or vapor	T65.4X-
dioxide (gas)	T59.7X-
medicinal	T41.5X-
nonmedicinal	T59.7X-
snow	T49.4X-
disulfide (liquid) or vapor	T65.4X-
monoxide (from incomplete combustion)	T58.9-
blast furnace gas	T58.8X-
butane (distributed in mobile container or through pipes)	T58.1-
charcoal fumes or coal	T58.2X-
coke (in domestic stoves, fireplaces)	T58.2X-
gas (piped)	T58.1-
solid (in domestic stoves, fireplaces)	T58.2X-
exhaust gas (motor)not in transit	T58.0-
combustion engine, any not in watercraft	T58.0-
farm tractor, not in transit	T58.0-
gas engine / motor pump	T58.01
motor vehicle, not in transit	T58.0-
fuel (in domestic use)	T58.2X-
gas (piped) (natural) or in mobile container	T58.1-
utility	T58.1-
in mobile container	T58.1-
illuminating gas	T58.1-
industrial fuels or gases, any	T58.8X-
kerosene (in domestic stoves, fireplaces)	T58.2X-
kiln gas or vapor	T58.8X-
motor exhaust gas, not in transit	T58.0-
piped gas (manufactured) (natural)	T58.1-
producer gas	T58.8X-
propane (distributed in mobile container)	T58.1-
distributed through pipes	T58.1-
specified source NEC	T58.8X-
stove gas (piped) / utility gas (piped) / water gas	T58.1-
wood (in domestic stoves, fireplaces)	T58.2X-
tetrachloride (vapor)NEC	T53.0X-
Carbonic acid gas	T59.7X-
anhydrase inhibitor NEC	T50.2X-
Carbophenothion	T60.0X-
Carboplatin	T45.1X-
Carboprost	T48.0X-
Carboquone	T45.1X-
Carbowax	T49.3X-
Carboxymethyl-cellulose	T47.4X-
S-Carboxymethyl-cysteine	T48.4X-

Drug/Chemical	Code
Carbrital	T42.3X-
Carbromal	T42.6X-
Carbutamide	T38.3X-
Carbuterol	T48.6X-
Cardiac medications (depressants) (rhythm regulater) NEC	T46.2X-
Cardiografin	T50.8X-
Cardio-green	T50.8X-
Cardiotonic (glycoside)NEC	T46.0X-
Cardiovascular drug NEC	T46.90-
Cardrase	T50.2X-
Carfecillin	T36.0X-
Carfenazine	T43.3X-
Carfusin	T49.0X-
Carindacillin	T36.0X-
Carisoprodol	T42.8X-
Carmellose	T47.4X-
Carminative	T47.5X-
Carmofur	T45.1X-
Carmustine	T45.1X-
Carotene	T45.2X-
Carphenazine	T43.3X-
Carpipramine	T42.4X-
Carprofen	T39.31-
Carpronium chloride	T44.3X-
Carrageenan	T47.8X-
Carteolol	T44.7X-
Carter's Little Pills	T47.2X-
Cascara (sagrada)	T47.2X-
Cassava	T62.2X-
Castellani's paint	T49.0X-
Castor (bean) (oil)	T62.2X-
Catalase	T45.3X-
Caterpillar (sting)	T63.431
Catha (edulis) (tea)	T43.69-
Cathartic NEC	T47.4X-
anthacene derivative	T47.2X-
bulk	T47.4X-
contact	T47.2X-
emollient NEC	T47.4X-
irritant NEC	T47.2X-
mucilage	T47.4X-
saline	T47.3X-
vegetable	T47.2X-
Cathine	T50.5X-
Cathomycin	T36.8X-
Cation exchange resin	T50.3X-

Drug/Chemical	Code
Caustic (s) NEC	T54.9-
alkali	T54.3X-
hydroxide	T54.3X-
potash	T54.3X-
soda	T54.3X-
specified NEC	T54.9-
Ceepryn	T49.0X-
ENT agent	T49.6X-
lozenges	T49.6X-
Cefacetrile	T36.1X-
Cefaclor	T36.1X-
Cefadroxil	T36.1X-
Cefalexin	T36.1X-
Cefaloglycin	T36.1X-
Cefaloridine	T36.1X-
Cefalosporins	T36.1X-
Cefalotin	T36.1X-
Cefamandole	T36.1X-
Cefamycin antibiotic	T36.1X-
Cefapirin	T36.1X-
Cefatrizine	T36.1X-
Cefazedone	T36.1X-
Cefazolin	T36.1X-
Cefbuperazone	T36.1X-
Cefetamet	T36.1X-
Cefixime	T36.1X-
Cefmenoxime	T36.1X-
Cefmetazole	T36.1X-
Cefminox	T36.1X-
Cefonicid	T36.1X-
Cefoperazone	T36.1X-
Ceforanide	T36.1X-
Cefotaxime	T36.1X-
Cefotetan	T36.1X-
Cefotiam	T36.1X-
Cefoxitin	T36.1X-
Cefpimizole	T36.1X-
Cefpiramide	T36.1X-
Cefradine	T36.1X-
Cefroxadine	T36.1X-
Cefsulodin	T36.1X-
Ceftazidime	T36.1X-
Cefteram	T36.1X-
Ceftezole	T36.1X-
Ceftizoxime	T36.1X-
Ceftriaxone	T36.1X-

Drug/Chemical	Code
Cefuroxime	T36.1X-
Cefuzonam	T36.1X-
Celestone	T38.0X-
topical	T49.0X-
Celiprolol	T44.7X-
Cell stimulants and proliferants	T49.8X-
Cellosolve	T52.9-
Cellulose	
cathartic	T47.4X-
hydroxyethyl	T47.4X-
nitrates (topical)	T49.3X-
oxidized	T49.4X-
Centipede (bite)	T63.41-
Central nervous system	
depressants	T42.71
anesthetic (general)NEC	T41.20-
gases NEC	T41.0X-
intravenous	T41.1X-
barbiturates	T42.3X-
benzodiazepines	T42.4X-
bromides	T42.6X-
cannabis sativa	T40.7X-
chloral hydrate	T42.6X-
ethanol	T51.0X-
hallucinogenics	T40.90-
hypnotics	T42.71
specified NEC	T42.6X-
muscle relaxants	T42.8X-
paraldehyde	T42.6X-
sedatives; sedative-hypnotics	T42.71
mixed NEC	T42.6X-
specified NEC	T42.6X-
muscle-tone depressants	T42.8X-
stimulants	T43.60-
amphetamines	T43.62-
analeptics	T50.7X-
antidepressants	T43.20-
opiate antagonists	T50.7X-
specified NEC	T43.69-
Cephalexin	T36.1X-
Cephaloglycin	T36.1X-
Cephaloridine	T36.1X-
Cephalosporins	T36.1X-
N (adicillin)	T36.0X-
Cephalothin	T36.1X-
Cephalotin	T36.1X-

Drug/Chemical	Code
Cephradine	T36.1X-
Cerbera (odallam)	T62.2X-
Cerberin	T46.0X-
Cerebral stimulants	T43.60-
psychotherapeutic	T43.60-
specified NEC	T43.69-
Cerium oxalate	T45.0X-
Cerous oxalate	T45.0X-
Ceruletide	T50.8X-
Cetalkonium (chloride)	T49.0X-
Cethexonium chloride	T49.0X-
Cetiedil	T46.7X-
Cetirizine	T45.0X-
Cetomacrogol	T50.99-
Cetotiamine	T45.2X-
Cetoxime	T45.0X-
Cetraxate	T47.1X-
Cetrimide	T49.0X-
Cetrimonium (bromide)	T49.0X-
Cetylpyridinium chloride	T49.0X-
ENT agent or lozenges	T49.6X-
Cevitamic acid	T45.2X-
Chalk, precipitated	T47.1X-
Chamomile	T49.0X-
Ch'an su	T46.0X-
Charcoal	T47.6X-
activated—see also Charcoal, medicinal	T47.6X-
fumes (Carbon monoxide)	T58.2X-
industrial	T58.8X-
medicinal (activated)	T47.6X-
antidiarrheal	T47.6X-
poison control	T47.8X-
specified use other than for diarrhea	T47.8X-
topical	T49.8X-
Chaulmosulfone	T37.1X-
Chelating agent NEC	T50.6X-
Chelidonium majus	T62.2X-
Chemical substance NEC	T65.9-
Chenodeoxycholic acid	T47.5X-
Chenodiol	T47.5X-
Chenopodium	T37.4X-
Cherry laurel	T62.2X-
Chinidin (e)	T46.2X-
Chiniofon	T37.8X-
Chlophedianol	T48.3X-

Drug/Chemical	Code
Chloral	T42.6X-
derivative	T42.6X-
hydrate	T42.6X-
Chloralamide	T42.6X-
Chloralodol	T42.6X-
Chloralose	T60.4X-
Chlorambucil	T45.1X-
Chloramine	T57.8X-
topical	T49.0X-
Chloramphenicol	T36.2X-
ENT agent	T49.6X-
ophthalmic preparation	T49.5X-
topical NEC	T49.0X-
Chlorate (potassium) (sodium)NEC	T60.3X-
herbicide	T60.3X-
Chlorazanil	T50.2X-
Chlorbenzene, chlorbenzol	T53.7X-
Chlorbenzoxamine	T44.3X-
Chlorbutol	T42.6X-
Chlorcyclizine	T45.0X-
Chlordan (e) (dust)	T60.1X-
Chlordantoin	T49.0X-
Chlordiazepoxide	T42.4X-
Chlordiethyl benzamide	T49.3X-
Chloresium	T49.8X-
Chlorethiazol	T42.6X-
Chlorethyl—see Ethyl chloride	
Chloretone	T42.6X-
Chlorex	T53.6X-
insecticide	T60.1X-
Chlorfenvinphos	T60.0X-
Chlorhexadol	T42.6X-
Chlorhexamide	T45.1X-
Chlorhexidine	T49.0X-
Chlorhydroxyquinolin	T49.0X-
Chloride of lime (bleach)	T54.3X-
Chlorimipramine	T43.01-
Chlorinated	
camphene	T53.6X-
diphenyl	T53.7X-
hydrocarbons NEC (solvents)	T53.9-
lime (bleach)	T54.3X-
and boric acid solution	T49.0X-
naphthalene (insecticide)	T60.1X-
industrial (non-pesticide)	T53.7X-
pesticide NEC	T60.8X-
solution	T49.0X-

CEPHRADINE–CHLORINATED

Drug/Chemical	Code
Chlorine (fumes) (gas)	T59.4X-
bleach	T54.3X-
compound gas NEC	T59.4X-
disinfectant	T59.4X-
releasing agents NEC	T59.4X-
Chlorisondamine chloride	T46.99-
Chlormadinone	T38.5X-
Chlormephos	T60.0X-
Chlormerodrin	T50.2X-
Chlormethiazole	T42.6X-
Chlormethine	T45.1X-
Chlormethylenecycline	T36.4X-
Chlormezanone	T42.6X-
Chloroacetic acid	T60.3X-
Chloroacetone	T59.3X-
Chloroacetophenone	T59.3X-
Chloroaniline	T53.7X-
Chlorobenzene, chlorobenzol	T53.7X-
Chlorobromomethane (fire extinguisher)	T53.6X-
Chlorobutanol	T49.0X-
Chlorocresol	T49.0X-
Chlorodehydro-methyltestosterone	T38.7X-
Chlorodinitrobenzene	T53.7X-
Chlorodiphenyl	T53.7X-
Chloroethane—see Ethyl chloride	
Chloroethylene	T53.6X-
Chlorofluorocarbons	T53.5X-
Chloroform (fumes) (vapor)	T53.1X-
anesthetic	T41.0X-
solvent	T53.1X-
water, concentrated	T41.0X-
Chloroguanide	T37.2X-
Chloromycetin	T36.2X-
ENT agent or otic solution	T49.6X-
ophthalmic preparation	T49.5X-
topical NEC	T49.0X-
Chloronitrobenzene	T53.7X-
Chlorophacinone	T60.4X-
Chlorophenol	T53.7X-
Chlorophenothane	T60.1X-
Chlorophyll	T50.99-
Chloropicrin (fumes)	T53.6X-
fumigant / pesticide	T60.8X-
fungicide	T60.3X-

Drug/Chemical	Code
Chloroprocaine (infiltration) (topical) (subcutaneous) (nerve block) (spinal)	T41.3X-
Chloroptic	T49.5X-
Chloropurine	T45.1X-
Chloropyramine	T45.0X-
Chloropyrifos	T60.0X-
Chloropyrilene	T45.0X-
Chloroquine	T37.2X-
Chlorothalonil	T60.3X-
Chlorothen	T45.0X-
Chlorothiazide	T50.2X-
Chlorothymol	T49.4X-
Chlorotrianisene	T38.5X-
Chlorovinyldichloro-arsine	T57.0X-
Chloroxine	T49.4X-
Chloroxylenol	T49.0X-
Chlorphenamine	T45.0X-
Chlorphenesin	T42.8X-
topical (antifungal)	T49.0X-
Chlorpheniramine	T45.0X-
Chlorphenoxamine	T45.0X-
Chlorphentermine	T50.5X-
Chlorproguanil	T37.2X-
Chlorpromazine	T43.3X-
Chlorpropamide	T38.3X-
Chlorprothixene	T43.4X-
Chlorquinaldol	T49.0X-
Chlorquinol	T49.0X-
Chlortalidone	T50.2X-
Chlortetracycline	T36.4X-
Chlorthalidone	T50.2X-
Chlorthiophos	T60.0X-
Chlortrianisene	T38.5X-
Chlor-Trimeton	T45.0X-
Chlorthion	T60.0X-
Chlorzoxazone	T42.8X-
Choke damp	T59.7X-
Cholagogues	T47.5X-
Cholebrine	T50.8X-
Cholecalciferol	T45.2X-
Cholecystokinin	T50.8X-
Cholera vaccine	T50.A9-
Choleretic	T47.5X-
Cholesterol-lowering agents	T46.6X-
Cholestyramine (resin)	T46.6X-
Cholic acid	T47.5X-

Drug/Chemical	Code
Choline	T48.6X-
chloride	T50.99-
dihydrogen citrate	T50.99-
salicylate	T39.09-
theophyllinate	T48.6X-
Cholinergic (drug)NEC	T44.1X-
muscle tone enhancer	T44.1X-
organophosphorus	T44.0X-
insecticide	T60.0X-
nerve gas	T59.89-
trimethyl ammonium propanediol	T44.1X-
Cholinesterase reactivator	T50.6X-
Cholografin	T50.8X-
Chorionic gonadotropin	T38.89-
Chromate	T56.2X-
dust or mist	T56.2X-
lead—see also lead	T56.0X-
paint	T56.0X-
Chromic	
acid	T56.2X-
dust or mist	T56.2X-
phosphate 32P	T45.1X-
Chromium	T56.2X-
compounds—see Chromate	
sesquioxide	T50.8X-
Chromomycin A3	T45.1X-
Chromonar	T46.3X-
Chromyl chloride	T56.2X-
Chrysarobin	T49.4X-
Chrysazin	T47.2X-
Chymar	T45.3X-
ophthalmic preparation	T49.5X-
Chymopapain	T45.3X-
Chymotrypsin	T45.3X-
ophthalmic preparation	T49.5X-
Cianidanol	T50.99-
Cianopramine	T43.01-
Cibenzoline	T46.2X-
Ciclacillin	T36.0X-
Ciclobarbital—see Hexobarbital	
Ciclonicate	T46.7X-
Ciclopirox (olamine)	T49.0X-
Ciclosporin	T45.1X-
Cicuta maculata or virosa	T62.2X-
Cicutoxin	T62.2X-
Cigarette lighter fluid	T52.0X-

Drug/Chemical	Code
Cigarettes (tobacco)	T65.22-
Ciguatoxin	T61.0-
Cilazapril	T46.4X-
Cimetidine	T47.0X-
Cimetropium bromide	T44.3X-
Cinchocaine	T41.3X-
Cinchona	T37.2X-
Cinchonine alkaloids	T37.2X-
Cinchophen	T50.4X-
Cinepazide	T46.7X-
Cinnamedrine	T48.5X-
Cinnarizine	T45.0X-
Cinoxacin	T37.8X-
Ciprofibrate	T46.6X-
Ciprofloxacin	T36.8X-
Cisapride	T47.8X-
Cisplatin	T45.1X-
Citalopram	T43.22-
Citanest (infiltration) (topical) (subcutaneous) (nerve block)	T41.3X-
Citric acid	T47.5X-
Citrovorum (factor)	T45.8X-
Claviceps purpurea	T62.2X-
Clavulanic acid	T36.1X-
Cleaner, cleansing agent, type not specified	T65.89-
of paint or varnish	T52.9-
specified type NEC	T65.89-
Clebopride	T47.8X-
Clefamide	T37.3X-
Clemastine	T45.0X-
Clematis vitalba	T62.2X-
Clemizole (penicillin)	T45.0X-
Clenbuterol	T48.6X-
Clidinium bromide	T44.3X-
Clindamycin	T36.8X-
Clinofibrate	T46.6X-
Clioquinol	T37.8X-
Cliradon	T40.2X-
Clobazam	T42.4X-
Clobenzorex	T50.5X-
Clobetasol	T49.0X-
Clobetasone	T49.0X-
Clobutinol	T48.3X-
Clocortolone	T38.0X-
Clodantoin	T49.0X-
Clodronic acid	T50.99-
Clofazimine	T37.1X-

Drug/Chemical	Code
Clofedanol	T48.3X-
Clofenamide	T50.2X-
Clofenotane	T49.0X-
Clofezone	T39.2X-
Clofibrate	T46.6X-
Clofibride	T46.6X-
Cloforex	T50.5X-
Clomethiazole	T42.6X-
Clometocillin	T36.0X-
Clomifene	T38.5X-
Clomiphene	T38.5X-
Clomipramine	T43.01-
Clomocycline	T36.4X-
Clonazepam	T42.4X-
Clonidine	T46.5X-
Clonixin	T39.8X-
Clopamide	T50.2X-
Clopenthixol	T43.4X-
Cloperastine	T48.3X-
Clophedianol	T48.3X-
Cloponone	T36.2X-
Cloprednol	T38.0X-
Cloral betaine	T42.6X-
Cloramfenicol	T36.2X-
Clorazepate (dipotassium)	T42.4X-
Clorexolone	T50.2X-
Clorfenamine	T45.0X-
Clorgiline	T43.1X-
Clorotepine	T44.3X-
Clorox (bleach)	T54.9-
Clorprenaline	T48.6X-
Clortermine	T50.5X-
Clotiapine	T43.59-
Clotiazepam	T42.4X-
Clotibric acid	T46.6X-
Clotrimazole	T49.0X-
Cloxacillin	T36.0X-
Cloxazolam	T42.4X-
Cloxiquine	T49.0X-
Clozapine	T42.4X-
Coagulant NEC	T45.7X-
Coal (carbon monoxide from)—*see also* Carbon, monoxide, coal	T58.2X-
oil—*see Kerosene*	
tar	T49.1X-
fumes	T59.89-
medicinal (ointment)	T49.4X-

Drug/Chemical	Code
Coal (carbon monoxide from), continued	
analgesics NEC	T39.2X-
naphtha (solvent)	T52.0X-
Cobalamine	T45.2X-
Cobalt (nonmedicinal) (fumes) (industrial)	T56.89-
medicinal (trace) (chloride)	T45.8X-
Cobra (venom)	T63.041
Coca (leaf)	T40.5X-
Cocaine	T40.5X-
topical anesthetic	T41.3X-
Cocarboxylase	T45.3X-
Coccidioidin	T50.8X-
Cocculus indicus	T62.1X-
Cochineal	T65.6X-
medicinal products	T50.99-
Codeine	T40.2X-
Cod-liver oil	T45.2X-
Coenzyme A	T50.99-
Coffee	T62.8X-
Cogalactoiso-merase	T50.99-
Cogentin	T44.3X-
Coke fumes or gas (carbon monoxide)	T58.2X-
industrial use	T58.8X-
Colace	T47.4X-
Colaspase	T45.1X-
Colchicine	T50.4X-
Colchicum	T62.2X-
Cold cream	T49.3X-
Colecalciferol	T45.2X-
Colestipol	T46.6X-
Colestyramine	T46.6X-
Colimycin	T36.8X-
Colistimethate	T36.8X-
Colistin	T36.8X-
sulfate (eye preparation)	T49.5X-
Collagen	T50.99-
Collagenase	T49.4X-
Collodion	T49.3X-
Colocynth	T47.2X-
Colophony adhesive	T49.3X-
Colorant—*see also Dye*	T50.99-
Combustion gas (after combustion) —*see Carbon, monoxide*	
prior to combustion	T59.89-
Compazine	T43.3X-

Drug/Chemical	Code
Compound	
42 (warfarin)	T60.4X-
269 (endrin)	T60.1X-
497 (dieldrin)	T60.1X-
1080 (sodium fluoroacetate)	T60.4X-
3422 (parathion)	T60.0X-
3911 (phorate)	T60.0X-
3956 (toxaphene)	T60.1X-
4049 (malathion)	T60.0X-
4069 (malathion)	T60.0X-
4124 (dicapthon)	T60.0X-
E (cortisone)	T38.0X-
F (hydrocortisone)	T38.0X-
Congener, anabolic	T38.7X-
Congo red	T50.8X-
Coniine, conine	T62.2X-
Conium (maculatum)	T62.2X-
Conjugated estrogenic substances	T38.5X-
Contac	T48.5X-
Contact lens solution	T49.5X-
Contraceptive (oral)	T38.4X-
vaginal	T49.8X-
Contrast medium, radiography	T50.8X-
Convallaria glycosides	T46.0X-
Convallaria majalis	T62.2X-
berry	T62.1X-
Copper (dust) (fumes) (nonmedicinal) NEC	T56.4X-
arsenate, arsenite	T57.0X-
insecticide	T60.2X-
emetic	T47.7X-
fungicide	T60.3X-
gluconate	T49.0X-
insecticide	T60.2X-
medicinal (trace)	T45.8X-
oleate	T49.0X-
sulfate	T56.4X-
cupric	T56.4X-
fungicide	T60.3X-
medicinal	
ear	T49.6X-
emetic	T47.7X-
eye	T49.5X-
cuprous	T56.4X-
fungicide	T60.3X-

Drug/Chemical	Code
Copper (dust) (fumes) (nonmedicinal) NEC, continued	
medicinal	
ear	T49.6X-
emetic	T47.7X-
eye	T49.5X-
Copperhead snake (bite) (venom)	T63.06-
Coral (sting)	T63.69-
snake (bite) (venom)	T63.02-
Corbadrine	T49.6X-
Cordite	T65.89-
vapor	T59.89-
Cordran	T49.0X-
Corn cures	T49.4X-
Corn starch	T49.3X-
Cornhusker's lotion	T49.3X-
Coronary vasodilator NEC	T46.3X-
Corrosive NEC	T54.9-
acid NEC	T54.2X-
aromatics	T54.1X-
disinfectant	T54.1X-
fumes NEC	T54.9-
specified NEC	T54.9-
sublimate	T56.1X-
Cortate	T38.0X-
Cort-Dome	T38.0X-
ENT agent	T49.6X-
ophthalmic preparation	T49.5X-
topical NEC	T49.0X-
Cortef	T38.0X-
ENT agent	T49.6X-
ophthalmic preparation	T49.5X-
topical NEC	T49.0X-
Corticosteroid	T38.0X-
ENT agent	T49.6X-
mineral	T50.0X-
ophthalmic	T49.5X-
topical NEC	T49.0X-
Corticotropin	T38.81-
Cortisol	T49.0X-
ENT agent	T49.6X-
ophthalmic preparation	T49.5X-
topical NEC	T49.0X-
Cortisone (acetate)	T38.0X-
ENT agent	T49.6X-
ophthalmic preparation	T49.5X-
topical NEC	T49.0X-

Drug/Chemical	Code
Cortivazol	T38.0X-
Cortogen	T38.0X-
ENT agent	T49.6X-
ophthalmic preparation	T49.5X-
Cortone	T38.0X-
ENT agent	T49.6X-
ophthalmic preparation	T49.5X-
Cortril	T38.0X-
ENT agent	T49.6X-
ophthalmic preparation	T49.5X-
topical NEC	T49.0X-
Corynebacterium parvum	T45.1X-
Cosmetic preparation	T49.8X-
Cosmetics	T49.8X-
Cosyntropin	T38.81-
Cotarnine	T45.7X-
Co-trimoxazole	T36.8X-
Cottonseed oil	T49.3X-
Cough mixture (syrup)	T48.4X-
containing opiates	T40.2X-
expectorants	T48.4X-
Coumadin	T45.51-
rodenticide	T60.4X-
Coumaphos	T60.0X-
Coumarin	T45.51-
Coumetarol	T45.51-
Cowbane	T62.2X-
Cozyme	T45.2X-
Crack	T40.5X-
Crataegus extract	T46.0X-
Creolin	T54.1X-
disinfectant	T54.1X-
Creosol (compound)	T49.0X-
Creosote (coal tar) (beechwood)	T49.0X-
medicinal (expectorant) (syrup)	T48.4X-
Cresol (s)	T49.0X-
and soap solution	T49.0X-
Cresyl acetate	T49.0X-
Cresylic acid	T49.0X-
Crimidine	T60.4X-
Croconazole	T37.8X-
Cromoglicic acid	T48.6X-
Cromolyn	T48.6X-
Cromonar	T46.3X-
Cropropamide	T39.8X-
with crotethamide	T50.7X-
Crotamiton	T49.0X-

Drug/Chemical	Code
Crotethamide	T39.8X-
with cropropamide	T50.7X-
Croton (oil)	T47.2X-
chloral	T42.6X-
Crude oil	T52.0X-
Cryogenine	T39.8X-
Cryolite (vapor)	T60.1X-
insecticide	T60.1X-
Cryptenamine (tannates)	T46.5X-
Crystal violet	T49.0X-
Cuckoopint	T62.2X-
Cumetharol	T45.51-
Cupric	
acetate	T60.3X-
acetoarsenite	T57.0X-
arsenate	T57.0X-
gluconate	T49.0X-
oleate	T49.0X-
sulfate	T56.4X-
Cuprous sulfate—see also Copper sulfate	T56.4X-
Curare, curarine	T48.1X-
Cyamemazine	T43.3X-
Cyamopsis tetragono-loba	T46.6X-
Cyanacetyl hydrazide	T37.1X-
Cyanic acid (gas)	T59.89-
Cyanide (s) (compounds) (potassium) (sodium)NEC	T65.0X-
dust or gas (inhalation)NEC	T57.3X-
fumigant	T65.0X-
hydrogen	T57.3X-
mercuric—see Mercury	
pesticide (dust) (fumes)	T65.0X-
Cyanoacrylate adhesive	T49.3X-
Cyanocobalamin	T45.8X-
Cyanogen (chloride) (gas)NEC	T59.89-
Cyclacillin	T36.0X-
Cyclaine	T41.3X-
Cyclamate	T50.99-
Cyclamen europaeum	T62.2X-
Cyclandelate	T46.7X-
Cyclazocine	T50.7X-
Cyclizine	T45.0X-
Cyclobarbital	T42.3X-
Cyclobarbitone	T42.3X-
Cyclobenzaprine	T48.1X-
Cyclodrine	T44.3X-
Cycloguanil embonate	T37.2X-
Cyclohexane	T52.8X-

Drug/Chemical	Code
Cyclohexanol	T51.8X-
Cyclohexanone	T52.4X-
Cycloheximide	T60.3X-
Cyclohexyl acetate	T52.8X-
Cycloleucin	T45.1X-
Cyclomethycaine	T41.3X-
Cyclopentamine	T44.4X-
Cyclopenthiazide	T50.2X-
Cyclopentolate	T44.3X-
Cyclophosphamide	T45.1X-
Cycloplegic drug	T49.5X-
Cyclopropane	T41.29-
Cyclopyrabital	T39.8X-
Cycloserine	T37.1X-
Cyclosporin	T45.1X-
Cyclothiazide	T50.2X-
Cycrimine	T44.3X-
Cyhalothrin	T60.1X-
Cymarin	T46.0X-
Cypermethrin	T60.1X-
Cyphenothrin	T60.2X-
Cyproheptadine	T45.0X-
Cyproterone	T38.6X-
Cysteamine	T50.6X-
Cytarabine	T45.1X-
Cytisus	T62.2X-
Cytochrome C	T47.5X-
Cytomel	T38.1X-
Cytosine arabinoside	T45.1X-
Cytoxan	T45.1X-
Cytozyme	T45.7X-
2,4-D	T60.3X-
Dacarbazine	T45.1X-
Dactinomycin	T45.1X-
DADPS	T37.1X-
Dakin's solution	T49.0X-
Dalapon (sodium)	T60.3X-
Dalmane	T42.4X-
Danazol	T38.6X-
Danilone	T45.51-
Danthron	T47.2X-
Dantrolene	T42.8X-
Dantron	T47.2X-
Daphne (gnidium) (mezereum)	T62.2X-
berry	T62.1X-
Dapsone	T37.1X-
Daraprim	T37.2X-

Drug/Chemical	Code
Darnel	T62.2X-
Darvon	T39.8X-
Daunomycin	T45.1X-
Daunorubicin	T45.1X-
DBI	T38.3X-
D-Con	T60.9-
insecticide	T60.2X-
rodenticide	T60.4X-
DDAVP	T38.89-
DDE (bis (chlorophenyl)-dichloroethylene)	T60.2X-
DDS	T37.1X-
DDT (dust)	T60.1X-
Deadly nightshade	T62.2X-
berry	T62.1X-
Deamino-D-arginine vasopressin	T38.89-
Deanol (aceglumate)	T50.99-
Debrisoquine	T46.5X-
Decaborane	T57.8X-
fumes	T59.89-
Decadron	T38.0X-
topical NEC	T49.0X-
Decahydronaphthalene	T52.8X-
Decalin	T52.8X-
Decamethonium (bromide)	T48.1X-
Decholin	T47.5X-
Declomycin	T36.4X-
Decongestant, nasal (mucosa)	T48.5X-
Deet	T60.8X-
Deferoxamine	T45.8X-
Deflazacort	T38.0X-
Deglycyrrhizinized extract of licorice	T48.4X-
Dehydrocholic acid	T47.5X-
Dehydroemetine	T37.3X-
Dekalin	T52.8X-
Delalutin	T38.5X-
Delorazepam	T42.4X-
Delphinium	T62.2X-
Deltamethrin	T60.1X-
Deltasone	T38.0X-
Deltra	T38.0X-
Delvinal	T42.3X-
Demecarium (bromide)	T49.5X-
Demeclocycline	T36.4X-
Demecolcine	T45.1X-
Demegestone	T38.5X-
Demelanizing agents	T49.8X-
Demephion -O and -S	T60.0X-

Drug/Chemical	Code
Demerol	T40.2X-
Demethylchlortetracycline	T36.4X-
Demethyltetracycline	T36.4X-
Demeton -O and -S	T60.0X-
Demulcent (external)	T49.3X-
Demulen	T38.4X-
Denatured alcohol	T51.0X-
Dendrid	T49.5X-
Dental drug, topical application NEC	T49.7X-
Dentifrice	T49.7X-
Deodorant spray (feminine hygiene)	T49.8X-
Deoxycortone	T50.0X-
2-Deoxy-5-fluorouridine	T45.1X-
5-Deoxy-5-fluorouridine	T45.1X-
Deoxyribonuclease (pancreatic)	T45.3X-
Depilatory	T49.4X-
Deprenalin	T42.8X-
Deprenyl	T42.8X-
Depressant, appetite	T50.5X-
Depressant	
appetite (central)	T50.5X-
cardiac	T46.2X-
central nervous system (anesthetic)—*see also Central nervous system, depressants*	T42.7-
general anesthetic	T41.20-
muscle tone	T42.8X-
muscle tone, central	T42.8X-
psychotherapeutic	T43.50-
Deptropine	T45.0X-
Dequalinium (chloride)	T49.0X-
Derris root	T60.2X-
Deserpidine	T46.5X-
Desferrioxamine	T45.8X-
Desipramine	T43.01-
Deslanoside	T46.0X-
Desloughing agent	T49.4X-
Desmethylimipramine	T43.01-
Desmopressin	T38.89-
Desocodeine	T40.2X-
Desogestrel	T38.5X-
Desomorphine	T40.2X-
Desonide	T49.0X-
Desoximetasone	T49.0X-
Desoxycorticosteroid	T50.0X-
Desoxycortone	T50.0X-
Desoxyephedrine	T43.62-
Detaxtran	T46.6X-

Drug/Chemical	Code
Detergent	T49.2X-
external medication	T49.2X-
local	T49.2X-
medicinal	T49.2X-
nonmedicinal	T55.1X-
specified NEC	T55.1X-
Deterrent, alcohol	T50.6X-
Detoxifying agent	T50.6X-
Detrothyronine	T38.1X-
Dettol (external medication)	T49.0X-
Dexamethasone	T38.0X-
ENT agent	T49.6X-
ophthalmic preparation	T49.5X-
topical NEC	T49.0X-
Dexamfetamine	T43.62-
Dexamphetamine	T43.62-
Dexbrompheniramine	T45.0X-
Dexchlorpheniramine	T45.0X-
Dexedrine	T43.62-
Dexetimide	T44.3X-
Dexfenfluramine	T50.5X-
Dexpanthenol	T45.2X-
Dextran (40) (70) (150)	T45.8X-
Dextriferron	T45.4X-
Dextro calcium pantothenate	T45.2X-
Dextro pantothenyl alcohol	T45.2X-
Dextroamphetamine	T43.62-
Dextromethorphan	T48.3X-
Dextromoramide	T40.4X-
topical	T49.8X-
Dextropropoxyphene	T40.4X-
Dextrorphan	T40.2X-
Dextrose	T50.3X-
concentrated solution, intravenous	T46.8X-
Dextrothyroxin	T38.1X-
Dextrothyroxine sodium	T38.1X-
DFP	T44.0X-
DHE	T37.3X-
45	T46.5X-
Diabinese	T38.3X-
Diacetone alcohol	T52.4X-
Diacetyl monoxime	T50.99-
Diacetylmorphine	T40.1X-
Diachylon plaster	T49.4X-
Diaethylstilboestrolum	T38.5X-
Diagnostic agent NEC	T50.8X-

Drug/Chemical	Code
Dial (soap)	T49.2X-
sedative	T42.3X-
Dialkyl carbonate	T52.9-
Diallylbarbituric acid	T42.3X-
Diallymal	T42.3X-
Dialysis solution (intraperitoneal)	T50.3X-
Diaminodiphenylsulfone	T37.1X-
Diamorphine	T40.1X-
Diamox	T50.2X-
Diamthazole	T49.0X-
Dianthone	T47.2X-
Diaphenylsulfone	T37.0X-
Diasone (sodium)	T37.1X-
Diastase	T47.5X-
Diatrizoate	T50.8X-
Diazepam	T42.4X-
Diazinon	T60.0X-
Diazomethane (gas)	T59.89-
Diazoxide	T46.5X-
Dibekacin	T36.5X-
Dibenamine	T44.6X-
Dibenzepin	T43.01-
Dibenzheptropine	T45.0X-
Dibenzyline	T44.6X-
Diborane (gas)	T59.89-
Dibromochloropropane	T60.8X-
Dibromodulcitol	T45.1X-
Dibromoethane	T53.6X-
Dibromomannitol	T45.1X-
Dibromopropamidine isethionate	T49.0X-
Dibrompropamidine	T49.0X-
Dibucaine	T41.3X-
Dibunate sodium	T48.3X-
Dibutoline sulfate	T44.3X-
Dicamba	T60.3X-
Dicapthon	T60.0X-
Dichlobenil	T60.3X-
Dichlone	T60.3X-
Dichloralphenozone	T42.6X-
Dichlorbenzidine	T65.3X-
Dichlorhydrin	T52.8X-
Dichlorhydroxyquinoline	T37.8X-
Dichlorobenzene	T53.7X-
Dichlorobenzyl alcohol	T49.6X-
Dichlorodifluoromethane	T53.5X-
Dichloroethane	T52.8X-
Sym-Dichloroethyl ether	T53.6X-

Drug/Chemical	Code
Dichloroethyl sulfide, not in war	T59.89-
Dichloroethylene	T53.6X-
Dichloroformoxine, not in war	T59.89-
Dichlorohydrin, alpha-dichlorohydrin	T52.8X-
Dichloromethane (solvent) (vapor)	T53.4X-
Dichloronaphthoquinone	T60.3X-
Dichlorophen	T37.4X-
2,4-Dichlorophenoxyacetic acid	T60.3X-
Dichloropropene	T60.3X-
Dichloropropionic acid	T60.3X-
Dichlorphenamide	T50.2X-
Dichlorvos	T60.0X-
Diclofenac	T39.39-
Diclofenamide	T50.2X-
Diclofensine	T43.29-
Diclonixine	T39.8X-
Dicloxacillin	T36.0X-
Dicophane	T49.0X-
Dicoumarol, dicoumarin, dicumarol	T45.51-
Dicrotophos	T60.0X-
Dicyanogen (gas)	T65.0X-
Dicyclomine	T44.3X-
Dicycloverine	T44.3X-
Dideoxycytidine	T37.5X-
Dideoxyinosine	T37.5X-
Dieldrin (vapor)	T60.1X-
Diemal	T42.3X-
Dienestrol	T38.5X-
Dienoestrol	T38.5X-
Dietetic drug NEC	T50.90-
Diethazine	T42.8X-
Diethyl	
barbituric acid / carbinol	T42.3X-
carbamazine	T37.4X-
carbonate / oxide	T52.8X-
ether (vapor)—*see also ether*	T41.0X-
propion	T50.5X-
stilbestrol	T38.5X-
toluamide (nonmedicinal)	T60.8X-
medicinal	T49.3X-
Diethylcarbamazine	T37.4X-
Diethylene	
dioxide	T52.8X-
glycol (monoacetate) (monobutyl ether) (monoethyl ether)	T52.3X-
Diethylhexylphthalate	T65.89-
Diethylpropion	T50.5X-
Diethylstilbestrol	T38.5X-

DIETHYLSTILBOESTROL–DIMETHYLAMINE SULFATE

Drug/Chemical	Code
Diethylstilboestrol	T38.5X-
Diethylsulfone-diethylmethane	T42.6X-
Diethyltoluamide	T49.0X-
Diethyltryptamine (DET)	T40.99-
Difebarbamate	T42.3X-
Difencloxazine	T40.2X-
Difenidol	T45.0X-
Difenoxin	T47.6X-
Difetarsone	T37.3X-
Diffusin	T45.3X-
Diflorasone	T49.0X-
Diflos	T44.0X-
Diflubenzuron	T60.1X-
Diflucortolone	T49.0X-
Diflunisal	T39.09-
Difluoromethyldopa	T42.8X-
Difluorophate	T44.0X-
Digestant NEC	T47.5X-
Digitalin (e)	T46.0X-
Digitalis (leaf) (glycoside)	T46.0X-
Digitoxin	T46.0X-
Digitoxose	T46.0X-
Digoxin	T46.0X-
Digoxine	T46.0X-
Dihydralazine	T46.5X-
Dihydrazine	T46.5X-
Dihydrocodeine	T40.2X-
Dihydrocodeinone	T40.2X-
Dihydroergocornine	T46.7X-
Dihydroergocristine (mesilate)	T46.7X-
Dihydroergokryptine	T46.7X-
Dihydroergotamine	T46.5X-
Dihydroergotoxine (mesilate)	T46.7X-
Dihydrohydroxycodeinone	T40.2X-
Dihydrohydroxymorphinone	T40.2X-
Dihydroisocodeine	T40.2X-
Dihydromorphine	T40.2X-
Dihydromorphinone	T40.2X-
Dihydrostreptomycin	T36.5X-
Dihydrotachysterol	T45.2X-
Dihydroxyaluminum aminoacetate	T47.1X-
Dihydroxyaluminum sodium carbonate	T47.1X-
Dihydroxyanthraquinone	T47.2X-
Dihydroxycodeinone	T40.2X-
Dihydroxypropyl theophylline	T50.2X-

Drug/Chemical	Code
Diiodohydroxyquin	T37.8X-
topical	T49.0X-
Diiodohydroxyquinoline	T37.8X-
Diiodotyrosine	T38.2X-
Diisopromine	T44.3X-
Diisopropylamine	T46.3X-
Diisopropylfluorophos-phonate	T44.0X-
Dilantin	T42.0X-
Dilaudid	T40.2X-
Dilazep	T46.3X-
Dill	T47.5X-
Diloxanide	T37.3X-
Diltiazem	T46.1X-
Dimazole	T49.0X-
Dimefline	T50.7X-
Dimefox	T60.0X-
Dimemorfan	T48.3X-
Dimenhydrinate	T45.0X-
Dimercaprol (British anti-lewisite)	T45.8X-
Dimercaptopropanol	T45.8X-
Dimestrol	T38.5X-
Dimetane	T45.0X-
Dimethicone	T47.1X-
Dimethindene	T45.0X-
Dimethisoquin	T49.1X-
Dimethisterone	T38.5X-
Dimethoate	T60.0X-
Dimethocaine	T41.3X-
Dimethoxanate	T48.3X-
Dimethyl	
arsine, arsinic acid	T57.0X-
carbinol	T51.2X-
carbonate	T52.8X-
diguanide	T38.3X-
ketone (vapor)	T52.4X-
meperidine	T40.2X-
parathion	T60.0X-
phthlate	T49.3X-
polysiloxane	T47.8X-
sulfate (fumes)	T59.89-
liquid	T65.89-
sulfoxide (nonmedicinal)	T52.8X-
medicinal	T49.4X-
tryptamine	T40.99-
tubocurarine	T48.1X-
Dimethylamine sulfate	T49.4X-

Drug/Chemical	Code
Dimethylformamide	T52.8X-
Dimethyltubocurarinium chloride	T48.1X-
Dimeticone	T47.1X-
Dimetilan	T60.0X-
Dimetindene	T45.0X-
Dimetotiazine	T43.3X-
Dimorpholamine	T50.7X-
Dimoxyline	T46.3X-
Dinitrobenzene	T65.3X-
vapor	T59.89-
Dinitrobenzol	T65.3X-
vapor	T59.89-
Dinitrobutylphenol	T65.3X-
Dinitro (-ortho-) cresol (pesticide) (spray)	T65.3X-
Dinitrocyclohexylphenol	T65.3X-
Dinitrophenol	T65.3X-
Dinoprost	T48.0X-
Dinoprostone	T48.0X-
Dinoseb	T60.3X-
Dioctyl sulfosuccinate (calcium) (sodium)	T47.4X-
Diodone	T50.8X-
Diodoquin	T37.8X-
Dionin	T40.2X-
Diosmin	T46.99-
Dioxane	T52.8X-
Dioxathion	T60.0X-
Dioxin	T53.7X-
Dioxopromethazine	T43.3X-
Dioxyline	T46.3X-
Dipentene	T52.8X-
Diperodon	T41.3X-
Diphacinone	T60.4X-
Diphemanil	T44.3X-
metilsulfate	T44.3X-
Diphenadione	T45.51-
rodenticide	T60.4X-
Diphenhydramine	T45.0X-
Diphenidol	T45.0X-
Diphenoxylate	T47.6X-
Diphenylamine	T65.3X-
Diphenylbutazone	T39.2X-
Diphenylchloroarsine, not in war	T57.0X-
Diphenylhydantoin	T42.0X-
Diphenylmethane dye	T52.1X-
Diphenylpyraline	T45.0X-

Drug/Chemical	Code
Diphtheria	
antitoxin	T50.Z1-
vaccine — *See also* Vaccines	T50.A9-
Diphylline	T50.2X-
Dipipanone	T40.4X-
Dipivefrine	T49.5X-
Diplovax	T50.B9-
Diprophylline	T50.2X-
Dipropyline	T48.29-
Dipyridamole	T46.3X-
Dipyrone	T39.2X-
Diquat (dibromide)	T60.3X-
Disinfectant	T65.89-
alkaline	T54.3X-
aromatic	T54.1X-
intestinal	T37.8X-
Disipal	T42.8X-
Disodium edetate	T50.6X-
Disoprofol	T41.29-
Disopyramide	T46.2X-
Distigmine (bromide)	T44.0X-
Disulfamide	T50.2X-
Disulfanilamide	T37.0X-
Disulfiram	T50.6X-
Disulfoton	T60.0X-
Dithiazanine iodide	T37.4X-
Dithiocarbamate	T60.0X-
Dithranol	T49.4X-
Diucardin	T50.2X-
Diupres	T50.2X-
Diuretic NEC	T50.2X-
benzothiadiazine	T50.2X-
carbonic acid anhydrase inhibitors	T50.2X-
furfuryl NEC	T50.2X-
loop (high-ceiling)	T50.1X-
mercurial NEC or osmotic	T50.2X-
purine or saluretic NEC	T50.2X-
sulfonamide	T50.2X-
thiazide NEC or xanthine	T50.2X-
Diurgin	T50.2X-
Diuril	T50.2X-
Diuron	T60.3X-
Divalproex	T42.6X-
Divinyl ether	T41.0X-
Dixanthogen	T49.0X-
Dixyrazine	T43.3X-

D-LYSERGIC ACID DIETHYLAMIDE–EMBRAMINE

Drug/Chemical	Code
D-lysergic acid diethylamide	T40.8X-
DMCT	T36.4X-
DMSO—*see Dimethyl sulfoxide*	
DNBP	T60.3X-
DNOC	T65.3X-
Dobutamine	T44.5X-
DOCA	T38.0X-
Docusate sodium	T47.4X-
Dodicin	T49.0X-
Dofamium chloride	T49.0X-
Dolophine	T40.3X-
Doloxene	T39.8X-
Domestic gas (after combustion)—*see Gas, utility*	
prior to combustion	T59.89-
Domiodol	T48.4X-
Domiphen (bromide)	T49.0X-
Domperidone	T45.0X-
Dopa	T42.8X-
Dopamine	T44.99-
Doriden	T42.6X-
Dormiral	T42.3X-
Dormison	T42.6X-
Dornase	T48.4X-
Dorsacaine	T41.3X-
Dosulepin	T43.01-
Dothiepin	T43.01-
Doxantrazole	T48.6X-
Doxapram	T50.7X-
Doxazosin	T44.6X-
Doxepin	T43.01-
Doxifluridine	T45.1X-
Doxorubicin	T45.1X-
Doxycycline	T36.4X-
Doxylamine	T45.0X-
Dramamine	T45.0X-
Drano (drain cleaner)	T54.3X-
Dressing, live pulp	T49.7X-
Drocode	T40.2X-
Dromoran	T40.2X-
Dromostanolone	T38.7X-
Dronabinol	T40.7X-
Droperidol	T43.59-
Dropropizine	T48.3X-
Drostanolone	T38.7X-
Drotaverine	T44.3X-
Drotrecogin alfa	T45.51-

Drug/Chemical	Code
Drug NEC	T50.90-
specified NEC	T50.99-
DTIC	T45.1X-
Duboisine	T44.3X-
Dulcolax	T47.2X-
Duponol (C) (EP)	T49.2X-
Durabolin	T38.7X-
Dyclone	T41.3X-
Dyclonine	T41.3X-
Dydrogesterone	T38.5X-
Dye NEC	T65.6X-
antiseptic	T49.0X-
diagnostic agents	T50.8X-
pharmaceutical NEC	T50.90-
Dyflos	T44.0X-
Dymelor	T38.3X-
Dynamite	T65.3X-
fumes	T59.89-
Dyphylline	T44.3X-
Ear drug NEC	T49.6X-
Ear preparations	T49.6X-
Echothiophate, echothiopate, ecothiopate	T49.5X-
Econazole	T49.0X-
Ecothiopate iodide	T49.5X-
Ecstasy	T43.62-
Ectylurea	T42.6X-
Edathamil disodium	T45.8X-
Edecrin	T50.1X-
Edetate, disodium (calcium)	T45.8X-
Edoxudine	T49.5X-
Edrophonium	T44.0X-
chloride	T44.0X-
EDTA	T50.6X-
Eflornithine	T37.2X-
Efloxate	T46.3X-
Elase	T49.8X-
Elastase	T47.5X-
Elaterium	T47.2X-
Elcatonin	T50.99-
Elder	T62.2X-
berry, (unripe)	T62.1X-
Electrolyte balance drug	T50.3X-
Electrolytes NEC	T50.3X-
Electrolytic agent NEC	T50.3X-
Elemental diet	T50.90-
Elliptinium acetate	T45.1X-
Embramine	T45.0X-

Drug/Chemical	Code
Emepronium (salts) (bromide)	T44.3X-
Emetic NEC	T47.7X-
Emetine	T37.3X-
Emollient NEC	T49.3X-
Emorfazone	T39.8X-
Emylcamate	T43.59-
Enalapril	T46.4X-
Enalaprilat	T46.4X-
Encainide	T46.2X-
Endocaine	T41.3X-
Endosulfan	T60.2X-
Endothall	T60.3X-
Endralazine	T46.5X-
Endrin	T60.1X-
Enflurane	T41.0X-
Enhexymal	T42.3X-
Enocitabine	T45.1X-
Enovid	T38.4X-
Enoxacin	T36.8X-
Enoxaparin (sodium)	T45.51-
Enpiprazole	T43.59-
Enprofylline	T48.6X-
Enprostil	T47.1X-
ENT preparations (anti-infectives)	T49.6X-
Enterogastrone	T38.89-
Enviomycin	T36.8X-
Enzodase	T45.3X-
Enzyme NEC	T45.3X-
depolymerizing	T49.8X-
fibrolytic	T45.3X-
gastric / intestinal	T47.5X-
local action / proteolytic	T49.4X-
thrombolytic	T45.3X-
EPAB	T41.3X-
Epanutin	T42.0X-
Ephedra	T44.99-
Ephedrine	T44.99-
Epichlorhydrin, epichlorohydrin	T52.8X-
Epicillin	T36.0X-
Epiestriol	T38.5X-
Epimestrol	T38.5X-
Epinephrine	T44.5X-
Epirubicin	T45.1X-
Epitiostanol	T38.7X-
Epitizide	T50.2X-
EPN	T60.0X-
EPO	T45.8X-

Drug/Chemical	Code
Epoetin alpha	T45.8X-
Epomediol	T50.99-
Epoprostenol	T45.521
Epoxy resin	T65.89-
Eprazinone	T48.4X-
Epsilon amino-caproic acid	T45.62-
Epsom salt	T47.3X-
Eptazocine	T40.4X-
Equanil	T43.59-
Equisetum	T62.2X-
diuretic	T50.2X-
Ergobasine	T48.0X-
Ergocalciferol	T45.2X-
Ergoloid mesylates	T46.7X-
Ergometrine	T48.0X-
Ergonovine	T48.0X-
Ergot NEC	T64.81
derivative or medicinal (alkaloids) or prepared	T48.0X-
Ergotamine	T46.5X-
Ergotocine	T48.0X-
Ergotrate	T48.0X-
Eritrityl tetranitrate	T46.3X-
Erythrityl tetranitrate	T46.3X-
Erythrol tetranitrate	T46.3X-
Erythromycin (salts)	T36.3X-
ophthalmic preparation	T49.5X-
topical NEC	T49.0X-
Erythropoietin	T45.8X-
human	T45.8X-
Escin	T46.99-
Esculin	T45.2X-
Esculoside	T45.2X-
ESDT (ether-soluble tar distillate)	T49.1X-
Eserine	T49.5X-
Esflurbiprofen	T39.31-
Eskabarb	T42.3X-
Eskalith	T43.8X-
Esmolol	T44.7X-
Estanozolol	T38.7X-
Estazolam	T42.4X-
Estradiol	T38.5X-
with testosterone	T38.7X-
benzoate	T38.5X-
Estramustine	T45.1X-
Estriol	T38.5X-
Estrogen	T38.5X-
Estrone	T38.5X-

Drug/Chemical	Code
Estropipate	T38.5X-
Etacrynate sodium	T50.1X-
Etacrynic acid	T50.1X-
Etafedrine	T48.6X-
Etafenone	T46.3X-
Etambutol	T37.1X-
Etamiphyllin	T48.6X-
Etamivan	T50.7X-
Etamsylate	T45.7X-
Etebenecid	T50.4X-
Ethacridine	T49.0X-
Ethacrynic acid	T50.1X-
Ethadione	T42.2X-
Ethambutol	T37.1X-
Ethamide	T50.2X-
Ethamivan	T50.7X-
Ethamsylate	T45.7X-
Ethanol (beverage)	T51.0X-
Ethanolamine oleate	T46.8X-
Ethaverine	T44.3X-
Ethchlorvynol	T42.6X-
Ethebenecid	T50.4X-
Ether (vapor)	T41.0X-
anesthetic	T41.0X-
divinyl	T41.0X-
ethyl (medicinal)	T41.0X-
nonmedicinal	T52.8X-
solvent	T52.8X-
Ethiazide	T50.2X-
Ethidium chloride (vapor)	T59.89-
Ethinamate	T42.6X-
Ethinylestradiol, ethinyloestradiol	T38.5X-
with	
levonorgestrel or norethisterone	T38.4X-
Ethiodized oil (131 I)	T50.8X-
Ethion	T60.0X-
Ethionamide	T37.1X-
Ethioniamide	T37.1X-
Ethisterone	T38.5X-
Ethobral	T42.3X-
Ethocaine (infiltration) (topical) (nervel block) (spinal)	T41.3X-
Ethoheptazine	T40.4X-
Ethopropazine	T44.3X-
Ethosuximide	T42.2X-
Ethotoin	T42.0X-
Ethoxazene	T37.9-
Ethoxazorutoside	T46.99-

Drug/Chemical	Code
2-Ethoxyethanol	T52.3X-
Ethoxzolamide	T50.2X-
Ethyl	
acetate	T52.8X-
alcohol (beverage)	T51.0X-
aldehyde (vapor)	T59.89-
liquid	T52.8X-
aminobenzoate	T41.3X-
aminophenothiazine	T43.3X-
benzoate	T52.8X-
biscoumacetate	T45.51-
bromide (anesthetic)	T41.0X-
carbamate	T45.1X-
carbinol	T51.3X-
carbonate	T52.8X-
chaulmoograte	T37.1X-
chloride (anesthetic)	T41.0X-
anesthetic (local)	T41.3X-
inhaled	T41.0X-
local	T49.4X-
solvent	T53.6X-
dibunate	T48.3X-
dichloroarsine (vapor)	T57.0X-
estranol	T38.7X-
ether—see also ether	T52.8X-
formate NEC (solvent)	T52.0X-
fumarate	T49.4X-
hydroxyisobutyrate NEC (solvent)	T52.8X-
iodoacetate	T59.3X-
lactate NEC (solvent)	T52.8X-
loflazepate	T42.4X-
mercuric chloride	T56.1X-
methylcarbinol	T51.8X-
morphine	T40.2X-
noradrenaline	T48.6X-
oxybutyrate NEC (solvent)	T52.8X-
Ethylene (gas)	T59.89-
anesthetic (general)	T41.0X-
chlorohydrin	T52.8X-
vapor	T53.6X-
dichloride	T52.8X-
vapor	T53.6X-
dinitrate	T52.3X-
glycol (s)	T52.8X-
dinitrate	T52.3X-
monobutyl ether	T52.3X-
imine	T54.1X-

Drug/Chemical	Code
Ethylene (gas), continued	
oxide (fumigant) (nonmedicinal)	T59.89-
medicinal	T49.0X-
Ethylenediamine theophylline	T48.6X-
Ethylenediaminetetra-acetic acid	T50.6X-
Ethylenedinitrilotetra-acetate	T50.6X-
Ethylestrenol	T38.7X-
Ethylhydroxycellulose	T47.4X-
Ethylidene	
chloride NEC	T53.6X-
diacetate	T60.3X-
dicoumarin / dicoumarol	T45.51-
diethyl ether	T52.0X-
Ethylmorphine	T40.2X-
Ethylnorepinephrine	T48.6X-
Ethylparachlorophen-oxyisobutyrate	T46.6X-
Ethynodiol	T38.4X-
with mestranol diacetate	T38.4X-
Etidocaine (infiltration) (subcutaneous) (nerve block)	T41.3X-
Etidronate	T50.99-
Etidronic acid (disodium salt)	T50.99-
Etifoxine	T42.6X-
Etilefrine	T44.4X-
Etilfen	T42.3X-
Etinodiol	T38.4X-
Etiroxate	T46.6X-
Etizolam	T42.4X-
Etodolac	T39.39-
Etofamide	T37.3X-
Etofibrate	T46.6X-
Etofylline	T46.7X-
clofibrate	T46.6X-
Etoglucid	T45.1X-
Etomidate	T41.1X-
Etomide	T39.8X-
Etomidoline	T44.3X-
Etoposide	T45.1X-
Etorphine	T40.2X-
Etoval	T42.3X-
Etozolin	T50.1X-
Etretinate	T50.99-
Etryptamine	T43.69-
Etybenzatropine	T44.3X-
Etynodiol	T38.4X-
Eucaine	T41.3X-
Eucalyptus oil	T49.7X-
Eucatropine	T49.5X-

Drug/Chemical	Code
Eucodal	T40.2X-
Euneryl	T42.3X-
Euphthalmine	T44.3X-
Eurax	T49.0X-
Euresol	T49.4X-
Euthroid	T38.1X-
Evans blue	T50.8X-
Evipal	T42.3X-
sodium	T41.1X-
Evipan	T42.3X-
sodium	T41.1X-
Exalamide	T49.0X-
Exalgin	T39.1X-
Excipients, pharmaceutical	T50.90-
Exhaust gas (engine) (motor vehicle)	T58.0-
Ex-Lax (phenolphthalein)	T47.2X-
Expectorant NEC	T48.4X-
Extended insulin zinc suspension	T38.3X-
External medications (skin) (mucous membrane)	T49.9-
dental agent	T49.7X-
ENT agent	T49.6X-
ophthalmic preparation	T49.5X-
specified NEC	T49.8X-
Extrapyramidal antagonist NEC	T44.3X-
Eye agents (anti-infective)	T49.5X-
Eye drug NEC	T49.5X-
FAC (fluorouracil + doxorubicin + cyclophosphamide)	T45.1X-
Factor	
I (fibrinogen)	T45.8X-
III (thromboplastin)	T45.8X-
VIII (antihemophilic Factor) (concentrate)	T45.8X-
IX complex	T45.7X-
human	T45.8X-
Famotidine	T47.0X-
Fat suspension, intravenous	T50.99-
Fazadinium bromide	T48.1X-
Febarbamate	T42.3X-
Fecal softener	T47.4X-
Fedrilate	T48.3X-
Felodipine	T46.1X-
Felypressin	T38.89-
Femoxetine	T43.22-
Fenalcomine	T46.3X-
Fenamisal	T37.1X-
Fenazone	T39.2X-
Fenbendazole	T37.4X-
Fenbutrazate	T50.5X-

Drug/Chemical	Code
Fencamfamine	T43.69-
Fendiline	T46.1X-
Fenetylline	T43.69-
Fenflumizole	T39.39-
Fenfluramine	T50.5X-
Fenobarbital	T42.3X-
Fenofibrate	T46.6X-
Fenoprofen	T39.31-
Fenoterol	T48.6X-
Fenoverine	T44.3X-
Fenoxazoline	T48.5X-
Fenproporex	T50.5X-
Fenquizone	T50.2X-
Fentanyl	T40.4X-
Fentazin	T43.3X-
Fenthion	T60.0X-
Fenticlor	T49.0X-
Fenylbutazone	T39.2X-
Feprazone	T39.2X-
Fer de lance (bite) (venom)	T63.06-
Ferric—see also Iron	
chloride	T45.4X-
citrate	T45.4X-
hydroxide	T45.4X-
pyrophosphate	T45.4X-
Ferritin	T45.4X-
Ferrocholinate	T45.4X-
Ferrodextrane	T45.4X-
Ferropolimaler	T45.4X-
Ferrous—see also Iron	T45.4X-
Ferrous fumerate, gluconate, lactate, salt NEC, sulfate (medicinal)	T45.4X-
Ferrovanadium (fumes)	T59.89-
Ferrum—see Iron	
Fertilizers NEC	T65.89-
with herbicide mixture	T60.3X-
Fetoxilate	T47.6X-
Fiber, dietary	T47.4X-
Fiberglass	T65.831
Fibrinogen (human)	T45.8X-
Fibrinolysin (human)	T45.69-
Fibrinolysis	
affecting drug	T45.60-
inhibitor NEC	T45.62-
Fibrinolytic drug	T45.61-
Filix mas	T37.4X-
Filtering cream	T49.3X-

Drug/Chemical	Code
Fiorinal	T39.01-
Firedamp	T59.89-
Fish, noxious, nonbacterial	T61.9-
ciguatera	T61.0-
scombroid	T61.1-
shell	T61.781
specified NEC	T61.771
Flagyl	T37.3X-
Flavine adenine dinucleotide	T45.2X-
Flavodic acid	T46.99-
Flavoxate	T44.3X-
Flaxedil	T48.1X-
Flaxseed (medicinal)	T49.3X-
Flecainide	T46.2X-
Fleroxacin	T36.8X-
Floctafenine	T39.8X-
Flomax	T44.6X-
Flomoxef	T36.1X-
Flopropione	T44.3X-
Florantyrone	T47.5X-
Floraquin	T37.8X-
Florinef	T38.0X-
ENT agent	T49.6X-
ophthalmic preparation	T49.5X-
topical NEC	T49.0X-
Flowers of sulfur	T49.4X-
Floxuridine	T45.1X-
Fluanisone	T43.4X-
Flubendazole	T37.4X-
Fluclorolone acetonide	T49.0X-
Flucloxacillin	T36.0X-
Fluconazole	T37.8X-
Flucytosine	T37.8X-
Fludeoxyglucose (18F)	T50.8X-
Fludiazepam	T42.4X-
Fludrocortisone	T50.0X-
ENT agent	T49.6X-
ophthalmic preparation	T49.5X-
topical NEC	T49.0X-
Fludroxycortide	T49.0X-
Flufenamic acid	T39.39-
Fluindione	T45.51-
Flumequine	T37.8X-
Flumethasone	T49.0X-
Flumethiazide	T50.2X-
Flumidin	T37.5X-
Flunarizine	T46.7X-

FENCAMFAMINE–FLUNARIZINE

Drug/Chemical	Code
Flunidazole	T37.8X-
Flunisolide	T48.6X-
Flunitrazepam	T42.4X-
Fluocinolone (acetonide)	T49.0X-
Fluocinonide	T49.0X-
Fluocortin (butyl)	T49.0X-
Fluocortolone	T49.0X-
Fluohydrocortisone	T38.0X-
ENT agent	T49.6X-
ophthalmic preparation	T49.5X-
topical NEC	T49.0X-
Fluonid	T49.0X-
Fluopromazine	T43.3X-
Fluoracetate	T60.8X-
Fluorescein	T50.8X-
Fluorhydrocortisone	T50.0X-
Fluoride (nonmedicinal) (pesticide) (sodium) NEC	T60.8X-
medicinal NEC	T50.99-
dental use	T49.7X-
not pesticide NEC	T54.9-
stannous	T49.7X-
Fluorinated corticosteroids	T38.0X-
Fluorine (gas)	T59.5X-
Fluoristan	T49.7X-
Fluormetholone	T49.0X-
Fluoroacetate	T60.8X-
Fluorocarbon monomer	T53.6X-
Fluorocytosine	T37.8X-
Fluorodeoxyuridine	T45.1X-
Fluorometholone	T49.0X-
ophthalmic preparation	T49.5X-
Fluorophosphate insecticide	T60.0X-
Fluorosol	T46.3X-
Fluorouracil	T45.1X-
Fluorphenylalanine	T49.5X-
Fluothane	T41.0X-
Fluoxetine	T43.22-
Fluoxymesterone	T38.7X-
Flupenthixol	T43.4X-
Flupentixol	T43.4X-
Fluphenazine	T43.3X-
Fluprednidene	T49.0X-
Fluprednisolone	T38.0X-
Fluradoline	T39.8X-
Flurandrenolide	T49.0X-
Flurandrenolone	T49.0X-
Flurazepam	T42.4X-

Drug/Chemical	Code
Flurbiprofen	T39.31-
Flurobate	T49.0X-
Fluroxene	T41.0X-
Fluspirilene	T43.59-
Flutamide	T38.6X-
Flutazolam	T42.4X-
Fluticasone propionate	T49.1X-
Flutoprazepam	T42.4X-
Flutropium bromide	T48.6X-
Fluvoxamine	T43.22-
Folacin	T45.8X-
Folic acid	T45.8X-
with ferrous salt	T45.2X-
antagonist	T45.1X-
Folinic acid	T45.8X-
Folium stramoniae	T48.6X-
Follicle-stimulating hormone, human	T38.81-
Folpet	T60.3X-
Fominoben	T48.3X-
Food, foodstuffs, noxious, nonbacterial, NEC	T62.9-
berries	T62.1X-
mushrooms	T62.0X-
plants	T62.2X-
seafood	T61.9-
specified NEC	T61.8X-
seeds	T62.2X-
shellfish	T61.781
specified NEC	T62.8X-
Fool's parsley	T62.2X-
Formaldehyde (solution), gas or vapor	T59.2X-
fungicide	T60.3X-
Formalin	T59.2X-
fungicide	T60.3X-
vapor	T59.2X-
Formic acid	T54.2X-
vapor	T59.89-
Foscarnet sodium	T37.5X-
Fosfestrol	T38.5X-
Fosfomycin	T36.8X-
Fosfonet sodium	T37.5X-
Fosinopril	T46.4X-
sodium	T46.4X-
Fowler's solution	T57.0X-
Foxglove	T62.2X-
Framycetin	T36.5X-
Frangula	T47.2X-
extract	T47.2X-

Drug/Chemical	Code
Frei antigen	T50.8X-
Freon	T53.5X-
Fructose	T50.3X-
Frusemide	T50.1X-
FSH	T38.81-
Ftorafur	T45.1X-
Fuel	
automobile	T52.0X-
exhaust gas, not in transit	T58.0-
vapor NEC	T52.0X-
gas (domestic use) / utility / in mobile container / piped	T59.89-
industrial, incomplete combustion	T58.8X-
Fugillin	T36.8X-
Fulminate of mercury	T56.1X-
Fulvicin	T36.7X-
Fumadil	T36.8X-
Fumagillin	T36.8X-
Fumaric acid	T49.4X-
Fumes (from)	T59.9-
corrosive NEC	T54.9-
freons	T53.5X-
hydrocarbons (all types)	T59.89-
nitrogen dioxide	T59.0X-
petroleum (liquefied) (distributed)	T59.89-
polyester	T59.89-
specified source NEC	T59.89-
sulfur dioxide	T59.1X-
Fumigant NEC	T60.9-
Fungi, noxious, used as food	T62.0X-
Fungicide NEC (nonmedicinal)	T60.3X-
Fungizone	T36.7X-
topical	T49.0X-
Furacin	T49.0X-
Furadantin	T37.9-
Furazolidone	T37.8X-
Furazolium chloride	T49.0X-
Furfural	T52.8X-
Furnace (coal burning) (domestic), gas from	T58.2X-
industrial	T58.8X-
Furniture polish	T65.89-
Furosemide	T50.1X-
Furoxone	T37.9-
Fursultiamine	T45.2X-
Fusafungine	T36.8X-
Fusel oil (any) (amyl) (butyl) (propyl), vapor	T51.3X-
Fusidate (ethanolamine) (sodium)	T36.8X-
Fusidic acid	T36.8X-

Drug/Chemical	Code
Fytic acid, nonasodium	T50.6X-
GABA	T43.8X-
Gadopentetic acid	T50.8X-
Galactose	T50.3X-
b-Galactosidase	T47.5X-
Galantamine	T44.0X-
Gallamine (triethiodide)	T48.1X-
Gallium citrate	T50.99-
Gallopamil	T46.1X-
Gamboge	T47.2X-
Gamimune	T50.Z1-
Gamma globulin	T50.Z1-
Gamma-aminobutyric acid	T43.8X-
Gamma-benzene hexachloride (medicinal)	T49.0X-
nonmedicinal, vapor	T53.6X-
Gamma-BHC (medicinal)	T49.0X-
Gamulin	T50.Z1-
Ganciclovir (sodium)	T37.5X-
Ganglionic blocking drug NEC	T44.2X-
specified NEC	T44.2X-
Ganja	T40.7X-
Garamycin	T36.5X-
ophthalmic preparation	T49.5X-
topical NEC	T49.0X-
Gardenal	T42.3X-
Gardepanyl	T42.3X-
Gas	T59.9-
acetylene	T59.89-
incomplete combustion of	T58.1-
air contaminants, source or type not specified	T59.9-
anesthetic	T41.0X-
blast furnace	T58.8X-
chlorine	T59.4X-
coal	T58.2X-
cyanide	T57.3X-
dicyanogen	T65.0X-
exhaust	T58.0-
prior to combustion	T59.89-
from wood- or coal-burning stove or fireplace	T58.2X-
industrial use	T58.8X-
prior to combustion	T59.89-
utility (in mobile container or piped)	T59.89-
garage	T58.0-
hydrocarbon NEC (piped)	T59.89-
hydrocyanic acid	T65.0X-

Drug/Chemical	Code
Gas, continued	
illuminating (after combustion)	T58.1-
prior to combustion	T59.89-
kiln	T58.8X-
lacrimogenic	T59.3X-
marsh	T59.89-
motor exhaust, not in transit	T58.0-
natural	T59.89-
oil	T52.0X-
petroleum (liquefied) (distributed in mobile containers) (piped)	T59.89-
producer	T58.8X-
refrigerant (chlorofluoro-carbon)	T53.5X-
not chlorofluoro-carbon	T59.89-
sewer	T59.9-
specified source NEC	T59.9-
stove (after combustion)	T58.1-
prior to combustion	T59.89-
tear	T59.3X-
therapeutic	T41.5X-
utility (for cooking, heating, or lighting) (piped) (mobile container) NEC	T59.89-
water	T58.1-
Gasoline	T52.0X-
vapor	T52.0X-
Gastric enzymes	T47.5X-
Gastrografin	T50.8X-
Gastrointestinal drug	T47.9-
biological	T47.8X-
specified NEC	T47.8X-
Gaultheria procumbens	T62.2X-
Gefarnate	T44.3X-
Gelatin (intravenous)	T45.8X-
absorbable (sponge)	T45.7X-
Gelfilm	T49.8X-
Gelfoam	T45.7X-
Gelsemine	T50.99-
Gelsemium (sempervirens)	T62.2X-
Gemeprost	T48.0X-
Gemfibrozil	T46.6X-
Gemonil	T42.3X-
Gentamicin	T36.5X-
ophthalmic preparation	T49.5X-
topical NEC	T49.0X-
Gentian	T47.5X-
violet	T49.0X-
Gepefrine	T44.4X-
Gestonorone caproate	T38.5X-

Drug/Chemical	Code
Gexane	T49.0X-
Gila monster (venom)	T63.11-
Ginger	T47.5X-
Gitalin	T46.0X-
Gitaloxin	T46.0X-
Gitoxin	T46.0X-
Glafenine	T39.8X-
Glandular extract (medicinal)NEC	T50.Z9-
Glaucarubin	T37.3X-
Glibenclamide	T38.3X-
Glibornuride	T38.3X-
Gliclazide	T38.3X-
Glimidine	T38.3X-
Glipizide	T38.3X-
Gliquidone	T38.3X-
Glisolamide	T38.3X-
Glisoxepide	T38.3X-
Globin zinc insulin	T38.3X-
Globulin (antilymphocytic) (antirhesus) (antivenin) (antiviral)	T50.Z1-
Glucagon	T38.3X-
Glucocorticoids	T38.0X-
Glucocorticosteroid	T38.0X-
Gluconic acid	T50.99-
Glucosamine sulfate	T39.4X-
Glucose	T50.3X-
with sodium chloride	T50.3X-
Glucosulfone sodium	T37.1X-
Glucurolactone	T47.8X-
Glue NEC	T52.8X-
Glutamic acid	T47.5X-
Glutaral (medicinal)	T49.0X-
nonmedicinal	T65.89-
Glutaraldehyde (nonmedicinal)	T65.89-
medicinal	T49.0X-
Glutathione	T50.6X-
Glutethimide	T42.6X-
Glyburide	T38.3X-
Glycerin	T47.4X-
Glycerol	T47.4X-
borax	T49.6X-
intravenous	T50.3X-
iodinated	T48.4X-
Glycerophosphate	T50.99-
Glyceryl	
gualacolate	T48.4X-
nitrate	T46.3X-

Drug/Chemical	Code
Glyceryl, continued	
triacetate (topical)	T49.0X-
trinitrate	T46.3X-
Glycine	T50.3X-
Glyclopyramide	T38.3X-
Glycobiarsol	T37.3X-
Glycols (ether)	T52.3X-
Glyconiazide	T37.1X-
Glycopyrrolate	T44.3X-
Glycopyrronium (bromide)	T44.3X-
Glycoside, cardiac (stimulant)	T46.0X-
Glycyclamide	T38.3X-
Glycyrrhiza extract	T48.4X-
Glycyrrhizic acid	T48.4X-
Glycyrrhizinate potassium	T48.4X-
Glymidine sodium	T38.3X-
Glyphosate	T60.3X-
Glyphylline	T48.6X-
Gold	
colloidal (I98Au)	T45.1X-
salts	T39.4X-
Golden sulfide of antimony	T56.89-
Goldylocks	T62.2X-
Gonadal tissue extract	T38.90-
female	T38.5X-
male	T38.7X-
Gonadorelin	T38.89-
Gonadotropin	T38.89-
chorionic	T38.89-
pituitary	T38.81-
Goserelin	T45.1X-
Grain alcohol	T51.0X-
Gramicidin	T49.0X-
Granisetron	T45.0X-
Gratiola officinalis	T62.2X-
Grease	T65.89-
Green hellebore	T62.2X-
Green soap	T49.2X-
Grifulvin	T36.7X-
Griseofulvin	T36.7X-
Growth hormone	T38.81-
Guaiac reagent	T50.99-
Guaiacol derivatives	T48.4X-
Guaifenesin	T48.4X-
Guaimesal	T48.4X-
Guaiphenesin	T48.4X-
Guamecycline	T36.4X-

Drug/Chemical	Code
Guanabenz	T46.5X-
Guanacline	T46.5X-
Guanadrel	T46.5X-
Guanatol	T37.2X-
Guanethidine	T46.5X-
Guanfacine	T46.5X-
Guano	T65.89-
Guanochlor	T46.5X-
Guanoclor	T46.5X-
Guanoctine	T46.5X-
Guanoxabenz	T46.5X-
Guanoxan	T46.5X-
Guar gum (medicinal)	T46.6X-
Hachimycin	T36.7X-
Hair	
dye	T49.4X-
preparation NEC	T49.4X-
Halazepam	T42.4X-
Halcinolone	T49.0X-
Halcinonide	T49.0X-
Halethazole	T49.0X-
Hallucinogen NEC	T40.90-
Halofantrine	T37.2X-
Halofenate	T46.6X-
Halometasone	T49.0X-
Haloperidol	T43.4X-
Haloprogin	T49.0X-
Halotex	T49.0X-
Halothane	T41.0X-
Haloxazolam	T42.4X-
Halquinols	T49.0X-
Hamamelis	T49.2X-
Haptendextran	T45.8X-
Harmonyl	T46.5X-
Hartmann's solution	T50.3X-
Hashish	T40.7X-
Hawaiian Woodrose seeds	T40.99-
HCB	T60.3X-
HCH	T53.6X-
medicinal	T49.0X-
HCN	T57.3X-
Headache cures, drugs, powders NEC	T50.90-
Heavenly Blue (morning glory)	T40.99-
Heavy metal antidote	T45.8X-
Hedaquinium	T49.0X-
Hedge hyssop	T62.2X-
Heet	T49.8X-

Drug/Chemical	Code
Helenin	T37.4X-
Helium (nonmedicinal)NEC	T59.89-
medicinal	T48.99-
Hellebore (black) (green) (white)	T62.2X-
Hematin	T45.8X-
Hematinic preparation	T45.8X-
Hematological agent	T45.9-
specified NEC	T45.8X-
Hemlock	T62.2X-
Hemostatic	T45.62-
drug, systemic	T45.62-
Hemostyptic	T49.4X-
Henbane	T62.2X-
Heparin (sodium)	T45.51-
action reverser	T45.7X-
Heparin-fraction	T45.51-
Heparinoid (systemic)	T45.51-
Hepatic secretion stimulant	T47.8X-
Hepatitis B	
immune globulin	T50.Z1-
vaccine	T50.B9-
Hepronicate	T46.7X-
Heptabarb	T42.3X-
Heptabarbital	T42.3X-
Heptabarbitone	T42.3X-
Heptachlor	T60.1X-
Heptalgin	T40.2X-
Heptaminol	T46.3X-
Herbicide NEC	T60.3X-
Heroin	T40.1X-
Herplex	T49.5X-
HES	T45.8X-
Hesperidin	T46.99-
Hetacillin	T36.0X-
Hetastarch	T45.8X-
HETP	T60.0X-
Hexachlorobenzene (vapor)	T60.3X-
Hexachlorocyclohexane	T53.6X-
Hexachlorophene	T49.0X-
Hexadiline	T46.3X-
Hexadimethrine (bromide)	T45.7X-
Hexadylamine	T46.3X-
Hexaethyl tetraphos-phate	T60.0X-
Hexafluorenium bromide	T48.1X-
Hexafluronium (bromide)	T48.1X-
Hexa-germ	T49.2X-
Hexahydrobenzol	T52.8X-

Drug/Chemical	Code
Hexahydrocresol(s)	T51.8X-
arsenide	T57.0X-
arseniurated	T57.0X-
cyanide	T57.3X-
gas	T59.89-
Fluoride (liquid)	T57.8X-
vapor	T59.89-
phophorated	T60.0X-
sulfate	T57.8X-
sulfide (gas)	T59.6X-
arseniurated	T57.0X-
sulfurated	T57.8X-
Hexahydrophenol	T51.8X-
Hexalen	T51.8X-
Hexamethonium bromide	T44.2X-
Hexamethylene	T52.8X-
Hexamethylmelamine	T45.1X-
Hexamidine	T49.0X-
Hexamine (mandelate)	T37.8X-
Hexanone, 2-hexanone	T52.4X-
Hexanuorenium	T48.1X-
Hexapropymate	T42.6X-
Hexasonium iodide	T44.3X-
Hexcarbacholine bromide	T48.1X-
Hexemal	T42.3X-
Hexestrol	T38.5X-
Hexethal (sodium)	T42.3X-
Hexetidine	T37.8X-
Hexobarbital	T42.3X-
rectal	T41.29-
sodium	T41.1X-
Hexobendine	T46.3X-
Hexocyclium (metilsulfate)	T44.3X-
Hexoestrol	T38.5X-
Hexone	T52.4X-
Hexoprenaline	T48.6X-
Hexylcaine	T41.3X-
Hexylresorcinol	T52.2X-
HGH (human growth hormone)	T38.81-
Hinkle's pills	T47.2X-
Histalog	T50.8X-
Histamine (phosphate)	T50.8X-
Histoplasmin	T50.8X-
Holly berries	T62.2X-
Homatropine	T44.3X-
methylbromide	T44.3X-

Drug/Chemical	Code
Homochlorcyclizine	T45.0X-
Homosalate	T49.3X-
Homo-tet	T50.Z1-
Hormone	T38.80-
adrenal cortical steroids	T38.0X-
androgenic	T38.7X-
anterior pituitary NEC	T38.81-
antidiabetic agents	T38.3X-
antidiuretic	T38.89-
cancer therapy	T45.1X-
follicle stimulating	T38.81-
gonadotropic	T38.89-
pituitary	T38.81-
growth	T38.81-
luteinizing	T38.81-
ovarian	T38.5X-
oxytocic	T48.0X-
parathyroid (derivatives)	T50.99-
pituitary (posterior)NEC	T38.89-
anterior	T38.81-
specified, NEC	T38.89-
thyroid	T38.1X-
Hornet (sting)	T63.451
Horse anti-human lymphocytic serum	T50.Z1-
Horticulture agent NEC	T65.9-
with pesticide	T60.9-
Human	
albumin	T45.8X-
growth hormone (HGH)	T38.81-
immune serum	T50.Z1-
Hyaluronidase	T45.3X-
Hyazyme	T45.3X-
Hycodan	T40.2X-
Hydantoin derivative NEC	T42.0X-
Hydeltra	T38.0X-
Hydergine	T44.6X-
Hydrabamine penicillin	T36.0X-
Hydralazine	T46.5X-
Hydrargaphen	T49.0X-
Hydrargyri amino-chloridum	T49.0X-
Hydrastine	T48.29-
Hydrazine	T54.1X-
monoamine oxidase inhibitors	T43.1X-
Hydrazoic acid, azides	T54.2X-
Hydriodic acid	T48.4X-
Hydrocarbon gas	T59.89-

Drug/Chemical	Code
Hydrochloric acid (liquid)	T54.2X-
medicinal (digestant)	T47.5X-
vapor	T59.89-
Hydrochlorothiazide	T50.2X-
Hydrocodone	T40.2X-
Hydrocortisone (derivatives)	T49.0X-
aceponate	T49.0X-
ENT agent	T49.6X-
ophthalmic preparation	T49.5X-
topical NEC	T49.0X-
Hydrocortone	T38.0X-
ENT agent	T49.6X-
ophthalmic preparation	T49.5X-
topical NEC	T49.0X-
Hydrocyanic acid (liquid)	T57.3X-
gas	T65.0X-
Hydroflumethiazide	T50.2X-
Hydrofluoric acid (liquid)	T54.2X-
vapor	T59.89-
Hydrogen	T59.89-
arsenide	T57.0X-
arseniureted	T57.0X-
chloride	T57.8X-
cyanide (salts) (gas)	T57.3X-
Fluoride (vapor)	T59.5X-
peroxide	T49.0X-
phosphureted	T57.1X-
sulfide (sulfureted)	T59.6X-
arseniureted	T57.0X-
Hydromethylpyridine	T46.7X-
Hydromorphinol	T40.2X-
Hydromorphinone	T40.2X-
Hydromorphone	T40.2X-
Hydromox	T50.2X-
Hydrophilic lotion	T49.3X-
Hydroquinidine	T46.2X-
Hydroquinone	T52.2X-
vapor	T59.89-
Hydrosulfuric acid (gas)	T59.6X-
Hydrotalcite	T47.1X-
Hydrous wool fat	T49.3X-
Hydroxide, caustic	T54.3X-
Hydroxocobalamin	T45.8X-
Hydroxyamphetamine	T49.5X-
Hydroxycarbamide	T45.1X-
Hydroxychloroquine	T37.8X-
Hydroxydihydrocodeinone	T40.2X-

Drug/Chemical	Code
Hydroxyestrone	T38.5X-
Hydroxyethyl starch	T45.8X-
Hydroxymethylpenta-none	T52.4X-
Hydroxyphenamate	T43.59-
Hydroxyphenylbutazone	T39.2X-
Hydroxyprogesterone	T38.5X-
caproate	T38.5X-
Hydroxyquinoline (derivatives)NEC	T37.8X-
Hydroxystilbamidine	T37.3X-
Hydroxytoluene (nonmedicinal)	T54.0X-
medicinal	T49.0X-
Hydroxyurea	T45.1X-
Hydroxyzine	T43.59-
Hyoscine	T44.3X-
Hyoscyamine	T44.3X-
Hyoscyamus	T44.3X-
dry extract	T44.3X-
Hypaque	T50.8X-
Hypertussis	T50.Z1-
Hypnotic	T42.71
anticonvulsant	T42.71
specified NEC	T42.6X-
Hypochlorite	T49.0X-
Hypophysis, posterior	T38.89-
Hypotensive NEC	T46.5X-
Hypromellose	T49.5X-
Ibacitabine	T37.5X-
Ibopamine	T44.99-
Ibufenac	T39.31-
Ibuprofen	T39.31-
Ibuproxam	T39.31-
Ibuterol	T48.6X-
Ichthammol	T49.0X-
Ichthyol	T49.4X-
Idarubicin	T45.1X-
Idrocilamide	T42.8X-
Ifenprodil	T46.7X-
Ifosfamide	T45.1X-
Iletin	T38.3X-
Ilex	T62.2X-
Illuminating gas (after combustion)	T58.1-
prior to combustion	T59.89-
Ilopan	T45.2X-
Iloprost	T46.7X-
Ilotycin	T36.3X-
ophthalmic preparation	T49.5X-
topical NEC	T49.0X-

Drug/Chemical	Code
Imidazole-4-carboxamide	T45.1X-
Imipenem	T36.0X-
Imipramine	T43.01-
Iminostilbene	T42.1X-
Immu-G	T50.Z1-
Immuglobin	T50.Z1-
Immune (globulin) (serum)	T50.Z1-
Immunoglobin human (intravenous) (normal)	T50.Z1-
Immunosuppressive drug	T45.1X-
Immu-tetanus	T50.Z1-
Indalpine	T43.22-
Indanazoline	T48.5X-
Indandione (derivatives)	T45.51-
Indapamide	T46.5X-
Indendione (derivatives)	T45.51-
Indenolol	T44.7X-
Inderal	T44.7X-
Indian	
hemp	T40.7X-
tobacco	T62.2X-
Indigo carmine	T50.8X-
Indobufen	T45.521
Indocin	T39.2X-
Indocyanine green	T50.8X-
Indometacin	T39.39-
Indomethacin	T39.39-
farnesil	T39.4X-
Indoramin	T44.6X-
Industrial	
alcohol	T51.0X-
fumes	T59.89-
solvents (fumes) (vapors)	T52.9-
Influenza vaccine	T50.B9-
Ingested substance NEC	T65.9-
INH	T37.1X-
Inhibitor	
angiotensin-converting enzyme	T46.4X-
carbonic anhydrase	T50.2X-
fibrinolysis	T45.62-
monoamine oxidase NEC	T43.1X-
hydrazine	T43.1X-
postsynaptic	T43.8X-
prothrombin synthesis	T45.51-
Ink	T65.89-
Inorganic substance NEC	T57.9-
Inosine pranobex	T37.5X-

Drug/Chemical	Code
Inositol	T50.99-
nicotinate	T46.7X-
Inproquone	T45.1X-
Insect (sting), venomous	T63.481
ant	T63.421
bee	T63.441
caterpillar	T63.431
hornet	T63.451
wasp	T63.461
Insecticide NEC	T60.9-
carbamate	T60.0X-
chlorinated	T60.1X-
mixed	T60.9-
organochlorine	T60.1X-
organophosphorus	T60.0X-
Insular tissue extract	T38.3X-
Insulin (amorphous) (globin) (isophane) (Lente) (NPH) (Semilente) (Ultralente)	T38.3X-
defalan	T38.3X-
human	T38.3X-
injection, soluble (biphasic)	T38.3X-
intermediate acting	T38.3X-
protamine zinc	T38.3X-
slow acting	T38.3X-
zinc protamine injection/suspension (amorphous) (crystalline)	T38.3X-
Interferon (alpha) (beta) (gamma)	T37.5X-
Intestinal motility control drug	T47.6X-
biological	T47.8X-
Intranarcon	T41.1X-
Intravenous	
amino acids or fat suspensions	T50.99-
Inulin	T50.8X-
Invert sugar	T50.3X-
Iobenzamic acid	T50.8X-
Iocarmic acid	T50.8X-
Iocetamic acid	T50.8X-
Iodamide	T50.8X-
Iodide NEC—*see also Iodine*	T49.0X-
mercury (ointment)	T49.0X-
methylate	T49.0X-
potassium (expectorant)NEC	T48.4X-
Iodinated	
contrast medium	T50.8X-
glycerol	T48.4X-
human serum albumin (131I)	T50.8X-

Drug/Chemical	Code
Iodine (antiseptic, external) (tincture) NEC	T49.0X-
125—*see also Radiation sickness, and Exposure to radioactivce isotopes*	T50.8X-
therapeutic	T50.99-
131—*see also Radiation sickness, and Exposure to radioactivce isotopes*	T50.8X-
therapeutic	T38.2X-
diagnostic	T50.8X-
for thyroid conditions (antithyroid)	T38.2X-
solution	T49.0X-
vapor	T59.89-
Iodipamide	T50.8X-
Iodized (poppy seed)oil	T50.8X-
Iodobismitol	T37.8X-
Iodochlorhydroxyquin	T37.8X-
topical	T49.0X-
Iodochlorhydroxyquinoline	T37.8X-
Iodocholesterol (131I)	T50.8X-
Iodoform	T49.0X-
Iodohippuric acid	T50.8X-
Iodopanoic acid	T50.8X-
Iodophthalein (sodium)	T50.8X-
Iodopyracet	T50.8X-
Iodoquinol	T37.8X-
Iodoxamic acid	T50.8X-
Iofendylate	T50.8X-
Ioglycamic acid	T50.8X-
Iohexol	T50.8X-
Ion exchange resin	
anion	T47.8X-
cation	T50.3X-
cholestyramine	T46.6X-
intestinal	T47.8X-
Iopamidol	T50.8X-
Iopanoic acid	T50.8X-
Iophenoic acid	T50.8X-
Iopodate, sodium	T50.8X-
Iopodic acid	T50.8X-
Iopromide	T50.8X-
Iopydol	T50.8X-
Iotalamic acid	T50.8X-
Iothalamate	T50.8X-
Iothiouracil	T38.2X-
Iotrol	T50.8X-
Iotrolan	T50.8X-
Iotroxate	T50.8X-
Iotroxic acid	T50.8X-

Drug/Chemical	Code
Ioversol	T50.8X-
Ioxaglate	T50.8X-
Ioxaglic acid	T50.8X-
Ioxitalamic acid	T50.8X-
Ipecac	T47.7X-
Ipecacuanha	T48.4X-
Ipodate, calcium	T50.8X-
Ipral	T42.3X-
Ipratropium (bromide)	T48.6X-
Ipriflavone	T46.3X-
Iprindole	T43.01-
Iproclozide	T43.1X-
Iprofenin	T50.8X-
Iproheptine	T49.2X-
Iproniazid	T43.1X-
Iproplatin	T45.1X-
Iproveratril	T46.1X-
Iron (compounds) (medicinal) NEC	T45.4X-
ammonium/dextran injection/salts/sorbitex/sorbitol citric acid complex	T45.4X-
nonmedicinal	T56.89-
Irrigating fluid (vaginal)	T49.8X-
eye	T49.5X-
Isepamicin	T36.5X-
Isoaminile (citrate)	T48.3X-
Isoamyl nitrite	T46.3X-
Isobenzan	T60.1X-
Isobutyl acetate	T52.8X-
Isocarboxazid	T43.1X-
Isoconazole	T49.0X-
Isocyanate	T65.0X-
Isoephedrine	T44.99-
Isoetarine	T48.6X-
Isoethadione	T42.2X-
Isoetharine	T44.5X-
Isoflurane	T41.0X-
Isoflurophate	T44.0X-
Isomaltose, ferric complex	T45.4X-
Isometheptene	T44.3X-
Isoniazid	T37.1X-
with	
rifampicin	T36.6X-
thioacetazone	T37.1X-
Isonicotinic acid hydrazide	T37.1X-
Isonipecaine	T40.4X-
Isopentaquine	T37.2X-
Isophane insulin	T38.3X-

Drug/Chemical	Code
Isophorone	T65.89-
Isophosphamide	T45.1X-
Isopregnenone	T38.5X-
Isoprenaline	T48.6X-
Isopromethazine	T43.3X-
Isopropamide	T44.3X-
iodide	T44.3X-
Isopropanol	T51.2X-
Isopropyl	
acetate	T52.8X-
alcohol	T51.2X-
medicinal	T49.4X-
ether	T52.8X-
Isopropylaminophenazone	T39.2X-
Isoproterenol	T48.6X-
Isosorbide dinitrate	T46.3X-
Isothipendyl	T45.0X-
Isotretinoin	T50.99-
Isoxazolyl penicillin	T36.0X-
Isoxicam	T39.39-
Isoxsuprine	T46.7X-
Ispagula	T47.4X-
husk	T47.4X-
Isradipine	T46.1X-
I-thyroxine sodium	T38.1X-
Itraconazole	T37.8X-
Itramin tosilate	T46.3X-
Ivermectin	T37.4X-
Izoniazid	T37.1X-
with thioacetazone	T37.1X-
Jalap	T47.2X-
Jamaica	
dogwood (bark)	T39.8X-
ginger	T65.89-
root	T62.2X-
Jatropha	T62.2X-
curcas	T62.2X-
Jectofer	T45.4X-
Jellyfish (sting)	T63.62-
Jequirity (bean)	T62.2X-
Jimson weed (stramonium)	T62.2X-
Josamycin	T36.3X-
Juniper tar	T49.1X-
Kallidinogenase	T46.7X-
Kallikrein	T46.7X-
Kanamycin	T36.5X-
Kantrex	T36.5X-

Drug/Chemical	Code
Kaolin	T47.6X-
light	T47.6X-
Karaya (gum)	T47.4X-
Kebuzone	T39.2X-
Kelevan	T60.1X-
Kemithal	T41.1X-
Kenacort	T38.0X-
Keratolytic drug NEC	T49.4X-
anthracene	T49.4X-
Keratoplastic NEC	T49.4X-
Kerosene, kerosine (fuel) (solvent)NEC	T52.0X-
insecticide	T52.0X-
vapor	T52.0X-
Ketamine	T41.29-
Ketazolam	T42.4X-
Ketazon	T39.2X-
Ketobemidone	T40.4X-
Ketoconazole	T49.0X-
Ketols	T52.4X-
Ketone oils	T52.4X-
Ketoprofen	T39.31-
Ketorolac	T39.8X-
Ketotifen	T45.0X-
Khat	T43.69-
Khellin	T46.3X-
Khelloside	T46.3X-
Kiln gas or vapor (carbon monoxide)	T58.8X-
Kitasamycin	T36.3X-
Konsyl	T47.4X-
Kosam seed	T62.2X-
Krait (venom)	T63.09-
Kwell (insecticide)	T60.1X-
anti-infective (topical)	T49.0X-
Labetalol	T44.8X-
Laburnum (seeds)	T62.2X-
leaves	T62.2X-
Lachesine	T49.5X-
Lacidipine	T46.5X-
Lacquer	T65.6X-
Lacrimogenic gas	T59.3X-
Lactated potassic saline	T50.3X-
Lactic acid	T49.8X-
Lactobacillus (all forms or compounds)	T47.6X-
Lactoflavin	T45.2X-
Lactose (as excipient)	T50.90-
Lactuca (virosa) (extract)	T42.6X-
Lactucarium	T42.6X-

Drug/Chemical	Code
Lactulose	T47.3X-
Laevo—see Levo-	
Lanatosides	T46.0X-
Lanolin	T49.3X-
Largactil	T43.3X-
Larkspur	T62.2X-
Laroxyl	T43.01-
Lasix	T50.1X-
Lassar's paste	T49.4X-
Latamoxef	T36.1X-
Latex	T65.81-
Lathyrus (seed)	T62.2X-
Laudanum	T40.0X-
Laudexium	T48.1X-
Laughing gas	T41.0X-
Laurel, black or cherry	T62.2X-
Laurolinium	T49.0X-
Lauryl sulfoacetate	T49.2X-
Laxative NEC	T47.4X-
osmotic	T47.3X-
saline	T47.3X-
stimulant	T47.2X-
L-dopa	T42.8X-
Lead (dust) (fumes) (vapor) NEC	T56.0X-
acetate	T49.2X-
alkyl (fuel additive)	T56.0X-
anti-infectives	T37.8X-
antiknock compound (tetraethyl)	T56.0X-
arsenate, arsenite (dust) (herbicide) (insecticide) (vapor)	T57.0X-
carbonate (paint)	T56.0X-
chromate (paint)	T56.0X-
dioxide	T56.0X-
inorganic	T56.0X-
iodide (pigment) (paint)	T56.0X-
monoxide (dust) (paint)	T56.0X-
organic	T56.0X-
oxide (paint)	T56.0X-
salts	T56.0X-
specified compound NEC	T56.0X-
tetra-ethyl	T56.0X-
Lebanese red	T40.7X-
Lefetamine	T39.8X-
Lenperone	T43.4X-
Lente lietin (insulin)	T38.3X-
Leptazol	T50.7X-
Leptophos	T60.0X-
Leritine	T40.2X-

Drug/Chemical	Code
Letosteine	T48.4X-
Letter	T38.1X-
Lettuce opium	T42.6X-
Leucinocaine	T41.3X-
Leucocianidol	T46.99-
Leucovorin (factor)	T45.8X-
Leukeran	T45.1X-
Leuprolide	T38.89-
Levalbuterol	T48.6X-
Levallorphan	T50.7X-
Levamisole	T37.4X-
Levanil	T42.6X-
Levarterenol	T44.4X-
Levdropropizine	T48.3X-
Levobunolol	T49.5X-
Levocabastine (hydrochloride)	T45.0X-
Levocarnitine	T50.99-
Levodopa (w carbidopa)	T42.8X-
Levo-dromoran	T40.2X-
Levoglutamide	T50.99-
Levoid	T38.1X-
Levo-iso-methadone	T40.3X-
Levomepromazine	T43.3X-
Levonordefrin	T49.6X-
Levonorgestrel	T38.4X-
with ethinylestradiol	T38.5X-
Levopromazine	T43.3X-
Levoprome	T42.6X-
Levopropoxyphene	T40.4X-
Levopropylhexedrine	T50.5X-
Levoproxyphylline	T48.6X-
Levorphanol	T40.4X-
Levothyroxine	T38.1X-
sodium	T38.1X-
Levsin	T44.3X-
Levulose	T50.3X-
Lewisite (gas), not in war	T57.0X-
Librium	T42.4X-
Lidex	T49.0X-
Lidocaine	T41.3X-
regional	T41.3X-
spinal	T41.3X-
Lidofenin	T50.8X-
Lidoflazine	T46.1X-
Lighter fluid	T52.0X-
Lignin hemicellulose	T47.6X-

Drug/Chemical	Code
Lignocaine	T41.3X-
regional	T41.3X-
spinal	T41.3X-
Ligroin (e) (solvent)	T52.0X-
vapor	T59.89-
Ligustrum vulgare	T62.2X-
Lily of the valley	T62.2X-
Lime (chloride)	T54.3X-
Limonene	T52.8X-
Lincomycin	T36.8X-
Lindane (insecticide) (nonmedicinal) (vapor)	T53.6X-
medicinal	T49.0X-
Liniments NEC	T49.9-
Linoleic acid	T46.6X-
Linolenic acid	T46.6X-
Linseed	T47.4X-
Liothyronine	T38.1X-
Liotrix	T38.1X-
Lipancreatin	T47.5X-
Lipo-alprostadil	T46.7X-
Lipo-Lutin	T38.5X-
Lipotropic drug NEC	T50.90-
Liquefied petroleum gases	T59.89-
piped (pure or mixed with air)	T59.89-
Liquid	
paraffin	T47.4X-
petrolatum	T47.4X-
topical	T49.3X-
specified NEC	T65.89-
substance	T65.9-
Liquor creosolis compositus	T65.89-
Liquorice	T48.4X-
extract	T47.8X-
Lisinopril	T46.4X-
Lisuride	T42.8X-
Lithane	T43.8X-
Lithium	T56.89-
gluconate	T43.59-
salts (carbonate)	T43.59-
Lithonate	T43.8X-
Liver	
extract	T45.8X-
for parenteral use	T45.8X-
fraction 1	T45.8X-
hydrolysate	T45.8X-
Lizard (bite) (venom)	T63.121
LMD	T45.8X-

Drug/Chemical	Code
Lobelia	T62.2X-
Lobeline	T50.7X-
Local action drug NEC	T49.8X-
Locorten	T49.0X-
Lofepramine	T43.01-
Lolium temulentum	T62.2X-
Lomotil	T47.6X-
Lomustine	T45.1X-
Lonidamine	T45.1X-
Loperamide	T47.6X-
Loprazolam	T42.4X-
Lorajmine	T46.2X-
Loratidine	T45.0X-
Lorazepam	T42.4X-
Lorcainide	T46.2X-
Lormetazepam	T42.4X-
Lotions NEC	T49.9-
Lotusate	T42.3X-
Lovastatin	T46.6X-
Lowila	T49.2X-
Loxapine	T43.59-
Lozenges (throat)	T49.6X-
LSD	T40.8X-
L-Tryptophan—*see amino acid*	
Lubricant, eye	T49.5X-
Lubricating oil NEC	T52.0X-
Lucanthone	T37.4X-
Luminal	T42.3X-
Lung irritant (gas)NEC	T59.9-
Luteinizing hormone	T38.81-
Lutocylol	T38.5X-
Lutromone	T38.5X-
Lututrin	T48.29-
Lye (concentrated)	T54.3X-
Lygranum (skin test)	T50.8X-
Lymecycline	T36.4X-
Lymphogranuloma venereum antigen	T50.8X-
Lynestrenol	T38.4X-
Lyovac Sodium Edecrin	T50.1X-
Lypressin	T38.89-
Lysergic acid diethylamide	T40.8X-
Lysergide	T40.8X-
Lysine vasopressin	T38.89-
Lysol	T54.1X-
Lysozyme	T49.0X-
Lytta (vitatta)	T49.8X-
Mace	T59.3X-

Drug/Chemical	Code
Macrogol	T50.99-
Macrolide	
anabolic drug	T38.7X-
antibiotic	T36.3X-
Mafenide	T49.0X-
Magaldrate	T47.1X-
Magic mushroom	T40.99-
Magnamycin	T36.8X-
Magnesia magma	T47.1X-
Magnesium NEC	T56.89-
carbonate	T47.1X-
citrate	T47.4X-
hydroxide (oxide)	T47.1X-
peroxide	T49.0X-
salicylate	T39.09-
silicofluoride	T50.3X-
sulfate	T47.4X-
thiosulfate	T45.0X-
trisilicate	T47.1X-
Malathion (medicinal) (insecticide)	T49.0X-
insecticide	T60.0X-
Male fern extract	T37.4X-
M-AMSA	T45.1X-
Mandelic acid	T37.8X-
Manganese (dioxide) (salts)	T57.2X-
medicinal	T50.99-
Mannitol	T47.3X-
hexanitrate	T46.3X-
Mannomustine	T45.1X-
MAO inhibitors	T43.1X-
Mapharsen	T37.8X-
Maphenide	T49.0X-
Maprotiline	T43.02-
Marcaine (infiltration) (subcutaneous) (nerve block)	T41.3X-
Marezine	T45.0X-
Marihuana	T40.7X-
Marijuana	T40.7X-
Marine (sting)	T63.69-
animals (sting)	T63.69-
plants (sting)	T63.71-
Marplan	T43.1X-
Marsh gas	T59.89-
Marsilid	T43.1X-
Matulane	T45.1X-
Mazindol	T50.5X-
MCPA	T60.3X-
MDMA	T43.62-

Drug/Chemical	Code
Meadow saffron	T62.2X-
Measles virus vaccine (attenuated)	T50.B9-
Meat, noxious	T62.8X-
Meballymal	T42.3X-
Mebanazine	T43.1X-
Mebaral	T42.3X-
Mebendazole	T37.4X-
Mebeverine	T44.3X-
Mebhydrolin	T45.0X-
Mebumal	T42.3X-
Mebutamate	T43.59-
Mecamylamine	T44.2X-
Mechlorethamine	T45.1X-
Mecillinam	T36.0X-
Meclizine (hydrochloride)	T45.0X-
Meclocycline	T36.4X-
Meclofenamate	T39.39-
Meclofenamic acid	T39.39-
Meclofenoxate	T43.69-
Meclozine	T45.0X-
Mecobalamin	T45.8X-
Mecoprop	T60.3X-
Mecrilate	T49.3X-
Mecysteine	T48.4X-
Medazepam	T42.4X-
Medicament NEC	T50.90-
Medinal	T42.3X-
Medomin	T42.3X-
Medrogestone	T38.5X-
Medroxalol	T44.8X-
Medroxyprogesterone acetate (depot)	T38.5X-
Medrysone	T49.0X-
Mefenamic acid	T39.39-
Mefenorex	T50.5X-
Mefloquine	T37.2X-
Mefruside	T50.2X-
Megahallucinogen	T40.90-
Megestrol	T38.5X-
Meglumine	
antimoniate	T37.8X-
diatrizoate	T50.8X-
iodipamide	T50.8X-
iotroxate	T50.8X-
MEK (methyl ethyl ketone)	T52.4X-
Meladinin	T49.3X-
Meladrazine	T44.3X-
Melaleuca alternifolia oil	T49.0X-

Drug/Chemical	Code
Melanizing agents	T49.3X-
Melanocyte-stimulating hormone	T38.89-
Melarsonyl potassium	T37.3X-
Melarsoprol	T37.3X-
Melia azedarach	T62.2X-
Melitracen	T43.01-
Mellaril	T43.3X-
Meloxine	T49.3X-
Melperone	T43.4X-
Melphalan	T45.1X-
Memantine	T43.8X-
Menadiol (sodium sulfate)	T45.7X-
Menadione	T45.7X-
sodium bisulfite	T45.7X-
Menaphthone	T45.7X-
Menaquinone	T45.7X-
Menatetrenone	T45.7X-
Meningococcal vaccine	T50.A9-
Menningovax (-AC) (-C)	T50.A9-
Menotropins	T38.81-
Menthol	T48.5X-
Mepacrine	T37.2X-
Meparfynol	T42.6X-
Mepartricin	T36.7X-
Mepazine	T43.3X-
Mepenzolate	T44.3X-
bromide	T44.3X-
Meperidine	T40.4X-
Mephebarbital	T42.3X-
Mephenamin (e)	T42.8X-
Mephenesin	T42.8X-
Mephenhydramine	T45.0X-
Mephenoxalone	T42.8X-
Mephentermine	T44.99-
Mephenytoin	T42.0X-
with phenobarbital	T42.3X-
Mephobarbital	T42.3X-
Mephosfolan	T60.0X-
Mepindolol	T44.7X-
Mepiperphenidol	T44.3X-
Mepitiostane	T38.7X-
Mepivacaine (epidural)	T41.3X-
Meprednisone	T38.0X-
Meprobam	T43.59-
Meprobamate	T43.59-
Meproscillarin	T46.0X-
Meprylcaine	T41.3X-

MEPTAZINOL–METHEDRINE

Drug/Chemical	Code
Meptazinol	T39.8X-
Mepyramine	T45.0X-
Mequitazine	T43.3X-
Meralluride	T50.2X-
Merbaphen	T50.2X-
Merbromin	T49.0X-
Mercaptobenzothiazole salts	T49.0X-
Mercaptomerin	T50.2X-
Mercaptopurine	T45.1X-
Mercumatilin	T50.2X-
Mercuramide	T50.2X-
Mercurochrome	T49.0X-
Mercurophylline	T50.2X-
Mercury, mercurial, mercuric, mercurous (compounds) (cyanide) (fumes) (nonmedicinal) (vapor) NEC	T56.1X-
ammoniated	T49.0X-
anti-infective	
local	T49.0X-
systemic	T37.8X-
topical	T49.0X-
chloride (ammoniated)	T49.0X-
diuretic NEC	T50.2X-
fungicide (organic)	T56.1X-
oxide, yellow	T49.0X-
Mersalyl	T50.2X-
Merthiolate	T49.0X-
ophthalmic preparation	T49.5X-
Meruvax	T50.B9-
Mesalazine	T47.8X-
Mescal buttons	T40.99-
Mescaline	T40.99-
Mesna	T48.4X-
Mesoglycan	T46.6X-
Mesoridazine	T43.3X-
Mestanolone	T38.7X-
Mesterolone	T38.7X-
Mestranol	T38.5X-
Mesulergine	T42.8X-
Mesulfen	T49.0X-
Mesuximide	T42.2X-
Metabutethamine	T41.3X-
Metactesylacetate	T49.0X-
Metacycline	T36.4X-
Metaldehyde (snail killer) NEC	T60.8X-

Drug/Chemical	Code
Metals (heavy) (nonmedicinal)	T56.9-
dust, fumes, or vapor NEC	T56.9-
light NEC	T56.9-
dust, fumes, or vapor NEC	T56.9-
specified NEC	T56.89-
thallium	T56.81-
Metamfetamine	T43.62-
Metamizole sodium	T39.2X-
Metampicillin	T36.0X-
Metamucil	T47.4X-
Metandienone	T38.7X-
Metandrostenolone	T38.7X-
Metaphen	T49.0X-
Metaphos	T60.0X-
Metapramine	T43.01-
Metaproterenol	T48.29-
Metaraminol	T44.4X-
Metaxalone	T42.8X-
Metenolone	T38.7X-
Metergoline	T42.8X-
Metescufylline	T46.99-
Metetoin	T42.0X-
Metformin	T38.3X-
Methacholine	T44.1X-
Methacycline	T36.4X-
Methadone	T40.3X-
Methallenestril	T38.5X-
Methallenoestril	T38.5X-
Methamphetamine	T43.62-
Methampyrone	T39.2X-
Methandienone	T38.7X-
Methandriol	T38.7X-
Methandrostenolone	T38.7X-
Methane	T59.89-
Methanethiol	T59.89-
Methaniazide	T37.1X-
Methanol (vapor)	T51.1X-
Methantheline	T44.3X-
Methanthelinium bromide	T44.3X-
Methaphenilene	T45.0X-
Methapyrilene	T45.0X-
Methaqualone (compound)	T42.6X-
Metharbital	T42.3X-
Methazolamide	T50.2X-
Methdilazine	T43.3X-
Methedrine	T43.62-

Drug/Chemical	Code
Methenamine (mandelate)	T37.8X-
Methenolone	T38.7X-
Methergine	T48.0X-
Methetoin	T42.0X-
Methiacil	T38.2X-
Methicillin	T36.0X-
Methimazole	T38.2X-
Methiodal sodium	T50.8X-
Methionine	T50.99-
Methisazone	T37.5X-
Methisoprinol	T37.5X-
Methitural	T42.3X-
Methixene	T44.3X-
Methobarbital, methobarbitone	T42.3X-
Methocarbamol	T42.8X-
skeletal muscle relaxant	T48.1X-
Methohexital	T41.1X-
Methohexitone	T41.1X-
Methoin	T42.0X-
Methopholine	T39.8X-
Methopromazine	T43.3X-
Methorate	T48.3X-
Methoserpidine	T46.5X-
Methotrexate	T45.1X-
Methotrimeprazine	T43.3X-
Methoxa-Dome	T49.3X-
Methoxamine	T44.4X-
Methoxsalen	T50.99-
Methoxyaniline	T65.3X-
Methoxybenzyl penicillin	T36.0X-
Methoxychlor	T53.7X-
Methoxy-DDT	T53.7X-
2-Methoxyethanol	T52.3X-
Methoxyflurane	T41.0X-
Methoxyphenamine	T48.6X-
Methoxypromazine	T43.3X-
5-Methoxypsoralen (5-MOP)	T50.99-
8-Methoxypsoralen (8-MOP)	T50.99-
Methscopolamine bromide	T44.3X-
Methsuximide	T42.2X-
Methyclothiazide	T50.2X-
Methyl	
acetate	T52.4X-
acetone	T52.4X-
acrylate	T65.89-
alcohol	T51.1X-
aminophenol	T65.3X-

Drug/Chemical	Code
Methyl, continued	
amphetamine	T43.62-
androstanolone	T38.7X-
atropine	T44.3X-
benzene	T52.2X-
benzoate	T52.8X-
benzol	T52.2X-
bromide (gas)	T59.89-
fumigant	T60.8X-
butanol	T51.3X-
carbinol	T51.1X-
carbonate	T52.8X-
CCNU	T45.1X-
cellosolve	T52.9-
cellulose	T47.4X-
chloride (gas)	T59.89-
chloroformate	T59.3X-
cyclohexane	T52.8X-
cyclohexanol	T51.8X-
cyclohexanone	T52.8X-
cyclohexyl acetate	T52.8X-
demeton	T60.0X-
dihydromorphinone	T40.2X-
ergometrine	T48.0X-
ergonovine	T48.0X-
ethyl ketone	T52.4X-
glucamine antimonate	T37.8X-
hydrazine	T65.89-
iodide	T65.89-
isobutyl ketone	T52.4X-
isothiocyanate	T60.3X-
mercaptan	T59.89-
morphine NEC	T40.2X-
nicotinate	T49.4X-
paraben	T49.0X-
parafynol	T42.6X-
parathion	T60.0X-
peridol	T43.4X-
phenidate	T43.631
ENT agent	T49.6X-
ophthalmic preparation	T49.5X-
topical NEC	T49.0X-
propylcarbinol	T51.3X-
rosaniline NEC	T49.0X-
salicylate	T49.2X-
sulfate (fumes)	T59.89-
liquid	T52.8X-

Drug/Chemical	Code
Methyl, continued	
sulfonal	T42.6X-
testosterone	T38.7X-
thiouracil	T38.2X-
Methylamphetamine	T43.62-
Methylated spirit	T51.1X-
Methylatropine nitrate	T44.3X-
Methylbenactyzium bromide	T44.3X-
Methylbenzethonium chloride	T49.0X-
Methylcellulose	T47.4X-
laxative	T47.4X-
Methylchlorophenoxy-acetic acid	T60.3X-
Methyldopa	T46.5X-
Methyldopate	T46.5X-
Methylene	
blue	T50.6X-
chloride or dichloride (solvent)NEC	T53.4X-
Methylenedioxyamphetamine	T43.62-
Methylenedioxymethamphetamine	T43.62-
Methylergometrine	T48.0X-
Methylergonovine	T48.0X-
Methylestrenolone	T38.5X-
Methylethyl cellulose	T50.99-
Methylhexabital	T42.3X-
Methylmorphine	T40.2X-
Methylparaben (ophthalmic)	T49.5X-
Methylparafynol	T42.6X-
Methylpentynol, methylpenthynol	T42.6X-
Methylphenidate	T43.631
Methylphenobarbital	T42.3X-
Methylpolysiloxane	T47.1X-
Methylprednisolone	T38.0X-
Methylrosaniline	T49.0X-
Methylrosanilinium chloride	T49.0X-
Methyltestosterone	T38.7X-
Methylthionine chloride	T50.6X-
Methylthioninium chloride	T50.6X-
Methylthiouracil	T38.2X-
Methyprylon	T42.6X-
Methysergide	T46.5X-
Metiamide	T47.1X-
Meticillin	T36.0X-
Meticrane	T50.2X-
Metildigoxin	T46.0X-
Metipranolol	T49.5X-
Metirosine	T46.5X-
Metisazone	T37.5X-

Drug/Chemical	Code
Metixene	T44.3X-
Metizoline	T48.5X-
Metoclopramide	T45.0X-
Metofenazate	T43.3X-
Metofoline	T39.8X-
Metolazone	T50.2X-
Metopon	T40.2X-
Metoprine	T45.1X-
Metoprolol	T44.7X-
Metrifonate	T60.0X-
Metrizamide	T50.8X-
Metrizoic acid	T50.8X-
Metronidazole	T37.8X-
Metycaine (infiltration) (topical) (subcutaneous) (nerve block)	T41.3X-
Metyrapone	T50.8X-
Mevinphos	T60.0X-
Mexazolam	T42.4X-
Mexenone	T49.3X-
Mexiletine	T46.2X-
Mezereon	T62.2X-
berries	T62.1X-
Mezlocillin	T36.0X-
Mianserin	T43.02-
Micatin	T49.0X-
Miconazole	T49.0X-
Micronomicin	T36.5X-
Midazolam	T42.4X-
Midecamycin	T36.3X-
Mifepristone	T38.6X-
Milk of magnesia	T47.1X-
Millipede (tropical) (venomous)	T63.41-
Miltown	T43.59-
Milverine	T44.3X-
Minaprine	T43.29-
Minaxolone	T41.29-
Mineral	
acids	T54.2X-
oil (laxative) (medicinal)	T47.4X-
emulsion	T47.2X-
nonmedicinal	T52.0X-
topical	T49.3X-
salt NEC	T50.3X-
spirits	T52.0X-
Mineralocorticosteroid	T50.0X-
Minocycline	T36.4X-
Minoxidil	T46.7X-
Miokamycin	T36.3X-

Drug/Chemical	Code
Miotic drug	T49.5X-
Mipafox	T60.0X-
Mirex	T60.1X-
Mirtazapine	T43.02-
Misonidazole	T37.3X-
Misoprostol	T47.1X-
Mithramycin	T45.1X-
Mitobronitol	T45.1X-
Mitoguazone	T45.1X-
Mitolactol	T45.1X-
Mitomycin	T45.1X-
Mitopodozide	T45.1X-
Mitotane	T45.1X-
Mitoxantrone	T45.1X-
Mivacurium chloride	T48.1X-
Miyari bacteria	T47.6X-
Moclobemide	T43.1X-
Moderil	T46.5X-
Mofebutazone	T39.2X-
Molindone	T43.59-
Molsidomine	T46.3X-
Mometasone	T49.0X-
Monistat	T49.0X-
Monkshood	T62.2X-
Monoamine oxidase inhibitor NEC	T43.1X-
hydrazine	T43.1X-
Monobenzone	T49.4X-
Monochloroacetic acid	T60.3X-
Monochlorobenzene	T53.7X-
Monoethanolamine (oleate)	T46.8X-
Monooctanoin	T50.99-
Monophenylbutazone	T39.2X-
Monosodium glutamate	T65.89-
Monosulfiram	T49.0X-
Monoxidine hydrochloride	T46.1X-
Monuron	T60.3X-
Moperone	T43.4X-
Mopidamol	T45.1X-
MOPP (mechloreth-amine + vincristine + prednisone + procarbazine)	T45.1X-
Morfin	T40.2X-
Morinamide	T37.1X-
Morning glory seeds	T40.99-
Moroxydine	T37.5X-
Morphazinamide	T37.1X-
Morphine	T40.2X-
antagonist	T50.7X-

Drug/Chemical	Code
Morpholinylethylmorphine	T40.2X-
Morsuximide	T42.2X-
Mosapramine	T43.59-
Moth balls (naphthalene)	T60.2X-
paradichlorobenzene	T60.1X-
Motor exhaust gas	T58.0-
Mouthwash (antiseptic)	T49.6X-
Moxastine	T45.0X-
Moxaverine	T44.3X-
Moxisylyte	T46.7X-
Mucilage, plant	T47.4X-
Mucolytic drug	T48.4X-
Mucomyst	T48.4X-
Mucous membrane agents (external)	T49.9-
specified NEC	T49.8X-
Mumps	
immune globulin (human)	T50.Z1-
skin test antigen	T50.8X-
vaccine	T50.B9-
Mupirocin	T49.0X-
Muromonab-CD3	T45.1X-
Muscle-action drug NEC	T48.20-
Muscle affecting agents NEC	T48.20-
oxytocic	T48.0X-
relaxants	T48.20-
central nervous system	T42.8X-
skeletal	T48.1X-
smooth	T44.3X-
Mushroom, noxious	T62.0X-
Mussel, noxious	T61.781
Mustard (emetic) (black)	T47.7X-
gas, not in war	T59.9-
nitrogen	T45.1X-
Mustine	T45.1X-
M-vac	T45.1X-
Mycifradin	T36.5X-
topical	T49.0X-
Mycitracin	T36.8X-
ophthalmic preparation	T49.5X-
Mycostatin	T36.7X-
topical	T49.0X-
Mycotoxins (NEC)	T64.81
aflatoxin	T64.0-
Mydriacyl	T44.3X-
Mydriatic drug	T49.5X-
Myelobromal	T45.1X-
Myleran	T45.1X-

MYOCHRYSIN (E)-NICKEL (CARBONYL) (TETRA-CARBONYL) (FUMES) (VAPOR)

Drug/Chemical	Code
Myochrysin (e)	T39.2X-
Myoneural blocking agents	T48.1X-
Myralact	T49.0X-
Myristica fragrans	T62.2X-
Myristicin	T65.89-
Mysoline	T42.3X-
Nabilone	T40.7X-
Nabumetone	T39.39-
Nadolol	T44.7X-
Nafcillin	T36.0X-
Nafoxidine	T38.6X-
Naftazone	T46.99-
Naftidrofuryl (oxalate)	T46.7X-
Naftifine	T49.0X-
Nail polish remover	T52.9-
Nalbuphine	T40.4X-
Naled	T60.0X-
Nalidixic acid	T37.8X-
Nalorphine	T50.7X-
Naloxone	T50.7X-
Naltrexone	T50.7X-
Namenda	T43.8X-
Nandrolone	T38.7X-
Naphazoline	T48.5X-
Naphtha (painters') (petroleum)	T52.0X-
solvent	T52.0X-
vapor	T52.0X-
Naphthalene (non-chlorinated)	T60.2X-
chlorinated	T60.1X-
vapor	T60.1X-
insecticide or moth repellent	T60.2X-
chlorinated	T60.1X-
vapor	T60.2X-
chlorinated	T60.1X-
Naphthol	T65.89-
Naphthylamine	T65.89-
Naphthylthiourea (ANTU)	T60.4X-
Naproxen (Naprosyn)	T39.31-
Narcotic (drug)	T40.60-
analgesic NEC	T40.60-
antagonist	T50.7X-
specified NEC	T40.69-
synthetic	T40.4X-
Narcotine	T48.3X-
Nardil	T43.1X-
Nasal drug NEC	T49.6X-
Natamycin	T49.0X-

Drug/Chemical	Code
Natural	
blood (product)	T45.8X-
gas (piped)	T59.89-
incomplete combustion	T58.1-
Nealbarbital	T42.3X-
Nectadon	T48.3X-
Nedocromil	T48.6X-
Nefopam	T39.8X-
Nematocyst (sting)	T63.69-
Nembutal	T42.3X-
Nemonapride	T43.59-
Neoarsphenamine	T37.8X-
Neocinchophen	T50.4X-
Neomycin (derivatives)	T36.5X-
with bacitracin	T49.0X-
with neostigmine	T44.0X-
ENT agent	T49.6X-
ophthalmic preparation	T49.5X-
topical NEC	T49.0X-
Neonal	T42.3X-
Neoprontosil	T37.0X-
Neosalvarsan	T37.8X-
Neosilversalvarsan	T37.8X-
Neosporin	T36.8X-
ENT agent	T49.6X-
opthalmic preparation	T49.5X-
topical NEC	T49.0X-
Neostigmine bromide	T44.0X-
Neraval	T42.3X-
Neravan	T42.3X-
Nerium oleander	T62.2X-
Nerve gas, not in war	T59.9-
Nesacaine (infiltration) (subcutaneous) (nerve block)	T41.3X-
Netilmicin	T36.5X-
Neurobarb	T42.3X-
Neuroleptic drug NEC	T43.50-
Neuromuscular blocking drug	T48.1X-
Neutral insulin injection	T38.3X-
Neutral spirits (beverage)	T51.0X-
Niacin	T46.7X-
Niacinamide	T45.2X-
Nialamide	T43.1X-
Niaprazine	T42.6X-
Nicametate	T46.7X-
Nicardipine	T46.1X-
Nicergoline	T46.7X-
Nickel (carbonyl) (tetra-carbonyl) (fumes) (vapor)	T56.89-

Drug/Chemical	Code
Nickelocene	T56.89-
Niclosamide	T37.4X-
Nicofuranose	T46.7X-
Nicomorphine	T40.2X-
Nicorandil	T46.3X-
Nicotiana (plant)	T62.2X-
Nicotinamide	T45.2X-
Nicotine (insecticide) (spray) (sulfate) NEC	T60.2X-
from tobacco	T65.29-
cigarettes	T65.22-
not insecticide	T65.29-
Nicotinic acid	T46.7X-
Nicotinyl alcohol	T46.7X-
Nicoumalone	T45.51-
Nifedipine	T46.1X-
Nifenazone	T39.2X-
Nifuraldezone	T37.9-
Nifuratel	T37.8X-
Nifurtimox	T37.3X-
Nifurtoinol	T37.8X-
Nightshade, deadly (solanum)	T62.2X-
berry	T62.1X-
Nikethamide	T50.7X-
Nilstat	T36.7X-
topical	T49.0X-
Nilutamide	T38.6X-
Nimesulide	T39.39-
Nimetazepam	T42.4X-
Nimodipine	T46.1X-
Nimorazole	T37.3X-
Nimustine	T45.1X-
Niridazole	T37.4X-
Nisentil	T40.2X-
Nisoldipine	T46.1X-
Nitramine	T65.3X-
Nitrate, organic	T46.3X-
Nitrazepam	T42.4X-
Nitrefazole	T50.6X-
Nitrendipine	T46.1X-
Nitric	
acid (liquid)	T54.2X-
vapor	T59.89-
oxide (gas)	T59.0X-
Nitrimidazine	T37.3X-
Nitrite, amyl (medicinal) (vapor)	T46.3X-
Nitroaniline	T65.3X-
vapor	T59.89-

Drug/Chemical	Code
Nitrobenzene, nitrobenzol (vapor)	T65.3X-
Nitrocellulose	T65.89-
lacquer	T65.89-
Nitrodiphenyl	T65.3X-
Nitrofural	T49.0X-
Nitrofurantoin	T37.8X-
Nitrofurazone	T49.0X-
Nitrogen	T59.0X-
mustard	T45.1X-
Nitroglycerin, nitro-glycerol (medicinal)	T46.3X-
nonmedicinal	T65.5X-
fumes	T65.5X-
Nitroglycol	T52.3X-
Nitrohydrochloric acid	T54.2X-
Nitromersol	T49.0X-
Nitronaphthalene	T65.89-
Nitrophenol	T54.0X-
Nitropropane	T52.8X-
Nitroprusside	T46.5X-
Nitrosodimethylamine	T65.3X-
Nitrothiazol	T37.4X-
Nitrotoluene, nitrotoluol	T65.3X-
vapor	T65.3X-
Nitrous	
acid (liquid)	T54.2X-
fumes	T59.89-
ether spirit	T46.3X-
oxide	T41.0X-
Nitroxoline	T37.8X-
Nitrozone	T49.0X-
Nizatidine	T47.0X-
Nizofenone	T43.8X-
Noctec	T42.6X-
Noludar	T42.6X-
Nomegestrol	T38.5X-
Nomifensine	T43.29-
Nonoxinol	T49.8X-
Nonylphenoxy (polyethoxy-ethanol)	T49.8X-
Noptil	T42.3X-
Noradrenaline	T44.4X-
Noramidopyrine	T39.2X-
methanesulfonate sodium	T39.2X-
Norbormide	T60.4X-
Nordazepam	T42.4X-
Norepinephrine	T44.4X-
Norethandrolone	T38.7X-
Norethindrone	T38.4X-

Drug/Chemical	Code
Norethisterone (acetate) (enantate)	T38.4X-
with ethinylestradiol	T38.5X-
Noretynodrel	T38.5X-
Norfenefrine	T44.4X-
Norfloxacin	T36.8X-
Norgestrel	T38.4X-
Norgestrienone	T38.4X-
Norlestrin	T38.4X-
Norlutin	T38.4X-
Normal serum albumin (human), salt-poor	T45.8X-
Normethandrone	T38.5X-
Normorphine	T40.2X-
Norpseudoephedrine	T50.5X-
Nortestosterone (furanpropionate)	T38.7X-
Nortriptyline	T43.01-
Noscapine	T48.3X-
Nose preparations	T49.6X-
Novobiocin	T36.5X-
Novocain (infiltration) (topical) (spinal)	T41.3X-
Noxious foodstuff	T62.9-
specified NEC	T62.8X-
Noxiptiline	T43.01-
Noxytiolin	T49.0X-
NPH Iletin (insulin)	T38.3X-
Numorphan	T40.2X-
Nunol	T42.3X-
Nupercaine (spinal anesthetic)	T41.3X-
topical (surface)	T41.3X-
Nutmeg oil (liniment)	T49.3X-
Nutritional supplement	T50.90-
Nux vomica	T65.1X-
Nydrazid	T37.1X-
Nylidrin	T46.7X-
Nystatin	T36.7X-
topical	T49.0X-
Nytol	T45.0X-
Obidoxime chloride	T50.6X-
Octafonium (chloride)	T49.3X-
Octamethyl pyrophos-phoramide	T60.0X-
Octanoin	T50.99-
Octatropine methyl-bromide	T44.3X-
Octotiamine	T45.2X-
Octoxinol (9)	T49.8X-
Octreotide	T38.99-
Octyl nitrite	T46.3X-
Oestradiol	T38.5X-
Oestriol	T38.5X-

Drug/Chemical	Code
Oestrogen	T38.5X-
Oestrone	T38.5X-
Ofloxacin	T36.8X-
Oil (of)	T65.89-
bitter almond	T62.8X-
cloves	T49.7X-
colors	T65.6X-
fumes	T59.89-
lubricating	T52.0X-
Niobe	T52.8X-
vitriol (liquid)	T54.2X-
fumes	T54.2X-
wintergreen (bitter)NEC	T49.3X-
Oily preparation (for skin)	T49.3X-
Ointment NEC	T49.3X-
Olanzapine	T43.59-
Oleander	T62.2X-
Oleandomycin	T36.3X-
Oleandrin	T46.0X-
Oleic acid	T46.6X-
Oleovitamin A	T45.2X-
Oleum ricini	T47.2X-
Olive oil (medicinal)NEC	T47.4X-
Olivomycin	T45.1X-
Olsalazine	T47.8X-
Omeprazole	T47.1X-
OMPA	T60.0X-
Oncovin	T45.1X-
Ondansetron	T45.0X-
Ophthaine	T41.3X-
Ophthetic	T41.3X-
Opiate NEC	T40.60-
antagonists	T50.7X-
Opioid NEC	T40.2X-
Opipramol	T43.01-
Opium alkaloids (total)	T40.0X-
Oracon	T38.4X-
Oragrafin	T50.8X-
Oral contraceptives	T38.4X-
Oral rehydration salts	T50.3X-
Orazamide	T50.99-
Orciprenaline	T48.29-
Organidin	T48.4X-
Organonitrate NEC	T46.3X-
Organophosphates	T60.0X-
Orimune	T50.B9-
Orinase	T38.3X-

Drug/Chemical	Code
Ormeloxifene	T38.6X-
Ornidazole	T37.3X-
Ornithine aspartate	T50.99-
Ornoprostil	T47.1X-
Orphenadrine (hydrochloride)	T42.8X-
Ortal (sodium)	T42.3X-
Orthoboric acid	T49.0X-
ENT agent	T49.6X-
ophthalmic preparation	T49.5X-
Orthocaine	T41.3X-
Orthodichlorobenzene	T53.7X-
Ortho-Novum	T38.4X-
Orthotolidine (reagent)	T54.2X-
Osmic acid (liquid) (fumes)	T54.2X-
Osmotic diuretics	T50.2X-
Otilonium bromide	T44.3X-
Otorhinolaryngological drug NEC	T49.6X-
Ouabain (e)	T46.0X-
Ovarian (hormone) (stimulant)	T38.5X-
Ovral	T38.4X-
Ovulen	T38.4X-
Oxacillin	T36.0X-
Oxalic acid	T54.2X-
ammonium salt	T50.99-
Oxamniquine	T37.4X-
Oxanamide	T43.59-
Oxandrolone	T38.7X-
Oxantel	T37.4X-
Oxapium iodide	T44.3X-
Oxaprotiline	T43.02-
Oxaprozin	T39.31-
Oxatomide	T45.0X-
Oxazepam	T42.4X-
Oxazimedrine	T50.5X-
Oxazolam	T42.4X-
Oxazolidine derivatives	T42.2X-
Oxazolidinedione (derivative)	T42.2X-
Oxcarbazepine	T42.1X-
Oxedrine	T44.4X-
Oxeladin (citrate)	T48.3X-
Oxendolone	T38.5X-
Oxetacaine	T41.3X-
Oxethazine	T41.3X-
Oxetorone	T39.8X-
Oxiconazole	T49.0X-
Oxidizing agent NEC	T54.9-
Oxipurinol	T50.4X-

Drug/Chemical	Code
Oxitriptan	T43.29-
Oxitropium bromide	T48.6X-
Oxodipine	T46.1X-
Oxolamine	T48.3X-
Oxolinic acid	T37.8X-
Oxomemazine	T43.3X-
Oxophenarsine	T37.3X-
Oxprenolol	T44.7X-
Oxsoralen	T49.3X-
Oxtriphylline	T48.6X-
Oxybate sodium	T41.29-
Oxybuprocaine	T41.3X-
Oxybutynin	T44.3X-
Oxychlorosene	T49.0X-
Oxycodone	T40.2X-
Oxyfedrine	T46.3X-
Oxygen	T41.5X-
Oxylone	T49.0X-
ophthalmic preparation	T49.5X-
Oxymesterone	T38.7X-
Oxymetazoline	T48.5X-
Oxymetholone	T38.7X-
Oxymorphone	T40.2X-
Oxypertine	T43.59-
Oxyphenbutazone	T39.2X-
Oxyphencyclimine	T44.3X-
Oxyphenisatine	T47.2X-
Oxyphenonium bromide	T44.3X-
Oxypolygelatin	T45.8X-
Oxyquinoline (derivatives)	T37.8X-
Oxytetracycline	T36.4X-
Oxytocic drug NEC	T48.0X-
Oxytocin (synthetic)	T48.0X-
Ozone	T59.89-
PABA	T49.3X-
Packed red cells	T45.8X-
Padimate	T49.3X-
Paint NEC	T65.6X-
cleaner	T52.9-
fumes NEC	T59.89-
lead (fumes)	T56.0X-
solvent NEC	T52.8X-
stripper	T52.8X-
Palfium	T40.2X-
Palm kernel oil	T50.99-
Paludrine	T37.2X-
PAM (pralidoxime)	T50.6X-

Drug/Chemical	Code
Pamaquine (naphthoute)	T37.2X-
Panadol	T39.1X-
Pancreatic	
digestive secretion stimulant	T47.8X-
dornase	T45.3X-
Pancreatin	T47.5X-
Pancrelipase	T47.5X-
Pancuronium (bromide)	T48.1X-
Pangamic acid	T45.2X-
Panthenol	T45.2X-
topical	T49.8X-
Pantopon	T40.0X-
Pantothenic acid	T45.2X-
Panwarfin	T45.51-
Papain (digestant)	T47.5X-
Papaveretum	T40.0X-
Papaverine	T44.3X-
Para-acetamidophenol	T39.1X-
Para-aminobenzoic acid	T49.3X-
Para-aminophenol derivatives	T39.1X-
Para-aminosalicylic acid	T37.1X-
Paracetaldehyde	T42.6X-
Paracetamol	T39.1X-
Parachlorophenol (camphorated)	T49.0X-
Paracodin	T40.2X-
Paradione	T42.2X-
Paraffin (s) (wax)	T52.0X-
liquid (medicinal)	T47.4X-
nonmedicinal	T52.0X-
Paraformaldehyde	T60.3X-
Paraldehyde	T42.6X-
Paramethadione	T42.2X-
Paramethasone	T38.0X-
acetate	T49.0X-
Paraoxon	T60.0X-
Paraquat	T60.3X-
Parasympatholytic NEC	T44.3X-
Parasympathomimetic drug NEC	T44.1X-
Parathion	T60.0X-
Parathormone	T50.99-
Parathyroid extract	T50.99-
Paratyphoid vaccine	T50.A9-
Paredrine	T44.4X-
Paregoric	T40.0X-
Pargyline	T46.5X-
Paris green (insecticide)	T57.0X-
Parnate	T43.1X-

Drug/Chemical	Code
Paromomycin	T36.5X-
Paroxypropione	T45.1X-
Parzone	T40.2X-
PAS	T37.1X-
Pasiniazid	T37.1X-
PBB (polybrominated biphenyls)	T65.89-
PCB	T65.89-
PCP	
meaning pentachlorophenol	T60.1X-
fungicide / herbicide	T60.3X-
insecticide	T60.1X-
meaning phencyclidine	T40.99-
Peach kernel oil (emulsion)	T47.4X-
Peanut oil (emulsion)NEC	T47.4X-
topical	T49.3X-
Pearly Gates (morning glory seeds)	T40.99-
Pecazine	T43.3X-
Pectin	T47.6X-
Pefloxacin	T37.8X-
Pegademase, bovine	T50.Z9-
Pelletierine tannate	T37.4X-
Pemirolast (potassium)	T48.6X-
Pemoline	T50.7X-
Pempidine	T44.2X-
Penamecillin	T36.0X-
Penbutolol	T44.7X-
Penethamate	T36.0X-
Penfluridol	T43.59-
Penflutizide	T50.2X-
Pengitoxin	T46.0X-
Penicillamine	T50.6X-
Penicillin (any)	T36.0X-
Penicillinase	T45.3X-
Penicilloyl polylysine	T50.8X-
Penimepicycline	T36.4X-
Pentachloroethane	T53.6X-
Pentachloronaphthalene	T53.7X-
Pentachlorophenol (pesticide)	T60.1X-
fungicide / herbicide	T60.3X-
insecticide	T60.1X-
Pentaerythritol	T46.3X-
chloral	T42.6X-
tetranitrate NEC	T46.3X-
Pentaerythrityl tetranitrate	T46.3X-
Pentagastrin	T50.8X-
Pentalin	T53.6X-
Pentamethonium bromide	T44.2X-

Drug/Chemical	Code
Pentamidine	T37.3X-
Pentanol	T51.3X-
Pentapyrrolinium (bitartrate)	T44.2X-
Pentaquine	T37.2X-
Pentazocine	T40.4X-
Pentetrazole	T50.7X-
Penthienate bromide	T44.3X-
Pentifylline	T46.7X-
Pentobarbital (sodium)	T42.3X-
Pentobarbitone	T42.3X-
Pentolonium tartrate	T44.2X-
Pentosan polysulfate (sodium)	T39.8X-
Pentostatin	T45.1X-
Pentothal	T41.1X-
Pentoxifylline	T46.7X-
Pentoxyverine	T48.3X-
Pentrinat	T46.3X-
Pentylenetetrazole	T50.7X-
Pentylsalicylamide	T37.1X-
Pentymal	T42.3X-
Peplomycin	T45.1X-
Peppermint (oil)	T47.5X-
Pepsin (digestant)	T47.5X-
Pepstatin	T47.1X-
Peptavlon	T50.8X-
Perazine	T43.3X-
Percaine (spinal)	T41.3X-
topical (surface)	T41.3X-
Perchloroethylene	T53.3X-
medicinal	T37.4X-
vapor	T53.3X-
Percodan	T40.2X-
Percogesic	T45.0X-
Percorten	T38.0X-
Pergolide	T42.8X-
Pergonal	T38.81-
Perhexilene	T46.3X-
Perhexiline (maleate)	T46.3X-
Periactin	T45.0X-
Periciazine	T43.3X-
Periclor	T42.6X-
Perindopril	T46.4X-
Perisoxal	T39.8X-
Peritoneal dialysis solution	T50.3X-
Peritrate	T46.3X-
Perlapine	T42.4X-
Permanganate	T65.89-

Drug/Chemical	Code
Permethrin	T60.1X-
Pernocton	T42.3X-
Pernoston	T42.3X-
Peronine	T40.2X-
Perphenazine	T43.3X-
Pertofrane	T43.01-
Pertussis	
immune serum (human)	T50.Z1-
vaccine (DTP)	T50.A1-
Peruvian balsam	T49.0X-
Peruvoside	T46.0X-
Pesticide (dust) (fumes) (vapor)NEC	T60.9-
arsenic	T57.0X-
chlorinated	T60.1X-
cyanide / kerosene	T65.0X-
mixture (of compounds)	T60.9-
naphthalene	T60.2X-
organochlorine (compounds)	T60.1X-
petroleum (distillate) (products)NEC	T60.8X-
specified ingredient NEC	T60.8X-
strychnine	T65.1X-
thallium	T60.4X-
Pethidine	T40.4X-
Petrichloral	T42.6X-
Petrol	T52.0X-
vapor	T52.0X-
Petrolatum	T49.3X-
hydrophilic	T49.3X-
liquid	T47.4X-
topical	T49.3X-
nonmedicinal	T52.0X-
red veterinary	T49.3X-
white	T49.3X-
Petroleum (products) NEC	T52.0X-
jelly	T49.3X-
pesticide	T60.8X-
solids	T52.0X-
solvents	T52.0X-
vapor	T52.0X-
Peyote	T40.99-
Phanodorm, phanodorn	T42.3X-
Phanquinone	T37.3X-
Phanquone	T37.3X-
Pharmaceutical (adjunct) (excipient) (sweetner) NEC	
Phemitone	T42.3X-
Phenacaine	T41.3X-
Phenacemide	T42.6X-

Drug/Chemical	Code
Phenacetin	T39.1X-
Phenadoxone	T40.2X-
Phenaglycodol	T43.59-
Phenantoin	T42.0X-
Phenaphthazine reagent	T50.99-
Phenazocine	T40.4X-
Phenazone	T39.2X-
Phenazopyridine	T39.8X-
Phenbenicillin	T36.0X-
Phenbutrazate	T50.5X-
Phencyclidine	T40.99-
Phendimetrazine	T50.5X-
Phenelzine	T43.1X-
Phenemal	T42.3X-
Phenergan	T42.6X-
Pheneticillin	T36.0X-
Pheneturide	T42.6X-
Phenformin	T38.3X-
Phenglutarimide	T44.3X-
Phenicarbazide	T39.8X-
Phenindamine	T45.0X-
Phenindione	T45.51-
Pheniprazine	T43.1X-
Pheniramine	T45.0X-
Phenisatin	T47.2X-
Phenmetrazine	T50.5X-
Phenobal	T42.3X-
Phenobarbital	T42.3X-
with mephenytoin	T42.3X-
with phenytoin	T42.3X-
sodium	T42.3X-
Phenobarbitone	T42.3X-
Phenobutiodil	T50.8X-
Phenoctide	T49.0X-
Phenol	T49.0X-
disinfectant	T54.0X-
in oil injection	T46.8X-
medicinal	T49.1X-
nonmedicinal NEC	T54.0X-
pesticide	T60.8X-
red	T50.8X-
Phenolic preparation	T49.1X-
Phenolphthalein	T47.2X-
Phenolsulfonphthalein	T50.8X-
Phenomorphan	T40.2X-
Phenonyl	T42.3X-
Phenoperidine	T40.4X-

Drug/Chemical	Code
Phenopyrazone	T46.99-
Phenoquin	T50.4X-
Phenothiazine (psychotropic)NEC	T43.3X-
insecticide	T60.2X-
Phenothrin	T49.0X-
Phenoxybenzamine	T46.7X-
Phenoxyethanol	T49.0X-
Phenoxymethyl penicillin	T36.0X-
Phenprobamate	T42.8X-
Phenprocoumon	T45.51-
Phensuximide	T42.2X-
Phentermine	T50.5X-
Phenthicillin	T36.0X-
Phentolamine	T46.7X-
Phenyl	
butazone	T39.2X-
enediamine	T65.3X-
hydrazine	T65.3X-
antineoplastic	T45.1X-
salicylate	T49.3X-
Phenylalanine mustard	T45.1X-
Phenylbutazone	T39.2X-
Phenylenediamine	T65.3X-
Phenylephrine	T44.4X-
Phenylethylbiguanide	T38.3X-
Phenylmercuric (acetate) (borate) (nitrate)	T49.0X-
Phenylmethylbarbitone	T42.3X-
Phenylpropanol	T47.5X-
Phenylpropanolamine	T44.99-
Phenylsulfthion	T60.0X-
Phenyltoloxamine	T45.0X-
Phenyramidol, phenyramidon	T39.8X-
Phenytoin	T42.0X-
with Phenobarbital	T42.3X-
pHisoHex	T49.2X-
Pholcodine	T48.3X-
Pholedrine	T46.99-
Phorate	T60.0X-
Phosdrin	T60.0X-
Phosfolan	T60.0X-
Phosgene (gas)	T59.89-
Phosphamidon	T60.0X-
Phosphate	T65.89-
laxative	T47.4X-
organic	T60.0X-
solvent	T52.9-
tricresyl	T65.89-

Drug/Chemical	Code
Phosphine (fumigate)	T57.1X-
Phospholine	T49.5X-
Phosphoric acid	T54.2X-
Phosphorus (compound)NEC	T57.1X-
pesticide	T60.0X-
Phthalates	T65.89-
Phthalic anhydride	T65.89-
Phthalimidoglutarimide	T42.6X-
Phthalylsulfathiazole	T37.0X-
Phylloquinone	T45.7X-
Physeptone	T40.3X-
Physostigma venenosum	T62.2X-
Physostigmine	T49.5X-
Phytolacca decandra	T62.2X-
berries	T62.1X-
Phytomenadione	T45.7X-
Phytonadione	T45.7X-
Picoperine	T48.3X-
Picosulfate (sodium)	T47.2X-
Picric (acid)	T54.2X-
Picrotoxin	T50.7X-
Piketoprofen	T49.0X-
Pilocarpine	T44.1X-
Pilocarpus (jaborandi)extract	T44.1X-
Pilsicainide (hydrochloride)	T46.2X-
Pimaricin	T36.7X-
Pimeclone	T50.7X-
Pimelic ketone	T52.8X-
Pimethixene	T45.0X-
Piminodine	T40.2X-
Pimozide	T43.59-
Pinacidil	T46.5X-
Pinaverium bromide	T44.3X-
Pinazepam	T42.4X-
Pindolol	T44.7X-
Pindone	T60.4X-
Pine oil (disinfectant)	T65.89-
Pinkroot	T37.4X-
Pipadone	T40.2X-
Pipamazine	T45.0X-
Pipamperone	T43.4X-
Pipazetate	T48.3X-
Pipemidic acid	T37.8X-
Pipenzolate bromide	T44.3X-
Piperacetazine	T43.3X-
Piperacillin	T36.0X-

Drug/Chemical	Code
Piperazine	T37.4X-
estrone sulfate	T38.5X-
Piper cubeba	T62.2X-
Piperidione	T48.3X-
Piperidolate	T44.3X-
Piperocaine (all types)	T41.3X-
Piperonyl butoxide	T60.8X-
Pipethanate	T44.3X-
Pipobroman	T45.1X-
Pipotiazine	T43.3X-
Pipoxizine	T45.0X-
Pipradrol	T43.69-
Piprinhydrinate	T45.0X-
Pirarubicin	T45.1X-
Pirazinamide	T37.1X-
Pirbuterol	T48.6X-
Pirenzepine	T47.1X-
Piretanide	T50.1X-
Piribedil	T42.8X-
Piridoxilate	T46.3X-
Piritramide	T40.4X-
Piromidic acid	T37.8X-
Piroxicam	T39.39-
beta-cyclodextrin complex	T39.8X-
Pirozadil	T46.6X-
Piscidia (bark) (erythrina)	T39.8X-
Pitch	T65.89-
Pitkin's solution	T41.3X-
Pitocin	T48.0X-
Pitressin (tannate)	T38.89-
Pituitary extracts (posterior)	T38.89-
anterior	T38.81-
Pituitrin	T38.89-
Pivampicillin	T36.0X-
Pivmecillinam	T36.0X-
Placental hormone	T38.89-
Placidyl	T42.6X-
Plague vaccine	T50.A9-
Plant	
food or fertilizer NEC	T65.89-
containing herbicide	T60.3X-
noxious, used as food	T62.2X-
berries	T62.1X-
seeds	T62.2X-
specified type NEC	T62.2X-
Plasma	T45.8X-
Plasmanate	T45.8X-

Drug/Chemical	Code
Plasminogen (tissue) activator	T45.61-
Plaster dressing	T49.3X-
Plastic dressing	T49.3X-
Plegicil	T43.3X-
Plicamycin	T45.1X-
Podophyllotoxin	T49.8X-
Podophyllum (resin)	T49.4X-
Poison NEC	T65.9-
Poisonous berries	T62.1X-
Pokeweed (any part)	T62.2X-
Poldine metilsulfate	T44.3X-
Polidexide (sulfate)	T46.6X-
Polidocanol	T46.8X-
Poliomyelitis vaccine	T50.B9-
Polish (car) (floor) (furniture) (metal) (porcelain) (silver)	T65.89-
Poloxalkol	T47.4X-
Poloxamer	T47.4X-
Polyaminostyrene resins	T50.3X-
Polycarbophil	T47.4X-
Polychlorinated biphenyl	T65.89-
Polycycline	T36.4X-
Polyester fumes	T59.89-
Polyester resin hardener	T52.9-
fumes	T59.89-
Polyestradiol phosphate	T38.5X-
Polyethanolamine alkyl sulfate	T49.2X-
Polyethylene adhesive	T49.3X-
Polyferose	T45.4X-
Polygeline	T45.8X-
Polymyxin	T36.8X-
B	T36.8X-
ENT agent	T49.6X-
ophthalmic preparation	T49.5X-
topical NEC	T49.0X-
E sulfate (eye preparation)	T49.5X-
Polynoxylin	T49.0X-
Polyoestradiol phosphate	T38.5X-
Polyoxymethyleneurea	T49.0X-
Polysilane	T47.8X-
Polytetrafluoroethylene (inhaled)	T59.89-
Polythiazide	T50.2X-
Polyvidone	T45.8X-
Polyvinylpyrrolidone	T45.8X-
Pontocaine (hydrochloride) (infiltration) (topical)	T41.3X-
Porfiromycin	T45.1X-
Posterior pituitary hormone NEC	T38.89-
Pot	T40.7X-

Drug/Chemical	Code
Potash (caustic)	T54.3X-
Potassic saline injection (lactated)	T50.3X-
Potassium (salts)NEC	T50.3X-
aminobenzoate	T45.8X-
aminosalicylate	T37.1X-
antimony ' tartrate'	T37.8X-
arsenite (solution)	T57.0X-
bichromate	T56.2X-
bisulfate	T47.3X-
bromide	T42.6X-
canrenoate	T50.0X-
carbonate	T54.3X-
chlorate NEC	T65.89-
chloride	T50.3X-
citrate	T50.99-
cyanide	T65.0X-
ferric hexacyanoferrate (medicinal)	T50.6X-
nonmedicinal	T65.89-
Fluoride	T57.8X-
glucaldrate	T47.1X-
hydroxide	T54.3X-
iodate	T49.0X-
iodide	T48.4X-
nitrate	T57.8X-
oxalate	T65.89-
perchlorate (nonmedicinal)NEC	T65.89-
antithyroid	T38.2X-
medicinal	T38.2X-
Permanganate (nonmedicinal)	T65.89-
medicinal	T49.0X-
sulfate	T47.2X-
Potassium-removing resin	T50.3X-
Potassium-retaining drug	T50.3X-
Povidone	T45.8X-
iodine	T49.0X-
Practolol	T44.7X-
Prajmalium bitartrate	T46.2X-
Pralidoxime (iodide) (chloride)	T50.6X-
Pramiverine	T44.3X-
Pramocaine	T49.1X-
Pramoxine	T49.1X-
Prasterone	T38.7X-
Pravastatin	T46.6X-
Prazepam	T42.4X-
Praziquantel	T37.4X-
Prazitone	T43.29-
Prazosin	T44.6X-

Drug/Chemical	Code
Prednicarbate	T49.0X-
Prednimustine	T45.1X-
Prednisolone	T38.0X-
ENT agent	T49.6X-
ophthalmic preparation	T49.5X-
steaglate	T49.0X-
topical NEC	T49.0X-
Prednisone	T38.0X-
Prednylidene	T38.0X-
Pregnandiol	T38.5X-
Pregneninolone	T38.5X-
Preludin	T43.69-
Premarin	T38.5X-
Premedication anesthetic	T41.20-
Prenalterol	T44.5X-
Prenoxdiazine	T48.3X-
Prenylamine	T46.3X-
Preparation H	T49.8X-
Preparation, local	T49.4X-
Preservative (nonmedicinal)	T65.89-
medicinal	T50.90-
wood	T60.9-
Prethcamide	T50.7X-
Pride of China	T62.2X-
Pridinol	T44.3X-
Prifinium bromide	T44.3X-
Prilocaine	T41.3X-
Primaquine	T37.2X-
Primidone	T42.6X-
Primula (veris)	T62.2X-
Prinadol	T40.2X-
Priscol, Priscoline	T44.6X-
Pristinamycin	T36.3X-
Privet	T62.2X-
berries	T62.1X-
Privine	T44.4X-
Pro-Banthine	T44.3X-
Probarbital	T42.3X-
Probenecid	T50.4X-
Probucol	T46.6X-
Procainamide	T46.2X-
Procaine	T41.3X-
benzylpenicillin	T36.0X-
nerve block (periphreal) (plexus)	T41.3X-
penicillin G	T36.0X-
regional / spinal	T41.3X-
Procalmidol	T43.59-

Drug/Chemical	Code
Procarbazine	T45.1X-
Procaterol	T44.5X-
Prochlorperazine	T43.3X-
Procyclidine	T44.3X-
Producer gas	T58.8X-
Profadol	T40.4X-
Profenamine	T44.3X-
Profenil	T44.3X-
Proflavine	T49.0X-
Progabide	T42.6X-
Progesterone	T38.5X-
Progestin	T38.5X-
oral contraceptive	T38.4X-
Progestogen NEC	T38.5X-
Progestone	T38.5X-
Proglumide	T47.1X-
Proguanil	T37.2X-
Prolactin	T38.81-
Prolintane	T43.69-
Proloid	T38.1X-
Proluton	T38.5X-
Promacetin	T37.1X-
Promazine	T43.3X-
Promedol	T40.2X-
Promegestone	T38.5X-
Promethazine (teoclate)	T43.3X-
Promin	T37.1X-
Pronase	T45.3X-
Pronestyl (hydrochloride)	T46.2X-
Pronetalol	T44.7X-
Prontosil	T37.0X-
Propachlor	T60.3X-
Propafenone	T46.2X-
Propallylonal	T42.3X-
Propamidine	T49.0X-
Propane (in mobile container)	T59.89-
distributed through pipes	T59.89-
incomplete combustion	T58.1-
Propanidid	T41.29-
Propanil	T60.3X-
1-Propanol	T51.3X-
2-Propanol	T51.2X-
Propantheline (bromide)	T44.3X-
Proparacaine	T41.3X-
Propatylnitrate	T46.3X-
Propicillin	T36.0X-
Propiolactone	T49.0X-

Drug/Chemical	Code
Propiomazine	T45.0X-
Propionaidehyde (medicinal)	T42.6X-
Propionate (calcium) (sodium)	T49.0X-
Propion gel	T49.0X-
Propitocaine	T41.3X-
Propofol	T41.29-
Propoxur	T60.0X-
Propoxycaine (infiltration) (spinal) (subcutaneous) (nerve block) (topical)	T41.3X-
Propoxyphene	T40.4X-
Propranolol	T44.7X-
Propyl	
alcohol	T51.3X-
carbinol	T51.3X-
hexadrine	T44.4X-
iodone	T50.8X-
thiouracil	T38.2X-
Propylaminopheno-thiazine	T43.3X-
Propylene	T59.89-
Propylhexedrine	T48.5X-
Propyliodone	T50.8X-
Propylparaben (ophthalmic)	T49.5X-
Propylthiouracil	T38.2X-
Propyphenazone	T39.2X-
Proquazone	T39.39-
Proscillaridin	T46.0X-
Prostacyclin	T45.521
Prostaglandin (I2)	T45.521
E1	T46.7X-
E2	T48.0X-
F2 alpha	T48.0X-
Prostigmin	T44.0X-
Prosultiamine	T45.2X-
Protamine sulfate	T45.7X-
zinc insulin	T38.3X-
Protease	T47.5X-
Protectant, skin NEC	T49.3X-
Protein hydrolysate	T50.99-
Prothiaden—see Dothiepin hydrochloride	
Prothionamide	T37.1X-
Prothipendyl	T43.59-
Prothoate	T60.0X-
Prothrombin	
activator	T45.7X-
synthesis inhibitor	T45.51-
Protionamide	T37.1X-
Protirelin	T38.89-

Drug/Chemical	Code
Protokylol	T48.6X-
Protopam	T50.6X-
Protoveratrine (s) (A) (B)	T46.5X-
Protriptyline	T43.01-
Provera	T38.5X-
Provitamin A	T45.2X-
Proxibarbal	T42.3X-
Proxymetacaine	T41.3X-
Proxyphylline	T48.6X-
Prozac—see Fluoxetine hydrochloride	
Prunus	
laurocerasus	T62.2X-
virginiana	T62.2X-
Prussian blue	
commercial	T65.89-
therapeutic	T50.6X-
Prussic acid	T65.0X-
vapor	T57.3X-
Pseudoephedrine	T44.99-
Psilocin	T40.99-
Psilocybin	T40.99-
Psilocybine	T40.99-
Psoralene (nonmedicinal)	T65.89-
Psoralens (medicinal)	T50.99-
PSP (phenolsulfonphthalein)	T50.8X-
Psychodysleptic drug NEC	T40.90-
Psychostimulant	T43.60-
amphetamine	T43.62-
caffeine	T43.61-
methylphenidate	T43.631
specified NEC	T43.69-
Psychotherapeutic drug NEC	T43.9-
antidepressants	T43.20-
specified NEC	T43.8X-
tranquilizers NEC	T43.50-
Psychotomimetic agents	T40.90-
Psychotropic drug NEC	T43.9-
specified NEC	T43.8X-
Psyllium hydrophilic mucilloid	T47.4X-
Pteroylglutamic acid	T45.8X-
Pteroyltriglutamate	T45.1X-
PTFE—see Polytetrafluoroethylene	
Pulp	
devitalizing paste	T49.7X-
dressing	T49.7X-
Pulsatilla	T62.2X-
Pumpkin seed extract	T37.4X-

Drug/Chemical	Code
Purex (bleach)	T54.9-
Purgative NEC—*see also Cathartic*	T47.4X-
Purine analogue (antineoplastic)	T45.1X-
Purine diuretics	T50.2X-
Purinethol	T45.1X-
PVP	T45.8X-
Pyrabital	T39.8X-
Pyramidon	T39.2X-
Pyrantel	T37.4X-
Pyrathiazine	T45.0X-
Pyrazinamide	T37.1X-
Pyrazinoic acid (amide)	T37.1X-
Pyrazole (derivatives)	T39.2X-
Pyrazolone analgesic NEC	T39.2X-
Pyrethrin, pyrethrum (nonmedicinal)	T60.2X-
Pyrethrum extract	T49.0X-
Pyribenzamine	T45.0X-
Pyridine	T52.8X-
aldoxime methiodide	T50.6X-
aldoxime methyl chloride	T50.6X-
vapor	T59.89-
Pyridium	T39.8X-
Pyridostigmine bromide	T44.0X-
Pyridoxal phosphate	T45.2X-
Pyridoxine	T45.2X-
Pyrilamine	T45.0X-
Pyrimethamine (w/ sulfadoxine)	T37.2X-
Pyrimidine antagonist	T45.1X-
Pyriminil	T60.4X-
Pyrithione zinc	T49.4X-
Pyrithyldione	T42.6X-
Pyrogallic acid	T49.0X-
Pyrogallol	T49.0X-
Pyroxylin	T49.3X-
Pyrrobutamine	T45.0X-
Pyrrolizidine alkaloids	T62.8X-
Pyrvinium chloride	T37.4X-
PZI	T38.3X-
Quaalude	T42.6X-
Quarternary ammonium	
anti-infective	T49.0X-
ganglion blocking	T44.2X-
parasympatholytic	T44.3X-
Quazepam	T42.4X-
Quicklime	T54.3X-
Quillaja extract	T48.4X-
Quinacrine	T37.2X-

Drug/Chemical	Code
Quinaglute	T46.2X-
Quinalbarbital	T42.3X-
Quinalbarbitone sodium	T42.3X-
Quinalphos	T60.0X-
Quinapril	T46.4X-
Quinestradiol	T38.5X-
Quinestradol	T38.5X-
Quinestrol	T38.5X-
Quinethazone	T50.2X-
Quingestanol	T38.4X-
Quinidine	T46.2X-
Quinine	T37.2X-
Quiniobine	T37.8X-
Quinisocaine	T49.1X-
Quinocide	T37.2X-
Quinoline (derivatives)NEC	T37.8X-
Quinupramine	T43.01-
Quotane	T41.3X-
Rabies	
immune globulin (human)	T50.Z1-
vaccine	T50.B9-
Racemoramide	T40.2X-
Racemorphan	T40.2X-
Racepinefrin	T44.5X-
Raclopride	T43.59-
Radiator alcohol	T51.1X-
Radioactive drug NEC	T50.8X-
Radio-opaque (drugs) (materials)	T50.8X-
Ramifenazone	T39.2X-
Ramipril	T46.4X-
Ranitidine	T47.0X-
Ranunculus	T62.2X-
Rat poison NEC	T60.4X-
Rattlesnake (venom)	T63.01-
Raubasine	T46.7X-
Raudixin	T46.5X-
Rautensin	T46.5X-
Rautina	T46.5X-
Rautotal	T46.5X-
Rauwiloid	T46.5X-
Rauwoldin	T46.5X-
Rauwolfia (alkaloids)	T46.5X-
Razoxane	T45.1X-
Realgar	T57.0X-
Recombinant (R)—*see specific protein*	
Red blood cells, packed	T45.8X-
Red squill (scilliroside)	T60.4X-

Drug/Chemical	Code
Reducing agent, industrial NEC	T65.89-
Refrigerant gas (CFC)	T53.5X-
not chlorofluoro-carbon	T59.89-
Regroton	T50.2X-
Rehydration salts (oral)	T50.3X-
Rela	T42.8X-
Relaxant, muscle	
anesthetic	T48.1X-
central nervous system	T42.8X-
skeletal NEC	T48.1X-
smooth NEC	T44.3X-
Remoxipride	T43.59-
Renese	T50.2X-
Renografin	T50.8X-
Replacement solution	T50.3X-
Reproterol	T48.6X-
Rescinnamine	T46.5X-
Reserpin (e)	T46.5X-
Resorcin, resorcinol (nonmedicinal)	T65.89-
medicinal	T49.4X-
Respaire	T48.4X-
Respiratory drug NEC	T48.90-
antiasthmatic NEC	T48.6X-
anti-common-cold NEC	T48.5X-
expectorant NEC	T48.4X-
stimulant	T48.90-
Retinoic acid	T49.0X-
Retinol	T45.2X-
Rh (D) immune globulin (human)	T50.Z1-
Rhodine	T39.01-
RhoGAM	T50.Z1-
Rhubarb	
dry extract	T47.2X-
tincture, compound	T47.2X-
Ribavirin	T37.5X-
Riboflavin	T45.2X-
Ribostamycin	T36.5X-
Ricin	T62.2X-
Ricinus communis	T62.2X-
Rickettsial vaccine NEC	T50.A9-
Rifabutin	T36.6X-
Rifamide	T36.6X-
Rifampicin	T36.6X-
with isoniazid	T37.1X-
Rifampin	T36.6X-
Rifamycin	T36.6X-
Rifaximin	T36.6X-

Drug/Chemical	Code
Rimantadine	T37.5X-
Rimazolium metilsulfate	T39.8X-
Rimifon	T37.1X-
Rimiterol	T48.6X-
Ringer (lactate)solution	T50.3X-
Ristocetin	T36.8X-
Ritalin	T43.631
Ritodrine	T44.5X-
Rociverine	T44.3X-
Rocky Mtn spotted fever vaccine	T50.A9-
Rodenticide NEC	T60.4X-
Rohypnol	T42.4X-
Rokitamycin	T36.3X-
Rolaids	T47.1X-
Rolitetracycline	T36.4X-
Romilar	T48.3X-
Ronifibrate	T46.6X-
Rosaprostol	T47.1X-
Rose bengal sodium (131I)	T50.8X-
Rose water ointment	T49.3X-
Rosoxacin	T37.8X-
Rotenone	T60.2X-
Rotoxamine	T45.0X-
Rough-on-rats	T60.4X-
Roxatidine	T47.0X-
Roxithromycin	T36.3X-
Rt-PA	T45.61-
Rubbing alcohol	T51.2X-
Rubefacient	T49.4X-
Rubella vaccine	T50.B9-
Rubeola vaccine	T50.B9-
Rubidium chloride Rb82	T50.8X-
Rubidomycin	T45.1X-
Rue	T62.2X-
Rufocromomycin	T45.1X-
Russel's viper venin	T45.7X-
Ruta (graveolens)	T62.2X-
Rutinum	T46.99-
Rutoside	T46.99-
Sabadilla (plant) (pesticide)	T62.2X-
Saccharated iron oxide	T45.8X-
Saccharin	T50.90-
Saccharomyces boulardii	T47.6X-
Safflower oil	T46.6X-
Safrazine	T43.1X-
Salazosulfapyridine	T37.0X-
Salbutamol	T48.6X-

Drug/Chemical	Code
Salicylamide	T39.09-
Salicylate NEC	T39.09-
methyl	T49.3X-
theobromine calcium	T50.2X-
Salicylazosulfapyridine	T37.0X-
Salicylhydroxamic acid	T49.0X-
Salicylic acid	T49.4X-
with benzoic acid	T49.4X-
congeners/derivatives/salts	T39.09-
Salinazid	T37.1X-
Salmeterol	T48.6X-
Salol	T49.3X-
Salsalate	T39.09-
Salt substitute	T50.90-
Salt-replacing drug	T50.90-
Salt-retaining mineralocorticoid	T50.0X-
Saluretic NEC	T50.2X-
Saluron	T50.2X-
Salvarsan 606 (neosilver) (silver)	T37.8X-
Sambucus canadensis	T62.2X-
berry	T62.1X-
Sandril	T46.5X-
Sanguinaria canadensis	T62.2X-
Saniflush (cleaner)	T54.2X-
Santonin	T37.4X-
Santyl	T49.8X-
Saralasin	T46.5X-
Sarcolysin	T45.1X-
Sarkomycin	T45.1X-
Saroten	T43.01-
Savin (oil)	T49.4X-
Scammony	T47.2X-
Scarlet red	T49.8X-
Scheele's green	T57.0X-
insecticide	T57.0X-
Schizontozide (blood) (tissue)	T37.2X-
Schradan	T60.0X-
Schweinfurth green	T57.0X-
insecticide	T57.0X-
Scilla, rat poison	T60.4X-
Scillaren	T60.4X-
Sclerosing agent	T46.8X-
Scombrotoxin	T61.1-
Scopolamine	T44.3X-
Scopolia extract	T44.3X-
Scouring powder	T65.89-

Drug/Chemical	Code
Sea	
anemone (sting)	T63.631
cucumber (sting)	T63.69-
snake (bite) (venom)	T63.09-
urchin spine (puncture)	T63.69-
Seafood	T61.9-
specified NEC	T61.8X-
Secbutabarbital	T42.3X-
Secbutabarbitone	T42.3X-
Secnidazole	T37.3X-
Secobarbital	T42.3X-
Seconal	T42.3X-
Secretin	T50.8X-
Sedative NEC	T42.71
mixed NEC	T42.6X-
Sedormid	T42.6X-
Seed disinfectant or dressing	T60.8X-
Seeds (poisonous)	T62.2X-
Selegiline	T42.8X-
Selenium NEC (fumes)	T56.89-
disulfide or sulfide	T49.4X-
Selenomethionine (75Se)	T50.8X-
Selsun	T49.4X-
Semustine	T45.1X-
Senega syrup	T48.4X-
Senna	T47.2X-
Sennoside A+B	T47.2X-
Septisol	T49.2X-
Seractide	T38.81-
Serax	T42.4X-
Serenesil	T42.6X-
Serenium (hydrochloride)	T37.9-
Serepax—see Oxazepam	
Sermorelin	T38.89-
Sernyl	T41.1X-
Serotonin	T50.99-
Serpasil	T46.5X-
Serrapeptase	T45.3X-
Serum	
antibotulinus	T50.Z1-
anticytotoxic	T50.Z1-
antidiphtheria	T50.Z1-
antimeningococcus	T50.Z1-
anti-Rh	T50.Z1-
anti-snake-bite	T50.Z1-
antitetanic	T50.Z1-
antitoxic	T50.Z1-

SERUM–SODIUM

Drug/Chemical	Code
Serum, continued	
complement (inhibitor)	T45.8X-
convalescent	T50.Z1-
hemolytic complement	T45.8X-
immune (human)	T50.Z1-
protective NEC	T50.Z1-
Setastine	T45.0X-
Setoperone	T43.59-
Sewer gas	T59.9-
Shampoo	T55.0X-
Shellfish, noxious, nonbacterial	T61.781
Sildenafil	T46.7X-
Silibinin	T50.99-
Silicone NEC	T65.89-
medicinal	T49.3X-
Silvadene	T49.0X-
Silver	T49.0X-
anti-infectives	T49.0X-
arsphenamine	T37.8X-
colloidal	T49.0X-
nitrate	T49.0X-
ophthalmic preparation	T49.5X-
toughened (keratolytic)	T49.4X-
nonmedicinal (dust)	T56.89-
protein	T49.5X-
salvarsan	T37.8X-
sulfadiazine	T49.4X-
Silymarin	T50.99-
Simaldrate	T47.1X-
Simazine	T60.3X-
Simethicone	T47.1X-
Simfibrate	T46.6X-
Simvastatin	T46.6X-
Sincalide	T50.8X-
Sinequan	T43.01-
Singoserp	T46.5X-
Sintrom	T45.51-
Sisomicin	T36.5X-
Sitosterols	T46.6X-
Skeletal muscle relaxants	T48.1X-
Skin	
agents (external)	T49.9-
specified NEC	T49.8X-
test antigen	T50.8X-
Sleep-eze	T45.0X-
Sleeping draught, pill	T42.71
Smallpox vaccine	T50.B1-

Drug/Chemical	Code
Smelter fumes NEC	T56.9-
Smog	T59.1X-
Smoke NEC	T59.81-
Smooth muscle relaxant	T44.3X-
Snail killer NEC	T60.8X-
Snake venom or bite	T63.00-
hemocoagulase	T45.7X-
Snuff	T65.21-
Soap (powder) (product)	T55.0X-
enema	T47.4X-
medicinal, soft	T49.2X-
superfatted	T49.2X-
Sobrerol	T48.4X-
Soda (caustic)	T54.3X-
bicarb	T47.1X-
Sodium	
acetosulfone	T37.1X-
acetrizoate	T50.8X-
acid phosphate	T50.3X-
alginate	T47.8X-
amidotrizoate	T50.8X-
aminopterin	T45.1X-
amylosulfate	T47.8X-
amytal	T42.3X-
antimony gluconate	T37.3X-
arsenate	T57.0X-
aurothiomalate	T39.4X-
aurothiosulfate	T39.4X-
barbiturate	T42.3X-
basic phosphate	T47.4X-
bicarbonate	T47.1X-
bichromate	T57.8X-
biphosphate	T50.3X-
bisulfate	T65.89-
borate	
cleanser	T57.8X-
eye	T49.5X-
therapeutic	T49.8X-
bromide	T42.6X-
cacodylate (nonmedicinal)NEC	T50.8X-
anti-infective	T37.8X-
herbicide	T60.3X-
calcium edetate	T45.8X-
carbonate NEC	T54.3X-
chlorate NEC	T65.89-
herbicide	T54.9-
chloride	T50.3X-

Drug/Chemical	Code
Sodium, continued	
with glucose	T50.3X-
chromate	T65.89-
citrate	T50.99-
cromoglicate	T48.6X-
cyanide	T65.0X-
cyclamate	T50.3X-
dehydrocholate	T45.8X-
diatrizoate	T50.8X-
dibunate	T48.4X-
dioctyl sulfosuccinate	T47.4X-
dipantoyl ferrate	T45.8X-
edetate	T45.8X-
ethacrynate	T50.1X-
feredetate	T45.8X-
Fluoride—*see Fluoride*	
fluoroacetate (dust) (pesticide)	T60.4X-
free salt	T50.3X-
fusidate	T36.8X-
glucaldrate	T47.1X-
glucosulfone	T37.1X-
glutamate	T45.8X-
hydrogen carbonate	T50.3X-
hydroxide	T54.3X-
hypochlorite (bleach)NEC	T54.3X-
disinfectant	T54.3X-
medicinal (anti-infective) (external)	T49.0X-
vapor	T54.3X-
hyposulfite	T49.0X-
indigotin disulfonate	T50.8X-
iodide	T50.99-
I-131	T50.8X-
therapeutic	T38.2X-
iodohippurate (131I)	T50.8X-
iopodate	T50.8X-
iothalamate	T50.8X-
iron edetate	T45.4X-
lactate (compound solution)	T45.8X-
lauryl (sulfate)	T49.2X-
L-triiodothyronine	T38.1X-
magnesium citrate	T50.99-
mersalate	T50.2X-
metasilicate	T65.89-
metrizoate	T50.8X-
monofluoroacetate (pesticide)	T60.1X-
morrhuate	T46.8X-
nafcillin	T36.0X-

Drug/Chemical	Code
Sodium, continued	
nitrate (oxidizing agent)	T65.89-
nitrite	T50.6X-
nitroferricyanide	T46.5X-
nitroprusside	T46.5X-
oxalate	T65.89-
oxide/peroxide	T65.89-
oxybate	T41.29-
para-aminohippurate	T50.8X-
perborate (nonmedicinal)NEC	T65.89-
medicinal	T49.0X-
soap	T55.0X-
percarbonate—*see Sodium, perborate*	
pertechnetate Tc99m	T50.8X-
phosphate	
cellulose	T45.8X-
dibasic	T47.2X-
monobasic	T47.2X-
phytate	T50.6X-
picosulfate	T47.2X-
polyhydroxyaluminium monocarbonate	T47.1X-
polystyrene sulfonate	T50.3X-
propionate	T49.0X-
propyl hydroxybenzoate	T50.99-
psylliate	T46.8X-
removing resins	T50.3X-
salicylate	T39.09-
salt NEC	T50.3X-
selenate	T60.2X-
stibogluconate	T37.3X-
sulfate	T47.4X-
sulfoxone	T37.1X-
tetradecyl sulfate	T46.8X-
thiopental	T41.1X-
thiosalicylate	T39.09-
thiosulfate	T50.6X-
tolbutamide	T38.3X-
(L)-triiodothyronine	T38.1X-
tyropanoate	T50.8X-
valproate	T42.6X-
versenate	T50.6X-
Sodium-free salt	T50.90-
Sodium-removing resin	T50.3X-
Soft soap	T55.0X-
Solanine	T62.2X-
berries	T62.1X-

Drug/Chemical	Code
Solanum dulcamara	T62.2X-
berries	T62.1X-
Solapsone	T37.1X-
Solar lotion	T49.3X-
Solasulfone	T37.1X-
Soldering fluid	T65.89-
Solid substance	T65.9-
specified NEC	T65.89-
Solvent, industrial NEC	T52.9-
naphtha	T52.0X-
petroleum	T52.0X-
specified NEC	T52.8X-
Soma	T42.8X-
Somatorelin	T38.89-
Somatostatin	T38.99-
Somatotropin	T38.81-
Somatrem	T38.81-
Somatropin	T38.81-
Sominex	T45.0X-
Somnos	T42.6X-
Somonal	T42.3X-
Soneryl	T42.3X-
Soothing syrup	T50.90-
Sopor	T42.6X-
Soporific	T42.71
Soporific drug	T42.71
specified type NEC	T42.6X-
Sorbide nitrate	T46.3X-
Sorbitol	T47.4X-
Sotalol	T44.7X-
Sotradecol	T46.8X-
Soysterol	T46.6X-
Spacoline	T44.3X-
Spanish fly	T49.8X-
Sparine	T43.3X-
Sparteine	T48.0X-
Spasmolytic	
anticholinergics	T44.3X-
autonomic	T44.3X-
bronchial NEC	T48.6X-
quaternary ammonium	T44.3X-
skeletal muscle NEC	T48.1X-
Spectinomycin	T36.5X-
Speed	T43.62-
Spermicide	T49.8X-
Spider (bite) (venom)	T63.39-
antivenin	T50.Z1-

Drug/Chemical	Code
Spigelia (root)	T37.4X-
Spindle inactivator	T50.4X-
Spiperone	T43.4X-
Spiramycin	T36.3X-
Spirapril	T46.4X-
Spirilene	T43.59-
Spirit (s) (neutral)NEC	T51.0X-
beverage / industrial/ mineral/surgical	T51.0X-
Spironolactone	T50.0X-
Spiroperidol	T43.4X-
Sponge, absorbable (gelatin)	T45.7X-
Sporostacin	T49.0X-
Spray (aerosol)	T65.9-
cosmetic	T65.89-
medicinal NEC	T50.90-
Spurge flax	T62.2X-
Spurges	T62.2X-
Sputum viscosity-lowering drug	T48.4X-
Squill	T46.0X-
rat poison	T60.4X-
Squirting cucumber (cathartic)	T47.2X-
Stains	T65.6X-
Stannous fluoride	T49.7X-
Stanolone	T38.7X-
Stanozolol	T38.7X-
Staphisagria or stavesacre (pediculicide)	T49.0X-
Starch	T50.90-
Stelazine	T43.3X-
Stemetil	T43.3X-
Stepronin	T48.4X-
Sterculia	T47.4X-
Sternutator gas	T59.89-
Steroid	T38.0X-
anabolic	T38.7X-
androgenic	T38.7X-
antineoplastic, hormone	T38.7X-
estrogen	T38.5X-
ENT agent	T49.6X-
ophthalmic preparation	T49.5X-
topical NEC	T49.0X-
Stibine	T56.89-
Stibogluconate	T37.3X-
Stibophen	T37.4X-
Stilbamidine (isetionate)	T37.3X-
Stilbestrol	T38.5X-
Stilboestrol	T38.5X-

SOLANUM DULCAMARA–STILBOESTROL

Drug/Chemical	Code
Stimulant	
central nervous system	T43.60-
analeptics / opiate antagonist	T50.7X-
psychotherapeutic NEC	T43.60-
specified NEC	T43.69-
respiratory	T48.90-
Stone-dissolving drug	T50.90-
Storage battery (cells) (acid)	T54.2X-
Stovaine (infiltration) (topical) (subcutaneous) (nerve block) (spinal)	T41.3X-
Stovarsal	T37.8X-
Stoxil	T49.5X-
Stramonium	T48.6X-
natural state	T62.2X-
Streptodornase	T45.3X-
Streptoduocin	T36.5X-
Streptokinase	T45.61-
Streptomycin (derivative)	T36.5X-
Streptonivicin	T36.5X-
Streptovarycin	T36.5X-
Streptozocin	T45.1X-
Streptozotocin	T45.1X-
Stripper (paint) (solvent)	T52.8X-
Strobane	T60.1X-
Strofantina	T46.0X-
Strophanthin (g) (k)	T46.0X-
Strophanthus	T46.0X-
Strophantin	T46.0X-
Strophantin-g	T46.0X-
Strychnine (nonmedicinal) (pesticide) (salts)	T65.1X-
medicinal	T48.29-
Styramate	T42.8X-
Styrene	T65.89-
Succinimide, antiepileptic or anticonvulsant	T42.2X-
Succinylcholine	T48.1X-
Succinylsulfathiazole	T37.0X-
Sucralfate	T47.1X-
Sucrose	T50.3X-
Sufentanil	T40.4X-
Sulbactam	T36.0X-
Sulbenicillin	T36.0X-
Sulbentine	T49.0X-
Sulfacetamide	T49.0X-
ophthalmic preparation	T49.5X-
Sulfachlorpyridazine	T37.0X-
Sulfacitine	T37.0X-
Sulfadiasulfone sodium	T37.0X-

Drug/Chemical	Code
Sulfadiazine	T37.0X-
silver (topical)	T49.0X-
Sulfadimethoxine	T37.0X-
Sulfadimidine	T37.0X-
Sulfadoxine	T37.0X-
with pyrimethamine	T37.2X-
Sulfaethidole	T37.0X-
Sulfafurazole	T37.0X-
Sulfaguanidine	T37.0X-
Sulfalene	T37.0X-
Sulfaloxate	T37.0X-
Sulfaloxic acid	T37.0X-
Sulfamazone	T39.2X-
Sulfamerazine	T37.0X-
Sulfameter	T37.0X-
Sulfamethazine	T37.0X-
Sulfamethizole	T37.0X-
Sulfamethoxazole	T37.0X-
with trimethoprim	T36.8X-
Sulfamethoxydiazine	T37.0X-
Sulfamethoxypyridazine	T37.0X-
Sulfamethylthiazole	T37.0X-
Sulfametoxydiazine	T37.0X-
Sulfamidopyrine	T39.2X-
Sulfamonomethoxine	T37.0X-
Sulfamoxole	T37.0X-
Sulfamylon	T49.0X-
Sulfan blue (diagnostic dye)	T50.8X-
Sulfanilamide	T37.0X-
Sulfanilylguanidine	T37.0X-
Sulfaperin	T37.0X-
Sulfaphenazole	T37.0X-
Sulfaphenylthiazole	T37.0X-
Sulfaproxyline	T37.0X-
Sulfapyridine	T37.0X-
Sulfapyrimidine	T37.0X-
Sulfarsphenamine	T37.8X-
Sulfasalazine	T37.0X-
Sulfasuxidine	T37.0X-
Sulfasymazine	T37.0X-
Sulfated amylopectin	T47.8X-
Sulfathiazole	T37.0X-
Sulfatostearate	T49.2X-
Sulfinpyrazone	T50.4X-
Sulfiram	T49.0X-
Sulfisomidine	T37.0X-

STIMULANT–SULFISOMIDINE

SULFISOXAZOLE–TANNIC ACID (TANNIN)

Drug/Chemical	Code
Sulfisoxazole	T37.0X-
ophthalmic preparation	T49.5X-
Sulfobromophthalein (sodium)	T50.8X-
Sulfobromphthalein	T50.8X-
Sulfogaiacol	T48.4X-
Sulfomyxin	T36.8X-
Sulfonal	T42.6X-
Sulfonamide NEC	T37.0X-
eye	T49.5X-
Sulfonazide	T37.1X-
Sulfones	T37.1X-
Sulfonethylmethane	T42.6X-
Sulfonmethane	T42.6X-
Sulfonphthal, sulfonphthol	T50.8X-
Sulfonylurea derivatives, oral	T38.3X-
Sulforidazine	T43.3X-
Sulfoxone	T37.1X-
Sulfur, sulfurated, sulfuric, (compounds NEC) (medicinal)	T49.4X-
acid	T54.2X-
dioxide (gas)	T59.1X-
hydrogen	T59.6X-
ointment	T49.0X-
pesticide (vapor)	T60.9-
vapor NEC	T59.89-
Sulfuric acid	T54.2X-
Sulglicotide	T47.1X-
Sulindac	T39.39-
Sulisatin	T47.2X-
Sulisobenzone	T49.3X-
Sulkowitch's reagent	T50.8X-
Sulmetozine	T44.3X-
Suloctidil	T46.7X-
Sulphadiazine	T37.0X-
Sulphadimethoxine	T37.0X-
Sulphadimidine	T37.0X-
Sulphadione	T37.1X-
Sulphafurazole	T37.0X-
Sulphamethizole	T37.0X-
Sulphamethoxazole	T37.0X-
Sulphan blue	T50.8X-
Sulphaphenazole	T37.0X-
Sulphapyridine	T37.0X-
Sulphasalazine	T37.0X-
Sulphinpyrazone	T50.4X-
Sulpiride	T43.59-
Sulprostone	T48.0X-
Sulpyrine	T39.2X-

Drug/Chemical	Code
Sultamicillin	T36.0X-
Sulthiame	T42.6X-
Sultiame	T42.6X-
Sultopride	T43.59-
Sumatriptan	T39.8X-
Sunflower seed oil	T46.6X-
Superinone	T48.4X-
Suprofen	T39.31-
Suramin (sodium)	T37.4X-
Surfacaine	T41.3X-
Surital	T41.1X-
Sutilains	T45.3X-
Suxamethonium (chloride)	T48.1X-
Suxethonium (chloride)	T48.1X-
Suxibuzone	T39.2X-
Sweet niter spirit	T46.3X-
Sweet oil (birch)	T49.3X-
Sweetener	T50.90-
Sym-dichloroethyl ether	T53.6X-
Sympatholytic NEC	T44.8X-
haloalkylamine	T44.8X-
Sympathomimetic NEC	T44.90-
anti-common-cold	T48.5X-
bronchodilator	T48.6X-
specified NEC	T44.99-
Synagis	T50.B9-
Synalar	T49.0X-
Synthroid	T38.1X-
Syntocinon	T48.0X-
Syrosingopine	T46.5X-
Systemic drug	T45.9-
specified NEC	T45.8X-
2,4,5-T	T60.3X-
Tablets—see also specified substance	T50.90-
Tace	T38.5X-
Tacrine	T44.0X-
Tadalafil	T46.7X-
Talampicillin	T36.0X-
Talbutal	T42.3X-
Talc powder	T49.3X-
Talcum	T49.3X-
Taleranol	T38.6X-
Tamoxifen	T38.6X-
Tamsulosin	T44.6X-
Tandearil, tanderil	T39.2X-
Tannic acid (Tannin)	T49.2X-
medicinal (astringent)	T49.2X-

Drug/Chemical	Code
Tansy	T62.2X-
TAO	T36.3X-
Tapazole	T38.2X-
Tar NEC	T52.0X-
camphor	T60.1X-
distillate	T49.1X-
fumes	T59.89-
medicinal (ointment)	T49.1X-
Taractan	T43.59-
Tarantula (venomous)	T63.321
Tartar emetic	T37.8X-
Tartaric acid	T65.89-
Tartrate, laxative	T47.4X-
Tartrated antimony (anti-infective)	T37.8X-
Tauromustine	T45.1X-
TCA—see Trichloroacetic acid	
TCDD	T53.7X-
TDI (vapor)	T65.0X-
Teclothiazide	T50.2X-
Teclozan	T37.3X-
Tegafur	T45.1X-
Tegretol	T42.1X-
Teicoplanin	T36.8X-
Telepaque	T50.8X-
Tellurium	T56.89-
TEM	T45.1X-
Temazepam	T42.4X-
Temocillin	T36.0X-
Tenamfetamine	T43.62-
Teniposide	T45.1X-
Tenitramine	T46.3X-
Tenoglicin	T48.4X-
Tenonitrozole	T37.3X-
Tenoxicam	T39.39-
TEPA	T45.1X-
TEPP	T60.0X-
Teprotide	T46.5X-
Terazosin	T44.6X-
Terbufos	T60.0X-
Terbutaline	T48.6X-
Terconazole	T49.0X-
Terfenadine	T45.0X-
Teriparatide (acetate)	T50.99-
Terizidone	T37.1X-
Terlipressin	T38.89-
Terodiline	T46.3X-
Teroxalene	T37.4X-

Drug/Chemical	Code
Terpin (cis)hydrate	T48.4X-
Terramycin	T36.4X-
Tertatolol	T44.7X-
Tessalon	T48.3X-
Testolactone	T38.7X-
Testosterone	T38.7X-
Tetanus toxoid or vaccine	T50.A9-
antitoxin	T50.Z1-
immune globulin (human)	T50.Z1-
toxoid	T50.A9-
with diphtheria toxoid	T50.A2-
with pertussis	T50.A1-
Tetrabenazine	T43.59-
Tetracaine	T41.3X-
Tetrachlorethylene—see Tetrachloroethylene	
Tetrachlormethiazide	T50.2X-
2,3,7,8-Tetrachlorodibenzo-p-dioxin	T53.7X-
Tetrachloroethane	T53.6X-
vapor	T53.6X-
paint or varnish	T53.6X-
Tetrachloroethylene (liquid)	T53.3X-
medicinal	T37.4X-
vapor	T53.3X-
Tetracosactide	T38.81-
Tetracosactrin	T38.81-
Tetracycline	T36.4X-
ophthalmic preparation	T49.5X-
topical NEC	T49.0X-
Tetradifon	T60.8X-
Tetradotoxin	T61.771
Tetraethyl	
lead	T56.0X-
pyrophosphate	T60.0X-
Tetraethylammonium chloride	T44.2X-
Tetraethylthiuram disulfide	T50.6X-
Tetrahydroaminoacridine	T44.0X-
Tetrahydrocannabinol	T40.7X-
Tetrahydrofuran	T52.8X-
Tetrahydronaphthalene	T52.8X-
Tetrahydrozoline	T49.5X-
Tetralin	T52.8X-
Tetramethrin	T60.2X-
Tetramethylthiuram (disulfide)NEC	T60.3X-
medicinal	T49.0X-
Tetramisole	T37.4X-
Tetranicotinoyl fructose	T46.7X-
Tetrazepam	T42.4X-

Drug/Chemical	Code
Tetronal	T42.6X-
Tetryl	T65.3X-
Tetrylammonium chloride	T44.2X-
Tetryzoline	T49.5X-
Thalidomide	T45.1X-
Thallium (compounds) (dust)NEC	T56.81-
pesticide	T60.4X-
THC	T40.7X-
Thebacon	T48.3X-
Thebaine	T40.2X-
Thenoic acid	T49.6X-
Thenyldiamine	T45.0X-
Theobromine (calcium salicylate)	T48.6X-
sodium salicylate	T48.6X-
Theophyllamine	T48.6X-
Theophylline	T48.6X-
Thiabendazole	T37.4X-
Thialbarbital	T41.1X-
Thiamazole	T38.2X-
Thiambutosine	T37.1X-
Thiamine	T45.2X-
Thiamphenicol	T36.2X-
Thiamylal (sodium)	T41.1X-
Thiazesim	T43.29-
Thiazides (diuretics)	T50.2X-
Thiazinamium metilsulfate	T43.3X-
Thiethylperazine	T43.3X-
Thimerosal	T49.0X-
ophthalmic preparation	T49.5X-
Thioacetazone	T37.1X-
Thiobarbital sodium	T41.1X-
Thiobarbiturate anesthetic	T41.1X-
Thiobismol	T37.8X-
Thiobutabarbital sodium	T41.1X-
Thiocarbamate (insecticide)	T60.0X-
Thiocarbamide	T38.2X-
Thiocarbarsone	T37.8X-
Thiocarlide	T37.1X-
Thioctamide	T50.99-
Thioctic acid	T50.99-
Thiofos	T60.0X-
Thioglycolate	T49.4X-
Thioglycolic acid	T65.89-
Thioguanine	T45.1X-
Thiomercaptomerin	T50.2X-
Thiomerin	T50.2X-
Thiomersal	T49.0X-

Drug/Chemical	Code
Thionazin	T60.0X-
Thiopental (sodium)	T41.1X-
Thiopentone (sodium)	T41.1X-
Thiopropazate	T43.3X-
Thioproperazine	T43.3X-
Thioridazine	T43.3X-
Thiosinamine	T49.3X-
Thiotepa	T45.1X-
Thiothixene	T43.4X-
Thiouracil (benzyl) (methyl) (propyl)	T38.2X-
Thiourea	T38.2X-
Thiphenamil	T44.3X-
Thiram	T60.3X-
medicinal	T49.2X-
Thonzylamine (systemic)	T45.0X-
mucosal decongestant	T48.5X-
Thorazine	T43.3X-
Thorium dioxide suspension	T50.8X-
Thornapple	T62.2X-
Throat drug NEC	T49.6X-
Thrombin	T45.7X-
Thrombolysin	T45.61-
Thromboplastin	T45.7X-
Thurfyl nicotinate	T46.7X-
Thymol	T49.0X-
Thymopentin	T37.5X-
Thymoxamine	T46.7X-
Thymus extract	T38.89-
Thyreotrophic hormone	T38.81-
Thyroglobulin	T38.1X-
Thyroid (hormone)	T38.1X-
Thyrolar	T38.1X-
Thyrotrophin	T38.81-
Thyrotropic hormone	T38.81-
Thyroxine	T38.1X-
Tiabendazole	T37.4X-
Tiamizide	T50.2X-
Tianeptine	T43.29-
Tiapamil	T46.1X-
Tiapride	T43.59-
Tiaprofenic acid	T39.31-
Tiaramide	T39.8X-
Ticarcillin	T36.0X-
Ticlatone	T49.0X-
Ticlopidine	T45.521
Ticrynafen	T50.1X-
Tidiacic	T50.99-

TETRONAL–TIDIACIC

Drug/Chemical	Code
Tiemonium	T44.3X-
iodide	T44.3X-
Tienilic acid	T50.1X-
Tifenamil	T44.3X-
Tigan	T45.0X-
Tigloidine	T44.3X-
Tilactase	T47.5X-
Tiletamine	T41.29-
Tilidine	T40.4X-
Timepidium bromide	T44.3X-
Timiperone	T43.4X-
Timolol	T44.7X-
Tin (chloride) (dust) (oxide) NEC	T56.6X-
anti-infectives	T37.8X-
Tindal	T43.3X-
Tinidazole	T37.3X-
Tinoridine	T39.8X-
Tiocarlide	T37.1X-
Tioclomarol	T45.51-
Tioconazole	T49.0X-
Tioguanine	T45.1X-
Tiopronin	T50.99-
Tiotixene	T43.4X-
Tioxolone	T49.4X-
Tipepidine	T48.3X-
Tiquizium bromide	T44.3X-
Tiratricol	T38.1X-
Tisopurine	T50.4X-
Titanium (compounds) (vapor)	T56.89-
dioxide/ointment/oxide	T49.3X-
tetrachloride	T56.89-
Titanocene	T56.89-
Titroid	T38.1X-
Tizanidine	T42.8X-
TMTD	T60.3X-
TNT (fumes)	T65.3X-
Toadstool	T62.0X-
Tobacco NEC	T65.29-
cigarettes	T65.22-
Indian	T62.2X-
smoke, second-hand	T65.22-
Tobramycin	T36.5X-
Tocainide	T46.2X-
Tocoferol	T45.2X-
Tocopherol (acetate)	T45.2X-
Tocosamine	T48.0X-
Todralazine	T46.5X-

Drug/Chemical	Code
Tofisopam	T42.4X-
Tofranil	T43.01-
Toilet deodorizer	T65.89-
Tolamolol	T44.7X-
Tolazamide	T38.3X-
Tolazoline	T46.7X-
Tolbutamide (sodium)	T38.3X-
Tolciclate	T49.0X-
Tolmetin	T39.39-
Tolnaftate	T49.0X-
Tolonidine	T46.5X-
Toloxatone	T42.6X-
Tolperisone	T44.3X-
Tolserol	T42.8X-
Toluene (liquid)	T52.2X-
diisocyanate	T65.0X-
Toluidine (vapor)	T65.89-
Toluol (liquid)	T52.2X-
vapor	T52.2X-
Toluylenediamine	T65.3X-
Tolylene-2,4-diisocyanate	T65.0X-
Tonic NEC	T50.90-
Topical action drug NEC	T49.9-
ear, nose or throat	T49.6X-
eye	T49.5X-
skin	T49.9-
specified NEC	T49.8X-
Toquizine	T44.3X-
Toremifene	T38.6X-
Tosylchloramide sodium	T49.8X-
Toxaphene (dust) (spray)	T60.1X-
Toxin, diphtheria (Schick Test)	T50.8X-
Tractor fuel NEC	T52.0X-
Tragacanth	T50.99-
Tramadol	T40.4X-
Tramazoline	T48.5X-
Tranexamic acid	T45.62-
Tranilast	T45.0X-
Tranquilizer NEC	T43.50-
with hypnotic or sedative	T42.6X-
benzodiazepine NEC	T42.4X-
butyrophenone NEC	T43.4X-
carbamate	T43.59-
dimethylamine / ethylamine	T43.3X-
hydroxyzine	T43.59-
major NEC	T43.50-
penothiazine NEC / piperazine NEC	T43.3X-

Drug/Chemical	Code
Tranquilizer NEC, continued	
piperidine / propylamine	T43.3X-
specified NEC	T43.59-
thioxanthene NEC	T43.59-
Tranxene	T42.4X-
Tranylcypromine	T43.1X-
Trapidil	T46.3X-
Trasentine	T44.3X-
Travert	T50.3X-
Trazodone	T43.21-
Trecator	T37.1X-
Treosulfan	T45.1X-
Tretamine	T45.1X-
Tretinoin	T49.0X-
Tretoquinol	T48.6X-
Triacetin	T49.0X-
Triacetoxyanthracene	T49.4X-
Triacetyloleandomycin	T36.3X-
Triamcinolone	T49.0X-
ENT agent	T49.6X-
hexacetonide	T49.0X-
ophthalmic preparation	T49.5X-
topical NEC	T49.0X-
Triampyzine	T44.3X-
Triamterene	T50.2X-
Triazine (herbicide)	T60.3X-
Triaziquone	T45.1X-
Triazolam	T42.4X-
Triazole (herbicide)	T60.3X-
Tribenoside	T46.99-
Tribromacetaldehyde	T42.6X-
Tribromoethanol, rectal	T41.29-
Tribromomethane	T42.6X-
Trichlorethane	T53.2X-
Trichlorethylene	T53.2X-
Trichlorfon	T60.0X-
Trichlormethiazide	T50.2X-
Trichlormethine	T45.1X-
Trichloroacetic acid, Trichloracetic acid	T54.2X-
medicinal	T49.4X-
Trichloroethane	T53.2X-
Trichloroethanol	T42.6X-
Trichloroethyl phosphate	T42.6X-
Trichloroethylene (liquid) (vapor)	T53.2X-
anesthetic (gas)	T41.0X-
Trichlorofluoromethane NEC	T53.5X-
Trichloronate	T60.0X-

Drug/Chemical	Code
2,4,5-Trichlorophen-oxyacetic acid	T60.3X-
Trichloropropane	T53.6X-
Trichlorotriethylamine	T45.1X-
Trichomonacides NEC	T37.3X-
Trichomycin	T36.7X-
Triclobisonium chloride	T49.0X-
Triclocarban	T49.0X-
Triclofos	T42.6X-
Triclosan	T49.0X-
Tricresyl phosphate	T65.89-
solvent	T52.9-
Tricyclamol chloride	T44.3X-
Tridesilon	T49.0X-
Tridihexethyl iodide	T44.3X-
Tridione	T42.2X-
Trientine	T45.8X-
Triethanolamine NEC	T54.3X-
Triethanomelamine	T45.1X-
Triethylenemelamine	T45.1X-
Triethylenephosphoramide	T45.1X-
Triethylenethiophosphoramide	T45.1X-
Trifluoperazine	T43.3X-
Trifluoroethyl vinyl ether	T41.0X-
Trifluperidol	T43.4X-
Triflupromazine	T43.3X-
Trifluridine	T37.5X-
Triflusal	T45.521
Trihexyphenidyl	T44.3X-
Triiodothyronine	T38.1X-
Trilene	T41.0X-
Trilostane	T38.99-
Trimebutine	T44.3X-
Trimecaine	T41.3X-
Trimeprazine (tartrate)	T44.3X-
Trimetaphan camsilate	T44.2X-
Trimetazidine	T46.7X-
Trimethadione	T42.2X-
Trimethaphan	T44.2X-
Trimethidinium	T44.2X-
Trimethobenzamide	T45.0X-
Trimethoprim (w/ sulfamethoxazole)	T37.8X-
Trimethylcarbinol	T51.3X-
Trimethylpsoralen	T49.3X-
Trimeton	T45.0X-
Trimetrexate	T45.1X-
Trimipramine	T43.01-
Trimustine	T45.1X-

Drug/Chemical	Code	Drug/Chemical	Code
Trinitrine	T46.3X-	Tybamate	T43.59-
Trinitrobenzol	T65.3X-	Tyloxapol	T48.4X-
Trinitrophenol	T65.3X-	Tymazoline	T48.5X-
Trinitrotoluene (fumes)	T65.3X-	Tyropanoate	T50.8X-
Trional	T42.6X-	Tyrothricin	T49.6X-
Triorthocresyl phosphate	T65.89-	ENT agent	T49.6X-
Trioxide of arsenic	T57.0X-	ophthalmic preparation	T49.5X-
Trioxysalen	T49.4X-	Ufenamate	T39.39-
Tripamide	T50.2X-	Ultraviolet light protectant	T49.3X-
Triparanol	T46.6X-	Undecenoic acid	T49.0X-
Tripelennamine	T45.0X-	Undecoylium	T49.0X-
Triperiden	T44.3X-	Undecylenic acid (derivatives)	T49.0X-
Triperidol	T43.4X-	Unna's boot	T49.3X-
Triphenylphosphate	T65.89-	Unsaturated fatty acid	T46.6X-
Triple bromides	T42.6X-	Uracil mustard	T45.1X-
Triple carbonate	T47.1X-	Uramustine	T45.1X-
Triprolidine	T45.0X-	Urapidil	T46.5X-
Trisodium hydrogen edetate	T50.6X-	Urari	T48.1X-
Trisoralen	T49.3X-	Urate oxidase	T50.4X-
Trisulfapyrimidines	T37.0X-	Urea	T47.3X-
Trithiozine	T44.3X-	peroxide	T49.0X-
Tritiozine	T44.3X-	stibamine	T37.4X-
Tritoqualine	T45.0X-	topical	T49.8X-
Trofosfamide	T45.1X-	Urethane	T45.1X-
Troleandomycin	T36.3X-	Uric acid metabolism drug NEC	T50.4X-
Trolnitrate (phosphate)	T46.3X-	Uricosuric agent	T50.4X-
Tromantadine	T37.5X-	Urinary anti-infective	T37.8X-
Trometamol	T50.2X-	Urofollitropin	T38.81-
Tromethamine	T50.2X-	Urokinase	T45.61-
Tronothane	T41.3X-	Urokon	T50.8X-
Tropacine	T44.3X-	Ursodeoxycholic acid	T50.99-
Tropatepine	T44.3X-	Ursodiol	T50.99-
Tropicamide	T44.3X-	Urtica	T62.2X-
Trospium chloride	T44.3X-	Vaccine NEC	T50.Z9-
Troxerutin	T46.99-	antineoplastic	T50.Z9-
Troxidone	T42.2X-	bacterial NEC	T50.A9-
Tryparsamide	T37.3X-	with	
Trypsin	T45.3X-	other bacterial component	T50.A2-
Tryptizol	T43.01-	pertussis component	T50.A1-
TSH	T38.81-	viral-rickettsial component	T50.A2-
Tuaminoheptane	T48.5X-	mixed NEC	T50.A2-
Tuberculin, (PPD)	T50.8X-	BCG	T50.A9-
Tubocurare	T48.1X-	cholera	T50.A9-
Tubocurarine (chloride)	T48.1X-	diphtheria	T50.A9-
Tulobuterol	T48.6X-	with tetanus	T50.A2-
Turpentine (spirits of)	T52.8X-	and pertussis	T50.A1-
vapor	T52.8X-	influenza	T50.B9-

VACCINE NE–VENOM, VENOMOUS (BITE) (STING)

Drug/Chemical	Code
Vaccine NEC, continued	
measles, mumps and rubella	T50.B9-
meningococcal	T50.A9-
paratyphoid	T50.A9-
pertussis with diphtheria and tetanus	T50.A1-
with other component	T50.A1-
plague	T50.A9-
poliomyelitis	T50.B9-
rabies	T50.B9-
respiratory syncytial virus	T50.B9-
rickettsial NEC	T50.A9-
with	
bacterial component	T50.A2-
Rocky Mountain spotted fever	T50.A9-
rubella	T50.B9-
sabin oral	T50.B9-
smallpox	T50.B1-
TAB	T50.A9-
tetanus	T50.A9-
typhoid	T50.A9-
typhus	T50.A9-
viral NEC	T50.B9-
yellow fever	T50.B9-
Vaccinia immune globulin	T50.Z1-
Vaginal contraceptives	T49.8X-
Valerian (root) (tincture)	T42.6X-
tincture	T42.6X-
Valethamate bromide	T44.3X-
Valisone	T49.0X-
Valium	T42.4X-
Valmid	T42.6X-
Valnoctamide	T42.6X-
Valproate (sodium)	T42.6X-
Valproic acid	T42.6X-
Valpromide	T42.6X-
Vanadium	T56.89-
Vancomycin	T36.8X-
Vapor—see also Gas	T59.9-
kiln (carbon monoxide)	T58.8X-
specified source NEC	T59.89-
Vardenafil	T46.7X-
Varicose reduction drug	T46.8X-
Varnish	T65.4X-
cleaner	T52.9-
Vaseline	T49.3X-
Vasodilan	T46.7X-

Drug/Chemical	Code
Vasodilator	
coronary NEC	T46.3X-
peripheral NEC	T46.7X-
Vasopressin	T38.89-
Vasopressor drugs	T38.89-
Vecuronium bromide	T48.1X-
Vegetable extract, astringent	T49.2X-
Venlafaxine	T43.21-
Venom, venomous (bite) (sting)	T63.9-
amphibian NEC	T63.831
animal NEC	T63.89-
ant	T63.421
arthropod NEC	T63.481
bee	T63.441
centipede	T63.41-
fish	T63.59-
frog	T63.81-
hornet	T63.451
insect NEC	T63.481
lizard	T63.121
marine	
animals	T63.69-
bluebottle	T63.61-
jellyfish NEC	T63.62-
Portugese Man-o-war	T63.61-
sea anemone	T63.631
specified NEC	T63.69-
fish	T63.59-
plants	T63.71-
sting ray	T63.51-
millipede (tropical)	T63.41-
plant NEC	T63.79-
marine	T63.71-
reptile	T63.19-
gila monster	T63.11-
lizard NEC	T63.12-
scorpion	T63.2X-
snake	T63.00-
African NEC	T63.081
American (North) (South)NEC	T63.06-
Asian	T63.08-
Australian	T63.07-
cobra	T63.041
coral snake	T63.02-
rattlesnake	T63.01-
specified NEC	T63.09-
taipan	T63.03-

Drug/Chemical	Code
Venom, venomous (bite) (sting), continued	
specified NEC	T63.89-
spider	T63.30-
black widow	T63.31-
brown recluse	T63.33-
specified NEC	T63.39-
tarantula	T63.321
sting ray	T63.51-
toad	T63.821
wasp	T63.461
Venous sclerosing drug NEC	T46.8X-
Ventolin—see Albuterol	
Veramon	T42.3X-
Verapamil	T46.1X-
Veratrine	T46.5X-
Veratrum	
album	T62.2X-
alkaloids	T46.5X-
viride	T62.2X-
Verdigris	T60.3X-
Veronal	T42.3X-
Veroxil	T37.4X-
Versenate	T50.6X-
Versidyne	T39.8X-
Vetrabutine	T48.0X-
Vidarabine	T37.5X-
Vienna	
green	T57.0X-
insecticide	T60.2X-
red	T57.0X-
pharmaceutical dye	T50.99-
Vigabatrin	T42.6X-
Viloxazine	T43.29-
Viminol	T39.8X-
Vinbarbital, vinbarbitone	T42.3X-
Vinblastine	T45.1X-
Vinburnine	T46.7X-
Vincamine	T45.1X-
Vincristine	T45.1X-
Vindesine	T45.1X-
Vinesthene, vinethene	T41.0X-
Vinorelbine tartrate	T45.1X-
Vinpocetine	T46.7X-
Vinyl	
acetate	T65.89-
bital	T42.3X-
bromide	T65.89-

Drug/Chemical	Code
Vinyl, continued	
chloride	T59.89-
ether	T41.0X-
Vinylbital	T42.3X-
Vinylidene chloride	T65.89-
Vioform	T37.8X-
topical	T49.0X-
Viomycin	T36.8X-
Viosterol	T45.2X-
Viper (venom)	T63.09-
Viprynium	T37.4X-
Viquidil	T46.7X-
Viral vaccine NEC	T50.B9-
Virginiamycin	T36.8X-
Virugon	T37.5X-
Viscous agent	T50.90-
Visine	T49.5X-
Visnadine	T46.3X-
Vitamin NEC	T45.2X-
A, B, B1 or B2 or B6 or B12 or B15, C, D, D2, D3, E (acetate) NEC	T45.2X-
nicotinic acid	T46.7X-
hematopoietic	T45.8X-
K, K1, K2, NEC	T45.7X-
PP	T45.2X-
ulceroprotectant	T47.1X-
Vleminckx's solution	T49.4X-
Voltaren—see Diclofenac sodium	
Warfarin	T45.51-
rodenticide	T60.4X-
sodium	T60.4X-
Wasp (sting)	T63.461
Water	
balance drug	T50.3X-
distilled	T50.3X-
hemlock	T62.2X-
moccasin (venom)	T63.06-
purified	T50.3X-
Wax (paraffin) (petroleum)	T52.0X-
automobile	T65.89-
Weed killers NEC	T60.3X-
Welldorm	T42.6X-
White	
arsenic	T57.0X-
hellebore	T62.2X-
lotion (keratolytic)	T49.4X-
spirit	T52.0X-

Drug/Chemical	Code
Whitewash	T65.89-
Whole blood (human)	T45.8X-
Wild (black cherry) (poisonous plants NEC)	T62.2X-
Window cleaning fluid	T65.89-
Wintergreen (oil)	T49.3X-
Wisterine	T62.2X-
Witch hazel	T49.2X-
Wood alcohol or spirit	T51.1X-
Wool fat (hydrous)	T49.3X-
Woorali	T48.1X-
Wormseed, American	T37.4X-
Xamoterol	T44.5X-
Xanthine diuretics	T50.2X-
Xanthinol nicotinate	T46.7X-
Xanthotoxin	T49.3X-
Xantinol nicotinate	T46.7X-
Xantocillin	T36.0X-
Xenon (127Xe) (133Xe)	T50.8X-
Xenysalate	T49.4X-
Xibornol	T37.8X-
Xigris	T45.51-
Xipamide	T50.2X-
Xylene (vapor)	T52.2X-
Xylocaine (infiltration) (topical)	T41.3X-
Xylol (vapor)	T52.2X-
Xylometazoline	T48.5X-
Yeast (dried)	T45.2X-
Yellow (jasmine)	T62.2X-
phenolphthalein	T47.2X-
Yew	T62.2X-
Yohimbic acid	T40.99-
Zactane	T39.8X-
Zalcitabine	T37.5X-
Zaroxolyn	T50.2X-
Zephiran (topical)	T49.0X-
ophthalmic preparation	T49.5X-

Drug/Chemical	Code
Zeranol	T38.7X-
Zerone	T51.1X-
Zidovudine	T37.5X-
Zimeldine	T43.22-
Zinc (compounds) (fumes) (vapor)NEC	T56.5X-
anti-infectives (bacitracin)	T49.0X-
antivaricose	T46.8X-
chloride (mouthwash)	T49.6X-
chromate	T56.5X-
gelatin or oxide (plaster)	T49.3X-
peroxide	T49.0X-
pesticides	T56.5X-
phosphide or pyrithionate	T60.4X-
stearate	T49.3X-
sulfate	T49.5X-
ENT agent	T49.6X-
ophthalmic solution	T49.5X-
topical NEC	T49.0X-
undecylenate	T49.0X-
Zineb	T60.0X-
Zinostatin	T45.1X-
Zipeprol	T48.3X-
Zofenopril	T46.4X-
Zolpidem	T42.6X-
Zomepirac	T39.39-
Zopiclone	T42.6X-
Zorubicin	T45.1X-
Zotepine	T43.59-
Zovant	T45.51-
Zoxazolamine	T42.8X-
Zuclopenthixol	T43.4X-
Zygadenus (venenosus)	T62.2X-
Zyprexa	T43.59-

New 2017 pediatric-specific coding resources
from the AAP!

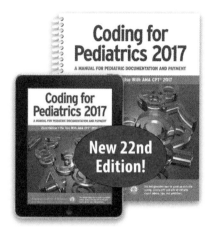

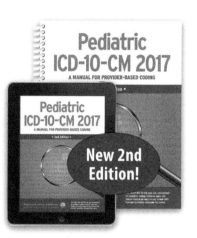

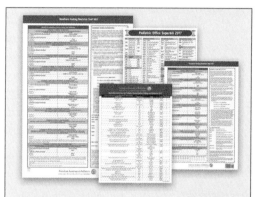

Coding for Pediatrics 2017, 22nd Edition
A Manual for Pediatric Documentation and Payment

This AAP exclusive complements standard coding manuals with pediatric-specific documentation and billing solutions for pediatricians, nurse practitioners, administration staff, and pediatric coders. Newly updated and revised for 2017!

Spiral-bound, 2016—443 pages • MA0798 • Price: $134.95 • *Member Price: $107.95*
Book ISBN 978-1-61002-039-8 • eBook ISBN 978-1-61002-040-4

Pediatric ICD-10-CM
A Manual for Provider-Based Coding, 2nd Edition

This coding manual strives to bring to the pediatric provider, coder, and biller the most accurate and easy-to use manual on *ICD-10-CM* yet. Composed entirely with a pediatrics focus, this manual exclusively features codes and guidelines for physician- and provider-based coding, all in a simplified yet familiar format.

Spiral-bound, 2016—532 pages • MA0800 • Price: 109.95 • *Member Price: $87.95*
Book ISBN 978-1-61002-042-8 • eBook ISBN 978-1-61002-043-5

Quick Reference Coding Tools

Pediatric Evaluation and Management Coding Card 2017
MA0801 • Price: $21.95 • *Member Price: $16.95*
ISBN: 978-1-61002-044-2

Quick Reference Guide to Coding Pediatric Vaccines 2017
MA0799 • Price: $21.95 • *Member Price: $16.95*
ISBN: 978-1-61002-041-1

Newborn Coding Decision Tool 2017
MA0802 • Price: $21.95 • *Member Price: $16.95*
ISBN: 978-1-61002-045-9

Pediatric Office Superbill 2017
MA0803 • Price: $21.95 • *Member Price: $16.95*
ISBN: 978-1-61002-046-6

AAP Pediatric Coding Webinars
presented by the American Academy of Pediatrics
DEDICATED TO THE HEALTH OF ALL CHILDREN

New 2016–2017 webinar topics include
- Coding Updates for 2017
- Hospital Services Coding for General Pediatrics
- Mental and Behavioral Health Coding

Register today at www.aap.org/webinars/coding.

AAP Pediatric Coding Newsletter™

This information-packed monthly publication brings you proven coding strategies, tips, and techniques you won't see on any other periodical.

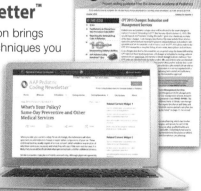

Featuring the "Maximizing 10" column with coding tips and tricks for successful *ICD-10-CM* utilization

SUB1005 **1-YEAR SUBSCRIPTION**
Price: $219.95
Member Price: $199.95

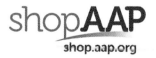
shop.aap.org

American Academy of Pediatrics
DEDICATED TO THE HEALTH OF ALL CHILDREN™